DEPARTMENT OF
ORTHOPAEDICS

THE UNIVERSITY OF TEXAS
HEALTH SCIENCE CENTER AT SAN ANTONIO

Sports-Induced Inflammation: Clinical and Basic Science Concepts

American Orthopaedic Society
for Sports Medicine
Symposium

Published by the
American Academy of Orthopaedic Surgeons

Dedication

This book is dedicated to the memory of George D. Rovere, MD. Dr. Rovere was a long-standing member of the American Orthopaedic Society for Sports Medicine. He served as chairman of the education committee of the Society from 1985 until his untimely death on November 24, 1988. Under Dr. Rovere's leadership, the education committee embarked on many innovative projects. Perhaps the most important and ambitious of these projects was the workshop on sports-induced soft-tissue inflammation. Through his inspiration and leadership this project was formulated. Dr. Rovere served as an inspiration to us all, and in so doing, made the workshop and this publication possible.

Sports-Induced Inflammation: Clinical and Basic Science Concepts

Edited by
Wayne B. Leadbetter, MD
Clinical Assistant Professor
Department of Surgery
Uniformed Services University of Health Sciences
F. Edward Hebert School of Medicine
Bethesda, Maryland

Joseph A. Buckwalter, MD
Professor
Department of Orthopaedic Surgery
The University of Iowa Hospitals and Clinics
Iowa City, Iowa

Stephen L. Gordon, PhD
Musculoskeletal Diseases Program Director
National Institute of Arthritis and
Musculoskeletal and Skin Diseases
National Institutes of Health
Bethesda, Maryland

with 175 illustrations

Workshop
Bethesda, Maryland
May 1989

Supported by the
Foundation for Sports Medicine Education and Research, an affiliate of the American Orthopaedic Society for Sports Medicine

and the
National Institute of Arthritis and Musculoskeletal and Skin Diseases

Published by the
American Academy of Orthopaedic Surgeons
222 South Prospect Avenue
Park Ridge, IL 60068

Sports-Induced Inflammation: Clinical and Basic Science Concepts

The American Academy of Orthopaedic Surgeons is pleased to publish this text in cooperation with the American Orthopaedic Society for Sports Medicine and to include this volume as the third in our Symposium Series and the first volume in the series to be produced by an orthopaedic specialty society.

Executive Director:
Thomas C. Nelson

Director of Communications and Publications:
Mark W. Wieting

Assistant Director, Publications:
Marilyn L. Fox, PhD

Senior Editor:
Wendy O. Schmidt

Medical Editor:
Bruce A. Davis

Library of Congress Cataloging-in-Publication Data

Sports-induced inflammation : clinical and basic science concepts / edited by Wayne B. Leadbetter, Joseph A. Buckwalter, Stephen L. Gordon.
p. cm.
"Workshop, Bethesda, Maryland, May 1989, supported by the Foundation for Sports Medicine Education and Research, an affiliate of the American Orthopaedic Society for Sports Medicine, and the National Institute of Arthritis and Musculoskeletal and Skin Diseases."
Includes bibliographical references.
Includes index.
ISBN 0-89203-037-2 : $75.00
1. Musculoskeletal system—Wounds and injuries—Congresses. 2. Inflammation—Congresses. 3. Sports—Physiological aspects—Congresses. I. Leadbetter, Wayne B., 1943- . II. Buckwalter, Joseph A. III. Gordon, Stephen L. IV. Foundation for Sports Medicine Education and Research. V. American Orthopaedic Society for Sports Medicine. VI. National Institute of Arthritis and Musculoskeletal and Skin Diseases (U.S.)
[DNLM: 1. Athletic Injuries—therapy—congresses. 2. Inflammation—etiology—congresses. QZ 150 S764 1989]
RC925.5.S66 1990
617.4'73044—dc20
DNLM/DLC
for Library of Congress 90-1055
CIP

Workshop Participants

Steven Abramson, MD
Associate Professor of Medicine
New York University School of Medicine
New York, New York

Steven P. Arnoczky, DVM
Director, Laboratory for Comparative Orthopaedic Research
The Hospital for Special Surgery
New York, New York

William J. Arnold, MD
Chairman, Department of Medicine
Lutheran General Hospital
Park Ridge, Illinois

Jeffrey R. Basford, MD, PhD
Consultant, Department of Physical Medicine and Rehabilitation
Mayo Clinic
Rochester, Minnesota

Louis U. Bigliani, MD
Assistant Professor of Orthopaedic Surgery
Columbia Presbyterian Medical Center
New York, New York

W. Watson Buchanan, MD, FRCP (Edin, Glasg, and C)
Professor
Department of Medicine
McMaster University Faculty of Health Sciences
Hamilton, Ontario

Joseph A. Buckwalter, MD
Professor
Department of Orthopaedic Surgery
Division of Oncology
The University of Iowa Hospitals and Clinics
Iowa City, Iowa

David L. Butler, PhD
Professor, Noyes-Giannestras Biomechanics Laboratories
Department of Aerospace Engineering
University of Cincinnati
Cincinnati, Ohio

William G. Clancy, Jr., MD
Clinical Professor of Orthopaedic Surgery
University of Virginia
Charlottesville, Virginia

Walton W. Curl, MD
Director, Sports Medicine Unit
Wake Forest University
Winston-Salem, North Carolina

Sandra L. Curwin, PhD
Assistant Professor
School of Physiotherapy
Dalhousie University
Halifax, Nova Scotia
Canada

Jesse C. DeLee, MD
Associate Clinical Professor
Department of Orthopaedic Surgery
University of Texas at San Antonio Health Science Center
San Antonio, Texas

David R. Eyre, PhD
Professor, Departments of Orthopaedics and Biochemistry
University of Washington
Seattle, Washington

Joseph C. Fantone, MD
Associate Professor
Department of Pathology
University of Michigan Medical School
Ann Arbor, Michigan

James A. Farmer, Jr, EdD
Associate Professor of Continuing Education
University of Illinois at Urbana-Champaign
Champaign, Illinois

Gerald A.M. Finerman, MD
Professor
Division of Orthopaedic Surgery
University of California at Los Angeles
Los Angeles, California

Evan L. Flatow, MD
Assistant Professor of Orthopaedic Surgery
New York Orthopaedic Hospital
Columbia-Presbyterian Medical Center
New York, New York

Cyril B. Frank, MD, FRCS (C)
Associate Professor
Department of Surgery
Facility of Medicine, University of Calgary
Calgary, Alberta
Canada

Gary E. Friedlaender, MD
Professor and Chairman
Department of Orthopaedics and Rehabilitation
Yale University School of Medicine
New Haven, Connecticut

Freddie H. Fu, MD
Blue Cross of Western Pennsylvania Professor
Department of Orthopaedic Surgery
University of Pittsburgh
Pittsburgh, Pennsylvania

William E. Garrett, Jr., MD, PhD
Assistant Professor
Division of Orthopaedic Surgery
Sports Medicine Section
Duke University Medical Center
Durham, North Carolina

James S. Goodwin, MD
Professor of Medicine and Chief
Division of Geriatrics
University of Wisconsin School of Medicine
Milwaukee, Wisconsin

Stephen L. Gordon, PhD
Musculoskeletal Diseases Program Director
National Institute of Arthritis and MUsculoskeletal and Skin Diseases
National Institutes of Health
Bethesda, Maryland

Kenneth M. Hargreaves, DDS, PhD
Associate Professor
Division of Endodontics
Department of Rehabilitative Sciences
University of Minnesota School of Dentistry
Minneapolis, Minnesota

Herbert A. Haupt, MD
Orthopaedic Surgeon
St. Louis, Missouri

Peter Jokl, MD
Professor of Orthopaedics and Rehabilitation
Yale University School of Medicine
New Haven, Connecticut

W. Ben Kibler, MD
Orthopaedic Surgeon
Lexington, Kentucky

Kenneth Knight, PhD, ATC
Director, Sports Injury Research Laboratory
Indiana State University
Terre Haute, Indiana

William J. Kraemer, PhD
Associate Professor of Applied Physiology
The Pennsylvania State University
University Park, Pennsylvania

Wayne B. Leadbetter, MD
Clinical Assistant Professor
Department of Surgery
Uniformed Services University of Health Sciences
F. Edward Hebert School of Medicine
Bethesda, Maryland

Barbara Loitz, PhD, PT
Postdoctoral fellow
Department of Kinesiology
University of California at Los Angeles
Los Angeles, California

Richard Lymn, PhD
Director, Muscle Biology Program
National Institute of Arthritis and Musculoskeletal and Skin Diseases
National Institutes of Health
Bethesda, Maryland

Terry R. Malone, EdD, PT, ATC
Associate Professor
Department of Physical Therapy
Duke University
Durham, North Carolina

Antonio Martinez-Hernandez, MD
Professor of Pathology and Cell Biology
Thomas Jefferson University
Philadelphia, Pennsylvania

Thomas M. Mohr, PT, PhD
Associate Professor
Department of Physical Therapy
University of North Dakota School of Medicine
Grand Forks, North Dakota

Van C. Mow, PhD
Professor of Mechanical Engineering and Orthopaedic Bioengineering
Department of Orthopaedic Surgery
Columbia University, New York

Fred Nelson, MD
Clinical Assistant Professor
Uniform Services University of the Health Sciences
Bethesda, Maryland

Walter Newman, PhD
Chief Scientist, Immunology
Otsuka America Pharmaceutical Company
Rockville, Maryland

James A. Nicholas, MD
Professor
Cornell University Medical College
York, New York

Robert P. Nirschl, MD
Assistant Clinical Professor
Department of Orthopaedic Surgery
Georgetown University School of Medicine
Arlington, Virginia

Frank R. Noyes, MD
Professor
Department of Orthopaedic Surgery
University of Cincinnati
Cincinnati, Ohio

Stephen J. O'Brien, MD
Assistant Professor of Surgery
Cornell University Medical College
New York, New York

Arthur J. Pearl, MD
Associate Professor
University of Missouri Health Sciences Center
Division of Orthopaedic Surgery
Columbia, Missouri

Edward C. Percy, MD, FRCS (C)
Associate Professor
Section of Orthopaedic Surgery
University of Arizona College of Medicine
Tucson, Arizona

Arnold E. Postlethwaite, MD
Professor
Department of Medicine
University of Tennessee
Memphis, Tennessee

William S. Quillen, PhD, PT, SCS
Assistant Head, Physical Therapy Department
National Naval Medical Center
Bethesda, Maryland

Per Renstrom, MD, PhD
Professor
Department of Orthopaedics and Rehabilitation
University of Vermont
Burlington, Vermont

William G. Rodkey, DVM
Chief, Division of Military Trauma Research
Letterman Army Institute of Research
San Francisco, California

Mark William Rodosky, MD
Orthopaedic Resident
Department of Orthopaedic Surgery
University of Pittsburgh School of Medicine
Pittsburgh, Pennsylvania

Ethan N. Saliba, MEd, ATC, PT
Instructor, Curry School of Education
University of Virginia
Charlottesville, Virginia

David J. Schurman, MD
Chief, Division of Orthopaedic Surgery
Stanford University
Stanford, California

Matthew S. Shapiro, MD
Assistant Clinical Professor
Division of Orthopaedic Surgery
University of California at Los Angeles
Los Angeles, California

Lawrence E. Shulman, MD, PhD
Director
National Institute of Arthritis and Musculoskeletal and Skin Diseases
National Institutes of Health
Bethesda, Maryland

Arthur J. Siegel, MD
Assistant Professor of Medicine
Harvard Medical School
Boston, Massachusetts

J. Richard Steadman, MD
Chairman and Chief Physician
Sports Medicine Council
United States Ski Team
South Lake Tahoe, California

William T. Stauber, PhD
Professor of Physiology and Neurology
West Virginia University
Health Sciences Center North
Morgantown, West Virginia

Lawrence V. Tkach, MD
Clinical Instructor
University of California at San Diego
San Diego, California

Arthur Vailas, PhD
Associate Professor, Director
Biodynamics Laboratory
University of Wisconsin
Madison, Wisconsin

James C. Vailas, MD
Assistant Professor of Orthopaedic Surgery
George Washington University
Washington, D.C.

Sharon M. Wahl, PhD
Chief, Cellular Immunology Section
National Institute of Dental Research
National Institutes of Health
Bethesda, Maryland

W. Michael Walsh, MD
Associate Professor and Director of Sports Medicine
Department of Orthopaedic Surgery and Rehabilitation
University of Nebraska Medical Center
Omaha, Nebraska

Peter A. Ward, MD
Chairman, Godfrey D. Stobbe Professor of Pathology
Department of Pathology
University of Michigan
Ann Arbor, Michigan

Ronald R. Watson, PhD
Research Professor
School of Medicine
Department of Family and Community Medicine
University of Arizona
Tucson, Arizona

Savio L-Y Woo, PhD
Professor of Surgery and Bioengineering
University of California, San Diego
La Jolla, California

Ronald F. Zernicke, PhD
Professor and Chairman
Department of Kinesiology
University of California at Los Angeles
Los Angeles, California

Preface

Inflammation is a commonly observed tissue response to musculoskeletal injury.[2,6] Sports-induced inflammation is unique, however, in the circumstances surrounding its etiology. Furthermore, the treatment of sports-induced inflammation must be given in the context of patients who are eager to regain and even exceed their pre-injury performance levels. Media coverage of professional sports has heightened public awareness of sports injuries. This concern is sharpened by the health profession's emphasis on the value of physical fitness and the general need for the psychological gratification, stress relief, and other rewards to be derived from athletic participation. Although the risk of injury is particularly important to the highly competitive athlete, a much larger number of persons are included in the population at risk for sports injury. According to the 1978 Perrier study on fitness in America,[5] exercise activities—tennis, football, archery, jogging, swimming, bowling, and others—involve almost 300 million Americans. There were only 150 million adult Americans in 1978, so it is obvious that many persons took part in more than one sport. Recent statistics show no slackening in that trend. It is currently estimated that 15% to 20% of our population (30 million to 40 million participants) either jog or run; 10 million to 20 million people swim; cycling now claims 75 million enthusiasts.[1] Such endurance sports place enormous demands on the body's connective tissues. These demands can be quantified in such terms as the 220 tons of impact force per mile absorbed by the marathoner, the 400,000 to 650,000 strokes required of the swimmer during an average training season, or the 30 to 40 hours of exhausting practice by the gymnast per week. Such soft-tissue overuse leads to an estimated 30% to 50% of all sports injuries.[1] Many of these complaints are identified without the benefit of rigorous assessment technology. Such terms as "myositis," "fibrositis," "fibrocystic nodule," and "tendinitis," are used to justify a therapeutic regimen, simultaneously satisfying the patient's expectations of a finite diagnosis and relieving the sports physician of admitting the limits of his knowledge.

Since Virchow, modern pathology has defined injury in terms of the cell.[3] The present study of sports injury is the study of cell and matrix injury and the expression of the preexisting capacity to adapt to such injury on the part of the injured or intact cell-matrix complex. This emphasis on understanding the pathophysiology of inflammation at the cellular level is in keeping with current trends throughout orthopaedic medicine.

The workshop on Sports-Induced Soft-Tissue Inflammation evolved from the ongoing efforts of the Education Committee of the American Orthopaedic Society for Sports Medicine (AOSSM) to seek the scientific rationale for current sports medicine diagnosis and treatment. The workshop and subsequent publication were conceived under the chairmanship of the late

George Rovere, MD. As the originator of the proposal, I served as chairman-editor, and Joseph A. Buckwalter, MD, and Stephen L. Gordon, PhD, were recruited as co-editors. A planning and editorial committee was established, which included William G. Clancy, MD, PhD; Frank R. Noyes, MD; Walton W. Curl, MD, subsequent chairman of the AOSSM's Education Committee; and Arthur Pearl, MD, chairman of the AOSSM's Publication Committee. James A. Farmer, Jr., EdD, served as educational consultant. Ultimately, the project involved the cooperation of the AOSSM and its Foundation for Sports Medicine Education and Research, the National Institute of Arthritis and Musculoskeletal and Skin Diseases, which contributed to the symposium, and the American Academy of Orthopaedic Surgeons, which served as publisher.

Initially, several questions were asked: (1) What constitutes a sports-induced inflammation, and under what circumstances is it initiated? (2) Are there differences between the macrotraumatic and microtraumatic inflammatory processes? (3) What promotes the direction and outcome of inflammation, that is, can it be beneficially modified? (4) What contributes to an insufficient or excessive fibrotic healing response? (5) What role does exercise have in controlling the onset or the course of an inflammatory response? These questions became the basis for the major sections of this publication in which are found a spectra of topics from the basic scientific to the clinical therapeutic level.

The specific goals of the workshop included reviewing the known mechanisms of injury in sports trauma with particular attention to the triggering mechanism of inflammatory response and repair, defining "sports-induced soft tissue inflammation" in the context of sports training and competitive demands, identifying a common base of knowledge, further defining the current rationale for diagnosis and treatment of sports-induced inflammation, understanding the implications of pain as a guide to the care of athletic injury and its correlation with structural injury, providing an interdisciplinary basis for further investigation, exchange of ideas, and encouragement of further study, and providing a framework of hypotheses about the basic scientific explanations of the observed clinical manifestations of sports-induced inflammation.

The multidisciplinary workshop was held in Bethesda, Maryland, May 22 to 24, 1989. Contributors provided manuscripts on an assigned topic within one of five subsections dealing with fundamental principles, pathophysiologic mechanisms, modifiers of inflammation, failed healing responses, or the protective role of training and conditioning. These manuscripts were sent to all participants six weeks before the meeting and formed the basis for further discussion. Evenings were devoted to addressing anomalous issues and provided time for free communication among the group as a whole. The authors were then requested to refine their manuscripts for final publication on the basis of their experience at the meeting.

At the onset, several constraints were apparent with regard to overuse or microtraumatically produced injury. Only a limited number of models existed for inflammation, and none of these was clearly applicable to the mechanisms of overuse. Little research on sports-induced injury existed regarding microtrauma at the cellular level. Lastly, there was a lack of biopsy material that could be correlated with a given stage of clinical diagnosis because many of these conditions are not treated surgically.

Given these constraints, the workshop

discussion of sports-induced inflammation relied, in part, on theoretical constructs. Such reliance, however, can ultimately lead to the systematic discovery of new facts through observation and experimentation, which will then confirm, modify, or refute the theory.[4] The history of science contains many examples of this process. Long before their physical existence could be observed, John Dalton theorized about atoms, and John Hunt Morgan based his genetic experiment on a theory of inheritance that posited genes as the basic hereditary units.

The workshop accomplished several important objectives. A multidisciplinary structure was created from a previously ill-defined area of knowledge. The known and the unknown were sorted out, and "facts" based on assumptions alone were challenged. Both cellular and matrix mechanisms of inflammation were posited, and hypotheses were suggested that might explain the observed clinical symptoms. There was valuable communication among basic scientists and sports medicine clinicians in areas formerly thought to be exclusively clinical. Many areas for new research were identified.[5]

Although a consensus was not achieved on all questions, the symposium called attention to a variety of myths about shortcomings of present diagnostic and therapeutic methods. Additionally, there was a growing sense that not all painful sports-induced conditions represent true inflammatory processes in the classic sense, and that other explanations involving different forms of biomechanical and biochemical mediation may have to be developed for the degenerative changes observed in overuse injuries, such as those that occur in tendon.

This book is intended to introduce to a broad readership a compendium of scientific and clinical observations of a subject about which much has been assumed, but much less verified. It is hoped that the familiarity so gained will create the starting point for more investigations.

WAYNE B. LEADBETTER, MD

References

1. Herring SA, Nilson KL: Introductions to overuse injuries. *Clin Sports Med* 1987;6:225–239.
2. Kellert J: Acute Soft Tissue Injuries—A Review of the Literature. *Med Science in Sports and Exercise* 1986;18(5):489–500.
3. Majno G: *The Healing Hand: Man and Wound in the Ancient World.* Cambridge, Harvard University Press, 1975.
4. Mazzeo ZJA: *The Design of Life—Major Theories in the Development of Biological Thought.* New York, Random House, 1967.
5. Mirkin G, Hoffman M: *The Sports Medicine Book.* Boston, Little Brown & Co, 1978.
6. Woo SL-Y, Buckwalter, JA: *Injury and Repair of the Musculoskeletal Soft Tissues.* Park Ridge, IL, American Academy of Orthopaedic Surgeons, 1988.

Acknowledgments

As in sport, life is often a team experience. The accomplishment of the workshop on sports-induced soft-tissue inflammation and this publication would not have been possible without a team to whom we remain grateful.

The American Orthopaedic Society for Sports Medicine and its Foundation for Sports Medicine Education and Research provided essential financial support and planning advice. The National Institute of Arthritis and Musculoskeletal and Skin Diseases added additional support. The timely encouragement of Lawrence E. Shulman, MD, PhD, Director of the Institute, was appreciated.

The earnest planning and on-site assistance of James A. Farmer Jr., EdD, educational consultant, and Arthur J. Pearl, MD, chairman of the publications committee of the Society, helped to focus our efforts.

We are most thankful for the hard work of our scientist and clinician colleagues, who were willing to share their insights, meet challenging deadlines, and shoulder considerable intellectual responsibilities. They have been called upon often and continue to serve so well.

The cooperation and technical help of the American Academy of Orthopaedic Surgeons and its publications staff have made this book a reality. In particular, Marilyn L. Fox, PhD, assistant director, publications, and Wendy O. Schmidt, senior editor, receive our praise for their professionalism and forbearance. In addition, Mark W. Wieting, director, communications and publications, and Thomas C. Nelson, executive director, provided overall direction and advice.

Finally, we would like to thank Mr. Sanford Hill, executive director of the American Orthopaedic Society for Sports Medicine, for his planning advice and efforts to make the workshop successful. Also, our workshop coordinator, Ms. Sharon Rolek, was a source of both spirited encouragement and pragmatism. Her efficiency and organization benefited us all. We also thank the untiring secretarial efforts of Deborah Whitehurst, Yvonne Copeland, Kathy Lacey, and Geraldine Dubberke.

Finally, to our families, a special thanks to the "home team."

Wayne B. Leadbetter, MD
Joseph A. Buckwalter, MD
Stephen L. Gordon, PhD

Contents

Section One
Fundamental Principles

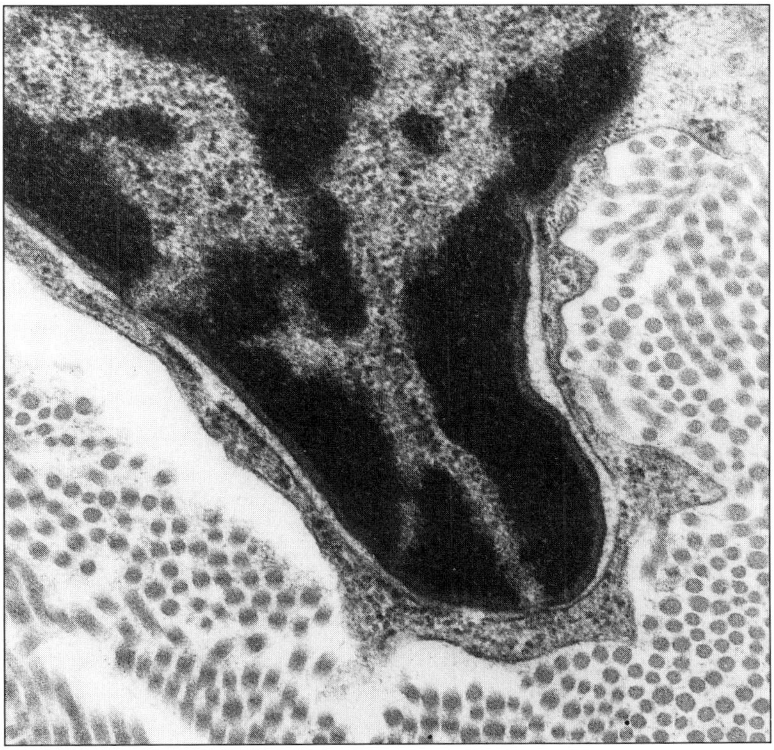

Group Leader

Wayne Leadbetter, MD

Group Participants

Sandra Curwin, PhD
Joseph Fantone, MD
Antonio Martinez-Hernandez, MD

Chapter 1

An Introduction to Sports-Induced Soft-Tissue Inflammation

Wayne B. Leadbetter, MD

> Healing is a matter of time, but is sometimes also a matter of opportunity.
>
> HIPPOCRATES

Inflammation is always a potential response to musculoskeletal injury. Sports and physical exercise invoke a variety of stress responses in the human body.[15,18,36,78] Many of these responses seem to be beneficial, such as improved cardiovascular function, decreased blood pressure, more efficient oxygen utilization (aerobic capacity), altered body composition, improved muscular strength, increased physical stamina, and a sense of well-being or fitness.[18,78]

As a signal of distress, inflammatory responses may be initiated whenever forces or loads applied to connective tissue structures exceed individual biomechanical and/or metabolic limits. Although commonly treated as an unwanted hindrance to athletic performance, inflammation is a complex vascular, cellular, and biochemical event necessary to the healing and repair process.[6,19,45] Sports medicine and sports science are engaged in efforts to reveal ways to modify the reparative process and potentially expedite the return to activity.

Historical Background

The history of inflammation in sport is an interwoven chronicle of the evolution of humanity's leisure time and sports play, the understanding of soft tissues and wound healing, and the growth of modern pathology.

Skeletal evidence has shown inflammation in human joint disease to be as old as humankind. Articular and periarticular changes have been seen in *Australopithecus afarensis,* other early hominids, Neanderthals, Neolithic humans, and ancient mummies.[16]

With regard to soft-tissue injury, only inferences made from changes in bones are possible since clearcut evidence from prehistoric times is absent because of the failure of these tissues to survive. No intact bodies or organs dating from earlier than 4000 BC have been discovered[41]

According to Majno,[43] written medical history began with the Sumerians around 3100 BC; the Sumerian term *ummu,* "the hot thing," is the first recorded equivalent of inflammation. The Egyptian papyri had much to say regarding the treatment of open wounds and inflammation. Seven of the 48 case reports included in the Smith Papyrus (1700 BC) describe wounds and their management. Principles of removing foreign bodies, suturing, and protection of wounds were recognized.[42] However, the use of nonsterile poultices gave rise to the concept of "laudable pus." The Egyptians documented what is thought to be the oldest contact sport, wrestling, with depictions on the walls of the tombs of Beni-Hassan (*c* 1991 to 1778 BC) located along the Nile between the ancient cities of Thebes and Gizeh. As many as 220 groups of wrestlers in various poses are displayed. It was during this period that boxing, polo, and an early form of soccer began.[20]

Sports trauma and medicine as the discipline of diagnosis and treatment have been by necessity closely associated throughout recorded history. The rise of the Greek city states in the fifth and fourth centuries BC with their emphasis on body improvement and "a sound mind in a healthy body" promoted this relationship.[3,54] The first Olympic games, according to McGregor,[46] were held in 776 BC, and the second games took place in 772 BC. Initially they consisted of running events, wrestling, boxing, racing, and chariot races.[4,46]

What the Greeks could not see with a microscope, they conceptualized: "What escapes the sight of the eyes can be seen with the sight of the mind."[43] For example, the Greeks used posttraumatic local compression to reduce excess hemorrhage and localized cell necrosis secondary to ischemia and proteolytic enzyme digestion ("rotting").

Hippocrates (*c* 460–380 BC), a pupil of Herodicus, the first advocate of therapeutic exercise, emphasized that the physician's chief responsibility was to make conditions favorable for the natural forces in the body to reach harmony and therefore health. His "method" emphasized a meticulous history and physical examination, recorded with accuracy and objectivity.[41] These tenets lie at the heart of modern sports medicine philosophy.

In the absence of new scientific knowledge, the management of open wounds changed little, but Hippocrates recognized that pus was not essential to successful wound healing. In response to the frequent disability caused by major joint dislocation, especially of the shoulders of wrestlers, Hippocrates not only emphasized restoration of normal alignment, but also provided the first recorded surgical success in the treatment of recurrent joint instability. He used the principles of scar formation and wound contraction by cauterization ("In this way, the cavity, into which the humerus is mostly displaced, is best scarred over and cut off").[27,43] However crude, this method represented the first attempt to direct and harness the pathophysiology of inflammation to achieve a specific therapeutic goal (Fig. 1).

It was a Roman encyclopaedist living at the time of Tiberius (ruled

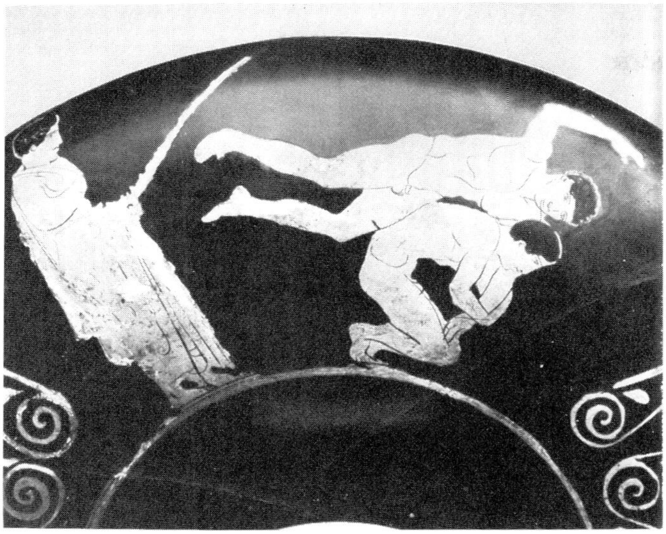

Fig. 1 *Greek wrestlers. This throw, the* se-oi-nage *of modern judo, contributed to the incidence of shoulder dislocation, leading to therapeutic intervention to harness the inflammatory process of scar formation by cauterization. (Reproduced with permission from Majno G:* The Healing Hand: Man and Wound in the Ancient World. *Cambridge, Harvard University Press, 1975.)*

AD 14 to 37), who provided the classic description of inflammation. Writing about the characteristics of disease in the chest in *De Medicina*, Cornelius Celsus[8] reported the four cardinal signs of acute inflammation: *"Rubor et tumor cum calore et dolore"* (redness and swelling with heat and pain). Majno[43] believed this may have applied to the end stages of empyema and fistula.

The prominent Roman physician, Galen (AD 138–200) has been called the father of sports medicine.[64,65] This reputation is derived primarily from his much glamorized role as physician to the gladiators, the first professional sports competitors (Fig. 2). Although he never wrote a book on surgery, his experience during three years as surgeon to the gladiators is well recorded.[22] Practicing 500 years after his idol Hippocrates, Galen reiterated that inflammation was not always required for successful wound healing. "Those who believe that inflammation necessarily follows a wound show great ignorance, since it is possible for anyone to see even large ones reach the stage of being practically healed in two to four days without inflammation."[43]

During the medieval period, the science of wound healing stagnated. The principles of gentle wound treatment were abandoned and applications of boiling oil, burning oil, hot cautery, and scalding water were substituted.[42]

The Renaissance saw several important milestones. French war sur-

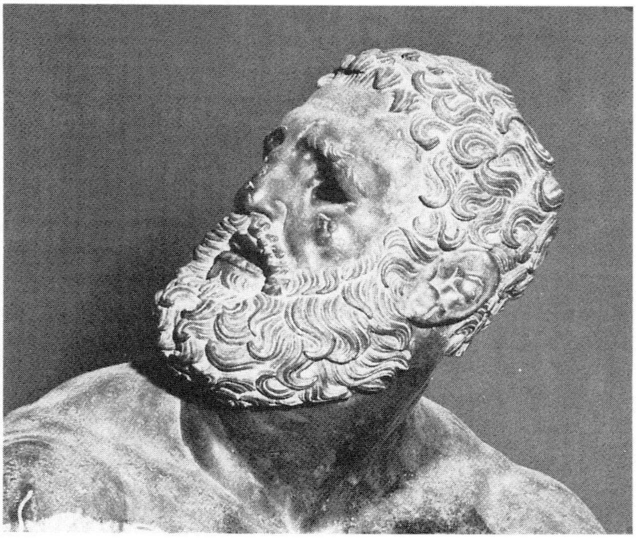

Fig. 2 *Hellenistic pugilist demonstrating a typical "cauliflower ear," an early example of the fibrotic response to injury and inflammation. (Reproduced with permission from Majno G:* The Healing Hand: Man and Wound in the Ancient World. *Cambridge, Harvard University Press, 1975.)*

geon Ambroise Pare (1517–1590) made a landmark, albeit accidental, discovery when he ran out of boiling oil during the battle of Villaine and found that wounds that were simply cleansed and dressed healed better, heralding the beginning of a new era.[30]

The invention of the first objective measurement of inflammation, the thermometer, is credited to Galileo in 1592.[41] In 1870, Thomas Clifford Albutt designed the modern thermometer.[41]

However, it was the microscope that allowed the science of cellular pathology to advance. Although its origins probably date back to the middle ages, it was Antony Van Leeuwenhoek (1632–1723), a cloth merchant from Delft, Holland, who refined the instrument and discovered blood corpuscles, spermatozoa, and the striated characteristics of skeletal muscle. The botanist Robert Hook (1635–1703) is credited with the first reference in science to the cell. He described "little boxes or cells distinct from one another."[22] Marcello Malpighi (1628–1694), regarded as the founder of biologic microscopy, demonstrated the presence of capillaries in the lung of the frog in 1687, thereby verifying the blood circulation theory of William Harvey (1578–1657) and establishing the scientific basis for the vascular response of inflammation.[22,41]

An important transitional figure in this age was the English surgeon and experimenter, John Hunter (1729–1793) (Fig. 3). He is credited

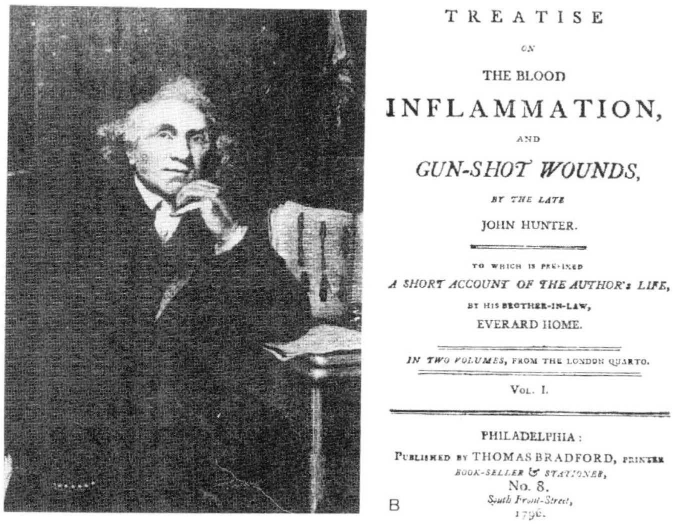

TREATISE

ON

THE BLOOD

INFLAMMATION,

AND

GUN-SHOT WOUNDS,

BY THE LATE

JOHN HUNTER.

TO WHICH IS PREFIXED

A SHORT ACCOUNT OF THE AUTHOR's LIFE,

BY HIS BROTHER-IN-LAW,

EVERARD HOME.

IN TWO VOLUMES, FROM THE LONDON QUARTO.

VOL. I.

PHILADELPHIA:

PUBLISHED BY THOMAS BRADFORD, PRINTER

BOOK-SELLER & STATIONER,

No. 8.

South Front-Street,

1796.

B

Fig. 3 *John Hunter (1729–1793). This English surgeon and experimenter established the beneficial role of inflammation in wound healing. He is shown with the title page of his book, which was published three years after his death. (Reproduced with permission from Perez-Tamayo R:* Mechanisms of Disease: An Introduction to Pathology, *ed 2. Chicago, Year Book Medical Publishers, 1985, p 182.)*

with calling attention to the nonspecificity of the process of inflammation and, more importantly, clearly established that the traumatic inflammatory process is essentially protective in nature and the initiator of wound repair.[55] "The operation in the body called inflammation is one of the most common and extensive in its effects . . . and in so many diseases is the first step to a cure. . . ."[30]

Modern medicine and modern sports began in the 19th century. During the 1800s there were unprecedented scientific discoveries in cellular biology. Most modern recreational competitive sports were invented during this period. Rudolph Virchow (1821–1902), the father of modern pathology, announced that "all cells come from other cells," thus directing medical science to the concept that disease was produced by disturbances in the structure and function of the body's cells.[22,41] He thought the primary disturbance in inflammation was the cellular edema (cloudy swelling) produced by noxious substances. Most importantly, it is now recognized that it was Virchow, not Galen, who described the so-called fifth cardinal sign of inflammation—*functi laesa* or "disturbed function."[43] Describing this sign, which is now paramount in sports medicine treatment and rehabilitation, Virchow[73] wrote, "Nobody would expect a muscle that is inflamed to perform its function normally."

Virchow's pupil, Julius Cohnheim (1839–1884) identified the role of vascular permeability in early inflammation and the process of extravascular cellular migration.[55] In 1892, Meshikoff described phagocytosis and lymphocytic migration, further emphasizing the defensive role of inflammation.[17,55]

At this time, the modern controversy regarding the definition of soft-tissue inflammation had its beginnings. In 1852, Virchow attributed syndromes of muscle pains or soreness to muscular rheumatism or rheumatic fever. In 1904, in a paper on lumbago, Gowers formally introduced the term "fibrositis," as a name more specific than muscular rheumatism, the term used by Virchow.[71] He theorized that local areas of tenderness in regions of palpable hardness in muscle resulted from underlying inflammation of fibrous tissue. He described this as the underlying pathologic response involved in sciatica, frozen shoulder, and other disorders. As Travell and Simons[71] noted, modern biopsy specimens did not substantiate the existence of inflammation in most cases of fibrositis, which led to the description of fibrositis as "a wastebasket term useful to describe pain of nonorganic origin." They pointed out, "Fibrositis (and other musculoskeletal pain syndromes generally assumed to involve classic inflammation) remains a term in search of redefinition and continues to welcome diagnoses by default."[71] Goldenberg[24] concurred.

Since the beginning of the 1900s, the role of mediators has been investigated. This search for mediators of the various "tissue responses and structural changes" in acute inflammation was initiated to explain the various vascular reactions of the skin to injury.

Lewis and Grant postulated in 1924 the existence of a humeral factor (H substance) that was released in the tissues and that increased capillary permeability.[55] Mencken is credited with drawing attention to inflammatory exudates by the first isolation of a chemical mediator.[55] This was "leukotaxine," named for its stimulation of chemotactic behavior in leukocytes. Mencken's work has led to the discovery of several hundred endogenous chemical substances, the biologic value of which is "so fundamental that nature has woven around it [*sic*] a very complicated and reiterated web of mediators and controls in order to guarantee its preservation."[55]

In 1870, consistent with the protective role being assigned to inflammation, the French physiologist Claude Bernard (1813–1878) emphasized "the constancy of the internal environment (*milieu interieur*) is the condition that life should be free and independent."[70] To describe the process by which the internal environment is kept constant, American physiologist Walter Cannon coined the term "homeostasis." Stress was defined as any stimulus that created an imbalance in the internal environment.[70] The Canadian behavioral scientist Hans Selye later refined the concept of stress response to physical activity and not only created a whole diagnostic category of illness—psychosomatic disease—but also laid the foundation for modern athletic sports and physical training. This culminated with Allman's[1] pronunciation of the SAID principle (Specific Adaption to Imposed Demands), which states that the body responds to a given physical demand with a specific predictable adaptation.

A growing urban middle class with increasing resources and leisure spearheaded the growth of modern sports in both Britain[47] and the United States. The 1800s saw the growth of cricket from an exclusively aristocratic sport to a middle-class pastime and the organization of rugby and association football under national rules. Lawn tennis and polo also originated in Great Britain as leisure increased. The United States contributed its own brand of football, baseball, and basketball. Canada saw the emergence of ice hockey. The rise of these commercially successful sports created a surge in spectatorship. The preeminence of American football as a collision sport conscripted the orthopaedic surgeon as a team physician, much as Galen was drawn to the gladiators.

The advent of private and public transportation brought a paradoxical decrease in daily exercise. A hundred years ago, nearly everyone walked to work; Dickens' Mr. Pickwick and his friends took a walk of 25 miles to help them digest a Christmas meal.[47] During the Industrial Revolution, human labor accounted for 30% of the energy used in factories and farms. Now it accounts for less than 1%.[31] This sedentary trend did not reverse itself dramatically until the advent of cardiologist Kenneth Cooper's aerobic exercise and fitness philosophy. Jogging and aerobic dance became household words in the 1970s. A consequence of what Roger Bannister dubbed the "sports for all" philosophy in the 1970s and 1980s has been an epidemic of soft-tissue aches and pains and inflammations loosely defined as "sports injuries." In 1968, in an article on running and the causes of shin splints, Slocum and James[63] originated the term "overuse injury."

In England, the Central Council of Physical Recreation was founded in 1935 to promote physical fitness in the general population in response to the increasing concern about the inadequate physical fitness of young men recruited into the Armed Forces.[47] The American College of Sports Medicine was formally organized in 1954. In the early 1950s, the National Athletic Trainers Association (NATA) was founded. In 1960, the American Medical Association appointed a committee on the medical aspects of sports. The President's Council on Physical Fitness was initiated in 1956.[31] The International Federation of Sports Medicine was created at the 1958 Winter Olympics in St. Moritz.[62] Orthopaedic sports medicine was officially established in 1972, when the American Orthopaedic Society for Sports Medicine was founded.[31] Similar sports medicine organizations have been established in recent years in almost every area of health care, including family medicine, pediatrics, physical therapy, and athletic training. These national organizations continue to focus attention on the question of inflammation and healing.

Although the vast difference between the modern Olympiad and the Olympic games of the ancient world typifies the evolution of sport, biologic evolution has not kept pace. The modern athlete is not invulnerable. It is likely, therefore, that the association of sport with medicine that has been so prominent throughout history will continue to be important, not only in treating injury but, it is hoped, in preventing it.

Soft-Tissue Response to Sports Trauma

It is important to have a working definition of the variables involved in soft-tissue response to physical injury. Although all attempts at definition encourage challenge, the following discussion provides a framework from which to formulate further opinion.

Sports Trauma

Sports trauma implies an injury from a mechanical force applied externally, causing structural stress or strain that results in a cellular or tissue response.[68] Load is a measure of external mechanical force. Use implies the accumulation of load over time, that is, a rate. Such repetition is seen in endurance sports in the form of cyclic loading and overuse. The effect of load on tissue is described by the terms "strain" and "stress." Strain is the deformation of a structure in response to an external load, whereas stress is its internal resistance to such deformation. The role of such load-generated stress and strain responses in promoting cellular and matrix responses such as inflammation or degeneration is the subject of further discussion throughout this volume. Sports trauma may be thought of as the mechanism by which injury occurs.

Sports Injury Injury (from the Latin *injure,* to make unjust, not right) is the loss of cells and/or extracellular matrix resulting from sports-induced trauma.[90] Injuries are divided into acute or chronic injuries according to rate of onset and the mechanism. Acute injury is characterized by a rapid-onset, macrotraumatic event and has a clearly identifiable initiating cause or moment of onset. Acute injuries are typified by a sudden crisis followed by a fairly predictable, although often lengthy, resolution. Ligament sprains, fractures, and sudden muscle strains exemplify this form of injury. Chronic injury is characterized by a slow, insidious onset, implying an antecedent subthreshold spectrum of structural damage leading to a crisis episode that is often heralded by pain and/or signs of inflammation. Chronic injury lasts months or even years, and is distinguished by a persistence of symptoms without resolution. Tendinitis, bursitis, and fasciitis are typical of chronic complaints. There appears to be some overlap between acute and chronic injuries, with the bridging stage at four to six weeks, termed the subacute stage of injury.[38]

It is difficult to define injury clinically. From the athlete's point of view, an injury is any condition that prevents participation or desired level of performance, which may or may not be accompanied by all of the signs of inflammation. From an epidemiologic point of view, the definition of injury continues to cause much argument. Sports injury has been defined as "injury or illness causing cessation of an athlete's customary participation throughout the participation day following the day of onset," and "any injury or illness that requires subsequent professional attention before that athlete's return to participation."[52]

The Research Committee of the American Orthopaedic Society for Sports Medicine recently reviewed the definitions of injury used by several sports medicine facilities throughout the United States. They determined that no one definition of injury was being used, and therefore, that injury rates between studies and between sports could not be compared accurately. Anatomic tissue diagnosis is considered the most objective method to determine if an injury has occurred. However, although the severity of tissue injury can be assessed by mechanical methods such as stress roentgenograms or magnetic resonance imaging, a significant number of early-onset soft-tissue inflammations, particularly those of synovial structures, do not at present have a means of objective assessment nor do they warrant biopsy to establish their existence. In an effort to define injuries other than "lumps, bumps and bruises" as distinguished from structurally threatening injuries, Noyes and associates[52] proposed the following clinical definition: "Sports-related injury or illness prevents the player from practicing or competing on the day after the injury and requires medical or dental care beyond icing or wrapping. All concussions, nerve injuries and eye injuries, no matter how transient, are included." However, this is not a pathologic definition.

Rovere and associates'[59] definition of tendinitis exemplifies the difficulty of clinically defining soft-tissue sports abnormalities. In a study of theatrical dance students, they defined tendinitis as "a syndrome of pain and tenderness localized over a tendon, usually aggravated by activities that bring the particular muscle tendon unit into play (usually against resistance). We recognize that the syndrome is inclusive of tenosynovitis and tenovaginitis as well as actual inflammation of the tendon substance itself."[59]

Since Virchow, modern pathology has defined injury in terms of the cell. It may be said, therefore, that the study of sports injury is in part the study of cell injury and the expression of preexisting capacity to adapt to such injury on the part of the injured or intact cell.[60] Today, sport injury is further defined by the degree to which normal mechanical properties and function are lost as a consequence of both cell and matrix injury.

Terms such as "rheumatism," "myositis," "fibrositis," "arthritis," "tension or spasm state," "fibrocystic nodule," and "tendinitis" are frequently used to justify a therapeutic regimen, simultaneously satisfying the patient's expectation of a definite diagnosis and relieving the sports physician of admitting the limits of his knowledge. Yet, without a clearer understanding of the pathobiology of these "syndromes," both effective therapy and the proper preventative measures remain obscure.[7]

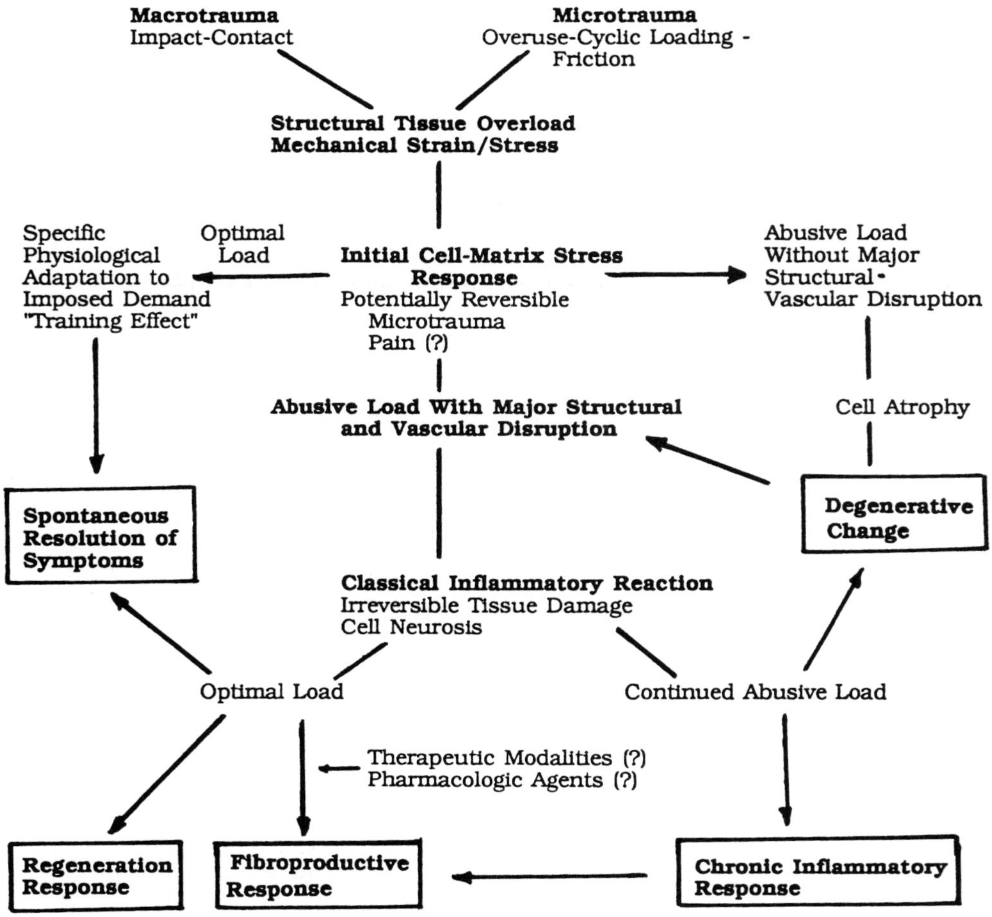

Fig. 4 *Schema demonstrating theoretical pathways of sports-induced inflammation.*

Sports-Induced Inflammation

Sports-induced inflammation (from the Latin *inflammare,* to set on fire) is a localized tissue response initiated by injury or destruction of vascularized tissues exposed to excessive mechanical load. It is a time-dependent, evolving process characterized by vascular, chemical, and cellular events leading to tissue repair or regeneration or to scar formation.[26,38,55,60] Clinically observed pathways of sports-induced soft-tissue inflammation include spontaneous resolution, fibroproductive healing, regeneration, or a chronic inflammatory response (Fig. 4).

Although the various stages of inflammation and wound repair are dealt with elsewhere in this volume, attention must be given to the phenomenon of pain, for it is often pain that announces and defines the state of injury (see Figure 1 in Chapter 39). Among the so-called cardinal signs, pain is of a dual nature in that it is recognized as both a symptom or "hurt" that the athlete experiences subjectively and as a sign of physical diagnosis in the form of local tenderness.[74] Because an inflamed structure may be difficult to palpate, the diagnosis rests purely on subjective opinion. Whether classic inflammation is present in every painful athletic injury remains unknown. Clancy[10] found little evidence of inflammation in chronic overuse injuries of the Achilles' tendon; Colosimo and Bassett[12] also noted a distinct absence of acute or chronic inflammation in patellar tendinitis. One explanation for such findings may be that the classic inflammatory process is only set into action after sufficient structural disruption and microvascular damage occur.

Repair and Regeneration

Repair of soft-tissue injury has been defined as replacement of damaged or lost cells and extracellular matrices with new cells and matrices.[80]

Regeneration is a form of repair that produces new tissue that is structurally and functionally identical to normal tissue.[80] It has been said that inflammation can occur without healing, but healing cannot occur without inflammation. Peacock[53] noted that during the course of human evolution, a valuable defense mechanism—the ability to regenerate compound tissues—was replaced by healing, a much less complicated and far less valuable process. Amphibians are the most advanced animals in which regeneration of a lost extremity occurs; in humans, limited regeneration of epithelium and endothelium and partial regeneration of the liver have been observed.[29] As Hunt and Dunphy[29] noted, "the major mysteries of repair have always been and continue to be: what in the injury stimulates repair, and how does the wound recognize that it is no longer needed, and why does healing stop?"

Degeneration

Degeneration describes a change of a tissue from a higher to a lower or less functionally active form.[60] Such weakened structures are then more vulnerable to sudden dynamic overload or cyclic overloading, leading to mechanical fatigue and failure. Degeneration is the end result of cell atrophy, which is the decrease in the size and function of a cell in response to an environmental signal.[60] Such downregulation involves decreased protein synthesis and a decrease in such activities as energy production, replication, storage, or contractility. In sports injury, immobilization is a prominent cause of cell atrophy.[51,69,81] Additional causes include decreased nutrition, diminished endocrine hormonal influence, persistent inflammation, and aging. Under conditions of overload or overuse, various forms of cellular response and adaptation may be overtaxed, resulting in cell death and a loss of matrix integrity. Matrix breakdown products may play a feedback role in regulating or possibly inhibiting cell function, ultimately resulting in alterations in proteoglycan content and variation in collagen synthesis. As weakening and mechanical disruption progress, vascular injury is produced, and initiation of a renewed inflammatory process may appear. Rest may permit an atrophied cell to recover but a lack of physical stimulation, such as in immobilization or complete rest, may also prevent a sufficient healing response. In the absence of adequate tissue integrity, a return to sports activity carries the risk of reinjury. The clinical observation that complete rest is often an incomplete therapeutic solution and that protected activity or therapeutic exercise provides a better remedy tend to support such theories.[61]

Chronic Inflammation

Chronic inflammation involves the replacement of leukocytes by macrophages, plasma cells, and lymphocytes in a highly vascularized and enervated loose connective tissue milieu at the site of injury.[60] Histologic findings typical of chronic inflammation have been noted in lateral epicondylar injuries of the elbow, that is, tennis elbow. Such chronic inflammatory tissue responses are not found in all chronic sports injuries. The mechanisms that convert an acute inflammation to a chronic inflammatory process are not known, but seem to be promoted by circumstances of overuse or overload with what may represent cumulative structural microtrauma. Chronic inflammatory abnormalities may coincide with atrophy and degeneration at the site of injury.

Epidemiology of Sports-Induced Soft-Tissue Injuries

Injury to the soft connective tissues is the most common disability associated with athletic competition and recreational athletics. The "connecting tissues" represent the largest tissue component of the body and include muscle, tendon, ligament, joint capsule, fascia, meniscus, articular cartilage, synovium, intervertebral disk, and adipose tissue.[2] Sports differ in risk because of the quantitative differences in stresses to different anatomic areas, but soft-tissue injuries make up the majority of complaints in all sports at all levels of competition.[14,21,76,82] It is estimated that 30% to 50% of all sports injuries are caused by soft-tissue overuse.[26] Most of these complaints are diagnosed by the symptoms of inflammation.

Sites of Injury

The sites of injury vary according to the sport. Garrick and Requa[21] pointed out that most sports injuries involve the lower extremities, reflecting the strenuous running, jumping, and cutting maneuvers common to the most popular sports. As many as 90% of sports injuries are sustained by the hip, thigh, knee, leg, ankle, and foot. Shoulder and upper-extremity complaints predominate in racket, throwing, and swimming sports. DeHaven and Lintner[14] found that 48.1% of baseball injuries involved the shoulder and upper extremity and that 57% of world-class swimmers have experienced shoulder pain. Ligament sprains, the most common injuries to joints in general and to the knee in particular, account for 25% to 40% of all knee injuries in most studies.[80] Witman and associates,[79] in a review of 1,280 urban sports-medicine patients with an average age of 30.2 years, found the most frequently injured areas to be the knee (45.5%), the ankle (9.8%), and the shoulder (7.7%). Of these injuries, 53.9% involved soft tissue.

Gender

Chandy and Grana,[9] in a three-year study of seven paired sports in 130 Oklahoma secondary schools involving 24,485 boys and 18,289 girls, found a significant difference in rate of injury only in basketball, in which the girls had significantly more injuries and more severe injuries. Overall, the girls had more sprains and dislocations whereas the boys had more strains and fractures. There was a significant variance in the sites of injuries—boys had significantly more shoulder complaints and girls had more knee injuries. DeHaven and Lintner[14] found patellofemoral pain to be more prevalent in women (19.6% of women vs 7.4% of men). Sprains and strains occurred in 33.4% of men and in 28.7% of women. They also confirmed the higher rate of knee injuries among injured female athletes (20.7% vs 8.5%). In a study of four Seattle high schools, Garrick and Requa[21] found the average injury rate for all athletes in ten sports was 5.2%. The rate for girls was 3.5% and the adjusted rate (excluding football and wrestling) for boys was 3%. Again, although the injury rate for all girls' sports was lower, a higher percentage of the girls' injuries required a loss of five days or more (52% of girls vs 44% of boys).[21] These studies point to a difference in the severity and types of injuries in male and female athletes, but they do not resolve such variables as level of conditioning, performance technique, anatomic predisposition, or coaching.

Age

In the United States, one half of boys and one fourth of girls from 8 to 16 years old (7 million students) engage in some type of organized competitive sports programs during the school year.[23] Of all children participating in sports programs in the United States, 3% to 11% are injured. In a survey of Irish high-school children between the ages of 10 and 18 years, the overall incidence of injury was found to be 2.94 injuries per 100 children per calendar year. More than one half of these were sprains, strains, and contusions.[75] The rarer occurrences of tendinitis or inflammatory changes at the musculotendinous junction in children have been attributed to the transfer of forces to the attendant apophysis.[13,67] Hoffman and Lyman,[28] assessing sideline injuries in high-school football, found that contusions (26.6%), sprains (21.6%), strains (8.6%), and suspected fractures (8.6%) accounted for most of the injuries. The knee (14.4%), the lower leg (13.7%), and the ankle

(11.5%) were the most common sites of injuries. Keller and associates[37] found 15 to 30 times as many soccer injuries in senior and professional athletes as in youths. Hip and thigh injuries were also more common in senior and professional athletes. Notable exceptions were knee and ligament strains, which accounted for one third of soccer injuries regardless of age. Contusions were most often significant in youths.

These differences can be accounted for in part by the intensity of the game. Menard and Stanish[48] noted that "The Masters athlete is often the victim of two sets of injuries; those that they incurred in their youth and those that result from their current training regimen." Inflammatory problems such as tendinitis or bursitis gradually increase in importance. Three of the top five maladies are inflammatory in nature by the seventh decade of life.[14] Grossman and Nicholas[25] have called attention to the changing pattern of knee injuries with age. Chondromalacia patellae, patellar tendon rupture, and degenerative arthritis are common knee injuries in aging athletes.

Choice of Sport

Both collision and endurance sports are characterized by the predominance of soft-tissue injury. DeHaven and Lintner[14] found 12 times as many injuries in football as in the next sport, basketball. Football accounted for 63.9% of all injuries as well as 60% of all knee injuries, which were primarily internal derangements and medial collateral ligament injuries. Total injury rates among high-school football players ranged from 25% to 65% depending on the definition of injury and the method of data collection.

Rates of significant injury ranged from 15% to 18%. Sprains and strains were the most common injuries.[21] Requa and Garrick[57] found wrestling second only to football in knee injuries requiring surgery. Rovere and associates[59] studied soft-tissue inflammation in theatrical dance students. Hip tendinitis produced a 6.9-day average loss of participation. For ankle sprain, the average loss was 2.1 days. Soccer caused two to five times fewer injuries in young athletes than American football. Sprains, strains, contusions, and tendinitis dominate the injury patterns. Knee and ankle injuries represent about 20% of all soccer injuries regardless of age.

In downhill skiing, a collision-prone recreational sport, soft-tissue injury still predominates. In an analysis of 2,596 skiing injuries, Johnson and Pope[35] found that soft-tissue injuries accounted for 53.4% of the total. The five most frequent diagnoses were knee sprains (20.9%), thumb sprains (10.2%), leg contusions (8.7%), lacerations (7.8%), and ankle sprains (5.8%).[37]

Endurance sports include jogging, running, swimming, cycling, rowing, and race-walking. An estimated 30 to 40 million Americans now jog regularly.[5,26,32,66] Of these, approximately 10 million run regularly, and 800,000 to 1 million enter competitive races.[33] The incidence of running injuries has ranged from 46.6% to an estimated 70% over the past decade.[33,40,56,66] Inflammatory disorders of soft tissues accounted for five of the six most common problems in the series of James and associates.[33] Musculotendinous injuries predominate in track and field.[56] Knee pain, representing a broad spectrum of overuse soft-tissue complaints, occurs in 23% to 40% of all runners.[50] Clement and associates[11] noted a decrease in the prevalence of Achilles peritendinitis from 11% of all injuries, as reported by James and associates,[33] to 6%. Historically, Achilles tendinitis has been a difficult lesion for runners. Welsh and Clodman[77] reported in 1980 that 16% of those involved had abandoned running and 54% still participated despite discomfort. The prevalence of injury in running is directly proportional to the load exposure. Mann[44] calculated that the ground-reaction force at mid-stance in running is equal to two to three times body weight. A 70-kg runner at 1,175 steps per mile absorbs at least 220 tons of force per mile.

Swimming is another endurance sport characterized by excessive cumulative load. Competitive swimmers swim 8,000 to 20,000 yards per day, five to seven days per week. This distance is the equivalent of running up to 45 miles daily. It is estimated that during a ten-month swimming season, a male swimmer performs 400,000 strokes and that a female swimmer performs 660,000 strokes.[58] Shoulder pain secondary to glenohumeral instability, secondary subacromial impingement, muscle fatigue, and tendinitis are typical causes of "swimmer's shoulder." Soft-tissue overuse of the medial aspect of the knee secondary to incorrect mechanics in the whip kick in the breast stroke and inflammation of the extensor tendons of the dorsum of the foot have also been reported.[34]

Level of Participation

Keller and associates,[37] in a study of soccer injuries, concluded that professionals sustain a higher rate of injury because of the greater intensity of play. Leach's[39] description of the Major League baseball pitcher's typical throwing rotation is another example of the different intensity of soft-tissue stress between amateurs and professionals. A Major League baseball pitcher usually pitches every four days and throws 110 to 130 pitches in the course of a regular game. The next day his arm is so sore that it is difficult to raise. The second day is characterized by recovery and easy throwing, and the third day by a normal workout. The pitcher returns to starting on either the fourth or fifth day.

An injury analysis of the Olympic games of 1968 and 1972 revealed that sprains, strains, and contusions were the most common soft-tissue injuries treated, accounting for 61% to 96% of soft-tissue problems. Thus, the Olympic experience parallels the rest of sport.[82]

Clinical Observations

From the previous discussion, it is apparent that sports-induced soft-tissue inflammation is not only a clinical problem, but that it is one that has plagued clinicians throughout recorded history. Although it is claimed that most soft-tissue sports injuries are not "serious," even a subcutaneous bruise can prove painful enough to inhibit normal performance, and many injures are potentially career-ending, for example, rotator cuff tendinitis in a baseball pitcher, degenerative disk disease in a golfer, or chronic synovitis of the knee in a football player.[49]

The "injured" athlete with soft-tissue complaints has pain and an inability to perform. Classic signs of inflammation are not always present or identifiable. The complaint is not so much identified with a specific structure as with an anatomic area. It is a "painful shoulder," not a painful biceps tendon; it is a "painful knee," not a painful medial meniscus tear. The immediate onus on the examiner is to be competent and accurate in making the physical diagnosis.

Principle of Transition

A prominent cause of sports injury is transition. The principle of transition states that sports injury is most likely to occur when the athlete experiences any change in mode or use of the involved part. Sudden, ill-timed activity changes, whether in training or in injury recovery, result in an undesired breakdown response and may outstrip tissue morphostatic efforts by imposing overload and/or overuse demands on the cell matrix environment. Examples of transitional risks include any attempts to increase performance level, improper training, changes in equipment, environmental changes (such as new surfaces, different training altitudes), alterations in frequency, intensity, or duration of training, attempts to master new techniques, and even body growth itself.

It is the history that plays an important role in determining the occurrence of abusive training, that is, overuse. In this respect, a comparison of the historical characteristics of acute and chronic injury is useful in further defining the interrelationships of the variables influencing healing and the timing of returning to sports play.

Acute vs Chronic Injury Pattern

The acute injury pattern is characterized by a defined time of onset in that the trauma is generally observed as a sudden catastrophic occurrence, such as a collision or contact injury to the knee in football or a sudden ankle sprain. At the moment of injury, pain is likely to be severe; this is typically followed by a period of gradually decreasing pain as inflammation is treated intensively. Pain eventually falls below an arbitrary threshold, at which time the patient will feel "well." When pain is no longer inhibiting, the athlete may request a return to activity. However, when the biologic curve of wound healing is plotted vs healing rate on the same graph, a period of potential vulnerability to reinjury appears. The length of this period of vulnerability is proportional to the original severity of structural damage, the rate of healing of the given individual, which is likely to be longer with age, the nature of the target tissue that is injured (differences in intrinsic rates of healing have been documented in ligament compared with other connective tissues), and, lastly, by the expected demand or load exposure. The period of vulnerability after an acute injury would, in theory, be lengthened by any intrinsic raising of the arbitrary pain threshold of the athlete, or by any rapid removal of the pain (for example, with aggressive anti-inflammatory treatment such as corticosteroids). It would be lengthened by the adverse effects of inappropriate immobilization but would be shortened by functional rehabilitation that expedited wound fibrogenesis and increased tensile strength. Because research has suggested that injured ligaments may attain only 70% of their original structural and tensile integrity after as much as 12 months,[80] the period of vulnerability in such injuries could be lengthy, implying the need for protective activity despite the absence of pain and an ongoing rehabilitative program to recruit extrinsic muscular support.

Chronic soft-tissue injuries differ from acute injuries in several important ways. The moment of injury will, in the athlete's perception, be a moment of noxious pain. This often occurs after an exertion such as a long-distance run or intense throwing after which the pain either becomes insidiously inhibiting over a period of time or becomes explosively disabling hours or days after the event. Muscle, tendon, and synovial structures typically evidence this type of stress response to sports activity. The examiner's ability to ask about the preinjury training patterns and cumulative load exposures is critical to understanding why this type of inflammation has been triggered. For instance, a careful history in a marathon distance runner might reveal that an inadequate amount of time was spent in prerace preparation and that several weeks of mild, but not inhibiting, pain symptoms had been generated by abusive training before the actual moment of injury, that is, a transitional injury pattern. In theory, subclinical injury and dysfunction, that is, microtrauma, precede the moment of recognizable injury. The implication is that damage has been accumulating for a long time before the first opportunity for medical treatment. This is a distinct difference from acute injury, in which the onset of injury and the initial treatment often coincide closely. The accumulation of repetitive scar adhesions, degenerative change, and adverse effects in chronic inflammation imply that a recovery will be slower. Again, a period of vulnerability to reinjury results when conventional anti-inflammatory measures reduce the pain of injury without necessarily adding to structural integrity. In chronic inflammatory injury, it is the history that allows a proper recommendation and adjustment of activity.

Therapeutic Guidelines

In diagnosing and treating sports injury, van der Meulen[72] identified at least three important questions that help determine the therapeutic approach and the timing of return to athletic activity. First, a definition of the injury must be established. Early mobilization of an isolated medial collateral ligament injury of the knee may be acceptable, whereas early weightbearing in the anterior cruciate ligament injury would be less favorable because of the different stresses on the structures. Muscle healing and recovery vary from those of tendon. Secondly, the seriousness of the injury must be assessed. Methods of objective soft-tissue assessment are limited, but include stress radiographs of a joint and magnetic resonance imaging. Assessing the degree of structural damage remains a clinical dilemma in many cases. Thirdly, the relationship between the cause of the injury and its effect must be determined. When a slight load creates serious soft-tissue damage, it may be assumed that the damaged tissue was less resistant or had increased vulnerability. This defines the overuse syndrome and explains the occurrence of sudden dynamic rupture of a structure such as a patellar tendon during a routine sports activity as a result of abusive accumulative training with subclinical tissue damage. The implication of disproportionate injury is that a training error has occurred and must be rectified to avoid a recurrence.

The ideal goals of sports injury treatment include (1) positively influencing the process of inflammation and repair and expediting recovery of function (defined not simply as increased tensile strength, but also in terms of range of motion, endurance, neuromuscular coordination, metabolic capacity, reduction of atrophy, and flexibility); (2) reducing the ill effects of early excessive inflammatory processes such as severe pain, edema, and associated muscle spasm with loss of joint motion or contracture; (3) returning the athlete or exerciser to the former level of activity; and (4) preventing the recurrence of injury by influencing the structural ability of the target tissue to resist future overloads by such measures as training, equipment change, and improving technique.

The philosophy of sports medicine in the care of soft-tissue inflammation and injury is the philosophy of all wound care—to assist the natural processes of the body while doing no harm. This is not a matter of telling athletes what they want to hear, but rather of focusing our present knowledge of wound healing and its therapeutic modifiers on the problem and telling athletes what they need to hear. It is, as Hippocrates stated, a matter of not only timing, but also of "opportunity" to direct, guide, and stimulate the recovery of structural integrity and function of the injured part. In this regard, sports-induced soft-tissue inflammation provides a stimulating challenge, for as Bowerman[4] so aptly stated, "It is the circumstances of the injury, the risk taking involved, and the continued exposure to risk that produce interesting characteristics of the injury in sport."

References

1. Allman FL: Exercise in sports medicine, in Basmajian JV (ed): *Therapeutic Exercise*, ed 4. Baltimore, Williams & Wilkins, 1984, pp 485–509.
2. Arey LB: *Human Histology: A Textbook in Outline Form*, ed 2. Philadelphia, WB Saunders, 1963.
3. Aristotle: *Nichomachean Ethics*, 112b.5.

4. Bowerman JW: *Radiology and Injury in Sport*. New York, Appleton-Century-Crofts, 1977.
5. Brody DM: Techniques in the evaluation and treatment of the injured runner. *Orthop Clin North Am* 1982;13:541–558.
6. Bryant WM: Wound healing. *Clin Symp* 1977;29:1–36.
7. Cailliet R: *Soft Tissue Pain and Disability*. Philadelphia, FA Davis, 1977, pp 8 and 9.
8. Celsus AC: *De Medicina, with an English Translation by W.G. Spencer*, III 10.2/LB 1273. Cambridge, Loeb Classical Library, 1935–1938.
9. Chandy DA, Grana WA: Secondary school athletic injury in boys and girls: A three-year comparison. *Phys Sportsmed* 1985;13:106–111.
10. Clancy WG Jr: Tendinitis and plantar fasciitis in runners, in D'Ambrosia R, Drez D Jr (eds): *Prevention and Treatment of Running Injuries.* Thorofare, Charles B Slack, 1982, pp 77–87.
11. Clement DB, Taunton JE, Smart GW, et al: A survey of overuse running injuries. *Phys Sportsmed* 1981;9:47–58.
12. Colosimo AJ, Bassett FH: Jumper's knee: Diagnosis and treatment. *Orthop Rev* 1990;19:139–149.
13. Curwin S, Stanish WD: *Tendinitis, Its Etiology and Treatment.* Lexington, Collamore Press, 1984.
14. DeHaven KE, Lintner DM: Athletic injuries: Comparison by age, sport, and gender. *Am J Sports Med* 1986;14:218–224.
15. De Vries HA: *Physiology of Exercise for Physical Education and Athletics*, ed 3. Dubuque, WC Brown, 1980.
16. Dieppe P, Rogers JM: Skeletal paleopathology of rheumatic disorders, in McCarty DJ (ed): *Arthritis and Allied Conditions: A Textbook of Rheumatology*, ed 11. Philadelphia, Lea & Febiger, 1989, pp 8–15.
17. DiSabatino CA Jr: Inflammation, in Albright JA, Brand RA (eds): *The Scientific Basis of Orthopaedics.* New York, Appleton-Century-Crofts, 1979, pp 415–436.
18. Fox EL, Bowers RW, Foss ML: *The Physiological Basis of Physical Education and Athletics*, ed 4. Philadelphia, Saunders College Publishing, 1989.
19. Gamble JG: *The Musculoskeletal System: Physiological Basics.* New York, Raven Press, 1988.
20. Gardiner EN: *Athletics of the Ancient World.* Oxford, Clarendon Press, 1930.
21. Garrick JG, Requa RK: The epidemiology of foot and ankle injuries in sports. *Clin Sports Med* 1988;7:29–36.
22. Garrison FH: *An Introduction to the History of Medicine, With Medical Chronology, Suggestions for Study and Bibliographic Data*, ed 4. Philadelphia, WB Saunders, 1963, p 225.
23. Goldberg B: Injury patterns in youth sports. *Phys Sportsmed* 1989;17:175–184.
24. Goldenberg DL: Fibromyalgia syndrome (fibrositis), in Goodwin JS (ed): *Mediguide to Inflammatory Diseases.* New York, Lawrence Dellacorte, 1988, vol 7, pp 1–6.
25. Grossman RB, Nicholas JA: Common disorders in the knee. *Orthop Clin North Am* 1977;8:619–640.
26. Herring SA, Nilson KL: Introduction to overuse injuries. *Clin Sports Med* 1987;6:225–239.
27. Hippocrates: Writings on the articulations, in Hutchins RM (ed): *Great Books of the Western World.* Chicago, Encyclopaedia Britannica, 1952, vol 10, pp 91–121.
28. Hoffman MD, Lyman KA: Medical needs at high school football games in Milwaukee. *J Orthop Sports Phys Ther* 1988;10:167–171.

29. Hunt TK, Dunphy JE (eds): *Fundamentals of Wound Management*. New York, Appleton-Century-Crofts, 1979.
30. Hunter J: Lectures on the principles of surgery, in Palmer JF (ed): *The Works of John Hunter*. London, Longman, 1835, vol 1, p 265.
31. Jackson DW: The history of sports medicine: Part 2. *Am J Sports Med* 1984;12:255–257.
32. Jacobs SJ, Berson BL: Injuries to runners: A study of entrants to a 10,000 meter race. *Am J Sports Med* 1986;14:151–155.
33. James SL, Bates BT, Osternig LR: Injuries to runners. *Am J Sports Med* 1978;6:40–50.
34. Johnson JE, Sim FH, Scott SG: Musculoskeletal injuries in competitive swimmers. *Mayo Clin Proc* 1987;62:289–304.
35. Johnson RJ, Pope MH: Safety in skiing, in Scott WN, Nisonson B, Nicholas JA (eds): *Principles of Sports Medicine*. Baltimore, Williams & Wilkins, 1984, pp 367–374.
36. Katch FI, Freedson PS (eds): Training. *Clin Sports Med* 1986;5:1–619.
37. Keller CS, Noyes FR, Buncher CR: The medical aspects of soccer injury epidemiology. *Am J Sports Med* 1987;15:230–237.
38. Kellett J: Acute soft tissue injuries: A review of the literature. *Med Sci Sports Exerc* 1986;18:489–500.
39. Leach R: Tennis serving compared with baseball pitching, in Zarins B, Andrews JR, Carson WG: *Injuries to the Throwing Arm*. Philadelphia, WB Saunders, 1985, p 308.
40. Leadbetter WB: Getting ahead of running injury. *Emerg Med*, June 15, 1979, pp 27–39.
41. Lyons AS, Petrucelli RJ II: *Medicine: An Illustrated History*. New York, Harry N Abrams, 1978, p 217.
42. Madden JW, Arem AJ: Wound healing: Biological and clinical features, in Schwartz SI (ed): *Principles of Surgery*. New York, McGraw-Hill, 1969.
43. Majno G: *The Healing Hand: Man and Wound in the Ancient World*. Cambridge, Harvard University Press, 1975, pp 29, 102, 165, and 373.
44. Mann RA: Biomechanics of running, in Mack RP (ed): American Academy of Orthopaedic Surgeons *Symposium on the Foot and Leg in Running Sports*. St. Louis, CV Mosby, 1982, pp 1–29.
45. Martinez-Hernandez A: Repair, degeneration, and fibrosis, in Rubin E, Farber JL (eds): *Pathology*. Philadelphia, JB Lippincott, 1988, pp 68–95.
46. McGregor MF: *The Story of Greece*. Edinburgh, Wilson, 1960, pp 84–96.
47. McIntosh PC: Chapter one, in Williams JGP, Sperrys PN (eds): *Sports Medicine*, ed 2. London, Edward Arnold, 1979, p 1.
48. Menard D, Stanish WD: The aging athlete. *Am J Sports Med* 1989;17:187–196.
49. Mirkin G, Hoffman M: *The Sports Medicine Book*. Boston, Little Brown & Co, 1978.
50. Newell SG, Bramwell ST: Overuse injuries to the knee in runners. *Phys Sportsmed* 1984;12:80–92.
51. Noyes FR: Functional properties of knee ligaments and alterations induced by immobilization: A correlative biomechanical and histological study in primates. *Clin Orthop* 1977;123:210–242.
52. Noyes FR, Lindenfeld TN, Marshall MT: What determines an athletic injury (definition)? Who determines an injury (occurrence)? *Am J Sports Med* 1988;16(suppl 1):S65-S66.
53. Peacock EE: *Wound Repair*, ed 3. Philadelphia, WB Saunders, 1984, p 289.
54. Peltier LF: The classic: Geronimo Mercuriali (1530–1606) and the first illustrated book on sports medicine. *Clin Orthop* 1985;198:21–24.
55. Perez-Tamayo R: *Mechanisms of Disease: An Introduction to Pathology*, ed 2. Chicago, Year Book Medical Publishers, 1985, p 182.

56. Requa RK, Garrick JG: Injuries in interscholastic track and field. *Phys Sportsmed* 1981;9:42–49.
57. Requa RK, Garrick JG: Injuries in interscholastic wrestling. *Phys Sportsmed* 1981;9:44–51.
58. Richardson AB, Jobe FW, Collins HR: The shoulder in competitive swimming. *Am J Sports Med* 1980;8:159–163.
59. Rovere GD, Webb LX, Gristina AG, et al: Musculoskeletal injuries in theatrical dance students. *Am J Sports Med* 1983;11:195–198.
60. Rubin E, Farber JL (eds): *Pathology.* Philadelphia, JB Lippincott, 1988, p 4.
61. Saal JA: General principles of sports injury rehabilitation. *Phys Med Rehabil* 1987;1:523–536.
62. Schneider RC, Kennedy JC, Plant ML: *Sports Injuries: Mechanics, Prevention, and Treatment.* Baltimore, Williams & Wilkins, 1985.
63. Slocum DB, James SL: Biomechanics of running. *JAMA* 1968;205:721–728.
64. Snook GA: The father of sports medicine (Galen). *Am J Sports Med* 1978;6:128–131.
65. Snook GA: The history of sports medicine: Part I. *Am J Sports Med* 1984;12:252–254.
66. Stanish WD: Overuse injuries in athletes: A perspective. *Med Sci Sports Exerc* 1984;16:1–7.
67. Stanitski CL: Management of sports injuries in children and adolescents. *Orthop Clin North Am* 1988;19:689–698.
68. Teitz CC: *Scientific Foundations of Sports Medicine.* Philadelphia, BC Decker, 1989.
69. Tipton CM, James SL, Mergner W, et al: Influence of exercise on strength of medial collateral knee ligaments of dogs. *Am J Physiol* 1970;218:894–902.
70. Tortora GJ, Evans RL: *Principles of Human Physiology*, ed 2. New York, Harper & Row, 1986, pp 2 and 3.
71. Travell JG, Simons DG: *Myofascial Pain and Dysfunction: The Trigger Point Manual.* Baltimore, Williams & Wilkins, 1983, pp 6 and 7.
72. van der Meulen JC: Present state of knowledge on processes of healing in collagen structures. *Int J Sports Med* 1982;3(suppl 1):4–8.
73. Virchow RLK: *Cellular Pathology As Based Upon Physiological and Pathological Histology.* New York, Donen, 1971.
74. Wall PD, Melzack R: *Textbook of Pain.* Edinburgh, Churchill Livingstone, 1984.
75. Watson AW: Sports injuries during one academic year in 6799 Irish school children. *Am J Sports Med* 1984;12:65–71.
76. Webber A: Acute soft-tissue injuries in the young athlete. *Clin Sports Med* 1988;7:611–624.
77. Welsh RP, Clodman J: Clinical survey of Achilles tendinitis in athletes. *Can Med Assoc J* 1980;122:193–195.
78. Wilmore JH: *Training for Sport and Activity: The Physiological Basis of the Conditioning Process*, ed 2. Boston, Allyn & Bacon, 1982.
79. Witman PA, Melvin M, Nicholas JA: Common problems seen in a metropolitan sports injury clinic. *Phys Sportsmed* 1981;9:105–110.
80. Woo SL-Y, Buckwalter JA (eds): *Injury and Repair of the Musculoskeletal Soft Tissues.* Park Ridge, American Academy of Orthopaedic Surgeons, 1988.
81. Woo SL-Y, Matthews JV, Akeson WH, et al: Connective tissue response to immobility: Correlative study of biomechanical and biochemical measurements of normal and immobilized rabbit knees. *Arthritis Rheum* 1975;18:257–264.
82. Zarins B, Ciullo JV: Acute muscle and tendon injuries in athletes. *Clin Sports Med* 1983;2:167–182.

Chapter 2

Basic Concepts in Inflammation

Joseph C. Fantone, MD

Introduction

The development of an inflammatory reaction to tissue injury involves a dynamic and complex series of cellular and biochemical reactions manifested by structural and functional changes in the tissue. The ultimate goal of these reactions is to eliminate the pathologic insult, remove injured tissue, and promote regeneration of normal tissue structure with return of physiologic function. However, depending on the tissue affected and the nature of the pathologic insult, irreversible injury may occur, along with scar formation. Further, alterations in the regulatory mechanisms of the inflammatory response or associated immune responses to microbial products, foreign materials, or to altered tissue components may trigger excessive tissue destruction and a chronic inflammatory reaction. Thus, a persistent, uncontrolled inflammatory response may be harmful to the host. In sports-induced soft-tissue inflammation, many questions regarding the mechanisms of induction, regulation, and resolution remain unresolved. These questions are the crux of the dilemma for both the injured athlete and the clinician.

In considering a specific pathologic condition and its clinical manifestation, it is important to understand the complexity of the cellular and molecular mechanisms that may be functioning and that the host's response to tissue injury is a dynamic and evolving process. This is typified by the multiple pathophysiologic mechanisms functioning in bacterial endotoxin-mediated shock. In addition, it is clear that parenchymal and vascular cells (for example, endothelium) are more active in regulating the inflammatory response than was initially thought.

The purpose of this chapter is to lay a foundation for understanding the pathophysiologic mechanisms functioning during the host's response to tissue injury and to direct attention to possible correlates with the sports-induced injuries described in other chapters.

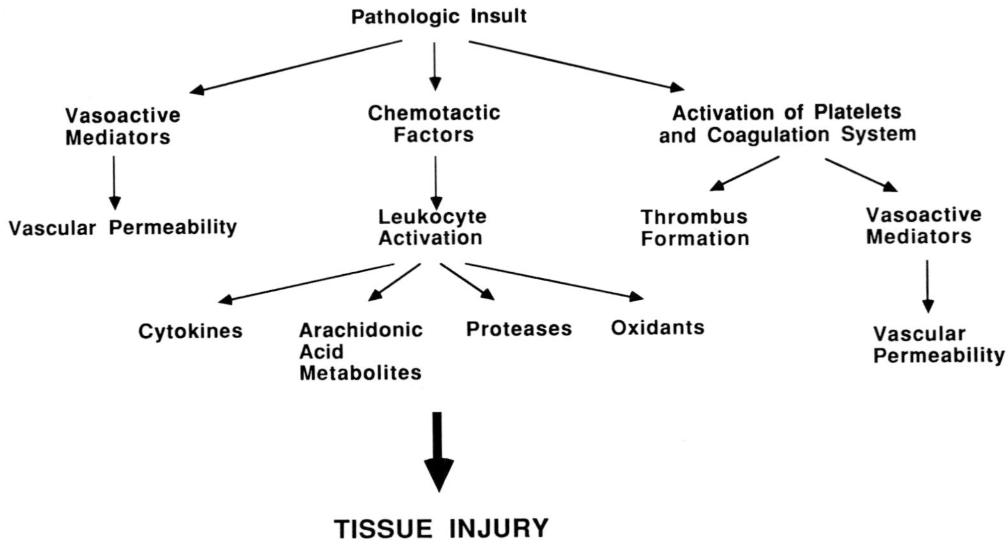

Fig. 1 *Mediators of the inflammatory response.*

Vascular Response to the Injury

After tissue injury, the primary sites at which the initial events of the inflammatory response occur are capillaries and postcapillary venules.[7,12,16,25] Under normal conditions, circulating erythrocytes, leukocytes, and plasma components are confined within the vasculature and separated from the tissue by a continuous layer of endothelium connected by tight junctions and a limiting basement membrane composed of a complex macromolecular matrix of type IV collagen, glycoproteins (fibronectin, laminin), and glycosaminoglycans. After injury, the structure of the vascular wall changes, leading to a loss of endothelial integrity, alterations in the structure and function of the basement membrane, local platelet activation, leakage of plasma components, and emigration of erythrocytes and leukocytes into the extravascular tissue (Fig. 1).

The response of the vasculature to injury is a dynamic process characterized by a sequential series of physiologic and pathologic changes (Fig. 2). At sites of tissue injury, vasoactive mediators, generated from both plasma and cellular sources, bind to specific receptors on vascular endothelium and smooth-muscle cells, and induce either vasoconstriction or vasodilation. When the role of a specific vasoactive mediator is evaluated, the effects of the mediator on specific components of the vasculature must be identified. Arteriolar vasoconstriction decreases blood flow to a tissue, whereas vasodilation increases blood flow, potentially exacerbating fluid leakage into the target tissue. Vasoconstric-

Ag + IgE →	Mast Cell/Basophil →	Histamine, PAF, LTC_4, D_4, E_4
Thrombin, Collagen →	Platelet →	Histamine, Serotonin
Phagocytic Chemotactic Stimulus →	Leukocytes →	PAF, Leukotrienes, Prostaglandins

Fig. 2 *Cell-derived vasoactive mediators. LT, leukotriene; PAF, platelet-activating factor.*

tion of venules increases the hydrostatic pressure in the capillary bed and thereby potentiates edema formation, whereas vasodilation of venules decreases capillary hydrostatic pressure.

Many vasoactive mediators induce primary endothelial changes at the level of the postcapillary venule.[16] Stimulation of endothelial cells by vasoactive mediators initiates a complex series of biochemical events, causing cell contraction, loss of tight junctions, and gap formation, with extravasation of intravascular fluids. The response of the vasculature to stimulation by vasoactive mediators is a reversible process, typically characterized by a maximum change in vascular permeability between ten and 30 minutes after the stimulation and a return to normal vascular integrity by one hour. This contrasts with the response of the microvasculature to thermal or chemical injuries. Mild injury to endothelium results in a biphasic response, with an early change in permeability occurring 15 to 30 minutes after injury, and a second increase in vascular permeability occurring three to five hours after injury. Severe injury results in a progressive increase in the exudation of intravascular fluid that reaches a peak between three and four hours after injury.

Sources of Vasoactive Mediators

There are two primary sources of vasoactive mediators: cells and plasma.[12,25] Important cellular sources of vasoactive mediators include the circulating platelets, leukocytes, and tissue mast cells (Fig. 2). In addition to its important role in normal homeostasis and in the initiation and regulation of thrombus and clot formation, the platelet is an important source of inflammatory mediators. These include potent vasoactive substances (for example, serotonin, histamine, and thromboxane A_2) and growth factors. These mediators are either preformed within cytoplasmic lysosomes and granules or generated on stimulation. After vascular injury, with exposure of basement membrane, or after activation of the coagulation system, platelet adherence, aggre-

Table 1 Biologic activity of lipid inflammatory mediators

Mediating Agent	Action
Prostaglandins D_2, E_2, and I_2	Vasodilation; bronchodilation; inhibition of inflammatory cell function
Prostaglandin $F_2\alpha$	Vasodilation; bronchoconstriction; vasoconstriction; enhancement of inflammatory cell functions (especially platelets)
Leukotriene B_4	Chemotactic for phagocytic cells; stimulation of phagocytic cell adherence; enhancement of microvascular permeability
Leukotrienes C_4, D_4, and E_4	Smooth-muscle contraction; constriction of pulmonary airways; increase in microvascular permeability
Platelet-activating factor	Platelet and neutrophil activation; peripheral vasodilation; hypotension; bronchial smooth-muscle contraction; pulmonary vasoconstriction; pulmonary hypertension; increase in vascular permeability

gation, and degranulation may occur in response to contact with fibrillar collagen or thrombin. Serotonin and histamine, mediators that directly induce vascular permeability changes, are released from cytosolic granules, while the arachidonic acid metabolite thromboxane A_2 is generated from membrane phospholipids. Thromboxane A_2 is an important mediator of the "second wave" of platelet aggregation and is a potent smooth-muscle constrictor.

Additional cellular sources of vasoactive mediators include tissue mast cells and circulating basophils. Both cell types, as a result of their ability to secrete specific mediators after stimulation, play an important role in the regulation of vascular permeability and smooth-muscle tone, especially in many forms of allergic hypersensitivity reactions. Stimulation of IgE-sensitized cells with antigen or the complement anaphylatoxins C3a and C5a releases histamine from electron-dense granules.[2,12,25] Histamine and serotonin induce reversible endothelial cell contraction, gap formation, and edema when injected into skin. The effects of histamine on the vasculature are mediated by H1 histamine receptors and blocked by H1 receptor antagonists. Other stimuli of mast cell and basophil degranulation include physical agonists (cold and trauma) and cationic proteins secreted by activated platelets and neutrophils.

The release of products of arachidonic acid metabolism, including the so-called slow-reacting substances of anaphylaxis (SRS-As) by stimulated mast cells, also functions to modulate vascular responses.[11,17,21] The SRS-As are lipoxygenase products of arachidonic acid metabolism and consist of three sulfidopeptide leukotrienes (leukotrienes C_4, D_4, and E_4). They bind to specific receptors on target cells, induce smooth-muscle contraction, and increase vascular permeability in the skin.

In recent years, much attention has focused on the role of an additional group of inflammatory mediators, termed platelet-activating factor, which is generated primarily by activated mast cells and leukocytes.[17] Its biochemical structure is an acetylated lysophospholipid

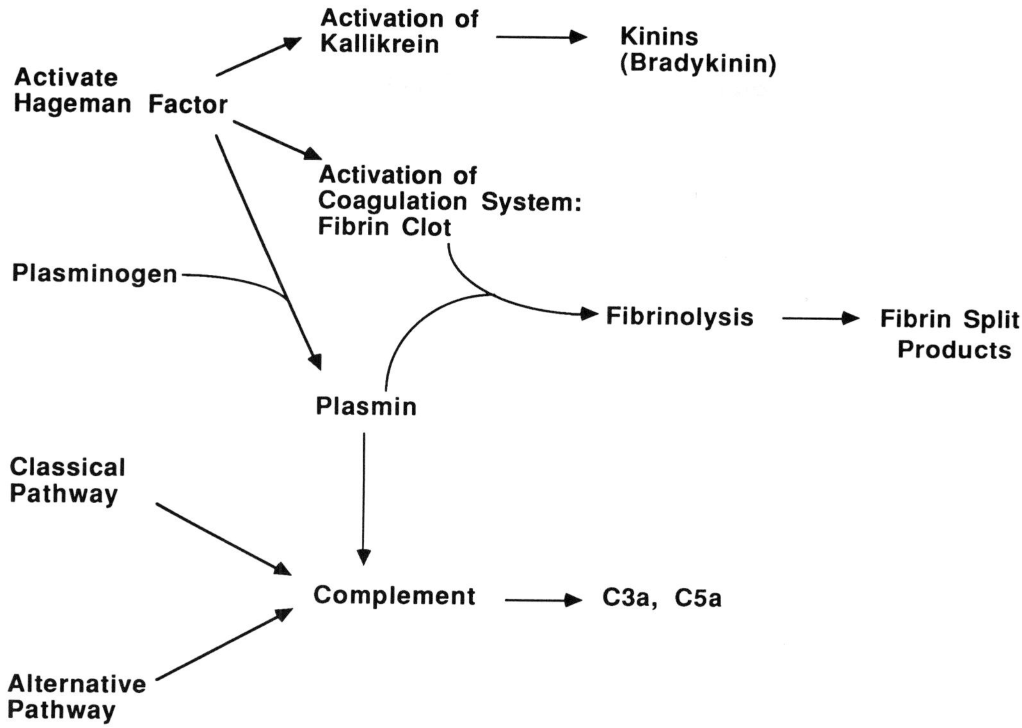

Fig. 3 *Plasma-derived vasoactive mediators.*

and in the rabbit is characterized as 1-0-hexadecyl/octyldecyl-2-acetyl-sn-glycero-3-phosphocholine (AGEPC). The biologic effects of platelet-activating factor are diverse, and include platelet aggregation and degranulation as well as stimulation of leukocyte chemotaxis and degranulation. Platelet-activating factor also has direct effects on the microvasculature, causing vasodilation and enhancing vascular permeability at sites of tissue injury.

Platelet-activating factor has been implicated as an important pathophysiologic mediator in a variety of experimental disease models, including immune complex-mediated vasculitis, IgE-mediated anaphylactic shock, septic shock, and necrotizing enterocolitis. Several of the effects of platelet-activating factor have been shown to be mediated by either lipoxygenase or cyclo-oxygenase products of arachidonic acid metabolism, demonstrating an important interrelationship between the two lipid mediator systems in the pathogenesis of tissue injury (Table 1).

Several components of plasma are known to be important sources of vasoactive mediators (Fig. 3). These include fibrin, the complement system, and high-molecular-weight kininogen. After proteolytic activation, low-molecular-weight peptides with potent vasoactive properties are generated. One mechanism for their generation involves the activation of clotting factor XII (Hageman factor) after exposure to negatively charged surfaces such as basement-membrane collagen, proteolytic enzymes, bacterial lipopolysaccharides, and foreign materials. Activated factor XII cleaves plasminogen and prekallikrein, generating plasmin and kallikrein, respectively; it also activates the alternative complement pathway.

Plasmin, a serine protease, promotes fibrinolysis, generating fibrin-degradation products that are capable of inducing vascular permeability. Plasmin may also utilize components of the complement system as substrates, generating biologically active products, including the anaphylatoxins C3a and C5a. C3a and C5a induce changes in microvascular permeability via both direct and indirect (for example, mast-cell dependent) mechanisms.

Kallikrein, a second product of factor XII activation, generates low-molecular-weight peptides collectively referred to as kinins, secondary to cleavage of high-molecular-weight kininogen. The best characterized of the vasoactive kinins is bradykinin, a nanopeptide that elicits reversible changes of the endothelium and edema formation within the microvasculature. Two enzymes present in plasma, carboxypeptidase N (kininase I) and angiotensin-converting enzyme (kininase II), inhibit the biologic activity of bradykinin secondary to proteolytic cleavage of the carboxy terminal peptide and dipeptides, respectively.

The permeability changes induced by vasoactive mediators may also be modulated by the local production of vasodilatory compounds. Specific prostaglandins (prostaglandins I_2, E_2, and D_2) increase edema formation when injected locally at sites of tissue injury. The anti-inflammatory effects of aspirin and indomethacin are believed to be, in part, secondary to the inhibition of local prostaglandin production with reduction of edema at sites of inflammation.

Complement System

The complement system is a group of 20 plasma proteins that play an important role in host defense against bacterial infection and are an integral component of the body's immune system.[2] Two distinct pathways, "classic" and "alternative," exist for activation (Fig. 4). The classic complement pathway may be activated by several inflammatory mediators, including immune complexes and microbial products. The process of activation of the classic pathway involves recognition of the inflammatory agent by the first component of complement (C1). C1 consists of three separate proteins, C1q, C1r, and C1s. C1q binds to the Fc component of immunoglobulin molecules of specific IgG subclasses or IgM when bound to soluble or fixed antigens. Sequential enzymatic activation of C1r and C1s occurs. Activated C1r and C1s react with C4 and C2, generating the soluble anaphylatoxin C4a and the biomolecular complex C4b, C2a. This complex, referred to as C3

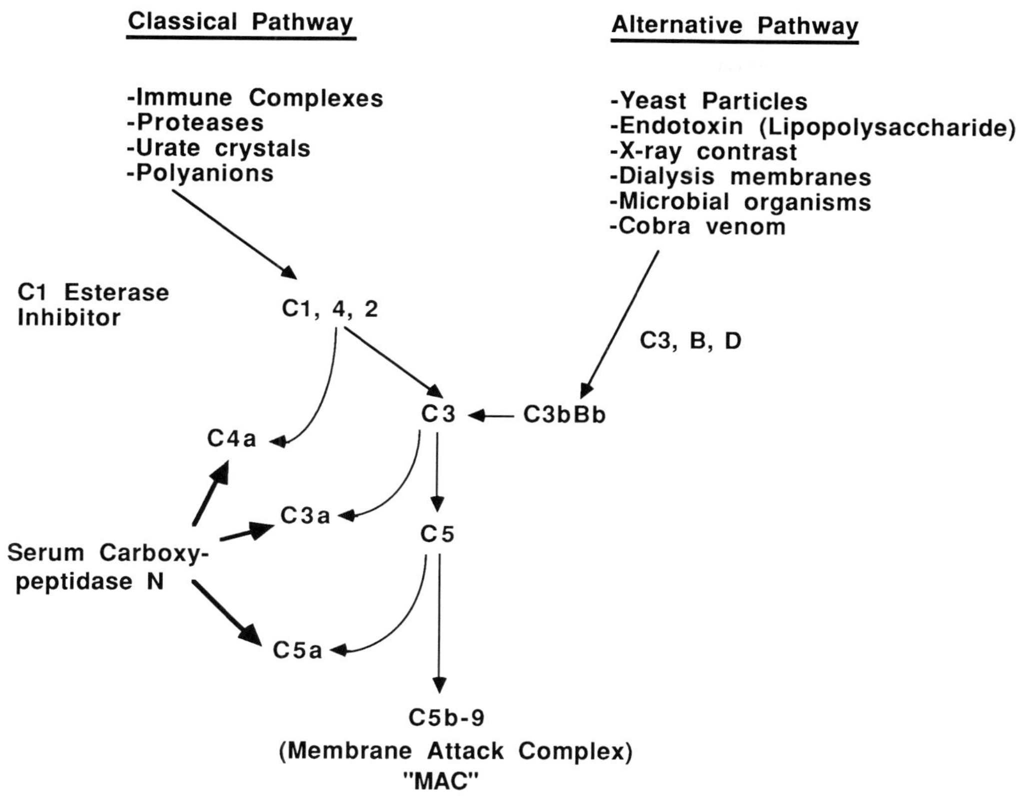

Fig. 4 *The complement system.*

convertase, is proteolytic for the C3 molecule, generating a second soluble anaphylatoxin molecule, C3a, and C3b. The resulting multimolecular complex binds C5 and initiates enzymatic hydrolysis of the C5 molecule, generating a third complement-derived anaphylatoxin, C5a, and a residual component of C5 cleavage, C5b. The C5b molecule serves as a nucleus on target cell membranes and surfaces for the sequential binding of C6, C7, and C8 and the polymerization of multiple C9 molecules, forming a macromolecular complex referred to as the membrane attack complex. Assembly of the membrane attack complex on a cell surface results in the formation of cylindrical holes in the cell membrane with loss of membrane integrity and cell lysis.

The alternative complement pathway may be activated by a variety of microbial and cell products as well as by foreign material. This results in the binding of C3 with two plasma proteins, factor B and factor D, and the subsequent formation of an enzymatically active derivative of factor B, Bb, that catalyzes the conversion of C3 to C3b

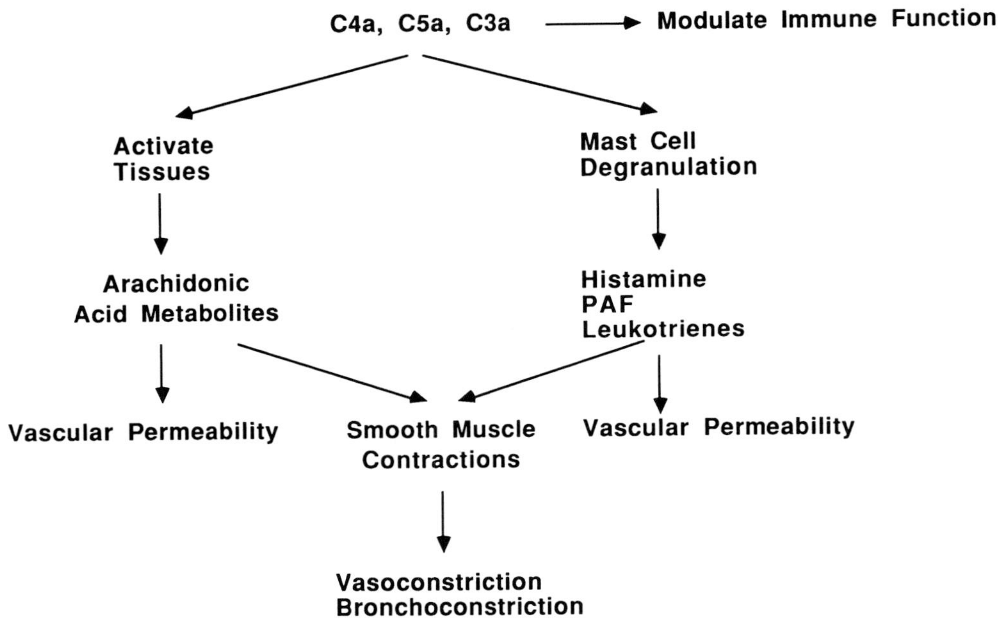

Fig. 5 *Biologic activity of anaphylatoxins.*

and C3a. When bound to Bb, C3b functions as C3 convertase, generating additional C3b and C3a in an amplification step. Subsequently, C5 convertase is formed with the sequential generation of C5b (and soluble C5a), followed by assembly of the membrane attack complex. In contrast to their role in the classic pathway, C1, C4, and C2 are not involved in the alternative pathway.

The results of activation of either the alternative or classic complement pathways are similar: the generation of a C3 convertase, the generation of the biologically active anaphylatoxins, C3a and C5a, and formation of a membrane attack complex capable of inducing cell lysis.

Three important products of classic pathway complement activation include the anaphylatoxins C3a, C4a, and C5a. Each of these molecules is capable of causing smooth-muscle contraction and increasing vascular permeability (Fig. 5). Both C3a and C5a also induce mast-cell and basophil degranulation, causing release of histamine, platelet-activating factor, and leukotrienes that further potentiate vascular permeability changes. The anaphylatoxins have also been shown to induce contraction of bronchial smooth muscle and to cause airway narrowing. This effect is mediated by at least two pathways; the first depends on arachidonic acid metabolite formation in lung tissue and the second is mediated by the stimulated release of mast cell products. One of the most important roles of C5a is that of chemotactic factor for leukocytes. The local production of C5a has been shown to be critical for the recruitment of neutrophils and monocytes to sites of tissue injury in a number of experimental disease models. In addition, C5a has been shown both to induce low levels of neutrophil degranulation and superoxide anion production and to enhance the phagocytic response and the extent of degranulation and superoxide anion production in response to a second stimulus. This enhancement effect has been referred to as "cell priming." C3a and C5a function to modulate certain immune responses: whereas C3a inhibits T-lymphocyte proliferation, C5a has been shown to promote immune reactions.

Several mechanisms regulate complement activation. These include (1) spontaneous decay of individual enzymatically active complexes (C4b, C2a, C3b, Bb) or cleavage products (C3b and C4b); (2) proteolytic inactivation of specific components, and (3) the binding of active components by plasma proteins. The plasma protein, factor I, inhibits the activity of C3b and C4b, while serum carboxypeptidase N cleaves the carboxy terminal arginine from the anaphylatoxins C4a, C3a, and C5a in a manner similar to bradykinin, decreasing their biologic activity. A third plasma protein, C1 esterase inhibitor, regulates the activation of the classic pathway by binding to C1r and C1s, forming an irreversible, inactive complex. Additional binding proteins present in plasma include factor H and C4b binding protein. These proteins form complexes with C3b and C4b, respectively, and enhance their susceptibility to proteolytic cleavage by factor I.

The complement system functions as a defense against bacterial infection by several mechanisms. Bacteria may activate the complement system either by direct activation of the alternative pathway or as a result of antibody binding to the surface of the bacterium with activation of the classic pathway. This may cause the initiation of bacteriolysis via the assembly of the membrane attack complex or enhanced clearance of bacteria by phagocytic cells through opsonization. Bacterial opsonization is the process by which a specific molecule (IgG or C3b) binds to the surface of the bacterium (Fig. 6), resulting in enhanced phagocytosis, as the opsonized bacteria are bound to receptors (Fc or C3b receptor) on phagocytic cell membranes. Viruses, parasites, and transformed cells may also activate the complement system by similar mechanisms, resulting in their inactivation or death.

The importance to the host of an intact and functional complement system is exemplified by persons who have acquired or congenital deficiencies of specific complement components or regulatory proteins. Acquired deficiencies of early complement components are observed in patients with certain autoimmune diseases, including specific forms of membranous glomerulonephritis and systemic lupus erythematosus. Patients with congenital deficiencies in the early components of the complement system express clinical syndromes similar to systemic lupus erythematosus. The importance of selective components of the complement system in host surveillance against bacterial infection is manifest in patients with deficiencies in the middle (C3, C5) and terminal (C6, C7, or C8) complement components by increased suscep-

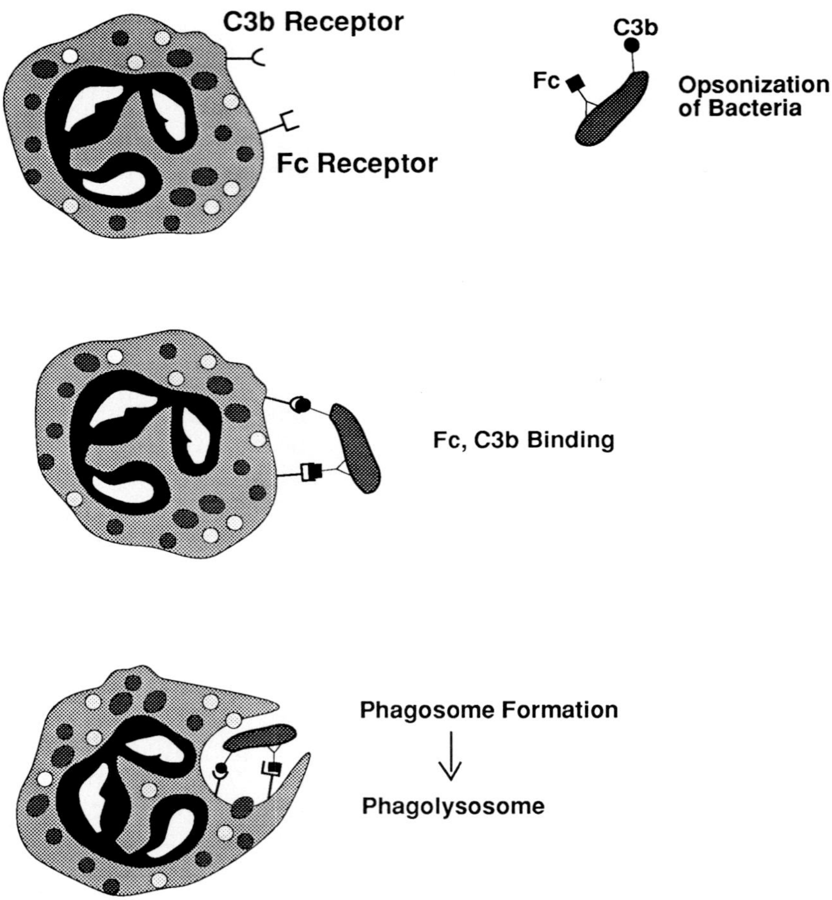

Fig. 6 *Neutrophil phagocytosis of opsonized bacteria.*

tibility to pyogenic bacterial and Neisserial infections. The C2 deficiency is the most common congenital complement defect, although congenital defects in the regulatory proteins of the complement system (C1 esterase inhibitor and serum carboxypeptidase N) have also been reported. The syndrome of hereditary angioedema is characterized by episodic, painless, nonpitting edema of soft tissues, most pronounced in the subepithelial areas, gastrointestinal tract, and upper respiratory tract. If involvement of the larynx occurs, it may become life-threatening and it is associated with a deficiency of C1 esterase inhibitor.

Arachidonic Acid Metabolites

One class of biologically active mediators generated by inflammatory cells and injured tissues includes specific enzymatic derivatives of

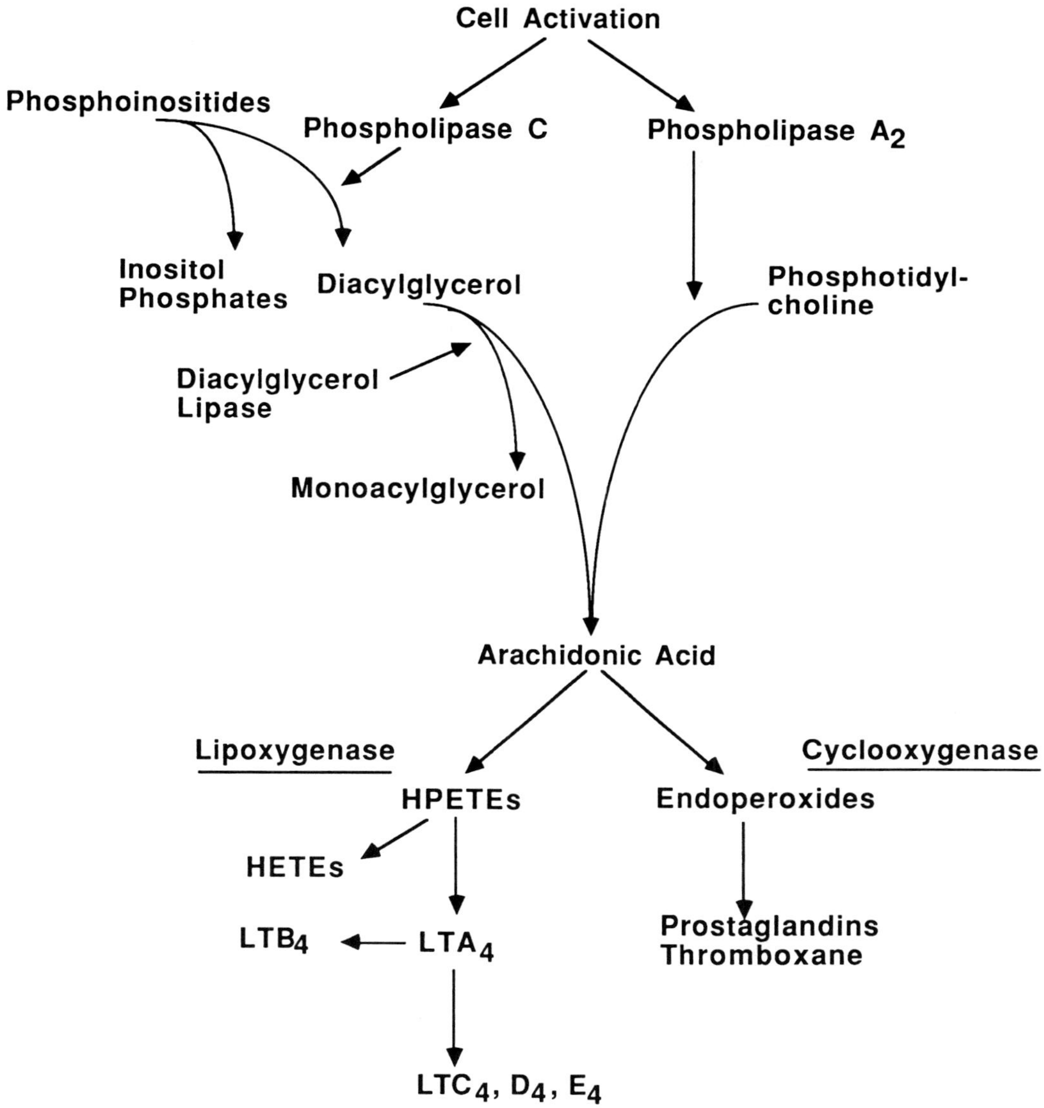

Fig. 7 *Generation of arachidonic acid metabolites. HETEs, hydroxyeicosatetranoic acids; HPETEs, hydroperoxyeicosatetranoic acid compounds; LT, leukotriene.*

phospholipids and fatty acids.[11,14,17,21] Depending on the specific inflammatory cell and stimulus, activated cells generate significant quantities of arachidonic acid (Fig. 7). Arachidonic acid can be released from cell membrane phospholipids by at least two distinct metabolic pathways. The first involves stimulus-induced activation of phospholipase A_2 with the hydrolysis of arachidonic acid from the second carbon of the glycerol backbone. In particular, phosphatidylcholine is an important substrate of phospholipase A_2 and a source of arachidonic acid in inflammatory cells. A second mechanism by which arachidonic acid can be generated is via the metabolism of phosphatidylinositides by phospholipase C to diacylglycerol and inositol phosphates. Diacylglycerol is a substrate for diacylglycerol lipase, which cleaves arachidonic acid from the second position of the glycerol backbone. Once generated, arachidonic acid, a polyunsaturated fatty acid consisting of 20 carbons and four conjugated double bonds, can be metabolized by cyclo-oxygenase and lipoxygenase enzymes. Specific cyclo-oxygenase enzymes in inflammatory cells generate unstable endoperoxide derivatives of arachidonic acid, including prostaglandin G_2 and prostaglandin H_2. Depending on the cell and tissue, the endoperoxides are metabolized to more stable prostaglandins, including prostaglandin I_2 (also known as prostacyclin), prostaglandin F_2, prostaglandin E_2, and thromboxane A_2. In platelets the primary cyclo-oxygenase metabolite is thromboxane A_2, whereas endothelial cells secrete principally prostaglandin I_2. Macrophages, depending on their state of activation, produce varying amounts of each product.

At sites of inflammation, prostaglandins I_2 and E_2 are associated with enhanced vascular permeability because they are vasodilators. Thromboxane A_2 is a potent vasoconstrictor and plays an important role in the mediation of the "second wave" of platelet aggregation. Prostaglandin I_2 has also been shown to bind to specific receptors on inflammatory cells, resulting in the activation of adenylate cyclase and an increase in intracellular cyclic adenosine monophosphate (cAMP) levels. In addition, prostaglandin E_2 increases cAMP levels in neutrophils and macrophages and inhibits their functional responses to other inflammatory stimuli.

A second pathway by which arachidonic acid can be metabolized in inflammatory cells and tissue is via lipoxygenation and the formation of hydroperoxyeicosatetranoic acid compounds. Hydroperoxy compounds can be metabolized to hydroxyeicosatetranoic acids or leukotriene A_4. In the neutrophil and certain macrophage populations, leukotriene A_4 is metabolized to leukotriene B_4, a compound with potent chemotactic activity for neutrophils, monocytes, and macrophages. In other cell types, especially mast cells, basophils, and macrophages, the addition of glutathione to leukotriene A_4 results in the formation of leukotriene C_4. After sequential removal of the amino acids glycine and glutamine, leukotrienes D_4 and E_4 are formed, respectively. Leukotrienes C_4, D_4, and E_4, collectively known as the SRS-As, have potent smooth-muscle contracting activity, and are capable of enhancing vascular permeability changes. At sites of tissue injury, leukotriene B_4 plays an important role in the recruitment of polymorphonuclear leukocytes, whereas leukotrienes C_4, D_4, and E_4 mediate many of the clinical symptoms associated with allergic reactions.

The importance of arachidonic acid metabolite production in mediating many of the effects of the inflammatory response is demonstrated by the ability of inhibitors of arachidonic acid metabolism to attenuate both the pathologic changes and the clinical symptoms of inflammatory-cell-mediated tissue injury. Corticosteroids have been widely used to inhibit the tissue destruction associated with many inflammatory diseases, including allergic responses, rheumatoid arthritis, and systemic lupus erythematosus. One mechanism by which corticosteroids function is to induce the synthesis of lipocortin, an inhibitor of phospholipase A_2 that blocks the release of arachidonic acid in inflammatory cells. Originally described as two different proteins, lipomodulin and macrocortin, these regulatory proteins are now known to be similar in derivation.

Additional anti-inflammatory agents widely used in the treatment of inflammatory diseases are the nonsteroidal anti-inflammatory drugs (NSAIDs), including aspirin, indomethacin, ibuprofen, and piroxicam. The effects of these compounds are thought to be secondary to inhibition of the cyclo-oxygenase enzyme and the synthesis of prostaglandins and thromboxanes. Compounds that inhibit specific lipoxygenase activities in inflammatory cells are not yet available for clinical use, but it is anticipated that their development will provide an additional pharmacologic approach to the effective, specific modulation of the inflammatory response.

Cellular Recruitment

Neutrophils, monocytes, and lymphocytes are recruited to inflammatory sites as the result of the local generation of specific soluble chemotactic factors. Chemotactic factors are generated in relatively high concentrations at sites of tissue injury, and in a decreasing gradient of concentration away from the injured tissue. The physiologic responses of the circulating leukocytes after exposure to chemotactic factors include margination of the cells along the vascular wall, adherence of the leukocytes to the endothelium or vascular basement membrane, emigration through the vascular wall, and unidirectional migration, or chemotaxis, toward increasing concentrations of the chemotactic agent (Fig. 8).

The most important chemotactic factors for neutrophils generated in vivo include the complement-derived chemotactic factor C5a, bacteria- and mitochondria-derived low-molecular-weight N-formylated peptides, such as N-formyl-methionyl-leucyl-phenylalanine; and specific products of lipid metabolism, including leukotriene B_4. Additional sources of chemotactic factors include low-molecular-weight cell-derived products (cytokines). Recently, a novel peptide chemotactic factor for neutrophils (interleukin-8) has been shown to be produced by a variety of activated cells, including monocytes, fibroblasts, and endothelial cells. Finally, proteases from phagocytic cells and plasma (plasmin) can generate C5a or C5a-related chemotactic peptides secondary to proteolytic cleavage.

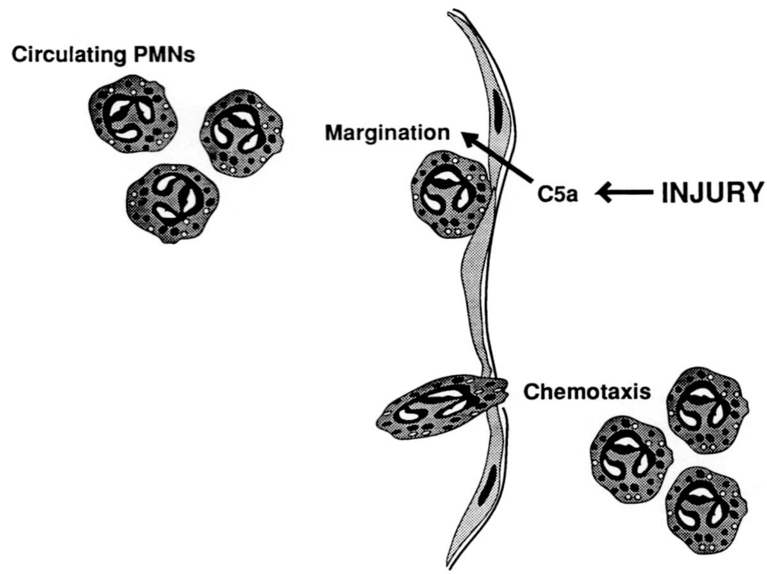

Fig. 8 *The chemotactic response of neutrophils. PMNs, polymorphonuclear leukocytes.*

Inflammatory Cell Activation

The neutrophil, mast cell, and platelet are important cellular components of acute inflammatory reactions. After stimulation, specific inflammatory mediators released by these cells can cause tissue injury. The neutrophil may be activated in response to phagocytic stimuli or after the binding of chemotactic mediators or immune complexes to specific receptors on the cell membrane. In a similar manner, receptor-specific activation of mast cells, platelets, mononuclear phagocytic cells, lymphocytes, and endothelial cells occurs in response to inflammatory mediators. The biochemical processes associated with stimulation of inflammatory cells leading to functional responses of these cells (degranulation, aggregation) has been referred to as stimulus-response coupling.[1,4,23] Although the biochemical processes after stimulation of each of the cell types are different, several common pathways are associated with inflammatory cell activation (Fig. 9).

After contact, the stimulus is bound to a specific receptor on the cell membrane, resulting in the formation of a ligand-receptor complex. The ligand-receptor complex is coupled via a guanine-nucleotide regulatory protein to a specific phosphodiesterase associated with the inflammatory cell membrane, which activates this enzyme. In the neutrophil, this phosphodiesterase activation is that of phospholipase C. Stimulus-induced activation of phospholipase C results in enhanced phosphoinositide turnover with the formation of two potent metab-

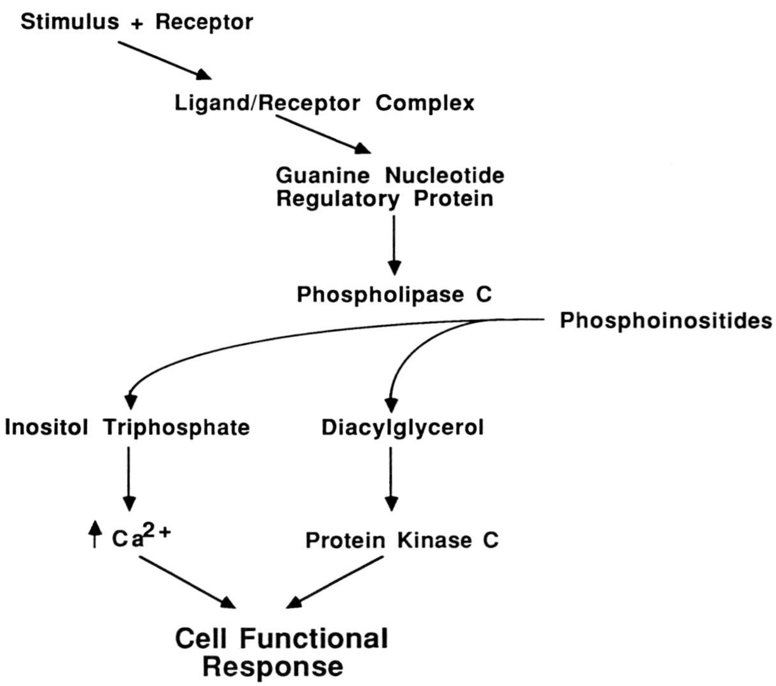

Platelet	Aggregation, degranulation
Mast Cell	Degranulation, arachidonic acid metabolism
Neutrophil	Chemotaxis, O_2^- production, degranulation

Fig. 9 *Early events of inflammatory cell activation (stimulus-response coupling).*

olites, diacylglycerol and inositol triphosphate. Inositol triphosphate releases calcium from intracellular stores.[3] In addition to this release, there is an influx of calcium ions from the extracellular environment. Together, these two sources contribute to a net increase in free intracellular calcium. This increase in free intracellular calcium is a critical component in the activation of most inflammatory cells by physiologic stimuli. The increase in free intracellular calcium can have many effects on the biochemical processes of the cell, including the potentiation of phospholipase A_2 activity and activation of various protein kinases capable of phosphorylating and altering the activity of specific cell-associated proteins. Also, the critical role of calmodulin (a high-affinity, calcium-binding protein of nonmuscle cells) in the activation of inflammatory cells has been established. The mobilization of intracellular calcium is also closely linked to the activation of cytoskeletal elements. Assembly of the microtubular system and activation of actin-myosin complexes are critical for secretion of cytoplasmic granules and chemotaxis of neutrophils and other inflammatory cells.

Diacylglycerol, the second product of phospholipase C, is important in mediating additional response within the cell, including the activation of protein kinase C. Protein kinase C functions to phosphorylate several substrate proteins within the cell, including cytoskeletal elements, altering their functional properties. However, the precise mechanism by which protein phosphorylation regulates functional responses of the cell is not clearly defined.

Stimulation of inflammatory cells also activates phospholipase A_2. Phospholipase A_2 is a calcium-dependent enzyme that hydrolyzes the ester bond at the second carbon of the glycerol backbone of phospholipids, releasing fatty acids. In inflammatory cells, phosphatidylcholine is an important substrate for phospholipase A_2 and a source of arachidonic acid. The release of arachidonic acid from membrane phospholipids and its subsequent metabolism to biologically active compounds are important in both inflammatory cell activation and the development of the inflammatory response. Integrity of the lipoxygenase system appears necessary for full expression of chemotactic-factor-induced neutrophil activation, while the integrity of the cyclooxygenase system and production of thromboxane A_2 is critical for certain forms of platelet activation.

Although increases in phospholipid metabolism, changes in intracellular calcium levels, and activation of specific protein kinases are known to be important intermediate steps in the stimulus-induced functional responses of inflammatory cells, we have only a primitive understanding of how specific functional responses are elicited. Additional study will provide insights important for the development of new strategies for therapeutic modulation of inflammatory responses in human disease. An example is the ongoing development of specific lipoxygenase and phospholipase inhibitors that have the potential to inhibit the early activation processes of inflammatory cells and suppress the tissue injury associated with certain diseases.

Modulation of Inflammatory Cell Function

The modulation of inflammatory cell activation by pharmacologic means can be demonstrated by the inhibitory effects of prostaglandins of the E series and prostaglandin I_2 on the functional responses of the mast cell, neutrophil, macrophage, and platelet.[14] Prostaglandins of the E series and prostaglandin I_2 inhibit inflammatory cell function secondary to their ability to activate adenylate cyclase and increase intracellular cAMP levels. Additional agents that stimulate adenylate cyclase activity, including β-adrenergic agonists and cholera toxin, have also been shown to inhibit inflammatory cell function. Further, treatment of inflammatory cells with cyclic nucleotide phosphodiesterase inhibitors such as theophylline potentiates increased cAMP levels within the cell and enhanced the inhibition of their functional responses by adenylate cyclase agonists. Adenylate cyclase agonists and phosphodiesterase inhibitors may also have effects on target tissues of inflammatory mediators. For instance, increased cAMP levels in bronchiole smooth-muscle cells causes relaxation and blocks the effects of mediators that promote bronchoconstriction. This is the biochemical basis of phosphodiesterase inhibition (by theophylline, for example) of mast cell degranulation and of the clinical symptoms associated with certain allergic reactions. In contrast, those biologic mediators, including thromboxane and acetylcholine, that function to activate guanylate cyclase and increase intracellular cyclic guanosine monophosphate levels enhance inflammatory cell function. Therefore, the ability of both the inflammatory cell and the target tissue to respond to a specific inflammatory mediator is modulated by intracellular cyclic nucleotides and is subject to pharmacologic modulation and alteration of the inflammatory response.

The ability of prostaglandin I_2, a secretory product of endothelial cells, to inhibit neutrophil and platelet activation is critical for the maintenance of vascular integrity and the modulation of the recruitment of neutrophils to sites of inflammation. Under normal conditions, prostaglandin I_2 secreted by endothelial cells functions to increase intracellular cAMP levels and suppress platelet and neutrophil activation within the vascular compartment. However, any pathologic insult that decreases the production of prostaglandin I_2 by endothelium decreases the sensitivity of platelets and neutrophils to prostaglandin I_2 or presents an overwhelming inflammatory stimulus that promotes functional responses of both cell types. Alterations in the homeostatic balance between platelet stimulation and suppression by endothelial-cell-derived prostaglandin I_2 has been postulated as significant in the development of atherosclerotic vascular disease and thrombus formation (Fig. 10). Similar alterations in the regulation of neutrophil activation of prostaglandin I_2 are thought to underlie the initiation of acute inflammatory reactions.

Mechanisms of Neutrophil Cell and Tissue Injury

One of the important functions of phagocytic cells is the clearance of foreign agents or injured tissues.[10,25] Phagocytosis of a bacterium or foreign material may be enhanced by the opsonization of that particle by antibody and/or the fixation of C3b on the surface (Fig. 6). Phagocytic cells, including the neutrophil, monocyte, and macrophage, possess specific receptors on their cell membrane surfaces that recognize C3b, C3bi, and the Fc fragment of immunoglobulin molecules to enhance the phagocytic process. The engulfment of a foreign agent by the cell membrane results in the formation of a phagosome within the cytoplasm. Lysosomal granules are directed by cytoskeletal elements within the cell to the phagosome. Fusion of lysosomes with the phagosomes results in the formation of phagolysosome. Release of lyso-

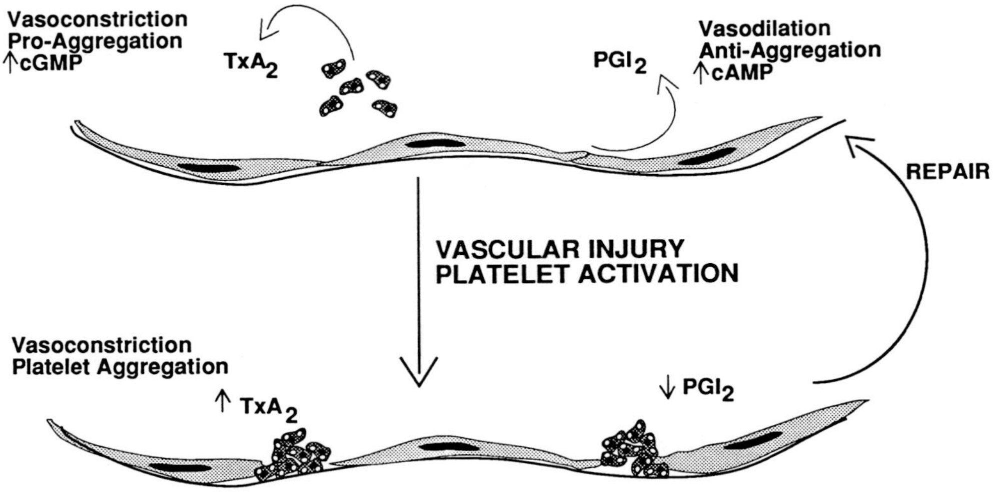

Fig. 10 *Role of thromboxane A_2 (TxA_2) and prostaglandin I_2 (PGI_2) in platelet and endothelial cell interactions.*

somal granule contents into the phagolysosome occurs, exposing the engulfed particle to the degradative properties of these enzymes.

Neutrophils contain three distinct cytoplasmic granules: primary, secondary, and tertiary. Primary granules contain potent acid hydrolases capable of digesting mucopolysaccharide substances and serine protease (elastase and cathespin G) that degrade structural proteins of tissues, including elastin and collagen. Also in these granules are several cationic proteins that function to promote neutrophil adherence to targets and to initiate cytotoxic injury of certain cell types; both these functions are important in killing bacteria. Additional enzymes in the primary granule with known bactericidal activity include lysozyme and phospholipase A_2. These enzymes degrade bacterial cell walls and membranes, respectively. Phospholipase A_2 also promotes changes in the vascular permeability of the skin and is important in the degradation of eukaryotic cell membranes at sites of tissue injury. Myeloperoxidase, another enzyme in these granules, enhances cell cytotoxicity by metabolizing hydrogen peroxide in the presence of halide ions (eg, Cl^-, I^-) to form hypochlorous acid. Secondary granules also contain phospholipase A_2, lysozyme, the cationic protein lactoferrin, a vitamin B_{12}-binding protein, and a collagenase active against type IV collagen. Tertiary granules contain acid hydrolases and gelatinase, a metalloprotease capable of digesting basement membrane and denatured collagen. Release of tertiary granules has been observed at the leading front of neutrophils during chemotaxis and is thought to be the source of enzymes that promote the migration of cells through basement membrane and tissues. Similar granules are present in mon-

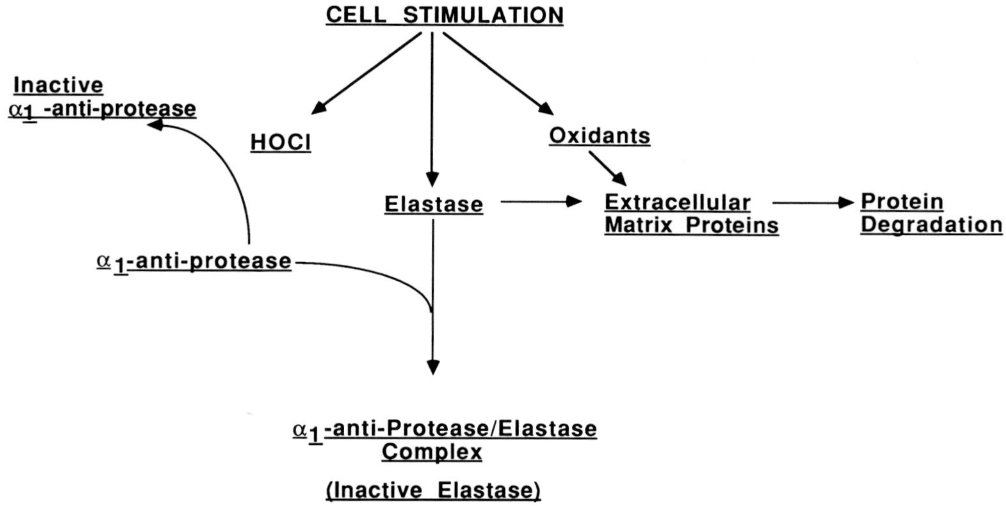

Fig. 11 *Regulation of neutrophil-dependent degradation of extracellular matrix proteins.*

ocytes and macrophages, although their enzyme content differs. Although monocytes possess myeloperoxidase, myeloperoxidase is absent in tissue macrophages. Both monocytes and macrophages contain acid hydrolase activity, collagenase, and gelatinase. However, there is a relative scarcity of elastase and cathespin G within both cell types. An additional neutral protease, plasminogen activator, is also secreted by both neutrophils and mononuclear phagocytic cells. Plasmin, the product of plasminogen-activator-mediated cleavage of plasminogen, is enzymatically active against several biologic substrates, including fibrin, complement, and fibronectin. Therefore, under appropriate conditions, both neutrophils and mononuclear phagocytic cells can promote fibrin degradation at sites of tissue injury as well as activate the complement system.

The biologic activities of proteases, such as elastase and cathespin G, are regulated by the presence of inhibitors in serum and tissue fluids (Fig. 11). α_1-Antiprotease is synthesized by hepatocytes and is the primary inhibitor of neutrophil elastase. The importance of its inhibitory activity is evident in patients with genetic deficiency of α_1-antiprotease, who have an increased incidence of pulmonary emphysema, presumably as a result of the lack of elastase inhibitory activity. A second antiprotease present in serum is α_2-macroglobulin. This protein will also inhibit elastase and cathespin G activity. Both α_1-antiprotease, and α_2-macroglobulin also inhibit plasmin, trypsin, and chymotrypsin activity. Therefore, circulating serum inhibitors exist that not only

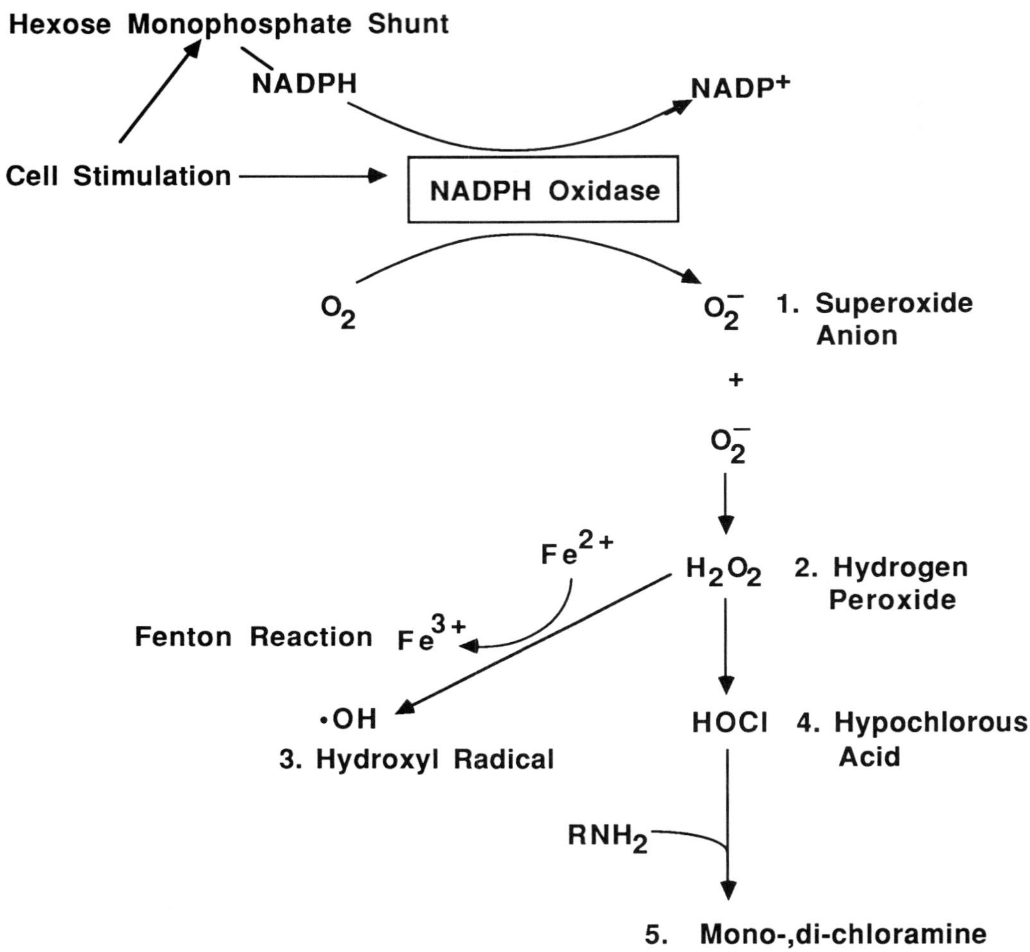

Fig. 12 *Reactive oxygen metabolites generated by neutrophils.*

block phagocytic-cell-derived protease activity but also inhibit protease activity generated within the plasma and tissues.

In addition to the release of granular enzymes into the phagolysosome, an NADPH oxidase enzyme present in the cell membrane of phagocytic cells is activated after phagocytosis (Fig. 12). This activation is associated with a "respiratory burst" characterized by an increase in cell oxygen consumption, chemiluminescence, and activation of the hexose monophosphate shunt.[6,8,9,24] The primary function of the NADPH oxidase is to reduce molecular oxygen forming the superoxide anion, O_2^-. More than 90% of the oxygen consumed after initiation of the respiratory burst in neutrophils can be accounted for by the generation of O_2^-. NADPH generated from the hexose monophosphate shunt is the primary source of electrons for the reduction of O_2^-.

This superoxide anion can be converted to additional reactive oxygen species at the cell surface and within phagolysosomes. Hydrogen peroxide can be generated by either spontaneous or enzymatic dismutation of O_2. Hydrogen peroxide may subsequently react with reduced transition metals in a Fenton-type reaction (for example, Fe^{2+}) to form the highly reactive hydroxyl radical ·OH, or with myeloperoxidase (a component of neutrophil primary granules) to form hypochlorous acid. Hypochlorous acid is a potent bactericidal agent that has been shown to activate neutrophil-derived metalloproteinases, collagenase, and gelatinase. Reaction of hypochlorous acid with molecules containing free amino acid groups produces monochloramine and dichloramine compounds. These compounds are relatively stable and are capable of oxidizing sulfhydryl residues to dialdehydes and thioethers to sulfoxides. Reactive oxygen metabolites can potentially react with all cell and tissue components. Both in vivo and in vitro studies have demonstrated the ability of specific oxygen reactive metabolites to promote lipid peroxidation, DNA scission and cross-linking, sulfhydryl group oxidation and peptide bond cleavage in proteins, and depolymerization of glycosaminoglycans.

There is also a synergistic effect between reactive oxygen metabolites and lysosomal enzyme in mediating tissue injury. Exposure of proteins and glycosaminoglycans to oxidants renders the molecules more susceptible to degradation by proteases and acid hydrolases, respectively. Oxidant present in cigarette smoke and generated by activated phagocytic cells oxidizes a methionine residue on α_1-antiprotease and renders it biologically inactive. The oxidant-dependent inactivation of α_1-antiprotease leads to an enhancement of elastase activity at sites of tissue injury.

Monocytes, macrophages, and eosinophils are also capable of producing significant quantities of superoxide anion and hydrogen peroxide, depending on their state of activation and the stimulus to which they are exposed. The production of reactive oxygen metabolites by these cells has been implicated in their bactericidal and fungicidal activity as well as in their ability to kill certain parasites.

The importance of oxygen-dependent mechanisms in phagocytic cell function is demonstrated in patients who suffer from a defect in NADPH oxidase. Chronic granulomatous disease of childhood is characterized by an inherited enzymatic defect in NADPH oxidase or in its expression and by a failure of production of superoxide anion and hydrogen peroxide during phagocytosis. Patients with this disorder are susceptible to recurrent infections, especially gram-positive cocci.

Depending on the nature of the tissue injury and the size of the phagocytic particle, lysosomal enzymes may be released into the extracellular milieu, and prolonged activation of NADPH oxidase may release significant quantities of hydrogen peroxide and superoxide anion into the adjacent tissues. These products can act on tissue substrates and cells to promote injury and alter the physiologic function of a tissue. Under these conditions, the activation of phagocytic cells may prove harmful to the host organism, damaging or destroying the tissue. Such mechanisms of tissue injury are associated with certain forms of necrosis and play an important role in the pathogenesis of several diseases, including pulmonary emphysema, rheumatoid arthritis, and other immune complex diseases, as well as adult respiratory distress syndrome.

Cell Adherence and Tissue Injury

One of the critical events required for the recruitment of circulating inflammatory cells to sites of tissue injury is the adherence of the cells to endothelium or vascular basement membrane (Outline 1). Under normal physiologic conditions, both cell membranes and vascular basement membrane possess a mutually repulsive negative charge. After injury to endothelial cells or basement membrane, there may be a decrease in the number of anionic sites and net negative charge on the surfaces. This decreases the repulsion between the circulating cells and the vascular wall. Other components of plasma, vascular wall, and phagocytic cell membranes participate in modulating cell adherence reactions. Fibronectin, a glycoprotein present in plasma, in basement membranes, and to a lesser degree in phagocytic cell membranes, has been shown to play a critical role in modulating phagocytic cell attachment to vascular walls. After injury to the vascular wall or tissues, increased amounts of fibronectin are deposited. In addition, fibronectin is a potent opsonin that enhances phagocytosis of bacteria and phagocytic cell adherence. Laminin, a glycoprotein present in the basement membrane, is also important in modulating phagocytic cell function via receptor-specific mechanisms.

Additional factors functioning to enhance phagocytic cell attachment to vascular walls and phagocytic particles include a group of cell membrane glycoproteins that promote adherence.[13] The adherence glycoproteins of human leukocytes constitute a family of molecules consisting of alpha and beta subunits. The three best studied molecules are designated Mo-1, leukocyte function antigen-1, and glycoprotein

Outline 1 Mechanisms of leukocyte adhesion

- Charge effect
- Receptor binding to extracellular matrix proteins (integrins)
  - Fibronectin
  - Laminin
  - Collagens
- Leukocyte adhesion protein
  - Leukocyte function antigen-1
  - Mo-1
  - Glycoprotein 150,95
- Endothelial cell adhesion proteins
  - Endothelial leukocyte adhesion molecule-1
  - Intercellular adhesion molecule-1

150,95. In each of these molecules the beta chain is conserved and specificity of the molecule for adherence properties is conferred by the alpha chain. Activation of phagocytic cells with chemotactic stimuli increases expression of these adherence molecules on the cell surface. The importance of these glycoproteins in the adherence responses of phagocytic cells is demonstrated by two observations. When normal phagocytic cells are treated with antibodies to block the expression of the adherence glycoproteins Mo-1 and glycoprotein 150,95, on their cell surface, there is an inhibition of chemotactic-factor-induced adherence to endothelial cells and foreign surfaces. In addition, a group of patients who possess deficiencies of specific adherence glycoproteins has been identified. Patients deficient in Mo-1 or glycoprotein 150,95 are susceptible to recurrent bacterial infection. Thus, it appears that the expression of these glycoproteins on phagocytic cell surfaces plays an important role in the host defense against bacterial infection and the localization of cells within the vasculature at sites of tissue injury.

Further, endothelial cells can be induced by cytokines secreted by activated macrophages and lymphocytes to express a distinct set of glycoproteins that promote inflammatory cell adherence and localization to sites of inflammation.[19] Increased expression of endothelial leukocyte adhesion molecule-1 (ELAM-1) occurs on the surface of endothelial cells after stimulation with either interleukin-1 or tumor necrosis factor. ELAM-1 binds neutrophils and in organ culture is selectively increased in postcapillary venules. A second endothelial cell glycoprotein, intercellular adhesion molecule-1 (ICAM-1), is also expressed at increased levels after endothelial cell activation by tumor necrosis factor, interleukin-1, and interferon gamma. ICAM-1 functions as a ligand for the leukocyte adhesion protein described. Thus, at sites of inflammation, cytokines potentially function to amplify the inflammatory response through "activation" of endothelial cells and increased expression of proteins that promote leukocyte localization to sites of injury.

The adherence of phagocytic cells to their target is associated with increased cytotoxicity and degradation of substrates.[8] The ability of a phagocytic cell to recognize its target and to adhere serves to "focus" the functional responses of the cell along the adherent surface. When stimulated phagocytic cells adhere to basement membrane, the production of reactive oxygen is greatest along the adherent surface. This is also the site of greatest lysosomal degranulation, indicating that these potentially injurious agents are about to be released nearby. In addition, close approximation of the phagocytic cell with its target serves to exclude macromolecular inhibitors such as α_1-antiprotease from the cell-substrate interface. Thus, phagocytic cell adherence, secretion of reactive oxygen metabolites, and the release of lysosomal enzymes may function in a synergistic manner to enhance cytotoxicity and tissue degradation.

Chronic Inflammation

When there is an immune response to altered host tissue or foreign materials, or when the inflammatory response is unable to eliminate the injurious agent and restore injured tissue to its normal physiologic state, there may be a progression to chronic inflammation. The primary cellular components of the chronic inflammatory response are lymphocytes, macrophages, plasma cells, and, sometimes, eosinophils. The progression of the response to chronic inflammation may use both immunologic and nonimmunologic mechanisms and is frequently observed in conjunction with granulation tissue. The macrophage is an important source of inflammatory and immunologic mediators and is the pivotal cell in regulating these reactions. The accumulation of macrophages occurs primarily as a consequence of recruitment of circulating monocytes by chemotactic stimuli and their differentiation in tissues. However, the local proliferation and differentiation of resident tissue macrophages may also occur, contributing to the net increase in total mononuclear phagocytes. Many of the inflammatory mediators generated by macrophages are similar to those of the neutrophil and include reactive oxygen metabolites, proteases, acid hydrolases, and biologically active lipids, including platelet-activating factor and leukotrienes. Further, macrophages also regulate lymphocyte responses to antigen and secrete several mediators (cytokines) that function to modulate mesenchymal cell (for example, fibroblast and endothelial cell) proliferation and function.

Eosinophils may also be prominent in chronic inflammatory tissue injury. However, they are most evident during allergic reactions and parasitic infection. Eosinophils share many common functional characteristics with the neutrophil and contain granules with a distinctive rhomboid crystalloid granular structure. These granules are rich in acid phosphatase, peroxidase activity, and a unique eosinophil basic protein that is toxic to certain parasites and to normal host cells. The precise role of eosinophils in chronic inflammatory reactions is less clear.

Depending on the inflammatory stimulus, a distinctive pattern of chronic inflammation defined as granulomatous inflammation may develop. This inflammatory response is typical of the tissue response associated with fungal infection, tuberculosis, leprosy, schistosomiasis, and foreign materials (sutures, talc). Granulomas are frequently associated with a cell-mediated hypersensitivity reaction and consist of collections of modified macrophages called epithelioid cells, usually surrounded by a rim of lymphocytes. In contrast to circulating monocytes, these cells have abundant cytoplasm and numerous lysosomal granules. An additional feature of granulomas is the presence of multinucleated giant cells. Either the foreign pathogenic agent (silica, histoplasmosis) or other indigestible material is frequently identifiable within the cytoplasm of a multinucleated giant cell. Giant cells are relatively inactive, especially when compared with macrophages.

Cell-Mediated Immune Hypersensitivity Reactions

Depending on the nature of the antigen associated with a pathologic insult, a distinctive cell-mediated immune hypersensitivity response may occur with associated tissue damage (Fig. 13). In delayed hypersensitivity reactions, macrophages exposed to a specific antigen internalize and process the antigen and subsequently "present" the antigen in association with class II major histocompatibility complex (MHC) molecules. Antigen-specific T lymphocytes are activated after binding to the antigen class II MHC complex. Macrophages also secrete cytokines, including interleukin-1, that promote T-lymphocyte responses. After activation, T lymphocytes synthesize and release soluble mediators (collectively referred to as lymphokines) that react with additional inflammatory and parenchymal cells. One primary effect of lymphokines is the additional recruitment of inflammatory cells and activation of macrophages and fibroblasts. This represents the amplification phase of delayed hypersensitivity reactions.

A second cell-mediated hypersensitivity reaction involves T-lymphocyte-mediated cytotoxicity. This immune mechanism aids in the elimination of virus-infected cells, specific tumor cells that express neoantigens, and acute graft rejection in which foreign MHC antigens are present. In contrast to the delayed hypersensitivity reaction, specific cytotoxic or killer T cells interact with the target and class I MHC antigens. In certain instances, these cells may recognize "self" MHC antigens in addition to viral antigens or tumor neoantigens. After activation of cytotoxic T lymphocytes, the immune response is amplified by T-helper lymphocytes through the secretion of lymphokines, especially interleukin-1. The mechanisms by which cytotoxic T cells initiate cell injury are not well defined.

The cellular and molecular mechanisms that regulate the interactions of immune and inflammatory cells with the vasculature and tissue parenchyma at sites of cell-mediated hypersensitivity reactions are complex. Principally, these mechanisms involve direct interactions of the cell membrane components of a cell with specific binding sites, antigens, or receptors on tissue matrix components (laminin, fibronectin) or a second cell. The number of cell-derived soluble mediators (cytokines) identified as regulating the function of not only immune and inflammatory cells but also parenchymal cells is increasing.[5,13,15,18,20,22] In particular, the function of mononuclear phagocytic cells and subpopulations of T and B lymphocytes is tightly regulated by the secretion of cytokines. At present, several cytokines have been characterized by their molecular and functional features. They include at least eight distinct interleukins, tumor necrosis factors alpha and beta, interferons alfa, beta, and gamma, and many distinct growth factors.

Two of the better characterized cytokines important in inflammatory reactions are interleukin-1 and tumor necrosis factor.[5,13,15,20] Secretion of interleukin-1, previously called endogenous pyrogen or lymphocyte-activating factor, is critical in the host response to injury. Produced primarily by monocytes and macrophages, it is synthesized by a variety of stimulated parenchymal cells, including synovial cells, epithelial cells, fibroblasts, endothelial cells, mesangial cells, and several tumor cell lines. The effects of interleukin-1 include the induction of synthesis of acute-phase hepatic proteins and fever response as well as local

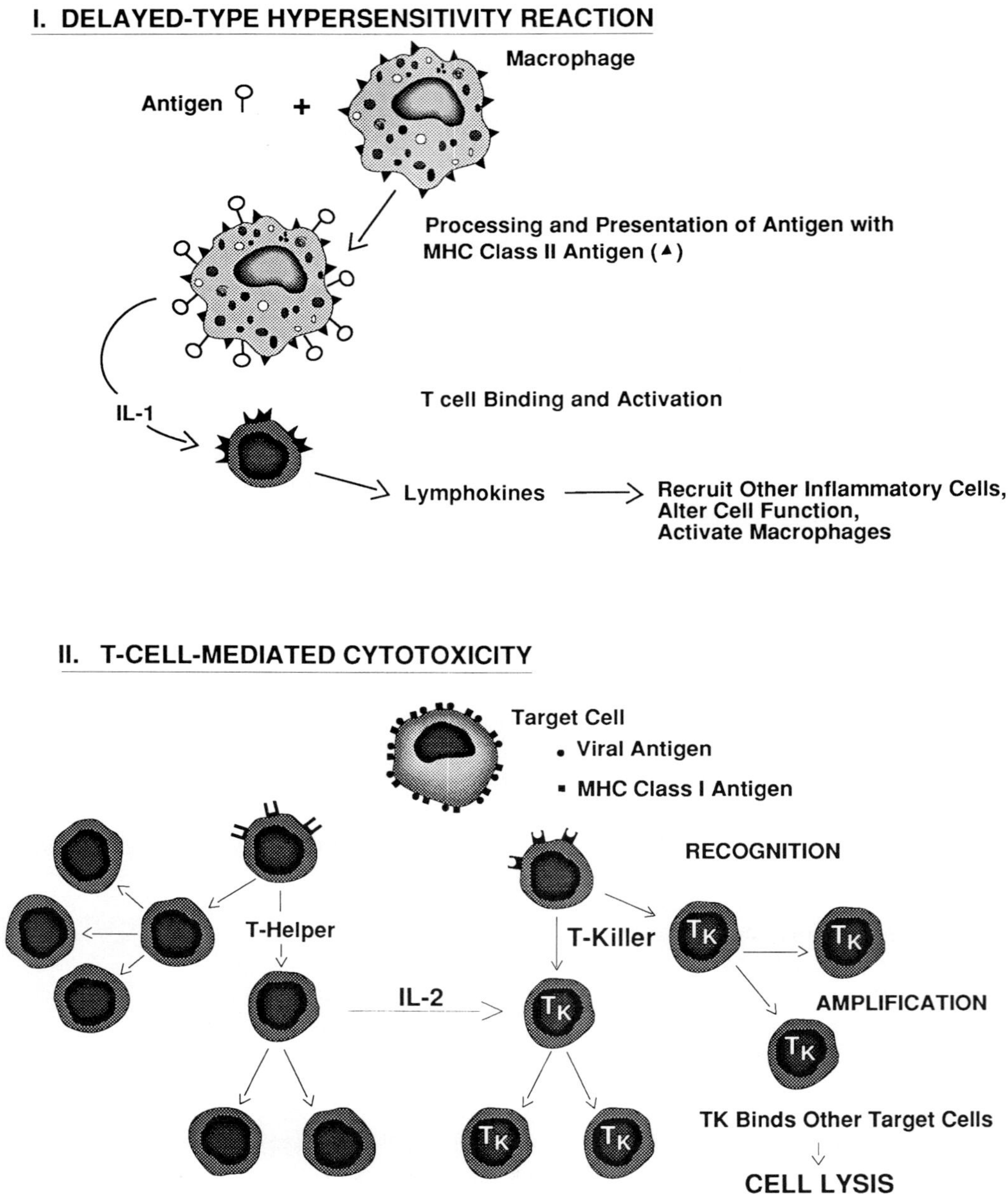

Fig. 13 *Mechanisms of cell-mediated hypersensitivity reactions. MHC, major histocompatibility complex; IL-2, interleukin-2.*

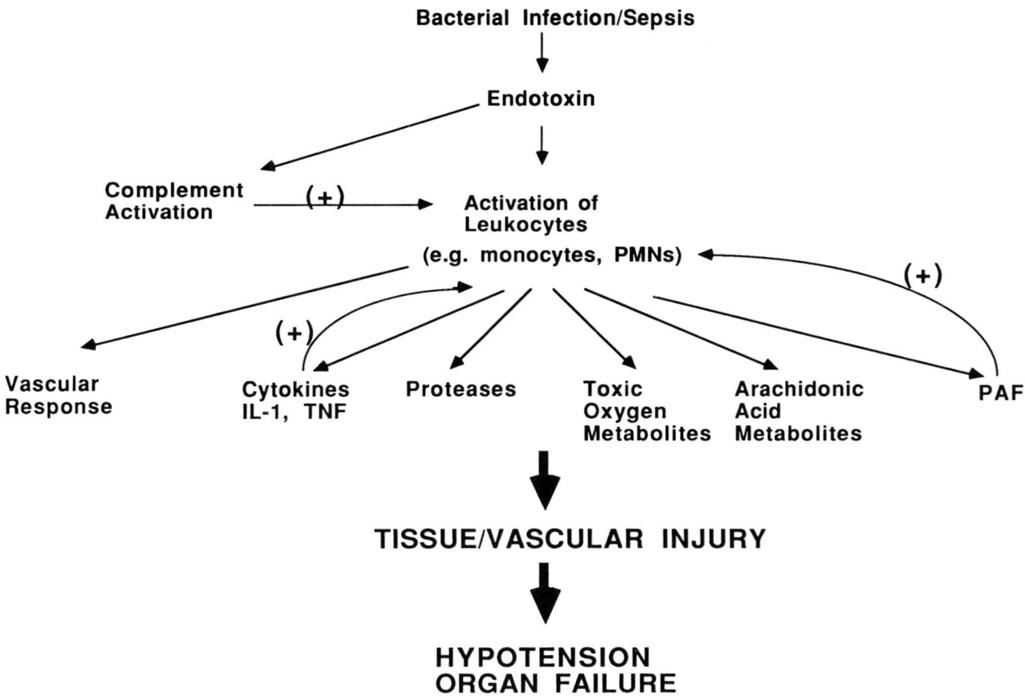

Fig. 14 *Proposed mechanisms of endotoxin shock. IL-1, interleukin-1; PAF, platelet-activating factor; PMNs, polymorphonuclear leukocytes; TNF, tumor necrosis factor.*

immune and inflammatory reactions. Interleukin-1 promotes the induction of several proteins by endothelial cells and thereby modulates thrombus formation and the activation of immune-inflammatory cells. These proteins include plasminogen activator inhibitor; a tissue factor-like procoagulant activity; adhesive factors for neutrophils, monocytes, and lymphocytes; and interleukin-8 (a chemotactic factor for neutrophils). Interleukin-1 also stimulates endothelial cell arachidonic acid metabolism and synthesis of prostaglandins E_2 and I_2.

Effects of interleukin-1 on other cells include stimulation of bone absorption and fibroblast proliferation. Interleukin-1 is also important in several shock states and is an important mediator of the fibrous response associated with many inflammatory conditions. Interleukin-1 acts on the thermoregulatory centers within the hypothalamus to initiate the fever response, which depends on interleukin-1-stimulated production of cyclo-oxygenase products of arachidonic acid (especially prostaglandin E_2) within the hypothalamus and is inhibited by cyclo-oxygenase inhibitors such as aspirin.

A second important product of stimulated mononuclear phagocytic cells is tumor necrosis factor. First recognized for its cytolytic effect on murine tumor cells, tumor necrosis factor has since been demonstrated to be an important mediator of immune and inflammatory reactions, including reactions to bacterial endotoxin (as in toxic shock syndromes) (Fig. 14). Tumor necrosis factor binds to specific receptors on endothelial cells and stimulates production of procoagulant activity, neutrophil chemotactic factor interleukin-8, and specific adherence proteins for granulocytes.[19,22] Tumor necrosis factor also directly activates polymorphonuclear leukocytes and stimulates the production of interleukin-1 and prostaglandin E_2 by human monocytes. Further evidence of a critical role for tumor necrosis factor in inflammatory reactions is demonstrated by its ability to promote fibroblast production of interferon gamma and to affect other parenchymal cell functions.

It is probable that additional cell-derived mediators with potent biologic effects will be identified. This should provide further insights into the complex cellular and molecular mechanisms by which the inflammatory response is regulated.

Acknowledgment

This chapter was adapted with permission from Fantone JC, Ward PA: Inflammation, in Rubin E, Farber JL (eds): *Pathology*. Philadelphia, JB Lippincott, 1988, pp 34–64.

References

1. Becker EL: Leukocyte stimulation: Receptor, membrane, and metabolic events. *Fed Proc* 1986;45:2148–2150.
2. Bellanti JA (ed): *Immunology III*, ed 3. Philadelphia, WB Saunders, 1985.
3. Berridge MJ: Inositol triphosphate and diacylglycerol as second messengers. *Biochem J* 1984;220:345–360.
4. Cochrane CG: Mechanisms coupling stimulation and function in leukocytes. *Fed Proc* 1984;43:2729–2731.
5. Dinarello CA: Biology of interleukin 1. *FASEB J* 1988;2:108–115.
6. Elsbach P, Weiss J: Oxygen-dependent and oxygen-independent mechanisms of microbicidal activity of neutrophils. *Immunol Lett* 1985;11:159-163.
7. Fantone JC, Ward PA: Inflammation, in Rubin E, Farber JL (eds): *Pathology*. Philadelphia, JB Lippincott, 1988, pp 34–64.
8. Fantone JC, Ward PA: Polymorphonuclear leukocyte-mediated cell and tissue injury: Oxygen metabolites and their relations to human diseases. *Hum Pathol* 1985;16:973–978.
9. Fantone JC, Ward PA: Role of oxygen-derived free radicals and metabolites in leukocyte-dependent inflammatory reactions. *Am J Pathol* 1982;107:395–418.
10. Gallin JI, Fauci AS (eds): *Advances in Host Defense Mechanisms*. New York, Raven Press, 1982.
11. Goetzl EJ, Payan DG, Goldman DW: Immunopathogenetic roles of leukotrienes in human diseases. *J Clin Immunol* 1984;4:79–84.
12. Houck JC (ed): *Chemical Messengers of the Inflammatory Process*. Amsterdam, Elsevier/North Holland Biomedical Press, 1979.

13. Ikejima T, Okusawa S, Van Der Meer JWM, et al: Toxic shock syndrome is mediated by interleukin 1 and tumor necrosis factor. *Rev Infect Dis* 1989;12(suppl 1):S316-S317.
14. Marcus AJ: The eicosanoids in biology and medicine. *J Lipid Res* 1984;25:1511–1516.
15. Movat HZ: Tumor necrosis factor and interleukin-1: Role in acute inflammation and microvascular injury. *J Lab Clin Med* 1987;110:668–681.
16. Movat HZ (ed): *Inflammation, Immunity, and Hypersensitivity: Cellular and Molecular Mechanisms*, ed 2. Hagerstown, Harper & Row, 1979.
17. O'Flaherty JT: Lipid mediators of inflammation and allergy. *Lab Invest* 1982;47:314–329.
18. Peveri P, Walz A, Dewald B, et al: A novel neutrophil-activating factor produced by human mononuclear phagocytes. *J Exp Med* 1988;167:1547–1559.
19. Pober JS: Cytokine-mediated activation of vascular endothelium: Physiology and pathology. *Am J Pathol* 1988;133:426–433.
20. Remick DG, Scales WE, Chensue SW, et al: The pathophysiology of interleukins and tumor necrosis factor, in Sayeed M (ed): *Focus on Cellular Pathophysiology*. Boca Raton, CRC Press, 1989.
21. Samuelsson B: Leukotrienes: Mediators of immediate hypersensitivity reactions and inflammation. *Science* 1983;220:568–575.
22. Strieter RM, Kunkel SL, Showell HJ, et al: Endothelial cell gene expression of a neutrophil chemotactic factor by TNF-α, LPS, and IL-1β. *Science* 1989;243:1467–1469.
23. Synderman R, Pike MC: Chemoattractant receptors on phagocytic cells. *Annu Rev Immunol* 1984;2:257–281.
24. Weiss SJ: Tissue destruction by neutrophils. *N Engl J Med* 1989;320:365–376.
25. Weissman G (ed): *The Cell Biology of Inflammation*. Amsterdam, Elsevier/North Holland Biomedical Press, 1980.

Chapter 3

Basic Concepts in Wound Healing

Antonio Martinez-Hernandez, MD
Peter S. Amenta, MD, PhD

Introduction

A wound can be defined as the disruption of cellular and anatomic continuity, and wound healing as the restoration of that continuity.[1] Healing, a basic response of an organism to injury, is the process by which dead or lost tissue is replaced by living tissue. Long-lived organisms require processes and mechanisms to replace obsolete components and to maintain their structural and functional constancy. These processes constitute morphostasis. Examples of morphostasis are the continuous renewal of the gastrointestinal lining and bone remodeling. Ideally, the dead or lost tissue is replaced by tissue with identical morphologic characteristics and function, resulting in regeneration. If every lost cell could be replaced, organisms would be immortal; if no lost cell could be replaced, few would survive embryonic development. In general, the lower an organism is on the phylogenetic ladder, the greater is its regenerative capacity.

Healing requires complex interactions between cells, between extracellular matrix components, and between cells and extracellular matrix. For optimal repair, these interactions must occur in the proper spatial and temporal sequence. The extent of the injury and the balance and timing of the interactions between cells, matrix, and regulatory factors determine the outcome of the healing process—restoration of function or scarring and dysfunction.

The Extracellular Matrix

The extracellular matrix is a complex of macromolecules surrounding stromal cells and underlying most epithelia.[37,38,49,67,98,145,186] More than simply an inert structural support, it contains information that modulates cell behavior, migration, attachment, and differentiation. Thus, it has profound effects on morphogenesis and repair.[32,67,145,186] The extracellular matrix consists of three major classes of macromolecules: the collagens, the noncollagenous structural glycoproteins, and the proteoglycans. Basement membranes are specialized extracellular matrices that exist between most epithelial cells, some mesenchymal cells, and the adjacent interstitium. Basement membranes also contain components of the three major macromolecular groups.[45,120,181]

For the extracellular matrix to influence adjacent cells, the intracellular and extracellular compartments must be able to communicate with each other, although the mechanisms of communication are not yet clear. The extracellular matrix may bind to specific sites on the cell surface via a family of receptors, the integrins, and thus convey information to cells.[17,160,176] The integrins are transmembrane proteins that interact with both the extracellular matrix and the intracellular compartment.[17,68,69,160,177] Through these interactions, the extracellular matrix modulates cell behavior and the repair reaction. This modulation depends on the synthesis and deposition of individual extracellular matrix components in a specific temporal and spatial sequence that integrates cells and matrix into a functional unit.[99,119]

Components of the Extracellular Matrix

Collagens

The major structural constituent of the extracellular matrix is the protein family known as the collagens (*koila,* glue), which constitute approximately 30% of the total protein in an adult man.[16,19,27,54,96,115,128,129] The collagens are a complex, heterogeneous family of macromolecules that share common characteristics such as resistance to proteases, tensile strength, their primary amino acid sequence, long helical domains, and a basic constituent polypeptide, the alpha chain.[16,19,27,54,96,115,129] Each alpha chain has approximately 1,000 amino acid residues, generally in a Gly-X-Y sequence (X and Y are often proline and lysine). The primary sequence of each alpha chain gives the individual collagen type its characteristic features. Several of the collagens contain intrahelical globular regions, often called noncollagenous domains. In these regions, the typical Gly-X-Y sequence is absent and the region is susceptible to nonspecific proteases.[27,130] A collagen molecule is formed by the association of three alpha chains coiled in a right-handed helix, with a left-handed supercoil (Fig. 1). Currently, 13 different collagen types are known, coded for by over 20 distinct genes.[10,20,27,147]

Each collagen type is identified by its respective alpha chain or chains. The chains are designated with arabic numerals followed by the collagen type in roman numerals. For example, collagen type I is typically heterotrimeric and consists of two identical alpha chains, $\alpha 1(I)$, and a dissimilar chain, $\alpha 2(I)$. These form the collagen molecule, $[\alpha 1(I)]_2\ \alpha 2(I)$. Type III collagen, on the other hand, is homotrimeric $[\alpha 1(III)]_3$. Individual collagen molecules may aggregate into larger groups of fibrils, fibers, and bundles through the process of fibrillogenesis.[13,14,48,50,87] The characteristic associations and tissue distribu-

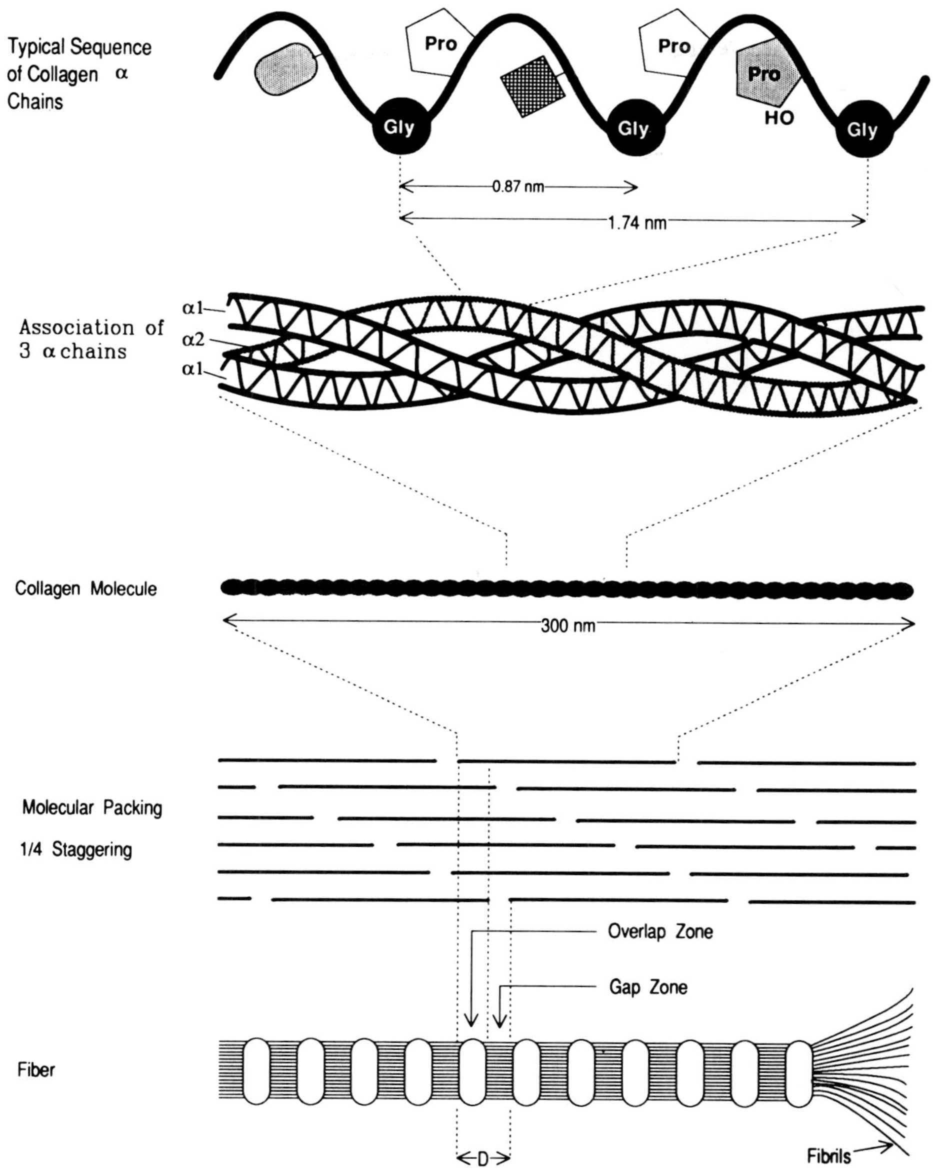

Fig. 1 *Collagen alpha chains have a Gly-X-Y amino-acid sequence. Glycine is found in every third position and proline is often at the X position. Each glycine rotates the polypeptide chain 120 degrees; three glycine residues complete the rotation. Three alpha chains associate to form a collagen molecule. For some collagen types (for example, types II and III) the three chains are identical (homotrimers). Other types (for example, type I) have different alpha chains (heterotrimers). Collagen fibers are formed by association of individual collagen chains. The chains are side-to-side in a quarter-stagger array. The space between the ends of two molecules (gap zone) permits penetration of heavy metals; the overlap zone excludes them. The result is the characteristic cross-banding of some collagen fibers on electron microscopy. The association of several molecules results in fibril formation; several fibrils form a fiber, and several fibers make a bundle.*

Type	Chains	Macromolecular Association	Aggregate Form	Localization
I	α 1(I), α 2(I)			Most abundant collagen: Ubiquitous —Bone, Tendon, Capsules, Muscle, etc.
II	α 1(II)			Major cartilage collagen: Cartilage, Nucleus pulposus, Vitreous humor.
III	α 1(III)			Found in pliable tissues: Blood vessels, Muscle, Uterus, etc.
IV	α 1(IV), α 2(IV)			Component of all Basement Membranes
V	α 1(V), α 2(V), α 3(V)	???		Minor component in most interstitial tissues
VI	α 1(VI), α 2(VI)			Abundant in most interstitial tissues
VII	α 1(VII)			Anchoring fibrils
VIII	α 1(VIII)*	???		Secreted by some endothelia
IX	α 1(IX), α 2(IX), α 3(IX)	???		Minor cartilage collagen
X	α 1(X)	???		Present in mineralizing cartilage

Fig. 2 *Distinct genetic collagen types. Collagen types I to X are shown with their chain compositions, macromolecular associations, aggregate forms, and major tissue distributions.*

tions of each collagen type are summarized in Figure 2 and reviewed elsewhere in this volume.

Collagen Biosynthesis Collagen biosynthesis is similar to that for all proteins (including other components of the extracellular matrix) targeted for export (Fig. 3), with translation on membrane-bound ribosomes, transport into the cisternae of the rough endoplasmic reticulum, to the Golgi complex, and then to the extracellular space.[16,87] Each polypeptide chain has a signal sequence at the amino terminal (N-terminal), which is severed shortly after translation. The result is the procollagen chain, consisting of three major regions: the nonhelical N-terminal, the carboxy terminal (C-terminal), and the central helical domain (Fig. 1). While in the cisternae of the endoplasmic reticulum, the respective procollagen alpha chains aggregate to form the procollagen molecule. The molecule undergoes additional posttranslational modifications, including hydroxylation of proline and lysine residues, glycosylation, and disulfide bonding. The latter events are critical if the fibers are to attain their maximum tensile strength.[16,87] Procollagen hydroxylation is accomplished by two enzymes, lysyl hydroxylase and prolyl hydroxylase. It also depends on vitamin C or ascorbic acid, a reducing agent, as a cofactor, and on α-ketoglutarate, ferrous iron, and oxygen. Vitamin C deficiency results in scurvy, with deficient collagen

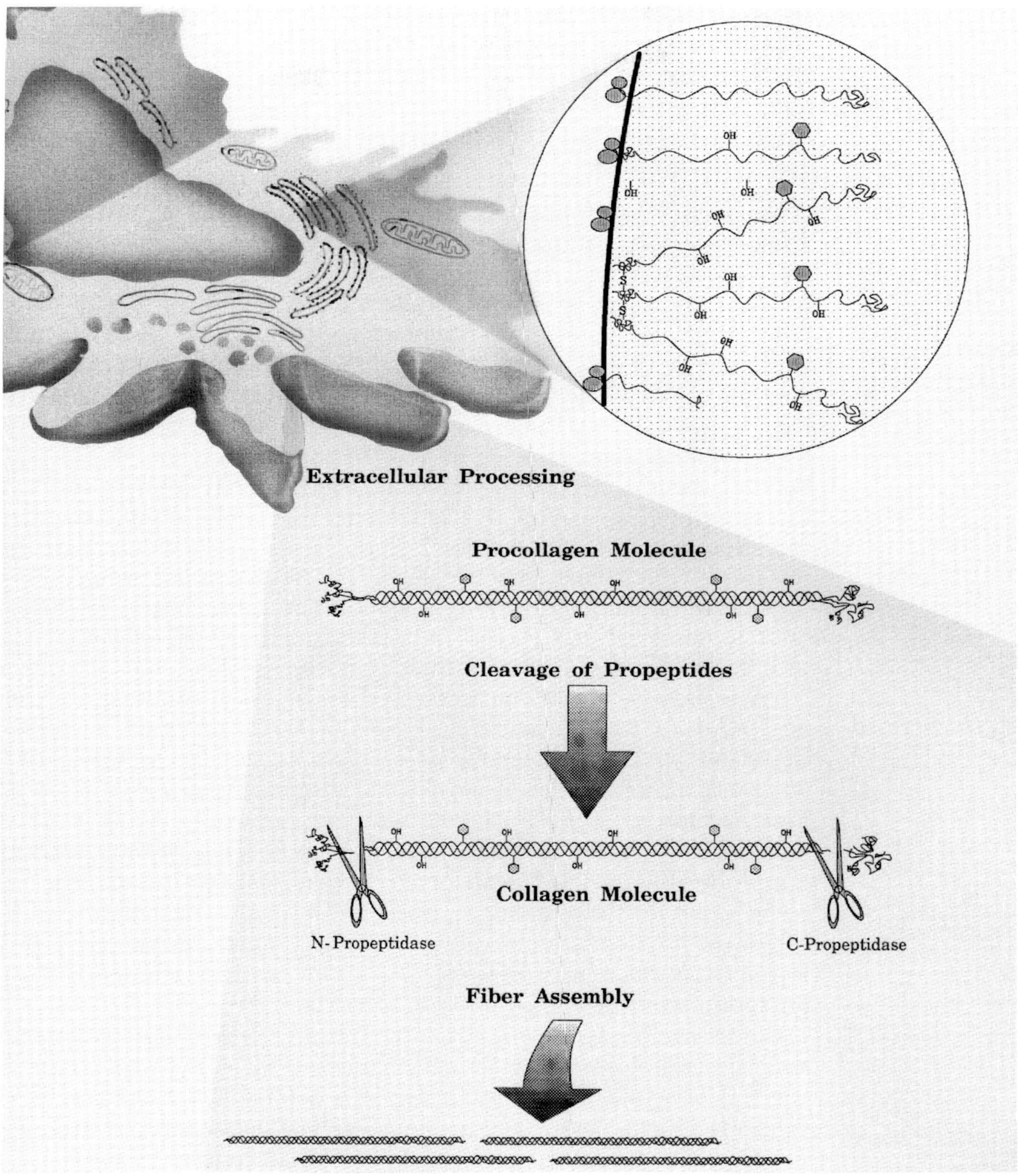

Fig. 3 *Collagen biosynthesis. Collagen alpha chains synthesized in ribosomes enter the rough endoplasmic reticulum. Both ends of the chain have regions (the propeptides) with sequences other than Gly-X-Y. As chain elongation proceeds, several posttranslational modifications, including hydroxylation and glycosylation, occur. While in the endoplasmic reticulum, three alpha chains associate and become disulfide-bonded at the C-terminal, forming a procollagen molecule. Procollagen molecules enter the Golgi complex where further glycosylation and packing takes place. They are then secreted into the extracellular space. In the confines of cellular infoldings, specific proteases sever both propeptides, resulting in the definitive collagen molecule. Association of collagen molecules results in fiber formation. (Modified with permission from Prockop D, Guzman NA: Collagen diseases and the biosynthesis of collagen.* Hosp Pract *1977;12:61–68.)*

formation, vascular fragility, hemorrhage, and poor healing. From the endoplasmic reticulum, the procollagen molecule is transported to the Golgi complex, where further glycosylation takes place. The extent of glycosylation varies for each collagen type.[85,129] After glycosylation, the procollagen chains are packaged into secretory vesicles in the Golgi complex, transported to the plasma membrane, and secreted into the extracellular environment.[16,87]

Collagen Fibrillogenesis Extracellular processing within the confined space (Fig. 3) formed by deep plasmalemmal invaginations is a prerequisite for fiber formation.[13,14] Before fiber formation, the nonhelical ends of the procollagen molecule are removed by extracellular N-terminal and C-terminal propeptidases. Individual collagen molecules, now with only short, straight, nonhelical extension peptides (telopeptides), associate through covalent bonds (Fig. 1) in a quarter-stagger array.[50,95,107,129] This aggregation forms gaps in the fiber that can be penetrated by metallic stains, resulting in the characteristic collagen banding seen on electron microscopy. The covalent bonding results in the cross-linking of collagen and depends on the copper-requiring metalloenzyme lysyl oxidase.[87] The resultant intermolecular and intramolecular bonds are necessary if the collagen fiber is to reach its maximum tensile strength. Some collagen fibers may be heteropolymeric[11,12,86,108]; if this is so, interactions between collagen molecules of different types will be required for fibrillogenesis.[19]

With such a complex process preceding fiber formation, a variety of conditions can affect various stages of fibrillogenesis and result in defective collagen formation.[94] Marfan's syndrome is characterized by structural abnormalities of the skeletal system, the cardiovascular system, and the eye.[27,94,148] Although the exact molecular defect is not yet defined, it is similar to that of a well-known lysyl oxidase inhibitor, β-aminopropionitrile, found in sweet clover (*Lathyrus odoratus*) and responsible for lathyrism.[28] Copper chelation or other abnormalities of copper metabolism interfere with collagen cross-linking and fibrillogenesis. Menkes' syndrome is an example, with its abnormal copper absorption and defective collagen formation.

Ehlers-Danlos syndrome is another group of hereditary disorders of collagen and elastin biosynthesis characterized by hyperelasticity, tissue fragility, joint hypermobility, and a hemorrhagic diathesis.[21,76] In type VII Ehlers-Danlos syndrome, there is a deficiency of N-terminal propeptidase. Thus, the nonhelical N-terminal is retained and collagen fiber formation inhibited. Osteogenesis imperfecta, another hereditary disorder, is characterized by abnormal collagen synthesis.[22,42,146,148–150] These conditions may impair wound healing. Therefore, defining the regulatory mechanisms of collagen fibrillogenesis is essential to understanding repair. Local and systemic (hormonal) influences have a role in collagen deposition, but their mechanisms for regulating collagen synthesis, secretion, deposition, and fiber diameter are unknown.

Collagen Functions The tensile strength of collagen is the result of the associations of molecules into fibers and bundles linked by intramolecular and intermolecular bonds.[16,107,129,130] The orientation of these collagen fibers is critical to their function. For example, in tendon the linear array of the collagen type I bundles produces a resilient structure; in the cornea, the arrangement of the same collagen type into orthogonal lamellae produces a transparent structure.[13,14,189]

Type I collagen is the major structural buttress of the extracellular matrix.[3,4] Other collagen types, including types III, V, VI, and XI, are associated with the surface of the fibers and may be partially responsible for the integration of the extracellular matrix. The prominent structural properties of the collagens should not mask their functions in platelet aggregation, cell attachment, migration, and morphogenesis.[90,138,175]

Noncollagenous Structural Glycoproteins

Fibronectin The fibronectins are a class of noncollagenous glycoproteins that exist as immunologically distinct, soluble (plasma) and insoluble (cellular) forms.[75,158,161,195,196] Soluble fibronectin is present in many body fluids, including plasma, urine, amniotic fluid, and cerebrospinal fluid. Fibronectin consists of two 250-kd polypeptide chains connected by disulfide bonds at the C-terminal (Fig. 4). Under rotary shadowing, plasma fibronectin appears as a V-shaped molecule with 80-nm arms.[133] Fibronectin binds or interacts with several macromolecules, bacteria, other extracellular matrix components, and cells. These interactions occur through specific, globular domains located along the molecule (Fig. 4) and indicate that fibronectin is an adhesive molecule, integrating the extracellular matrix.[158,159,161]

Although there are immunologic and structural differences between plasma fibronectin and cellular fibronectin, both are the product of a single gene located on human chromosome 2.[73,74,92,93] DNA sequencing has demonstrated three distinct, partially homologous (25% to 50%) domains. The first two domains each contain 45 to 50 amino acid residues; the third has 90 amino acid residues. These domains are repeated throughout the fibronectin subunits. For example, type I domains are repeated in the collagen- and fibrin-binding regions and the type III domains are prevalent in cell- and heparin-binding regions. In addition, cellular fibronectin contains an additional type III domain, the extradomain, absent from plasma fibronectin. Therefore, the differences between cellular fibronectin and plasma fibronectin result from posttranscriptional modification.[167,178] Differential splicing of mRNA can create at least six different fibronectin molecules, but the significance of this heterogeneous population is not clearly understood.[73,74,92,93,137,166,179] Posttranslational modifications such as glycosylation are also important. N-terminal-linked glycosylation is critical in protecting the collagen-binding domain from proteolysis.[53]

Fibronectins are widespread in the extracellular matrix where they form either fine filaments (6 to 10 nm) or granular deposits.[2,3,35,36,40,51,105,106,116,118,119,122,168,172,185,194] Fibronectin often coats the surface of various collagen types and is found adjacent to, but not within,

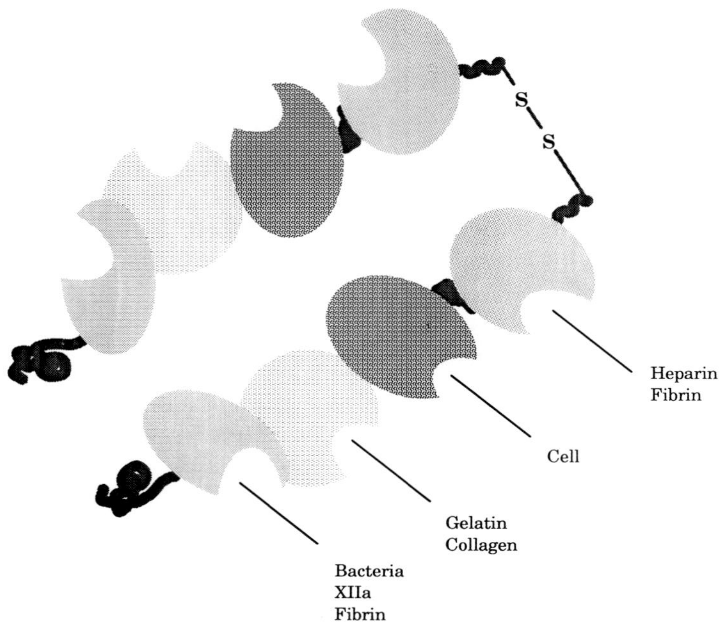

Fig. 4 *Schema of a fibronectin molecule. Fibronectin has two similar polypeptide chains, linked at the C-terminal by disulfide bonds. The individual chains have discrete globular domains, each with specific binding properties. These binding sites allow fibronectin to interact with cells, extracellular matrix, and plasma components.*

the basement membranes. Fibronectin is not found in mature cartilage, and only traces are found in tendons; however, it is abundant in the extracellular matrix of most soft tissues and skeletal muscle.

Fibronectins have critical roles in development and in wound healing.[43,44,99,185,189] During development, many mesenchymal cells initially deposit a fibronectin-rich extracellular matrix. As the cells differentiate toward their definitive phenotypes, they produce a more specialized extracellular matrix. For instance, in developing cartilage, the switch from fibronectin secretion to collagen type II secretion marks the differentiation of mesenchymal cell to chondroblast[191,192]; similarly, the switch from fibronectin secretion to laminin secretion marks the differentiation of mesenchymal cell to renal tubular cell.[43,44] In wound healing, plasma fibronectin is a component of the initial clot.[99] The glutamine in fibronectin enables it to be cross-linked to fibrin or collagen by transglutaminases.[131] This cross-linking of plasma and tissue components forms the initial primitive matrix that is eventually replaced by the definitive scar.

Studies on the cell-binding properties of fibronectin have isolated a specific domain responsible for this action. Later studies determined

BASEMENT MEMBRANE COMPONENTS

COMPONENT	CONSTITUENT CHAINS	MOLECULAR COMPOSITION	SUPRAMOLECULAR AGGREGATE	FUNCTION
TYPE IV COLLAGEN	$\alpha 1(IV), \alpha 2(IV)$	3 αChains	Network	Structural
LAMININ	A, B_1, B_2	1 A and 2 B Chains	Cross Shaped	Cell Attachement
ENTACTIN	Single Polypeptide Chain	Single Polypeptide Chain	Globular	Unknown
HEPARAN SULFATE PROTEOGLYCAN	Polypeptide Chain Glycosaminoglycan Side Chains	Protein Core Glycosaminoglycan Side Chains		Electrostatic Charge

Fig. 5 *The four major components of basement membranes are depicted with their chain compositions, macromolecular associations, aggregate forms, and proposed functions.*

that this cell-binding property resided in the amino acid sequence arginine-glycine-asparagine (RGD).[142–144] The RGD sequence is not unique to fibronectin; other proteins with cell-binding properties, such as vitronectin, fibrinogen, osteopontin, and collagen, have this sequence.[17,143,160] After the RGD sequence was defined, a corresponding family of cell-surface receptors, the integrins, was discovered.

Laminin Laminin is the most abundant and best characterized of the noncollagenous glycoproteins of the basement membranes.[88,114,120,134,135,181,184,190] It has a molecular weight of 800,000 and consists of three distinct polypeptide chains, A, B1, and B2 (Fig. 5). The B1 and B2 chains have homologous nucleotide sequences.[114] Under rotary shadowing, laminin displays a cruciate configuration. It can interact with itself and with other molecules, including collagen type IV, heparan sulfate, proteoglycans, and entactin. These interactions occur at specific binding domains on the laminin molecule. The B1 and B2 chains each have globular domains at the N-terminal and an α-helical configuration extending to the long arm of the cross, where the interaction with the helical region of the A chain occurs.[8,114] The A chain has two globular domains, one at or near the N-terminal and the other at the C-terminal.[8,114] The cell-attachment region is at the intersection of the three arms. A pentapeptide, the YIGSR sequence, may be responsible for cell attachment and receptor binding.[58] Domains responsible for neurite outgrowth and heparin binding are present in the C-terminal of the A chain.[114] Several regions with homology to epidermal growth factor have been described on the B1 chains.[114]

Laminin has been found in all basement membranes studied and is present in both the lamina rara and the lamina densa, with a preferential distribution in the lamina rara.[2,3,45,83,101,102,114,118–120] Traces of laminin have been identified in the hepatic and splenic sinusoids unassociated with basement membranes. Laminin is secreted in the early stages of embryogenesis, suggesting a role for this protein in ontogenesis.

The ability of laminin to bind to cells and to increase cell motility and migration led to the discovery of a 68-kd receptor protein on the plasmalemma of several cell types. How the laminin receptor modulates these cellular events is unknown; however, it may be through transmembrane proteins and connection with the cytoskeleton.[192]

Entactin Entactin, which has a molecular weight of 150,000, was originally isolated from a murine cell line producing copious amounts of basement membrane.[24,114,121] Also referred to as nidogen, entactin is a highly sulfated, dumbbell-shaped glycoprotein (Fig. 5) restricted to basement membranes. It interacts at one globular domain with the center of the laminin cross. The functions of entactin are unknown; perhaps its interaction with the cell attachment site of laminin modifies the cell-binding activity of that component.[114]

Osteonectin Osteonectin is a 32-kd bone-associated glycoprotein, first identified from guanidine extracts of mineralized calf bone.[180] Osteonectin binds to type I collagen and hydroxyapatite. Its name reflects its ability to bind the mineral and collagen components of bone. It is also found in dentin, but not in enamel or calcified cartilage. The binding of extracellular matrix with hydroxyapatite by osteonectin suggests an important function for this glycoprotein in initiating mineralization. Osteonectin is found immediately subjacent to the zone of calcified cartilage on new bone surfaces, and on mineralized metaphyseal and subperiosteal trabeculae in long and membranous bones.

Recent studies found osteonectin in nonosseus tissues rich in basement membrane. Further, the cDNA and amino acid sequence of osteonectin is more than 90% homologous with that of another protein found in some murine neoplastic basement membranes. This 43-kd protein is called SPARC, for secreted protein rich in cysteine.[123,165] Osteopontin and osteocalcin are other structural glycoproteins in osseous tissues.[66,136]

Tenascin Recently, another extracellular matrix glycoprotein has been characterized, tenascin (*tenere*, to hold; *nasci*, to be born), consisting of 240-kd disulfide-linked subunits.[29,30,110] This protein has been found in perichondrium, in developing and mature tendon, in myotendinous junctions, and in association with chondroitin sulfate proteoglycans in skeletal muscle cell cultures. Tenascin may also have a role in chrondrogenesis and osteogenesis.[110] Tenascin persists in perichondrium and periostium, tissues that contain stem cells capable of chrondrogenic or osteogenic differentiation. This may mean that tenascin has a modulatory function in limb development. Tenascin is also

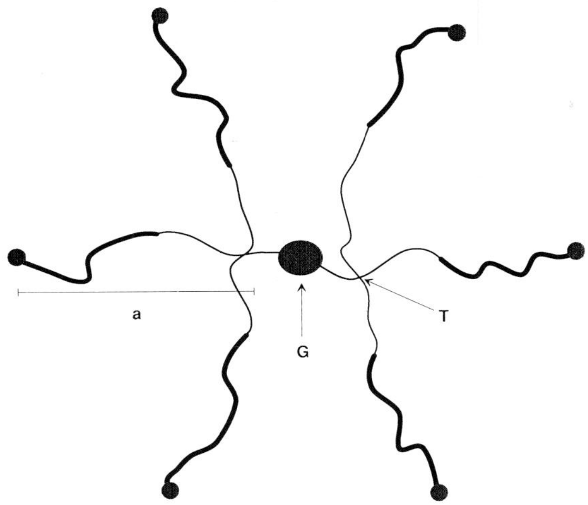

Fig. 6 *Tenascin. This glycoprotein was formerly called hexabrachion because it contains six identical arms. Each arm has a thinner proximal part (30 nm long), a thicker distal part (55 nm), and a terminal globular region. The arms join in two groups of three at the T-junction (T). The two groups then join at the central globular particle (G). (Modified with permission from Erickson HP, Iglesias JL: A six-armed oligomer isolated from cell surface fibronectin preparations.* Nature *1984;311:267–269.)*

found in the dense extracellular matrix adjacent to developing tooth buds, hair follicles, and mammary glands, suggesting a role in mesenchymal condensation and epithelial growth.

Tenascin, like fibronectin, has been discovered many times and renamed each time. It has been called cytotactin, myotendinous antigen, glioma mesenchymal extracellular matrix protein, J1, and hexabrachion.[29,46] It is a six-armed protein (Fig. 6) that may interact with the extracellular matrix and cells by means of its spidery configuration.

Elastin Elastic fibers are wavy and eosinophilic; electron microscopy (Fig. 7) shows two components, a central amorphous core and a peripheral rim of microfibrils, the elastic microfibril.[33,39,56] The central core is made of elastin. The composition of the microfibrils is not completely defined, but they do contain the protein fibrillin.[162]

Elastin is highly insoluble and is a widespread component of connective tissues. It is rich in glycine, proline, desmosine, and isodesmosine. The latter two are responsible for the covalent cross-links and the insolubility of elastin. The precursor protein of elastin, tropoelastin, was first identified from swine aorta. It consists of a single polypeptide chain of approximately 800 amino acid residues, with a molecular weight of 70,000. Its amino acid composition is similar to that of collagen, because approximately one third of the residues are glycine

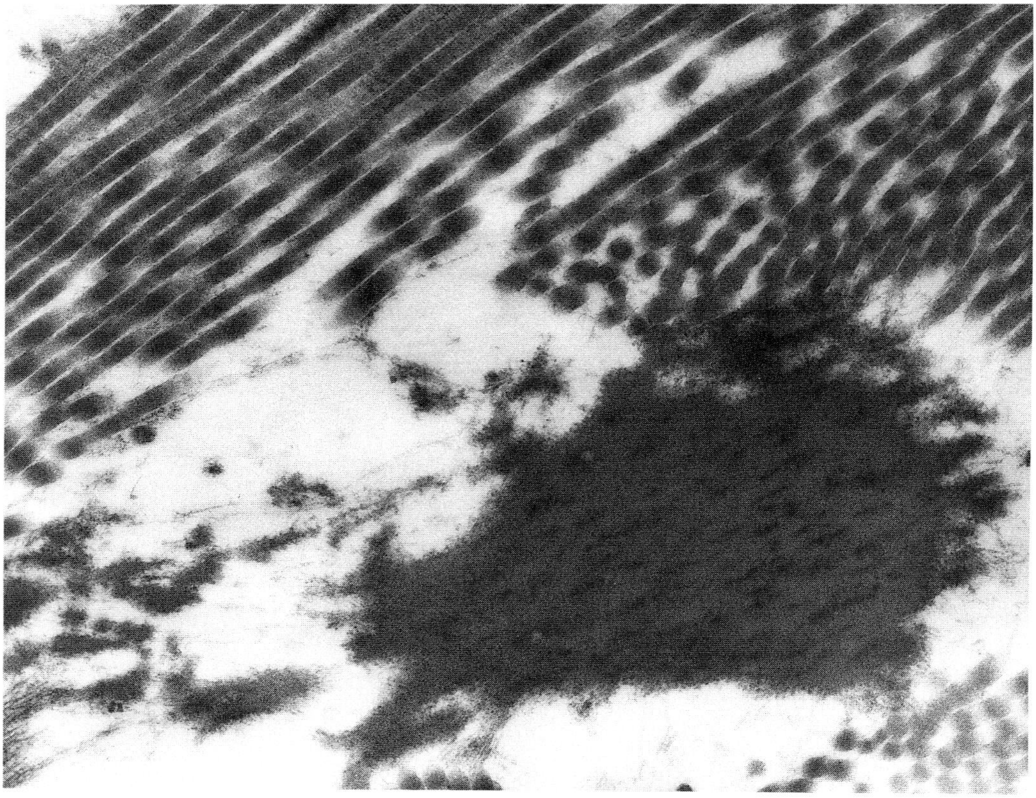

Fig. 7 *Electron micrograph of subcutaneous tissue shows an elastic fiber in cross section in the midst of collagen bundles. Elastic fibers have two distinct components: a central homogenous core and the peripheral microfibrils. The central core is made of elastin; the composition of the microfibrils is not clear, but they do contain fibrillin.*

and proline. However, unlike collagen, elastin has little OH-proline or OH-lysine and glycine is randomly distributed. The unique cross-linking of elastin occurs between four lysine molecules that form pyridine nuclei.[33,56]

A number of cell types are capable of elastin synthesis, including smooth muscle cells, fibroblasts, and myofibroblasts.[26,56,163] Like other extracellular matrix components, elastin is synthesized in the rough endoplasmic reticulum, secreted into the extracellular space, and then cross-linked into the elastic fiber. The microfibrillar components are apparently present in the extracellular matrix before the deposition of the amorphous central core and may be necessary for orderly fiber formation. Elastin is highly flexible because of its tortuous nature and the cross-links between individual chains. It is found in abundance in

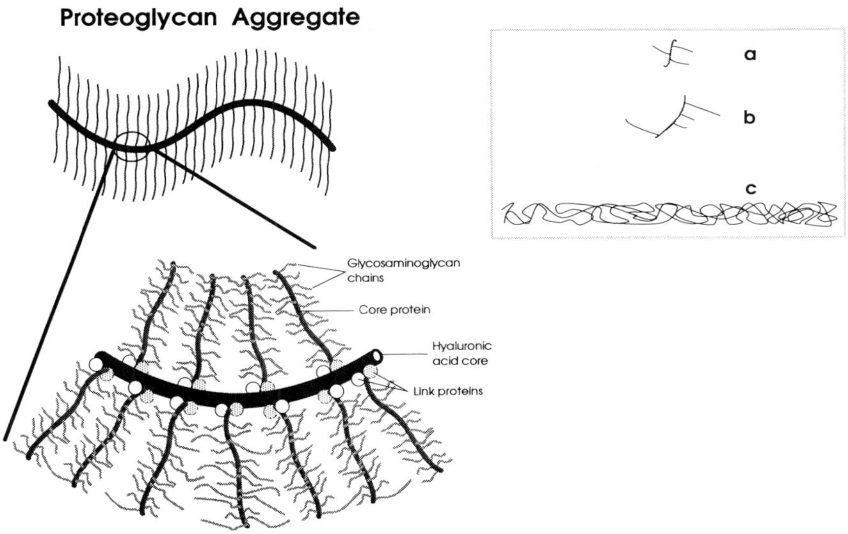

Fig. 8 *Schema of a typical cartilage proteoglycan aggregate. Individual proteoglycans are attached to a central chain of hyaluronic acid. The attachment of the core protein to the hyaluronic acid is mediated by the link proteins. The glycosaminoglycan side chains are typically extended and occupy a large volume relative to their mass. Their strong hydrophilicity creates a highly hydrated gel in which the other extracellular matrix components are embedded. The inset depicts the relative sizes of three molecules: a, cell-surface heparan sulfate proteoglycan; b, dermatan sulfate proteoglycan; c, hyaluronic acid glycosaminoglycan.*

several pliable tissues, but its role in the healing process remains to be defined.

Proteoglycans

Proteoglycans (Figs. 8 and 9) are a heterogeneous group of proteins that have a variable number (one to 100) of glycosaminoglycan side chains, covalently linked to a core protein.[65,70,78,157] Glycosaminoglycans (formerly called mucopolysaccharides) are linear arrays of repeating disaccharides that contain hexosamine and either a carboxylate or sulfate ester and provide anionic groups to the chain.[65,70,78,157] There are seven known glycosaminoglycan chains: chondroitin-4-sulfate, chondroitin-6-sulfate, dermatan sulfate, heparin, heparan sulfate, hyaluronic acid, and keratan sulfate. The proteoglycans have been named according to their glycosaminoglycan side chains. However, the respective core proteins are the product of distinct genes. Therefore, different gene products may have the same name, despite the nature of the core protein. To avoid confusion, when the same glycosaminoglycan is present on a different core protein, a modifier should be used, as in cell-surface heparan sulfate proteoglycan or basement-membrane heparan sulfate proteoglycan.[71,173,174]

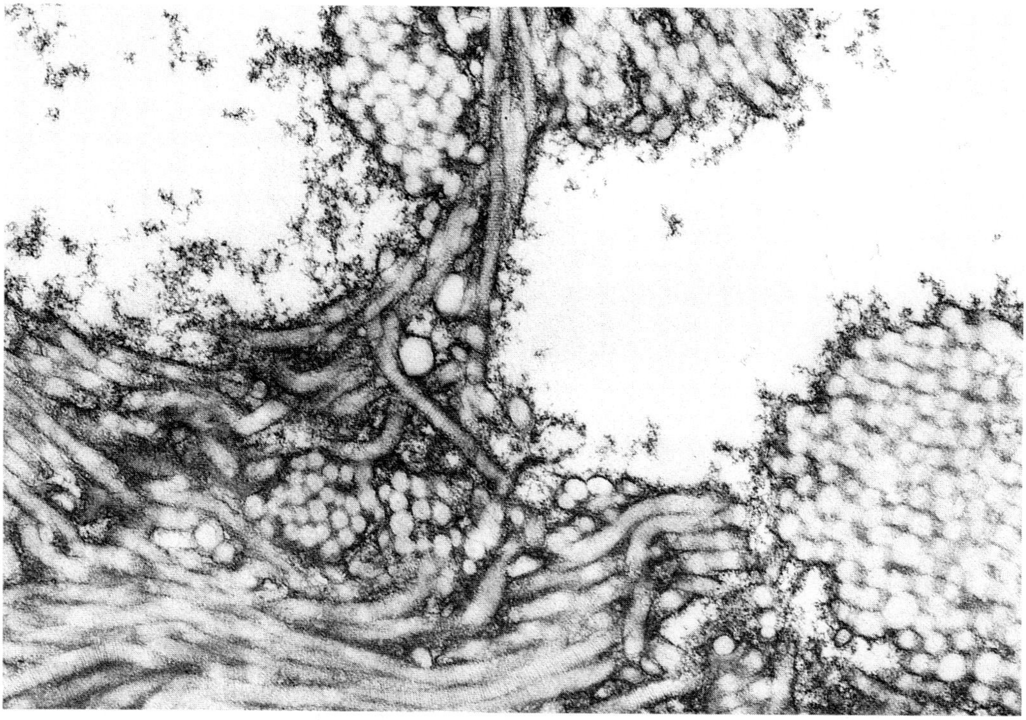

Fig. 9 *Dermis reacted with ruthenium red. This electron micrograph shows collagen fibers, in longitudinal and cross sections, embedded in a dense matrix of proteoglycan (electron-dense floccular material). Reaction with ruthenium red collapses the hydrophilic gel; therefore, the space occupied by the proteoglycan is artifactually reduced by this technique.*

Basement Membranes

Basement membranes are extracellular matrices located at the boundary between cells and adjacent stroma.[85,89,95,117,120,141,181] Basement membranes separate epithelial cells of most organs, such as the gastrointestinal tract, thyroid gland, and skin, from the adjacent connective tissues. They also separate many mesenchymal cells, such as lipocytes and skeletal, smooth, and cardiac muscle cells, and epithelial and endothelial cells, such as in the glomerulus and alveolus. The central nervous system has only vascular basement membranes; in the peripheral nervous system, Schwann cells are encased by basement membranes. All endothelial cells except the sinusoids in the liver, spleen, lymph nodes, and bone marrow are lined by basement membranes. Synovial cells, fibroblasts, and histiocytes lack a basement membrane.[85,89,95,119,120,141,181]

On light microscopy, basement membranes are pale, eosinophilic

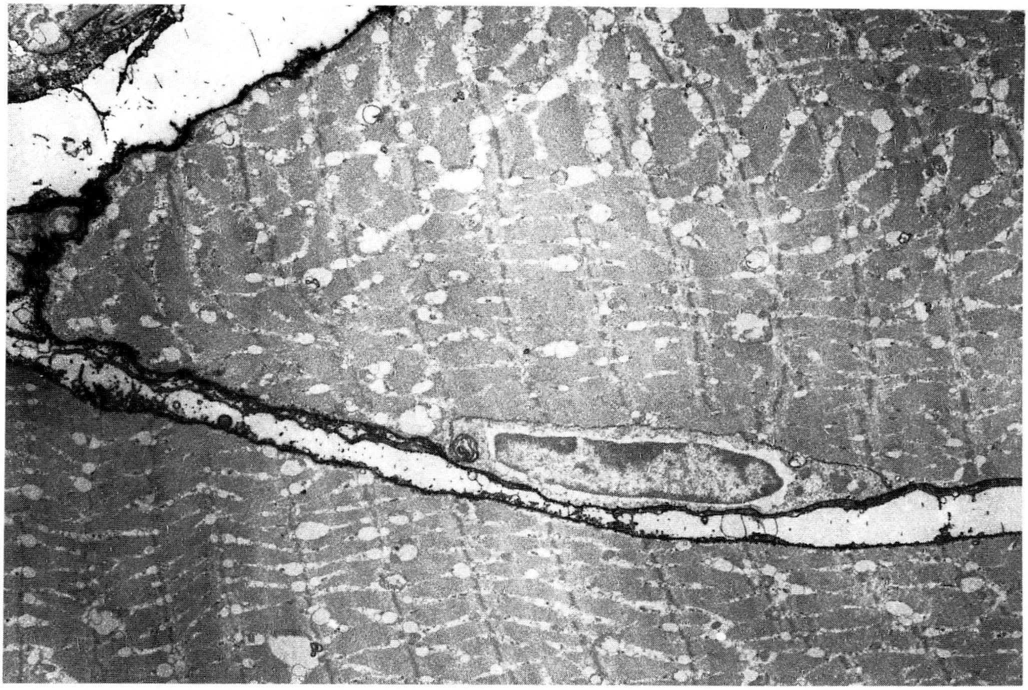

Fig. 10 *Skeletal muscle reacted with ruthenium red. Each skeletal muscle cell is enveloped by a delicate basement membrane (ruthenium-red positive). There is a satellite cell within the basement membrane of a differentiated skeletal muscle cell.*

structures that react with a variety of histochemical stains, including PAS,[125] reflecting their carbohydrate content. On conventional electron microscopy (Fig. 10), most basement membranes are 60 to 90 nm wide with two distinct layers.[95,120,181] The region adjacent to the cell membrane, the lamina rara (or lucida), is electron-lucent. The region adjacent to the interstitium, the lamina densa, is electron-dense. Exceptions are the endothelial basement membranes of the cornea and the lens capsule, which have a single lamina densa.[164] The glomerular basement membrane and segments of the alveolar basement membrane are trilaminar, with two 30-nm laminae rarae sandwiching a 60-nm lamina densa.[164]

Basement membranes are composed of the major macromolecular groups of the extracellular matrix (Fig. 5), including type IV collagen, noncollagenous structural glycoproteins (laminin and entactin), and proteoglycans (heparan sulfate).[77,84,97,114,120,183]

Type IV collagen was first identified in basement membranes and is a constituent of all basement membranes studied.[3,4,59,83,84,89,91,118,119,156,182,183] It has at least two distinct alpha chains,

α1(IV) and α2(IV). The first has a molecular weight of 185,000 and the second has a molecular weight of 170,000. The ratio of the type IV collagen alpha chains in each basement membrane is not known; however, heteropolymeric and homopolymeric molecules may exist.[64] Collagen type IV is the prototypical group 2 collagen molecule. In some group 2 molecules, unlike group 1 collagen molecules, the amino- and carboxy-propeptides are not removed after secretion but are incorporated into the basement membrane network.[31] Rotary shadowing shows that collagen type IV consists of threads, with a globular NC1 domain at the C-terminal and a tightly helical 7S domain at the N-terminal. Adjacent to the 7S region is the nonhelical NC2 domain. Tetramers of type IV collagen are connected at the 7S region, and dimers are attached at the globular NC1 domain. This relationship forms the basis for the proposed "chicken wire" arrangement of type IV collagen as the structural backbone of basement membranes. More recent studies have proposed a side-to-side arrangement of collagen type IV in basement membranes.[197,198]

Laminin and entactin are the major noncollagenous structural glycoproteins in basement membranes. Heparan sulfate proteoglycans are present in basement membranes, the core protein being specific for these structures.[47,65,79–81,126,174,193] These proteoglycans are located in discrete clusters in the lamina rara. The negative charge imparted to the basement membrane by the proteoglycans is critical to the selective filtration of glomerular basement membrane.[25,80–82,101,102,126,140,151,152,174] The proteoglycans are reportedly decreased in experimentally induced nephrotic syndrome[132] and in children with the Finnish type of congenital nephrotic syndrome. A similar decrease may explain the nephrotic syndrome of diabetes.[139,154,155]

Basement membranes have important roles in biologic processes such as differentiation, development, and wound repair.[95,120,181] Many of these functions are a consequence of the properties of the individual basement membrane components. Basement membrane functions can be classified under three major categories: tensile strength, cell attachment, and ultrafiltration. Much of the tensile strength of basement membrane is probably provided by the collagenous network of collagen type IV, which supports epithelia, vascular structures, and mesenchymal cells. Basement membranes are resilient structures that can withstand significant changes in shape when surrounding cells, such as cardiac, skeletal, and smooth muscle cells, undergo contraction. Laminin and type IV collagen have cell-binding properties for most epithelial cells and for some mesenchymal cells. Laminin has a variety of effects on cells through its interactions, depending on the cell type involved, and can cause glandular cells to assume a columnar configuration and neuronal cells to sprout axonal projections.[1,62,63,188] Type IV collagen also promotes cell attachment.[172] The presence of heavily charged molecules, proteoglycans, in the basement membrane determines the selective filtration capacity of these structures.

Extracellular Matrix Degradation

Normal morphostasis and repair require constant remodeling of tissue structure, with changes in the synthesis, secretion, and degradation of extracellular matrix. This degradation is carried out by a host of enzymes with broad range and specific activities. Several enzymes are particularly important in extracellular matrix degradation.[127]

Plasminogen Activators

Plasminogen activators convert the inactive zymogen plasminogen to the active enzyme plasmin by proteolytic action. These serine proteinases are well-known fibrinolytic agents that can degrade many proteins, although not native collagen or elastin.[100,127] Plasminogen activators include the enzymes urokinase and extrinsic plasminogen activator.[127] Among the cell types that produce these enzymes are keratinocytes, fibroblasts, endothelial cells, granulocytes, and macrophages. Plasmin can degrade the extracellular matrix components laminin, fibronectin, and the noncollagenous (globular) domains of the collagens.[127] In addition, plasminogen activators stimulate zymogens of other degradative enzymes, such as the procollagenases and elastases.[170]

Collagenases

Collagenases are calcium-dependent metalloproteinases that split native, helical collagen molecules under physiologic conditions.[60,111] This enzyme family is divided into subgroups according to the type of collagen degraded. For example, interstitial collagenases degrade group 1 collagens, basement membrane collagenase degrades type IV collagen,[109,112] and another collagenase degrades type V collagen.[113] Collagenases cleave a single peptide bond, three-fourths along the length of a collagen molecule from the N-terminal at an $\alpha 2$ Gly-Leu or $\alpha 1$ Gly-Ile sequence.[60] After the alpha chains are split at these points, the remaining fragments of the molecule unwind and become susceptible to a number of proteinases. Collagenases are produced by several cell types, including fibroblasts, neutrophils (stored in the primary granules), smooth muscle cells, and macrophages.[127]

Hyaluronidase

Hyaluronate, a glycosaminoglycan abundant in the extracellular matrix, is a prominent component of the initial matrix of wound healing, where it facilitates cell migration and imparts the hydrophobicity of the wound. As the wound matures, the amount of hyaluronate decreases and sulfated proteoglycans and cell differentiation increase. Hyaluronidase is an endoglycosidase, capable of cleaving hyaluronate at low pH (4.5). Neutrophils, macrophages, fibroblasts, and other cells secrete hyaluronidases with activity at a much lower pH.[127] The degradation of hyaluronate may be needed for cell differentiation at the wound site.

Elastases

Elastases are serine proteases present in various tissues. They can degrade elastin and other extracellular matrix components such as type IV collagen and fibronectin. An elastase is present in the azurophilic granules of neutrophils.[112]

Cells of the Repair Reaction

Fibroblasts

Fibroblast is a term used to refer to cells with different functions but similar morphologies. Tendon fibroblasts have functions and properties different from those of skeletal muscle or liver fibroblasts but the same term is applied to these diverse populations of cells because they have similar morphologic characteristics. Just as "lymphocyte" describes cells with such diverse functions as antibody production, cell killing, cell activation, and cell suppression, "fibroblast" may refer to connective-tissue stem cells, phagocytic cells (histiocytes), protein-secreting cells (fibrocytes), and contractile cells (myofibroblasts).

Fibrocytes

Fibrocytes are differentiated connective tissue cells that electron microscopy (Fig. 11) shows as elongated, with a prominent rough endoplasmic reticulum, a perinuclear Golgi complex, and an elaborate system of cell infoldings. They can synthesize most extracellular matrix components including collagens, fibronectin, and proteoglycans. They are prominent at a wound site six to 12 days after an injury.

Myofibroblasts

By light microscopy, myofibroblasts are indistinguishable from fibrocytes. Electron microscopy, however, shows that myofibroblasts have an abundance of contractile elements (actin-myosin filaments) in the peripheral cytoplasm, a concentration of synthetic organelles (rough endoplasmic reticulum and Golgi complex) in the perinuclear region and an indented nucleus. In contrast to fibrocytes, myofibroblasts are often surrounded by an incomplete basement membrane.[103] They are prominent at the wound site three to ten days after injury.

Macrophages

Although macrophages are better known for their role in inflammation, they are active participants in wound healing. Macrophages are derived either from circulating monocytes or by proliferation of local macrophages.[9] Activated macrophages can phagocytize extracellular matrix components and secrete growth factors (macrophage-derived growth factor) that stimulate proliferation of several mesenchymal cells, including smooth muscle and endothelial cells.[15,103]

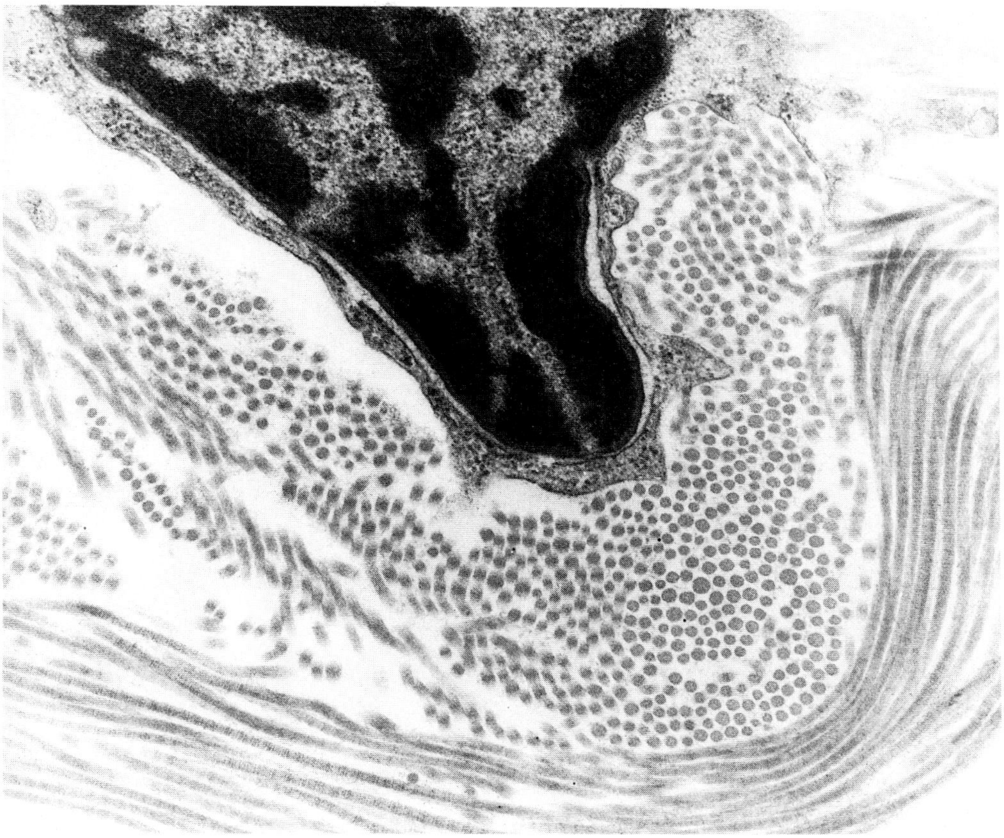

Fig. 11 *Electron micrograph of fibroblast and collagen bundles. Collagen fibers are present within a cell recess.*

Macrophages may also be able to regulate synthesis of extracellular matrix by other cell types. They are prominent at the wound site from two to ten days after injury.

Endothelial Cells

The repair reaction depends on the growth of new capillaries into the fibrin-extracellular matrix-fibroblast meshwork of the wound space. Because endothelial cells can respond to specific stimuli, migrate, divide, and differentiate, the wound is transformed into a richly vascularized tissue. As the wound matures and the metabolic needs of the tissue decrease, many capillary sprouts are reabsorbed, and the rich vascularized granulation tissue becomes a pale, avascular scar.

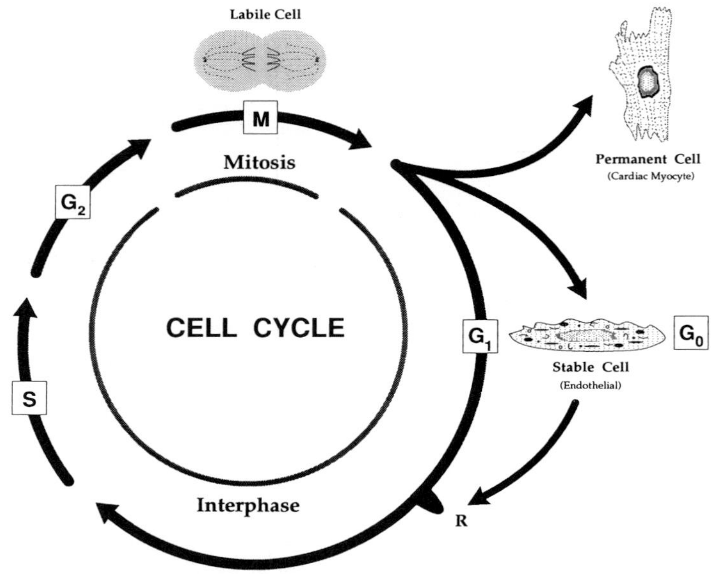

Fig. 12 *The cell cycle. Labile cells (such as bone marrow stem cells) undergo continuous replication. The interval between two consecutive mitoses is designated the cell cycle. After division, the cells enter a gap phase (G_1) in which they pursue their own specialized activities.*

Regenerative Capabilities of Cell Types

The Cell Cycle

Controlled proliferation is necessary to replace dead or injured cells.[124] For example, constant division and differentiation of the stem cells of the epidermis, gastrointestinal tract, and genitourinary tract replace the desquamated surface cells. Tissues with stem cells can replace large defects by regeneration. For any cell type, the interval between successive cell divisions is called the cell cycle.[124] Understanding of the factors controlling this cycle is necessary to understand tissue repair and neoplasia.

The cell cycle is divided into four unequal phases (Fig. 12). The M phase is the mitotic phase. After the M phase, the daughter cells enter the interphase, which is further divided into the G_1, S, and G_2 phases. The interphase accounts for 90% of the entire cell cycle. In the G_1 phase, the cells perform their specialized synthetic and biologic activities. Some cells, such as hepatocytes and endothelial cells, exit the cycle, become mitotically inactive, and only reenter the cycle if stimulated (G_0). DNA is synthesized during the S phase. The G_2 phase is a short phase preceding cell division or mitosis. Different cell types proceed through the cell cycle at varying rates; some never divide again after reaching maturation.

Cell Types

Tissues can be classified according to the proportion of cells in mitosis normally present.[176] Cells that continuously repeat the cell cycle are called labile. Cells that have lost the capacity for physiologic regeneration but can proliferate if stimulated in adulthood are called stable. Cells that completely lose the ability to divide after birth are called permanent.

Labile Cells When more than 1.5% of the cells in a tissue are in mitosis, the tissue is made of labile cells. Labile cells are found in the epidermis, in the gastrointestinal, genitourinary, and respiratory tracts, and in bone marrow. This population of dividing stem cells is often basally located and continually divides. After division, one of the daughter cells remains a stem cell and the other undergoes differentiation to the tissue-specific phenotype. Depending on the tissue, these cells may be either unipotent, as in the squamous epithelium of the skin, or pluripotent, as in the epithelium of the gastrointestinal tract or in bone marrow. Tissues composed of labile cells have excellent regenerative potential.

Stable Cells When fewer than 1.5% of a tissue's cells are in mitosis, the tissue is made of stable cells. Examples include the parenchymal cells of the endocrine glands, the liver, the kidney, and the pancreas, as well as mesenchymal cells such as fibroblasts, osteocytes, endothelial cells, and chondrocytes. Although they have a low mitotic rate, tissues of stable cells have excellent regenerative potential under the proper stimulus.

Permanent Cells Permanent cells totally lose their capacity to proliferate soon after birth. These cells include neurons, those in the lens of the eye, and those in cardiac muscle. Differentiated skeletal myocytes are also incapable of dividing. Skeletal muscle is replaced only if stem cells (satellite cells) differentiate into myoblasts and later fuse into multinucleated cells that differentiate into mature myocytes. Tissues composed of permanent cells have no regenerative capacity.

Cell Migration in Repair

Wound repair requires the orderly accumulation of both cells and matrix. The interaction of extracellular matrix and cells is critical to the migration of the cell types in the area of injury. Soluble chemotactic factors attract cells to the wound site, and signals in the insoluble matrix direct the distribution of these cells.

Haptotaxis is the migration of cells along an adhesion gradient on a substratum.[144] During haptotaxis, cells randomly extend processes in all directions; those that reach a proper substratum (Fig. 13) adhere to it and spread, preventing other processes from adhering. The binding

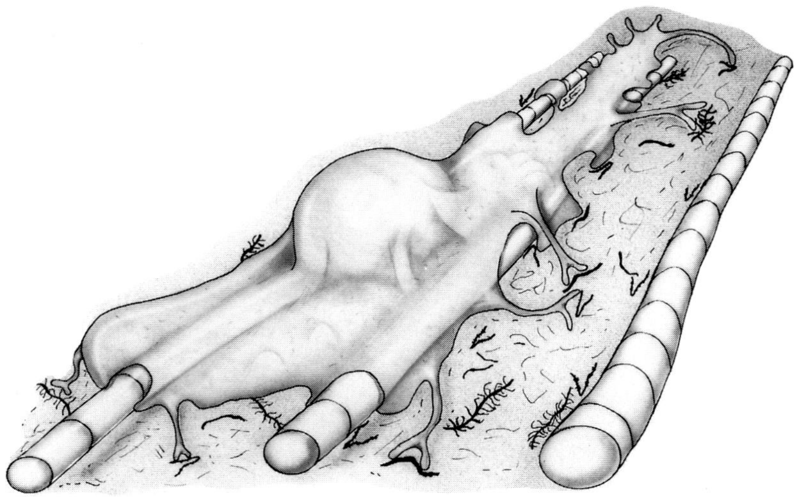

Fig. 13 *Haptotaxis. Haptotaxis is the migration of cells along an adhesion gradient on a substratum.*

of the plasmalemma to a specific extracellular matrix component creates an anchor for other cells. The unattached portions of the membrane form new processes and help create a new advancing edge. Depending on the cell type, extracellular matrix components such as fibronectin and laminin can enhance haptotaxis.[17,160]

Cell-Matrix Interactions

The extracellular matrix contains information that modifies cell behavior, and the extracellular matrix itself is modified by adjacent cells. The modulation of cell behavior by the extracellular matrix is apparently mediated by specific components that interact or bind to the cell surface.[17,142,144,160] Many adhesive extracellular matrix proteins contain the cell-adhesion tripeptide RGD, first identified on fibronectin.[176] This sequence, and perhaps others, bind to a family of cell surface receptors, the integrins.[104]

Integrins

The integrins were first isolated from cells in culture by using affinity chromatography on Sepharose linked to the extracellular matrix component containing the cell-attachment ligand RGD. Fibronectin, vitronectin, and type I collagen used as ligands have their own distinct

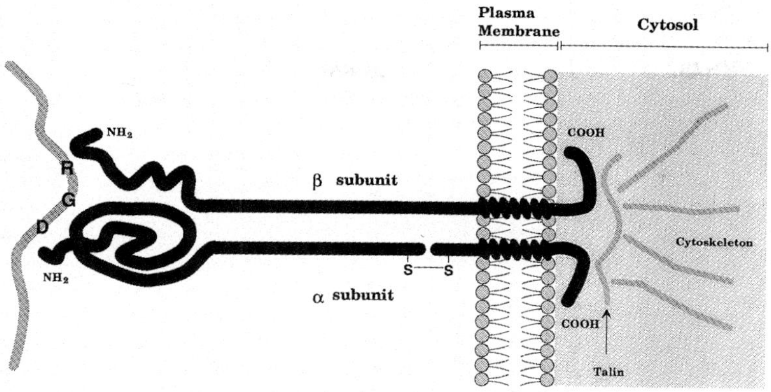

Fig. 14 *Integrins are a family of cell-surface proteins, containing two polypeptide chains: alpha and beta. The alpha chain consists of two subunits connected by disulfide bonds, whereas the beta chain is a single polypeptide. The integrins span the extracellular, intramembranous, and intracellular compartments. The N-terminal contains the matrix-binding site, which often recognizes the RGD sequence (although some integrins bind to other sequences). Interaction of the integrins with the subplasmalemmal protein talin, itself connected to cytoplasmic filaments, results in the exchange of information between the extracellular and intracellular compartments.*

receptors. Similarly, platelets contain a fourth receptor for fibrinogen. All these extracellular matrix binding proteins are similar to other surface adhesive proteins and compose the integrin family.[153]

The structures of various integrins are similar. All are heterodimeric and consist of alpha and beta polypeptide chains (Fig. 14). The alpha chain consists of two disulfide-bonded polypeptides, which together have a molecular weight of 140,000. The beta chain is a single polypeptide. The integrins can be grouped on the basis of their beta chains. For example, fibronectin, vitronectin, and platelet receptor (groups IIb and IIIa) all have the same beta chains.

The association of the extracellular matrix-cell receptors with cytoskeletal filaments may provide a communication route between the matrix and the intracellular compartments.[153] Each integrin subunit contains a large extracellular (calcium-dependent) domain, a transmembrane segment near the C-terminal, and an intracytoplasmic region (Fig. 13). The integrins bind to intracytoplasmic proteins such as talin and actin. Sequences on the intracytoplasmic portion of these receptors also have phosphorylating capacity. These receptors may be responsible for the transfer of information between the extracellular matrix and cells.

Growth Factors in Wound Healing

Cellular migration, activation, and proliferation are essential for wound healing. Several proteins that bind to specific cell-surface re-

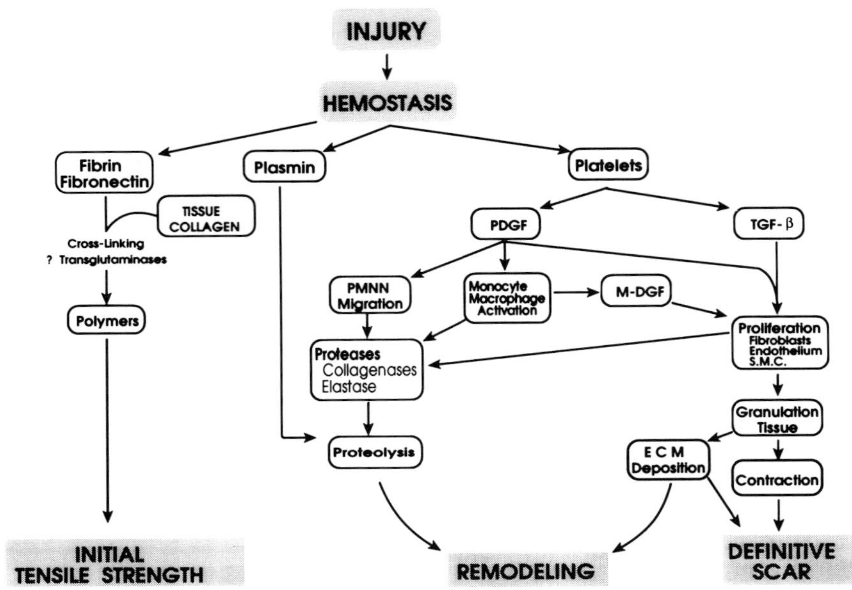

Fig. 15 *Diagram of possible interactions among components of hemostasis, growth factors, extracellular matrix, and cells during the repair reaction. The actual interactions taking place in an individual injury determine the outcome of healing.*

ceptors and are mitogenic (growth factors) are known. Many of these growth factors are secreted as part of the response to injury and, by modifying cell behavior, they modulate the healing response (Fig. 15).

Macrophage-Derived Growth Factor

In vivo, the depletion of circulating monocytes inhibits fibroblast proliferation and connective tissue formation[153] while macrophages produce a factor that stimulates proliferation of quiescent fibroblasts. The exact nature of this macrophage-derived growth factor remains to be determined but stimulating macrophages by fibronectin fragments, endotoxin, phorbol, and concavalin A enhances its secretion.[6] Macrophage-derived growth factor also stimulates the in vitro proliferation of endothelial and smooth muscle cells.[72] Similarities among macrophage-derived growth factor, platelet-derived growth factor, and interleukin-1 have been reported.[72]

Platelet-Derived Growth Factor

Cultured fibroblasts require serum to proliferate.[72] This fact led to the identification of platelet-derived growth factor. Platelet-derived growth factor is localized in the α-granules of platelets and is released as part of the hemostatic response. It contains two disulfide-bonded polypeptide chains (A and B).[72] Several cells, including macrophages, endothelial cells, smooth muscle cells, and transformed fibroblasts, produce similar molecules.[72]

Platelet-derived growth factor is a potent mitogen for mesodermal-derived cells such as microglia, smooth muscle cells, and fibroblasts.[34] Its activity is mediated by a specific receptor on the cell membrane. This receptor is an 18-kd glycoprotein with tyrosine kinase activity.[7] In addition to its mitogenic activity, platelet-derived growth factor is a potent chemotactic signal for inflammatory cells. Monocytes and neutrophils responding to its chemotactic stimulus may have a different receptor than cells that respond to its mitogenic properties.[7]

These chemotactic and mitogenic properties may have an important role in healing. They may recruit inflammatory cells, fibroblasts, endothelial cells, and smooth muscle cells to the wound site, activate neutrophils and monocytes, and induce proliferation of connective tissue cells (Fig. 15).

Epidermal Growth Factor

Epidermal growth factor is a single-chain polypeptide that contains 53 amino acid residues and has a wide range of physiologic effects.[7] It binds to a heavily glycosylated, transmembrane protein receptor present in most mammalian cell types, and most abundant on epithelial cells. Its receptor complex is internalized, triggering a complex sequence of events. On internalization, the receptor becomes a tyrosine kinase, phosphorylating itself and other intracellular proteins. The cells become less differentiated and divide rapidly.[57] In vivo, epidermal growth factor accelerates the healing of corneal and skin wounds and gastrointestinal ulcers.[52] In wound chambers, epidermal growth factor stimulates collagen deposition and increases the organization of granulation tissue,[52] suggesting that it may be therapeutic in wound healing. There is, however, little evidence of a physiologic role.

Fibroblast Growth Factor

Brain or pituitary gland extracts stimulate fibroblast growth.[52] The factors responsible for this activity have been isolated and named fibroblast growth factor. Fibroblast growth factor exists in two forms, basic and acidic; the basic form is ten times more active than the acidic form. Both are the product of a single gene located on chromosome 4. Both forms are single-chain 16-kd nonglycosylated proteins.[41] Fibroblast growth factor is angiogenic in vitro and in vivo. It is also mitogenic for fibroblasts, endothelial cells, smooth muscle cells, and several mesenchymal cells.[5] In experimental wounds, fibroblast growth factor increased the rate of healing as well as collagen, protein, and DNA content.[5]

Transforming Growth Factor Beta

Assoian[5] showed that transformed cells in culture released a growth factor.[41] Two proteins were responsible for this activity, transforming growth factors alpha and beta (TGF-α and TGF-β). TGF-β is more important in wound healing. It is a 25-kd dimer of two apparently identical subunits held together by disulfide bonds. TGF-β binds to a cell receptor distinct from the epidermal growth factor receptor.[5] TGF-β is not exclusive to transformed cells; platelets have high concentrations of TGF-β in their α-granules,[61] and activation of lymphocytes induces transcription of the TGF-β gene.[170] In vivo, TGF-β increases the amount of fibroblasts, collagen, and protein at the wound site. Further, the delay in healing induced by doxorubicin can be reversed by TGF-β, and daily subcutaneous injections of purified TGF-β induces formation of granulation tissue within three days.[18]

The presence of TGF-β in platelets and lymphocytes, the enhancement of experimental wound healing, the mitogenic action on fibroblasts, and the induction of collagen and protein synthesis strongly suggest that TGF-β has an important role in wound healing.

Wound Healing

Phases of Wound Healing

Any stimulus, external or internal, physical or chemical, can result in cell and tissue injury if it is severe enough. The process that restores tissue continuity is called healing. Healing can proceed by regeneration, which replaces lost tissue with tissue of similar functional and morphologic characteristics, or by repair, which replaces lost tissue by granulation tissue that matures to form a scar.

Strictly speaking, inflammation and repair are parts of a single process, the response to injury. For the first week after the injury, inflammation and repair coexist and overlap at the wound site. Healing itself is usually divided into three major phases (Fig. 16): the inflammatory phase, the proliferative phase, and the maturation phase.[18] This division into three distinct phases is arbitrary; further, the time sequence presented in Figure 16 refers to an ideal wound that has clean, sharp edges, is aseptic, and has perfect sutures. The time sequences differ for infected wounds, immunodeficient hosts, and other problem situations.

The Inflammatory Phase This phase starts immediately after injury and completely overlaps the inflammatory response. There is either hemorrhage or exudation of plasma into the wound site. Activation of the coagulation cascade results in the formation of a fibrin clot that incorporates fibronectin. Fibrin and fibronectin can be cross-linked by transglutaminases and fibronectin can be cross-linked to tissue collagens. This cross-linking of plasma proteins to tissue components provides the initial tensile strength. The activation of the coagulation cascade simultaneously activates the plasminogen system to generate plasmin. Polymorphonuclear neutrophils attracted to the wound site release several proteolytic enzymes that degrade the damaged extra-

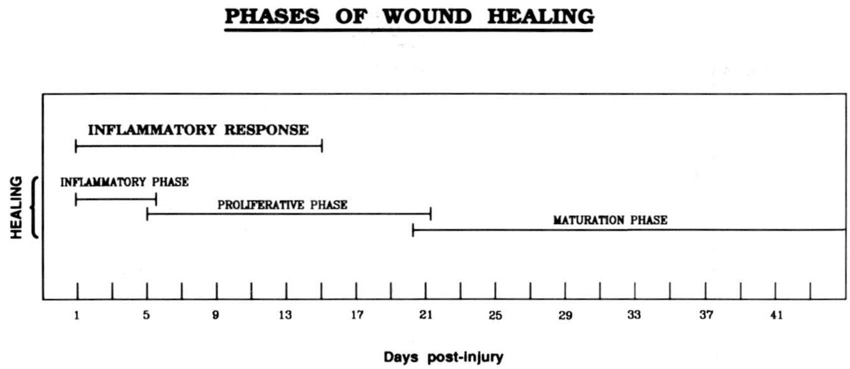

Fig. 16 *Wound healing can be divided into three overlapping phases: inflammation, proliferation, and maturation. The inflammatory phase of healing overlaps the inflammatory response.*

cellular matrix. Platelets and macrophages at the wound site release platelet-derived and macrophage-derived growth factors that are chemoattractant and mitogenic for pericytes and fibroblasts.

There are three major consequences of the inflammatory phase. First, some initial wound strength is provided by the cross-linking of fibrin, fibronectin, and collagen. Next, the removal of damaged tissue components is initiated by plasmin, elastase, and collagenases. Finally, endothelial cells, pericytes, and fibroblasts are recruited and stimulated to divide. In this manner, the initial inflammatory phase prepares the stage for the proliferative phase. The tensile strength provided by fibrin-fibronectin-collagen cross-links is the only source of tensile strength during the inflammatory phase; there is no further increase. Indeed, the proteolytic enzymes released may reduce the initial tensile strength.

Proliferative Phase This phase is characterized by the accumulation of endothelial cells, myofibroblasts, and fibroblasts at the wound site. Platelet-derived and macrophage-derived growth factors, TGF-β, angiogenesis factor, and the low oxygen tension at the center of the wound stimulate the migration of these cells to the wound site and their subsequent proliferation. Fibronectin, the breakdown products of collagens, and other extracellular matrix components are chemotactic for macrophages and other cells. The capillaries adjacent to the wound sprout, and the wound site has a rich capillary network within days. The direction and flow in these capillaries fluctuate continuously. As the capillaries grow into the wound, fibroblasts and myofibroblasts also accumulate at the wound site. Typically, these cells arrange themselves perpendicular to the capillaries. The combination of a rich cap-

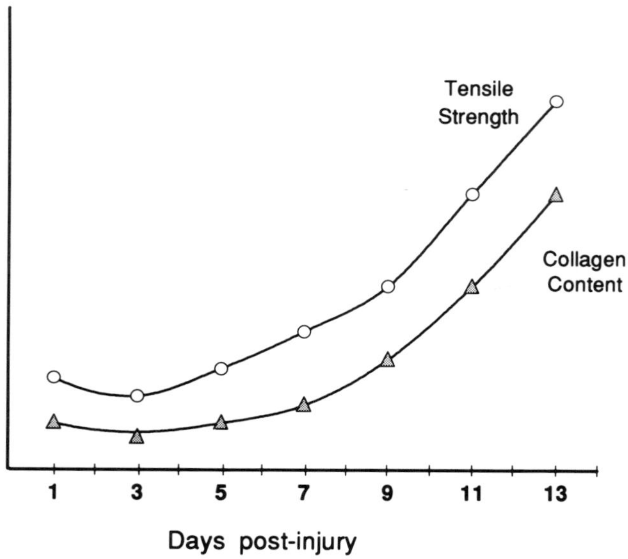

Fig. 17 *During the first weeks, the increase in a wound's tensile strength parallels the increase in collagen content.*

illary network with abundant myofibroblasts and fibroblasts is called granulation tissue.

Both myofibroblasts and fibroblasts secrete extracellular matrix components, initially fibronectin and proteoglycans. By day 6 or 7, some type III collagen begins to accumulate at the wound site, and the wound's tensile strength steadily increases, paralleling the total collagen content in the wound (Fig. 17). By day 12, type I collagen becomes prominent and, from then on, the ratio of type I to type III increases. In addition to secreting extracellular matrix components, the myofibroblasts are contractile. The coordinated contraction of these cells at the edges of the wound reduces the size of the wound. Along with the deposition of new extracellular matrix, capillary ingrowth, and cell proliferation, there is continuous breakdown of the initial clot, of damaged extracellular matrix, and of the newly deposited extracellular matrix. This continuous deposition and removal of extracellular matrix (with the balance toward deposition) results in the remodeling of the wound.

Maturation Phase The definitive tissue structure is established in this phase. The number of macrophages at the wound site declines sharply, a definitive pattern of blood flow is established in the capillaries, and capillaries with minimal flow are reabsorbed. The myofibroblasts and fibroblasts also decrease. The fibroblasts that remain are active in the synthesis and deposition of extracellular matrix components. The predominant collagen deposited is type I. Dense collagen bundles begin to appear, and the definitive scar forms. Extracellular matrix degradation continues, but again the balance favors synthesis. Tensile strength increases at a rate greater than the net collagen increase, as intramolecular and intermolecular cross-links are formed in collagen. It is difficult to define precisely when the maturation phase ends. The increases in collagen and tensile strength can continue for months or years.

Each phase of the healing response is essential to the subsequent one. Inadequacies in any phase interfere with proper healing. For instance, if the initial injury results in minimal hemorrhage at the wound site, little fibronectin and few platelets accumulate. As a result, few macrophages are attracted, there is a deficiency of growth factors, the resulting granulation tissue is scarce, and the scar is weak.

Healing Mechanisms

After the initial injury, the cells of the inflammatory response remove the damaged tissue components by a combination of extracellular and intracellular degradation. The task of the healing response is to replace the dead tissue by living tissue through three basic mechanisms: contraction, repair, and regeneration. These three basic mechanisms play a role in every wound, and the exact contribution of each determines the eventual outcome of the healing reaction. For instance, removal of 70% of the liver elicits a healing reaction dominated by regeneration, and the outcome is a normal liver in a matter of days. Injury to the esophagus may result in an exuberant proliferation of myofibroblasts, excessive wound contraction, and contracture. A wound on the anterior tibial surface, where the skin's attachment to the periosteum prevents contraction, forces healing almost exclusively by repair, and a large scar results.

Contraction Contraction is the inward movement of the wound edges by the action of myofibroblasts. Although the origin of the myofibroblasts is still debated, they are probably derived from mesenchymal stem cells or from perivascular cells (pericytes).[18] Whatever their origin, they appear at the wound site three to four days after injury and become prominent after six or seven days. Their contraction can reduce the size of the wound by as much as 70%, greatly facilitating healing. However, excessive contraction leads to contractures; conversely, inhibiting contraction (as with skin grafts prematurely placed on rapidly contracting wounds) results in large scars.

Repair Repair is the replacement of dead tissue by granulation tissue that eventually matures into a scar. Injury to vascular tissues triggers the hemostatic response. As part of this response, fibrin, fibronectin, platelets, and monocytes (macrophages) accumulate at the wound site. This results in an accumulation of chemoattractant and mitogenic factors that stimulate the migration and proliferation of specific cells of repair, such as myofibroblasts, fibroblasts, and capillary endothelial cells.

The effect of these stimuli becomes obvious three to five days after injury when endothelial cells near the wound divide and emit sprouts from the preexisting capillaries. Often, these sprouting capillaries protrude from the wound surface as red granules, thus, the term granulation tissue (Fig. 18). The vascular sprouts anastomose with each other, forming a network with a frequently changing direction of flow. There is a simultaneous influx of myofibroblasts and fibroblasts, which respond to various chemotactic stimuli, including growth factors, fibronectin, collagen, and other tissue-breakdown products. The signals controlling the path, spread, and orientation of the cells are not clearly understood; however, the specific binding sites in many of the extracellular matrix components are likely to have a major role in regulating cell locomotion, attachment, and orientation through their interactions with specific cell receptors (integrins). This regulation of cell motion by the extracellular matrix has been termed haptotaxis (Fig. 13).

As myofibroblasts and fibroblasts accumulate at the wound site, they secrete extracellular matrix components. The initial extracellular matrix contains mostly fibronectin and proteoglycans. By day 6 or 7, type III collagen begins to accumulate; by days 10 to 12, type I becomes predominant. This sequence is not unique to wound healing. A similar sequence occurs in embryonic development as proteoglycans and fibronectin form the initial undifferentiated matrix that is eventually replaced by the tissue-specific, differentiated matrix, that is, type I collagen in bone, type II collagen in cartilage, and laminin and type IV collagen around renal tubules. Collagen synthesis and degradation continue at the wound site for several months. Several enzymes, including lysyl oxidase, contribute to the formation of stable intramolecular and intermolecular cross-links that impart definitive tensile strength to the scar (Fig. 19).

Regeneration Injury to tissues composed of labile or stable cells triggers cell proliferation and the formation of a new extracellular matrix scaffold. Regeneration replaces lost cells and tissues with cells and tissues with similar functional and morphologic characteristics. Factors other than cell type regulate the extent of regeneration. In general, epithelia have good regenerative capacity if the extracellular matrix scaffold is not extensively damaged. For example, the lung can achieve a complete restoration of form and function after lobar pneumonia, if the scaffold has not been severely damaged. A single episode of massive hepatic necrosis can result in the regeneration of a normal liver. In contrast, in organs containing permanent cells, such as the heart and central nervous system, not even a single myocardial cell or neuron can be replaced. The regenerative potential of the constituent cells is one crucial determinant of the healing response.

The specific signals that trigger regeneration in a given organ are poorly understood. In endocrine organs, the decreased output of the glands triggers the feedback loop that results in regeneration of the

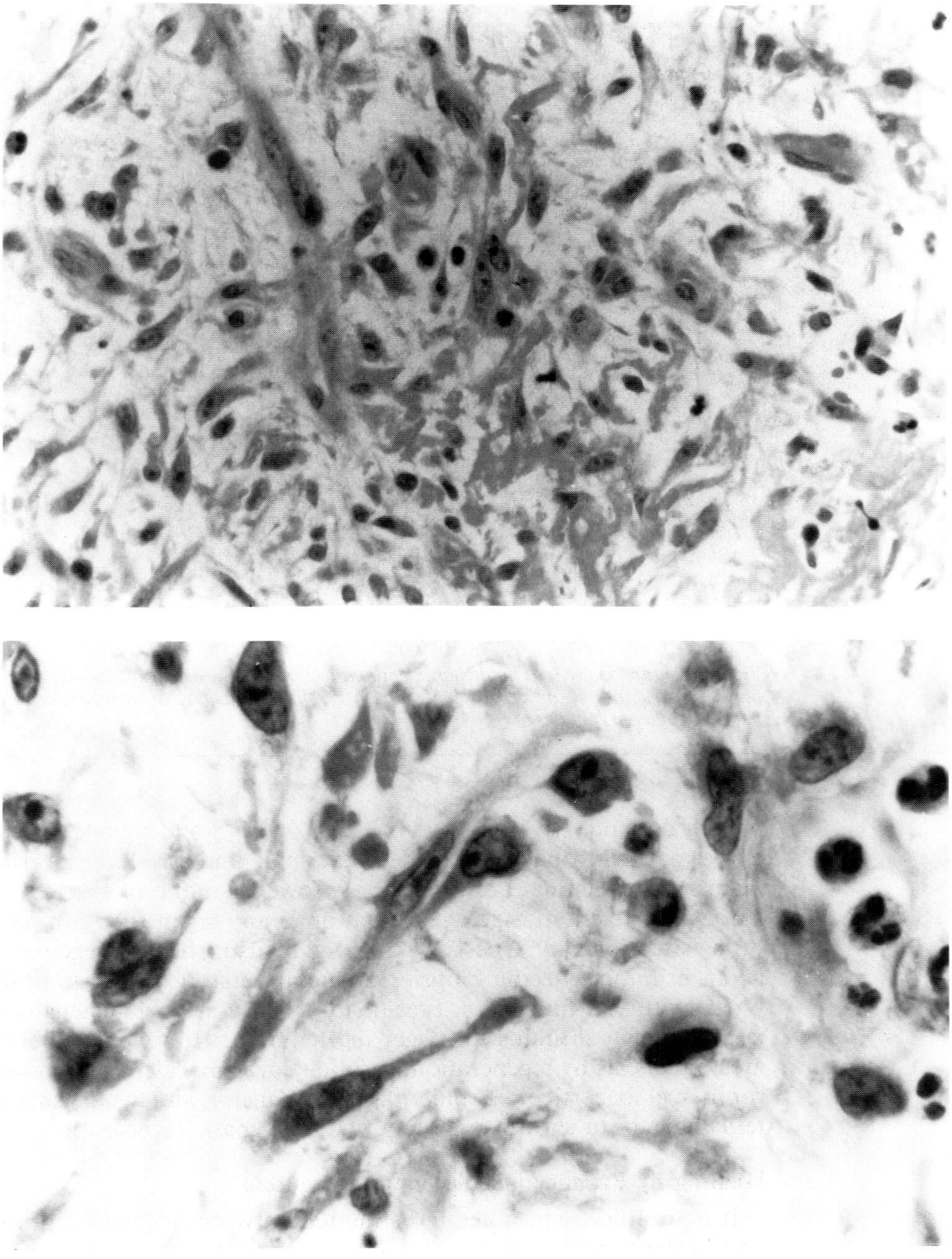

Fig. 18 ***Top,*** *Granulation tissue consists of a loose, connective-tissue matrix with fibrin, newly formed capillaries, numerous spindle cells (fibroblasts, fibrocytes, and myofibroblasts), and acute and chronic inflammatory cells.* ***Bottom,*** *Higher-magnification view of granulation tissue shows details of the spindle cells embedded in a loose matrix. A newly formed capillary contains neutrophils.*

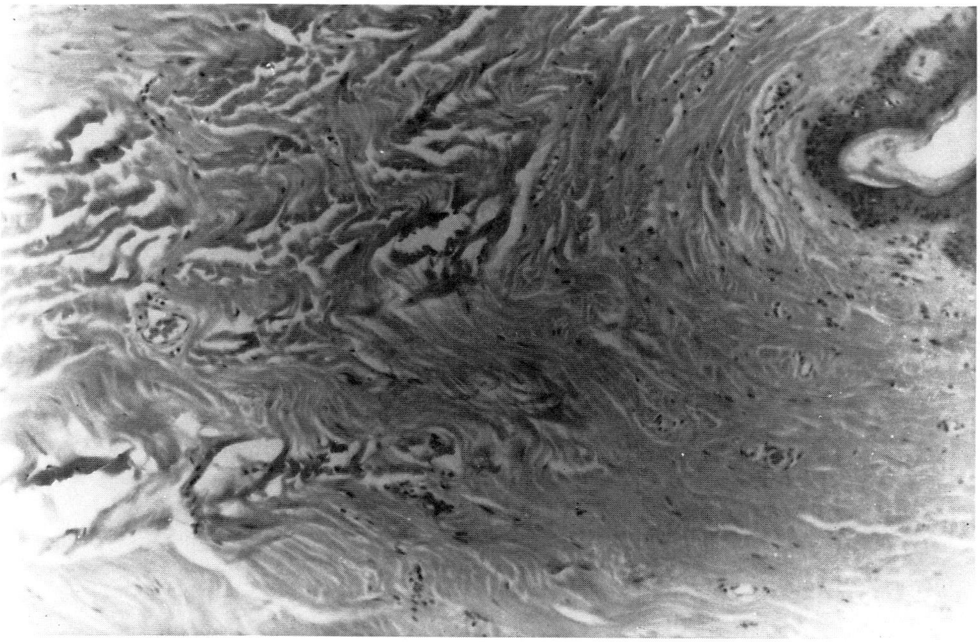

Fig. 19 *Cutaneous scar. The atrophic epithelium lacks adnexal structures. The papillary structure of the dermis is lost, as it is relatively avascular and contains dense parallel collagen bundles.*

damaged gland. Several growth factors (TGF-β and platelet-derived, epidermal macrophage-derived, epidermal, and insulin-like growth factors) can stimulate cell division. However, none of these factors alone is sufficient to trigger regeneration in any organ. The complexity of the situation can be best summarized by using hepatic regeneration as an example. Needle biopsies or granulomas in the liver heal by repair with scar formation. Presumably, the loss of a few hepatocytes is not enough stimulus to trigger regeneration. However, a 60% hepatectomy heals by regeneration. Insulin, glucagon, calcitonin, iodothyronines, glucocorticoids, epidermal growth factor, and two plasma proteins have been shown to be required for hepatic regeneration.

Healing by Primary and Secondary Intention

It is traditional to make a distinction between healing by primary and healing by secondary intention. In the first case, a wound with clean, closely apposed edges is sutured and minimal scarring ensues. In the second case, the distal edges of a gouged wound cannot be approximated and granulation tissue must fill the defect, resulting in extensive scarring. Although the end result is different, both wounds heal by an identical mechanism—repair.

Factors Modifying Wound Healing

The eventual outcome of a given injury depends not only on the type of injury (sharp or blunt trauma, extent of necrosis, and the like) but also on other factors. Ideally, these factors should be classified according to which of the basic healing mechanisms they influence: contraction, repair, or regeneration. However, current knowledge permits them to be classified only as local or systemic.

Local Factors

Type, Size, and Location of the Injury A clean, aseptic wound produced by a sharp scalpel heals faster than a wound produced by trauma with a contaminated, blunt instrument. Small wounds heal faster than large ones; wounds in richly vascularized areas (face or skeletal muscle) heal faster than those in poorly vascularized areas (foot or tendon). Adhesion to bony surfaces prevents contraction and adequate apposition of the wound edges.

Vascular Supply Wounds in tissues with a poor vascular supply heal slowly and poorly. This probably results from the lack of a strong initial stimulus (few platelets and macrophages result in low growth-factor concentrations; low fibrin and fibronectin contents result in low rates of chemotaxis and haptotaxis). A blood supply inadequate for the high metabolic needs of granulation tissue further complicates healing.

Infection Wounds are a potential entry point for microorganisms. Infection prevents or delays healing, encourages excessive granulation tissue, and often results in large, deforming scars.

Movement Early motion subjects the wound to new trauma and delays healing.

Ionizing Radiation Irradiation often results in arteritis that interferes with blood supply and results in slow healing. Irradiation of the wound site also blocks cell division.

Ultraviolet Light Moderate exposure of wounds to ultraviolet light accelerates the healing rate.

Systemic Factors

Circulatory Status The circulatory status determines the blood supply to the wound site and thus is important to wound healing. The poor healing usually attributed to old age is mostly the result of compromised circulation.

Nutrition Malnutrition hampers wound healing. Methionine is needed for good healing. Zinc, a cofactor of several enzymes, promotes faster healing in experimental wounds. Vitamin C is required for collagen secretion. A lack of vitamin C (scurvy) results in deficient wound healing, with inferior vascularization and scanty collagen deposition.

Despite these facts, nutritional status is seldom a significant factor in wound healing, except in extreme cases such as in concentration camp inmates or patients with anorexia or neoplastic cachexia.

Hormones Inadequate control of diabetes mellitus prevents wound healing. Further, wounds in diabetic patients often become infected; in turn, the infection makes controlling the diabetes more difficult. The result is severely delayed healing or failure to heal.

Glucocorticoids impair wound healing. The multiple actions of these hormones as anti–inflammatories, immunosuppressants, and general depressors of protein synthesis makes it difficult to attribute their effects on wound healing to any specific property. Thyroid hormones, androgens, estrogens, and growth hormone promote wound healing. Their influence is probably more related to their effects on general metabolic status than to any specific effect on healing.

Complications of Wound Healing

Abnormalities in any of the three basic healing mechanisms—regeneration, contraction, and repair—result in complications of healing.

Deficient Regeneration

Tissues containing permanent cells such as the central nervous system and myocardium, can heal only by scar formation. However, even in tissues capable of regeneration, such as the peripheral nervous system and skeletal muscle, regeneration is often incomplete or defective.

Excessive Regeneration

Chronic injury to tissues with excellent regenerative capacity may result in excessive regeneration or hyperplasia. Such is the case in gastrointestinal and genitourinary mucosae. In these tissues, excessive regeneration leads to hyperplastic polyps. In the liver, excessive regeneration results in regenerating nodules or, occasionally, in diffuse regenerative hyperplasia.

Deficient Scar Formation

Inadequate formation of granulation tissue or inability to form an appropriate extracellular matrix results in deficient scar formation. Wound dehiscence and ulceration are the consequences of deficient scar formation.

Excessive Scar Formation

An excessive number of active fibroblasts and excessive deposition of extracellular matrix result in hypertrophic scars and keloids. Both of these processes are characterized by the presence of more fibroblasts, capillaries, and thick collagen bundles than would be expected in a scar of the same age. The rate of collagen synthesis, the number of reducible cross-links, and the ratio of type III to type I collagen remains high, indicating a block in the healing process or persistent stimulation.

Deficient Contraction

If the wound edges are attached to hard tissues, as in wounds to the anterior tibial surface, myofibroblast contraction cannot approximate the wound edges, resulting in excessive granulation tissue, deficient epithelialization, and large, gruesome scars.

Excessive Contraction

Exaggerated wound contraction results in contracture or cicatrization. Contracture is particularly prominent in the healing of skin burns and often severe enough to freeze joints and to close natural openings. Contractures in the gastrointestinal tract lead to strictures and constrictive rings. Interestingly, areas with minimal wound contraction (palms, soles, and anterior thoracic wall) are susceptible to contractures. Several diseases are characterized by contracture and progressive fibrosis of superficial fascias, including Dupuytren's (palmar) contracture, lederhosen disease (plantar contracture), and Peyronie's disease (contracture of the cavernous tissues of the penis). Although the precipitating causes of these diseases are unknown, the basic process seems identical to that of wound contracture.

Healing in Specific Tissues

The primary determinants of the outcome of any wound are the type and extent of injury, the regenerative capacity of the constituent cells, the vascularization of the injured tissue, and the extent of the damage to the extracellular matrix framework. The basic principles of wound healing apply to all tissues. However, each organ contains different specialized cells, distinctive extracellular matrix, and different vascular supplies. These variations modify healing and bestow some tissue specificity to the healing response. For example, after a 60% hepatectomy, a normal liver will be regenerated, but even the thinnest of fracture lines along an articular cartilage is likely to result in dysfunction.

Cartilage

Cartilage has limited healing capacity. Injuries that kill chondrocytes and disrupt the matrix heal differently when the cartilage alone is affected and when the cartilage and subchondral bone are affected. Injuries confined to articular cartilage fail to elicit clot formation or to recruit neutrophils and macrophages. Only those chondrocytes adjacent to the injury show some reaction with mild proliferation and increased matrix synthesis. This limited response fails to heal the defect. However, these lesions seldom progress.[55]

When injuries affect the articular cartilage and subchondral bone, the vascularization of the subchondral bone allows the formation of fibrin-fibronectin gels, gives access to the inflammatory cells, and permits the formation of granulation tissue. Under these circumstances, healing proceeds according to the general pattern and differentiation of granulation tissue cells into chondrocytes begins in two weeks.[23] Two months after the initial injury, an apparently normal cartilage has been formed, healing the original defect; however, this cartilage has a low proteoglycan content. Further, one year after the injury, the new cartilage usually undergoes extensive fibrillar degeneration and erosive changes and becomes greatly attenuated.[23]

Tendon

The repair potential of tendons is the subject of some controversy. Cells intrinsic and extrinsic to the tendon participate in tendon repair. The exact role played by these cells and the final outcome of the healing reaction depend on several factors, including type of tendon, extent of damage to the tendon sheath and to the vascular supply, and length of the immobilization period. Generally, during the first four days after injury, there is an inflammatory phase when the injured area is infiltrated by extrinsic (peritendinous) and intrinsic (epitendinous and endotendinous) cells. Many of the infiltrating cells develop phagocytic capacities, and others become fibroblastic. Collagen synthesis becomes evident in seven or eight days; 14 days after the injury, fibroblasts are the predominant cell type. At this stage, both cells and collagen fibers are oriented perpendicular to the tendon's long axis. For the next two months, cells and collagen are remodeled and reoriented along the longitudinal axis of the tendon. Ultimate maturation of the collagen and achievement of optimal tensile strength develop only after suitable physiologic loading occurs.

The surrounding structures provide the cellular and vascular components for granulation tissue formation. Initially, extrinsic fibroblasts and phagocytic cells play the major role in the repair reaction. However, three weeks after the injury, proliferation of endotenon cells becomes prominent; by six weeks, they play the most significant role in tendon healing. The continuous collagen synthesis and degradation by these fibroblasts results in the remodeling of the wound site. Four months after the injury, the maturation of the wound is complete and the active cells revert to quiescent tenocytes.

If the synovial sheath is absent or not injured, the relative contributions of the epitenon and the endotenon are balanced and adhesions are minimal. If the synovial sheath is injured, the contributions by extrinsic cells overwhelm the capacities of intrinsic tendon cells and adhesions become a prominent feature.

Skeletal Muscle

Skeletal muscle cells are permanent cells with no proliferative capacity; however, skeletal muscle is endowed with stem or reserve cells (satellite cells). Satellite cells are small, mononucleated cells enclosed within the basement membrane of the differentiated muscle fiber (Fig. 10). Under the proper circumstances, the satellite cells proliferate and differentiate to form new skeletal muscle cells after the death of the adult muscle fibers. Skeletal muscle regeneration has been documented in muscle biopsy specimens of patients with muscular dystrophy, polymyositis, and certain infectious diseases such as diphtheria and typhus. However, little information is available on skeletal muscle regeneration in humans after trauma. In studies on severed rabbit muscle, healing of the sutured ends was by dense scar tissue with only occasional myotubules embedded in the scar tissue.[23] Clinical experience with human muscle shows similar findings.

The importance of the hemostatic components (Fig. 15) in the repair reaction is clearly illustrated by blunt injuries to muscle. In severe contusions with considerable hematoma formation, as many as 20% of the cases form bone in the scar, a process known as myositis ossificans.[23] However, myositis ossificans is rare in surgical cases with well-controlled hemostasis. Therefore, the proliferative and differentiation potential of cells present in adult muscles is indisputable. Satellite cells can generate functional skeletal muscle cells and some cells present in muscle can differentiate into osteoblasts. The clinical challenge is to enhance the regenerative potential of skeletal muscle and channel it to achieve regeneration in a surgical setting.

Acknowledgment

Portions of this chapter have been adapted from Martinez-Hernandez A: Repair, regeneration, and fibrosis, in Rubin E, Farber JL (eds): *Pathology*. Philadelphia, JB Lippincott, 1988.

References

1. Adler R, Jerdan J, Hewitt AT: Responses of cultured neural retinal cells to substratum-bound laminin and other extracellular matrix molecules. *Dev Biol* 1985;112:100–114.
2. Amenta PS, Clark CC, Martinez-Hernandez A: Deposition of fibronectin and laminin in the basement membrane of the rat parietal yolk sac: Immunohistochemical and biosynthetic studies. *J Cell Biol* 1983;96:104–111.
3. Amenta PS, Gay S, Vaheri A, et al: The extracellular matrix is an integrated unit: Ultrastructural localization of collagen types I, III, IV, V, VI, fibronectin, and laminin in human term placenta. *Collagen Relat Res* 1986;6:125–152.
4. Amenta PS, Gil J, Martinez-Hernandez A: Connective tissue of rat lung: II. Ultrastructural localization of collagen types III, IV, and VI. *J Histochem Cytochem* 1988;36:1167–1173.
5. Assoian RK: The role of growth factors in tissue repair IV: Type β-transforming growth factor and stimulation of fibrosis, in Clark RAF, Henson PM (eds): *The Molecular and Cellular Biology of Wound Repair*. New York, Plenum Press, 1988, pp 273–280.
6. Balk SD: Calcium as a regulator of the proliferation of normal, but not of transformed, chicken fibroblasts in a plasma containing medium. *Proc Natl Acad Sci USA* 1981;78:271–275.

7. Banks AR: The role of growth factors in tissue repair: II. Epidermal growth factor, in Clark RAF, Henson PM (eds): *The Molecular and Cellular Biology of Wound Repair.* New York, Plenum Press, 1988, pp 253–263.
8. Barlow DP, Green NM, Kurkinen M, et al: Sequencing of laminin B chain cDNAs reveals C-terminal regions of coiled-coil alpha-helix. *EMBO J* 1984;3:2355–2362.
9. Baserga R: *The Biology of Cell Reproduction.* Cambridge, Mass, Harvard University Press, 1985.
10. Bentz H, Morris NP, Murray LW, et al: Isolation and partial characterization of a new human collagen with an extended triple-helical structural domain. *Proc Natl Acad Sci USA* 1983;80:3168–3172.
11. Birk DE, Fitch JM, Linsenmayer TF: Organization of collagen types I and V in the embryonic chicken cornea. *Invest Ophthalmol Vis Sci* 1986;27:1470–1477.
12. Birk DE, Fitch JM, Mayne R, et al: Localization of types I and V collagen in the chick cornea using immuno-electron microscopy. *J Cell Biol* 1985;101:93A.
13. Birk DE, Trelstad RL: Extracellular compartments in tendon morphogenesis: Collagen fibril, bundle, and macroaggregate formation. *J Cell Biol* 1986;103:231-240.
14. Birk DE, Trelstad RL: Extracellular compartments in matrix morphogenesis: Collagen fibril, bundle, and lamellar formation by corneal fibroblasts. *J Cell Biol* 1984;99:2024–2033.
15. Bizzozero G: Growth and regeneration of the organism. *Br Med J* 1894;1:728–732.
16. Bornstein P, Sage H: Structurally distinct collagen types. *Annu Rev Biochem* 1980;49:957–1003.
17. Buck CA, Horowitz AF: Cell surface receptors for extracellular matrix molecules. *Annu Rev Cell Biol* 1987;3:179–205.
18. Buckwalter J, Rosenberg L, Coutts R, et al: Articular cartilage: Injury and repair, in Woo SL-Y, Buckwalter JA (eds): *Injury and Repair of the Musculoskeletal Soft Tissues.* Park Ridge, Ill, American Academy of Orthopaedic Surgeons, 1988, pp 465–482.
19. Burgeson RE: New collagens, new concepts. *Annu Rev Cell Biol* 1988;4:551–577.
20. Burgeson RE, Morris NP, Murray LW, et al: The structure of type VII collagen. *Ann NY Acad Sci* 1985;460:47–57.
21. Byers PH, Barsh GS, Holbrook KA: Molecular mechanisms of connective tissue abnormalities in the Ehlers-Danlos syndrome. *Collagen Relat Res* 1981;1:475–489.
22. Byers PH, Holbrook KA: Molecular basis of clinical heterogeneity in the Ehlers-Danlos syndrome. *Ann NY Acad Sci* 1985;460:298–310.
23. Caplan A, Carlson B, Faulkner J, et al: Skeletal muscle, in Woo SL-Y, Buckwalter JA (eds): *Injury and Repair of the Musculoskeletal Soft Tissues.* Park Ridge, Ill, American Academy of Orthopaedic Surgeons, 1988, pp 213–291.
24. Carlin B, Jaffe R, Bender B, et al: Entactin, a novel basal lamina-associated sulfated glycoprotein. *J Biol Chem* 1981;256:5209–5214.
25. Caulfield JP, Farquhar MG: Loss of anionic sites from the glomerular basement membrane in aminonucleoside nephrosis. *Lab Invest* 1978;39:505–512.
26. Champagnone R, Regan J, Rich CB, et al: Pulmonary fibroblasts: A model system for studying elastin synthesis. *Lab Invest* 1987;56:224–230.
27. Cheah KS: Collagen genes and inherited connective tissue disease. *Biochem J* 1985;229:287–303.

28. Chichester CO, Palmer KC, Hayes JA, et al: Lung lysyl oxidase and prolyl hydroxylase: Increases induced by cadmium chloride inhalation and the effect of beta-aminopropionitrile in rats. *Am Rev Respir Dis* 1981;124:709–713.
29. Chiquet M, Fambrough DM: Chick myotendinous antigen: I. A monoclonal antibody as a marker for tendon and muscle morphogenesis. *J Cell Biol* 1984;98:1926–1936.
30. Chiquet-Ehrismann R, Mackie EJ, Pearson CA, et al: Tenascin: An extracellular matrix protein involved in tissue interactions during fetal development and oncogenesis. *Cell* 1986;47:131–139.
31. Clark CC, Kefalides NA: Partial characterization of collagenous and noncollagenous basement membrane proteins synthesized by the 14.5-day rat embryo parietal yolk sac in vitro. *Connect Tissue Res* 1982;10:303–318.
32. Clark RAF, Henson PM (eds): *The Molecular and Cellular Biology of Wound Repair.* New York, Plenum Press, 1988.
33. Cleary EG, Gibson MA: Elastin-associated microfibrils and microfibrillar proteins. *Int Rev Connect Tissue Res* 1983;10:97–209.
34. Cohen S: Isolation of a mouse submaxillary gland protein accelerating incisor eruption and eyelid opening in the new-born animal. *J Biol Chem* 1962;237:1555–1562.
35. Courtoy PJ, Kanwar YS, Hynes RO, et al: Fibronectin localization in the rat glomerulus. *J Cell Biol* 1980;87:691–696.
36. Courtoy PJ, Timpl R, Farquhar MG: Comparative distribution of laminin, type IV collagen, and fibronectin in the rat glomerulus. *J Histochem Cytochem* 1982;30:874–886.
37. Cunningham LW (ed): *Methods in Enzymology, Volume 144: Structural and Contractile Proteins. Part D. Extracellular Matrix.* Orlando, Academic Press, 1987.
38. Cunningham LW (ed): *Methods in Enzymology, Volume 145: Structural and Contractile Proteins. Part E. Extracellular Matrix.* Orlando, Academic Press, 1987.
39. Damiano VV, Tsang A, Christner P, et al: Immunologic localization of elastin by electron microscopy. *Am J Pathol* 1979;96:439–455.
40. D'Ardenne AJ, Burns J, Sykes BC, et al: Comparative distribution of fibronectin and type III collagen in normal human tissues. *J Pathol* 1983;141:55–69.
41. de Larco JE, Todaro GJ: Growth factors from murine sarcoma virus-transformed cells. *Proc Natl Acad Sci USA* 1978;75:4001–4005.
42. Dickson LA, Pihlajaniemi T, Deak S, et al: Nuclease S1 mapping of a homozygous mutation in the carboxyl-propeptide-coding region of the pro alpha 2(I) collagen gene in a patient with osteogenesis imperfecta. *Proc Natl Acad Sci USA* 1984;81:4524–4528.
43. Ekblom P: Formation of basement membranes in the embryonic kidney: An immunohistological study. *J Cell Biol* 1981;91:1–10.
44. Ekblom P, Alitalo K, Vaheri A, et al: Induction of a basement membrane glycoprotein in embryonic kidney: Possible role of laminin in morphogenesis. *Proc Natl Acad Sci USA* 1980;77:485–489.
45. Ekblom P, Miettinen M, Rapola J, et al: Demonstration of laminin, a basement membrane glycoprotein, in routinely processed formalin-fixed human tissues. *Histochemistry* 1982;75:301–307.
46. Erickson HP, Iglesias JL: A six-armed oligomer isolated from cell surface fibronectin preparations. *Nature* 1984;311:267–269.
47. Fenger M, Wewer U, Albrechtsen R: Basement membrane heparan sulfate proteoglycan from the L2 rat yolk sac carcinoma. *FEBS Lett* 1984;173:75–79.
48. Fleischmajer R: Collagen fibrillogenesis: A mechanism of structural biology. *J Invest Dermatol* 1986;87:553–554.

49. Fleischmajer R, Olsen BR, Kuhn K (eds): *Biology, Chemistry, and Pathology of Collagen.* New York, New York Academy of Sciences, 1986.
50. Fleischmajer R, Perlish JS, Timpl R: Collagen fibrillogenesis in human skin. *Ann NY Acad Sci* 1985;460:246–257.
51. Fleischmajer R, Timpl R: Ultrastructural localization of fibronectin to different anatomic structures of human skin. *J Histochem Cytochem* 1984;32:315–321.
52. Fox GM: The role of growth factors in tissue repair III: Fibroblast growth factor, in Clark RAF, Henson PM (eds): *The Molecular and Cellular Biology of Wound Repair.* New York, Plenum Press, 1988, pp 265–271.
53. Fukuda M, Levery SB, Hakomori S: Carbohydrate structure of hamster plasma fibronectin: Evidence for chemical diversity between cellular and plasma fibronectins. *J Biol Chem* 1982;257:6856–6860.
54. Gay S, Miller EJ: What is collagen, what is not. *Ultrastruct Pathol* 1983;4:365–377.
55. Gelberman R, Goldberg V, An K-N, et al: Tendon, in Woo SL-Y, Buckwalter JA (eds): *Injury and Repair of the Musculoskeletal Soft Tissues.* Park Ridge, Ill, American Academy of Orthopaedic Surgeons, 1988, pp 5–40.
56. Gosline MJ, Rosenbloom J: Elastin, in Piez KA, Reddi AH (eds): *Extracellular Matrix Biochemistry.* New York, Elsevier, 1984, pp 191–228.
57. Gospodarowicz D: Localisation of a fibroblast growth factor and its effect alone and with hydrocortisone on 3T3 cell growth. *Nature* 1974;249:123–127.
58. Graf J, Iwamoto Y, Sasaki M, et al: Identification of an amino acid sequence in laminin mediating cell attachment, chemotaxis, and receptor binding. *Cell* 1987;48:989–996.
59. Griffin CA, Emanuel BS, Hansen JR, et al: Human collagen genes encoding basement membrane alpha 1 (IV) and alpha 2 (IV) chains map to the distal long arm of chromosome 13. *Proc Natl Acad Sci USA* 1987;84:512–516.
60. Gross J, Harper E, Harris ED, et al: Animal collagenases: Specificity of action, and structures of the substrate cleavage site. *Biochem Biophys Res Commun* 1974;61:605–612.
61. Gupta S, Gupta SK: Wound healing in surgical practice. *Q Med Rev* 1985;36:1–43.
62. Hadley MA, Byers SW, Suárez-Quian CA, et al: Extracellular matrix regulates Sertoli cell differentiation, testicular cord formation, and germ cell development in vitro. *J Cell Biol* 1985;101:1511–1522.
63. Hammarback JA, Palm SL, Furcht LT, et al: Guidance of neurite outgrowth by pathways of substratum-adsorbed laminin. *J Neurosci Res* 1985;13:213–220.
64. Haralson MA, Federspiel SJ, Martinez-Hernandez A, et al: Synthesis of [pro alpha 1(IV)]3 collagen molecules by cultured embryo-derived parietal yolk sac cells. *Biochemistry* 1985;24:5792–5797.
65. Hascall VC, Hascall GK: Proteoglycans, in Hay ED (ed): *Cell Biology of Extracellular Matrix.* New York, Plenum Press, 1981, pp 39–64.
66. Hauschka PV, Lian JB, Gallop PM: Direct identification of the calcium-binding amino acid, gamma-carboxyglutamate, in mineralized tissue. *Proc Natl Acad Sci USA* 1975;72:3925–3929.
67. Hay ED: Matrix-cytoskeletal interactions in the developing eye. *J Cell Biochem* 1985;27:143–156.
68. Hay ED: Interaction of embryonic surface and cytoskeleton with extracellular matrix. *Am J Anat* 1982;165:1–12.
69. Hay ED (ed): *Cell Biology of Extracellular Matrix.* New York, Plenum Press, 1981.

70. Heinegard D, Paulsson M: Structure and metabolism of protetoglycans, in Piez KA, Reddi AH (eds): *Extracellular Matrix Biochemistry*. New York, Elsevier, 1984, pp 277–322.

71. Höök M, Kjellén L, Johansson S: Cell-surface glycosaminoglycans. *Annu Rev Biochem* 1984;53:847–869.

72. Huang JS, Olsen TJ, Huang SS: The role of growth factors in tissue repair I: Platelet-derived growth factor, in Clark RAF, Henson PM (eds): *The Molecular and Cellular Biology of Wound Repair*. New York, Plenum Press, 1988, pp 243–251.

73. Hynes RO: Molecular biology of fibronectin, in Palade GE, Alberts BM, Spudich JA (eds): *Annual Review of Cell Biology*. Palo Alto, Annual Reviews, 1985, vol 1.

74. Hynes RO, Schwarzbauer JE, Tamkun JW: Fibronectin: A versatile gene for a versatile protein. *Ciba Found Symp* 1984;108:75–92.

75. Hynes RO, Yamada KM: Fibronectins: Multifunctional modular glycoproteins. *J Cell Biol* 1982;95:369–377.

76. Ihme A, Krieg T, Nerlich A, et al: Ehlers-Danlos syndrome type VI: Collagen type specificity of defective lysyl hydroxylation in various tissues. *J Invest Dermatol* 1984;83:161–165.

77. Iozzo RV: Proteoglycans: Structure, function, and role in neoplasia. *Lab Invest* 1985;53:373–396.

78. Iozzo RV: Proteoglycans and neoplastic: Mesenchymal cell interactions. *Hum Pathol* 1984;15:2-10.

79. Kanwar YS, Farquhar MG: Presence of heparan sulfate in the glomerular basement membrane. *Proc Natl Acad Sci USA* 1979;76:1303–1307.

80. Kanwar YS, Farquhar MG: Isolation of glycosaminoglycans (heparan sulfate) from glomerular basement membranes. *Proc Natl Acad Sci USA* 1979;76:4493–4497.

81. Kanwar YS, Farquhar MG: Anionic sites in the glomerular basement membrane: In vivo and in vitro localization to the laminae rarae by cationic probes. *J Cell Biol* 1979;81:137–153.

82. Kanwar YS, Linker A, Farquhar MG: Increased permeability of the glomerular basement membrane to ferritin after removal of glycosaminoglycans (heparan sulfate) by enzyme digestion. *J Cell Biol* 1980;86:688–693.

83. Karkavelas G, Kefalides NA, Amenta PS, et al: Comparative ultrastructural localization of collagen types III, IV, VI, and laminin rat uterus and kidney. *J Ultrastructr Mol Structr Res* 1988;100:137–155.

84. Kefalides NA: Isolation of collagen from basement membranes containing three identical alpha chains. *Biochem Biophys Res Commun* 1971;45:226–234.

85. Kefalides NA, Alper R, Clark CC: Biochemistry and metabolism of basement membranes. *Int Rev Cytol* 1979;61:167–228.

86. Keene DR, Sakai LY, Bächinger HP, et al: Type III collagen can be present on banded collagen fibrils regardless of fibril diameter. *J Cell Biol* 1987;105:2393–2402.

87. Kivirikko KI, Myllyla R: Biosynthesis of the collagens, in Piez KA, Reddi AH (eds): *Extracellular Matrix Biochemistry*. New York, Elsevier, 1984, pp 83–118.

88. Kleinman HK, Cannon FB, Laurie GW, et al: Biological activities of laminin. *J Cell Biochem* 1985;27:317–325.

89. Kleinman HK, Graf J, Iwamoto Y, et al: Role of basement membranes in cell differentiation. *Ann NY Acad Sci* 1987;513:134–145.

90. Kleinman HK, Klebe RJ, Martin GR: Role of collagenous matrices in the adhesion and growth of cells. *J Cell Biol* 1981;88:473–485.

91. Konomi H, Hori H, Sano J, et al: Immunohistochemical localization of type I, II, III, and IV collagens in the lung. *Acta Pathol Jpn* 1981;31:601–610.
92. Kornblihtt AR, Umezawa K, Vibe-Pedersen K, et al: Primary structure of human fibronectin: Differential splicing may generate at least 10 polypeptides from a single gene. *EMBO J* 1985;4:1755–1759.
93. Kornblihtt AR, Vibe-Pedersen K, Baralle FE: Human fibronectin: Cell specific alternative mRNA splicing generates polypeptide chains differing in the number of internal repeats. *Nucleic Acids Res* 1984;12:5853–5868.
94. Krane SM: Genetic and acquired disorder of collagen deposition, in Piez KA, Reddi AH (eds): *Extracellular Matrix Biochemistry.* New York, Elsevier, 1984, pp 413–463.
95. Kuehn K, Schoene H-H, Timpl R (eds): *New Trends in Basement Membrane Research: 10th Workshop Conference HOECHST, Eibsee, May 11–14, 1981.* New York, Raven Press, 1982.
96. Kühn K: Structure and biochemistry of collagen. *Aesthetic Plast Surg* 1985;9:141–144.
97. Kühn K, Glanville RW, Babel W, et al: The structure of type IV collagen. *Ann NY Acad Sci* 1985;460:14–24.
98. Kuehn K, Krieg T (eds): *Connective Tissue: Biological and Clinical Aspects.* Basel, S Karger, 1986.
99. Kurkinen M, Vaheri A, Roberts PJ, et al: Sequential appearance of fibronectin and collagen in experimental granulation tissue. *Lab Invest* 1980;43:47–51.
100. Larsson LI, Skriver L, Nielsen LS, et al: Distribution of urokinase-type plasminogen activator immunoreactivity in the mouse. *J Cell Biol* 1984;98:894–903.
101. Laurie GW, Bing JT, Kleinman HK, et al: Localization of binding sites for laminin, heparan sulfate proteoglycan and fibronectin on basement membrane (type IV) collagen. *J Mol Biol* 1986;189:205–216.
102. Laurie GW, Leblond CP, Martin GR: Light microscopic immunolocalization of type IV collagen, laminin, heparan sulfate proteoglycan, and fibronectin in the basement membranes of a variety of rat organs. *Am J Anat* 1983;167:71–82.
103. Leblond CP, Walker BE: Renewal of cell populations. *Physiol Rev* 1956;36:255–276.
104. Leibovich SJ, Ross R: The role of the macrophage in wound repair: A study with hydrocortisone and antimacrophage serum. *Am J Pathol* 1975;78:71–100.
105. Linder E, Stenman S, Lehto VP, et al: Distribution of fibronectin in human tissues and relationship to other connective tissue components. *Ann NY Acad Sci* 1978;312:151–159.
106. Linder E, Vaheri A, Ruoslahti E, et al: Distribution of fibroblast surface antigen in the developing chick embryo. *J Exp Med* 1975;142:41–49.
107. Linsenmayer TF: Collagen, in Hay ED (ed): *Cell Biology of Extracellular Matrix.* New York, Plenum Press, 1981, pp 5–37.
108. Linsenmayer TF, Fitch JM, Gross J, et al: Are collagen fibrils in the developing avian cornea composed of two different collagen types? Evidence from monoclonal antibody studies. *Ann NY Acad Sci* 1985;460:232–245.
109. Liotta LA, Rao CN, Wewer UM: Biochemical interactions of tumor cells with the basement membrane. *Annu Rev Biochem* 1986;55:1037–1057.
110. Mackie EJ, Thesleff I, Chiquet-Ehrismann R: Tenascin is associated with chondrogenic and osteogenic differentiation in vivo and promotes chondrogenesis in vitro. *J Cell Biol* 1987;105:2569–2579.
111. Mainardi CL: Collagenase in rheumatoid arthritis. *Ann NY Acad Sci* 1985;460:345–354.

112. Mainardi CL, Dixit SN, Kang AH: Degradation of type IV (basement membrane) collagen by a proteinase isolated from human polymorphonuclear leukocyte granules. *J Biol Chem* 1980;255:5435–5441.
113. Mainardi CL, Hibbs MS, Hasty KA, et al: Purification of a type V collagen degrading metalloproteinase from rabbit alveolar macrophages. *Collagen Relat Res* 1984;4:479–492.
114. Martin GR, Timpl R: Laminin and other basement membrane components. *Annu Rev Cell Biol* 1987;3:57–85.
115. Martin GR, Timpl R, Muller PK, et al: The genetically distinct collagens. *TIBS* 1985;12:285–287.
116. Martinez-Hernandez A: Formation of basement membranes in the cirrhotic liver: Electron immunohistochemical studies, in Shibata S (ed): *Basement Membranes.* Amsterdam, Elsevier, 1986.
117. Martinez-Hernandez A: The basement membrane in the microcirculation, in Effros RM, Schonbein HS, Ditzel J (eds): *The Microcirculation: Current Physiologic, Medical and Surgical Concepts.* New York, Academic Press, 1981, pp 95–115.
118. Martinez-Hernandez A: The hepatic extracellular matrix: I. Electron immunohistochemical studies in normal rat liver. *Lab Invest* 1984;51:57–74.
119. Martinez-Hernandez A: The hepatic extracellular matrix: II. Electron immunohistochemical studies in rats with CC_{14}-induced cirrhosis. *Lab Invest* 1985;53:166–186.
120. Martinez-Hernandez A, Amenta PS: The basement membrane in pathology. *Lab Invest* 1983;48:656–677.
121. Martinez-Hernandez A, Chung AE: The ultrastructural localization of two basement membrane components: Entactin and laminin in rat tissues. *J Histochem Cytochem* 1984;32:289–298.
122. Martinez-Hernandez A, Marsh CA, Clark CC, et al: Fibronectin: Its relationship to basement membranes. II. Ultrastructural studies in rat kidney. *Collagen Relat Res* 1981;1:405-418.
123. Mason IJ, Taylor A, Williams JG, et al: Evidence from molecular cloning that SPARC, a major product of mouse embryo parietal endoderm, is related to an endothelial cell 'culture shock' glycoprotein of Mr 43,000. *EMBO J* 1986;5:1465–1472.
124. McCarthy JB, Sas DF, Furcht LT: Mechanisms of parenchymal cell migration into wounds, in Clark RAF, Henson PM (eds): *The Molecular and Cellular Biology of Wound Repair.* New York, Plenum Press, 1988, pp 281–319.
125. McManus LM, Naughton MA, Martinez-Hernandez A: Human chorionic gonadotropin in human neoplastic cells. *Cancer Res* 1976;36:3476–3481.
126. Miettinen A, Stow JL, Mentone S, et al: Antibodies to basement membrane heparan sulfate proteoglycans bind to the laminae rarae of the glomerular basement membrane (GBM) and induce subepithelial GBM thickening. *J Exp Med* 1986;163:1064–1084.
127. Mignatti P, Welgus HG, Rifkin DB: Role of degradative enzymes in wound healing, in Clark RAF, Henson PM (eds): *The Molecular and Cellular Biology of Wound Repair.* New York, Plenum Press, 1988, pp 497–523.
128. Miller EJ: The structure of fibril-forming collagens. *Ann NY Acad Sci* 1985;460:1-13.
129. Miller EJ, Gay S: The collagens: An overview and update. *Methods Enzymol* 1987;144:3–41.
130. Miller EJ, Gay S: Collagens: An overview. *Methods Enzymol* 1982;82:3–32.

131. Mosher DF, Schad PE, Vann JM: Cross-linking of collagen and fibronectin by factor XIIIa: Localization of participating glutaminyl residues to a tryptic fragment of fibronectin. *J Biol Chem* 1980;255:1181–1188.
132. Mynderse LA, Hassell JR, Kleinman HK, et al: Loss of heparan sulfate proteoglycan from glomerular basement membrane of nephrotic rats. *Lab Invest* 1983;48:292–302.
133. Odermatt E, Engle J, Richter H, et al: Shape, conformation and stability of fibronectin fragments determined by electron microscopy, circular dichroism and ultracentrifugation. *J Mol Biol* 1982;159:109–123.
134. Ohno M, Martinez-Hernandez A, Ohno N, et al: Comparative study of laminin found in normal placental membrane with laminin of neoplastic origin, in Shibata S (ed): *Basement Membranes*. Amsterdam, Elsevier, 1986.
135. Ohno M, Martinez-Hernandez A, Ohno N, et al: Isolation of laminin from human placental basement membranes: Amnion, chorion and chorionic microvessels. *Biochem Biophys Res Commun* 1983;112:1091–1098.
136. Oldberg A, Franzén A, Heinegård D: Cloning and sequence analysis of rat bone sialoprotein (osteopontin) cDNA reveals an Arg-Gly-Asp cell-binding sequence. *Proc Natl Acad Sci USA* 1986;83:8819–8823.
137. Oldberg A, Ruoslahti E: Evolution of the fibronectin gene: Exon structure of cell attachment domain. *J Biol Chem* 1986;261:2113–2116.
138. Packham MA, Mustard JF: The role of platelets in the development and complications of atherosclerosis. *Semin Hematol* 1986;23:8–26.
139. Parthasarathy N, Spiro RG: Isolation and characterization of the heparan sulfate proteoglycan of the bovine glomerular basement membrane. *J Biol Chem* 1984;259:12749–12755.
140. Parthasarathy N, Spiro RG: Effect of diabetes on the glycosaminoglycan component of the human glomerular basement membrane. *Diabetes* 1982;31:738–741.
141. Pierce GB, Nakane PK: Basement membranes: Synthesis and deposition in response to cellular injury. *Lab Invest* 1969;21:27–41.
142. Pierschbacher M, Hayman EG, Ruoslahti E: Synthetic peptide with cell attachment activity of fibronectin. *Proc Natl Acad Sci USA* 1983;80:1224–1227.
143. Pierschbacher MD, Hayman EG, Ruoslahti E: Location of the cell-attachment site in fibronectin using monoclonal antibodies and proteolytic fragments of the molecule. *Cell* 1981;26:259–267.
144. Pierschbacher MD, Ruoslahti E: Cell attachment activity of fibronectin can be duplicated by small synthetic fragments of the molecule. *Nature* 1984;309:30–33.
145. Piez KA, Reddi AH (eds): *Extracellular Matrix Biochemistry*. New York, Elsevier, 1984.
146. Pihlajaniemi T, Dickson LA, Pope FM, et al: Osteogenesis imperfecta: Cloning of a pro-alpha 2(I) collagen gene with a frameshift mutation. *J Biol Chem* 1984;259:12941–12944.
147. Pihlajaniemi T, Myllylä R, Seyer J, et al: Partial characterization of a low molecular weight human collagen that undergoes alternative splicing. *Proc Natl Acad Sci USA* 1987;84:940–944.
148. Pinnell SR, Bauer EA, Fleischmajer R, et al: Connective tissue diseases. *J Am Acad Dermatol* 1984;11:990–994.
149. Prockop DJ, Chu ML, de Wet W, et al: Mutations in osteogenesis imperfecta leading to the synthesis of abnormal type I procollagens. *Ann NY Acad Sci* 1985;460:289–297.
150. Pyeritz RE, Stolle CA, Parfrey NA, et al: Ehlers-Danlos syndrome IV due to a novel defect in type III procollagen. *Am J Med Genet* 1984;19:607–622.

151. Reeves WH, Kanwar YS, Farquhar MG: Assembly of the glomerular filtration surface: Differentiation of anionic sites in glomerular capillaries of newborn rat kidney. *J Cell Biol* 1980;85:735–753.
152. Rennke HG, Cotran RS, Venkatachalam MA: Role of molecular charge in glomerular permeability: Tracer studies with cationized ferritins. *J Cell Biol* 1975;67:638–646.
153. Riches DWH: The multiple roles of macrophages in wound healing, in Clark RAF, Henson PM (eds): *The Molecular and Cellular Biology of Wound Repair.* New York, Plenum Press, 1988, pp 213–239.
154. Rohrbach DH, Hassell JR, Kleinman HK, et al: Alterations in the basement membrane (heparan sulfate) proteoglycan in diabetic mice. *Diabetes* 1982;31:185–188.
155. Rohrbach DH, Wagner CW, Star VL, et al: Reduced synthesis of basement membrane heparan sulfate proteoglycan in streptozotocin-induced diabetic mice. *J Biol Chem* 1983;258:11672–11677.
156. Rojkind M, Kershenobich D: Extracellular matrix, fibrosis and cirrhosis, in Arias IM, Frenkel M, Wilson JHP (eds): *The Liver Annual, No. 5.* New York, Elsevier, 1986, pp 210–224.
157. Ruoslahti E: Structure and biology of proteoglycans. *Annu Rev Cell Biol* 1988;4:229–255.
158. Ruoslahti E, Hayman EG, Pierschbacher M, et al: Fibronectin: Purification, immunochemical properties, and biological activities. *Methods Enzymol* 1982;82:803–831.
159. Ruoslahti E, Pierschbacher MD: New perspectives in cell adhesion: RGD and integrins. *Science* 1987;238:491–497.
160. Ruoslahti E, Pierschbacher MD: Arg-Gly-Asp: A versatile cell recognition signal. *Cell* 1986;44:517–518.
161. Ruoslahti E, Pierschbacher M, Engvall E, et al: Molecular and biological interactions of fibronectin. *J Invest Dermatol* 1982;79(suppl 1):65s-68s.
162. Sakai LY, Keene DR, Engvall E: Fibrillin, a new 350-kD glycoprotein, is a component of extracellular microfibrils. *J Cell Biol* 1986;103:2499–2509.
163. Sandberg LB, Soskel NT, Leslie JG: Elastin structure, biosynthesis, and relation to disease states. *N Engl J Med* 1981;304:566–579.
164. Sariola H, Timpl R, von der Mark K, et al: Dual origin of glomerular basement membrane. *Dev Biol* 1984;101:86–96.
165. Schulz A, Jundt G, Berghäuser KH, et al: Immunohistochemical study of osteonectin in various types of osteosarcoma. *Am J Pathol* 1988;132:233–238.
166. Schwarzbauer JE, Tamkun JW, Lemischka IR, et al: Three different fibronectin mRNAs arise by alternative splicing within the coding region. *Cell* 1983;35:421–431.
167. Sekiguchi K, Klos AM, Kurachi K, et al: Human liver fibronectin complementary DNAs: Identification of two different messenger RNAs possibly encoding the alpha and beta subunits of plasma fibronectin. *Biochemistry* 1986;25:4936–4941.
168. Semoff S, Hogan BL, Hopkins CR: Localization of fibronectin, laminin-entactin, and entactin in Reichert's membrane by immunoelectron microscopy. *EMBO J* 1982;1:1171–1175.
169. Senior RM, Campbell EJ: Neutral proteinases from human inflammatory cells: A critical review of their role in extracellular matrix degradation. *Clin Lab Med* 1983;3:645–666.
170. Skalli O, Gabbiani G: The biology of the myofibroblast relationship to wound contraction and fibrocontractive diseases, in Clark RAF, Henson PM (eds): *The Molecular and Cellular Biology of Wound Repair.* New York, Plenum Press, 1988, pp 373–402.

171. Stanley JR, Foidart JM, Murray JC, et al: The epidermal cell which selectively adheres to a collagen substrate is the basal cell. *J Invest Dermatol* 1980;74:54–58.
172. Stenman S, Vaheri A: Distribution of a major connective tissue protein, fibronectin, in normal human tissues. *J Exp Med* 1978;147:1054–1064.
173. Stow JL, Kjellén L, Unger E, et al: Heparan sulfate proteoglycans are concentrated on the sinusoidal plasmalemmal domain and in intracellular organelles of hepatocytes. *J Cell Biol* 1985;100:975–980.
174. Stow JL, Sawada H, Farquhar MG: Basement membrane heparan sulfate proteoglycans are concentrated in the laminae rarae and in podocytes of the rat renal glomerulus. *Proc Natl Acad Sci USA* 1985;82:3296–3300.
175. Strom SC, Michalopoulos G: Collagen as a substrate for cell growth and differentiation. *Methods Enzymol* 1982;82:544–555.
176. Sugrue SP, Hay ED: The identification of extracellular matrix (ECM) binding sites on the basal surface of embryonic corneal epithelium and the effect of ECM binding on epithelial collagen production. *J Cell Biol* 1986;102:1907–1916.
177. Tamkun JW, DeSimone DW, Fonda D, et al: Structure of integrin, a glycoprotein involved in the transmembrane linkage between fibronectin and actin. *Cell* 1986;46:271–282.
178. Tamkun JW, Hynes RO: Plasma fibronectin is synthesized and secreted by hepatocytes. *J Biol Chem* 1983;258:4641–4647.
179. Tamkun JW, Schwarzbauer JE, Hynes RO: A single rat fibronectin gene generates three different mRNAs by alternative splicing of a complex exon. *Proc Natl Acad Sci USA* 1984;81:5140–5144.
180. Termine JD, Kleinman HK, Whitson SW, et al: Osteonectin, a bone-specific protein linking mineral to collagen. *Cell* 1981;26:99–105.
181. Timpl R, Dziadek M: Structure, development, and molecular pathology of basement membranes. *Int Rev Exp Pathol* 1986;29:1–112.
182. Timpl R, Martin GR, Bruckner P, et al: Nature of the collagenous protein in a tumor basement membrane. *Eur J Biochem* 1978;84:43–52.
183. Timpl R, Oberbäumer I, von der Mark H, et al: Structure and biology of the globular domain of basement membrane type IV collagen. *Ann NY Acad Sci* 1985;460:58–72.
184. Timpl R, Rohde H, Robey PG, et al: Laminin: A glycoprotein from basement membranes. *J Biol Chem* 1979;254:9933–9937.
185. Torikata C, Villiger B, Kuhn C III, et al: Ultrastructural distribution of fibronectin in normal and fibrotic human lung. *Lab Invest* 1985;52:399–408.
186. Trelstad RL (ed): *The Role of Extracellular Matrix in Development.* New York, AR Liss, 1984.
187. Trelstad RL, Coulumbre AJ: Problems in corneal morphogenesis. *Adv Morphog* 1965;4:81–109.
188. Van Evercooren A, Kleinman HK, Ohno S, et al: Nerve growth factor, laminin, and fibronectin promote neurite growth in human fetal sensory ganglia cultures. *J Neurosci Res* 1982;8:179–193.
189. Viljanto J, Penttinen R, Raekallio J: Fibronectin in early phases of wound healing in children. *Acta Chir Scand* 1981;147:7–13.
190. von der Mark K, Kühl U: Laminin and its receptor. *Biochim Biophys Acta* 1985;823:147–160.
191. Weiss RE, Reddi AH: Appearance of fibronectin during the differentiation of cartilage, bone, and bone marrow. *J Cell Biol* 1981;88:630–636.
192. Weiss RE, Reddi AH: Synthesis and localization of fibronectin during collagenous matrix-mesenchymal cell interaction and differentiation of cartilage and bone in vivo. *Proc Natl Acad Sci USA* 1980;77:2074–2078.

193. Wewer UM, Albrechtsen R, Hassell JR: Heparan sulfate proteoglycans made by different basement-membrane-producing tumors have immunological and structural similarities. *Differentiation* 1985;30:61–67.
194. Williams IF, McCullagh KG, Silver IA: The distribution of types I and III collagen and fibronectin in the healing equine tendon. *Connect Tissue Res* 1984;12:211–227.
195. Yamada KM: Fibronectin and other structural proteins, in Hay ED (ed): *Cell Biology of Extracellular Matrix.* New York, Plenum Press, 1981, pp 95–114.
196. Yamada KM, Akiyama SK, Hasegawa T, et al: Recent advances in research on fibronectin and other cell attachment proteins. *J Cell Biochem* 1985;28:79-97.
197. Yurchenco PD, Ruben GC: Type IV collagen lateral associations in the EHS tumor matrix: Comparison with amniotic and in vitro networks. *Am J Pathol* 1988;132:278–291.
198. Yurchenco PD, Ruben GC: Basement membrane structure in situ: Evidence for lateral associations in the type IV collagen network. *J Cell Biol* 1987;105:2559–2568.

Chapter 4

Models for Use in Studying Sports-Induced Soft-Tissue Inflammation

Sandra Curwin, PhD

Introduction

The study of inflammation encompasses a vast spectrum of tissues and techniques, with many important findings coming from the studies of skin, granulation tissue, and isolated cells. It is not always clear how—or indeed whether—these models are applicable to disorders involving musculoskeletal trauma. Typically, sports-induced soft-tissue inflammation involves load-bearing structures such as tendon, ligament, or muscle. The problem is usually chronic and is thought to be the result of cyclic loading (overuse syndrome). There are also more acute inflammatory situations involving synovial joints, bursae, ligaments (sprains), or muscle (strains). Because the extent of such injuries is difficult to determine in humans, animal models have been developed for a variety of healing situations. Most studies are of acute inflammatory conditions involving skin, tendon, muscle, or ligament. Chronic models have been developed to simulate arthritic conditions, but not the types of soft-tissue injuries commonly observed in sports. Naturally occurring animal models are rare, although tenosynovitis in chickens and tendon injuries in horses seem to be similar to injuries in humans. Tissue and cell culture techniques offer an opportunity to define the research protocol carefully and are, therefore, better suited to the examination of the effects of individual stimuli on healing and tissue physiology than in vivo studies.

This chapter examines models that have been used to address the nature of connective tissue injuries and their healing, discussing the advantages and drawbacks of each. The contribution of models from other systems is also discussed because these studies may contribute to the understanding of sports-related inflammation. The reader is referred to other parts of this volume or to several review articles for the basic concepts of inflammation in wound healing.[61,107,108,131,180]

Models used to study sports injuries can be divided into three categories: clinical models, biochemical and morphologic models, and mechanical models.

Clinical Models

These studies involve identification of problems primarily on the basis of findings such as pain, swelling, and degree of disability.[34,44] This approach has been used for supraspinatus tendinitis,[127,163] patellar tendinitis,[24,130] Achilles tendinitis,[37,62,115,151,155,161,166] tennis elbow,[40,150] and many other disorders.[13,82,110,129,164] Careful history-taking is essential and has led to two important concepts: (1) that most sports-induced inflammation is related to overuse; and (2) that eccentric muscle contraction is often involved in the pathogenesis of these disorders.[45,88,139,173] As discussed in Chapter 39, a variety of diagnostic criteria is used to distinguish tissues at fault and to monitor the severity of the problem. Clearly, clinical studies are pertinent, but they have serious limitations. The main drawback is that the exact nature and extent of the injury cannot be defined and measured accurately because in most cases tissue samples are unobtainable. There are some indications that techniques such as computed tomography,[144] magnetic resonance imaging,[16,25,177] ultrasound,[60,118,128,162,170] thermography,[157] scintigraphy,[101,132] radiography,[42] or blood serum measurements,[4,5,25,26,47,64,83,93,94,105,109,125,148,160,169,177] may be useful in diagnosing soft-tissue problems, but their ability to monitor clinical progression or regression is unknown.

Biochemical and Morphologic Models

If conservative treatment has failed, as may be the case in severe soft-tissue inflammation, surgery may be performed. Many techniques have been used,[24,115] but the basic approach involves excision of excessive scar tissue at the site of injury, followed either by repair of the surgically created defect or by allowing the tissue to heal in a lengthened position. Biochemical and histochemical studies of the excised tissue have revealed degenerative changes in collagen fibrils,[115] increased cellularity,[116] and changes suggestive of necrosis or hypoxia of tissues.[56,120] Findings limited to tendon sheaths or tendons alone have led to classification systems that differentiate between inflammatory and degenerative disorders.[161] These experimental findings were instrumental in formulating the current theory of sports-induced soft-tissue inflammation: that repeated loading leads to microscopic failure of collagen fibrils or bundles, provoking an inflammatory response that causes further tissue breakdown, thus perpetuating the problem. Again, the drawbacks of these studies are that the exact injury cannot be defined clearly and the sequence of events in the development of the abnormality cannot be determined. Further, these injuries, by definition, are atypical, because they have not responded to conservative therapy, and thus may not be entirely representative of more common disorders that do respond to conservative treatment.

Mechanical Models

The main goal of these studies is to estimate forces in soft tissues and compare the calculated values with known tensile strength measurements from isolated tissue specimens[1,17,23,55,143,187] in an effort to determine whether in vivo activities produce potentially damaging forces or stresses. Film and force platform data are collected simultaneously and used to calculate indirect estimates of muscle-tendon force and length.[182] This approach has yielded estimates that tendon forces in activities such as running, jumping, and kicking may approach maximum stress values for mammalian tendon[54] and are thus capable of tissue damage if repeated[194] (Table 1, p 110). Indeed, the filming of a weightlifter at the moment of patellar tendon rupture produced estimates of force that were in the range of 17 times body weight.[205] It is surmised that if such activities are capable of producing complete tendon rupture, which also occurs frequently in the Achilles tendon in badminton, then they are certainly capable of producing lesser injuries. The main question involves the nature of these lesser injuries.

The indirect approach to estimating muscle force necessarily leaves some uncertainty about the accuracy of values obtained. Direct force measurement requires placing a strain gauge transducer directly on the tendon. Strain values are recorded during activities, then later converted to force values using a calibration curve produced by applying known forces to the tendon-transducer system at or before the animal's death. Although this approach has been used frequently in animal studies,[14,79,104,124] only recently have buckle-type transducers been applied to human Achilles tendon and used to measure direct tendon forces during cycling.[78,113] Calibration was achieved with an external force application system.

In Vivo Models

The difficulties inherent in obtaining quantitative data in human subjects have led to the development of many animal models that can be applied to the study of sports-induced soft-tissue inflammation. In these cases, the interest is in the animal model itself because it represents a naturally occurring clinical disorder.

Complete Tissue Transection

The tissue, usually skin, tendon, or ligament, is completely divided and allowed to heal with or without intervention. Transection is most often accomplished by sharp excision with a scalpel, but wire cutting has also been used.[195] It has been suggested that collagen fibrils fail in tension even in these models. Because all tissue components are involved, a classic inflammatory response ensues.[35,70,74,75] Careful description of the incision makes the injury reproducible, an important consideration in experimental design. Such models, especially those used to study skin wound healing, have provided the majority of information currently available about acute inflammation and soft-tissue healing,[38,52,53,69,80,81,147,165,185,191] making them useful for studying the influence of various factors such as surgical repair,[32,35] exercise,[91,179,180,188,189] electrical stimulation,[154] and immobilization[8,9] on healing. Their applicability to chronic inflammation is not known. They are more representative of complete ligament or tendon rupture, and thus are most useful in simulating injuries such as anterior cruciate ligament disruption,[8,111] medial collateral ligament sprain,[76,188,190] or Achilles tendon rupture,[115,116,155] and evaluating therapies commonly used to treat these disorders.[158]

Partial Tissue Laceration

These models usually involve load-bearing structures and use a partial incision through the ligament or tendon. Again, careful anatomic definition is essential to ensure reproducibility. A method of creating reliable partial tendon laceration was described recently, and mechanical testing showed it to be more reliable than hand-produced scalpel cuts.[90]

The advantage of incomplete division is that the tissue is still partially continuous and thus can function in load-bearing. This simulates the clinical situation more closely than complete transection does but is still a model of the acute, rather than the chronic, inflammatory response. This model has been used to examine the effects of electrical stimulation on canine patellar tendon healing[136] and was a technique used for many years to treat equine tendinitis until it was recently shown to be of no benefit.[181]

Mechanical Overstretch

It is well-known that eccentric exercise is associated with muscle soreness, and that muscle "pulls" or strains are common athletic injuries.[34] Recently, models have been developed that simulate these injuries by pulling a muscle-tendon unit until failure, under either passive or stimulated conditions.[66,67,149] In all specimens examined so far, failure occurs through muscle fibers near their attachment to tendon. These models offer a good way of examining these common injuries. Stressing the muscle-tendon unit to less than failure load produces partial injuries.[149] The disadvantage of these models is that surgery is required because the tendon must be exposed and severed from its distal attachment to allow force application and then reattached for healing. This is a departure from the clinical scenario. These models will no doubt be further refined to provide even more realistic simulations of soft-tissue injuries.

Load Alteration

These models are often used in conjunction with complete or partial transection, but there are many new models of increased and decreased load that have not as yet been applied to injured tissues.[22,27,43,45,86,108,114,135,140,153,189,202] Because these models are described at length elsewhere in this volume, they are not discussed here except to say that models of isolated increases in load[43] may prove useful in simulating the load variable involved in sports injuries.

Blunt Trauma

Muscle contusions are also clinically common, and animal models have been developed to study their healing.[7,96] Using a spring-loaded hammer allows a reproducible injury to be delivered to the muscle of choice.[96] Lehto and associates,[120,121] using this model to study rat calf muscle, showed that the initial stages of healing were accompanied by hemorrhage and increased fibronectin levels. This model has also been used to evaluate the effects of dimethyl sulfoxide on healing of muscle injuries[145] and to examine the effects of anti-inflammatory drugs.[85,173]

Needle Puncture

This model is somewhat similar to partial laceration in that a mechanical disruption of a portion of the tissue is produced, in this case by inserting a standard 20-gauge needle.[65] This model is also interesting as a possible means of testing the theory that partial fibril disruption occurs, weakening the tissue and predisposing it to further injury. However, these partial injuries are thought to take place on a microscopic level, and a 20-gauge needle may therefore be too large. Liver biopsy needles,[123] microvascular surgery needles (5 to 50 μ in diameter),[39] or intracellular recording electrodes (0.25 to 0.50 μ in diameter)[93] may be more appropriate tools because collagen fibrils are usually 0.03 to 0.30 μ in diameter.[43,50]

Chemically Produced Injury

These models involve systemic or local chemical application. Systemic steroid injection has been shown to decrease the diameter of collagen fibrils in tendon, and fibril disruption is also evident on ultrastructural examination.[142,203] Direct steroid injection has been used to induce tendon injury.[46,106] Injection of collagenase into equine superficial digital flexor tendons has been used successfully as a model of both acute and chronic tendon inflammations.[181] Because connective tissues contain collagenase[84] and other proteases[156] and the levels of activity of these enzymes are increased after injury, this model seems to be appropriate. The major drawback appears to be that the tendon injury is severe, perhaps indicating that the amount of enzyme may need to be modified. Because the enzyme is injected directly into the tendon via needle puncture, a mechanical insult is also delivered. Again, smaller needles may prove useful.

Enzyme or chemical injection is also used to produce joint and skin inflammation[29] and is frequently used to simulate arthritic conditions.[48,204] These models may be useful in simulating joint sprains and evaluating methods used to treat such sprains.[51] Substances such as collagen or proteoglycans can also be injected into the circulatory system.[92] The latter techniques are used to produce animal models representative of rheumatoid arthritis,[12,92,172,206] and probably produce a response too widespread to be useful for studying sports-induced soft-tissue inflammation,[36] although it is possible that similar factors may be involved in some clinical cases.[12]

Ischemic Injury

It has been suggested that a decreased vascular supply may contribute to some forms of tendinitis. This was initially proposed as an explanation for supraspinatus tendinitis, because the region subject to compression below the acromion showed a decreased blood flow.[127,163] Similar tendinitis in young individuals[152] suggests that anatomic or physiologic features may also play a part. However, it is known that regions of tendon that are subjected to compression alter their biochemical composition, increasing glycosaminoglycan content[58,72] and becoming more cartilaginous in composition, and that this is readily reversible by changing the load on the tendon to a tensile force.[59,72] Because cartilage has a smaller blood supply than other tissues, it may be logical to assume that regions subjected to prolonged compression have a decreased blood supply. Because they lack the synovial environment and diffusion of nutrients that supply articular cartilage, degenerative changes may develop. The ready reversal of tendon composition when the load is changed to tensile may also have some clinical applications in treating tendinitis caused by excessive compression.

These clinical findings suggest that ischemia may play a role in overuse syndromes, perhaps via a mechanism similar to that responsible for compartment syndromes. This possibility has not yet been investigated, although there are reports that such a model is being developed in the horse. Avian flexor tendons deprived of a blood supply demonstrated a decreased healing response to incisional wound healing, but this was under in vitro conditions.[102,103]

Naturally Occurring Animal Models

There are very few naturally occurring animal models that simulate sports-induced soft-tissue inflammations. Such models are extremely useful because they represent a means of carefully examining the progression of a disorder and monitoring the effects of clinical intervention. Two animal models may be useful for studying overuse injuries.

Chicken

Certain broiler breeds of chicken (Cornish Rock) are predisposed to develop degenerative tendon disorders, including tenosynovitis and, occasionally, gastrocnemius tendon rupture.[196] White Leghorn chickens, which have been used in several experimental models,[43,45] are not susceptible. Because tenosynovitis and tendon degeneration are common in athletes,[37,56,71] this model may prove useful. To my knowledge, no such studies have yet been conducted. One disadvantage is that problems develop in only 10% of the poultry, so many animals would be required to carry out an experiment. This model, however, may afford a means of correlating external or serum measurements with the appearance of a soft-tissue disorder, which would be useful in diagnosis and monitoring.

Equine Models

Models of tendinitis in the horse deserve special mention because they probably represent the animal overuse model that most closely simulates the human clinical situation.[56,97,99,181,199–201] Tendinitis in race horses is a significant economic problem, because injuries that affect their racing careers develop in as many as 71% of horses.[99] This problem is being studied from many angles: identification of the clinical problem,[56,71] mechanical analysis,[124] therapeutic intervention,[199] noninvasive measurements,[186] and serum measurements.[181] The continued participation of these animals in racing is highly desirable, leading to comprehensive efforts to identify horses at risk and treat them appropriately. Because only objective data can be used to determine horses at risk for injury, elaborate techniques for assessing performance changes or gait asymmetries have been developed.[98] A recent statement about the operation of one training center serves to illustrate the point[99]:

> Horses in training are watched closely for signs of soreness, heat, and inflammation. Thermography is used to watch for hot joints and tendons. Heart rates during work are carefully considered in a continual effort to tell if a horse is experiencing overwork. Horses are weighed on a regular basis, with a scale which records the weight on each foot. Sometimes early lameness is picked up because a horse stands with less weight on a painful leg. Extensive information on every horse in training is put into the computer to be later analyzed . . .

A massive study on equine tendinitis was carried out by Silver and Rossdale.[181] It involved clinical, mechanical, biochemical, and immunohistologic studies of tendinitis and its treatment and has provided the most detailed information to date about this clinical problem.[56] Unfortunately, horses are expensive and difficult to maintain, so it is unlikely that their use as clinical models of overuse syndromes will become widespread.

In Vitro Models Related to Soft-Tissue Healing

Tissue and cell culture techniques make it possible to define the experimental environment clearly. Knowledge of the presence of many growth factors in serum has led to the development of a low-serum culture condition,[68] affording even greater control. These techniques explain how the effects observed in vivo are achieved.

Table 1 Stresses in tendons during sports activities

Tendon	Activity	Stress (MPa)*
Achilles	Walking	26 to 31
	Slow running	52 to 78
	Fast running	110 to 120
	Jumping	25 to 50
Patellar	Walking	2.5
	Running	37 to 45
	Kicking	26
	Jumping (takeoff)	13
	Jumping (landing)	40
Mammalian	Maximum tensile stress	50 to 100

*Estimated from force values from various sources using estimates of 75 mm^2 for Achilles tendon and 100 mm^2 for patellar tendon.

Tissue Culture

The technique of tissue culture requires the removal of part, or all, of a tissue and its maintenance under controlled conditions of nutrition, hydration, and chemical environment. These techniques have been used with cartilage,[100,174] muscle,[20,73] lung,[18] skin,[38] and tendon.[77,182] The advantage of these models is that the tissue environment can be controlled carefully, allowing manipulation of individual variables and measurement of their effect on tissue metabolism, composition, or mechanical behavior. This approach has yielded information about the effects of growth factors on patellar cartilage,[100] and provided an answer to the long-standing debate about the relative contributions of intrinsic and extrinsic factors in the healing of digital flexor tendons,[77] because healing under tissue culture conditions depends on intrinsic healing. Embryonic chick tendons being cultured have been subjected to cyclic loading to test the effects of load on tendon growth and metabolism.[182] Adult rabbit flexor tendons have been maintained in culture for as long as 42 days after surgical transection and repair to determine the effects of electrical stimulation on tendon healing.[2,146]

Tissue culture is superior to cell culture for studying most sports-related soft-tissue injuries because the extracellular matrix components of the tissue are often of particular interest. The controlled environment lends itself to answering research questions concerning the effects of growth factors, load changes, and nutritional variation. This technique has not been used to date on chronically injured or inflamed musculoskeletal tissues.

Cell Culture

These culture techniques represent the most effective way of determining how environmental change affects the physiology of the cell and have been used on cells from many tissues.[6,11] Factors of interest can be added to the cell culture media and the behavior of the cell monitored, often by measuring the synthesis of a particular protein (such as collagen), or enzyme activity, or mRNA production.[117] Separate culture of fibroblasts from different regions of the same tissue has shown that cells in different areas may have varying synthetic and metabolic capabilities.[167] Similarly, cells from injured and normal tissue show different patterns of activity, which can be useful in delineating the pathologic characteristics of various disorders. These techniques have provided almost all the information currently known about cell regulation,[193] the effects of growth factors on angiogenesis and collagen formation by fibroblasts,[31,63,126,168,184] fibroblast chemotaxis,[3,112,130,138,159,178] exercise activation of macrophages,[28,57,142] macrophage digestion of collagen and proteoglycans,[41,137] the mechanism of action of glucocorticoids,[33] and the effects of vitamin A on collagen production by fibroblasts.[87] This list could be extended greatly. This method has also been applied clinically.[30,171] The use of cell culture as a research model is widespread, and the findings of such experiments are covered in more detail elsewhere in this volume.

Implantation Models

The placement of tubes, sponges, or cages under the skin of animals provokes an inflammatory response.[49,89,119] The implanted structure becomes filled with inflammatory cells and granulation tissue, providing a convenient means of studying the early cellular response to injury.[133,134] It is also a means of collecting inflammatory cells for culture.[49,176] The implants can be removed without harm, allowing animals to be used for more than one experiment. When this method was used in horses and ponies, however, there was considerable variation in response to injury,[19] indicating that even closely related animal species can vary in healing response. Further, the tissue that filled the implants differed from that found in healing wounds,[175] limiting the usefulness of these techniques for studying sports-induced injuries.

This category also includes the transplantation of tissues from one location to another, such as replacing the anterior cruciate ligament with the patellar tendon,[14,111] the use of carbon fibers to repair or replace tendons,[10] or the use of collagen composites as ligament replacements.[197] These studies have provided information about the pattern of ligament and tendon healing in the most adverse clinical situations.[21]

Notes on Methodology and Study Design

It is increasingly clear that studies examining connective tissue physiology and behavior have become more sophisticated in both method and approach. The simple measurement of collagen content or total glycosaminoglycan concentration appears less valuable as studies show that changes in the types—rather than amounts—of collagen or proteoglycan, collagen fibril diameter, or collagen cross-link pattern may be the important results of experimental intervention. Similarly, the method chosen must suit the question being asked. For example, collagen types in tendon cannot be evaluated by standard electrophoresis of collagen chains[122] because of the small amounts of collagen types other than type I; more sophisticated methods must be chosen.[192]

The integrated approach to study design, with biochemical, histochemical, mechanical, and vascular studies combined, yields by far the most information about tissue response, because characteristics are measured rather than inferred. This approach has been used successfully by several groups[8,9,111] and should be encouraged. The addition of parallel clinical studies completes the picture.[181]

References

1. Abrahams M: Mechanical behaviour of tendon in vitro: A preliminary report. *Med Biol Engin* 1967;5:433–443.
2. Akai M, Oda H, Shirasaki Y, et al: Electrical stimulation of ligament healing: An experimental study of the patellar ligament of rabbits. *Clin Orthop* 1988;235:296–301.
3. Albini A, Adelmann-Grill BC: Collagenolytic cleavage products of collagen type I as chemoattractants for human dermal fibroblasts. *Eur J Cell Biol* 1985;36:104–107.
4. Alén M, Pakarinen A, Häkkinen K, et al: Responses of serum androgenic-anabolic and catabolic hormones to prolonged strength training. *Int J Sports Med* 1988;9:229–233.
5. Alén M, Rahkila P, Reinilä M, et al: Androgenic-anabolic steroid effects on serum thyroid, pituitary and steroid hormones in athletes. *Am J Sports Med* 1987;15:357–361.
6. Allen RE: Muscle cell culture as a tool in animal growth research. *Fed Proc* 1987;46:290–294.
7. Almekinders LC, Gilbert JA: Healing of experimental muscle strains and the effects of nonsteroidal antiinflammatory medication. *Am J Sports Med* 1986;14:303–308.
8. Amiel D, Kleiner JB: Biochemistry of ligament and tendon, in Nimni ME (ed): *Collagen: Biochemistry, Biomechanics, Biotechnology*. Boca Raton, CRC Press, 1988, vol 3, pp 224–251.
9. Amiel D, Woo SL, Harwood FL, et al: The effect of immobilization on collagen turnover in connective tissue: A biochemical-biomechanical correlation. *Acta Orthop Scand* 1982;53:325–332.
10. Amis AA, Campbell JR, Miller JH: Strength of carbon and polyester fibre tendon replacements: Variation after operation in rabbits. *J Bone Joint Surg* 1985;67B:829–834.
11. Andrews FJ, Morris CJ, Lewis EJ, et al: Effect of nutritional iron deficiency on acute and chronic inflammation. *Ann Rheum Dis* 1987;46:859–865.
12. Archer JR, Winrow VR, McLean IL: The role of HLA-B27 in arthritis. *Br J Rheumatol* 1988;27:306–309.
13. Armstrong TJ, Fine LJ, Goldstein SA, et al: Ergonomics considerations in hand and wrist tendinitis. *J Hand Surg* 1987;12A:830–837.
14. Arnoczky SP, Tarvin GB, Marshall JL: Anterior cruciate ligament replacement using patellar tendon: An evaluation of graft revascularization in the dog. *J Bone Joint Surg* 1982;64A:217–224.
15. Barnes GRG, Pinder DN: *In vivo* tendon tension and bone strain measurement and correlation. *J Biomech* 1974;7:35–42.
16. Beltran J, Noto AM, Herman LJ, et al: Tendons: High-field-strength, surface coil MR imaging. *Radiology* 1987;162:735–740.
17. Benedict JV, Walker LB, Harris EH: Stress-strain characteristics and tensile strength of unembalmed human tendon. *J Biomech* 1968;1:53–63.

18. Berg RA, Schwartz ML, Rome LH, et al: Lysosomal function in the degradation of defective collagen in cultured lung fibroblasts. *Biochemistry* 1984;23:2134–2138.
19. Bertone AL, Sullins KE, Stashak TS, et al: Effect of wound location and the use of topical collagen gel on exuberant granulation tissue formation and wound healing in the horse and pony. *Am J Vet Res* 1985;46:1438–1444.
20. Betz EH, Firket H, Reznik M: Some aspects of muscle regeneration. *Int Rev Cytol* 1966;19:203–227.
21. Birch JR, Lindsay WK: Histochemical studies of the fate of autologous digital flexor tendon grafts in the chicken. *Can J Surg* 1964;7:454–462.
22. Blanchard O, Cohen-Solal L, Tardieu C, et al: Tendon adaptation to different long term stresses and collagen reticulation in soleus muscle. *Connect Tissue Res* 1985;13:261–267.
23. Blanton PL, Biggs NL: Ultimate tensile strength of fetal and adult human tendons. *J Biomech* 1970;3:181–189.
24. Blazina ME, Kerlan RK, Jobe FW, et al: Jumper's knee. *Orthop Clin North Am* 1973;4:665–678.
25. Bodne D, Quinn SF, Murray WT, et al: Magnetic resonance images of chronic patellar tendinitis. *Skeletal Radiol* 1988;17:24–28.
26. Bonen A, Keizer HA: Pituitary, ovarian, and adrenal hormone responses to marathon running. *Int J Sports Med* 1987;8(suppl 3):161–167.
27. Booth FW, Gould EW: Effects of training and disuse on connective tissue. *Exerc Sport Sci Rev* 1975;3:83–107.
28. Bosenberg AT, Brock-Utne JG, Gaffin SL, et al: Strenuous exercise causes systemic endotoxemia. *J Appl Physiol* 1988;65:106–108.
29. Bouclier M, Luginbuhl B, Delamadeleine F, et al: Repeated application of arachidonic acid to the ear of mice: A model of chronic skin inflammation? *Agents Actions* 1989;26:227–228.
30. Brody GA, Eisinger M, Arnoczky SP, et al: In vitro fibroblast seeding of prosthetic anterior cruciate ligaments: A preliminary study. *Am J Sports Med* 1988;16:203–208.
31. Bronson RE, Bertolami CN, Siebert EP: Modulation of fibroblast growth and glycosaminoglycan synthesis by interleukin-1. *Coll Relat Res* 1987;7:323–332.
32. Brown TD, Fu FH, Hanley EN Jr: Comparative assessment of the early mechanical integrity of repaired tendon Achillis ruptures in the rabbit. *J Trauma* 1981;21:951–957.
33. Brune K: Ten years research on inflammation revisited. *Agents Action* 1989;26:4-8.
34. Burry HC: Soft tissue injury in sport. *Exerc Sport Sci Rev* 1975;3:275–298.
35. Carlstedt CA: Mechanical and chemical factors in tendon healing: Effects of indomethacin and surgery in the rabbit. *Acta Orthop Scand* 1987;224(suppl):1–75.
36. Cavender D, Haskard D, Yu CL, et al: Pathways to chronic inflammation in rheumatoid synovitis. *Fed Proc* 1987;46:113–117.
37. Clancy WG Jr, Neidhart D, Brand RL: Achilles tendonitis in runners: A report of five cases. *Am J Sports Med* 1976;4:46–57.
38. Clark RAF: Overview and general considerations of wound repair, in Clark RAF, Henson PM (eds): *The Molecular and Cellular Biology of Wound Repair*. New York, Plenum Press, 1988, pp 3–34.
39. Cook AF, Grossman JAI, Herpy ES, et al: The correlation of histology to needle type in microvascular anastomoses: A quantitative analysis. *Br J Plast Surg* 1982;35:156–157.
40. Coonrad RW, Hooper WR: Tennis elbow: Its course, natural history, conservative and surgical management. *J Bone Joint Surg* 1973;55A:1177–1182.

41. Couchman JR, Höök M: Proteoglycans and wound repair, in Clark RAF, Henson PM (eds): *The Molecular and Cellular Biology of Wound Repair.* New York, Plenum Press, 1988, pp 437–470.
42. Crass JR: Current concepts in the radiographic evaluation of the rotator cuff. *CRC Crit Rev Diagn Imaging* 1988;28:23–73.
43. Curwin SL: *The Effect of Increased Mechanial Load on Growing Tendon,* thesis, Los Angeles, 1988.
44. Curwin S, Stanish WD: *Tendinitis: Its Etiology and Treatment.* Lexington, Mass, Collamore Press, 1984.
45. Curwin SL, Vailas AC, Wood J: Immature tendon adaptation to strenuous exercise. *J Appl Physiol* 1988;65:2297–2301.
46. DaCruz DJ, Geeson M, Allen MJ, et al: Achilles paratendonitis: An evaluation of steroid injection. *Br J Sports Med* 1988;22:64–65.
47. Davis JM, Pate RR, Burgess WA, et al: Stress hormone response to exercise in elite female distance runners. *Int J Sports Med* 1987;8(suppl 2):132–135.
48. De Brito FB, Corry DG, Moore AR, et al: Polyarthritis and the air pouch reaction: Dissimilarity of adjuvant and collagen models. *Immunopharmacology* 1988;15:123–130.
49. Diegelmann RF, Kim JC, Lindblad WJ, et al: Collection of leukocytes, fibroblasts, and collagen within an implantable reservoir tube during tissue repair. *J Leukocyte Biol* 1987;42:667–672.
50. Doillon CJ, Dunn MG, Bender E, et al: Collagen fiber formation in repair tissue: Development of strength and toughness. *Coll Relat Res* 1985;5:481–492.
51. Dupont M, Béliveau P, Thériault G: The efficacy of antiinflammatory medication in the treatment of the acutely sprained ankle. *Am J Sports Med* 1987;15:41–45.
52. Ehrlich HP: Wound closure: Evidence of cooperation between fibroblasts and collagen matrix. *Eye* 1988;2:149–157.
53. Ehrlich HP: The role of connective tissue matrix in wound healing. *Prog Clin Biol Res* 1988;266:243–258.
54. Elliott DH: Structure and function of mammalian tendon. *Biol Rev* 1965;40:392–421.
55. Evans JH, Barbenel JC: Structural and mechanical properties of tendon related to function. *Equine Vet J* 1975;7:1–8.
56. Fackelman GE: The nature of tendon damage and its repair. *Equine Vet J* 1973;5:141–149.
57. Fehr HG, Lötzerich H, Michna H: The influence of physical exercise on peritoneal macrophage functions: Histochemical and phagocytic studies. *Int J Sports Med* 1988;9:77–81.
58. Flint MH, Gillard GC, Merrilees MJ: The effects of local physical environmental factors on connective tissue organization and glycosaminoglycan synthesis, in Parry D (ed): *Fibrous Proteins: Scientific, Industrial and Medical Aspects.* New York, Academic Press, 1980, pp 107–119.
59. Flint MH, Reilly HC: The effects of tensional forces on experimental wound healing: A biochemical study, abstract. *Connect Tissue Res* 1982;9:206.
60. Fornage BD, Rifkin MD: Ultrasound examination of tendons. *Radiol Clin North Am* 1988;26:87–107.
61. Forrest L: Current concepts in soft connective tissue wound healing. *Br J Surg* 1983;70:133–140.
62. Fox JM, Blazina ME, Jobe FW, et al: Degeneration and rupture of the Achilles tendon. *Clin Orthop* 1975;107:221–224.

63. Franchimont P, Reuter A, Vrindts-Gevaert Y, et al: Production of tumour necrosis factor-alpha, interferon, and interleukin-2 by peripheral blood mononuclear cells of subjects suffering from rheumatoid arthritis. *Scand J Rheumatol* 1988;17:203–212.
64. Friden J, Sfakianos PN, Hargens AR: Blood indices of muscle injury associated with eccentric muscle contractions. *J Orthop Res* 1989;7:142–145.
65. Frieder S, Weisberg J, Fleming B, et al: A pilot study: The therapeutic effect of ultrasound following partial rupture of Achilles tendons in male rats. *J Orthop Sports Phys Ther* 1988;10:39–46.
66. Garrett WE Jr, Safran MR, Seaber AV, et al: Biomechanical comparison of stimulated and nonstimulated skeletal muscle pulled to failure. *Am J Sports Med* 1987;15:448–454.
67. Garrett WE Jr, Tidball J: Myotendinous junction: Structure, function, and failure, in Woo SL-Y, Buckwalter JA (eds): *Injury and Repair of the Musculoskeletal Soft Tissues.* Park Ridge, Ill, American Academy of Orthopaedic Surgeons, 1988, pp 171–207.
68. Gauger A, Robertson C, Greenlee TK Jr, et al: A low-serum medium for tendon cells: Effects of growth factors on tendon cell growth and collagen production. *In Vitro Cell Dev Biol* 1985;21:291–296.
69. Gay S, Vijanto J, Raekallio J, et al: Collagen types in early phases of wound healing in children. *Acta Chir Scand* 1978;144:205–211.
70. Gelberman RH, Manske PR, Akeson WH, et al: Flexor tendon repair. *J Orthop Res* 1986;4:119–128.
71. Genovese RL, Simpson BS: Sports injuries: Tendon and ligament injuries, in Jones WE, et al (eds): *Equine Sports Medicine.* Philadelphia, Lea & Febiger, 1989, pp 241–248.
72. Gillard GC, Reilly HC, Bell-Booth PG, et al: The influence of mechanical forces on the glycosaminoglycan content of the rabbit flexor digitorum profundus tendon. *Connect Tissue Res* 1979;7:37–46.
73. Godman GC: On the regeneration and redifferentiation of mammalian striated muscle. *J Morphol* 1957;100:27–81.
74. Goldin B, Block WD, Pearson JR: Wound healing of tendon: I. Physical, mechanical and metabolic changes. *J Biomech* 1980;13:241–256.
75. Goldin B, Block WD, Pearson JR: Wound healing of tendon: II. A mathematical model. *J Biomech* 1980;13:257–264.
76. Gomez MA, Woo SL-Y, Inoue M, et al: Medial collateral ligament healing subsequent to different treatment regimens. *J Appl Physiol* 1989;66:245–252.
77. Graham MF, Becker H, Cohen IK, et al: Intrinsic tendon fibroplasia: Documentation by in vitro studies. *J Orthop Res* 1984;1:251–256.
78. Gregor RJ, Komi PV, Järvinen M: Achilles tendon forces during cycling. *Int J Sports Med* 1987;8(suppl 1):9–14.
79. Gregor RJ, Roy RR, Whiting WC, et al: Mechanical output of the cat soleus during treadmill locomotion: In vivo vs in situ characteristics. *J Biomech* 1988;21:721–732.
80. Grinnell F: Fibronectin and wound healing. *J Cell Biochem* 1984;26:107–116.
81. Grinnell F, Billingham RE, Burgess L: Distribution of fibronectin during wound healing *in vivo*. *J Invest Dermatol* 1981;76:181–189.
82. Hagberg M, Stenberg B, Sundelin G: The use of sign language as an aggravating factor in shoulder tendinitis: A case history of a deaf-mute cleaner. *J Hum Ergol (Tokyo)* 1987;16:173–178.
83. Hällgren R, Feltelius N, Lindh U: Redistribution of minerals and trace elements in chronic inflammation: A study on isolated blood cells from patients with ankylosing spondylitis. *J Rheumatol* 1987;14:548–553.

84. Harper J, Amiel D, Harper E: Collagenase production by rabbit ligaments and tendon. *Connect Tissue Res* 1988;17:253–259.
85. Heere LP: Piroxicam in acute musculoskeletal disorders and sports injuries. *Am J Med* 1988;84:50–55.
86. Heikkinen E, Vuori I: Effect of physical activity on the connective tissue metabolism in mice. *Scand J Clin Lab Invest* 1979;113(suppl):36–41.
87. Hein R, Mensing H, Müller PK, et al: Effect of vitamin A and its derivatives on collagen production and chemotactic response of fibroblasts. *Br J Dermatol* 1984;111:37–44.
88. Henke P: The painful tendon: A pathophysiological approach. *Aust Fam Physician* 1987;16:772–776.
89. Higgins AJ, Lees P, Sedgwick AD: Development of equine models of inflammation: The Ciba-Geigy Prize for Research in Animal Health. *Vet Rec* 1987;120:517–522.
90. Hitchcock TF, Candel AG, Light TR, et al: New technique for producing uniform partial lacerations of tendons. *J Orthop Res* 1989;7:451–455.
91. Hitchcock TF, Light TR, Bunch WH, et al: The effect of immediate constrained digital motion on the strength of flexor tendon repairs in chickens. *J Hand Surg* 1987;12A:590–595.
92. Hom JT, Bendele AM, Carlson DG: In vivo administration with IL-1 accelerates the development of collagen-induced arthritis in mice. *J Immunol* 1988;141:834–841.
93. Horikawa K, Armstrong WE: A versatile means of intracellular labeling: Injection of biocytin and its detection with avidin conjugates. *J Neurosci Methods* 1988;25:1–11.
94. Hørslev-Petersen K, Bentsen KD, Engström-Laurent A, et al: Serum amino terminal type III procollagen peptide and serum hyaluronan in arthritis: Relation to clinical and serological parameters of inflammation during 8 and 24 months' treatment with levamisole, penicillamine, or azathioprine. *Ann Rheum Dis* 1988;47:116–126.
95. Horswill CA, Layman DK, Boileau RA, et al: Excretion of 3-methylhistidine and hydroxyproline following acute weight-training exercise. *Int J Sports Med* 1988;9:245–248.
96. Järvinen M, Sorvari T: Healing of a crush injury in rat striated muscle: 1. Description and testing of a new method of inducing a standard injury to the calf muscle. *Acta Pathol Microbiol Scand* [A] 1975;83:259–265.
97. Jones WE: Equine athletic injuries. *Equine Sports Med News* 1988;7:49–50.
98. Jones WE: Putting it all together. *Equine Sports Med News* 1988;7:161–162.
99. Jones WE: Who is responsible for lameness? *Equine Sports Med News* 1988;7:177–178.
100. Joosten LAB, Schalkwijk J, van den Berg WB, et al: Chondrocyte unresponsiveness to insulin-like growth factor-1: A novel pathogenetic mechanism for cartilage destruction in experimental arthritis. *Agents Actions* 1989;26:193–195.
101. Kahn D, Wilson MA: Bone scintigraphic findings in patellar tendonitis. *J Nucl Med* 1987;28:1768–1770.
102. Kain CC, Russell JE, Burri R, et al: The effect of vascularization on avian flexor tendon repair: A biochemical study. *Clin Orthop* 1988;233:295–303.
103. Kain CC, Russell JE, Rouse AM, et al: Regional differences in matrix formation in the healing flexor tendon. *Clin Orthop* 1988;229:308–312.
104. Kear M, Smith RN: A method for recording tendon strain in sheep during locomotion. *Acta Orthop Scand* 1975;46:896–905.
105. Keizer HA, Kuipers H, de Haan J, et al: Multiple hormonal responses to physical exercise in eumenorrheic trained and untrained women. *Int J Sports Med* 1987;8(suppl 3):139–150.

106. Kennedy JC, Willis RB: The effects of local steroid injections on tendons: A biomechanical and microscopic correlative study. *Am J Sports Med* 1976;4:11–21.
107. Ketchum LD: Primary tendon healing: A review. *J Hand Surg* 1977;2:428–435.
108. Kiiskinen A: Physical training and connective tissues in young mice: Physical properties of Achilles tendons and long bones. *Growth* 1977;41:123–137.
109. Kjaer M: Epinephrine and some other hormonal responses to exercise in man: With special reference to physical training. *Int J Sports Med* 1989;10:2–15.
110. Kleiger B: The posterior calcaneal tubercule impingement syndrome. *Orthop Rev* 1988;17:487–493.
111. Kleiner JB, Amiel D, Harwood FL, et al: Early histologic, metabolic, and vascular assessment of anterior cruciate ligament autografts. *J Orthop Res* 1989;7:235–242.
112. Kleinman HK, Wilkes CM, Martin GR: Interaction of fibronectin with collagen fibrils. *Biochemistry* 1981;20:2325–2330.
113. Komi PV, Salonen M, Järvinen M, et al: In vivo registration of Achilles tendon forces in man: I. Methodological development. *Int J Sports Med* 1987;8(suppl 1):3–8.
114. Kovanen V, Suominen H, Heikkinen E: Mechanical properties of fast and slow skeletal muscle with special reference to collagen and endurance training. *J Biomech* 1984;17:725–735.
115. Kvist M, Józsa L, Järvinen MJ, et al: Chronic Achilles paratenonitis in athletes: A histological and histochemical study. *Pathology* 1987;19:1–11.
116. Kvist MH, Lehto MUK, Jozsa L, et al: Chronic Achilles paratenonitis: An immunohistologic study of fibronectin and fibrinogen. *Am J Sports Med* 1988;16:616–623.
117. La Fleur M, Beaulieu AD, Kreis C, et al: Fibronectin gene expression in polymorphonuclear leukocytes: Accumulation of mRNA in inflammatory cells. *J Biol Chem* 1987;262:2111–2115.
118. Laine HR, Harjula AL, Peltokallio P: Ultrasonography as a differential diagnostic aid in achillodynia. *J Ultrasound Med* 1987;6:351–362.
119. Lees P, Higgins AJ, Sedgwick AD, et al: Applications of equine models of acute inflammation: The Ciba-Geigy Prize for Research in Animal Health. *Vet Rec* 1987;120:522–529.
120. Lehto M, Duance VC, Restall D: Collagen and fibronectin in a healing skeletal muscle injury: An immunohistological study of the effects of physical activity on the repair of injured gastrocnemius muscle in the rat. *J Bone Joint Surg* 1985;67B:820–828.
121. Lehto M, Sims TJ, Bailey AJ: Skeletal muscle injury: Molecular changes in the collagen during healing. *Res Exp Med* 1985;185:95–106.
122. Light ND: Estimation of types I and III collagens in whole tissue by quantitation of CNBr peptides on SDS-polyacrylamide gels. *Biochim Biophys Acta* 1982;702:30–36.
123. Lin BP, Chu JM, Rose RA: Ultrasound-guided fine needle aspiration biopsy of the liver. *Pathology* 1987;19:173–177.
124. Lochner FK, Milne DW, Mills EJ, et al: In vivo and in vitro measurement of tendon strain in the horse. *Am J Vet Res* 1980;41:1929–1937.
125. Lohmander S: Proteoglycans of joint cartilage: Structure, function, turnover and role as markers of joint disease. *Baillieres Clin Rheumatol* 1988;2:37–62.
126. Lucas PA, Caplan AI: Chemotactic response of embryonic limb bud mesenchymal cells and muscle-derived fibroblasts to transforming growth factor-β. *Connect Tissue Res* 1988;18:1–7.

127. Macnab I: Rotator cuff tendinitis. *Ann R Coll Surg Engl* 1973;53:271–287.
128. Maffulli N, Regine R, Angelillo M, et al: Ultrasound diagnosis of Achilles tendon pathology in runners. *Br J Sports Med* 1987;21:158–162.
129. Martens MA, Hansen L, Mulier JC: Adductor tendinitis and musculus rectus abdominis tendopathy. *Am J Sports Med* 1987;15:353–356.
130. Martens M, Wouters P, Burssens A, et al: Patellar tendinitis: Pathology and results of treatment. *Acta Orthop Scand* 1982;53:445–450.
131. Martinez IR Jr: Wound healing: Ultrastructural aspects. *Clin Dermatol* 1987;5:37–56.
132. Matin P: Basic principles of nuclear medicine techniques for detection and evaluation of trauma and sports medicine injuries. *Semin Nucl Med* 1988;18:90–112.
133. May SA, Hooke RE, Lees P: Identification of a connective tissue degrading enzyme in bovine inflammatory exudate. *Res Vet Sci* 1988;45:259–261.
134. May SA, Lees P, Higgins AJ, et al: Inflammation: A clinical perspective. The Ciba-Geigy Prize for Research in Animal Health. *Vet Rec* 1987;120:514–517.
135. McGaw WT: The effect of tension on collagen remodelling by fibroblasts: A stereological ultrastructural study. *Connect Tissue Res* 1986;14:229–235.
136. McGillivary GR, Stanish WD: The effects of electrical stimulation on tendon healing. *Orthop Trans* 1984;8:65.
137. McGowan SE, Thompson RJ: Extracellular matrix proteoglycan degradation by human alveolar macrophages and neutrophils. *J Appl Physiol* 1989;66:400–409.
138. Mensing H, Pontz BF, Müller PK, et al: A study on fibroblast chemotaxis using fibronectin and conditioned medium as chemoattractants. *Eur J Cell Biol* 1983;29:268–273.
139. Messier SP, Pittala KA: Etiologic factors associated with selected running injuries. *Med Sci Sports Exerc* 1988;20:501-505.
140. Michna H: Morphometric analysis of loading-induced changes in collagen-fibril populations in young tendons. *Cell Tissue Res* 1984;236:465–470.
141. Michna H: The human macrophage system: Activity and functional morphology. *Bibl Anat* 1988;31:1–84.
142. Michna H: Tendon injuries induced by exercise and anabolic steroids in experimental mice. *Int Orthop* 1987;11:157–162.
143. Mohan D, Melvin JW: Failure properties of passive human aortic tissue: II. Biaxial tension tests. *J Biomech* 1983;16:31–44.
144. Mourad K, King J, Guggiana P: Computed tomography and ultrasound imaging of jumper's knee-patellar tendinitis. *Clin Radiol* 1988;39:162–165.
145. Myrer JW, Heckmann R, Francis RS: Topically applied dimethyl sulfoxide: Its effects on inflammation and healing of a contusion. *Am J Sports Med* 1986;14:165–169.
146. Nessler JP, Mass DP: Direct-current electrical stimulation of tendon healing in vitro. *Clin Orthop* 1987;217:303–312.
147. Nicoletis C, Bazin S, Lous ML: Clinical and biochemical features of normal, defective, and pathologic scars. *Clin Plast Surg* 1977;4:347–359.
148. Niebauer GW, Wolf B, Yarmush M, et al: Evaluation of immune complexes and collagen type-specific antibodies in sera and synovial fluids of horses with secondary osteoarthritis. *Am J Vet Res* 1988;49:1223–1227.
149. Nikolaou PK, Macdonald BL, Glisson RR, et al: Biomechanical and histological evaluation of muscle after controlled strain injury. *Am J Sports Med* 1987;15:9–14.
150. Nirschl RP: Prevention and treatment of elbow and shoulder injuries in the tennis player. *Clin Sports Med* 1988;7:289–308.
151. Nolla Sole JM, Juanola Roura X, Valverde Garcia J, et al: Isolated HLA-B27 cross reactive group (CREG) associated Achilles tendinitis, letter. *Ann Rheum Dis* 1988;47:615.

152. Nutton RW, Stothard J: Acute calcific supraspinatus tendinitis in a three-year-old child. *J Bone Joint Surg* 1987;69B:148.
153. Oakes BW, Parker AW, Norman J: Changes in collagen fiber populations in young rat cruciate ligaments in response to a one-month intensive exercise program, abstract. *Connect Tissue Res* 1982;9:212.
154. Owoeye I, Spielholz NI, Fetto J, et al: Low-intensity pulsed galvanic current and the healing of tenotomized rat Achilles tendons: Preliminary report using load-to-breaking measurements. *Arch Phys Med Rehabil* 1987;68:415–418.
155. Perugia L, Ippolitio E, Postacchini F: A new approach to the pathology, clinical features and treatment of stress tendinopathy of the Achilles tendon. *Ital J Orthop Traumatol* 1976;2:5–21.
156. Piening C, Riederer-Henderson MA: Neutral metalloprotease from tendons. *J Orthop Res* 1989;7:228–234.
157. Pochaczevsky R: Thermography in posttraumatic pain. *Am J Sports Med* 1987;15:243–250.
158. Porat S, Nyska M, Sofer B, et al: Increased collagenolytic activity in severed and sutured tendons following topical application of exogenous collagen in chickens. *J Orthop Res* 1985;3:43–48.
159. Postlethwaite AE, Seyer JM, Kang AH: Chemotactic attraction of human fibroblasts to type I, II, and III collagens and collagen-derived peptides. *Proc Natl Acad Sci USA* 1978;75:871–875.
160. Pountain GD, Keegan AL, Jayson MI: Impaired fibrinolytic activity in defined chronic back pain syndromes. *Spine* 1987;12:83–86.
161. Puddu G, Ippolito E, Postacchini F: A classification of Achilles tendon disease. *Am J Sports Med* 1976;4:145–150.
162. Rantanen NW, Gaines RD: The use of diagnostic ultrasound to detect structural damage to the soft tissues of the extremities of horses. *J Equine Vet Sci* 1983;13:134–135.
163. Rathbun JB, Macnab I: The microvascular pattern of the rotator cuff. *J Bone Joint Surg* 1970;52B:540–553.
164. Ray JM, Clancy WG Jr, Lemon RA: Semimembranosus tendinitis: An overlooked cause of medial knee pain. *Am J Sports Med* 1988;16:347–351.
165. Reid T, Flint MH: Changes in glycosaminoglycan content of healing rabbit tendon. *J Embryol Exp Morphol* 1974;31:489–495.
166. Riddle DL, Freeman DB: Management of a patient with a diagnosis of bilateral plantar fasciitis and Achilles tendinitis: A case report. *Phys Ther* 1988;68:1913–1916.
167. Riederer-Henderson MA, Gauger A, Olson L, et al: Attachment and extracellular matrix differences between tendon and synovial fibroblastic cells. *In Vitro* 1983;19:127–133.
168. Roberts AB, Sporn MB, Assoian RK, et al: Transforming growth factor type β: Rapid induction of fibrosis and angiogenesis in vivo and stimulation of collagen formation in vitro. *Proc Natl Acad Sci USA* 1986;83:4167–4171.
169. Roddie ME, Peters AM, Danpure HJ, et al: Inflammation: Imaging with Tc-99m HMPAO-labeled leukocytes. *Radiology* 1988;166:767–772.
170. Rubin CT, Pratt GW, Porter AL, et al: The use of ultrasound in vivo to determine acute change in the mechanical properties of bone following intense physical activity. *J Biomech* 1987;20:723-727.
171. Rubin K, Terracio L, Rönnstrand L, et al: Expression of platelet-derived growth factor receptors is induced on connective tissue cells during chronic synovial inflammation. *Scand J Immunol* 1988;27:285–294.
172. Sakata T, Scudamore RA, Cooke TD: Antigen-induced tenosynovitis in hypersensitized rabbits: A model for rheumatoid tenosynovitis. *Rheumatol Int* 1988;8:47–53.

173. Salminen A, Kihlström M: Protective effect of indomethacin against exercise-induced injuries in mouse skeletal muscle fibers. *Int J Sports Med* 1987;8:46–49.
174. Schalkwijk J, van den Berg WB, van de Putte LB, et al: An experimental model for hydrogen peroxide induced tissue damage: Effect on cartilage and other articular tissues. *Int J Tissue React* 1987;9:39–43.
175. Schreuders PD, Salthouse TN, von Recum AF: Normal wound healing compared to healing within porous Dacron implants. *J Biomed Mater Res* 1988;22:121–135.
176. Sedgwick AD, Lees P, Dawson J, et al: Cellular aspects of inflammation: The Ciba-Geigy Prize for Research in Animal Health. *Vet Rec* 1987;120:529–536.
177. Seeger LL, Gold RH, Bassett LW, et al: Shoulder impingement syndrome: MR findings in 53 shoulders. *AJR* 1988;150:343–347.
178. Seppä HE, Yamada KM, Seppä ST, et al: The cell binding fragment of fibronectin is chemotactic for fibroblasts. *Cell Biol Int Rep* 1981;5:813–819.
179. Seyfer AE, Bolger WE: Effects of unrestricted motion on healing: A study of posttraumatic adhesions in primate tendons. *Plast Reconstr Surg* 1989;83:122–128.
180. Shoshan S: Wound healing. *Int Rev Connect Tissue Res* 1981;9:1–26.
181. Silver IA, Rossdale PD: A clinical and experimental study of tendon injury, healing and treatment in the horse. *Equine Vet J* 1983;(suppl 1):1–43.
182. Slack C, Flint MH, Thompson BM: The effect of tensional load on isolated embryonic chicken tendons in organ culture. *Connect Tissue Res* 1984;12:229–247.
183. Smith AJ: Estimates of muscle and joint forces at the knee and ankle during a jumping activity. *J Hum Mvt Studies* 1975;1:78–86.
184. Sporn MB, Roberts AB: Peptide growth factors: Current status and therapeutic opportunities. *Important Adv Oncol* 1987;75–86.
185. Stein LE, Pijanowski GJ, Johnson AL: Collagen types in healing rabbit tendons: A biochemical assessment. *Vet Surg* 1985;14:149–152.
186. Strömberg B: Morphologic, thermographic and ^{133}Xe clearance studies on normal and diseased superficial digital flexor tendons in race horses. *Equine Vet J* 1973;5:156–161.
187. Svendsen KH, Thomson G: A new clamping and stretching procedure for determination of collagen fiber stiffness and strength relations upon maturation. *J Biomech* 1984;17:225–229.
188. Tipton CM, Tcheng T-K, Mergner W: Ligamentous strength measurements from hypophysectomized rats. *Am J Physiol* 1971;221:1144–1150.
189. Vailas AC, Deluna DM, Lewis LL, et al: Adaptation of bone and tendon to prolonged hindlimb suspension in rats. *J Appl Physiol* 1988;65:373–376.
190. Vailas AC, Tipton CM, Matthes RD, et al: Physical activity and its influence on the repair process of medial collateral ligaments. *Connect Tissue Res* 1981;9:25–31.
191. Viljanto J, Penttinen R, Raekallio J: Fibronectin in early phases of wound healing in children. *Acta Chir Scand* 1981;147:7–13.
192. von der Mark K: Localization of collagen types in tissues. *Int Rev Connect Tissue Res* 1981;9:265–324.
193. Wahl SM, Wahl LM: Regulation of macrophage collagenase, prostaglandin, and fibroblast-activating-factor production by anti-inflammatory agents: Different regulatory mechanisms for tissue injury and repair. *Cell Immunol* 1985;92:302-312.
194. Wahrenberg H, Lindbeck L, Ekholm J: Knee muscular moment, tendon tension force and EMG during a vigorous movement in man. *Scand J Rehabil Med* 1978;10:99–106.

195. Walsh S, Frank C: Two methods of ligament injury: A morphological comparison in a rabbit model. *J Surg Res* 1988;45:159–166.
196. Walsum JV, Vertommen MH, Laan AVD: Contribution to the aetiology of synovitis in chickens, with special reference to non-infective factors. *V Vet Q* 1981;3:111–117.
197. Wasserman AJ, Doillon CJ, Glasgold AI, et al: Clinical applications of electron microscopy in the analysis of collagenous biomaterials. *Scanning Microsc* 1988;2:1635–1646.
198. Watkins JP, Auer JA, Gau S, et al: Healing of surgically created defects in the equine superficial digital flexor tendon: Collagen-type transformation and tissue morphologic reorganization. *Am J Vet Res* 1985;46:2091–2096.
199. Watkins JP, Auer JA, Morgan SJ, et al: Healing of surgically created defects in the equine superficial digital flexor tendon: Effects of pulsing electromagnetic field therapy on collagen-type transformation and tissue morphologic reorganization. *Am J Vet Res* 1985;46:2097–2103.
200. Webbon PM: Equine tendon stress injuries. *Equine Vet J* 1973;5:58–64.
201. William IF, McCullagh KG, Silver IA: The distribution of types I and III collagen and fibronectin in the healing equine tendon. *Connect Tissue Res* 1984;12:211–227.
202. Wong TS, Booth FW: Skeletal muscle enlargement with weight-lifting exercise by rats. *J Appl Physiol* 1988;65:950–954.
203. Wood TO, Cooke PH, Goodship AE: The effect of exercise and anabolic steroids on the mechanical properties and crimp morphology of the rat tendon. *Am J Sports Med* 1988;16:153–158.
204. Yoo TJ, Kim S-Y, Stuart JM, et al: Induction of arthritis in monkeys by immunization with type II collagen. *J Exp Med* 1988;168:777–782.
205. Zernicke RF, Garhammer J, Jobe FW: Human patellar-tendon rupture. *J Bone Joint Surg* 1977;59A:179–183.
206. Zvaifler NJ: New perspectives on the pathogenesis of rheumatoid arthritis. *Am J Med* 1988;85(suppl 4A):12–17.

Section Two

Pathophysiologic Mechanisms

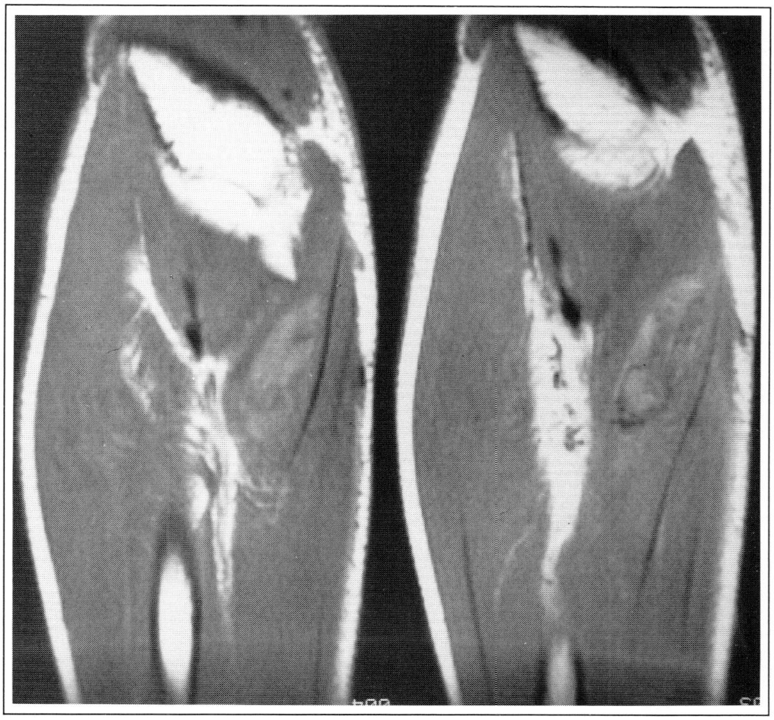

Group Leader

Joseph Buckwalter, MD

Group Participants

Steven Arnoczky, DVM
William Arnold, MD
Louis Bigliani, MD
Walton Curl, MD
David Eyre, PhD
Gerald Finerman, MD
Freddie Fu, MD
William Garrett, Jr, MD, PhD
Kenneth Hargreaves, DDS, PhD
Van Mow, PhD
Walter Newman, PhD
James Nicholas, MD
Stephen O'Brien, MD
Mark Rodosky, MD
David Schurman, MD
William Stauber, PhD
Lawrence Tkach, MD
W. Michael Walsh, MD
Peter Ward, MD
Savio Woo, PhD

Overview

Participation in vigorous sports frequently causes musculoskeletal soft-tissue inflammation. In many instances, inflammation results from mechanical loading of the soft tissues, through a single acute load or repetitive loads. An acute load that exceeds the strength of the tissue causes immediate detectable damage that activates the inflammatory response. In the typical sports-induced soft-tissue inflammation, the mechanism of tissue damage is known and the intensity of the inflammatory response is related to the extent and type of damage. Examples of this type of injury include acute tearing of tendon, ligament, muscle, or myotendinous junction. However, sports-induced soft-tissue inflammation may also result from repetitive loading that exceeds the capacity of the tissues to adapt. In this type of inflammation, significant tissue disruption may not be present or may be difficult to detect. The mechanism of tissue damage remains uncertain and the relationship between the tissue damage and the inflammation is unclear. Occasionally, a single load or repetitive loads may result in calcification of the affected tissue as well as inflammation.

The response of the musculoskeletal soft tissues to repetitive loading makes it possible to strengthen these tissues, thereby improving the performance of the musculoskeletal system, especially in young individuals. Under conditions of normal repetitive loading, the cells of tendon, ligament, joint capsule, myotendinous junction, and tendon and ligament insertions degrade and replace at least some components of their extracellular matrices, even in skeletally mature individuals. Quantitative studies on the rate of matrix turnover have not been reported; however, degradation and replacement must balance each other to maintain the structure and material properties of the tissue. Persistent changes in mechanical loading can alter this balance. Prolonged decreased loading may cause degradation to exceed replacement, causing a net decrease in tissue strength and possibly tissue volume. Prolonged or repetitive increased loading may cause replacement to exceed degradation, causing a net increase in tissue strength and possibly tissue volume. In addition to these mechanically induced changes, persistent changes in loading may affect the organization of the tissue. Some evidence suggests that decreased loading decreases the degree of orientation of matrix macromolecules, especially collagen fibrils, in relation to the applied loads. Similarly, increased loading may increase the degree of matrix orientation.

Although repetitive increased tissue loading caused by sports and other activities may have important beneficial effects, it may also have deleterious effects. Repetitive loads that exceed the capacity of the tissue to adapt may cause a cellular and vascular response that begins within the loaded tissue and extends to surrounding tissues. This response may include release of inflammatory mediators, increased vascular permeability, migration of inflammatory cells, and tissue edema. These events can cause the signs and symptoms of acute or chronic inflammation. Although the mechanism of this response remains poorly understood, the resulting clinical syndrome frequently impairs the performance of competitive and recreational athletes.

Diagnosis

The diagnosis of sports-induced soft-tissue inflammation is based on medical history and physical examination. Initially, most patients with sports-induced soft-tissue inflammation complain of pain or performance deficit. A thorough history usually provides the physician with information that can help define activities that cause or increase pain and that can allow the physician to determine the structures and tissues affected. The affected areas may demonstrate tenderness to palpation or increased pain and tenderness with loading. The extent and severity of an inflammation-induced performance deficit may be demonstrated by measuring muscle strength and range of motion.

The complex relationships between soft-tissue inflammation and clinically recognized signs and symptoms of inflammation are not well-defined. In some patients, the signs and symptoms of sports-induced soft-tissue inflammation include erythema, swelling, warmth, tenderness and performance deficit. Other individuals may have only pain and performance deficit. Because many variables affect the presentation of sports-induced soft-tissue inflammation, the intensity of the pain and the severity of the performance deficit may not correlate with the extent of tissue injury. That is, the degree or intensity of signs and symptoms may not be indicative of the extent of tissue inflammation. Even with similar degrees of tissue injury and inflammation, the signs and symptoms they induce may vary among patients, tissue types, and locations.

Other methods of diagnosing this condition and quantifying its severity are being investigated. These include electromyographic and dynamometric studies that can measure the performance deficit objectively. In some situations, diagnostic imaging studies, such as magnetic resonance imaging and bone scanning, may demonstrate the location and extent of tissue injury and inflammation. In the future, spectroscopy and positron emission tomography may be helpful. Thus far, serum and urine studies have not been useful in evaluating sports-induced soft-tissue inflammation. Most physicians currently use imaging and laboratory studies to eliminate the possibility of infection, tumor, or systemic rheumatologic disorder. Future research may show that systemic factors have a role in sports-induced soft- tissue inflammation and may reveal clinically useful serum, urine, and tissue markers.

Grading Severity

There is no consensus on the value of clinical grading of sports-induced soft-tissue inflammation. Principal methods of grading the severity of sports-induced inflammation include assessing the intensity of the associated pain and measuring the performance deficit. The tissue involved, the age of the individual, the chronicity of the problem, the degree of subjective and objective performance deficit, and the perception of pain intensity are among the factors that should be considered in applying current grading systems or in developing new systems. Combining pain measurement scales with measures of strength, endurance, flexibility, and range of motion may be the most effective method of developing clinical systems for grading sports-induced soft-tissue inflammation.

Mechanisms of Sports-Induced Inflammation

The mechanisms of musculoskeletal soft-tissue damage caused by acute loading that exceeds the strength of the tissue have been studied. To some extent, the relationships between the severity of acute tissue injury and the extent of inflammation and repair are known. Repetitive loading during sports activity can also induce soft-tissue inflammation, but these mechanisms have not been defined clinically or experimentally in terms of frequency, intensity, and type of loading. The mechanism of inflammation caused by repetitive loading can vary and the same mechanism may cause different patterns of inflammation in different individuals, tissues, and anatomic sites. Individual factors such as age, alignment of the tissues, previous injuries, conditioning, systemic disease, genetically determined differences, and environment may be important in defining the clinical mechanisms of sports-induced soft-tissue inflammation.

Effects on Soft-Tissue Cells and Matrices

Inflammation alters the structure and function of parenchymal tissues, such as heart, liver, kidney or brain. How acute or chronic sports-induced inflammation affects the cells and matrices of tissues such as tendon, ligament, joint capsule, tendon and ligament insertions into bone, and the myotendinous junction is not known. It seems likely that inflammation of the musculoskeletal soft tissues alters matrix synthesis, degradation, structure, and composition. However, these alterations have not been systematically investigated.

Effects on Soft-Tissue Material Properties

Clinical experience suggests that inflammation alters the material properties and biologic behavior of the soft tissues. Inflamed tissue often appears edematous and feels softer than uninflamed tissue. Chronic inflammation may decrease the tensile strength of the soft tissues. Perhaps chronic inflammation also alters cell metabolism and matrix composition and organization, and thereby adversely affects the material properties of the tissue but, at present, there is no clear evidence of a relationship between inflammation and altered soft-tissue material properties.

Pain Associated With Sports-Induced Soft-Tissue Inflammation

Sports-induced soft-tissue inflammation releases mediators that excite and sensitize peripheral nociceptive nerve fibers, thereby contributing to the perceptual state of hyperalgesia. In this state, the patient experiences persistent spontaneous pain, decreased pain threshold, and increased magnitude of pain after any stimulus. Clinically, the hyperalgesic state may involve production of pain by normally nonpainful activities, including stretching or mild exercise, and increased pain following normally painful stimuli, such as blunt trauma. In addition, the inflammatory mediators evoke secretion of neural peptides from nerve endings. The neural peptides can in turn promote the synthesis and release of inflammatory mediators. This positive-feedback cycle may prolong the inflammatory response and associated hyperalgesia. As these mediators are diffused away from the site of inflammation, the region of hyperalgesia expands. Although the magnitude of pain is generally proportional to the extent of tissue damage, such factors as the circumstances of the injury or the emotional state of the individual may obscure this relationship.

Chapter 5

Clinical Observations on Sports-Induced Soft-Tissue Injuries

James A. Nicholas, MD

Athletic activity makes special demands on the musculoskeletal soft tissues that may result in injuries. Mechanisms of injury vary and can cause different pathologic patterns at different anatomic sites.[39,41,42] The inflammatory response to injury may vary with the type of injury and the type of care received. Chronic tendon and joint inflammation may have its inception in mechanical overload of these tissues.[9,20,27]

With training and conditioning for sports, contractile forces generated by the linked muscle-tendon systems develop widespread combinations of rates of tension and peak tension and magnitudes up to prefailure and failure. Variables that influence the occurrence and severity of these injuries include performance demand,[35] the presence of preexisting injuries, and the nature of the athlete, such as the athlete's ability to be motivated in sports.[33]

Variables That Influence Frequency, Severity, and Type of Injury

Several variables influence the frequency, severity, and type of injuries that occur in sports.[23,31,32,35,45]

(1) The demands of the sport on an athlete. Pitching, for example, requires a precise, coordinated, balanced, rhythmic, strong, ballistic propulsion with precise control.[21] Injuries can occur if the athlete is unable to meet the demand at any point in the pitching motion. This property of sports relating to the athlete is called performance demand; each sport makes quantifiable demands on the performer (Outline 1).

(2) Previous injury. Weakness from previous injuries can facilitate reinjury.[51] These weaknesses impose different responses to load. In a study of preparticipation profiles of athletes in baseball, football, soccer, and hockey, more than 80% of the best professional players in the country were found to already have injuries that could shorten their careers.[19]

(3) The nature and characteristics of the athlete. Factors such as

Outline 1 Performance factors that impose demand in sports*

Neuromuscular and physical factors
- Strength
- Endurance
- Body type
- Flexibility
- Agility
- Balance
- Coordination
- Rhythm
- Timing
- Speed
- Accuracy
- Steadiness
- Reaction time

Mental and psychological factors
- Intelligence
- Creativity
- Alertness
- Motivation
- Discipline

Environmental factors
- Playing conditions
- Equipment
- Practice

*Reproduced with permission from Nicholas JA: Risk factors, sports medicine and the orthopedic system: An overview. *J Sports Med* 1975;3:243-259.

body build, state of fatigue, ability to control risk, motivation, and ability to meet the performance demand influence the injury pattern.

(4) Sports-specific motion and loading. Sports are characterized by motion, and different types of motion can produce forces that cause specific injuries. Six basic sports motions—walk, run, jump, throw, kick, and stance[31,32,35]—have been categorized and studied according to their qualitative use in sports. In each of these movements, overuse or overload can produce failure and injury. The effects of load on motion have not been sufficiently studied. The rate produced by such motion (sports), the cyclic patterns (sustained, intermittent, or slow), the onset stimulus, and the degree of load (shear, tension, compression) are part of how motion causes prefailure warnings with early injury as well as catastrophic acute failure.

(5) Playing surface and shoes. The playing surface has an important effect because of the ground reaction force it imposes on a player when there is foot fixation and velocity. The response in such cases may produce specific types of injury such as sprained ankles or knee instability from transmitted forces. The surfaces include turf, grass, hardwood floor, asphalt tracks, snow, ice, sand, and water. Footwear (such as boots, sneakers, skates, skis, spikes, or cleats) generates specific forces as it interacts with the surface and can cause injury from sliding on unstable ankles or fixed-foot knee injuries from high forces (Fig. 1).[47] The condition of the surface (dry, muddy, sticky, wet, or slippery) is a fundamental variable in producing athletic injuries. The great

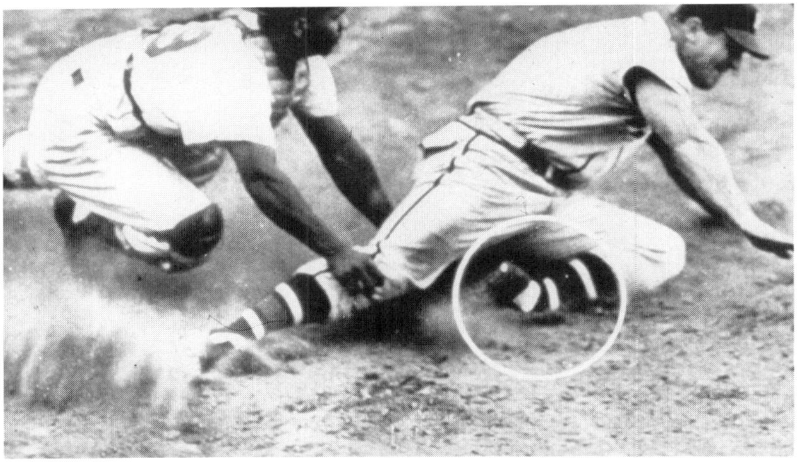

Fig. 1 *This baseball player with chronic sprains of the ankle dislocated his ankle while sliding. The photograph illustrates important causes of injury: foot fixation, ankle instability, the sliding moment, and the ground-shoe interface.*

variability in the intensity of these forces and the individual's ability to withstand them determines the pattern of injury to the foot or indirectly to the extremity.

(6) Force acting on the body. The type of force acting on an athlete is important. The forces may be direct or noncontact. They can be repetitive or multifrequency low-load types such as occur in overuse syndromes, or single-frequency high-load types caused by a direct blow.[38] The type of force is important in the type of injury. A high-frequency cyclic load or a high load with low frequency, in which the load is too great for bone and tissue to withstand, causes acute sudden disruptive injury. A low-load force with high repetition results in a gradual deterioration of tissue strength from strain to fatigue deformation (Fig. 2)[13,14,28] with prefailure symptoms such as pain on use, a common clinical sign of early inflammation from overuse. The transmission, direction, and type of force are extremely important. Is the force manifest as a shear, tensile, or compression phenomenon? From where and to where is it transmitted (leg, spine, upper extremity)? Lever length is a major determinant of the amount of force produced (Fig. 3).[38,40]

(7) Joint and body position. The joint position at time of contact is important in determining the moments of force and where they act. For example, a flexed knee is inherently more unstable than an extended knee when ground reaction forces pass through it. However, if the knee is hyperextended, the forces produce injuries different from those produced on the flexed knee. The pattern of athletic injury varies with the different angles of joint position. The torque generated in such

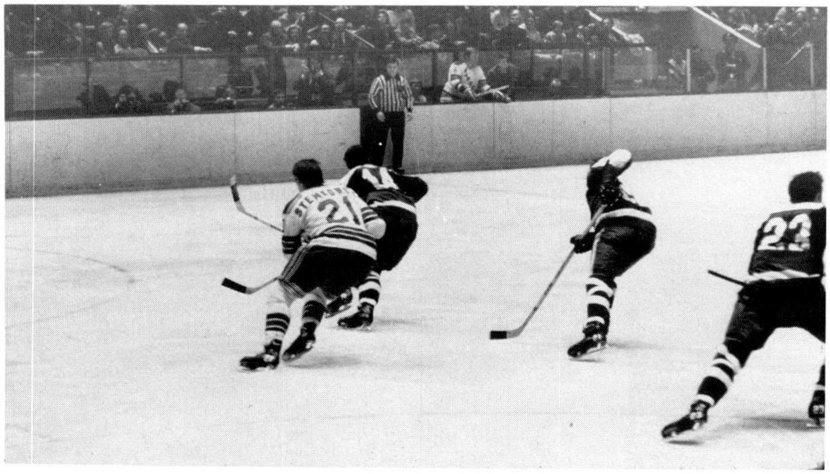

Fig. 2 *Notice the characteristic low-load, repetitious, multifrequency forces on ice in gliding and sliding. Motions are tandem. Number 14 is doing a crossover step. The mechanics of these movements frequently produce strains and chronic inflammation of the thigh and groin tendons caused by the lunging force of body against eccentric muscular propulsion.*

positions varies with the position of the limb. The type and extent of damaged tissue varies with such torque, and may involve multiple structures at a distance from one another. The linkage status of the elements transmitting the forces that cause injury is important. Forces pass not only from the ground to the lower extremity, but also to the pelvis and the spine (Fig. 4) as well as from the head and the hands to the spine and the lower extremity.[7] Therefore, linkage segment length is an important factor in generating torque at a joint, plays an important role in the type of injury that can occur, and is often a source of unrecognized inflammation from trauma.

Specific Sports-Injury Patterns

Ligaments (Sprains With or Without Avulsion)

Ligamentous tears of the substance are more common with rapid force application. Prefailure elongation with applied force to failure with avulsion of bone is more common in slowly applied loads, particularly about the knee joint at the tibial spine, the attachments of the muscles, and/or the collateral ligaments.[38] Partial ligament tears have not been studied extensively. Kennedy and associates[25] noted considerable ultrastructural disorganization in grossly intact anterior and posterior cruciate and medial collateral ligaments just before fail-

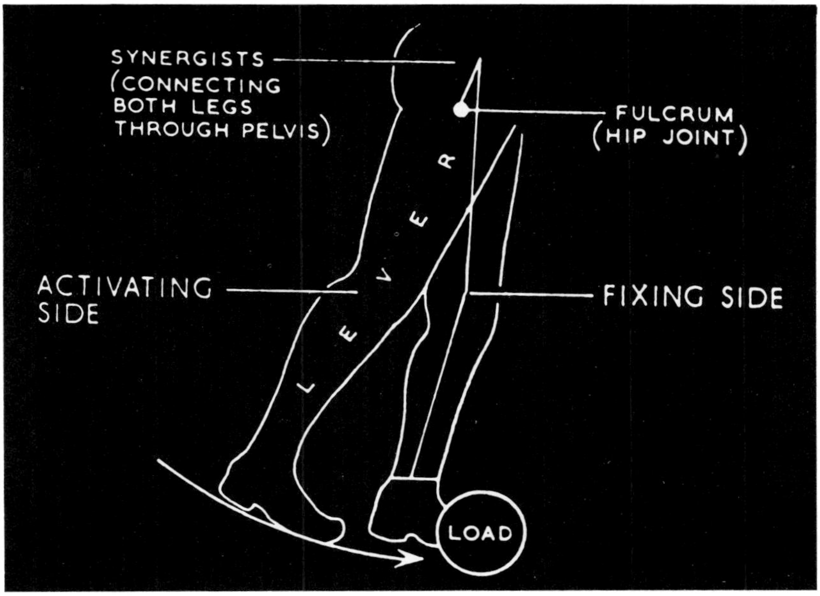

Fig. 3 *Lever length (along with joint position at the time of contact) is a major determinant of forces produced. Muscles develop force in two ways: passively by resistance to being stretched and by voluntary contraction.*

ure, showing that visual impressions can be deceptive. More study is needed, and a careful examination and history-taking are essential. Ligamentous injuries commonly occur in high-velocity, high-contact sports, in particular, football, soccer, skiing, basketball, hockey, tennis, and rugby. Among the vulnerable ligaments are the sternoclavicular ligaments, the acromioclavicular ligaments (shoulder), the wrist and thumb ligaments, the collateral and cruciate ligaments (knee), and ligaments about the arch of the foot (Chopart's joint of the first and second metatarsals).

Common causes of these injuries include twisting loads that produce large moments, overload from abnormal or unstable angular movements, and excessive stretching forces, usually in more than one and often in three axes of movement. Ligaments may stretch or elongate to prefailure or suddenly rupture to failure.[3,6] However, partial ligament tears and prefailure loading have not been studied extensively. Stretching the ligaments (grade I or II sprains) may slowly elongate them, with a considerable amount of force applied before rupture. Elongation to failure may produce an acute episode from a chronic sprain.

In the upper extremity, during a fall, the outstretched hand bears weight from the floor, with ground reaction forces transferred to the

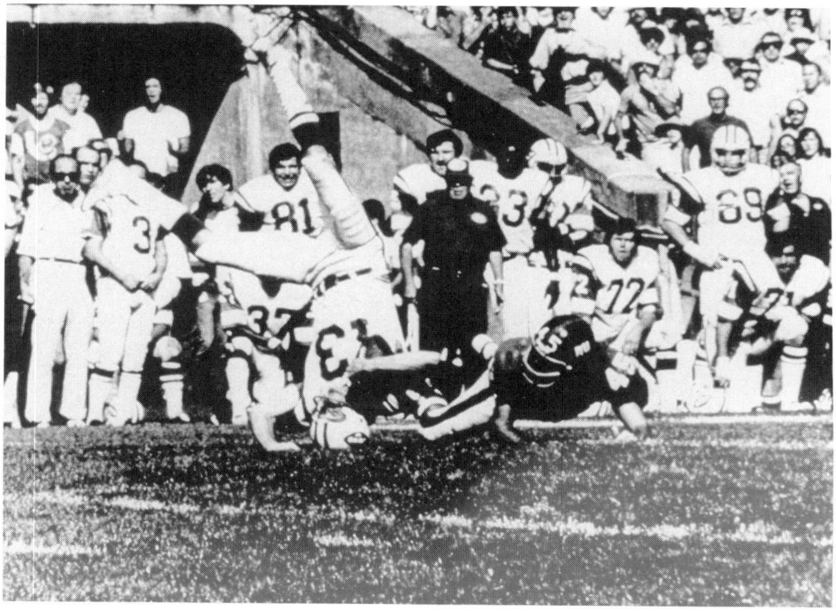

Fig. 4 *Linkage segment length is of elemental importance in the transmission of force from ground to arm, head, or knee, as shown.*

elbow and encountered by the body weight in an off-center position. The torque generated by this position is too great for the elbow to withstand; either the capsular ligaments tear and the elbow dislocates, or, if the wrist and elbow remain stable, the forces are transmitted to the shoulder. Direct falls on the tip of the acromion can also cause injury to the acromioclavicular joint and its ligaments, the glenoid, ribs, or scapula in a manner similar to ground force overload.

In the lower extremity, tears of the anterior cruciate ligament in combination with or without the medial collateral ligament or other capsular structures[22,50] may produce instability and increased laxity of the knee. Noncontact injuries often occur in ligaments from deceleration and change of direction, such as in the crossover step. When bearing weight, the anterior cruciate ligament can undergo fatigue to deformation and may tear in an isolated fashion without any contact other than the force of the foot striking the ground to change direction. There may be a lateral capsular tear and anterolateral instability. As the crossed-over foot decelerates and bears weight with the knee joint flexed, the tibia displaces anteriorly or the femur posteriorly.[2] This also happens during an outside cut or pivot (the athlete puts weight on the outside leg at a right angle and then turns away with the opposite foot). If external forces such as body contact are applied against the planted foot as it makes the right-angle cut with the leg held in valgus and

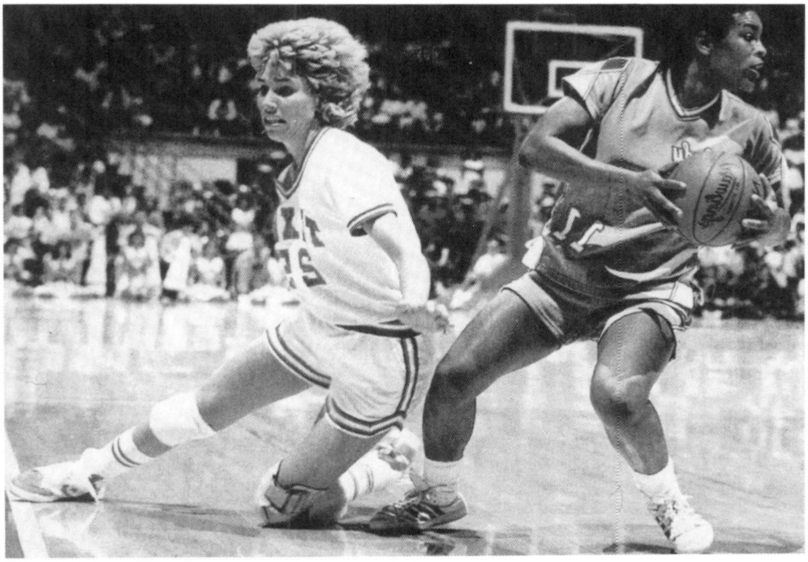

Fig. 5 *This photograph illustrates the many triaxial positions of the lower extremity. When it is stressed, major injuries can be produced by failure of different types, contusions, sprains, strains, and fractures.*

external rotation, severe bending, torsion, and failure at the ankle, the foot, the knee, or a combination of these can result.

In the lower extremity, cutting and change of direction are not the only causes of ligament tears. Deceleration (in which the hamstrings may be unable to absorb the load) and accelerated movements to gain speed suddenly can cause problems as well. Pivoting, jumping and landing off-balance, and sliding on footwear that catches on the surface with fixation of the foot can also cause substance tears from transmission of ground reaction forces through the everted foot in external rotation, or the inverted foot in internal rotation (Fig. 5).[29] Spiral tibial fractures can occur without the knee being involved.

Why and how some athletes prevent damage from prefailure loads and bypass loads to reach the relaxation state are still unanswered questions. There is much to learn about why some athletes never seem to get hurt, while others are frequently injured.

Knee Instabilities

Mechanisms Tears in knee ligaments produce instability of the knee joint in a number of directions depending upon how the knee was hit, how it was positioned at the time of the applied force, and whether the force was passed at the same time by the fixed foot and the body's lean into a vector of overloading force.[2,3,6,15–18,24,26,30,33,35,37,43,47,48,50,52] Me-

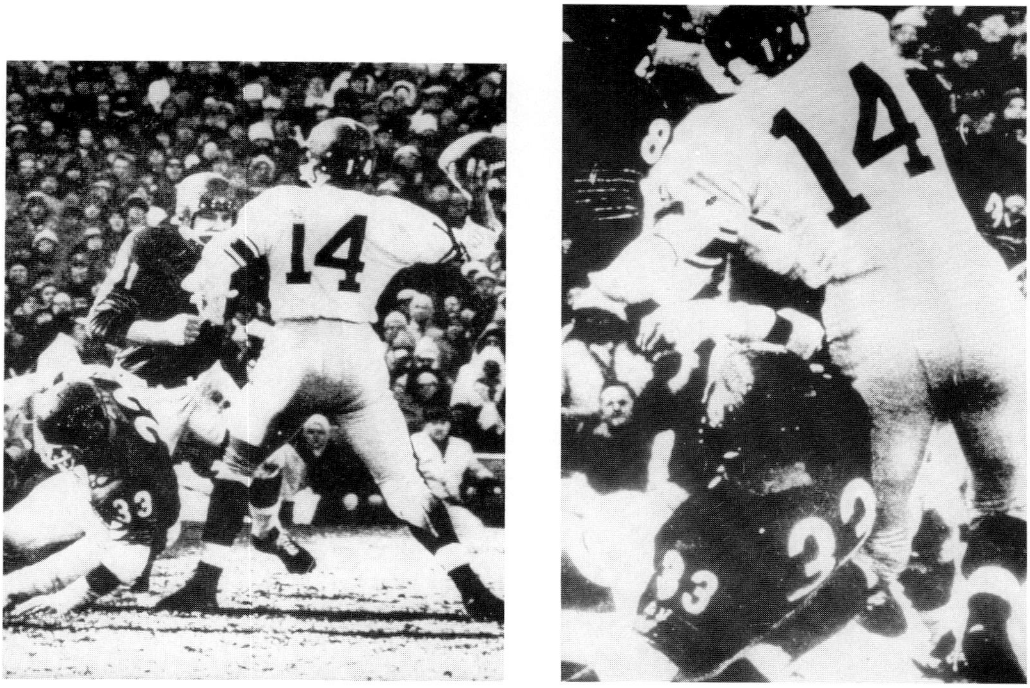

Fig. 6 *An example of both indirect and direct mechanisms of injury from a fixed valgus foot and an externally rotated, flexed leg with a direct blow. The result is anterior cruciate and medial collateral ligament-meniscus injury with an articular fracture. The organization of collagen may make the difference in stress tolerance to deformation in this frequent injury. (Reproduced with permission from Nicholas JA: The five-one reconstruction for anteromedial instability of the knee: Indications, technique, and the results in fifty-two patients.* J Bone Joint Surg *1973;55A:899–922.)*

niscus injury, patellofemoral and femoral-tibial bruising, and osteochondral fractures may occur. If these injuries are not treated properly, chronic symptoms may result, and instability and weakness will rapidly produce additional articular damage.

Anteromedial Instability If a blow occurs to the medial aspect of the tibia with the foot flexed and fixed, and the valgus stress is on the flexed, externally rotated knee, the medial tibial condyle may be forced forward (Fig. 6).[35] This displacement results from the rotation of the tibia about a vertical axis that has shifted forward and lateral to the normal axis. Anterior translation of the tibia occurs as the anterior cruciate ligament tears, while valgus movement tears the medial collateral ligament or posteromedial corner. If the knee is in varus, and the tibia is externally rotated, posterolateral rotary instability will develop, with posterior translation caused by elongation of the posterior cruciate ligament, varus caused by tears in the quadruple complex, and posterolateral dropback of the posterior tibial condyle.[4,29,37] Both anteromedial and posterolateral laxities are caused by externally rotating forces around the vertical axis.[29,37]

The most common type of internal rotation laxity is anterolateral instability. Posteromedial laxity is rare. Anterolateral instability occurs when the fixed, internally rotated foot decelerates with slight knee varus. Anterior cruciate ligament and lateral capsular elongation occur. Current arthroscopic methods for diagnosis and treatment of the acute anterior cruciate ligament tear often do not expose the posterolateral corner, just as posteromedial tears on the posteromedial corner are not recognized in patients who have arthroscopic diagnosis of the injury. This again underscores the importance of obtaining a careful history. A comprehensive examination of both extremities and the necessary radiographic images are important for diagnosis before an arthroscopy is performed.

If a fall on the flexed knee occurs, producing a blow to the tibia and tibial tubercle with the ankle and foot plantar flexed (a common mechanism),[24] and if the medial and lateral capsular stabilizers and the anterior cruciate ligament remain intact, the posterior cruciate ligament can tear from shear and compression (Fig. 7). If the knee is in valgus at the time and internally rotated, posteromedial instability occurs. Some observers have not seen this, but there are enough documented cases of posteromedial instabilities to consider it when there is posterior laxity. Another common way to "blow out" the knee occurs in a fall with the knee in hyperextension, which can tear both posterior and anterior cruciate ligaments as well as one of the other capsular complexes, depending on the position of the tibia in relation to the transverse and vertical axes with the ground.

It is important to learn from the patient, if possible, how these injuries occurred, for this information can be useful in making an accurate diagnosis and defining the clinical pattern of types of failure, as well as in determining the treatment, the long-term rehabilitation, and the types of inflammatory response and degenerative joint disease that may occur.[22,26]

Indirect blows to the foot while it is fixed may cause injuries anywhere in the ankle, tibial shaft, knee, or thigh. Chronic instability can cause chronic inflammation,[1] muscle weakness, periodic joint swelling and pain, and arthritic changes, which may ultimately produce a "benevolent" reduction in knee instability at the expense of the arthritis and increased stiffness.[32] A strong, comprehensively directed rehabilitation program and activity modification can help achieve a positive result and restoration, whether or not surgery is used.

Muscle-Tendon Unit (Strains)

These injuries[2,8,9,11,12,35,36,39,43,45,53] occur at the bone-tendon junction, at the myotendinous junction, and in the belly of the muscle. Tendons have very high tensile strength, minimal shear strength, and no resistance to compression. Tendons are frequently injured in jumping,

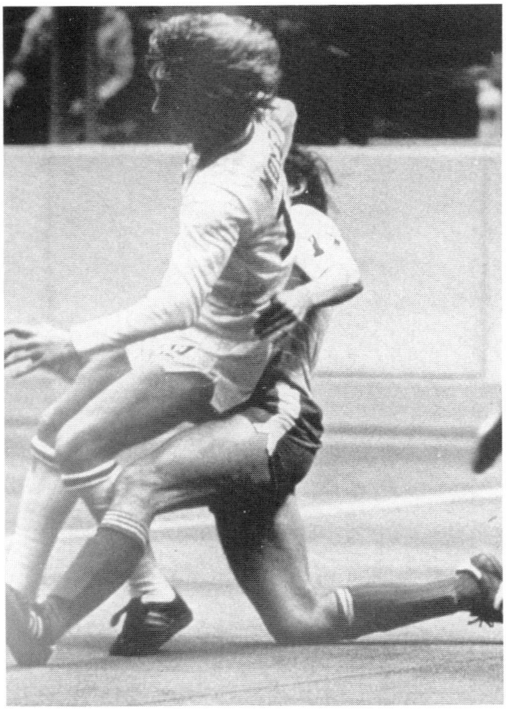

Fig. 7 *A mechanism by which the posterior cruciate ligament can tear or the patella can fracture. Note plantar-flexed foot and the direct blow to the knee. Also note, on the opposite leg, the calf elongation (eccentric) force working on the concentrically contracting hamstring. If the hamstring failed, the quadriceps could overpower it and allow anterior cruciate rupture.*

or with excessive acceleration/deceleration, particularly if the muscle has been fatigued or overloaded in contraction or overstretching,[12] such as in throwing. Strains represent fatigue reactions to low-load, repetitive stresses, with normal or less-than-normal forces required to tear tissue.[14] Strains commonly occur in sports in which throwing, jumping, and their variations are used, such as in ballet, baseball, gymnastics, golf, soccer, modern dance, running, basketball, figure skating, skiing, and hiking. Strains can occur with almost any type of mechanism. Among the vulnerable muscles are the pectoralis major, the rotator cuff, the biceps, the pronator teres, the epicondylar tendons of the elbow, the paraspinal muscles and tendinous attachments of the cervical and lumbar spine, the abdominal obliques, the abductors, the hamstrings, the quadriceps, the gastrocnemius/soleus, and the Achilles tendon.

A distinction should be made according to the injury site: did the forces act at the bone-tendon junction, at the muscle-tendon unit, or in the belly of the muscle?[12] Disruption can be complete and, if it is near the myotendinous junction (which is most common), can generate a profound inflammatory response.[13] The forces can be tensile and/or shear with concentric or (usually) eccentric muscle contraction at the time of load. Jumping is a movement commonly causing an eccentric load to failure. This may be an acute or chronic process and is especially disabling if it occurs in the quadriceps or in the hamstring tendons.[13,14] After injuries, the tensile strength of muscles decreases markedly and recurrence of the injury is common, often after weakened eccentric contraction, especially if the athlete returns to function without rehabilitation.

Overuse Injuries

Cabaud and associates[5] reported that endurance-type exercises increased strength and decreased stiffness, particularly in high-frequency, long-duration programs. However, overuse from overtraining occurs in many people because they are not ready to meet the demands of exercise. Overuse injuries are common in bones, tendons, and muscles. The role of prefailure injury needs to be elaborated, especially for tendon and ligament injury.

Severe pulls (strains) also result from chronic overuse syndromes and occur in hockey, football, rugby, horseback riding, cricket, and bowling. Excessive pulls and forces against contraction can cause lengthening of the muscles with tearing. In running, for example, thousands of deformations occur at at high load, producing tendon strain and microstress fractures.

As a result, a number of common injuries occur, manifested by pain and inflammation. These include "runner's knee," chondromalacia, patellar tendinitis, iliotibial band syndrome, tibial stress syndrome, anterior compartment syndrome, plantar fasciitis, and metatarsal stress syndrome.[9,39] Physical examinations of athletes with such problems are likely to reveal muscle weakness in other muscle groups in the hips or spine. Manual muscle tests can confirm this, as will dynamic tests such as single-leg hops, in which the body will lean to the weaker side.[37] In some cases, contracture may also be present.

In the throwing movement (as in all motions of sports using jumping, running, walking, and kicking), there is a complex interaction and adaptation to support joint functions in synergy with each other and in muscular contractions to produce movement in normal axes of motion. When repetitive loads fatigue muscles, the entire mechanism becomes subject to risk.

The hamstring muscles provide major deceleration forces to knee extension. Overuse can cause microscopic tears at the proximal or distal myotendinous junction. Tears of the muscle at the myotendinous junction, such as at the junction of the gastrocnemius/soleus muscle and the Achilles tendon, are uncommon. They are less common than tears through the Achilles itself, while tears of the belly or head of the gastrocnemius or plantaris are much more common ("tennis leg").

They occur in several ways. One common injury occurs when the heel is down and weightbearing while the athlete is making a charging movement (Fig. 7). The body leans forward in an accelerating movement. Strong gastrocnemius/soleus contractions under stretch eccentrically lengthen calf muscles, which can then tear the belly of the muscle proximally. They can also tear the myotendinous junction, although this is rare, and occasionally the Achilles tendon. Thus, the same eccentric loads can cause hip-flexor or knee-extension pulls.

With aging, the Achilles tendon weakens, so that Achilles tendon injuries occur in middle-aged athletes more frequently. This type of injury frequently occurs in badminton, tennis, and basketball. Patients feel a ripping sensation in either the calf or the lower leg. The same type of injury may occur in a tennis serve as well as in a golf swing when the arms are stretched on the backswing, causing rupture of the pronator teres muscle and retraction of the superficial head from concentric muscle contraction (Fig. 8). Because long-term weakness in proximal limb muscles of the appendicular skeleton is often present when injuries occur in peripheral and distal joints,[37] rehabilitation cannot be limited only to the injured site. With overuse syndromes in the lower extremity, comprehensive triaxial strengthening of muscles other than the quadriceps is important (for example, hip flexors, abductors, adductors, and rotators). Stretching the tight iliotibial band, quadriceps, and hamstrings in a three-plane manner is useful for acquiring the greatest degree of safety stress.

Sports commonly involved in overuse syndromes include baseball (pitching), racket sports, tennis, dance, basketball, volleyball, and swimming. Movements involving sudden acceleration and deceleration often cause reactions in muscles at the periosteal attachments (splints). Pulls may develop in repetitive, low-load movements. Delayed muscle soreness, cramps, or muscle damage, particularly in the hamstring or calf muscles, will occur in some cases as a result of the decelerating force, which acts against the quadriceps.

The Achilles, quadriceps, and patellar tendons are particular sites of overuse injuries because continual load with repetitious movement produces degeneration of the bone-tendon or the muscle-tendon attachment.

In the patella, the tip of the patellar tendon develops persistent pain on extension and flexion (jumper's knee). In time, a hyalinoid-type of reactive fibrous healing occurs. However, this is too weak to support the tendon and bone and causes the bone to be continuously loaded (Fig. 9). Rupture of the patellar tendon is then possible.

The same mechanism can apply to injuries to the quadriceps tendon at the superior pole of the patella, although this tendon is much stronger and rupture is less likely to occur in an active athlete. These tendons can actually fatigue to elongation, with tenosynovitis as the presenting early symptom.

In the upper extremity, the rotator cuff is readily overused as are the medial and lateral epicondylar tendons of the elbow, which can develop chronic tendinitis. The basis for these pathologic changes in

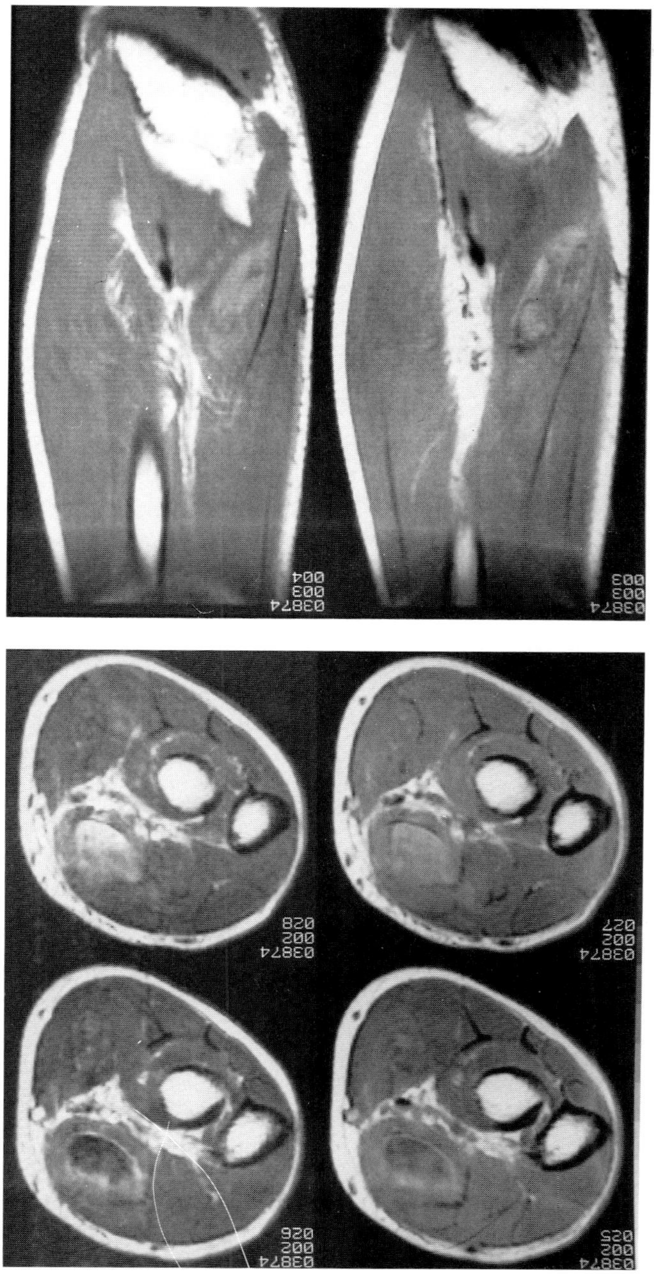

Fig. 8 *Magnetic resonance imaging shows a rupture of the superficial belly of the pronator teres from repetitive golf swings after months of overuse. Eccentric contraction in the hitting area caused this through mechanical overload from stretching the flexor pronator.*

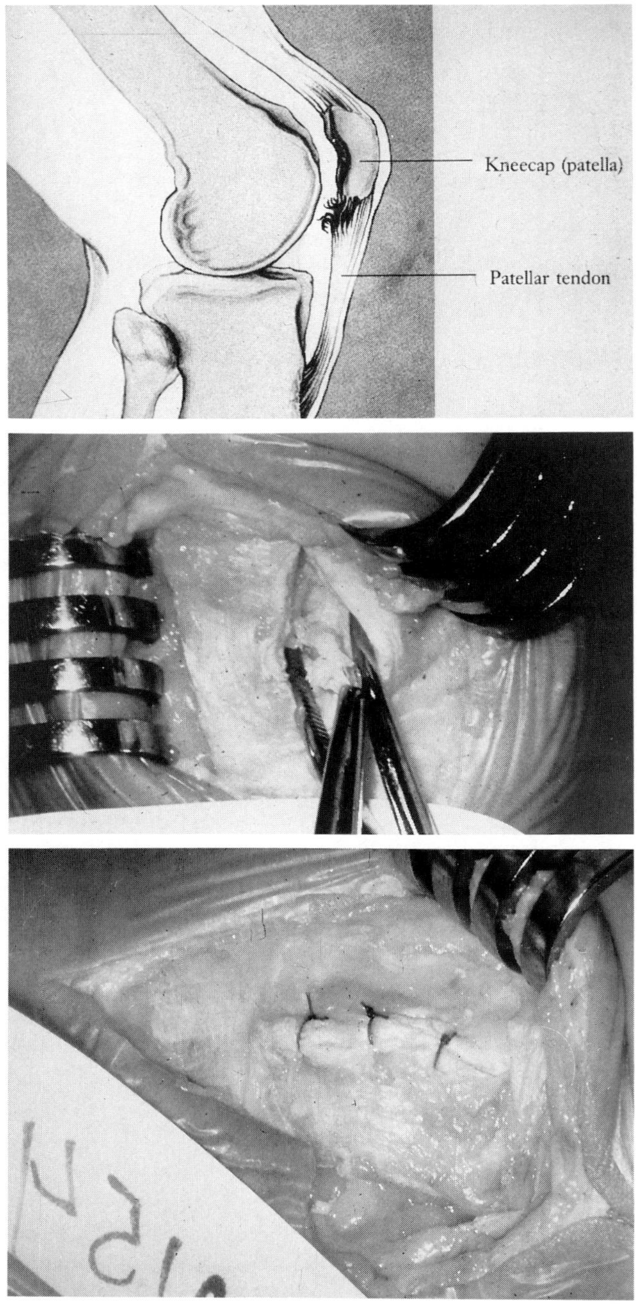

Fig. 9 *Jumper's knee is caused by overuse. Hyalinoid fibrous healing in tendon is too weak to support the patellar tendon on quadriceps activation, causing excessive loading. This is a highly stressed functional area in jumper's knee. Microfractures, cavities in collagen, and blue-line irregularities are common.*

the tendons is the demand the athlete puts on them. Selective muscle weakness such as in the rotator cuff, rather than general muscle impairment, leads to overuse in such instances.

The Throwing Mechanism

In studying inflammation and its causes in sports, it is useful to learn about the mechanics of throwing, one of the most important motions in sports.[11,20,21,23,36,42,43,46,49]

The mechanics of throwing are similar in tennis, swimming, pitching, and other throwing sports, and should be understood to see how they produce overuse injuries. Slocum,[44] Tullos and King,[50] and Jobe and Perry[20,21] have done considerable work in this area. The steps in throwing are as follows: (1) The windup ends when the ball leaves the gloved hand. (2) Early cocking is a period of shoulder abduction and external rotation that ends when the contralateral leg makes ground contact. (3) Late cocking is an arm position that continues until maximum external rotation of the shoulder occurs. (4) Acceleration starts with internal rotation of the humerus and ends with ball release. (5) Follow-through begins when the ball is released and ends when the motion is complete.

The deltoid and the rotator cuff have separate and independent actions. This is why there must be specific and comprehensive rehabilitation to strengthen the rotator cuff in order to prevent stress overload. The medial elbow is stressed by early cocking, as is the ligamentous tendon complex. The radiocapitellar joint is compressed in the late cocking phase, and the anterior capsule of the shoulder is stretched. Because the muscles of the scapula are contracting, origins of the shoulder tendons to the cuff are in contraction under the coracoacromial arch. As the arm comes forward in acceleration, the posterior capsule is stretched, while internal rotation of the humerus stresses the medial elbow pronators. As the arm comes into extension and internal rotation, flexor muscle action introduces a posterior-superior compressive force across the distal humerus. Because of the poor mechanical advantage the flexor muscles have with the elbow in extension, the isometric forces must be greatest in this position (Fig. 8).

Throwing athletes with impingement problems in the subacromial joint will have demonstrable discrepancies in the pattern of muscle action when compared with normal. The supraspinatus functions at a lower level and it is less able to assist the deltoid during wrist cock, resulting in reduced activity of the internal rotators (subcapularis), the pectoralis major, and the latissimus dorsi. This may contribute to the increased activity in external rotation (superior humeral migration) and faulty scapular rotation.

Swimming strokes have a "pull-through and recover phase."[21] The pull-through phase is similar to the cocking phase in pitching. To reduce the common phenomena of swimmer's shoulder and impingement, particular attention must be paid to the rotator cuff and serratus anterior. Scapular rotation must coincide with humeral abduction to prevent this problem. As the serratus anterior tires over a number of cycles (slow load), fatigue prevents it from completing an important function in recovery. Normally it allows the acromion to rotate clear of the abducting humerus under strong muscle control by the supraspinatus and infraspinatus and middle deltoid, which abduct and externally rotate the arm. With the whip kick, medial collateral ligament strain can occur, especially in the breaststroke.

The tennis serve requires complex muscle activities similar to those of baseball pitching. Like the phases of pitching, tennis has forehand, backhand, and ground strokes divided into three stages: racket preparation, acceleration, and follow-through. An imbalance of muscle strength in the throwing arc causes injuries and can lead to anatomic changes, as in proximal humeral migration or in medial stress overload at the elbow. Both of these are repetition, fatigue-type injuries of the muscle-tendon unit associated with a ballistic throwing movement. The make-up of the thrower's body (too tight or hypermobile) has an unexplained role in causing injury to the throwing arm. Presumably, if the glenohumeral joint is too tight, the load stresses different distribution points than when the joint is hypermobile. More studies are required in this area.

Athletes with impingement problems in the subacromial joint demonstrate discrepancies in the pattern of use when compared with normal patterns. Muscle weakness from the impingement problems occurs as far proximal as the neck and dorsal spinal musculature, as well as down to the hand. The supraspinatus functions at a lower level and is less able to assist the deltoid during wrist cock in throwing sports. Rehabilitation must involve retraining all the scapular musculature, as well as the rotator cuff, in a specific manner.

With reduced activity, the internal rotators (subscapularis, pectoralis major, and latissimus) may contribute to increased activity in external rotation, superior humeral migration, and faulty scapular rotation.

Articular Cartilage and Meniscal Injuries

"Endurance activities that require running and jumping may cause significantly more debilitating injuries to beginning exercisers than any other activity," stated the US Public Health Service in 1987.[10] These activities are likely to produce both meniscal and articular cartilage injuries. Articular cartilage injuries and meniscal tear injuries occur through compression and shear and through impingements and subluxations. The areas most affected are both menisci of the knee joint, the patellofemoral joint, and the lateral and medial condyles, especially with torsion and excessive impact forces. With throwing, these injuries also occur in the acromioclavicular joint and in the capitellum in the elbow. Articular cartilage injuries, such as chondromalacia, are also produced by the medial stress syndrome in pitchers. In young throwers, especially those in whom the epiphyses have not matured fully, osteochondritis is produced. When articular cartilage is injured, the surface may fibrillate and begin a process of incongruent joint motion.

Loose bodies may develop with the production of synovitis and intensify joint incongruity. In adolescents, fragmentation of the epiphysis of the elbow ("Little-League elbow") may develop. Direct trauma has been reported from running, jumping, and falling. Full-thickness lesions do not heal and will produce osteochondral fracture as part of the transmitted force of a direct trauma. Low loads with frequent repetitions at high speed are reported to cause articular cartilage damage. Meniscal injuries can occur as a result of both direct and indirect trauma. As previously noted, they may cause articular fractures or be part of a fracture. Repeated compression in extension and in flexion and shear with compression and rotation are most likely to cause meniscal injuries.

Particularly in running variations, such as cutting inside and outside, as well as with falls, twists, jumps, and deep-knee-bending with squatting, the posterior horns are impinged by the femoral condyles of the tibia as the latter drop back. Noncontact acceleration/deceleration injuries can produce torn menisci, particularly with twisting or repetitive sudden movements. Walking on uneven surfaces with twisting can cause such injuries in almost any sport in which wear and tear on articular cartilage can be demonstrated.

Increased patellofemoral joint compression is associated with damage to the patellofemoral joint. Degeneration in various stages will occur with "anterior knee pain" as a common complaint. Deformation with asynchronous patellar movement of all the aponeurotic attachments with their rich nerve supplies, with and without synovitis, can occur, although the articular cartilage itself is not painful. This often begins in adolescence. Jumping will irritate and twisting movements aggravate the pain. Persistent flexion in hamstring-calf contraction and hip flexion abductor-quadriceps weakness can also contribute to injury (Fig. 8). Quadriceps shortening increases patellofemoral compression in eccentric loading.

Poor patellar tracking and malalignment of the flexed knee in all axes contribute to knee pain ascribed to patellopathy. In growing children, long patellar tendons, excessive mobility, and apophysitis (Osgood-Schlatter disease) can cause pain.[52]

References

1. Akeson W, Amiel D, Woo SL-Y: Cartilage and ligaments: Physiology and repair process, in Nicholas JA, Hershman EB (eds): *The Lower Extremity and Spine in Sports Medicine.* St. Louis, CV Mosby, 1986, vol 1, pp 3–41.
2. Andriacchi TP, Kramer GM, Landon GC: The biomechanics of running and knee injuries, in Finerman G (ed): American Academy of Orthopaedic Surgeons *Symposium on Sports Medicine: The Knee.* St. Louis, CV Mosby, 1985, pp 23–32.
3. Brand RA: Knee ligaments: A new view. *J Biomech Eng* 1986;108:106–110.
4. Butler DL, Noyes FR, Grood ES: Ligamentous restraints to anterior-posterior drawer in the human knee: A biomechanical study. *J Bone Joint Surg* 1980;62A:259–270.

5. Cabaud HE, Chatty A, Gildengorin V, et al: Exercise effects on the strength of the rat anterior cruciate ligament. *Am J Sports Med* 1980;8:79–86.
6. Cabaud HE, Slocum DB: The diagnosis of chronic anterolateral rotary instability of the knee. *Am J Sports Med* 1977;5:99–105.
7. Carter DR, Frankel VH: Biomechanics of hyperextension injuries to the cervical spine in football. *Am J Sports Med* 1980;8:302–309.
8. Clancy WG Jr: Runners' injuries: Part 1. *Am J Sports Med* 1980;8:137–144.
9. Eichner ER: Does running cause osteoarthritis? An epidemiologic perspective. *Phys Sportsmed* 1989;17:147–154.
10. *The facts—Disease prevention and health promotion.* Office of Disease Prevention and Health Promotion, Public Health Service, US Department of Health and Human Services. Palo Alto, Brill Publishing, 1987.
11. Gainor BJ, Piotrowski G, Puhl J, et al: The throw: Biomechanics and acute injury. *Am J Sports Med* 1980;8:114–118.
12. Garrett WE Jr: Basic science of musculotendinous injuries, in Nicholas JA, Hershman EB (eds): *The Lower Extremity and Spine in Sports Medicine.* St. Louis, CV Mosby, 1986, vol 1, pp 42–58.
13. Garrett WE Jr, Almekinders LC, Seaber AV: Biomechanics of muscle tears in stretching injuries. *Trans Orthop Res Soc* 1984;9:384.
14. Garrett WE Jr, Tidball J: Myotendinous junction: Structure, function, and failure, in Woo SL-Y, Buckwalter JA (eds): *Injury and Repair of the Musculoskeletal Soft Tissues.* Park Ridge, Illinois, American Academy of Orthopaedic Surgeons, 1988, pp 171–207.
15. Gollehon DL, Torzilli PA, Warren RF: The role of the posterolateral and cruciate ligaments in the stability of the human knee: A biomechanical study. *J Bone Joint Surg* 1987;69A:233–242.
16. Grood ES, Noyes FR, Butler DL, et al: Ligamentous and capsular restraints preventing straight medial and lateral laxity in intact human cadaver knees. *J Bone Joint Surg* 1981;63A:1257–1269.
17. Grood ES, Stowers SF, Noyes FR: Limits of movement in the human knee: Effects of sectioning the posterior cruciate ligament and posterolateral structures. *J Bone Joint Surg* 1988;70A:88–97.
18. Hughston JC, Andrews JR, Cross MJ, et al: Classification of knee instabilities: Parts I and II. *J Bone Joint Surg* 1976:58A:159–179.
19. Hunter-Griffin LY (ed): Overuse injuries. *Clin Sports Med* 1987;6:1–470.
20. Jobe FW: Serious rotator cuff injuries. *Clin Sports Med* 1983;2:407–412.
21. Jobe FW, Perry J: The throwing mechanism, in Nicholas JA, Hershman EB (eds): *The Upper Extremity in Sports Medicine.* St. Louis, CV Mosby, in press.
22. Kennedy JC: Knee joint instability, in Nicholas JA: Report of the committee on research and education. *Am J Sports Med* 1978;6:295–306.
23. Kennedy JC: Orthopedic manifestations in swimming, in Erikson B, Furberg B (eds): *Medicine IV.* Stockholm, Swedish Medicine Press, 1978, pp 93–100.
24. Kennedy JC, Grainger RW: The posterior cruciate ligament. *J Trauma* 1967;7:367–377.
25. Kennedy JC, Roth JH, Mendenhall HV, et al: Intra-articular replacement in the anterior cruciate ligament-deficient knee: Presidential address. *Am J Sports Med* 1980;8:1–8.
26. Laros GS, Tipton CM, Cooper RR: Influence of physical activity on ligament insertions in the knees of dogs. *J Bone Joint Surg* 1971;53A:275–285.
27. Leach RE, James S, Wasilewski S: Achilles tendinitis. *Am J Sports Med* 1981;9:93–98.

28. Matheson GO, Clement DB, McKenzie DC, et al: Scintigraphic uptake of 99mTc at non-painful sites in athletes with stress fractures: The concept of bone strain. *Sports Med* 1987;4:65–75.
29. Nicholas JA: Acute and chronic lateral instabilities of the knee: Diagnosis, characteristics, and treatment, in Evarts CM (ed): American Academy of Orthopaedic Surgeons *Symposium on Reconstructive Surgery of the Knee.* St. Louis, CV Mosby, 1978, pp 187–206.
30. Nicholas JA: Injuries to knee ligaments: Relationship to looseness and tightness in football players. *JAMA* 1970;212:2236–2239.
31. Nicholas JA: Report of the committee on research and education. *Am J Sports Med* 1978;6:295–306.
32. Nicholas JA: Risk factors, sports medicine and the orthopedic system: An overview. *J Sports Med* 1975;3:243–259.
33. Nicholas JA: Sports medicine: Past, present, and future. *Am J Sports Med* 1980;8:389–394.
34. Nicholas JA: The five-one reconstruction for anteromedial instability of the knee: Indications, technique, and the results in fifty-two patients. *J Bone Joint Surg* 1973;55A:899–922.
35. Nicholas JA, Grossman RB, Hershman EB: The importance of a simplified classification of motion in sports in relation to performance. *Orthop Clin North Am* 1977;8:499–532.
36. Nicholas JA, Hershman EB (eds): Symposium on profiling. *Clin Sports Med* 1984;3:1–294.
37. Nicholas JA, Strizak A, Veras G: A study of thigh muscle weakness in different pathological states of the lower extremity. *Am J Sports Med* 1976;4:241–248.
38. Noyes FR: The Noyes knee rating system, in *Cincinnati Sports Medicine.* Cincinnati, Deaconess Hospital Sports Medicine and Cardiovascular Fitness Center, 1989.
39. *Orthopaedic Science: A Syllabus and Self-Study Guide for the Practitioner.* Park Ridge, Illinois, American Academy of Orthopaedic Surgeons, 1986, pp 134–182.
40. Pascale M, Grana WA: Does running cause osteoarthritis? An orthopedic perspective. *Phys Sportsmed* 1989;17:157–166.
41. Peterson L, Frankel VH: Biomechanics of the knee in athletes, in Nicholas JA, Hershman EB (eds): *The Lower Extremity and Spine in Sports Medicine.* St. Louis, CV Mosby, 1986, vol 1, pp 695–727.
42. Priest JD, Weise DJ: Elbow injury in women's gymnastics. *Am J Sports Med* 1981;9:288–295.
43. Richardson AB, Jobe FW, Collins HR: The shoulder in competitive swimming. *Am J Sports Med* 1980;8:159–163.
44. Slocum SD: The mechanics of some common injuries to the shoulder in sports. *Am J Surg* 1959;98:394–400.
45. Snyder RB, Lipscomb AB, Johnston RK: The relationship of tarsal coalitions to ankle sprains in athletes. *Am J Sports Med* 1981;9:313–317.
46. Steindler A: *Kinesiology of the Human Body Under Normal and Pathological Conditions.* Springfield, Charles C Thomas, 1955, pp 5–9.
47. Stulberg SD, Shulman K, Stuart S, et al: Breaststroker's knee: Pathology, etiology, and treatment. *Am J Sports Med* 1980;8:164–171.
48. Torg JS, Truex R Jr, Quedenfeld TC, et al: The National Football Head and Neck Injury Registry: Report and conclusions 1978. *JAMA* 1979;241:1477–1479.
49. Torzilli PA: Biomechanical analysis of knee stability, in Nicholas JA, Hershman EB (eds): *The Lower Extremity and Spine in Sports Medicine.* St. Louis, CV Mosby, 1986, vol 1, pp 728–764.

50. Tullos HS, King JW: Throwing mechanism in sports. *Orthop Clin North Am* 1973;4:709–720.
51. Weisman G, Pope MH, Johnson RJ: Cyclic loading in knee ligament injuries. *Am J Sports Med* 1980;8:24–30.
52. Whiteside JA, Fleagle SB, Kalenak A: Fractures and refractures in intercollegiate athletes: An eleven-year experience. *Am J Sports Med* 1981;9:369–377.
53. Wilkins KE: The uniqueness of the young athlete: Musculoskeletal injuries. *Am J Sports Med* 1980;8:377–382.

Chapter 6

Clinical Relevance of Sports-Induced Inflammation

Walton W. Curl, MD

The classic clinical manifestations of inflammation are swelling, increased temperature, erythema, pain, and loss of function. Unfortunately, they are not always reliable indicators of an underlying inflammatory condition, especially for chronic inflammation. Most inflammatory conditions, such as bursitis, synovitis, and tendinitis can be treated with rest, anti-inflammatory medications, and physical therapy modalities such as heat, ice, or ultrasound. The acute inflammatory response usually lasts for two or three days. The athlete can then resume protected activities. When the condition becomes chronic, however, the response to medication and physical therapy often diminishes and presents a more perplexing problem. Occasionally, surgery is needed to remove the inflamed tissues so that the chronic inflammatory process can heal, and the athlete can resume play.

Clinical Signs of Inflammation

Since 600 BC, physicians have known that swelling, increased warmth, erythema, pain, and loss of function are the characteristic signs of most inflammatory processes.[4] Only recently has the diagnostic significance of these classic signs been brought into question. Are swelling, increased warmth, erythema, pain, and loss of function always present with inflammation? Are they reliable indicators of the amount of inflammation present? In sports medicine, are they helpful in determining whether or not a person should be allowed to continue the sport? It has been stated that "pain should be interpreted as a warning sign of tissue injury, and should lead to a rest from activity."[6] Frequently pain, tenderness, and impaired function can prevent an athlete from performing at the highest level.

Inflammation occurring as the result of engaging in sports activities generally results from undue pressure on the soft tissue, friction between soft-tissue planes, repeated load or overload, or from external trauma.[6] A prolonged inflammatory condition can produce scar tissue that leads to decreased performance.

Pain is perhaps the most significant sign of inflammation and is often the athlete's presenting complaint. Generally, there is a high correlation between pain and the presence of inflammation; in fact, the presence or absence of pain is often the only indicator of the presence or absence of inflammation. How much inflammation is needed to produce pain is not known, but pain or tenderness usually signifies an underlying inflammatory response.

Athletic performance can be affected by several factors related to inflammation. Pain contributes to decreased performance by inhibiting the athlete's use of the inflamed area. This can lead to atrophy and weakness of the surrounding muscle, as well as to contracture of the involved soft tissue. As long as the inflammatory process continues, disuse is prolonged and performance suffers. Weakness and contracture can affect joint motion, leading to decreased performance and the possibility of further injury to the inflamed tissue and surrounding structures.

Performance and muscle strength can also be affected in other, more insidious ways. An effusion of the knee, for example, has a direct effect on quadriceps function[2] through the quadriceps reflex inhibition leading to disuse and atrophy. This increases the recovery time from injury because the weakened muscles must be rehabilitated before performance is resumed. An abnormal effusion in a joint from a traumatic hemarthrosis or synovial fluid has a deleterious effect on articular cartilage. The enzymatic components of the effusion contribute to cartilage breakdown, leading to an increased inflammatory response and setting the stage for a vicious cycle.

Although pain and altered function are the most common complaints of athletes with inflammation, other signs such as swelling, erythema, and increased warmth can sometimes be present by themselves. The presence of erythema, for example, implies an inflammatory response, but it is often difficult to determine the underlying cause of the erythema. Erythema without pain or swelling is not often associated with functional loss.

Increased warmth is a reliable indicator of an underlying inflammatory process, and when present, often correlates with an acute inflammatory process. However, in a chronic condition, increased warmth is not always present despite a significant loss of function. The absence of increased warmth does not indicate the absence of an inflammatory response.

Three areas of inflammation account for 80% to 90% of the inflammatory problems seen in sports medicine: bursitis; tendinitis and the inflammation of the peritendinous structures; and synovitis.

Bursitis

Bursitis can be classified into three categories. Septic bursitis caused by a bacterial infection usually results from an abrasion over a bursa that extends into the bursa, allowing bacterial contamination. Frictional bursitis can be caused by external trauma, such as rubbing of the shoe over the Achilles tendon. Chemical bursitis is generally caused by calcific or other material deposits in the bursa, usually through a metabolic process.[6]

The usual clinical presentation of bursitis includes swelling of the bursa, pain on motion of the joint, tenderness over the bursa, and erythema, which is generally accompanied by an increase in the temperature of the surrounding tissue. It may be difficult to differentiate septic, frictional, and chemical causes of an inflamed bursa. Often the inflammatory response can be dramatic, as in bursitis caused by direct trauma. The clinician cannot rule out septic bursitis, gout, or rheumatoid bursitis without aspirating the bursa.

The presence of bursitis, especially near nonweightbearing joints such as the olecranon bursa, does not generally prohibit participation in sports. It is necessary to protect the inflamed area and prevent aggravation, but often an individual with an inflamed bursa can play noncontact sports. In general, as the inflammation decreases in the bursa, the pain decreases and function increases. Anti-inflammatory medicines, aspiration, compression dressings, and heat can expedite resolution of the symptoms of acute bursitis. Generally, the tenderness and erythema of acute bursitis dissipate in one to two days but the swelling in the bursa may last for two to three weeks unless aspirated. While no real guidelines exist, to prevent repeated trauma to the bursa leading to a recurrent bursitis,[1] a person with bursitis should not return to play prematurely.

Recurrent or chronic bursitis can often be a problematic condition, especially in contact sports that subject the bursa to repetitive trauma. The bursa often has a thickened membrane, although, in general, chronic bursitis is not as painful as acute bursitis and it does not usually interfere with functioning. Recurrent bursitis generally does not respond as effectively as acute bursitis to conservative methods such as heat, anti-inflammatory medicines, and aspiration. Resection of the bursa is often needed to resolve the symptoms.

Synovitis

Synovitis is characterized by joint effusion, increased temperature, increased pain, and lack of erythema, and it generally interferes with the performance of the involved joint. Other clinical manifestations frequently seen with synovitis are pain on motion of the joint, pain on compression of the joint, as happens in the patellofemoral joint, and a synovial thickening that can be palpated in the joint, as in the synovial plica syndrome in the knee.

For most weightbearing joints, synovitis must be resolved almost completely before full activities can be resumed.[5] Quadriceps strength decreases with the presence of an effusion[6] and often, because of pain, an individual with synovitis cannot generate adequate force to maintain muscle strength. Aspiration of the joint may restore full, painless range of motion, and rehabilitation can increase muscle strength. During aspiration, all possible fluid is withdrawn from the joint to ameliorate the symptoms. Acute synovitis without a known history of trauma generally requires joint aspiration to rule out problems such as a hemarthrosis, infection, or a metabolic disorder such as gout. As the synovitis becomes more severe, function generally decreases, pain increases, and recurrent effusions become more common.

Recurrent synovitis of a joint may require a synovectomy to resolve the symptoms. However, synovitis in a joint can be secondary to multiple causes. In the knee, synovitis may be secondary to a torn meniscus, an osteochondral defect, a torn anterior cruciate ligament, a synovial plica, or a subluxating patella. In the shoulder, it may be secondary to a torn glenoid labrum or a rotator cuff impingement causing an inflammation of the underlying synovium in the glenohumeral joint. If the cause is found and resolved, the synovitis also subsides without any direct intervention to the synovium. A synovectomy may have to be performed in rare cases of recurrent synovitis that are recalcitrant to other types of treatment.

Tendinitis and Tenosynovitis

Tendinitis and tenosynovitis are common problems in sports medicine. They have been classified into three categories[8]: (1) Tenosynovitis and tenovaginitis: Inflammation of only the paratenon, whether or not a synovial lining is present. (2) Tendinitis: Injury or degeneration of the tendon resulting in an inflammatory reaction in the surrounding paratenon. Tendinitis may be acute (symptoms present for less than two weeks), subacute (symptoms present for two to six weeks), or chronic (symptoms present for six weeks or longer). Chronic tendon injuries may range from interstitial failure to complete tendon rupture. (3) Tendinosis: Asymptomatic tendon degeneration caused by aging or accumulated microtrauma, or both. These may also involve interstitial, partial, or complete ruptures.

Tenosynovitis

Tenosynovitis involves an inflammation of the tendon sheath when a true synovial lining is present, as occurs where the abductor pollicis longus and extensor pollicis brevis tendons cross in their tendon sheath and cause an inflammation known as de Quervain's syndrome.[7] A familiar clinical sign of tenosynovitis is crepitus along the tendon sheath with movement of the joint. Tenosynovitis is generally caused by overuse of the tendon, leading to inflammation and irritation of the tendon sheath.

Septic or suppurative tenosynovitis is classically characterized by Kanavel's cardinal signs: tenderness over the involved tendon sheath, pain on hyperextending the finger, flexion deformity, and fusiform swelling of the finger.[3] Septic tenosynovitis must be treated aggressively with antibiotics and surgical intervention to drain the tendon sheath of the purulent material. Without treatment the tendon sheath may scar, resulting in loss of function of the involved finger.

Tendinitis

Tendinitis generally occurs at the place where the tendon inserts into the bone. It is also called "tenoperiostitis" or an "enthesopathy."[7] There are many classifications of tendinitis. Patellar tendinitis, for example, has been divided into four phases, with phase 1 characterized by increasing pain and phase 4 by a complete disruption of the tendon.[1] Tendinitis is the most common inflammation about the tendons. It includes lateral epicondylitis or "tennis elbow," patellar tendinitis, or "jumper's knee," and plantar fasciitis, or "heel spurs." In these types of tendinitis, the player becomes more debilitated as the inflammation increases. Tendinitis can often be treated with anti-inflammatory medicine and heat before practice and ice afterwards to ameliorate some symptoms. Taping or bracing can also help to support the soft tissue and to retain some warmth about the tendon during workouts.

Recurrent tendinitis is particularly troublesome. Conservative measures are often unsuccessful in controlling recurrent tendinitis while the patient continues to play or work out. Surgery is recommended in some cases, such as jumper's knee and tennis elbow, to debride the chronically inflamed tissue. However, surgical exploration may not demonstrate an area of inflammation. It may be that surgically incising inflamed tendons produces a vascular response and induces an acute inflammatory response that eliminates a chronic inflammatory process. Inflammation of tendons, bursae, and synovia often produce few clinical findings. Tendinitis can be insidious in its onset; chronic patellar tendinitis, for example, can last for years, with only two clinical findings—tenderness directly over the patellar tendon and pain on extreme exercise such as running up and down stairs. For the most part, however, there is a high correlation between the physical signs of tenderness, pain, swelling, and erythema and the clinical symptoms of inflammation. Generally, when the physical signs diminish, the clinical symptoms also disappear.

References

1. Boland AL Jr: Soft tissue injuries of the knee, in Nicholas JA, Hershman EB (eds): *The Lower Extremity and Spine in Sports Medicine*. St. Louis, CV Mosby, 1986, vol 1, pp 983–1012.
2. Fahrer H, Rentsch HU, Gerber NJ, et al: Knee effusion and reflex inhibition of the quadriceps: A bar to effective retraining. *J Bone Joint Surg* 1988;70B:635–638.
3. Flynn JE: *Hand Surgery*. Baltimore, Williams & Wilkins, 1975, p 498.
4. Majno G: Infection: Inflammation and historic highlights, in Majno G, Cotran RS, Kaufman N (eds): *Current Topics in Inflammation and Infection*. Baltimore, Williams & Wilkins, 1982, p 1.
5. O'Donoghue DH: *Treatment of Injuries to Athletes*. Philadelphia, WB Saunders, 1976, p 661.
6. Peterson L, Renstrom P: *Sports Injuries: Their Prevention and Treatment*. Chicago, Year Book Medical Publishers, 1986, pp 42–48.

7. Williams JGP, Sperryn PN (eds): *Sports Medicine*, ed 2. Baltimore, Williams & Wilkins, 1976, pp 285–286.
8. Xethalis JL, Boiardo RA: Soccer injuries, in Nicholas JA, Hershman EB (eds): *The Lower Extremity and Spine in Sports Medicine*. St. Louis, CV Mosby, 1986, vol 2, p 1632.

Chapter 7

Clinical Methods of Measuring Inflammation

W. Michael Walsh, MD
Michele Helzer-Julin, MS, PA-C

Physicians and patients speak of inflammation in joints (arthritis, synovitis), soft tissues (tendinitis, bursitis), and internal organs (cholecystitis, meningitis). Yet, the inflammatory process resists accurate clinical quantification. How severe is the inflammation? What scale or meter for measurement is used? How practical is it to quantitate the inflammation? Clinical tests can measure severity of inflammation in internal organs as, for example, the use of serum amylase levels to detect pancreatitis. To detect inflammation in synovial joints, rheumatologists and orthopaedists resort to techniques based on physical examination alone. For soft-tissue inflammation, however, no single, practical technique measures the severity of inflammation when the soft tissue is injured or after the injury has been treated.

This chapter focuses on current and emerging techniques available to the clinician that may help in this regard. Two conceptual models are used: articular inflammation, as in the knee joint, and nonarticular soft-tissue inflammation, as in Achilles tendinitis.

The available methods of quantitation include physical examination, laboratory analysis, histologic examination, imaging techniques, and some miscellaneous techniques.

Physical Examination

The physical examination to detect inflammation focuses on the classic signs of inflammatory change: swelling, increased temperature, tenderness/pain, and redness of the overlying skin. Changes in temperature and skin color may be subtle. Skin erythema may be difficult to determine in dark-skinned persons. Temperature changes are best quantified by simple comparison with the temperature of the opposite extremity. The back of the examiner's hand may be the most effective detector of subtle temperature changes.

Swelling, tenderness, and limited motion (with joint involvement) are reliable indicators of inflammation. The inflammation may be "quantified" and tracked by systematic documentation of the degree

Table 1 "Quantification" of inflammation

Indicator	Physical Findings
Swelling	
S_1	Not apparent to the casual examiner
$S_{2,3,4}$	Increasing degrees of visible distension or thickening of synovial membrane
Tenderness	
T_1	Slight discomfort with palpation
T_2	Severe discomfort with normal palpation
T_3	Intolerable pain even with light palpation
T_4	Pain caused by mild stimulation (blowing onto skin, light touch, vibration of footsteps)
Loss of motion	
L_1	25%
L_2	50%
L_3	75%
L_4	100%

of each indicator. In the past, scale gradations ranged from 0 to 10. The current trend is toward a smaller scale, such as 0 to 4. A typical scheme might determine the degree of swelling, tenderness, and loss of motion, by using a quantitative scale of 0 through 4, with 0 as normal and 4 as maximally abnormal.[1] These gradations have a degree of subjectivity, but are still useful. Each indicator can then be quantified. Plus and minus signs can also be used for more exact gradations (Table 1).

Assessing tenderness, in particular, requires a great deal of subjective judgment. Patients' responses to local palpation vary greatly. To eliminate some of this subjectivity, a device known as a "dolorimeter" was developed. It consists of a pressure gauge attached to a tip and is used to apply direct pressure in patients with fibromyalgia. The gauge indicates the degree of pressure, but the pain level depends on the patient's subjective reporting, so even this involves a great deal of variability.

The patient can also report on the tenderness/pain component of inflammation. There are a number of visual analog scales that can be used for evaluating response in any given individual patient.

Laboratory Analysis

Not all pathologic products of inflammation are filtered out through the lymph tissues. Some products escape phagocytosis, and others are reabsorbed directly into the bloodstream. Thus, local inflammation may cause such systemic effects as fever, leukocytosis, and an elevated erythrocyte sedimentation rate (ESR).[11] These characterize the generalized effects of inflammation caused by infection or tissue damage and may aid in tracking and quantifying inflammation.

Fever is defined as a body temperature above 37 C, although the normal fluctuation may exceed 37 C. Fever is most commonly used to detect an infectious process, but it can indicate inflammation as well. The extent of temperature elevation generally reflects the severity of the infection or the inflammation. Body temperature has never been practical for measuring soft-tissue inflammation, but a more sensitive measurement technique such as the basal body temperature measurements used in infertility work might have some promise.

Alterations in leukocyte counts may also reflect the severity of inflammation. Normal leukocyte values may vary from laboratory to laboratory, but generally the greater the leukocytosis, the more severe the inflammation. However, no useful application of this analysis has been found for assessing sports-induced soft-tissue inflammation.

Although an ESR is most frequently used to evaluate inflammatory autoimmune diseases, it may be of some value in assessing inflammation secondary to tissue damage. Generally, the degree of elevation in the ESR correlates with the degree of inflammation. In the absence of clinical symptoms, however, an elevated ESR cannot be used as a reliable marker for inflammation.

Synovial fluid analysis is another method used to detect various forms of inflammation within a joint. The synovial fluid reflects alterations in the synovial tissue and intra-articular metabolism, and is therefore useful in detecting the presence of inflammation and in differentiating nontraumatic joint disease from traumatic arthritis.[10] Examination of the synovial fluid should yield information concerning the degree of inflammation in the synovium. However, this technique is inappropriate for a nonarticular soft-tissue inflammation such as that seen in Achilles tendinitis.

Histologic Examination

Histologic examination of soft tissue can prove or disprove the presence of inflammation. Biopsy can also differentiate between acute and chronic forms of inflammation. Depending on the stage and duration of inflammation, various forms and quantities of leukocytes appear. Macrophages and neutrophils appear in acute inflammation and persist throughout chronic inflammation. Plasma cells, eosinophils, and granulation tissue also appear in chronic inflammation.[4] Despite its diagnostic value, biopsy is invasive and uncomfortable and repeated biopsies might significantly weaken structures. As a result, current biopsy techniques are not practically applicable for grading the degree or amount of inflammation.

Imaging Techniques

Roentgenograms

The value of conventional radiography in demonstrating inflammation is limited. Soft-tissue swelling and effusions can be detected in many instances; however, a system for estimating the degree of inflammation is limited. Bone erosions are a specific radiologic sign that may indicate advanced or severe inflammation. A semiquantitative radiologic scale of 0 to 2 has been used to assess the overall severity of inflammatory changes, with 0 equaling no change, 1 indicating mild changes, and 2 indicating severe soft-tissue swelling, with or without bone alterations.[16]

Thermography

Soft-tissue trauma and inflammation can easily be detected and quantified by thermographic imaging.[12,14] After a soft-tissue injury, the vascular and metabolic systems alter the rate at which heat is generated at the site of injury, or the rate at which heat is transferred to and from the site. This changes the "normal" surface temperature distribution.

Joint inflammation, myositis, tenosynovitis, and tendinitis can be detected and monitored by thermography in a cold ambient temperature. After the body has adapted to an ambient temperature of 18 C, the increased convective heat transport from the body core can be quantified by several parameters that provide a method for monitoring inflammation and the effect of anti-inflammatory therapy.[8,9]

Under standard conditions, thermography is a valuable means of monitoring inflammation. The measurements are very sensitive. Healthy people exhibit symmetric thermal patterns. Research has shown that an asymmetry of 1 C is definitely abnormal.[8]

In the past, this technique has been criticized because an objective interpretation of the colored thermogram was lacking.[5] Newer techniques of computer-assisted calculation of temperature asymmetries may provide a means of objective and quantitative analysis, defining thermal asymmetry on the basis of a statistical criterion derived from the normal temperature difference for a specific area.[14,17,18]

Magnetic Resonance Imaging

The musculoskeletal system is particularly well-suited to study by magnetic resonance imaging because of its wide range of soft-tissue contrast.[15,16] Magnetic resonance imaging has an advantage over plain radiography because of its reproducibility and its ability to image soft-tissue changes.[2] Magnetic resonance imaging is valuable in identifying extra-articular structures such as muscles, tendons, and ligaments, and the various components of synovium, cartilage, and effusions.[3]

Magnetic resonance imaging can detect early soft-issue changes in rheumatoid arthritis more frequently than either conventional radiography or physical examination.[2,13,16] The goal of magnetic resonance imaging is not to make the diagnosis of rheumatoid arthritis, but to assess the extent of inflammation as manifested in the soft tissue and bone.[2] Magnetic resonance imaging can detect foci of inflammation in the synovial membrane.[16] Some quantification of the severity of the proliferative process seems possible, since diffuse inflammation shows characteristically different magnetic paramaters when compared with focal inflammation.

Research studies have developed a method of grading the severity of inflammatory lesions in joints on the basis of magnetic resonance imaging: grade 0, no detectable inflammatory lesion; grade I, local inflammatory lesion involving less than a cross-sectional area; grade II, diffuse inflammatory lesion; and grade III, late-stage arthritis. Magnetic resonance imaging can also quantify the volume of synovial fluid in joint effusions.

Magnetic resonance imaging is clearly superior to the other soft-tissue imaging techniques, and its future diagnostic possibilities for inflammation are promising. Studies are currently underway to evaluate whether paramagnetic contrast agents can further increase the usefulness of magnetic resonance imaging in arthritis. If magnetic resonance imaging can be used to quantify synovitis and relate it to the progression of erosions, it may yield significant information useful in treating rheumatologic disorders. It would also prove invaluable in tracking the effect or response to nonsteroidal anti-inflammatory drugs.

Ultrasonography

Some reports describe the use of diagnostic ultrasound to detect and quantify effusion within joints.[7] However, thus far its role has been limited, and it does not seem to have any current practical application in the clinical setting.

Miscellaneous Techniques

Magnetic resonance imaging proton spectroscopy can identify the presence or absence of specific metabolites in human tissues.[6] Most of the current literature deals with tumor work. Some reported extensions of this technique may prove useful in monitoring soft-tissue inflammation. However, from the practical standpoint, this technology is not yet usable.

Transcutaneous Po_2 measurements have been used for other purposes in orthopaedics and may be helpful in assessing soft-tissue inflammation. However, a practical application of this technique could not be found in the literature.

References

1. Beetham WP Jr, Polley HF, Slocumb CH, et al: *Physical Examination of the Joints.* Philadelphia, WB Saunders, 1965.
2. Beltran J, Caudill JL, Herman LA, et al: Rheumatoid arthritis: MR imaging manifestations. *Radiology* 1987;165:153–157.
3. Beltran J, Noto AM, Herman LJ, et al: Joint effusions: MR imaging. *Radiology* 1986;158:133–137.
4. Borysenko M, Beringer T: *Functional Histology,* ed 2. Boston, Little, Brown, 1984.
5. Frymoyer JW, Haugh LD: Thermography: A call for scientific studies to establish its diagnostic efficacy. *Orthopedics* 1986;9:699–700.

6. Kirn TF: Magnetic resonance spectroscopy may hold promise in studying metabolites, tissues. *JAMA* 1989;261:1103–1107.
7. Miralles M, Gonzalez G, Pulpeiro JR, et al: Sonography of the painful hip in children: 500 consecutive cases. *AJR* 1989;152:579–582.
8. Pochaczevsky R: Thermography in posttraumatic pain. *Am J Sports Med* 1987;15:243–250.
9. Ring EFJ, Phillips B (eds): International Congress of Thermology: *Recent Advances in Medical Thermology.* New York, Plenum Press, 1984.
10. Ropes MW, Bauer W: *Synovial Fluid Changes in Joint Disease.* Cambridge, Harvard University Press, 1953.
11. Ryan GB, Majno G: *Inflammation.* Kalamazoo, Upjohn Co, 1977.
12. Schumacher HR, Gall EP (eds): *Rheumatoid Arthritis: An Illustrated Guide To Pathology, Diagnosis, and Management.* Philadelphia, JB Lippincott, 1988.
13. Senac MO Jr, Deutsch D, Bernstein BH, et al: MR imaging in juvenile rheumatoid arthritis. *AJR* 1988;150:873–878.
14. Siegel MG, Siqueland KA, Noyes FR: The use of computerized thermography in the evaluation of non-traumatic anterior knee pain. *Orthopedics* 1987;10:825–830.
15. Sinclair HD: The attraction of magnetic resonance imaging. *Br J Rheumatol* 1988;27:68–71.
16. Terrier F, Hricak H, Revel D, et al: Magnetic resonance imaging and spectroscopy of the periarticular inflammatory soft-tissue changes in experimental arthritis of the rat. *Invest Radiol* 1985;20:813–823.
17. Uematsu S, Edwin DH, Jankel WR, et al: Quantification of thermal asymmetry: Part 1. Normal values and reproducibility. *J Neurosurg* 1988;69:552–555.
18. Uematsu S, Jankel WR, Edwin DH, et al: Quantification of thermal asymmetry: Part 2. Application in low-back pain and sciatica. *J Neurosurg* 1988;69:556–561.

Chapter 8

The Collagens of Musculoskeletal Soft Tissues

David R. Eyre, PhD

Introduction

Collagens form a critical matrix component of the musculoskeletal soft tissues. They give these tissues their basic form and tensile strength. They may be among the first matrix components to be damaged in sports-related injuries, and this molecular damage may contribute to sports-related soft-tissue inflammation. Failure to restore the matrix collagen framework after injury leaves the tissue weaker, whereas excessive collagen production after injury leaves the tissue stiffer and less mobile.

This chapter briefly reviews current knowledge of the structure, organization, and metabolism of collagen in musculoskeletal soft tissues. Changes in collagen metabolism that might result from or cause inflammation related to sports-induced injury are also considered.

Soft-Tissue Collagens—Current Concepts

Genetic Types

Thirteen types of collagen molecules, based on the products of more than 20 distinct genes, have now been named (Table 1).[13,21,38] By definition, each of these collagens counts as a structural protein in the extracellular matrix and has the collagen triple-helix structure for a major portion of its molecular conformation. (Other collagenous proteins that circulate or are less obviously structural, such as C1q, acetylcholinesterase, conglutinin, mannose-binding protein, and lung-surfactant protein, are not included in this table.)

The structural collagens can be grouped into subclasses based on their molecular topology and polymeric form. The most readily definable class, class 1, consists of those molecules that can form the typical banded fibrils seen in virtually all connective tissues.[24] Five molecular types are known in this group (types I, II, III, V, and XI) and all share essentially the same molecular form, which is a triple-helix domain

Table 1 Types of collagen

Type	Tissue	Polymeric Form
Class 1 (300-nm triple-helix)		
Type I	Skin, bone, etc	Banded fibril
Type II	Cartilage, disk	Banded fibril
Type III	Skin, blood vessels	Banded fibril
Type V	With type I	Banded fibril
Type XI (1α, 2α, 3α)	With type II	Banded fibril
Class 2 (basement membranes)		
Type IV	Basal lamina	Three-dimensional network
Type VII	Epithelial basement membrane	Anchoring fibril
Type VIII	Endothelial basement membrane	Unknown
Class 3 (short-chain)		
Type VI	Widespread	Microfilaments, 110-nm banded aggregates
Type IX	Cartilage (with type II)	Cross-linked to type II
Type X	Hypertrophic cartilage	Unknown
Type XII	Tendon, other?	Unknown
Type XIII	Endothelial cells	Unknown

composed of about 1,014 amino acid residues in each of the three polypeptide chains. Types I, II, and III make up the bulk of the collagen in the body. Type II is restricted to hyaline cartilage, the intervertebral disk, and the vitreous humor of the eye. Types V and XI are so-called "minor" fibrillar collagens. Type V is also distributed in small amounts (about 3% of type I) wherever type I collagen appears, and type XI is similarly distributed with type II collagen. Recent evidence suggests that hybrid molecules containing chains of both types V and XI collagens may also occur in bone and cartilage.[31] No distinguishing function linked to molecular structure is known for any of these fibrillar collagens. It is clear, however, that type I collagen is the structural workhorse of vertebrate connective tissue and predominates in all the tissues, apart from cartilage, under consideration in this chapter. Type III always occurs in association with type I collagen, possibly polymerized in the same fibrils,[19] and is present in most connective tissues, other than bone, that contain type I collagen. Its content can vary, however, with tissue type and stage of tissue maturity. For example, it is more enriched in developing dermis than in adult dermis.[5]

The remaining collagens can be lumped in a second class or subdivided somewhat arbitrarily into two classes, as shown in Table 1. Type IV collagen is the major structural component of basement membranes. Types VII and VIII can be grouped with it based on their apparent functions as an anchor filament (type VII)[34] or as a structural component (type VIII)[18] of certain types of basement membrane.

The short-helix collagens are the least understood molecules in terms of their individual polymeric forms and functions in the extracellular matrix. Little is known about evolutionary or functional relationships

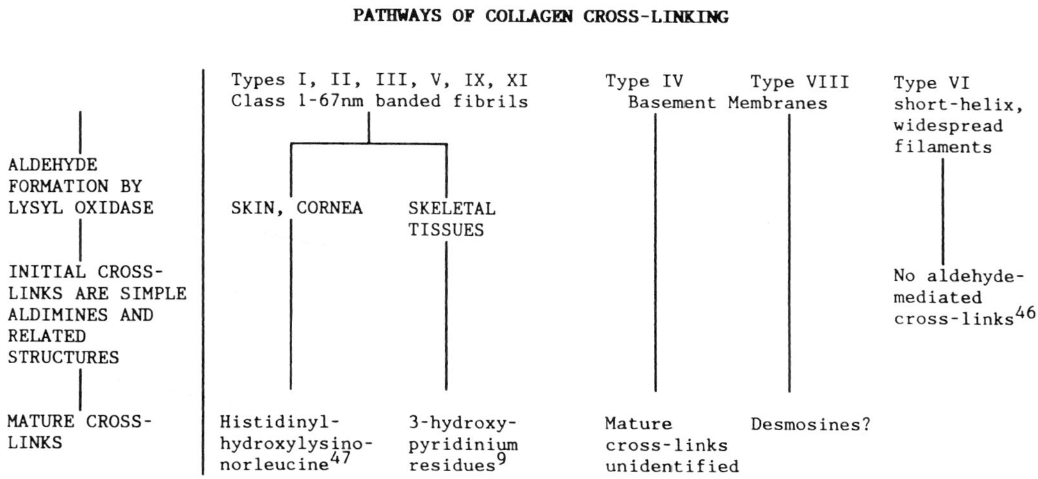

Fig. 1 *Summary overview of differences in intermolecular cross-linking evident among collagen types and between tissues for the same types of collagen.*

between these molecules. Some types are highly restricted in tissue distribution. For example, type X collagen appears exclusively in the calcified cartilage zones of the epiphyseal plate,[35] articular cartilage,[35] and bone fracture callus.[14] Other types are more widely distributed; type VI collagen, for example, appears in small amounts as filamentous material enriched around cells and between the banded collagen fibrils of most soft connective tissues.[39] Type VI collagen is, however, enriched in certain tissues, including the intervertebral disk[46] and the cornea.[48] It appears to act as a structural element between the cells and the matrix of soft connective tissues, and seems most concentrated in those tissues that readily deform as part of their normal functioning. Increased amounts of type VI collagen have been noted in inflamed skin,[12] in skin with certain forms of Ehlers-Danlos syndrome, and in the articular cartilage of patients with osteoarthrosis.[12,22]

Tissue-Specific Differences in Collagen Chemistry

The mechanical strength of the common collagens stems from the formation of two or three covalent intermolecular bonds (cross-links) per collagen molecule. Even though type I collagen predominates in all the musculoskeletal soft tissues (synovium, muscle, tendon, ligament) except cartilage, its posttranslational chemistry, particularly in the chemical type and extent of its intermolecular cross-linking, varies among tissues. The type and content of mature intermolecular cross-links in type I collagen seem to vary in a tissue-specific manner. Skin, cornea (Fig. 1), and rat-tail tendon have collagens that are largely cross-linked by lysine-derived aldehydes, whereas skeletal connective tissues use a pathway largely based on hydroxylysine-derived aldehydes.[9] Cross-links based on both pathways can be seen in some soft-connective tissues, such as tendon and muscle.[30,36] Tendons that transmit the highest forces in the body have the highest concentrations of trivalent, hydroxypyridinium cross-links compared with low-loadbearing tendons.[7] This finding has been corroborated in unpublished observations. Similarly, ligaments that bear high loads, such as the anterior cruciate ligament of the knee, contain the highest levels of such cross-links in any tissue samples of type I collagen (unpublished observations). Other tissues that dissipate or transmit high mechanical forces, such as fibrocartilages (knee meniscus, intervertebral disk), are also rich in mature hydroxypyridinium forms of collagen cross-linking amino acid.[7]

In summary, emerging data suggest that the quality of collagen cross-linking is associated with the degree of mechanical loading experienced by a particular skeletal connective tissue. This posttranslational protein quality is governed by the activity of intracellular enzymes responsible for processing the newly synthesized collagen polypeptide chains in the rough endoplasmic reticulum. This implies regulation of the chemical quality of the cross-linking in newly made collagen by a feedback control mechanism based on the mechanical loading experienced by the tissue during growth and development and perhaps even during adult remodeling of individual connective tissues.

Synovial membrane is rich in type III collagen. Nearly equal amounts of types I and III collagens have been recovered by pepsin from normal and rheumatoid human synovial-lining tissue.[8] Unpublished observations by Wu and Eyre indicate that type VI collagen may also be prominent in synovium. The significance of this finding is unknown, as no function has yet been defined for this protein. It is not covalently cross-linked by aldehyde-mediated bonds in the way that other collagens are.[46] This suggests that the polymeric filaments it forms in the extracellular matrix may be susceptible to disruption when connective tissues are strained mechanically. Thus, a speculative hypothesis is that type VI collagen can act as a "natural strain gauge" for cells in the matrix.

Supramolecular Assembly

Recent data based on studies of cartilage indicate that certain collagen types interact specifically with other fibrillar forms of collagen to create covalent, heterotypic polymers. Thus, type IX collagen, which is both a short-helix collagen and a proteoglycan molecule, exists exclusively in the extracellular matrix of cartilage and is covalently linked to the surface of type II collagen fibrils (Fig. 2).[6,28,40,41] It may function to couple the fibrils together mechanically and so form a cohesive network[6,45] or to link the fibrils to other components of the extracellular matrix.[28] It seems likely that other molecules, including the newly

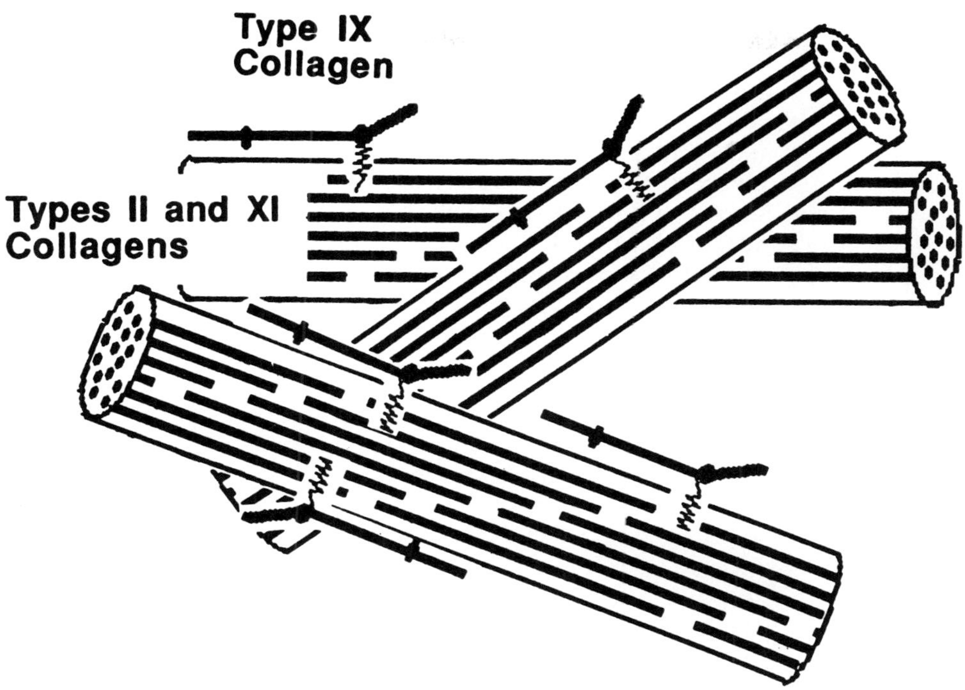

Fig. 2 *The distribution of collagen type IX molecules covalently linked to the surface of type II/type XI collagen fibrils in the extracellular matrix of hyaline cartilages.*

discovered collagen type XII,[13] may play related roles in skin, tendon, ligament, and other tissues.[4] Evidence also indicates that type V and type I collagen molecules may copolymerize to form hybrid fibrils,[2] as may type XI and type II collagens.[23] The exact form and purpose of such hybrid polymeric structures are still unknown.

In general, little is known about the molecular regulation of collagen polymer formation, the control of collagen fibril diameters, and the regulation of interactions and spatial relationships between fibrils. Perhaps there is a range of tissue-specific adhesion molecules, molecular lubricants, and flexible tethers that give each type of connective tissue the desired material properties. It will be important to define the molecular basis of the mechanical coupling of tendon collagen fibers to skeletal muscle fibers,[11] and of tendon, ligament, and capsule-insertion sites into bone,[44] because these are often the sites of traumatic injury and repetitive loading injuries.

Degradation and Turnover

Turnover rates of collagen in adult connective tissues are poorly documented. Bone turns over rapidly; articular cartilage collagen turns over slowly. Beyond these documented extremes, surprisingly little is known about the collagenous matrices of other connective tissues, such as tendon, ligament, capsule, fascia, and synovium. Knowing the turnover rates of skeletal soft-tissue collagens is important because outside influences (chronic mechanical overuse, stimulating cytokines and growth factors, and other inflammatory mediators) may alter the composition and properties of adult connective tissue that is remodeling at a significant rate.

Prolonged exercise results in a significant increase in two collagen markers in serum, type III collagen N-propeptide and the enzyme galactosylhydroxylysine glucosyltransferase.[37] This may be caused by injury to the connective tissue cells of the muscle-fascia-tendon complex, resulting in a short-term increase in type III collagen synthesis.

Collagen in Inflammation

Orthopaedic surgeons frequently divide patients into two categories: those with "stiff" shoulder joints and thickened, tough capsular collagen and those with lax joints and thin, weak capsular collagen. The "tight" patient often has diabetes and the stiff connective tissue may be a secondary effect of the disease, caused by increased cross-linking of collagen by an emerging nonenzymatic glycosylation mechanism.[26] In contrast, there is no clear explanation for "lax" patients. Some may have systemic laxity in their supporting tissues, suggesting a genetically based variation in their underlying connective tissue chemistry (perhaps mild variants of the Ehlers-Danlos syndrome). Others have no obvious systemic laxity. Clues about the underlying basis for such gross variations in supporting tissue anatomy and mechanical properties might come from seeking polymorphisms of structural collagen genes in the human population and from understanding rare inborn disorders of connective tissue (Ehlers-Danlos syndromes) and disorders resulting in connective tissue fibroses (systemic sclerosis).

Interleukin-1, which appears to play a key role in all inflammatory conditions, can directly affect the rates of synthesis and degradation of collagen by fibroblasts. Interleukin-1 alpha and beta increase the steady-state levels of the pro $\alpha 1$(I) and pro $\alpha 2$(I) mRNAs in fibroblasts, and so control the rate of collagen synthesis pretranslationally.[3] Two studies showed that interleukin-1 alpha and beta also stimulated synthesis of TIMP (a protein inhibitor of the metalloproteinases that is widely distributed in connective tissues), collagenase,[25] prostaglandin E_2,[25] and the growth of fibroblasts in vitro. In summary, therefore, interleukin-1 may be important in both collagen degradation and collagen formation at sites of tissue injury. How a natural interplay might be managed between these two seemingly conflicting effects of interleukin-1 remains to be seen.

Fibrotic Responses

An overdeposition of collagenous tissue is the cardinal feature of scleroderma (progressive systemic sclerosis). Studies of the disorder have focused on a faulty control of collagen production by the affected fibroblasts, resulting in their production of more collagen than by control cells.[20] Elevated levels of mRNA for the type I collagen proα1(I) chain have been reported.[17] Other reports indicate that certain lymphokines can inhibit the elevated collagen production of scleroderma fibroblasts.[16] The production and nature of the excess collagenous tissue formed in hypertrophic skin scars have also been studied. These results may help in understanding the fibrotic changes in skeletal soft-connective tissues after injury and in inflammation.[3,15,27]

Collagenolytic Responses

A family of neutral metalloproteinases is responsible for the degradation of extracellular collagens, proteoglycans, and associated matrix proteins during normal tissue growth and remodeling and during inflammatory responses to injury. These enzymes, which include tissue collagenase, stromelysin (identical to transin expressed by transformed fibroblasts), and gelatinase, are now being called matrix metalloendoproteinases. (MMP1 is collagenase, MMP2 is gelatinase, and MMP3 is stromelysin.[1,10,29,32,42,43])

A variety of cytokines and growth factors are known to affect the expression of these enzymes by fibroblasts, macrophages, polymorphonuclear leukocytes, and tumor cells. Their activities are also broadly controlled by TIMP. The major collagenolytic cathepsin, cathepsin L, is another secreted protease that may be responsible for connective tissue degradation and remodeling at inflammation sites.[32] Understanding how these degradative enzymes are coordinately regulated at sites of tissue injury and during remodeling in response to altered mechanical loading patterns is key to understanding collagen changes in injured and aging connective tissues.

References

1. Bejarano PA, Noelken ME, Suzuki K, et al: Degradation of basement membranes by human matrix metalloproteinase 3 (stromelysin). *Biochem J* 1988;256:413–419.
2. Birk DE, Fitch JM, Babiarz JP, et al: Collagen type I and type V are present in the same fibril in the avian corneal stroma. *J Cell Biol* 1988;106:999–1008.
3. Clore JN, Cohen IK, Diegelmann RF: Quantitative assay of types I and III collagen synthesized by keloid biopsies and fibroblasts. *Biochim Biophys Acta* 1979;586:384–390.
4. Dublet B, Dixon E, de Miguel E, et al: Bovine type XII collagen: Amino acid sequence of a 10 kDa pepsin fragment from periodontal ligament reveals a high degree of homology with the chicken alpha 1(XII) sequence. *FEBS Lett* 1988;233:177–180.
5. Epstein EH Jr: (Alpha 1(3))3 human skin collagen: Release by pepsin digestion and preponderance in fetal life. *J Clin Invest* 1974;53:3225–3231.
6. Eyre DR, Apone S, Wu JJ, et al: Collagen type IX: Evidence for covalent linkages to type II collagen in cartilage. *FEBS Lett* 1987;220:337–341.

7. Eyre DR, Koob TJ, Van Ness KP: Quantitation of hydroxypyridinium crosslinks in collagen by high-performance liquid chromatography. *Anal Biochem* 1984;137:380–388.
8. Eyre DR, Muir H: Type-III collagen in synovium, letter. *Lancet* 1975;2:609–610.
9. Eyre DR, Paz MA, Gallop PM: Cross-linking in collagen and elastin. *Annu Rev Biochem* 1984;53:717–748.
10. Frisch SM, Clark JE, Werb Z: Coordinate regulation of stromelysin and collagenase genes determined with cDNA probes. *Proc Natl Acad Sci USA* 1987;84:2600–2604.
11. Garrett W Jr, Tidball J: Myotendinous junction: Structure, function, and failure, in Woo SL-Y, Buckwalter JA (eds): *Injury and Repair of the Musculoskeletal Soft Tissues.* Park Ridge, Illinois, American Academy of Orthopaedic Surgeons, 1988, pp 171–207.
12. Garrone R, Tiollier J: Type VI collagen and inflammation, in Bienveu, Grimaud, Laurent (eds): *Marker Proteins in Inflammation, Volume 3.* Berlin, Walter de Gruyter & Co, 1986, pp 357–361.
13. Gordon MK, Gerecke DR, Olsen BR: Type XII collagen: Distinct extracellular matrix component discovered by cDNA cloning. *Proc Natl Acad Sci USA* 1987;84:6040–6044.
14. Grant WT, Wang GJ, Balian G: Type X collagen synthesis during endochondral ossification in fracture repair. *J Biol Chem* 1987;262:9844–9849.
15. Hembry RM, Ehrlich HP: Immunolocalization of collagenase and tissue inhibitor of metalloproteinases (TIMP) in hypertrophic scar tissue. *Br J Dermatol* 1986;115:409–420.
16. Jimenez SA, McArthur WM, Bashey RI, et al: Selective inhibition of excessive scleroderma fibroblast collagen production by lymphokines from normal human mononuclear cells. *Arthritis Rheum* 1985;28:502–510.
17. Kähäri VM, Multimäki P, Vuorio E: Elevated pro alpha 2(I) collagen mRNA levels in cultured scleroderma fibroblasts result from an increased transcription rate of the corresponding gene. *FEBS Lett* 1987;215:331–334.
18. Kapoor R, Bornstein P, Sage EH: Type VIII collagen from bovine Descemet's membrane: Structural characterization of a triple-helical domain. *Biochemistry* 1986;25:3930–3937.
19. Keene DR, Sakai LY, Bächinger HP, et al: Type III collagen can be present on banded collagen fibrils regardless of fibril diameter. *J Cell Biol* 1987;105:2393–2402.
20. LeRoy EC: Increased collagen synthesis by scleroderma skin fibroblasts in vitro: A possible defect in the regulation or activation of the scleroderma fibroblast. *J Clin Invest* 1974;54:880–889.
21. Mayne R, Burgeson RE (eds): *Structure and Function of Collagen Types.* Orlando, Academic Press, 1987.
22. McDevitt CA, Pahl JA, Ayad S, et al: Experimental osteoarthritic articular cartilage is enriched in guanidine-soluble type VI collagen. *Biochem Biophys Res Commun* 1988;157:250–255.
23. Mendler M, Eich-Bender SG, Vaughn L, et al: Cartilage contains mixed fibrils of collagen types II, IX, and XI. *J Cell Biol* 1989;108:191–197.
24. Miller EJ, Gay S: The collagens: An overview and update. *Methods Enzymol* 1987;144:3–41.
25. Mizel SB, Dayer JM, Krane SM, et al: Stimulation of rheumatoid synovial cell collagenase and prostaglandin production by partially purified lymphocyte-activating factor (interleukin 1). *Proc Natl Acad Sci USA* 1981;78:2474–2477.

26. Monnier VM, Vishwanath V, Frank KE, et al: Relation between complications of type I diabetes mellitus and collagen-linked fluorescence. *N Engl J Med* 1986;314:403–408.
27. Moriguchi T, Fujimoto D: Crosslink of collagen in hypertrophic scar. *J Invest Dermatol* 1979;72:143–145.
28. Müller-Glauser W, Humbel B, Glatt M, et al: On the role of type IX collagen in the extracellular matrix of cartilage: Type IX collagen is localized to intersections of collagen fibrils. *J Cell Biol* 1986;102:1931–1939.
29. Murphy G, Cawston TE, Galloway WA, et al: Metalloproteinases from rabbit bone culture medium degrade types IV and V collagens, laminin and fibronectin. *Biochem J* 1981;199:807–811.
30. Nakano T, Thompson JR, Aherne FX: Concentration of the collagen crosslink pyridinoline in porcine skeletal muscle epimysium. *Can Inst Food Sci Technol J* 1985;18:100–102.
31. Niyibizi C, Eyre DR: Identification of the cartilage a1(XI) chain in type V collagen from bovine bone. *FEBS Lett* 1989;242:314–318.
32. Overall CM, Wrana JL, Sodek J: Independent regulation of collagenase, 72 kDa progelatinase, and metalloendoproteinase inhibitor expression in human fibroblasts by transforming growth factor-B. *J Biol Chem* 1989;264:1860–1869.
33. Postlethwaite AE, Raghow R, Stricklin GP, et al: Modulation of fibroblast functions by interleukin 1: Increased steady-state accumulation of type I procollagen messenger RNAs and stimulation of other functions but not chemotaxis by human recombinant inerleukin 1 alpha and beta. *J Cell Biol* 1988;106:311–318.
34. Sakai LY, Keene DR, Morris NP, et al: Type VII collagen is a major structural component of anchoring fibrils. *J Cell Biol* 1986;103:1577–1586.
35. Schmid TM, Linsenmayer TF: Type X collagen, in Mayne R, Burgeson RE (eds): *Structure and Function of Collagen Types*. Orlando, Academic Press, 1987, pp 223–259.
36. Shimokomaki M, Elsden DF, Bailey AJ: Meat tenderness: Age related changes in bovine intramuscular collagen. *J Food Sci* 1972;37:892–896.
37. Takala TE, Vuori J, Anttinen H, et al: Prolonged exercise causes an increase in the activity of galactosylhydroxylysyl glucosyltransferase and in the concentration of type III procollagen aminopropeptide in human serum. *Pflügers Arch* 1986;407:500–503.
38. Tikka L, Pihlajaniemi T, Henttu P, et al: Gene structure for the a1 chain of a human short-chain collagen (type XIII) with alternatively spliced transcripts and translation termination codon at the 5' end of the last exon. *Proc Natl Acad Sci USA* 1988;85:7491–7495.
39. Timpl R, Engel J: Type VI collagen, in Mayne R, Burgeson RE (eds): *Structure and Function of Collagen Types*. Orlando, Academic Press, 1987, pp 105–143.
40. van der Rest M, Mayne R: Type IX collagen proteoglycan from cartilage is covalently cross-linked to type II collagen. *J Biol Chem* 1988;263:1615–1618.
41. Vaughn L, Mendler M, Huber S, et al: D-periodic distribution of collagen type IX along cartilage fibrils. *J Cell Biol* 1988;106:991–997.
42. Werb Z, Hembry RM, Murphy G, et al: Commitment to expression of the metalloendopeptidases, collagenase and stromelysin: Relationship of inducing events to changes in cytoskeletal architecture. *J Cell Biol* 1986;102:697–702.
43. Whitham SE, Murphy G, Angel P, et al: Comparison of human stromelysin and collagenase by cloning and sequence analysis. *Biochem J* 1986;240:913–916.

44. Woo SL-Y, Maynard J, Butler D, et al: Ligament, tendon, and joint capsule insertions to bone, in Woo SL-Y, Buckwalter JA (eds): *Injury and Repair of the Musculoskeletal Soft Tissues.* Park Ridge, Illinois, American Academy of Orthopaedic Surgeons, 1988, pp 133–166.
45. Wu JJ, Eyre DR: Cartilage type IX collagen is cross-linked by hydroxypyridinium residues. *Biochem Biophys Res Commun* 1984;123:1033–1039.
46. Wu JJ, Eyre DR, Slayter HS: Type VI collagen of the intervertebral disc. Biochemical and electron-microscopic characterization of the native protein. *Biochem J* 1987;248:373–381.
47. Yamauchi M, London RE, Guenat C, et al: Structure and formation of a stable histidine-based trifunctional cross-link in skin collagen. *J Biol Chem* 1987;262:11428–11434.
48. Zimmermann DR, Trüeb B, Winterhalter KH, et al: Type VI collagen is a major component of the human cornea. *FEBS Lett* 1986;197:55–58.

Chapter 9

Proteoglycans of Soft Connective Tissues

Lawrence Rosenberg, MD
Haing U. Choi, PhD
Peter J. Neame, PhD
Joachim Sasse, PhD
Peter J. Roughley, PhD
A. Robin Poole, PhD, DSc

Introduction

Collagens and proteoglycans are major extracellular components of many musculoskeletal tissues. Two forms of small interstitial dermatan sulfate proteoglycans, called DS-PGI and DS-PGII, are present in the extracellular matrices of tendon, ligament, meniscus, and articular cartilage. DS-PGI and DS-PGII have monomeric molecular weights of approximately 100,000 and 67,000 respectively. The identities of DS-PGI and DS-PGII have been established in terms of the amino acid sequences of their core proteins. DS-PGs have distinctive biochemical properties that affect the formation, organization, stability, and biologic properties of connective tissue extracellular matrices. For example, electron microscopic studies show that DS-PGs bind to the surfaces of collagen fibrils and form an interconnected network along the surface and around the circumference of collagen fibrils. Scott[31] showed that as the concentration of DS-PGs relative to collagen decreases during development, collagen fibril diameter increases, suggesting that the DS-PGs regulate the radial growth of collagen fibrils by impeding the accretion of collagen monomers onto growing fibrils.

Sports injuries of the musculoskeletal tissues interfere with the finely coordinated, intricately synchronized sequence of events involved in extracellular matrix formation. After injury, the chemical composition of the reparative tissue and the organization of its extracellular matrix in tendon, ligament, and articular cartilage are often abnormal. Matrix proteoglycans can be one of the matrix components affected by injury and have an important role in matrix formation after injury.

Soft connective tissues such as tendon, ligament, meniscus, and articular cartilage each contain two major classes of proteoglycans, which differ greatly in structure and function: the large cartilage-type proteoglycan monomer, and the small DS-PGs. The identities of these proteoglycans have been defined in terms of the amino acid sequences of their core proteins and the kinds of glycosaminoglycan chains that are attached to the core proteins.

The large cartilage-type proteoglycan monomer, which is synthesized

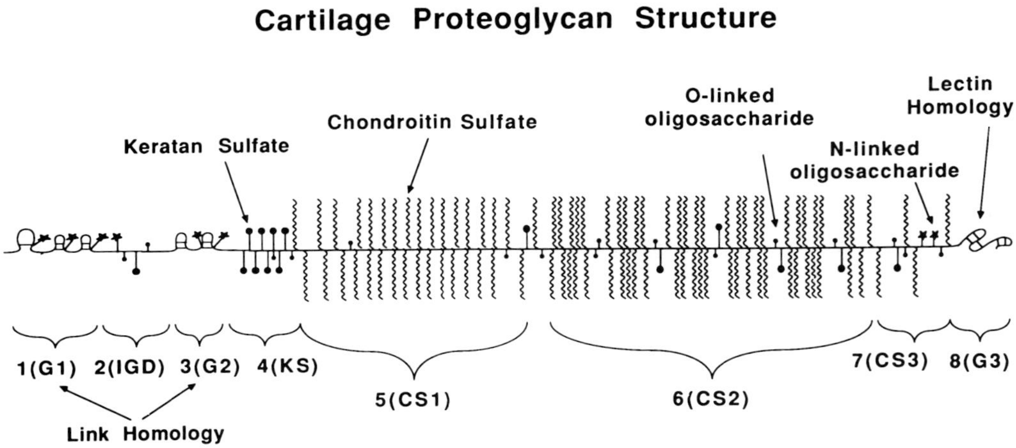

Fig. 1 *Model of the proteoglycan monomer from Swarm rat chondrosarcoma. The core protein consists of eight structural domains defined by their amino acid sequences. The hyaluronic-acid-binding region contains the G1 sequence. (Reproduced with permission from Doege K, Sasaki M, Horigan E, et al: Complete primary structure of the rat cartilage proteoglycan core protein deduced from cDNA clones.* J Biol Chem *1987;262:17757–17767.)*

and secreted into extracellular matrix, contains a core protein with a molecular weight of approximately 220,000, to which are attached more than 100 chondroitin sulfate (CS) and keratan sulfate (KS) chains.[9] The complete amino acid sequence of the core protein of the proteoglycan monomer from Swarm rat chondrosarcoma has been deduced from the nucleotide sequences of cDNA clones.[9] The core protein contains several regions with different functional properties (Fig. 1). A hyaluronic-acid-binding region is located at the NH_2 terminus, which mediates the binding of the proteoglycan monomer to hyaluronate. The hyaluronic-acid-binding region may be composed of two globular domains (G1 and G2), separated by an interglobular domain. A third globular domain (G3) is located at the COOH terminus, which has considerable homology with animal lectins. Between the hyaluronic-acid-binding region and the globular domain at the carboxy terminus are located the CS-rich region and the KS-rich region, which provide attachment sites for CS and KS chains.

After its synthesis and secretion into extracellular matrix, the cartilage-type proteoglycan monomer noncovalently associates with link protein and hyaluronate to form huge proteoglycan aggregates. As many as 100 proteoglycan monomers may bind at regular intervals to a single central filament of hyaluronic acid to form a proteoglycan aggregate with a molecular weight of 2×10^8.[4,5] The cartilage proteoglycan aggregates and monomers, which possess potent visceoelastic properties,[13,19] are located primarily in the spaces between collagen fibrils. They are elastic macromolecules that tend to expand into a maximum domain of solution until they are constrained by the surrounding network of collagen fibrils. The tendency of these proteoglycans to expand, absorb water, and exert a swelling pressure gives articular cartilage its special elastic properties.

In the extracellular matrices of articular cartilages, cartilage-type proteoglycans are present in high concentration and DS-PGs are present in relatively low concentration. In tendon, ligament, and meniscus, the small DS-PGs are present in high concentration and the cartilage-type proteoglycans are usually present in relatively low concentrations; however, in certain tendons that are subjected to compressive loads[40,42] and in certain parts of menisci,[2,3,18,27] the concentration of cartilage-type proteoglycans is increased significantly to provide these parts of the tissues with special biomechanical properties.

The cartilage-type proteoglycan monomer that is initially synthesized and secreted into extracellular matrix contains a core protein of uniform size, and monomer polydispersity is a result of variations in the sizes of its glycosaminoglycan chains. However, when cartilage proteoglycans reside in extracellular matrix for extended periods, proteolytic cleavages apparently occur in the CS-rich region of the proteoglycan monomer core protein. A population of monomers is created in which the monomer's molecular weight and the length of the CS-rich region vary greatly.[4] Proteoglycan monomers extracted from mature articular cartilage, tendons, menisci, and other connective tissues are, therefore, polydisperse in size and chemical composition and have molecular weights ranging from approximately 1,000,000 to 3,000,000.

Small interstitial DS-PGs are present in the extracellular matrices of skin,[7,20,22,23,38] tendon,[40,42] ligament,[24] meniscus,[1] fetal epiphyseal cartilage,[26] mature articular cartilage,[6,25] and a variety of other connective tissues. Unlike the large cartilage-type proteoglycans, which are localized in the extracellular matrix in the spaces between collagen fibrils, DS-PGs are present primarily on the surfaces of collagen fibrils. Most of the DS-PG molecules are oriented at right angles to the long axis of the collagen fibril and form rings around the circumference of the collagen fibril at its d bands.[31-37]

Biochemical Characteristics of DS-PGs

Two forms of small interstitial DS-PGs, DS-PGI and DS-PGII, have been found in each of the soft connective tissues examined.[6,25,41] DS-PGI and DS-PGII have monomeric molecular weights of approximately 100,000 and 67,000, respectively, in guanidine hydrochloride (4 mol/L) and Tris (50 mmol/L, pH7). The identities of DS-PGI and DS-PGII have been established in terms of the amino acid sequences of their core proteins. The DS-PGI core protein consists of 331 amino acids and has a molecular weight of 37,280. The DS-PGII core protein consists of 330 amino acids and has a molecular weight of 36,383. The two show considerable homology; but the sequences of the first 30

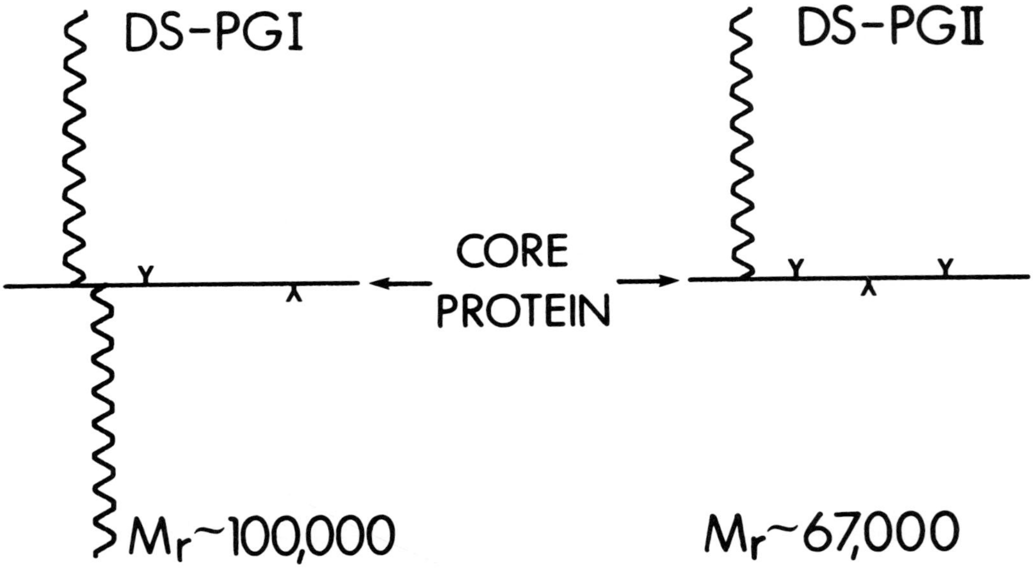

Fig. 2 *Model of the small interstitial DS-PGs.*

residues at the NH_2 termini are almost completely different. DS-PGI core protein contains the NH_2-terminal amino acid sequence

D E E A S G A E T T S G I P D L D S L P D T Y S A M

with two DS chains (molecular weight, 30,000) attached to serine residues at positions 5 and 11. DS-PGII core protein contains the NH_2-terminal amino acid sequence

D E A S G I G P E E H F D E V P E I E P M G P V

with one dermatan sulfate chain attached to the serine residue at position 4. The structures of DS-PGI and DS-PGII are summarized diagrammatically in Figure 2.

The existence of the two different types, DS-PGI and DS-PGII, went unrecognized until recently, primarily because the conventional methods used to isolate DS-PGs did not separate DS-PGI and DS-PGII. DS-PGs are frequently separated from cartilage-type proteoglycans and isolated by equilibrium density gradient centrifugation, ion-exchange chromatography, or gel chromatography. Figure 3 shows the DS-PGs from bovine articular cartilage, which have been separated from cartilage-type proteoglycans by equilibrium density gradient centrifugation, DEAE-Sephacel chromatography, and gel chromatography on Sepharose CL-4B in guanidine hydrochloride (4 mol/L), then recycled on Sepharose CL-4B in guanidine hydrochloride (4 mol/L). In this solution, DS-PGI and DS-PGII exist in their monomeric forms. Because DS-PGI and DS-PGII exist in guanidine hydrochloride (4 mol/

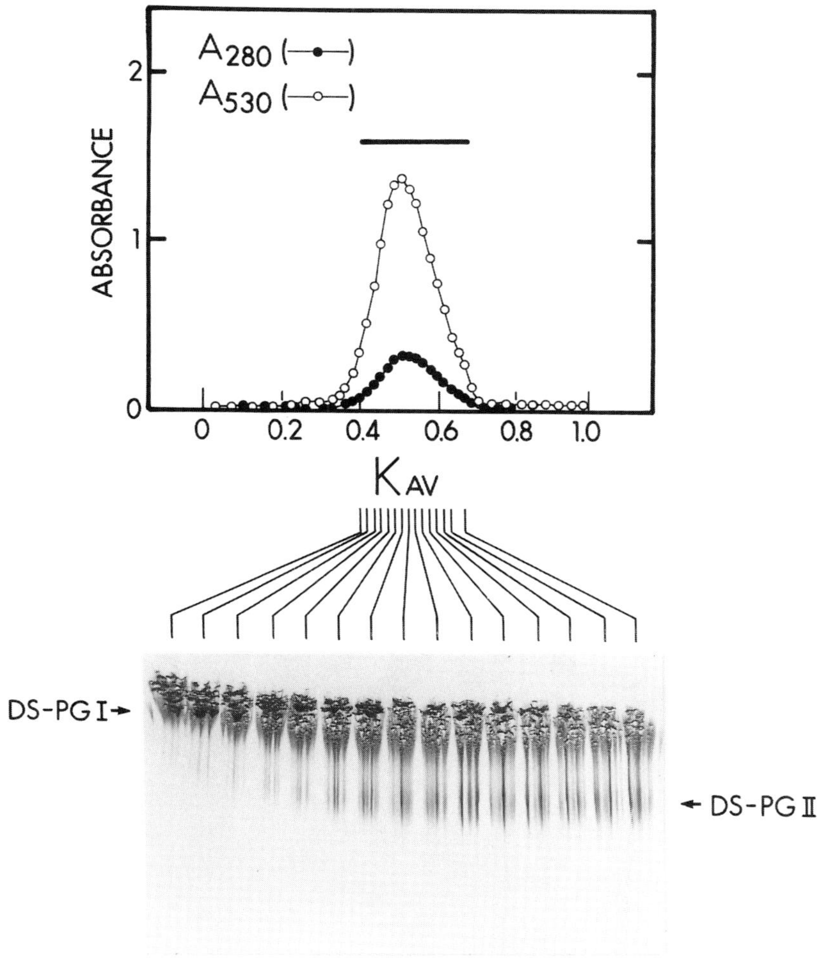

Fig. 3 *Gel chromatography on Sepharose CL-4B in guanidine hydrochloride (4 mol/L) of DS-PGs from calf articular cartilage. The chromatogram* ***(top)*** *does not suggest the existence of the two different types. However, the SDS-PAGE technique in Tris (0.375 mol/L) on a 4% to 20% gradient slab gel stained with toluidine blue clearly demonstrates the two* ***(bottom)****. (Reproduced with permission from Choi HU, Johnson TL, Pal S, et al: Characterization of the dermatan sulfate proteoglycans, DS-PGI and DS-PGII, from bovine articular cartilage and skin isolated by octyl-Sepharose chromatography.* J Biol Chem *1989;264:2876–2884.)*

L) as polydisperse monomers, the mixture of DS-PGs is eluted as a single unimodal peak. The appearance of the chromatogram does not suggest the existence of the two different proteoglycan types.

Furthermore, as shown in Figure 4, after chondroitinase ABC digestion, DS-PGI and DS-PGII both yield core proteins with a molecular weight of approximately 45,000. Thus, when the DS-PGI and DS-PGII

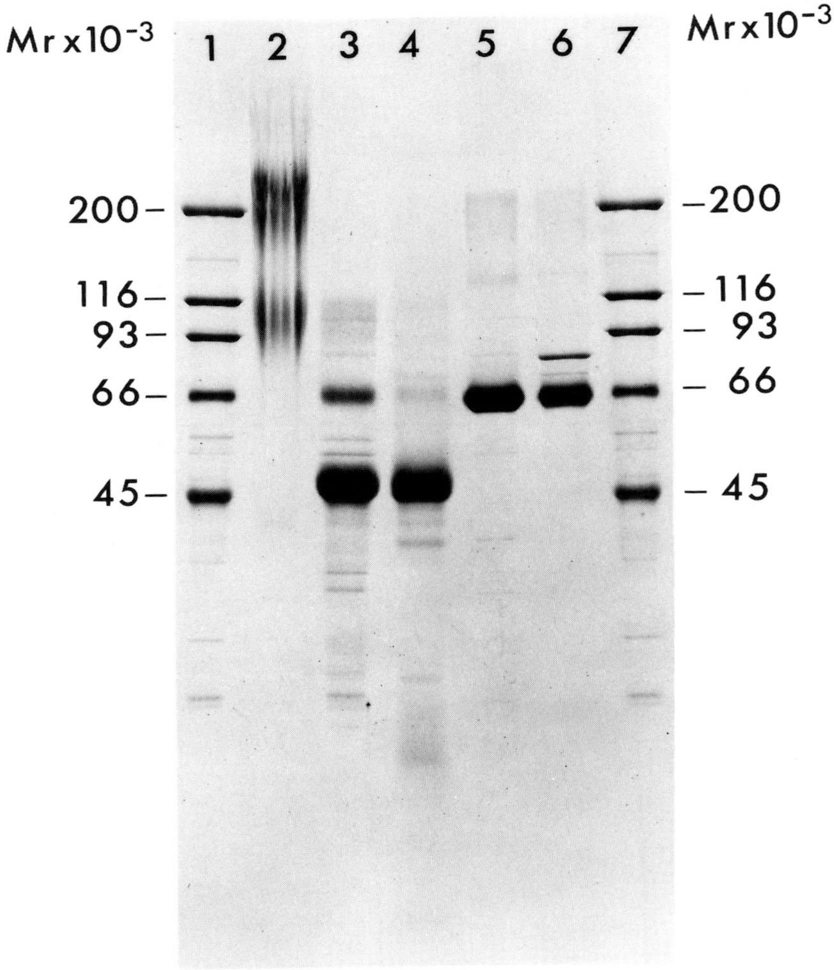

Fig. 4 *Demonstration of DS-PGs and their core proteins (prepared by chondroitinase digestion) by the SDS-PAGE technique in Tris (0.375 mol/L) on a 4% to 20% gradient slab gel. Lane 1 and 7 show molecular weight standards. Lane 2 shows the pooled DS-PGs after gel chromatography. The next two lanes show the core proteins obtained after digestion of the DS-PGs with chondroitinase AC (lane 3) or ABC (lane 4). The chondroitinase preparations contained carrier albumin. The SDS-PAGE technique was used on chondroitinase AC (lane 5) and ABC (lane 6) after DS-PG digestion. Both DS-PGI and DS-PGII yielded core proteins with molecular weights of 45,000; thus, there was no indication of the existence of two separate types. (Reproduced with permission from Rosenberg LC, Choi HU, Tang LH, et al: Isolation of dermatan sulfate proteoglycans from mature bovine articular cartilages.* J Biol Chem *1985;260:6304–6313.)*

eluted from Sepharose CL-4B (Fig. 3) are digested with chondroitinase ABC and subjected to the sodium dodecyl sulfate-polyacrylamide gel electrophoresis (SDS-PAGE) technique, there is no significant difference in the molecular weights of their core proteins to suggest that two different types possessing core proteins with different amino acid sequences have been isolated.

The discovery of the existence of the two types was fortuitous.[25] DS-PGI has a tendency to self-associate into oligomers of higher molecular weights in some high-ionic-strength buffers, such as the Tris used for the SDS-PAGE technique in the Laemmli procedure (0.375 mol/L).[25] In this solution, DS-PGI selectively self-associates into oligomers with molecular weights of about 300,000 whereas DS-PGII does not.

In our initial study,[25] this phenomenon was exploited to separate DS-PGI and DS-PGII by preparative electrophoresis on 5% to 20% gradient slab gels (Fig. 5). The immunologic identities of DS-PGI and DS-PGII were then examined. An antiserum to cartilage-type proteoglycan monomer from bovine articular cartilage reacted strongly on enzyme-linked immunosorbent assay (ELISA) with the cartilage-type proteoglycan monomer, but not at all with DS-PGI or DS-PGII, indicating that DS-PGI and DS-PGII possess core proteins different from that of the cartilage-type proteoglycan monomer. A polyclonal antiserum raised against the DS-PGs (mixture of DS-PGI and DS-PGII) reacted strongly against DS-PGII, but only weakly against DS-PGI. A monoclonal antibody prepared against DS-PGs reacted strongly with DS-PGII, but not at all against DS-PGI. These results were the first indication that DS-PGI and DS-PGII possess different core proteins and represent two different types of DS-PGs.

Two analogous types have since been identified in bovine tendon,[40,41] skin,[6] and bone.[10,11,41] PGI from bovine articular cartilage, skin, and bone possess the same core protein with the same amino acid sequence and contain two glycosaminoglycan chains; DS-PGII from bovine cartilage, tendon, skin, and bone possess the same core protein and contain one glycosaminoglycan chain. However, analogous types that possess the same core protein but are from different tissues (for example, DS-PGI from tendon, cartilage, skin, and bone) contain glycosaminoglycan chains that differ greatly in iduronic acid content and structure. The glycosaminoglycan chains of DS-PGs from skin, tendon, and articular cartilage contain 80%, 70%, and 40% iduronic acid, respectively. The glycosaminoglycan chains of DS-PGI and DS-PGII from bone appear to contain no iduronic acid and contain CS rather than DS chains.[10,11] Thus, DS-PGI and DS-PGII from the same tissue differ in the primary structure of their core proteins and the numbers of glycosaminoglycan chains attached to the core protein, but show little difference in the iduronic acid content of their glycosaminoglycan chains. Analogous, corresponding species from different tissues, such as DS-PGI from tendon and cartilage, possess the same core protein and the same number of glycosaminoglycan chains, but differ greatly in the composition and structure of these glycosaminoglycan chains.

It is not known how these differences in the primary structure of

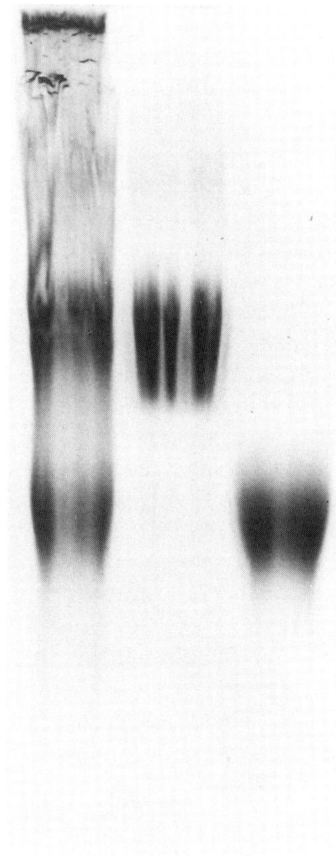

Fig. 5 *Appearance of DS-PGs from bovine articular cartilage after isolation to homogeneity by preparative electrophoresis on a 4% to 20% gradient slab stained with toluidine blue. The mixture of DS-PGs obtained after chromatography on Sepharose CL-4B in guanidine hydrochloride (4 mol/L) is shown at left. (Reproduced with permission from Rosenberg LC, Choi HU, Tang LH, et al: Isolation of dermatan sulfate proteoglycans from mature bovine articular cartilages.* J Biol Chem *1985;260:6304–6313.)*

the core proteins, the number of glycosaminoglycan chains, or the differences in composition and structure of the glycosaminoglycan chains affect the biochemical properties or the biologic functions of the DS-PGs, such as their binding to collagen fibrils or their effects on collagen fibril formation.

Isolation of DS-PGI and DS-PGII to Homogeneity

In our initial study,[25] DS-PGI and DGS-PGII were separated by the preparative SDS-PAGE technique, which provided only small amounts of homogeneous DS-PGI and DS-PGII. To provide DS-PGI and DS-PGII in amounts sufficient for extensive chemical and physical characterization and for studies of their biologic properties, methods were needed for the isolation of the types to homogeneity in milligram quantities.

Two methods have been developed.[6] The first depends on the propensity of DS-PGI to self-associate avidly into oligomers in sodium acetate (0.5 mol/L, pH 7) and involves gel chromatography on Sepharose CL-4B in this solvent.[6] The second method involves hydrophobic chromatography on octyl-Sepharose, which separates DS-PGI from DS-PGII by differences in the hydrophobic properties of their core proteins. Octyl-Sepharose chromatography should be particularly useful for the isolation of DS-PGI and DS-PGII from tendon, ligament, and meniscus, where small amounts of tissue are available and the two types differ greatly in their relative concentrations. For example, bovine fetal skin contains approximately 90% DS-PGII and only 10% DS-PGI. Although bovine fetal skin contains only small amounts of DS-PGI, octyl-Sepharose chromatography separates and concentrates it into a small number of fractions, making it possible to demonstrate its presence and isolate it to homogeneity (Fig. 6).

The primary structures of the core proteins of bovine DS-PGI[21] and PGII[8] are compared in Figure 7. The primary structures of the core proteins of human DS-PGI[12] and human DS-PGII[17] are compared in Figure 8. The primary structure of the core proteins of the human proteoglycans show extensive homology with those of the bovine proteoglycans, but there are also striking differences.

Immunologic Properties and Immunohistochemical Localization

Monospecific polyclonal and/or monoclonal antibodies to DS-PGI and DS-PGII are needed to demonstrate their immunohistochemical localization in normal tendon, ligament, meniscus, and articular cartilage, their degradation after injury, and their synthesis and assembly into extracellular matrices during repair. Monospecific polyclonal antibodies and monoclonal antibodies against DS-PGII have been prepared by several laboratories[24,25,28-30,43,44] but the preparation of monospecific polyclonal antibodies to DS-PGI has proven to be considerably more difficult. Although the immunohistochemical localization of DS-PGII in bovine tissues has been demonstrated,[24] to the best of our knowledge, no studies have demonstrated the immunohistochemical localization of DS-PGI in tendon, ligament, meniscus, or articular cartilage.

DS-PGI appears to be poorly immunogenic. When polyclonal antibodies were raised in rabbits against the matrix of bovine DS-PGI and DS-PGII, only antibodies to DS-PGII were obtained and these did not cross-react with DS-PGI.[25] Several attempts to raise polyclonal

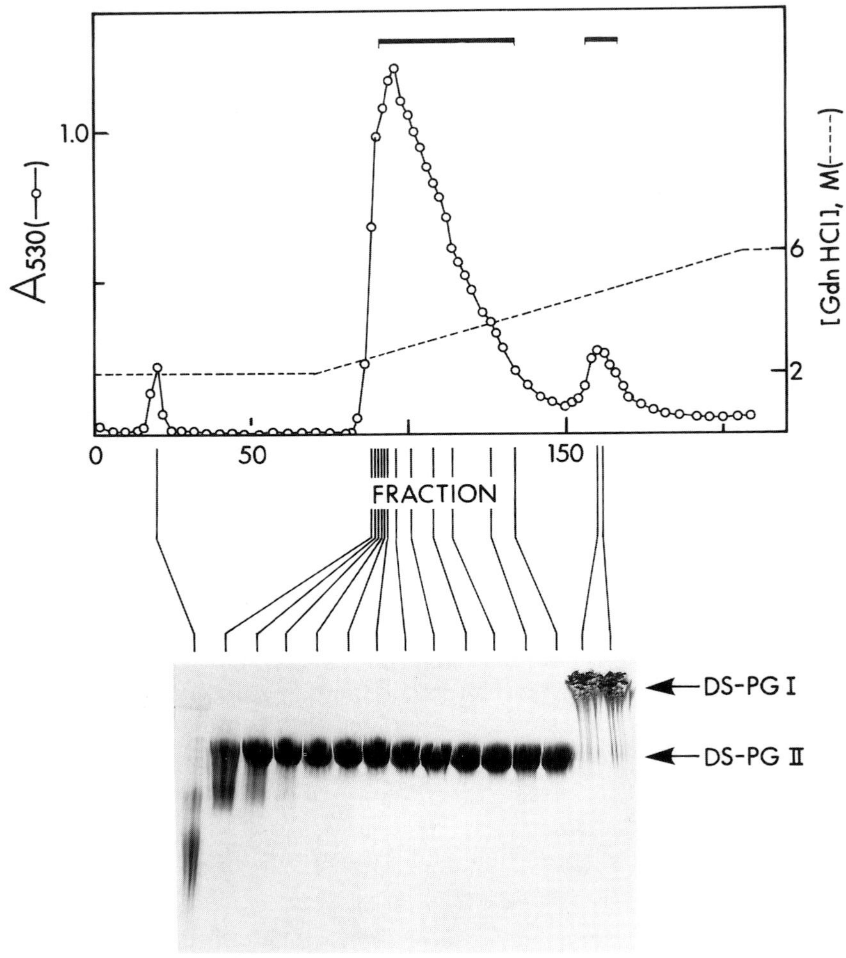

Fig. 6 *Isolation of DS-PGs from bovine fetal skin. The DS-PGs were applied to an octyl-Sepharose column in guanidine hydrochloride (2 mol/L) and then eluted with a guanidine hydrochloride linear gradient (2 to 6 mol/L). The fractions were analyzed for uronate and by the SDS-PAGE technique. (Reproduced with permission from Choi HU, Johnson TL, Pal S, et al: Characterization of the dermatan sulfate proteoglycans, DS-PGI and DS-PGII, from bovine articular cartilage and skin isolated by octyl-Sepharose chromatography.* J Biol Chem *1989;264:2876–2884.)*

antibodies in rabbits against homogenous DS-PGI have been unsuccessful (A.R. Poole, unpublished data; J. Sasse, unpublished data).

Fisher and associates,[12] however, prepared an antiserum in a single rabbit against a mixture of DS-PGI and DS-PGII and found that it contained antibodies against both. Thus, it is difficult but not impossible to raise polyclonal antibodies against DS-PGI in rabbits.

The degree of intertype cross-reactivity of polyclonal and mono-

```
DEEASGAETTSGIPDLDSLPPTYSAMCPFGCHCHLRVVQCSDLGLKAVPKEISPDTTLLDLQNNDISELRKDDFKGLQHL
  ::::                    ::: : :::::::::::::  ::: : ::: :::::::   :    ::: :  :
 DEASGIGPEEHFPEV PEIEPMGPVCPFRCQCHLRVVQCSDLGLEKVPKDLPPDTALLDLQNNKITEIKDGDFKNLKNL

YALVLVNNKISKIHEKAFSPLRKLQKLYISKNHLVEIPPNLPSSLVELRIHDNRIRKVPKGVFSGLRNMNEIEMGGNPLE
  : : :::::::   :: :: ::  :::::: : :::   :  : ::: : :   :: : :: ::  :   : : :::
HTLILINNKISKISPGAFAPLVKLERLYLSKNQLKELPEKMPKTLQELRVHENEITKVRKSVFNGLNQMIVVELGTNPLK

NSGFEPGAFDGLK LNYLRISEAKLTGIPKDLPETLNELHLDHNKIQAIELEDLLRYSKLYRLGLGHNQIRMIENGSLSF
 :: : ::: : : : : ::     : ::  ::  : ::::: :::       :     ::::  : :    ::::   :
SSGIENGAFQGMKKLSYIRIADTNITTIPQGLPPSLTELHLDGNKITKVDAASLKGLNNLAKLGLSFNSISAVDNGSLAN

LPTLRELHLDNNKLSRVPAGLPDLKLLQVVYLHTNNITKVGVNDFCPVGFGVKRAYYNGISLFNNPVPYWEVQPATFRCV
 :::::: ::::  :: :  : :  :::::: :::   : ::::: :   : : : : ::: ::: ::: :: :::::
TPHLRELHLNNNKLAKVPGGVADHKYIQVVYLHNNNISAIGSNDFCPPGYNTKKASYSGVSLFSNPVQYWEIQPSTFRCV

TDRLAIQFGNYY
: : ::::::
YVRAAVQLGNYK
```

Fig. 7 *Amino acid sequences of the core proteins of bovine PGI*[21] *and PGII.*[8]

```
DEEASGADTSGVLDPDSVTPTYSAMCPFGCHCHLRVVQCSDLGLKSVPKEISPDTTLLDLQNNDISELRKDDFKGLQHLY
  ::::     : :     :     ::: : :::::::::::::  ::: : ::::::::::: : :    ::: :  :
 DEASGIGPE VPDDRDFEPSLGPVCPFRCQCHLRVVQCSDLGLDKVPKDLPPDTTLLDLQNNKITEIKDGDFKNLKNLH

ALVLVNNKISKIHEKAFSPLRNVQKLYISKNHLVEIPPNLPSSLVDVRIHDNRIRKVPKGVFSGLRNMNCIEMGGNPLEN
:: ::::::::    ::  :     :::::: : :::   :  :   : : : : :: :  : ::  :  :: : :::
ALILVNNKISKVSPGAFTPLVKLERLYLSKNQLKELPEKMPKTLQELRAHENEITKVRKVTFNGLNQMIVIELGTNPLKS

SGFEPGAFDGL KLNYLRISEAKLTGIPKDLPETLNELHLDHNKIQAIELEDLRY SKLYRLGLGHNQIRMIENGSLSFL
:: : ::: :  :: : ::     : ::  ::  : ::::: :::       :     :  :::  : :    ::::
SGIENGAFQGMKKLSYIRIADTNITSIPQGLPPSLTELHLDGNKISRVDAASLKGLNNLAKLGLSFNSISAVDNGSLANT

PTLRELHLDNNKLARVPSGLPDLKLLQVVYLHSNNITKVGVNDFCPMGFGVKRAYYNGISLFNNPVPYVEVQPATFRCVT
: ::::::::::: ::: ::   :  :::::: :::  ::  :::: :   : : : : ::: ::: : : :: :::::
PHLRELHLDNNKLTRVPGGLAEHKYIQVVYLHNNNISVVGSSDFCPPGHNTKKASYSGVSLFSNPVQYWEIQPSTFRCVY

DRLAIQFGNYKK
 : ::::::::
VRSAIQLGNYK
```

Fig. 8 *Amino acid sequences of the core proteins of human PGI*[12] *and PGII.*[17]

clonal antibodies is extremely variable. In immunohistochemical studies,[24] antibodies against bovine DS-PGII stained DS-PGII in bovine tissues but did not stain DS-PGII in human or rat tissues. An antiserum raised in rabbits against bovine bone DS-PGII reacted strongly against DS-PGII from bovine bone and skin, but only weakly against DS-PGII from human cartilage on immunoblotting.[29] Schmidt and associates[30] prepared three monoclonal antibodies (LN1, LN3, LN4) against DS-PGII from human skin fibroblasts. Two of these (LN3 and LN4) reacted strongly against human articular cartilage DS-PGII, but very weakly or not at all against bovine skin DS-PGII[29]; however, LN1 reacted strongly against DS-PGII from both human articular cartilage and bovine skin. A monoclonal antibody against bovine skin DS-PGII reacted very strongly against both human articular cartilage DS-PGII and bovine skin DS-PGII. Thus, some antibodies to DS-PGII are type-specific whereas others show strong type cross-reactivity.

To the best of our knowledge, no studies have examined the type specificity or cross-reactivity of monospecific polyclonal or monoclonal antibodies to DS-PGI. Antibodies of high titer that react strongly with DS-PGI from human tissues are needed to study the distribution of this species in normal tissues and its changes in localization during injury and repair.

Biologic Functions of the DS-PGs

DS-PGs have distinctive biochemical properties that affect the formation, organization, stability, and biologic properties of connective tissue extracellular matrices. For example, DS-PGs appear to regulate the size of collagen fibrils formed during development and they may influence collagen fibril formation during tendon and ligament repair. DS-PGs also inhibit the adhesion and migration of fibroblasts on fibronectin substrata; this inhibitory capacity must be abolished temporarily if adhesion and migration of fibroblasts are to occur during the repair of tendon and ligament injuries.

Effect on Collagen Fibril Formation

Electron microscopic studies show that DS-PGs are distributed throughout the extracellular matrices of connective tissues in the spaces between collagen fibrils. However, DS-PGs are primarily found bound to the surfaces of collagen fibrils, where they form an interconnected network along the surface and around the circumference of collagen fibrils.[31-37] Scott and associates[31-37] systematically studied the localization of DS-PGs on the collagen fibrils of tendon by electron microscopy using the cationic dyes cuprolinic blue and cupromeronic blue. Tissue samples are first fixed in the presence of glutaraldehyde and cuprolinic blue or cupromeronic blue. Proteoglycans are lost from tissue samples during the fixation of connective tissues by conventional methods. These losses can be minimized or prevented by fixation in the presence of cationic dyes such as ruthenium hexamine trichloride[14–16] or cuprolinic blue or cupromeronic blue.

Cupromeronic blue has additional advantages.[31,33,36] It is a tetravalent copper-containing electron-dense cationic dye. When it is used in the presence of magnesium chloride (0.3 mol/L), only one of the positively charged groups of each molecule of cupromeronic blue binds to a negatively charged group in a DS chain, resulting in a high ratio of dye bound to polyanion and a high intensity of staining. Moreover, when connective tissues are stained first with cupromeronic blue and then with sodium tungstate, the tetravalent dye binds both to glycosaminoglycans and tungstate. This results in a still greater increase in the electron density of the stained proteoglycans, which are now clearly visible in electron micrographs, even when the collagen fibrils are subsequently positively stained with phosphotungstic acid and uranyl acetate.[36] Finally, cupromeronic blue is a relatively large, bulky dye molecule; when bound to glycosaminoglycans chains, it appears to maintain the chains in relatively extended configurations, rather than the collapsed formation seen when connective tissues are stained with lanthanum, toluidine blue, safranin O, and the like. DS-PGs stained with cupromeronic blue appear as elongated filamentous structures rather than matrix granules, and their ultrastructural morphologic characteristics are apparently better preserved.

In tendon stained with cupromeronic blue and sodium tungstate, DS-PGs are present on the surfaces of collagen fibrils (Fig. 9). Cross sections of tendon reveal no DS-PGs within collagen fibrils. The DS-PGs on the surface of the collagen fibrils appear as densely stained elongated filaments that form a network along the surface and around the circumference of collagen fibrils. Most of the DS-PGs appear as slender filaments orthogonally oriented at right angles to the long axis of the collagen fibrils (Fig. 9). These transversely oriented slender filaments are spaced at regular intervals approximately equal to the D periodicity of the collagen fibrils. In preparations that are positively stained with phosphotungstic acid and uranyl acetate[36] to demonstrate the bands of collagen fibrils from a to e, the orthogonally oriented DS-PGs are located predominantly at the d bands (Fig. 10).

A second type of DS-PG filament is randomly oriented on the collagen fibril surface. Because developing tendon contains both DS-PGI and DS-PGII, one type of DS-PG is probably transversely oriented and localized at the d bands and the other type is probably randomly oriented. Studies are indicated in which collagen fibrils are reassembled in the presence of homogeneous DS-PGI or DS-PGII and their orientation and localization are demonstrated by electron microscopy of the reassembled complexes. These studies should establish whether DS-PGI and DS-PGII are oriented and localized in specific patterns on collagen fibrils.

Effect of DS-PGs on Collagen Fibril Development

In electron microscopic studies of developing chick and calf flexor tendons, Scott[33,34] showed that there is an inverse relationship between

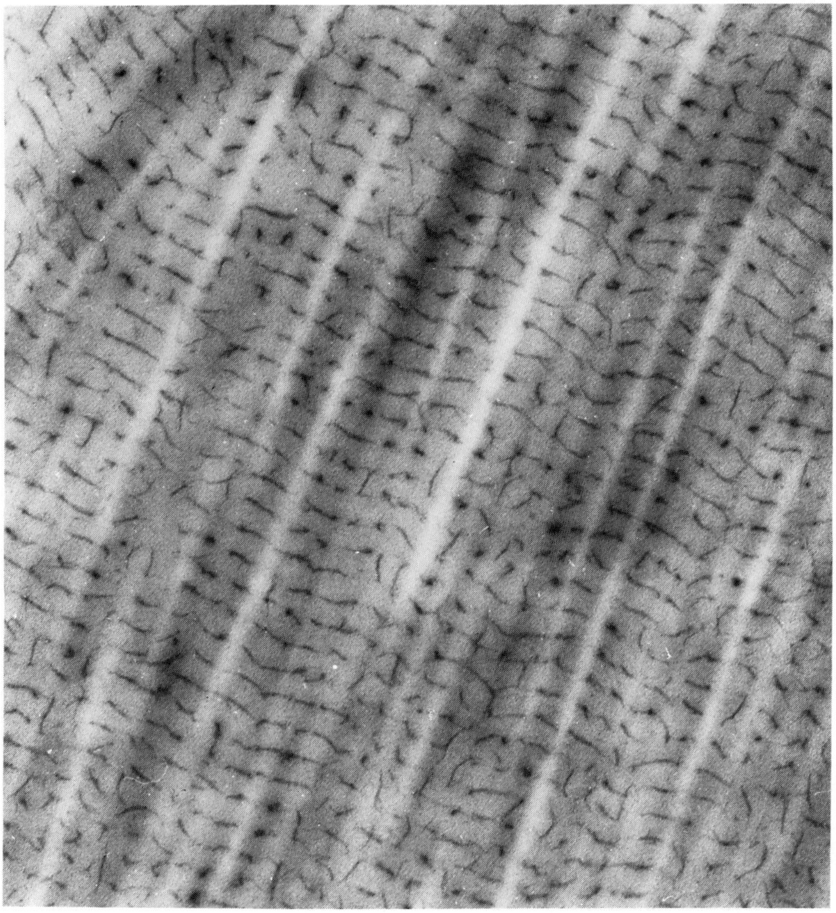

Fig. 9 *Electron micrograph of fetal calf flexor digitorum tendon stained with cupromeronic blue in magnesium chloride (0.3 mol/L) and sodium tungstate. Most of the DS-PGs are orthogonally oriented at right angles to the long axis of the collagen fibril. (Reproduced with permission from Scott JE: Proteoglycan-fibrillar collagen interactions.* Biochem J *1988;252:313–323.)*

collagen fibril diameter and the amount of DS-PGs present on the surface of collagen fibrils. As the concentration of DS-PGs relative to collagen decreases during development, collagen fibril diameter increases.[34] Scott has suggested that the DS-PGs inhibit the radial growth of collagen fibrils during fibrillogenesis by impeding the accretion of collagen monomers onto growing fibrils. Vogel and associates[43,44] showed that mixtures of DS-PGs from bovine tendon inhibit collagen fibrillogenesis and decrease collagen fibril diameters in vitro.[43,44] Uldbjerg and Danielsen,[39] however, obtained different results. They found that DS-PGs increased rather than decreased fibril formation

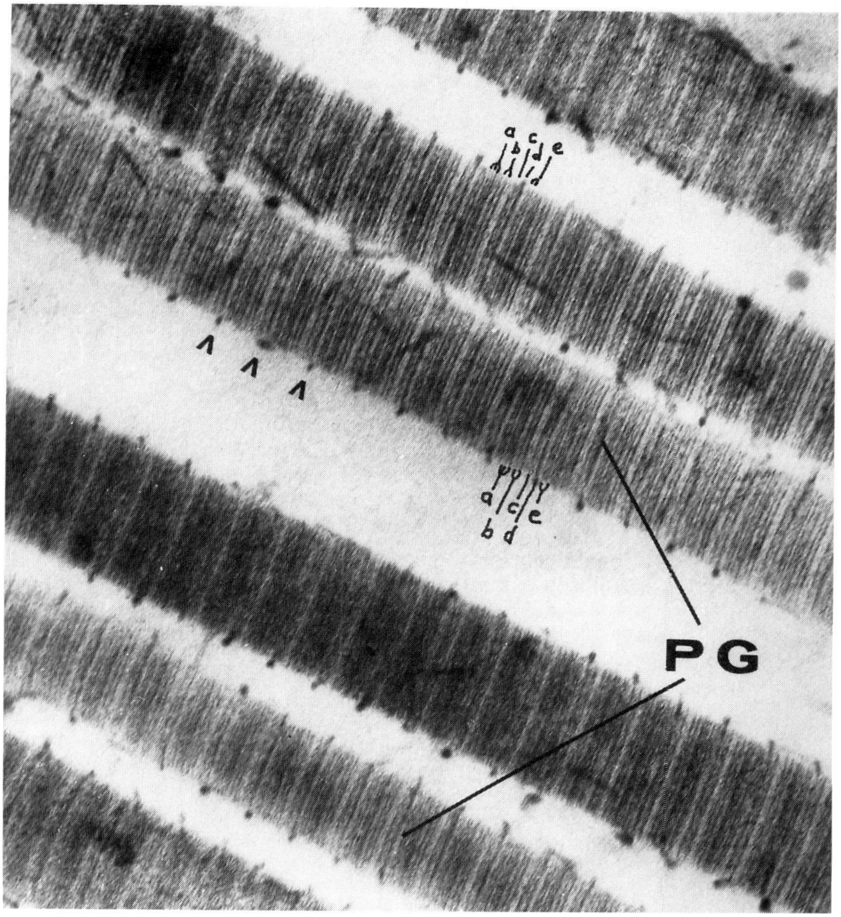

Fig. 10 *Electron micrograph of a tail tendon from a 25-day-old rat. The tendon was stained with cupromeronic blue in magnesium chloride (0.1 mol/L) and then positively stained with uranyl acetate to show the collagen bands from a to e. The DS-PGs are localized primarily at the d bands. (Reproduced with permission from Scott JE, Orford CR: Dermatan sulphate-rich proteoglycan associates with rat tail-tendon collagen at the d band in the gap region.* Biochem J *1981;197:213–216.)*

and that DS-PGs did not affect collagen fibril diameters. There are several possible explanations for these different results. Vogel and associates and Uldbjerg and Danielsen used mixtures of DS-PGs from different tissues. Different connective tissues contain markedly different proportions of DS-PGI and DS-PGII; also, DS-PGI and DS-PGII, which contain core proteins with different primary structures, may differ in their effects on collagen fibril formation. Moreover, different connective tissues contain DS-PGs that differ greatly in the iduronic acid content and composition of their glycosaminoglycan chains.[6] DS chains that differ in iduronic acid content and composition may have different effects on collagen fibril formation. To determine the effect of differences in core protein primary structure, studies of the effects of DS-PGI and DS-PGII collagen fibrillogenesis are required. To determine the effects of differences in the iduronic acid content and composition of the DS chains, studies of the effects of DS-PGs from tissues that differ in iduronic acid content and composition are indicated. These studies should make clear the effects of structural differences in the DS-PGs on their capacity to bind to collagen fibrils and influence collagen fibril formation.

References

1. Adams ME, Ho YA: Localization of glycosaminoglycans in human and canine menisci and their attachments. *Connect Tissue Res* 1987;16:269–279.
2. Adams ME, McDevitt CA, Ho A, et al: Isolation and characterization of high-buoyant-density proteoglycans from semilunar menisci. *J Bone Joint Surg* 1986;68A:55–64.
3. Adams ME, Muir H: The glycosaminoglycans of canine menisci. *Biochem J* 1981;197:385–389.
4. Buckwalter JA, Rosenberg LC: Electron microscopic studies of cartilage proteoglycans: Direct evidence for the variable length of the chondroitin sulfate-rich region of proteoglycan subunit core protein. *J Biol Chem* 1982;257:9830–9839.
5. Buckwalter JA, Rosenberg L: Structural changes during development in bovine fetal epiphyseal cartilage. *Collagen Relat Res* 1983;3:489–504.
6. Choi HU, Johnson TL, Pal S, et al: Characterization of the dermatan sulfate proteoglycans, DS-PGI and DS-PGII, from bovine articular cartilage and skin isolated by octyl-Sepharose chromatography. *J Biol Chem* 1989;264:2876–2884.
7. Damle SP, Coster L, Gregory JD: Proteodermatan sulfate isolated from pig skin. *J Biol Chem* 1982;257:5523–5527.
8. Day AA, McQuillan CI, Termine JD, et al: Molecular cloning and sequence analysis of the cDNA for small proteoglycan II of bovine bone. *Biochem J* 1987;248:801–805.
9. Doege K, Sasaki M, Horigan E, et al: Complete primary structure of the rat cartilage proteoglycan core protein deduced from cDNA clones. *J Biol Chem* 1987;262:17757–17767.
10. Fisher LW, Hawkins GR, Tuross N, et al: Purification and partial characterization of small proteoglycans I and II, bone sialoproteins I and II, and osteonectin from the mineral compartment of developing human bone. *J Biol Chem* 1987;262:9702–9708.
11. Fisher LW, Termine JD, Dejter SW Jr, et al: Proteoglycans of developing bone. *J Biol Chem* 1983;258:6588–6594.
12. Fisher LW, Termine JD, Young MF: Deduced protein sequence of bone small proteoglycan I (biglycan) shows homology with proteoglycan II (decorin) and several nonconnective tissue proteins in a variety of species. *J Biol Chem* 1989;264:4571–4576.
13. Hardingham TE, Muir H, Kwan MK, et al: Viscoelastic properties of proteoglycan solutions with varying proportions present as aggregates. *J Orthop Res* 1987;5:36–46.
14. Hunziker EB, Herrmann W: In situ localization of cartilage extracellular matrix components by immunoelectron microscopy after cryotechnical tissue processing. *J Histochem Cytochem* 1987;35:647–655.

15. Hunziker EB, Herrmann W, Schenk RK: Improved cartilage fixation by ruthenium hexammine trichloride (RHT): A prerequisite for morphometry in growth cartilage. *J Ultrastruct Res* 1982;81:1–12.
16. Hunziker EB, Herrmann W, Schenk RK: Ruthenium hexammine trichloride (RHT)-mediated interaction between plasmalemmal components and pericellular matrix proteoglycans is responsible for the preservation of chondrocytic plasma membranes in situ during cartilage fixation. *J Histochem Cytochem* 1983;31:717–727.
17. Krusius T, Ruoslahti E: Primary structure of an extracellular matrix proteoglycan core protein deduced from cloned cDNA. *Proc Natl Acad Sci USA* 1986;83:7683–7687.
18. McNicol D, Roughley PJ: Extraction and characterization of proteoglycan from human meniscus. *Biochem J* 1980;185:705–713.
19. Mow VC, Mak AF, Lai WM, et al: Viscoelastic properties of proteoglycan subunits and aggregates in varying solution concentrations. *J Biomech* 1984;17:325–338.
20. Nakamura T, Matsunaga E, Shinkai H: Isolation and some structural analyses of a proteodermatan sulphate from calf skin. *Biochem J* 1983;213:289–296.
21. Neame PJ, Choi HU, Rosenberg LC: The primary structure of the core protein of the small, leucine-rich proteoglycan (PG I) from bovine articular cartilage. *J Biol Chem* 1989;264:8653–8661.
22. Pearson CH, Gibson GJ: Proteoglycans of bovine periodontal ligament and skin: Occurrence of different hybrid-sulphated galactosaminoglycans in distinct proteoglycans. *Biochem J* 1982;201:27–37.
23. Pearson CH, Winterbottom N, Fackre DS, et al: The NH_2-terminal amino acid sequence of bovine skin proteodermatan sulfate. *J Biol Chem* 1983;258:15101–15104.
24. Poole AR, Webber C, Pidoux I, et al: Localization of a dermatan sulfate proteoglycan (DS-PGII) in cartilage and the presence of an immunologically related species in other tissues. *J Histochem Cytochem* 1986;34:619–625.
25. Rosenberg LC, Choi HU, Tang LH, et al: Isolation of dermatan sulfate proteoglycans from mature bovine articular cartilages. *J Biol Chem* 1985;260:6304–6313.
26. Rosenberg L, Tang L, Choi H, et al: Isolation, characterization and immunohistochemical localization of a dermatan sulfate-containing proteoglycan from bovine fetal epiphyseal cartilage, in Kelley RO, Goetinck PF, MacCabe JA (eds): *Limb Development and Regeneration: Part B*. New York, Alan R Liss, 1982, pp 67–84.
27. Roughley PJ, McNicol D, Santer V, et al: The presence of a cartilage-like proteoglycan in the adult human meniscus. *Biochem J* 1981;197:77–83.
28. Ruoslahti E: Structure and biology of proteoglycans. *Annu Rev Cell Biol* 1988;4:229–255.
29. Sampaio L de O, Bayliss MT, Hardingham TE, et al: Dermatan sulphate proteoglycan from human articular cartilage: Variation in its content with age and its structural comparison with a small chondroitin sulphate proteoglycan from pig laryngeal cartilage. *Biochem J* 1988;254:757–764.
30. Schmidt G, Robenek H, Harrach B, et al: Interaction of small dermatan sulfate proteoglycan from fibroblasts with fibronectin. *J Cell Biol* 1987;104:1683–1691.
31. Scott JE: Collagen-proteoglycan interactions: Localization of proteoglycans in tendon by electron microscopy. *Biochem J* 1980;187:887–891.
32. Scott JE: Proteoglycan-fibrillar collagen interactions. *Biochem J* 1988;252:313–323.
33. Scott JE: Proteoglycan histochemistry: A valuable tool for connective tissue biochemists. *Collagen Relat Res* 1985;5:541–575.

34. Scott JE: The periphery of the developing collagen fibril: Quantitative relationships with dermatan sulphate and other surface-associated species. *Biochem J* 1984;218:229–233.
35. Scott JE, Hughes EW: Proteoglycan-collagen relationships in developing chick and bovine tendons: Influence of the physiological environment. *Connect Tissue Res* 1986;14:267–278.
36. Scott JE, Orford CR: Dermatan sulphate-rich proteoglycan associates with rat tail-tendon collagen at the d band in the gap region. *Biochem J* 1981;197:213–216.
37. Scott JE, Orford CR, Hughes EW: Proteoglycan-collagen arrangements in developing rat tail tendon: An electron microscopical and biochemical investigation. *Biochem J* 1981;195:573–581.
38. Shinkai H, Nakamura T, Matsunaga E: Evidence for the presence and structure of asparagine-linked oligosaccharide units in the core protein of proteodermatan sulphate. *Biochem J* 1983;213:297–304.
39. Uldbjerg N, Danielsen CC: A study of the interaction in vitro between type I collagen and a small dermatan sulfate proteoglycan. *Biochem J* 1988;251:643–648.
40. Vogel KG, Evanko SP: Proteoglycans of fetal bovine tendon. *J Biol Chem* 1987;262:13607–13613.
41. Vogel KG, Fisher LW: Comparisons of antibody reactivity and enzyme sensitivity between small proteoglycans from bovine tendon, bone, and cartilage. *J Biol Chem* 1986;261:11334–11340.
42. Vogel KG, Heinegard D: Characterization of proteoglycans from adult bovine tendon. *J Biol Chem* 1985;260:9298–9306.
43. Vogel KG, Paulsson M, Heinegard D: Specific inhibition of type I and type II collagen fibrillogenesis by the small proteoglycan of tendon. *Biochem J* 1984;223:587–597.
44. Vogel KG, Trotter JA: The effect of proteoglycans on the morphology of collagen fibrils formed in vitro. *Collagen Relat Res* 1987;7:105–114.

Chapter 10

The Cellular and Matrix Response of Ligaments and Tendons to Mechanical Injury

Savio L-Y Woo, PhD
Lawrence V. Tkach, MD

Introduction

This chapter briefly describes the morphologic, anatomic, histologic, biochemical, and biomechanical properties of ligaments and tendons. These properties determine the strength of ligaments and tendons and their susceptibility to injury and subsequent repair. Partial tears and microinjuries may lead to more chronic injury. Recent advances in technology and methodology have permitted careful examination of these tissues' properties and have identified viscoelastic properties, temperature-dependent properties, and the effects of freezing, storage, strain rates, skeletal maturity, and aging on ligament and tendon. Quantitative information about the homeostasis of these tissues in response to exercise training and immobilization has been documented. The findings revealed that increasing the level of stress and motion in the tissues during exercise training results in relatively small changes in the mechanical properties of tendons and ligaments, as well as tissue hypertrophy, whereas stress deprivation, that is, lack of stress and motion, results in a rapid reduction in tissue mass and/or mechanical properties.

Relatively little information is available in terms of the responses of tendons and ligaments to stress and strain levels at or near the failure region. It has been demonstrated microscopically that there are ruptures of collagen fibers if these soft tissues are loaded to more than one third of the maximum load. For example, the loading of the tendon in vivo may not be pure uniaxial tension; therefore, nonuniform loading may cause some fibers to be overloaded and therefore fail, whereas the others are not loaded to the same extent. There is also speculation about the possibility of failure of collagen fibers because of interfibular shear stress that may exceed the elastic limit, which may result in partial failure of the ligaments and tendons. Such partial failure may be a source of tissue microinjury resulting in a phenomenon called chronic tendinosis, unless healing occurs. In addition, the bone-tendon junction and myotendinous junction are also easily subjected to microfractures and premature failures. Despite the fact that these junctions are well constructed to resist stress, the stress concentration resulting from tissue transition from soft to hard tissue in these areas could cause partial tissue failures. Unfortunately, understanding of the detailed mechanics involved in these complex regions is lacking.

Biology and Biomechanics of Tendons and Ligaments

On gross examination, tendons and ligaments are composed of dense connective tissues with closely packed, parallel collagenous fiber bundles with a glistening white appearance. Under microscopic examination, these tissues are seen to contain a meshwork of interlacing fibers, flattened and oval cells, and ground substance. Polarized light microscopy demonstrates an undulating pattern to the collagen fibers, and specialized stains can differentiate the fibrous elements as well as ground substance and fibroblasts in the interfibrillar spaces. The tendon and ligament insertions to bone are rather complex and generally can be categorized into two types. One is the direct insertion, in which the ligament and tendon fibrils pass into bone through zones of fibrocartilage (usually less than 0.6 mm), recognizable by round cells with lacunae organized in columnar arrangements, and through mineralized fibrocartilage (usually less than 0.4 mm). In this case, there is little interdigitation into the surrounding periosteum. The second type of tendon and ligament insertion to bone is more complex. The superficial fibrils course parallel with the bone and become confluent with the periosteum, while the deeper fibrils then course obliquely and insert directly into the underlying bone. Both insertion patterns serve to dissipate force and to enhance the strength of insertion sites; however, stress and motion are necessary to maintain their functional integrity.

In terms of blood supply, intraligamentous or intratendinous vessels are relatively sparse, which implies that at least some degree of diffusion is necessary for midsubstance cellular nutrition. The nerve supplies to the ligaments and tendons come from the nerves of the muscles acting on the joint. There are numerous free nerve endings in the ligaments, with both nonmyelinated and finely myelinated fibers that are believed to moderate pain sensation.

Biomechanically, tendons and ligaments consist of functional complexes of an interdependent aggregation of collagen, elastin, glycoproteins, protein polysaccharides, glycolipids, noncollagenous protein, and cells. Roughly 70% to 80% of the normal tissue is collagen by dry weight. The collagen is mainly type I and is the principal tensile-resistant substance present. The collagen also has the ability to form covalent intramolecular and intermolecular cross-links that contribute to both its tensile behavior and its resistance to chemical or enzymatic breakdown. About 1% of the total dry weight is the ground substance. Water, on the other hand, accounts for 65% to 75% of the total wet weight and a significant part of that water is associated with the ground substance. The water and proteoglycans probably provide lubrication and spacing that are crucial to the gliding function at intercept points where fibers cross in the tissue matrix. The proteoglycan subunit consists of a core protein with glycosaminoglycan side chains. Hyaluronic acid, chondroitin-4 sulfate, chondroitin-6 sulfate, and dermatan sulfate represent the majority of the glycosaminoglycans present. Except for the hyaluronic acid, the glycosaminoglycans are highly negatively charged; this negative charge confers predictable mechanical-chemical properties on the connective tissue.

The biomechanical behavior of ligaments and tendons demonstrates that they are well suited structurally and mechanically to the physical functions they perform. Different components of the tissue take up loads at different stress levels, thus contributing to a nonlinear, concave, upward stress-strain curve. The fibrillar components of ligaments and tendons are arranged in an undulating path between origin and insertion in their physiologically relaxed state. During normal movements in which tensile stretch is applied, progressive straightening and stretching of an increasing number of fibers occurs (recruitment). This mechanical behavior is designed generally to guide the joint into appropriate motion. Because the stress-strain curve is nonlinear (demonstrating increasing stiffness with increased deformation), the ligaments and tendons stiffen at higher loads and thus act as a "checkrein" to prevent excessive joint motion or displacement.

Ligaments and tendons also exhibit complex time- and history-dependent (rheologic) behavior, including creep (increased deformation with time under constant load) and stress relaxation (decreased stress with time under constant deformation). Because of these viscoelastic properties, repeated cyclic loading such as walking or jogging transiently softens (because of stress relaxation) the ligament and tendon substance as the number of cycles is increased. Such decreases in stress levels in the tissues can help to prevent fatigue failure of tendons and ligaments. On resting, the elastic behavior of ligaments and tendons allows them to recover their initial, unloaded state as the viscous behavior diminishes.

The tensile behavior of ligaments and tendons depends on the temperature. A linear inverse relationship can be established for the medial collateral ligament at a specified deformation between the tensile load and the temperature with a coefficient of 1% of load reduction per degree Celsius.[74] Therefore, in experiments on tendons and ligaments the temperature must be controlled and reported along with the mechanical properties because of this profound relationship. On the other hand, storage by freezing at -20 C for as long as several months has no appreciable effect on the mechanical properties of ligaments and tendons, especially if the tensile testing includes preconditioning.[75] However, crucial to this finding is the care taken in preparing the tissue sample before freezing, including ample care to prevent sample dehydration.

Skeletal maturation has important effects on the tendons and ligaments and their insertion sites. Specifically, the age of experimental animals has a significant effect on the relative strengths of the various components along the bone-ligament complex. In younger animals,

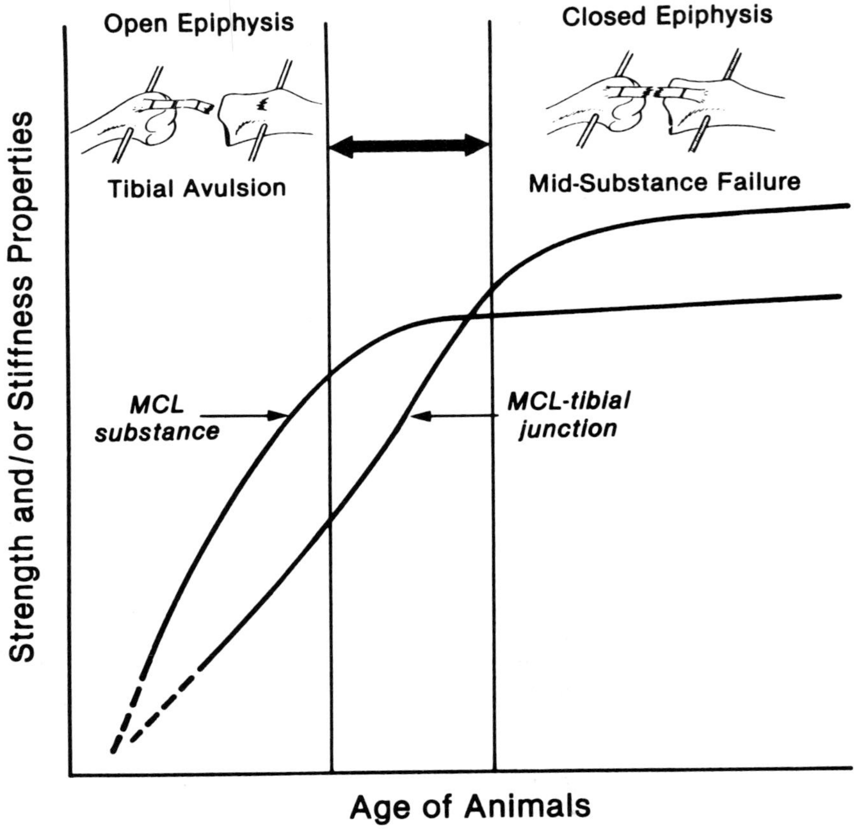

Fig. 1 *Schema of hypothesized asynchronous rates of maturation of the medial collateral ligament-tibia complex and the mechanical properties of the ligament's substance. (Reproduced with permission from Woo SL, Orlando CA, Gomez MA, et al: Tensile properties of the medial collateral ligament as a function of age.* J Orthop Res *1986;4:133–141.)*

before closure of the epiphyseal plate, the ligament tissue can closely approximate adult properties, whereas the bone at the attachment site is considerably weaker than in the adult. However, after epiphyseal plate closure, the insertion sites are affected directly by the activities of the growth plate and gain significant structural stiffness and strength that eventually surpass those of the ligament tissues (Fig. 1).

Recent studies have demonstrated that there are significant differences between the intra-articular ligaments, such as the anterior cruciate ligament, and the extra-articular ligaments, such as the medial collateral ligament of the knee. With the advent of new instruments, such as the laser micrometer,[34] for determining the complex cross-sectional area of these tissues, it was possible to demonstrate that the tangent modulus and tensile strength of the rabbit medial collateral ligament were significantly higher (approximately twofold) than those of the anterior cruciate ligament, although the strain at failure for both ligaments was about the same.[44] These findings are supported by histologic evaluation showing greater density of collagen fibers in the medial collateral ligament. Significant differences in matrix chemistry also exist between these two ligaments. The effects of age on these two tissues are also different. The medial collateral ligament seems to be able to maintain its mechanical characteristics until senescence, whereas the anterior cruciate ligament demonstrates significant deterioration in terms of strength characteristics with age. At senescence, the strength of the human anterior cruciate ligament has been demonstrated to be between one fourth and one third of that between the ages of 20 and 35 years.

Response to Exercise Training and Immobilization

The cellular and matrix components of tendons and ligaments have been found to respond to stress on a microscopic level in both pathologic and normative functioning states. Normal tendon has histologic and histochemical structural variations in areas subjected to different mechanical stresses. Banes and associates[5,6] demonstrated the preferential presence of synovial cells rich in the production of the cell attachment molecule fibronectin in the epitenon and endotenon. Fibronectin can, in turn, bind hyaluronic acid,[3] which can act as a boundary lubricant between tendon and surrounding structures. Fibroblasts populate the more central portion of the tendon between the collagen bundles. Regions of tendons that experience primarily tensile forces have a lower proteoglycan content and higher rates of collagen synthesis than areas that experience frictional and compressive forces as well as tensile forces.[6,33] These proteoglycans are more cartilage-like in areas of compressive loads.[38] Segmental variations in hydration, cellularity, collagen content, collagen fiber arrangement, and cross-sectional area have been found within individual flexor tendons, implying varying material properties.[1,38] It is not known whether nonsynovial tendons demonstrate similar biochemical and histologic variations, but Chun and associates[10] showed biomechanical differences in areas of the patellar tendon. The strain topography of other tendons is believed to be nonuniform as well.[72,78] Similarly, ligaments are nonuniform structures. Frank and associates[18] found differences in thickness, collagen content, hexosamine, and percentage of total water in different areas in the rabbit medial collateral ligament. Ligaments differ structurally and biochemically from each other to a degree (as do tendons), presumably because of the different mechanical demands and local nutritional environments.[11]

In the laboratory, the effect of increased tension in the rabbit medial collateral ligament was measured by inserting a stainless-steel pin underneath the ligament. The insertion of this pin increased the in situ load in the medial collateral ligament by 200% to 350%. With this quantitative increase in tension, the response of the ligament was studied in vivo. After 12 weeks, the strength of the bone-ligament complex for the group was slightly higher.[22] Woo and associates[71,76] found increases in strength, size, and collagen content in extensor tendons of exercised swine, but exercise had only a minimal effect on the mechanical properties of flexor tendons, and no increase in collagen content was observed. This was believed to be a result of the limiting effect of the tendon sheath and the inherently high collagen content per weight of the flexor tendon. Glycosaminoglycans remained unaffected.[54] Viidik[59] compared the properties of the peroneus brevis tendons from trained and nontrained rabbits and found the ultimate load was higher for the trained rabbits, but that the weight, water, and collagen content of these tendons were not significantly different. Others have noted enhanced tritiated hydroxyproline incorporation in the mouse Achilles tendon when exercised.[24,54] This implies that collagen metabolism is accelerated. Yet, if total collagen is unchanged, increased collagen degradation and reparative processes may be acting in response to the increase in mechanical stresses.

On an ultrastructural level, exercise loading of tendon in vivo increases the total number of collagen fibrils, producing an increased number of thinner fibrils and increasing their density.[39,40] Similar findings have been reported in the anterior cruciate ligament in response to physical loading.[78] Collagen fiber crimp angle is increased, while crimp length and elastic modulus are decreased in exercised rabbits.[78] Anabolic steroids accentuate these changes and increase ultrastructurally observed collagen dysplasia.[40,77]

Tipton and associates,[55] in their classic 1970 study of the canine medial collateral ligament, demonstrated that the exercised animals had significantly higher hydroxyproline concentrations representing the collagen content than did nontrained animals. Histologic measurements of the fiber bundles by light microscopy demonstrated that those in the trained group had the largest diameters. Conversely, collagen contents of the immobilized animals were found to be the lowest, and so were the fiber bundle diameters. In a follow-up study comparing the collagen content in ligaments from trained and untrained rats, it was demonstrated that there was no increase resulting from training, although the trained rats seemed to have wider, thicker, and heavier ligaments.[56] Part of the differences between the two studies may be attributed to the aging effect, as well as to the different species used. Using transmission electron microscopy to study the collagen fibril populations of the cruciate ligaments in response to short-term, intensive exercise programs, Oakes and associates[45] found that the number of smaller-diameter collagen fibril bundles in the anterior cruciate ligament of the rat increased with exercise.

A recent study by Wang and associates[62] illustrated the effect of lifelong duration of exercise training on the biomechanical properties of the medial collateral ligament in beagles. They found little or no effect on the structural properties of the bone-ligament complex (the tensile load-deformation curves were similar). Also, the mechanical properties of the medial collateral ligament substance were not statistically different, as the tangent modulus, tensile strength, and strain at failure for the trained dogs were similar to those of age-matched controls. Similar findings were obtained for the flexor tendons from the hindlimbs of these dogs. It is believed that the lack of differences associated with lifelong exercise training is a result of the aging process, which may have overcome the potential gains of exercise training.

The effect of immobilization on ligaments is profound. In addition to the findings of Tipton and associates[55] that immobilization of the canine knee resulted in smaller fiber-bundle diameters in the medial collateral ligament, Binkley and Peat[8] also found a decrease in collagen fibril density; however, the number of smaller-diameter collagen fibrils was found to be decreased, while the number of larger diameter fibrils was found to increase after immobilization. Biochemical analyses of the ligaments after immobilization showed that the collagen concentration was decreased in the canine medial collateral ligament. In rabbits, Amiel and associates[2] showed no decrease in collagen content but an increase in collagen turnover after nine weeks of immobilization; that is, both collagen synthesis and collagen degradation had increased. With longer periods of immobilization, up to 12 weeks, the collagen synthesis could not be maintained whereas degradation continued, and, as a result, decreases in total collagen mass and concentration were found. This result confirmed the findings of Klein and associates[31] in the canine anterior cruciate ligament. They found a 16% reduction in collagen mass and a 10% reduction in prelabeled tritiated hydroxyproline after 12 weeks of immobilization. Gamble and associates[20] found that the rabbit medial collateral ligament showed increased lysosomal activities leading to an increase in degradation of glycosaminoglycans after eight weeks of immobilization. This finding substantiated those from the Orthopaedic Bioengineering Laboratory, University of California, San Diego, that immobilization causes a 20% reduction in glycosaminoglycans in the medial collateral ligaments of the immobilized rabbit limb. Further, these investigators also demonstrated that the fibroblasts of the immobilized medial collateral ligament underwent an enzymatic adaptation into a catabolic state. Presumably, immobilization resulted in increased synthesis and degradation of collagen. This leads to newly synthesized collagen that is immature and not so well organized, and that therefore should be less capable of resisting tensile stresses. These observations have been confirmed by biomechanical studies indicating that the medial collateral ligament became less stiff as a result of immobilization.

Little is known regarding the effects of immobilization on nonsynovial tendons. This is an area in which additional investigations would be beneficial.

The most significant changes after immobilization of ligaments are at the soft tissue-bone junction. Histologically, the femoral and tibial insertion sites of the medial collateral ligament showed increased osteoclastic activity, resorption of bone, and disruption of the normal

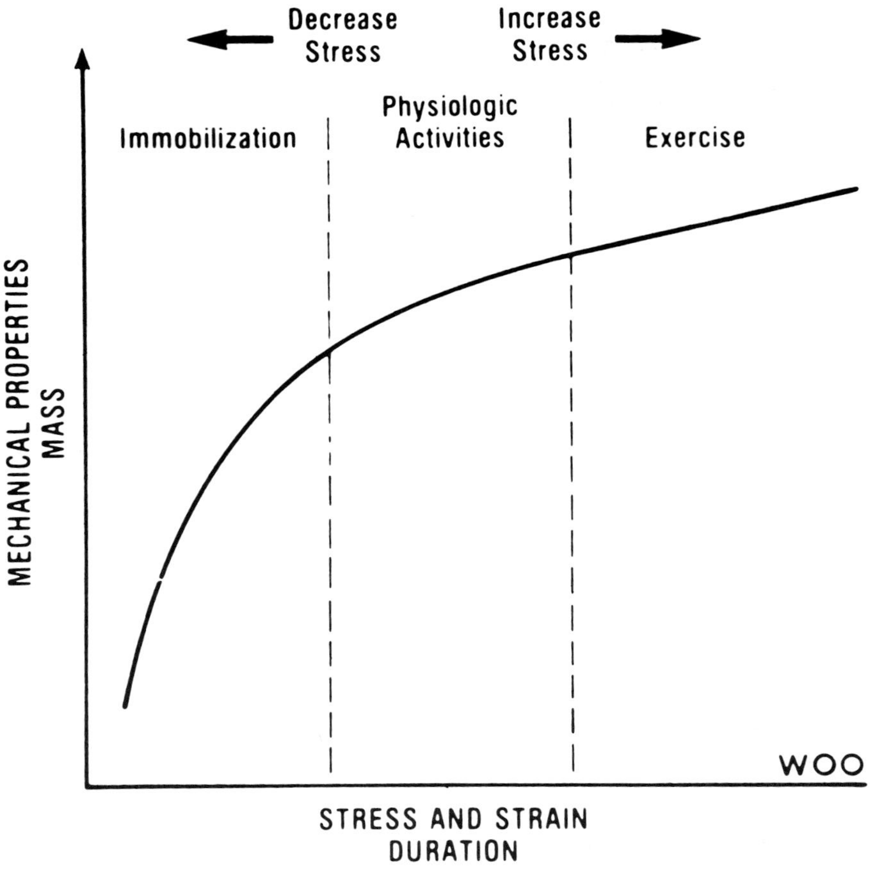

Fig. 2 *Hypothetical curve describing the nonlinear effects of stress and motion on the homeostatic responses of soft connective tissues. (Reproduced with permission from Woo SL, Gomez MA, Woo YK, et al: Mechanical properties of tendons and ligaments: II. The relationships of immobilization and exercise on tissue remodeling.* Biorheology *1982;19:397–408.)*

attachment between the bones and the ligament. Osteoclasts activated during immobilization resorbed the subperiosteal bone; thus, the ligament was secured by only a superficial periosteal attachment at the tibial end. As a result, significant reduction in the ultimate load-and energy-absorbing capability of the bone-ligament complex and an increase in the number of failures by tibial avulsion were found during tensile testing.[73]

On the basis of the above findings, a hypothetical curve to describe the homeostatic responses for ligaments and tendons is proposed (Fig. 2). The relationship between the level and duration of stress and motion and the resulting changes in tissue properties and tissue mass can be represented by a highly nonlinear curve. The normal range of physiologic activities is bracketed in the middle portion of the curve. With stress and motion deprivation, a rapid reduction in tissue properties and/or mass may occur, since the slope of the curve in this region is steep. For example, a short period of immobilization of the rabbit knee resulted in a significant alteration in the biomechanical characteristics of the bone-ligament complex. In contrast, with exercise training or increased levels of stress and motion, the resultant changes are less pronounced, because the slope for the curve in this region is relatively flat. Changes in the mechanical properties, collagen content, and other parameters are relatively moderate.

Response of Tendon and Ligament to Prefailure Injury

In vitro experiments have been performed on the microscopic and submicroscopic effects of prefailure loading on tendons. Tendon's microstructural viscoelasticity is similar to its macrostructural viscoelasticity.[41,43] Tendon collagen fibers can be stretched experimentally to a certain value while maintaining the tendon's elastic characteristics. Beyond this value (overstretching), irreversible loss of tendon crimp occurs.[12] Straightening out occurs nonuniformly, as it seems to occur a few bundles at a time and is more pronounced in the center of a cross section of the tendon.[60] This process is reversible until approximately one third of the maximum load of the tendon is reached; then irreversible changes occur[43,58] and microscopic failure of collagen fibers can be seen.

Just as crimp is eliminated within the tendon in a nonuniform fashion, so rupture of collagen fibers proceeds in a seemingly random fashion within the tendon. This is believed to be a result of nonuniform loading of individual fibers. Even in the case of relatively uniform loading, such as tensile testing of the femur-medial collateral ligament-tibia complex of the rabbit, it has been demonstrated that tensile loading to 50% and 75% of the expected failure load can cause partial failure of the ligament substance.[47] Histologic sections demonstrated that both the femoral and the tibial insertion sites had no visible failure whereas there were major tears of the collagen fiber bundles in the ligament substance.

Knörzer and associates,[32] Mosler and associates,[41] and Nemetschek and associates[42,43] have done extensive work on the ultrastructural changes in collagen caused by mechanical stress. They have demonstrated that collagen fibers are composed of subunits forming a system of overlapping, parallel-sliding, mechanically bridged linear fibrils or subfibrils. These fibrils are shorter than the actual length of the fibers, implying cross-linkages. Cyclical stretching of these fibrils leads to an improved arrangement of the helical molecular chains and is given as the explanation for the conditioning effect seen in collagenous tissue. A sudden initial stretch causes greater molecular deformation than further stretches of the same strength and may lead to fibril structural disruption. Normal wet collagen fibrils demonstrate a 67-nm banding pattern, called the D period, that is thought to be the result of the overlapping structure of collagen molecules making up the fibril. A constant stretch causes changes in the D-period characteristics of native collagen. This is thought to result from a sliding of the triple-helix collagen molecules relative to each other, resulting in an observed larger D period and an increased length in the gap region with shortening of the structural overlap region in collagen under strain. These findings imply that the cross-linked telopeptides between collagen molecules are stretched when a linear strain is applied. This ultrastructural process is rate-dependent. Ultimately, if a sufficient strain is applied, intrafibrillar slippage occurs. This immediately precedes microscopically observed interfibrillar slippage with its resultant observed decrease in tension on the stress-strain curve. Interestingly, slow overstretching, very fast loading (5,000%/sec), and very fast unloading (2,500%/sec) of a previously loaded tendon fiber can all lead to electron microscopic evidence of fibril splitting and so-called "kink" deformations.[31] These kink deformations are somewhat similar in appearance to the coiled, ruptured ends of collagen fibrils seen in totally ruptured tendons. The knotted and coiled ends represent ruptured and denatured collagen molecules because they are susceptible to trypsin digestion, whereas collagen in its normal triple-helix state is degradable only by collagenase.[52] Enzyme digestion studies such as this demonstrate that the mechanical damage to a collagen molecule is limited to the site of mechanical disruption and does not involve the entire molecule. The remainder of the disrupted collagen fibrils stay in their native intact state and are not susceptible to trypsin digestion.

The etiology of mechanical damage to tendon, whether complete or partial, can thus be related to intrafibrillar sliding beyond the elastic limit.[13,29,32] Initially, the most highly strained or weakest fibrils rupture, forcing increased loads on adjacent fibrils that can, if the force continues, rupture successively as well. This leads to fiber disruption and the loss of tendon composite structure. When such microscopic disruptions continue to accumulate, gross tendon rupture occurs. More commonly, the process is aborted before tendon rupture, but such microtrauma can lead to a weakened tendon. If healing processes are subsequently inadequate, or if additional microtrauma is superimposed, tendinosis may result.

The loading of tendons in vivo is often not just a purely tensile phenomenon restricted to the tendon. Barfred[7] demonstrated that rat Achilles tendon is more vulnerable to rupture when the tendon is loaded obliquely, when its muscle is in maximal contraction, when the muscle is exhausted, or when the initial length of the muscle-tendon unit is short. Thus, if the muscle portion of the muscle-tendon unit is fatigued, the muscle can no longer accept as much of the shock-absorbing function of the unit, and greater stresses are absorbed by the tendon. Fatigue failure of the tendon can ensue.

The relevance of the experimentally induced mechanical tendon injury to its physiologic counterpart in humans can be borne out by an analysis of the histopathologic findings in partial (tendinosis) and complete (rupture) tendon injury. The most consistent findings in partial injuries are fragmentation of collagen (including kink deformation), thinning and separation of collagen, edema with an increased ground substance separation of tenocytes in collagen, and proliferation of capillaries and small-walled vessels, often with mesenchymal tissue.[4,9,12,16,17,21,23,27,35–37,46,50,70] Less frequently, an increase in the number of fibroblasts can be seen, occasionally with hypoxic changes. If the process has been going on for some time, irregular, poorly oriented collagen with variations in fiber diameter and loss of periodicity can be seen. This may correspond to markedly increased formation of type III collagen.[11,28] An increase in type III collagen also has been noted in equine tendon scar.[67] Calcification, although rarely reported by radiographic criteria, is seen in as many as 25% of samples examined microscopically and in as many as 50% of samples seen under the electron microscope.[25,26] These calcific changes are thought to be hypoxic in nature and not related to necrosis or inflammation. Uhthoff and Sarkar[57] believed that calcification occurs in areas of cartilaginous transformation, whereas Józsa and associates[26] found such changes in noncartilaginous areas.

Inflammatory changes within the tendon are distinctly not a part of the histopathology of partial chronic tendon injury. Thus, the term "tendinosis" is more appropriate than the commonly used term "tendinitis" to denote this entity. Significant inflammatory changes become apparent within the tendon only when total tendon disruption occurs and major vascular disruption is present.[4,14]

On the other hand, significant inflammatory changes have been reported in peritendinous tissue. These may be important in the generation of pain in chronic tendinosis. In equine partial tendon injuries, marked peritendinous inflammation and thickening have been noted.[53,64] The most common and dramatic location in humans is in the tenosynovium of the pseudosheath of the Achilles tendon. Goldie[21] emphasized the importance of the granulation tissue in the subtendinous space immediately adjacent to the extensor carpi radialis brevis origin in the generation of pain in tennis elbow. Thickening and irregularities have been reported in the surrounding retinaculum of the patellar tendon in patellar tendinosis.[42] Inflammation and thickening of the subdeltoid bursa is a consistent finding in rotator cuff tears of the shoulder and is frequently present in partial cuff injuries.

Bone-tendon junctional changes have been reported, although this most commonly has been noted by certain authors in cases of "jumper's knee."[16,17,52] These include microfractures, increased thickness of the insertional fibrocartilage, blue-line irregularities, and pseudocystic cavities, along with collagen fiber disruption. Abnormalities of this highly stressed junctional area could well be expected, given the vast difference in mechanical properties between tendon and bone.

Various authors have attempted to study partial tendon injuries and tendinosis in animal models. Welsh and associates[65] performed biomechanical studies of various rabbit tendon (plantaris, gastrocnemius, soleus, and flexor digitorum longus) and also looked at the weakening effects of a small notched defect in these tendons. Postacchini and De Martino[48] studied the healing of such a defect. Initially they found a large increase in the number of small collagen fibrils and immature elastic fibers, but no inflammatory cells. Over the course of 16 weeks, the elastic fibers matured and collagen fibrils increased in size to approach normal diameters; however, even at the end of this period the tendon regeneration process appeared to be incomplete. Watkins and associates[63] investigated the healing of partial, central full-thickness defects in the equine superficial digital flexor tendon. A square, full-thickness defect was created surgically by excising the central third of the tendon. They believed that the gross histologic appearance of the tendon during healing was similar to that in naturally occurring partial injury. Kapetanos,[29] in an investigation of the effects of local corticosteroids on tendon healing, created what he believed was a partial injury by completely transecting one of the three approximately equal-sized tendons (gastrocnemius, soleus, and plantaris) making up the rabbit Achilles tendon. However, since each tendon has a distinct muscle belly and is clearly structurally distinguished from the two other tendons in the group, this seems to be a poor model of partial tendon injury to a specific tendon.

Silver and associates[51] and Williams and associates[68] proposed an equine tendon partial-injury model created by local injection of collagenase into the superficial digital flexor. They concluded that the enzyme-induced lesion clinically and histologically healed in a fashion similar to that of a naturally occurring tendon strain. As such, it was a good model of naturally occurring tendon strain and could be used as a model for a comparative study of treatment methods. Later, this same center used collagenase to create partial Achilles tendon injuries in rabbits, which subsequently demonstrated improved healing with heparin treatment.[51,68]

Wiig and associates[66] recently studied the healing of a variety of different partial anterior cruciate ligament lacerations. Improved healing was observed with the intra-articular injection of high-molecular-weight hyaluronic acid in central ligament defects. Kennedy and associates[30] demonstrated considerable ultrastructural disruption and disorganization of collagen fibrils throughout the substance of the anterior cruciate ligament, medial collateral ligament, and posterior cruciate ligament just before ultimate failure. These ligaments are still grossly intact to inspection at this point. Peterson[47] also demonstrated that failure of fiber bundles within the ligament substance can occur before complete ligamentous tear. Thus, clinical impressions of the amount of injury present in a ligament may be deceptive.

References

1. Amadio PC, Berglund LJ, An KN: Tensile properties of biochemically discrete zones of canine flexor tendon. *Trans Orthop Res Soc* 1989;14:251.
2. Amiel D, Akeson WH, Harwood FL, et al: Stress deprivation effect on metabolic turnover of the medial collateral ligament collagen: A comparison between nine- and 12-week immobilization. *Clin Orthop* 1983;172:265–270.

3. Amiel D, Frank C, Harwood F, et al: Tendons and ligaments: A morphological and biochemical comparison. *J Orthop Res* 1984;1:257–265.
4. Arner O, Lindholm Å, Orell SR: Histologic changes in subcutaneous rupture of the Achilles tendon: A study of 74 cases. *Acta Chir Scand* 1959;116:484–490.
5. Banes AJ, Donlon K, Link GW, et al: Cell populations of tendon: A simplified method for isolation of synovial cells and internal fibroblasts. Confirmation of origin and biologic properties. *J Orthop Res* 1988;6:83–94.
6. Banes AJ, Link GW, Bevin AG, et al: Tendon synovial cells secrete fibronectin in vivo and in vitro. *J Orthop Res* 1988;6:73–82.
7. Barfred T: Experimental rupture of the Achilles tendon: Comparison of various types of experimental rupture in rats. *Acta Orthop Scand* 1971;42:528–543.
8. Binkley JM, Peat M: The effect of immobilization on the ultrastructure and mechanical properties of the medial collateral ligament of rats. *Clin Orthop* 1986;203:301–308.
9. Brewer BJ: Aging of the rotator cuff. *Am J Sports Med* 1979;7:102–110.
10. Chun KJ, Butler DL, Stouffer DC, et al: Stress-strain relationships in fascicle-bone units from human patellar tendon and knee ligaments. *Trans Orthop Res Soc* 1988;13:82.
11. Coombs RRH, Klenerman L, Narcisi P, et al: Collagen typing in Achilles tendon rupture, abstract. *J Bone Joint Surg* 1980;62B:258.
12. Cotton RE, Rideout DF: Tears of the humeral rotator cuff: A radiological and pathological necropsy survey. *J Bone Joint Surg* 1964;46B:314–328.
13. Curwin S, Stanish WD: *Tendinitis: Its Etiology and Treatment.* Lexington, Collamore Press, 1984, pp 28–31.
14. Davidson L, Salo M: Pathogenesis of subcutaneous tendon ruptures. *Acta Chir Scand* 1969;135:209–212.
15. Diamant J, Keller A, Baer E, et al: Collagen: Ultrastructure and its relationship to mechanical properties as a function of ageing. *Proc R Soc Lond [Biol]* 1972;180:293–314.
16. Dupont M, Pasteels JL, Duchateau M, et al: Tendinites corporeales et osteotendinites, essai de definition des lesions et de leur traitement chirurgical. *Acta Orthop Belg* 1983;49:39–41.
17. Ferretti A, Ippolito E, Mariani P, et al: Jumper's knee. *Am J Sports Med* 1983;11:58–62.
18. Frank C, McDonald D, Lieber RL, et al: Biochemical heterogeneity within the maturing rabbit medial collateral ligament. *Clin Orthop* 1988;236:279–285.
19. Fritschy D, de Gautard R: Jumper's knee and ultrasonography. *Am J Sports Med* 1988;16:637–640.
20. Gamble JG, Edwards CC, Max SR: Enzymatic adaptation in ligaments during immobilization. *Am J Sports Med* 1984;12:221–228.
21. Goldie I: Epicondylitis lateralis humeri (epicondylalgia or tennis elbow): A pathogenetical study. *Acta Chir Scand* 1964;339(supp):1–119.
22. Gomez MA: *The Effect of Tension on Normal and Healing Medial Collateral Ligaments*, thesis. San Diego, University of California, 1988.
23. Gould N, Korson R: Stenosing tenosynovitis of the pseudosheath of the tendo Achilles. *Foot Ankle* 1980;1:179–187.
24. Heikkinen E, Vuori I: Effect of physical activity on the metabolism of collagen in aged mice. *Acta Physiol Scand* 1972;84:543–549.
25. Hörmann H, Jelinic V: Regulation by heparin and hyaluronic acid of the fibronectin-dependent association of collagen, type III, with macrophages. *Hoppe Seylers Z Physiol Chem* 1981;362:87–94.
26. Józsa L, Bálint BJ, Réffy A: Calcifying tendinopathy. *Arch Orthop Trauma Surg* 1980;97:305–307.

27. Józsa L, Bálint BJ, Réffy A, et al: Hypoxic alterations of tenocytes in degenerative tendinopathy. *Arch Orthop Trauma Surg* 1982;99:243–246.
28. Józsa L, Réffy A, Bálint BJ: Polarization and electron microscopic studies on the collagen of intact and ruptured human tendons. *Acta Histochem* 1984;74:209–215.
29. Kapetanos G: The effect of the local corticosteroids on the healing and biomechanical properties of the partially injured tendon. *Clin Orthop* 1982;163:170–179.
30. Kennedy JC, Hawkins RJ, Willis RB, et al: Tension studies of human knee ligaments: Yield point, ultimate failure, and disruption of the cruciate and tibial collateral ligaments. *J Bone Joint Surg* 1976;58A:350–355.
31. Klein L, Player JS, Heiple KG, et al: Isotopic evidence for resorption of soft tissues and bone in immobilized dogs. *J Bone Joint Surg* 1982;64A;225–230.
32. Knörzer E, Folkhard W, Geercken W, et al: New aspects of the etiology of tendon rupture: An analysis of time-resolved dynamic-mechanical measurements using synchrotron radiation. *Arch Orthop Trauma Surg* 1986;105:113–120.
33. Koob TJ, Vogel KG: Proteoglycan synthesis in organ cultures from regions of bovine tendon subjected to different mechanical forces. *Biochem J* 1987;246:589–598.
34. Lee TQ, Woo SL: A new method for determining cross-sectional shape and area of soft tissues. *J Biomech Eng* 1988;110:110–114.
35. Ljungqvist R: Subcutaneous partial rupture of the Achilles tendon. *Acta Orthop Scand* 1968;113(suppl):1–86.
36. Martens M, Wouters P, Burssens A, et al: Patellar tendinitis: Pathology and results of treatment. *Acta Orthop Scand* 1982;53:445–450.
37. Merkel KH, Hess H, Kunz M: Insertion tendopathy in athletes: A light microscopic, histochemical and electron microscopic examination. *Pathol Res Pract* 1982;173:303–309.
38. Merrilees MJ, Flint MH: Ultrastructural study of tension and pressure zones in a rabbit flexor tendon. *Am J Anat* 1980;157:87–106.
39. Michna H: Morphometric analysis of loading-induced changes in collagen-fibril populations in young tendons. *Cell Tissue Res* 1984;236:465–470.
40. Michna H: Tendon injuries induced by exercise and anabolic steroids in experimental mice. *Int Orthop* 1987;11:157–162.
41. Mosler E, Folkhard W, Knörzer E, et al: Stress-induced molecular rearrangement in tendon collagen. *J Mol Biol* 1985;182:589–596.
42. Nemetschek T, Jelinek K, Knörzer E, et al: Transformation of the structure of collagen: A time-resolved analysis of mechanochemical processes using synchrotron radiation. *J Mol Biol* 1983;167:461–479.
43. Nemetschek T, Riedl H, Jonak R, et al: Die Viskoelastizität parallelsträngigen Bindegewebes und ihre Bedeutung für die Funktion. *Virchows Arch [Pathol Anat]* 1980;386:125–151.
44. Newton PO, MacKenna DA, Lyon RM, et al: Comparison of the mechanical properties of medial collateral and anterior cruciate ligaments of the rabbit knee. Presented at the Third Joint ASCE/ASME Mechanics Conference, La Jolla, July 9–12, 1989.
45. Oakes BW, Parker AW, Norman J: Changes in collagen fiber populations in young rat cruciate ligaments in response to an intensive one month's exercise program, in Russo P, Gass G (eds): *Human Adaption.* Williamsberg, Kentucky, Cumberland College of Health Sciences, 1981, pp 223–230.
46. Perugia L, Ricciardi Pollini PT, Ippolito E: Ultrastructural aspects of degenerative tendinopathy. *Int Orthop* 1978;1:303–307.

47. Peterson RH: *The Effect of Strain Rate on Biomechanical Property of the Medial Collateral Ligament*, thesis. San Diego, University of California, 1986.
48. Postacchini F, De Martino C: Regeneration of rabbit calcaneal tendon maturation of collagen and elastic fibers following partial tenotomy. *Connect Tissue Res* 1980;8:41–47.
49. Refior HJ, Krödel A, Melzer C: Examinations of the pathology of the rotator cuff. *Arch Orthop Trauma Surg* 1987;106:301–308.
50. Sarkar K, Uhthoff HK: Ultrastructure of the common extensor tendon in tennis elbow. *Virchows Arch [Pathol Anat]* 1980;386:317–330.
51. Silver IA, Brown PN, Goodship AW, et al: A clinical and experimental study of tendon injury, healing and treatment in the horse. *Equine Vet J* 1983, suppl, pp 1–43.
52. Steven FS, Minns RJ, Finlay JB: Evidence for the local denaturation of collagen fibril during the mechanical rupture of human tendons. *Injury* 1975;6:317–319.
53. Strömberg B, Tufvesson G: Lesions of the superficial flexor tendon in race horses: A microangiographic and histopathologic study. *Clin Orthop* 1969;62:113–123.
54. Suominen H, Kiiskinen A, Heikkinen E: Effects of physical training on metabolism of connective tissues in young mice. *Acta Physiol Scand* 1980;108:17–22.
55. Tipton CM, James SL, Mergner W, et al: Influence of exercise on strength of medial collateral knee ligaments of dogs. *Am J Physiol* 1970;218:894–902.
56. Tipton CM, Martin RK, Mathes RD, et al: Hydroxyproline concentrations in ligaments from trained and nontrained rats, in Howald H, Poortmans JR (eds): *Metabolic Adaptation to Prolonged Physical Exercise.* Basel, Birkhauser Verlag, 1975, pp 262–267.
57. Uhthoff HK, Sarkar K: Calcifying tendinitis. *Int Orthop* 1978;2:187–193.
58. Viidik A: Simultaneous mechanical and light microscopic studies of collagen fibers. *Z Anat Entwicklungsgesch* 1972;136:204–212.
59. Viidik A: The effect of training on the tensile strength of isolated rabbit tendons. *Scand J Plast Reconstr Surg* 1967;1:141–147.
60. Viidik A, Ekholm R: Light and electron microscopic studies of collagen fibers under strain. *Anat Entwickl* 1968;127:154–164.
61. Vogel KG, Evanko SP: Proteoglycans of fetal bovine tendon. *J Biol Chem* 1987;262:13607–13613.
62. Wang CW, Weiss JA, Albright J, et al: Life-long exercise and aging effects on the canine medial collateral ligament. *Trans Orthop Res Soc* 1990;15:58.
63. Watkins JP, Auer JA, Gay S, et al: Healing of surgically created defects in the equine superficial digital flexor tendon: Collagen-type transformation and tissue morphologic reorganization. *Am J Vet Res* 1985;46:2091–2096.
64. Webbon PM: A post mortem study of equine digital flexor tendons. *Equine Vet J* 1977;9:61–67.
65. Welsh RP, Macnab I, Riley V: Biomechanical studies of rabbit tendon. *Clin Orthop* 1971;81:171–177.
66. Wiig ME, Amiel D, Harwood FL, et al: Anterior cruciate ligament healing: The effect of high molecular weight hyaluronan (hyaluronic acid). *Trans Orthop Res Soc* 1989;14:297.
67. Williams IF, Heaton A, McCullagh KG: Cell morphology and collagen types in equine tendon scar. *Res Vet Sci* 1980;28:302–310.
68. Williams IF, McCullagh KG, Goodship AE, et al: Studies on the pathogenesis of equine tendonitis following collagenase injury. *Res Vet Sci* 1984;36:326–338.

69. Williams IF, Nicholls JS, Goodship AE, et al: Experimental treatment of tendon injury with heparin. *Br J Plast Surg* 1986;39:367–372.
70. Wilson CL, Duff GL: Pathologic study of degeneration and rupture of the supraspinatus tendon. *Arch Surg* 1943;47:121–135.
71. Woo SL-Y, Gomez MA, Amiel D, et al: The effects of exercise on the biomechanical and biochemical properties of swine digital flexor tendons. *J Biomech Eng* 1981;103:51–56.
72. Woo SL-Y, Gomez MA, Seguchi Y, et al: Measurement of mechanical properties of ligament substance from a bone-ligament-bone preparation. *J Orthop Res* 1983;1:22–29.
73. Woo SL-Y, Gomez MA, Sites TJ, et al: The biomechanical and morphological changes in the medial collateral ligament of the rabbit after immobilization and remobilization. *J Bone Joint Surg* 1987;69A:1200–1211.
74. Woo SL-Y, Lee TQ, Gomez MA, et al: Temperature dependent behavior of the canine medial collateral ligament. *J Biomech Eng* 1987;109:68–71.
75. Woo SL-Y, Orlando CA, Camp J, et al: Effects of postmortem storage by freezing on ligament tensile behavior. *J Biomech* 1986;19:399–404.
76. Woo SL-Y, Ritter MA, Amiel D, et al: The biomechanical and biochemical properties of swine tendons: Long term effects of exercise on the digital extensors. *Connect Tissue Res* 1980;7:177–183.
77. Wood TO, Cooke PH, Goodship AE: The effect of exercise and anabolic steroids on the mechanical properties and crimp morphology of the rat tendon. *Am J Sports Med* 1988;16:153–158.
78. Zernicke RF, Butler DL, Grood ES, et al: Strain topography of human tendon and fascia. *J Biomech Eng* 1984;106:177–180.

Chapter 11

Repair Models and Specific Tissue Responses in Muscle Injury

William T. Stauber, PhD

Sports injuries that directly affect skeletal muscle involve either mechanical damage from the strain of the sport or energy depletion caused by the exhaustive nature of the activity. Laboratory procedures are available to study tissue responses to most muscle injuries. These injury models range from simple overuse, such as occurs during running activities, to complex overloading failure, which follows strain or impulse loading. Despite these useful research models, knowledge of injury mechanisms, inflammatory responses, and repair processes is limited because muscle has various different cell types and components, each of which may be important in repair and adaptation. Furthermore, muscle damage can result in myofiber breaks, fascial tears, or complete rupture of an entire muscle, each of which elicits different mechanisms of tissue response. The responses of muscle and related tissue to sports injuries are quite complex and require much interdisciplinary research.

Sports-related muscle injuries such as tears often occur as the result of specific muscle actions or when external forces directly traumatize muscle tissue and tear it. Muscles are susceptible to sports injuries because they perform multiple functions such as movement, stabilization, and shock absorption.[31] Sports injuries often involve mechanical strain or energy depletion.

Mechanical strain occurs when load overcomes a muscle's ability to resist it during deceleration; the shock absorber or spring-like function of the muscle fails.[36] The most dramatic illustration of such a deceleration injury is seen when an entire muscle (such as the hamstring) is torn in half. The least traumatic injury is one in which a single myofiber is broken, as might occur in walking downhill.

In the second type of muscle injury, energy depletion, exhaustive aerobic exercise or extensive anaerobic activity damages muscles. Running a marathon is an example of an exhaustive aerobic exercise; competitive wrestling is representative of an anaerobic sport. In both cases, but for different reasons, the muscle depletes its energy reserves and is damaged by processes resulting from the energy-deficient state. For example, muscle action by itself can occlude blood vessels and cause ischemic damage. The most severe injury of this type results in exercise-induced rhabdomyolysis[21,33] or compartment syndromes.[13] The energy-depletion injury is quite similar in its processes to the pathogenesis of the muscle abnormalities seen in mitochondrial myopathies. However, the muscle with an energy-depletion injury can return to a normal resting state by restorative physiologic processes.

Various experimental protocols have been used to study muscle injury and regeneration in animals and humans. These techniques include minced muscle grafting, free muscle grafting, ischemia (tourniquet application), toxin administration, and freezing. Although these protocols are useful in understanding the biology of muscle injury and repair,[6] they have little direct application to sport-induced muscle injuries. Instead, this chapter presents the experimental models used to stimulate sports-induced muscle injuries and discusses the specific tissue responses to mechanisms of inflammation and repair of damaged muscle.

Animal Models of Muscle Injury

Treadmill running is usually used in the study of exercise-induced injury in animals. In addition, mechanical strain and overload procedures that do not require the active cooperation of the animals have been developed to simulate muscle injuries occurring in various sports and exercises. Animals have been used to study muscle adaptation after downhill running,[2] drop-landing,[15] external trauma (crush, contusion, incision),[22,25] and controlled[24,29] or uncontrolled[37] mechanical strains.

During downhill running, the treadmill is elevated and the animal faces downhill. This orientation forces the front limbs to participate more vigorously in deceleration. In drop-landing, the animal lands on all four extremities and the impact shock of landing is absorbed by the muscles and connecting structures. Externally applied traumas (surgical incisions, impact contusion, and crushing with forceps) are used to study muscle injury and healing. Blunt trauma is common in contact sports, but in the laboratory it requires additional quantitation of the impact force absorbed.

Mechanical strains that occur regularly in sports can be duplicated to injure muscles in the laboratory. To measure the force (controlled strain) necessary to produce muscle damage or tendon rupture, it is necessary to externalize the muscle tendon through surgery.[24,29] In addition, experimental procedures often stretch the muscle beyond its physiologic working range, resulting in damage to blood vessels. In contrast, uncontrolled muscle strain[37] is simulated by activating the muscle with an external stimulator and pushing the limb through its normal range of motion while the muscle remains fully active (eccentric muscle action). This protocol results in damage more like that occurring naturally during locomotion, but it does not provide information about the amount of force required to damage a muscle or the amount of active force output lost as injury occurs. However, there is no capillary rupture, and thus this model most closely approximates the damage seen in weight training (performance of negative work).

With the exception of trauma, these protocols all use eccentric muscle action[7,36] (stretching of an active muscle) to produce the muscle injury. The muscle injury can occur after a single bout of muscle strain of sufficient magnitude to produce failure in an active muscle (breakage of some muscle component),[29] or after a series of small repeated loads during one session, which together produce failure as the tissue components become fatigued (as occurs in downhill running).[2] Most studies of muscle injury in animals focus on the response of the animal or of an individual muscle to one injury protocol. The animal's response to the injury is determined by measuring serum enzymes and evaluating muscle biopsy samples by biochemical and histologic techniques. The injury response, posttraumatic inflammatory state, and muscle repair processes have been studied to determine the length of time needed for complete healing.[37]

Drop-landing is an especially useful model. Animals used for jumping and humans engaged in exercise training often suffer injury from repetitive landing. Drop-landing[15] has several advantages; the animal does not undergo surgery as it must when strain devices are attached to an exposed muscle tendon,[24,29] and anesthesia is not necessary as it is in the studies of uncontrolled strains[37] or applications of trauma.[25] The impact force can be graded simply by varying the height of the drop. Different types of athletic injuries can be simulated by varying landing requirements or surfaces. More research with this model should be encouraged; the neuromuscular unit can be investigated as a unit rather than studying its components separately. In addition, large-impact loads can be applied over a period of days or weeks for study of the adaptations to repeated injury, such as occurs with exercise training.

Human Muscle Injury

The study of human muscle injury is difficult because injuries usually occur accidentally during a sports activity and are not controlled as part of a research design. Sports accidents do not allow repeated sampling at predetermined intervals with a control sample before injury. Nevertheless, sports-like injuries have been modeled in the laboratory to study human muscle damage, pain, inflammation, or adaptation after downhill running,[9,34] cycle ergometry (performing negative work),[11] repeated resisted muscle lengthening (eccentric muscle actions),[8] step test,[28] ischemic injury (tourniquet application[17]), and prolonged exercise (marathon).[18] Laboratory studies are also useful for patients with myopathic disorders in which exercise-induced damage reflects the fragility of the diseased muscle.[3]

Recently, a link was established between muscle injury during exercise and muscle inflammation in regard to the development of compartment syndromes.[16,17] Acute muscle damage and the resulting inflammation can lead to further muscle damage if the interstitial hydrostatic pressure is increased enough to impair local blood flow.[12] The reaction of muscle fibers within a compartment surrounded by the fascia resulting in a compartment syndrome is important in understanding chronic overuse syndromes and fibromyalgia.[4,5] Perhaps any fascicle within a given muscle might serve as a semirigid compartment and respond adversely to excessive use (a "microcompartment syndrome"). Repeated injury would lead to swelling and reduced blood flow within the fascicle. "Moth-eaten" type I fibers would be evident[4] because of reduced energy production[5,17] and lack of anaerobic capacity. However, these damaged fibers would be localized in one fascicle or a small region of the muscle. If the same muscles injured in sports are also required for posture, they may not receive enough rest to restore energy reserves or to complete the repair process. Thus, sometimes it may be difficult to separate the mechanical and energetic basis for muscle injury and inflammation—especially if the muscle fibers in the fascicle remain in spasm after the sports training ends but cannot be observed because the major portion of the muscle appears relaxed.

Components of Muscle Injury

Skeletal muscles can be injured by various techniques similar to sports activities. The simplest injury damages only one component, the myofiber, and results in leakage of the cytoplasmic enzyme, creatine kinase, and in a calcium influx caused by broken plasma membrane. However, such an injury does not necessarily produce pain.[36] Injury to the extracellular matrix[14] or to the fascia without myofiber rupture could result in the release of hydroxyproline from collagen disruption and degradation.[1] Collagen degradation products could signal the arrival of inflammatory cells[30] and there might be pain but without indication of muscle damage. Injury involving both myofiber and extracellular matrix damage is most common, resulting in leakage of muscle enzymes, collagen and proteoglycan degradation, and inflammation. In most muscle injuries, the capillaries, even in damaged areas, remain intact.[37] If the trauma involves complete muscle tears, bleeding and clotting occurs. The vascular disruption and clotting cause a state of local ischemia until normal blood flow has been restored. The response of a muscle as a unit to the different types of injury may vary if blood flow is arrested and clotting factors (proteases) are present. Thus, the cellular responses that characterize inflammation and repair can also differ.

The strain injury after downhill running is a useful example of a sports-induced injury. Running downhill at a constant speed causes increased oxygen consumption as existing motor units can no longer produce the necessary force as the result of cellular damage[9]. An increase in electromyographic activity shows that more motor units are necessary for the same work output. However, there may be no pain during or immediately after the exercise if the muscles were adequately oxygenated during the activity (that is, the exercise is not anaerobic in itself). Pain develops within 24 hours after exercise and may continue for days. The time lapse between the actual mechanical damage and the onset of pain is thought to be caused by inflammatory responses, which begin only after the tissue has been damaged. Nevertheless, increased indicators of muscle damage are present in the blood long after the exercise insult has been terminated.[32]

Inflammation

Inflammation has four components: (1) increased vascular permeability; (2) kallikrein action to produce kinins; (3) histamine release from mast cells; and (4) macrophage invasion to remove dead cells and debris. In the absence of capillary rupture, all these components can be observed in injured muscle, except the increase in macrophages,[37] possibly because most muscle cells do not become necrotic after injury but repair themselves within ten days. When macrophages are present, as after a marathon, there is often evidence of blood vessel damage, including extravascular localization of erythrocytes[18] and engulfment of some of these cells by the macrophages. Thus, a limited type of inflammatory response seems to follow most exercise-induced injuries.

If the soleus muscle of a rat is injured, increased vascular permeability can be observed for some plasma constituents that are not ordinarily transcytosed across the capillary endothelium; this is the case with the complement components, fibrinogen, and one plasma protease.[37] This alteration in vascular permeability increases the osmotic force in the interstitial fluid, attracts water, and results in swelling—a common feature of any exercise-induced injury.[13] Arrival of a plasma protease or the leakage of intracellular lysosomal proteases[37] into the extracellular space could act as tissue kallikreins and produce kinins from the kininogen present. The response of kinins to muscle injury has not been given much study. Bradykinin has been implicated as a mediator of muscle pain[26] and inflammation in other tissue.[38]

The significance of mast cell degranulation,[37] another component of inflammation, is also poorly understood. Histamine can mediate pain, but many other compounds are released with it when a mast cell degranulates. These include hydrolytic enzymes that can damage the extracellular matrix by protease, sulfatase, and exoglycosidase action.[27] In addition, there may be cell-mediated processes which continue to injure additional muscle cells even after the mechanical insult has been removed. Perhaps the inflammatory state of muscle is unique and would not respond to classical treatments and medications.

Lymphoid cells have been identified in myopathic muscle samples from patients with inflammatory myopathies.[10] Few studies using lymphoid markers after exercise-induced injury have been reported, and the preliminary results of these studies appear contradictory. In rats, lymphoid cells, presumably natural killer cells, have been observed invading muscle about 48 hours after injury.[37] These cells, if cytotoxic, could continue to produce muscle damage and result in continued elevation of serum muscle enzymes not related to the initial mechanical event. In human muscle samples from exercise-induced injuries, lymphoid markers were reportedly absent,[20] but the biopsy sample examined was extremely small. If the cytotoxic response was present but infrequent, it could easily have been missed considering the length of a myofiber and the small size of one lymphoid cell. Yet, only one natural killer cell may be required to injure a myofiber. The surveillance role of the immune system, in response to muscle injury and subsequent inflammation, remains poorly documented and understood.

Cell Death

In most inflammatory conditions there is some cellular death; muscle is no exception. Some necrotic fibers can be seen after any type of muscle injury. The mechanism of cell death seems to be the same whether from mechanical strain or energy depletion. A calcium overload develops[19,40] as the result of a damaged cell membrane or insufficient energy to regulate calcium homeostasis. The calcium accumulates in mitochondria and reduces their ability to produce energy. It also activates calcium-dependent proteases, causing further damage to the myofiber. Calcium also produces a focal hypercontraction of myofibrils, perhaps contributing to reduced blood flow in a single fascicle. Under such conditions, calcium could be toxic to the cell and cell death might result.

Some studies have used calcium-blocking drugs to reduce the influx of calcium into the injured myofibers and to prevent the adverse responses of myofiber damage. In animals, histologic evidence of muscle damage was observed after the application of calcium ionophores, which injured the muscle by allowing calcium entry.[19] In patients with exertional muscle pain, verapamil produced a striking improvement in pain-free exercise performance.[39] Unfortunately, these drugs have multiple effects and may even produce local anesthesia. Thus, the effect of calcium blockers such as verapamil remains poorly understood.

Muscle Repair

Muscle regeneration following exercise-induced damage to muscle has been reviewed in detail by Carlson and Faulkner.[6] For optimal regeneration, a functional nerve, an adequate blood supply, and an intact basal lamina are required. If any of these components are themselves damaged by the injury (such as rupture of the entire muscle), regeneration proceeds at a much slower rate. If the basal lamina remains intact, the remaining muscle uses it as a scaffold and remodels by budding or growing attachments from the remaining myofiber to connect the broken ends. This repair process reestablishes an intact myofiber within seven to 14 days depending on the species. Thus, muscle function can be preserved in the face of external forces that occasionally produce partial failure of the muscle.

The connective tissue of the sarcolemma also responds to injury by remodeling to assist in shock absorption and to provide structural and environmental factors necessary for regeneration. Without the presence of a properly aligned extracellular matrix, correct myofiber orientation may not occur and fibrosis may result. After long-term training in animals and humans, the connective tissue surrounding muscle[23] thickens, but the microfibrosis does not appear to be dysfunctional. Runners have no more dysfunction than persons who are inactive even though the runners have incurred multiple microtraumas and repeated inflammations.[35] Some persons may respond to repeated muscle damage by developing a fibrotic condition. Fibrosis as a response to even limited tissue damage seems to be a universal characteristic of the repair process, occurring in the liver, lungs, and skin, among other sites. When this adaptation becomes pathologic for skeletal muscles has not been investigated.

There are various laboratory models to simulate exercise damage, inflammation, and repair in both human and animal muscles. Studies should be done to determine the roles of lymphoid cells, pain mediators, and the extracellular matrix in the inflammatory response of muscles.

References

1. Abraham WM: Factors in delayed muscle soreness. *Med Sci Sports* 1977;9:11–20.
2. Armstrong RB, Ogilvie RW, Schwane JA: Eccentric exercise-induced injury to rat skeletal muscle. *J Appl Physiol* 1983;54:80–93.
3. Bär PR, Amelink GJ, Jennekens FGI: Carrier detection for muscular dystrophies after exercise-induced muscle leakage of creatine kinase and myoglobin, abstract. *Neurosci Lett* 1985;62(suppl 22):288.
4. Bengtsson A, Henriksson KG, Larsson J: Muscle biopsy in primary fibromyalgia: Light-microscopical and histochemical findings. *Scand J Rheumatol* 1986;15:1–6.
5. Bengtsson A, Henriksson KG, Larsson J: Reduced high-energy phosphate levels in the painful muscles of patients with primary fibromyalgia. *Arthritis Rheum* 1986;29:817–821.
6. Carlson BM, Faulkner JA: The regeneration of skeletal muscle fibers following injury: A review. *Med Sci Sports Exerc* 1983;15:187–198.
7. Cavanagh PR: On "muscle action" vs "muscle contraction." *J Biomech* 1988;21:69.
8. Clarkson PM, Tremblay I: Exercise-induced muscle damage, repair, and adaptation in humans. *J Appl Physiol* 1988;65:1–6.
9. Dick RW, Cavanagh PR: An explanation of the upward drift in oxygen uptake during prolonged sub-maximal downhill running. *Med Sci Sports Exerc* 1987;19:310–317.

10. Engel AG, Arahata K: Mononuclear cells in myopathies: Quantitation of functionally distinct subsets, recognition of antigen-specific cell-mediated cytotoxicity in some diseases, and implications for the pathogenesis of the different inflammatory myopathies. *Hum Pathol* 1986;17:704–721.
11. Evans WJ, Meredith CN, Cannon JG, et al: Metabolic changes following eccentric exercise in trained and untrained men. *J Appl Physiol* 1986;61:1864–1868.
12. Fridén J, Sfakianos PN, Hargens AR: Muscle soreness and intramuscular fluid pressure: Comparison between eccentric and concentric load. *J Appl Physiol* 1986;61:2175–2179.
13. Fridén J, Sfakianos PN, Hargens AR, et al: Residual muscular swelling after repetitive eccentric contractions. *J Orthop Res* 1988;6:493–498.
14. Fritz VK, Stauber WT: Characterization of muscles injured by forced lengthening: II. Proteoglycans. *Med Sci Sports Exerc* 1988;20:354–361.
15. Hauschka EO, Roy RR, Edgerton VR: Size and metabolic properties of single muscle fibers in rat soleus after hindlimb suspension. *J Appl Physiol* 1987;62:2338–2347.
16. Heppenstall RB, Sapega AA, Scott R, et al: The compartment syndrome: An experimental and clinical study of muscular energy metabolism using phosphorus nuclear magnetic resonance spectroscopy. *Clin Orthop* 1988;226:138–155.
17. Heppenstall RB, Scott R, Sapega AA, et al: A comparative study of the tolerance of skeletal muscle to ischemia: Tourniquet application compared with acute compartment syndrome. *J Bone Joint Surg* 1986;68A:820–828.
18. Hikida RS, Staron RS, Hagerman FC, et al: Muscle fiber necrosis associated with human marathon runners. *J Neurol Sci* 1983;59:185–203.
19. Jones DA, Jackson MJ, McPhail G, et al: Experimental mouse muscle damage: The importance of external calcium. *Clin Sci* 1984;66:317–322.
20. Jones DA, Newham DJ, Round JM, et al: Experimental human muscle damage: Morphological changes in relation to other indices of damage. *J Physiol (Lond)* 1986;375:435–448.
21. Knochel JP: Rhabdomyolysis and myoglobinuria. *Annu Rev Med* 1982;33:435–443.
22. Lehto M, Järvinen M, Nelimarkka O: Scar formation after skeletal muscle injury: A histological and autoradiographical study in rats. *Arch Orthop Trauma Surg* 1986;104:366–370.
23. MacDougall JD, Sale DG, Alway SE, et al: Muscle fiber number in biceps brachii in bodybuilders and control subjects. *J Appl Physiol* 1984;57:1399–1403.
24. McCully KK, Faulkner JA: Injury to skeletal muscle fibers of mice following lengthening contractions. *J Appl Physiol* 1985;59:119–126.
25. McGeachie JK, Grounds MD: Initiation and duration of muscle precursor replication after mild and severe injury to skeletal muscle of mice: An autoradiographic study. *Cell Tissue Res* 1987;248:125–130.
26. Mense S: Reduction of the bradykinin-induced activation of feline group III and IV muscle receptors by acetylsalicylic acid. *J Physiol (Lond)* 1982;326:269–283.
27. Metcalfe DD, Kaliner M, Donlon MA: The mast cell. *CRC Crit Rev Immunol* 1981;3:23–74.
28. Newham DJ, Mills KR, Quigley BM, et al: Pain and fatigue after concentric and eccentric muscle contractions. *Clin Sci* 1983;64:55–62.
29. Nikolaou PK, Macdonald BL, Glisson RR, et al: Biomechanical and histological evaluation of muscle after controlled strain injury. *Am J Sports Med* 1987;15:9–14.
30. Postlethwaite AE, Kang AH: Collagen- and collagen peptide-induced chemotaxis of human blood monocytes. *J Exp Med* 1976;143:1299–1307.

31. Radin EL: Role of muscles in protecting athletes from injury. *Acta Med Scand* 1986;711(suppl):143–137.
32. Round JM, Jones DA, Cambridge G: Cellular infiltrates in human skeletal muscle: Exercise induced damage as a model for inflammatory muscle disease? *J Neurol Sci* 1987;82:1–11.
33. Schmitt HP, Bersch W, Feustel HP: Acute abdominal rhabdomyolysis after body building exercise: Is there a "rectus abdominus syndrome"? *Muscle Nerve* 1983;6:228–232.
34. Schwane JA, Johnson SR, Vandenakker CB, et al: Delayed-onset muscular soreness and plasma CPK and LDH activities after downhill running. *Med Sci Sports Exerc* 1983;15:51–56.
35. Siegel AJ, Warhol MJ, Lang G: Muscle injury and repair in ultra-long distance runners, in Sutton JR, Brock RM (eds): *Sports Medicine for the Mature Athlete*. Indianapolis, Benchmark Press, 1984, pp 35–43.
36. Stauber WT: Eccentric action of muscles: Physiology, injury and adaptation, in Pandolf K (ed): *Exercise and Sports Sciences Reviews*. Baltimore, Williams & Wilkins, 1989, vol 17, pp 157–185.
37. Stauber WT, Fritz VK, Vogelbach DW, et al: Characterization of muscles injured by forced lengthening: I. Cellular infiltrates. *Med Sci Sports Exerc* 1988;20:345–353.
38. Taylor JE, DeFeudis FV, Moreau JP: Bradykinin-antagonists: Therapeutic perspectives. *Drug Dev Res* 1989;16:1–11.
39. Walton J: Diffuse exercise-induced muscle pain of undetermined causes relieved by verapamil. *Lancet* 1981;1:993.
40. Wrogemann K, Pena SD: Mitochondrial calcium overload: A general mechanism for cell-necrosis in muscle diseases. *Lancet* 1976;1:672–674.

Chapter 12

Cellular and Matrix Response to Mechanical Injury at the Myotendinous Junction

William E. Garrett, Jr, MD, PhD
John Lohnes, PA-C

Injuries to the muscle-tendon unit are common but poorly understood. Clinical and laboratory investigations of the morphology of muscle strains have indicated that the injury occurs at the myotendinous junction and is characterized primarily by inflammation and edema and to a lesser extent by hemorrhage.

Histologically, partial rupture of distal fibers and hemorrhage occur immediately after injury, followed by a proliferation of inflammatory cells and fibroblastic activity during the first 24 to 48 hours. A fibrotic response ensues as the inflammatory reaction resolves.

Nonsteroidal anti-inflammatory drugs (NSAIDs) have been shown to reduce the inflammation and pain associated with muscle strain without impairing the restoration of tensile strength.

Exercise-induced muscle soreness is of shorter duration and is completely reversible. It is also characterized by an inflammatory response that may respond to NSAIDs.

Sports-related muscle-tendon unit injuries are among the most frequent causes of pain and decreased performance. Muscles can be injured by a variety of mechanisms.[9] Direct trauma or blunt injury usually involves the fleshy part of the muscle or the muscle belly. Also common are indirect or strain injuries, which usually occur in response to powerful contractions combined with forced lengthening of the muscle. This mechanism usually produces a sudden, acutely painful injury near the myotendinous junction. Another common mechanism of injury to muscle involves intense exercise, which causes pain and soreness after a delay of some time, usually 12 to 24 hours. Exercise-induced muscle soreness is a painful but fully reversible injury lasting two to four days. Ongoing studies are attempting to identify the pathologic changes associated with such injuries; at present, such changes are believed to be scattered throughout the length of the muscle fibers.

This review considers in detail the processes involved in the indirect or strain injuries of muscle.

Muscle Strain Injuries

In contrast to injuries of ligament, bone, and tendon, muscle strain injuries are seldom treated surgically; therefore, most clinicians lack a basic knowledge of the nature of these injuries. Injuries that have been explored surgically are usully described as occurring near the bone-tendon junction or the myotendinous junction[9]; for example, the medial head of the gastrocnemius frequently ruptures at its junction with the Achilles tendon.[8] Similarly, pectoralis major ruptures have been described as occurring near the myotendinous junction.[21] High-resolution radiographic imaging studies may be useful in defining the location and nature of muscle strain injuries. For example, a study of hamstring muscle strains using computed tomography demonstrated that most of the injuries occurred near the proximal myotendinous junction of the bicep femoris.[11] Studies using magnetic resonance imaging are now under way. Imaging studies have been useful not only in localizing the injuries, but also in defining their nature. Computed tomography shows the injuries as low-density reactions within the muscle, characteristic of inflammation or edema. In contrast, a high-density radiographic appearance indicates a large hematoma within the injured muscle. The clinical manifestations of many muscle injuries include significant bleeding, with subcutaneous evidence of bleeding marked by skin discoloration. Obviously, such a clinical manifestation indicates that the hematoma has escaped from the confines of the muscle to the subcutaneous space.

Although few data are available from clinical studies, there is information from experimental studies of muscle strain injuries.[10,17] Muscles stretched to failure show disruption near the myotendinous junction; however, the disruption does not occur precisely at the junction. The muscle fibers rupture a short distance away from the tendon. The distance can range from 0.1 mm to several millimeters. Nondisruptive injuries have also been examined in some detail. Rabbit hindlimb muscles were stretched far enough to produce a plastic deformation in the muscle, as evidenced by the load-deformation curve[17] (Fig. 1). Nondisruptive injuries required a strain equal to 80% of the force required to disrupt the contralateral muscle completely. The injured muscles produced approximately 70% of normal tension in response to tetanic stimulation (Fig. 2). This value dropped to 50% by day 2 and recovered to 90% by day 7.

The tensile strength of injured muscles has also been evaluated in rats. The tensile strength of strained muscles initially declined to less than 50% of normal by day 2; this was followed by a return to near normal by 11 days. These experiments demonstrate that recovery to near-normal strengths can follow muscle strain injury.

The process of recovery has been demonstrated histologically.[17] The fibers became disrupted near the myotendinous junction (Fig. 3). Not all fibers were injured; only the fibers near the myotendinous junction showed disruption. Histologic changes were not seen farther away from the junction, eg, at the middle of the fiber, even when the distal fiber was disrupted. The syncytial nature of muscle fibers must ensure fiber viability, even when the terminal portions of the fibers are disrupted. Hemorrhage surrounding the ruptured ends of the fibers was also evident in the acute phase. No sizable hematoma developed, although

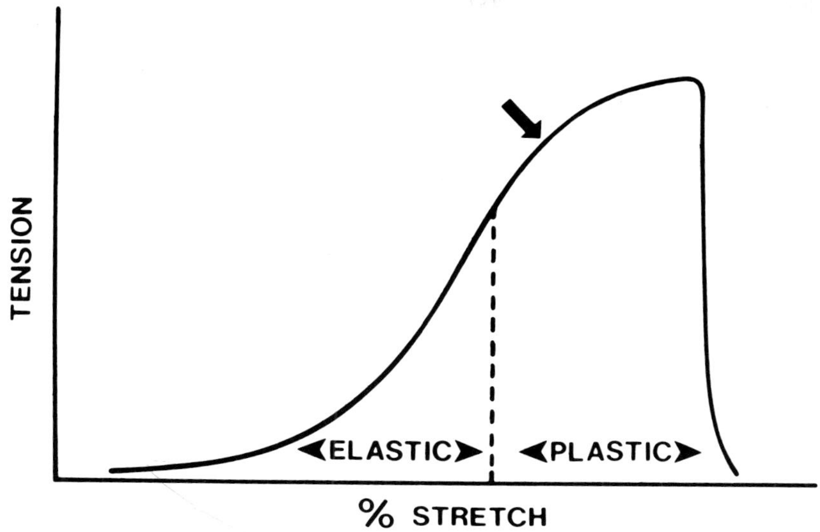

Fig. 1 *Deformation curve for muscle-tendon unit. Arrow indicates 80% failure force. (Reproduced with permission from Nikolaou PK, Macdonald BL, Glisson RR, et al: Biomechanical and histological evaluation of muscle after controlled strain injury.* Am J Sports Med *1987;15:9–14.)*

blood can escape from between the muscle fibers to elevate and collect under the epimysium.

During the next few days a typical cellular response to injury occurred. The disrupted fibers showed necrotic changes near the myotendinous junction. Macrophages could be seen within the disruptive fibers (Fig. 4). Inflammatory cells were prominent one day after injury and became more so by day 2 (Fig. 5). The inflammatory reaction was most intense near the region of muscle fiber disruption; the edema was more widespread. In rats, the wet weight of the injured muscle increased as much as 20% by day 2 because of the significant increase in tissue edema. In both rat and rabbit models the inflammatory response seemed most marked at day 2.

After the initial inflammatory changes, the cellular processes showed a clearing of the necrotic muscle fibers and a proliferation of granulation tissue with fibroblasts, capillaries, and residual inflammatory cells (Fig. 6). Muscle regeneration processes were evident with myotubal formation. A significant fibrotic response was most prominent. An increase in fibrosis became more prominent between days 4 and 11 with an increase in the connective tissue between the fibers and near the myotendinous junction. The fibrosis prevented restoration of the normal muscle structure within the periods of these studies.

These experimental studies demonstrated previously unrecognized

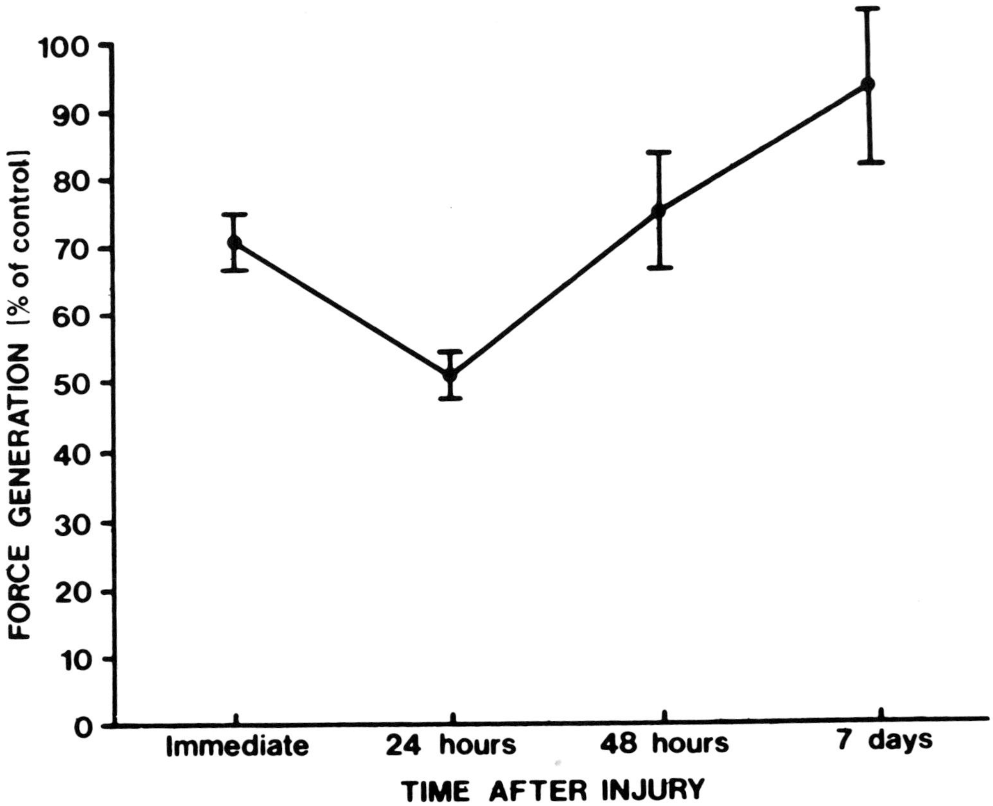

Fig. 2 *Percent of control force generation averaged over all frequencies tested vs time after injury. (Reproduced with permission from Nikolaou PK, Macdonald BL, Glisson RR, et al: Biomechanical and histological evaluation of muscle after controlled strain injury.* Am J Sports Med *1987;15:9–14.)*

properties of muscle injury. The injuries were not associated with a significant hematoma within the muscle. Small hemorrhages were seen but there was no large collection of blood within the muscle belly. In addition, the almost uniform localization of muscle injury to the region of the fibers near the myotendinous junction had not been appreciated.

There are many empiric approaches to the treatment of muscle strain injuries, but little consensus exists regarding how much activity is beneficial, which medications should be used, and what therapies should be employed. Few experimental studies have been performed. Basic studies have demonstrated an inflammatory response to muscle injury and common clinical practice has been the use of anti-inflammatory medications. There have been two basic investigations into the healing of muscle strain injuries treated with NSAIDs.

In a study using rat anterior tibialis, the healing process after ex-

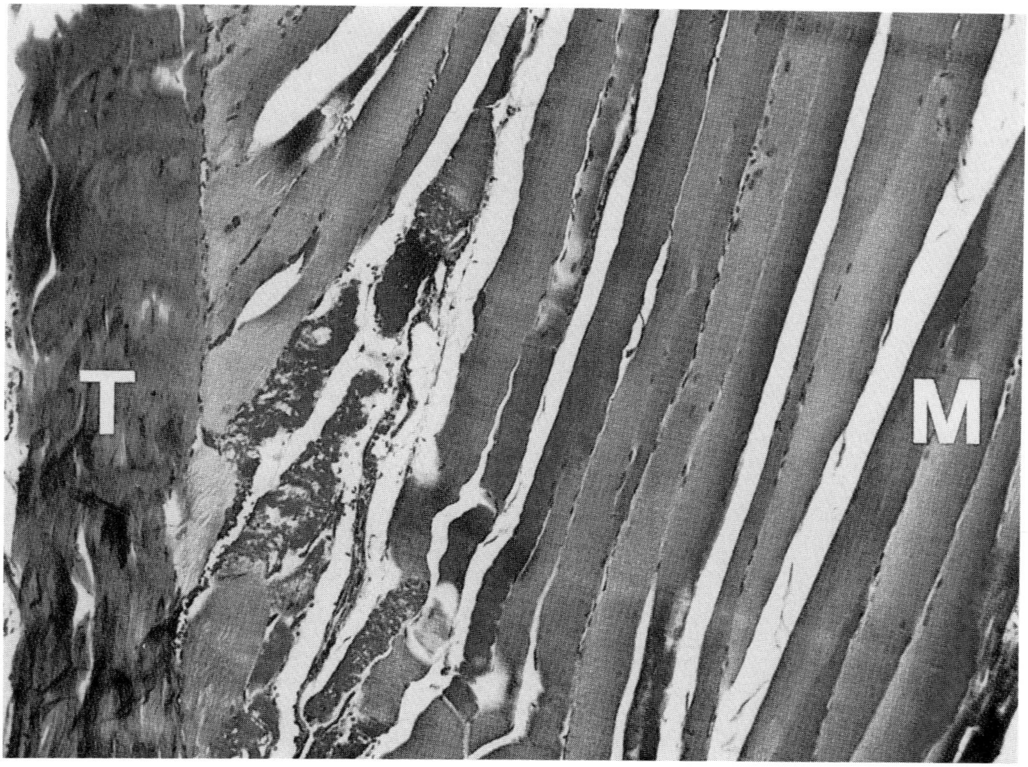

Fig. 3 *Histologic appearance of anterior tibialis muscle immediately after strain injury. Limited rupture of distal fibers is apparent along with hemorrhage. M, intact muscle fiber; T, tendon. (Reproduced with permission from Nikolaou PK, Macdonald BL, Glisson RR, et al: Biomechanical and histological evaluation of muscle after controlled strain injury.* Am J Sports Med *1987;15:9–14.)*

perimental strain injuries was evaluated with and without a treatment regimen involving the NSAID piroxicam.[2] Both the treated and the untreated groups were immobilized after the injury. At 11 days, piroxicam treatment had not significantly altered the tensile strength. The histologic findings were that the inflammatory response was delayed in the animals treated with piroxicam. It is interesting that tensile strength was not influenced by piroxicam, although the histologic studies showed clear differences between the treated and the untreated groups.

A second study evaluated recovery from muscle strains in rabbits.[18] The tensile strength at seven days was not significantly affected by treatment. The ability of the muscle to contract in response to nerve stimulation was improved one day after creation of the strain injury in the treatment group, possibly because of decreased edema. The histologic changes were similar to those seen in the rat model.

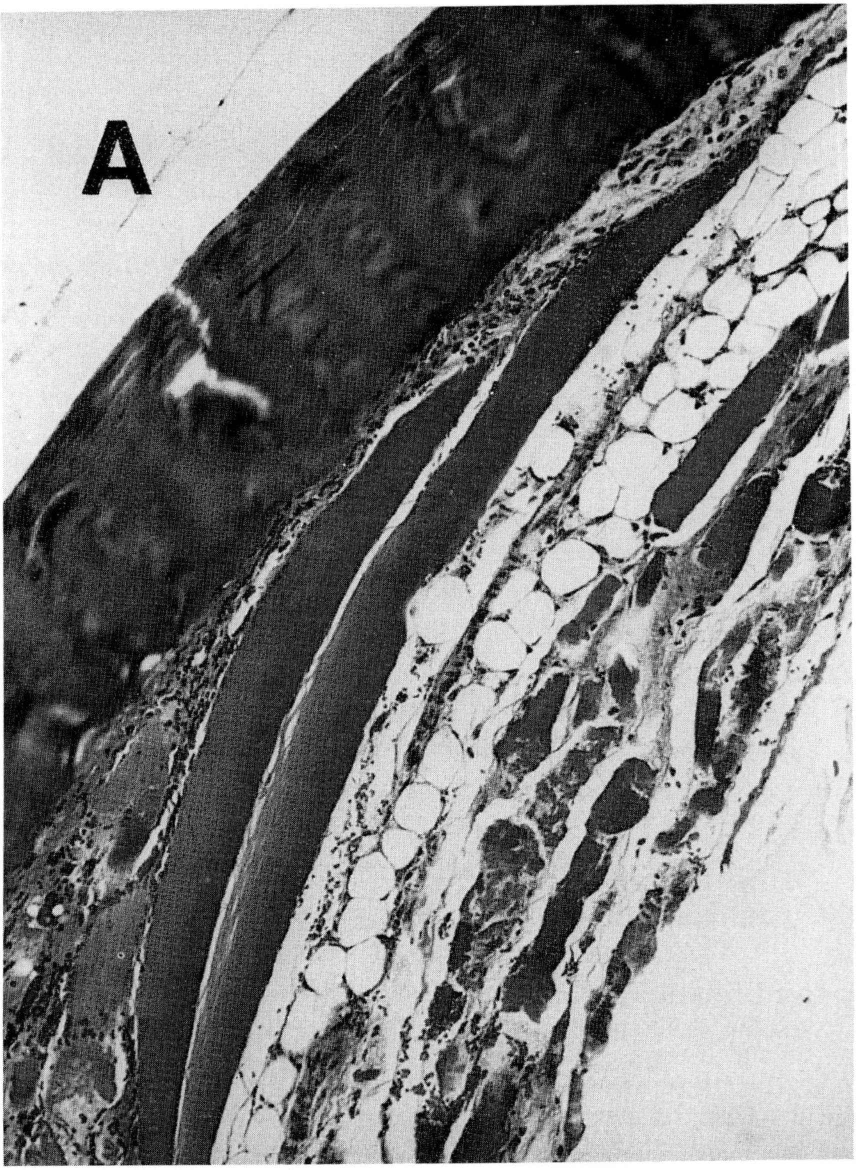

Fig. 4 *Histologic appearance of anterior tibialis muscle (A) 24 hours after controlled strain injury, showing complete breakdown of muscle fibers and a proliferation of inflammatory cells and fibroblastic activity at the myotendinous junction. (Reproduced with permission from Nikolaou PK, Macdonald BL, Glisson RR, et al: Biomechanical and histological evaluation of muscle after controlled strain injury.* Am J Sports Med *1987;15:9–14.)*

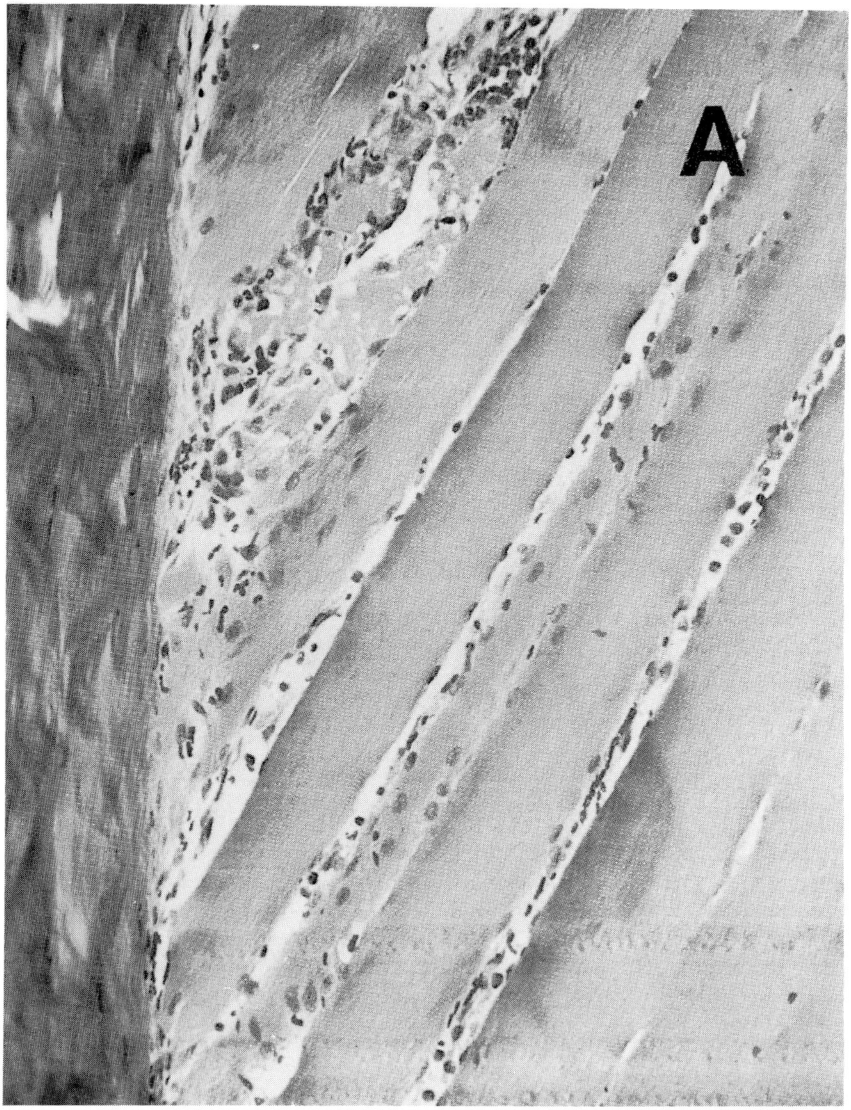

Fig. 5 *Histologic appearance of anterior tibialis muscle (A) 48 hours after controlled strain injury, showing complete breakdown of muscle fibers and a proliferation of inflammatory cells and fibroblastic activity at the myotendinous junction. (Reproduced with permission from Nikolaou PK, Macdonald BL, Glisson RR, et al: Biomechanical and histological evaluation of muscle after controlled strain injury.* Am J Sports Med *1987;15:9–14.)*

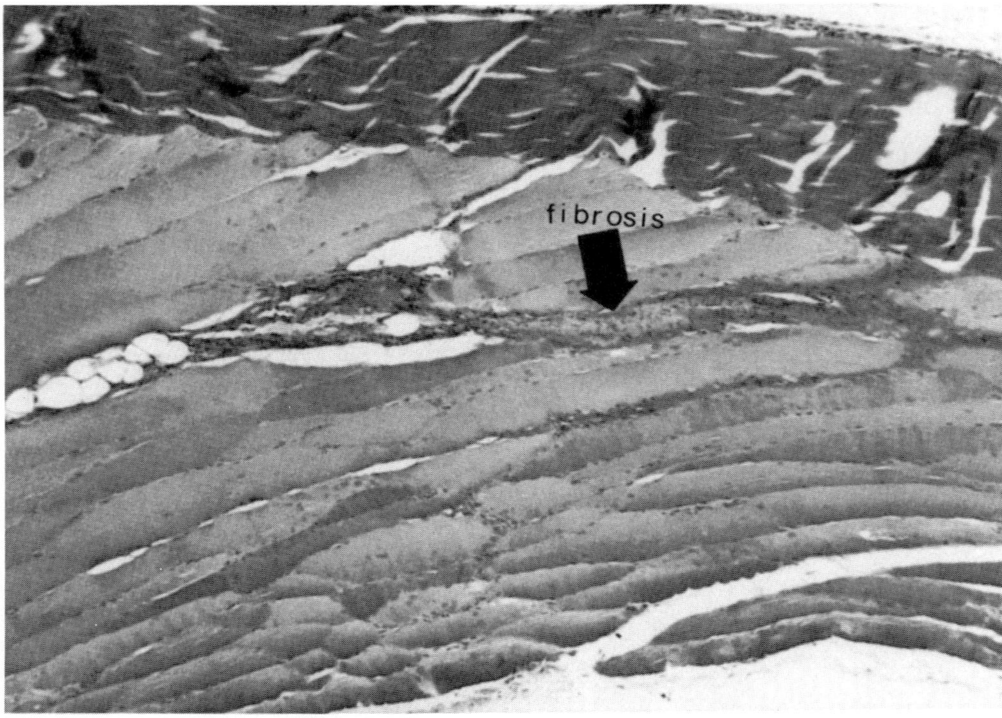

Fig. 6 *Muscles seven days after controlled strain, showing resolution of edema, hemorrhage, and inflammation with striking fibrotic changes localized to the site of injury. (Reproduced with permission from Nikolaou PK, Macdonald BL, Glisson RR, et al: Biomechanical and histological evaluation of muscle after controlled strain injury.* Am J Sports Med *1987;15:9–14.)*

Therefore, in both rat and rabbit models of muscle injury, the tensile strength of the muscle was not affected by piroxicam treatment, although there were definite changes showing a delay in the normal histologic processes of recovery from injury. In the rabbit model, the ability to contract actively was improved in the treated group on day 1 but at no other time. These animal studies cannot address the primary reason NSAIDs are used for muscle injury: ie, pain relief owing to their analgesic and anti-inflammatory effects. They do demonstrate that there is no significant deleterious effect on tensile strength and strength of muscle contraction in animals treated with piroxicam for seven to 11 days. Studies using longer intervals would be helpful, as would studies of the effects of dose-dependency. In addition, it is also very important to study the effects of corticosteroids, which have an even more pronounced effect on the inflammatory process.

Clinical studies evaluating the effect of NSAIDs on acute muscle strains are few. Several studies have evaluated the effects of various

NSAIDs on soft-tissue trauma in general, without specifying acute muscle strains as separate entities.[12,14,15] In separate studies, ibuprofen, piroxicam, indomethacin, and flurbiprofen have all been shown to be good analgesic medications with the ability to reduce swelling after injury. These medications allowed a quicker return to sports or to the activities of daily living. No studies have specifically investigated the harmful effects of NSAIDs in clinical trials.

Exercise-Induced Muscle Soreness and Injury

In addition to acute muscle injuries with significant disruption of fibers near the myotendinous junction, another common injury to muscle occurs after intense exercise. Athletes suffering from this condition usually do not experience a single acute injury, but instead have engaged in an extended period of unaccustomed heavy exercise. Very often this exercise is eccentric in nature[4,20]; ie, the muscles are forcibly lengthened while they contract. There are animal models of delayed muscle soreness and there are clinical studies evaluating human muscle after activities such as marathon running. In his early studies Hough[13] concluded that delayed muscle soreness was associated more with the amount of tension developed in the muscle than with fatigue. He proposed that the diminution of the muscle's ability to produce tension and the increased soreness could be explained by small ruptures within the muscle. More recent studies have supported this theory[1,3,5,7,16] and have shown that the weakness is transient, with the muscle returning to normal in a few days.

Serologic studies have demonstrated an increase in intramuscular enzymes (notably hydroxyproline) during the period of muscle soreness,[1] indicating the degradation of collagen. In contrast, serum lactic acid concentration is not related to delayed-onset muscle soreness.[6]

Histologic studies demonstrate an acute inflammatory response one to three days after injury.[3] A substantial number of necrotic muscle fibers are seen, as well as consistent inflammatory reactions. These changes are present diffusely through the muscle fibers. Clinical studies have shown similar changes in human muscles after very intense exercise such as marathon running or heavy eccentric exercise. Therefore, both clinical and animal studies support the involvement of an acute inflammatory response in the presence of exercise-induced muscle soreness.

Treatment of exercise-induced muscle soreness with NSAIDs has clinical and experimental support. Indomethacin was administered before, during, and after exercise in mouse hindlimb muscles and muscle damage was decreased as measured histologically and by serum enzymatic studies of skeletal muscle fiber damage.[19]

References

1. Abraham WM: Factors in delayed muscle soreness. *Med Sci Sports* 1977;9:11–20.
2. Almekinders LC, Gilbert JA: Healing of experimental muscle strains and the effects of nonsteroidal anti-inflammatory medication. *Am J Sports Med* 1986;14:303–308.

3. Armstrong RB, Garshnek V, Schwane JA: Muscle inflammation: Response to eccentric exercise, abstract. *Med Sci Sports Exerc* 1980;12:94–95.
4. Armstrong RB, Ogilvie RW, Schwane JA: Eccentric exercise-induced injury to rat skeletal muscle. *J Appl Physiol* 1983;54:80–93.
5. Asmussen E: Observations on experimental muscular soreness. *Acta Rheum Scand* 1956;2:109–116.
6. Besson C, Rochcongar P, Beauverger Y, et al: Etude des variations des taux seriques des enzymes musculaires et de la myoglobine apres epreuve d'effort maximale et au cours des 24 heures suivantes [Study of the valuations of serum muscular enzymes and myoglobin after maximal exercise test and during the next 24 hours]. *Eur J Appl Physiol* 1981;47:47–56.
7. Davies CT, White MJ: Muscle weakness following eccentric work in man. *Pflügers Arch* 1981;392:168–171.
8. Dürig M, Schuppisser JP, Gauer EF, et al: Spontaneous rupture of the gastrocnemius muscle. *Injury* 1977;9:143–145.
9. Garrett WE Jr: Injuries to the muscle-tendon unit, in Bassett FH III (ed): American Academy of Orthopaedic Surgeons *Instructional Course Lectures, XXXVII.* Park Ridge, Illinois, American Academy of Orthopaedic Surgeons, 1988, pp 275–282.
10. Garrett WE Jr, Nikolaou PK, Ribbeck BM, et al: The effect of muscle architecture on the biomechanical failure properties of skeletal muscle under passive extension. *Am J Sports Med* 1988;16:7–12.
11. Garrett WE Jr, Rich FR, Nikolaou PK, et al: Computed tomography of hamstring muscle strains. *Med Sci Sports Exerc* 1989;21:506–514.
12. Heere LP: Piroxicam in acute musculoskeletal disorders and sports injuries. *Am J Med* 1988;84:50–55.
13. Hough T: Ergographic studies in muscular soreness. *Am J Physiol* 1902;7:76–92.
14. Muckle DS: Comparative study of ibuprofen and aspirin in soft tissue injuries. *Rheumatol Rehabil* 1974;13:141–147.
15. Muckle DS: Flurbiprofen for the treatment of soft tissue trauma. *Am J Med* 1986;80:76–80.
16. Newham DJ, Mills KR, Quigley BM, et al: Pain and fatigue after concentric and eccentric muscle contractions. *Clin Sci* 1983;64:55–62.
17. Nikolaou PK, Macdonald BL, Glisson RR, et al: Biomechanical and histological evaluation of muscle after controlled strain injury. *Am J Sports Med* 1987;15:9–14.
18. Obremskey WT, Seaber AV, Ribbeck BM, et al: Biomechanical and histological assessment of a controlled muscle strain injury treated with piroxicam. *Trans Orthop Res Soc* 1988;13:338.
19. Salminen A, Kihlström M: Protective effect of indomethacin against exercise-induced injuries in mouse skeletal muscle fibers. *Int J Sports Med* 1987;8:46–49.
20. Tiidus PM, Ianuzzo CD: Effects of intensity and duration of muscular exercise on delayed soreness and serum enzyme activities. *Med Sci Sports Exerc* 1983;15:461–465.
21. Zeman SC, Rosenfeld RT, Lipscomb PR: Tears of the pectoralis major muscle. *Am J Sports Med* 1979;7:343–347.

Chapter 13

Inflammation and Healing of Meniscal Injury

Stephen J. O'Brien, MD
Steven P. Arnoczky, DVM

Introduction

Although meniscal injuries constitute one of the most common clinical entities in orthopaedics, the study of meniscal healing, regeneration, and repair is quite recent. The surgical management of meniscal lesions in the latter half of this century has shifted from the complete removal of "functionless remains of leg muscle," via arthrotomy, to standard arthroscopic meniscal suture repair in the vascular portions of the meniscus and the use of a fibrin clot derived from the patient's blood by venipuncture for repair of the avascular portions of the meniscus. This transformation of practice is the result of improved knowledge of meniscal composition, structure, and function and its potential for healing.

Anatomy

Menisci are C-shaped, biconcave disks of fibrocartilage interspaced between the condyles of the femur and tibia (Fig. 1). Phylogenetically, the meniscus represents an adaptation to the arthrograde position in which it extends the tibial condyles, matching the tibial plateau to the femoral condyle. At birth, the meniscus is almost entirely vascular, consists largely of fibroblasts without much intracellular matrix, and grossly resembles the shape of the adult meniscus.[12,23] By late adolescence, the vascular supply is more limited to the periphery of the meniscus, creating vascular and avascular zones. A detailed understanding of this vascular supply is essential to understanding the potential for meniscal healing.

The vascular supply to the medial and lateral meniscus originates primarily from the medial and lateral genicular arteries (both superior and inferior). Branches from these vessels give rise to a perimeniscal capillary plexus within the synovial and capsular tissues of the knee. This plexus is a branching network of vessels that supplies the peripheral border of the meniscus throughout its attachment to the joint capsule. These perimeniscal vessels are oriented in a predominantly circumferential pattern, with radial branches directed toward the center of the joint (Fig. 2). Microvascular studies[4] have shown that blood vessels penetrate the outer 10% to 30% of the medial meniscus and the outer 10% to 25% of the lateral meniscus. The anterior and posterior horn attachments have increased vascularity through vascular synovial coverings supplied by terminal branches of the middle genicular artery in addition to the medial and lateral genicular vessels. The lateral meniscus, however, has a relatively avascular zone surrounding the popliteal tendon as it courses through the knee (Fig. 3).

A "synovial fringe," containing small, terminally looped vessels, extends for 1 to 3 mm over the superior and inferior articular surfaces of the meniscus (Fig. 4). Although this vascular synovial fringe adheres to the surface of the meniscus, it does not directly contribute vessels into the meniscal tissue. Knowledge of this vascular anatomy enables us to determine which tears have a blood supply capable of supporting the inflammatory response necessary for the soft-tissue repair that occurs in other connective tissues.

The principal orientation of the collagen fibers in the meniscus is circumferential (Fig. 5). However, radially disposed fibers also exist, particularly on the tibial surface but also in the midzone and femoral surface (Fig. 6). Some of these radial fibers curl and change direction, becoming perpendicular to the surface. This arrangement allows the fibers to withstand the circumferential tension of normal loading conditions. Under large compressive loads, the radially disposed fibers act as tie fibers to resist longitudinal splitting. This distinctive orientation of the collagen fiber network, together with the proteoglycan and interstitial water components of the extracellular matrix, gives the meniscus its mechanical properties.

Although the meniscus is known to be viscoelastic and anisotropic, the exact responses of the tissue to compression, tension, and shear have yet to be elucidated. The precise mechanisms by which the menisci perform their functions within the joint and how the meniscal cells maintain their matrix are also unknown.

Two basic cell types exist within the meniscus: fusiform cells in the superficial zone of the meniscus and ovoid or polygonal cells throughout the remainder of the tissue.[17] These cells produce the collagen network described above. Light and electron microscopic examinations[9,43] reveal three collagen layers: (1) a superficial layer of collagen fibrils in a mesh-like matrix, (2) a surface layer of irregularly aligned collagen bundles, and (3) a middle layer of large, coarse fibers oriented parallel to each other in a circumferential fashion (Fig. 7). The overall composition of adult meniscal tissue is 75% collagen, 8% to 13% noncollagenous protein, and 1% hexosamine.

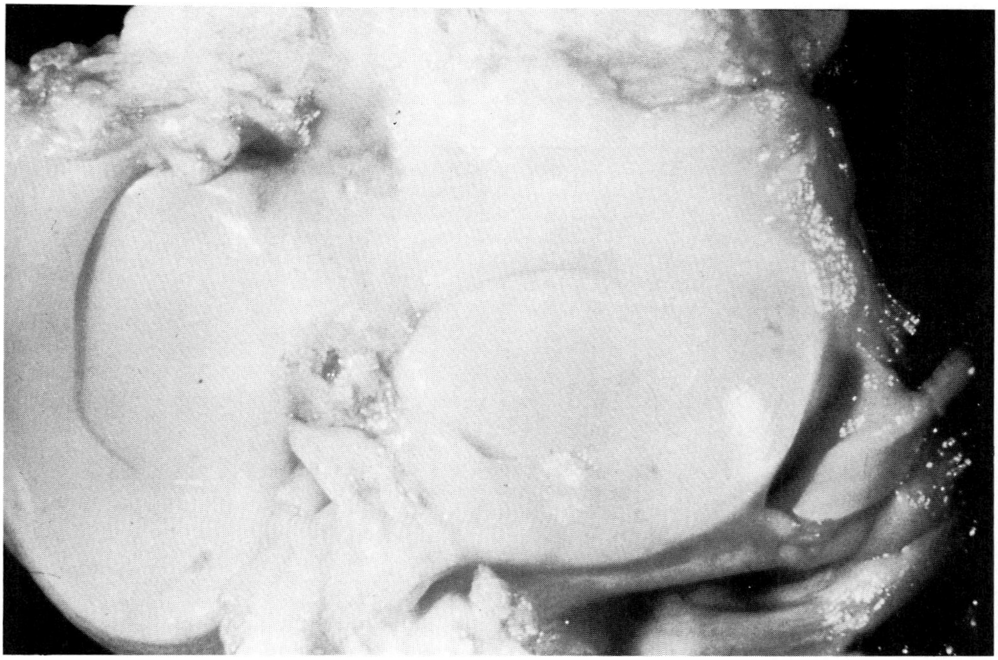

Fig. 1 *Transaxial view of medial and lateral menisci at rest on the tibial articular surface, showing their tibial attachments. The medial meniscus is longer anteroposteriorly and the lateral meniscus is more circular. Also, the posterior portion of the medial meniscus is longer than the anterior portion. (Reproduced with permission from Warren RP, Arnoczky SP, Wickiewicz TL: Anatomy of the knee, in Nicholas JA, Hershman EB (eds):* The Lower Extremity and Spine in Sports Medicine. *St. Louis, CV Mosby, 1986, vol 1.)*

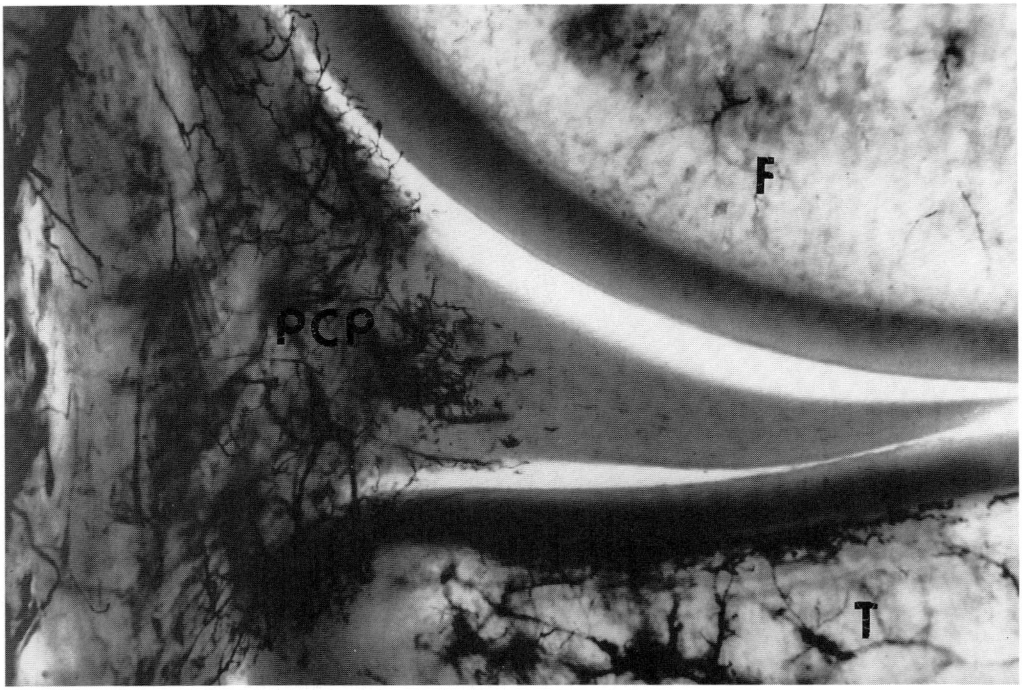

Fig. 2 *Frontal section of the medial compartment of the knee using the Spalteholtz technique. Branching radial vessels from the perimeniscal capillary plexus penetrate the peripheral border of the medial meniscus. F, femur; T, tibia. (Reproduced with permission from Arnoczky SP, Warren RF: Microvasculature of the human meniscus.* Am J Sports Med *1982;10:90–95.)*

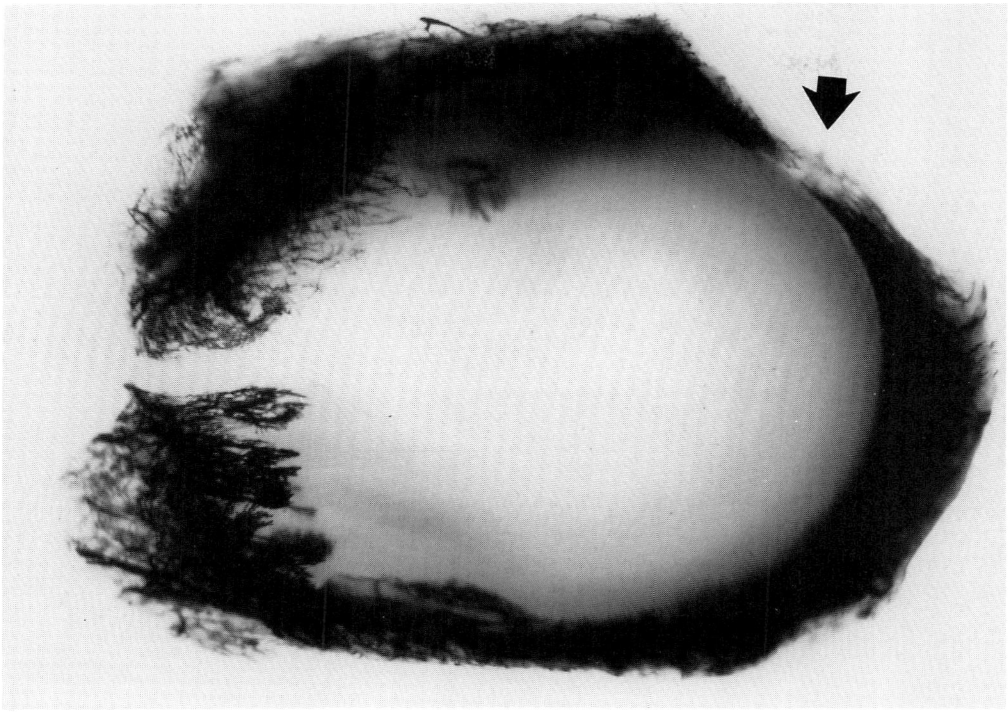

Fig. 3 *Superior view of lateral meniscus after vascular perfusion with india ink using the Spalteholtz technique demonstrates vascularity at the periphery of the meniscus as well as increased vascularity at the anterior and posterior horns. The peripheral vasculature is absent at the posterolateral corner (arrow). This represents the region through which the popliteal tendon passes. (Reproduced with permission from Arnoczky SP, Warren RF: Microvasculature of the human meniscus.* Am J Sports Med *1982;10:90–95.)*

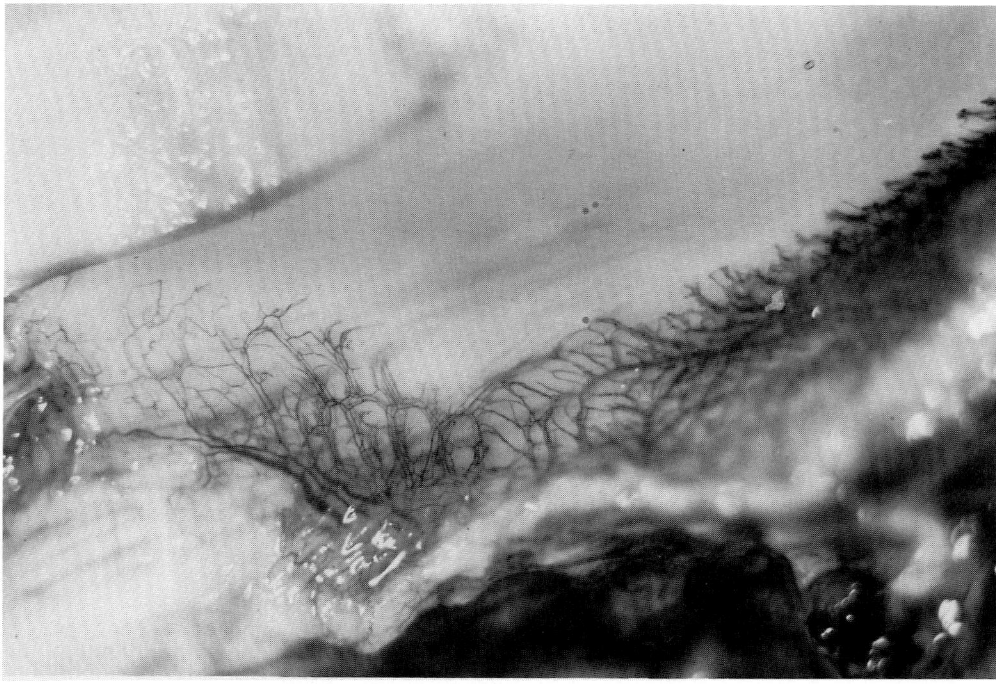

Fig. 4 *View of the anterior horn of the medial meniscus showing the extension of the vascular synovial fringe into the synovial covering of the anterior horn attachment. (Reproduced with permission from Arnoczky SP, Warren RF: Microvasculature of the human meniscus.* Am J Sports Med *1982;10:90–95.)*

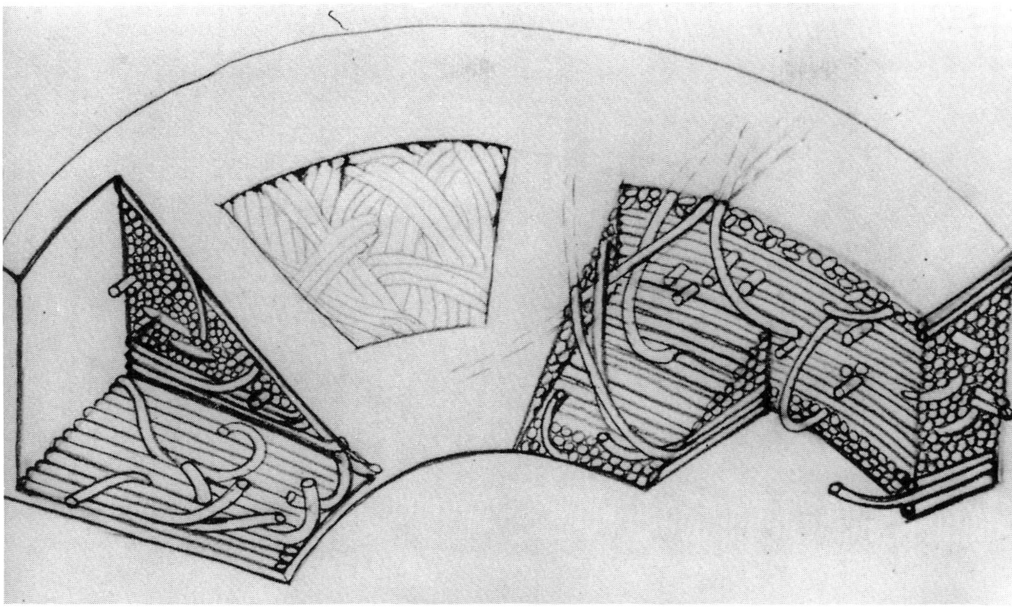

Fig. 5 *Collagen fiber pattern of the meniscus. (Reproduced with permission from Bullough PG, Munuera L, Murphy J, et al: The strength of the menisci of the knee as it relates to their fine structure.* J Bone Joint Surg *1970;52B:564–570.)*

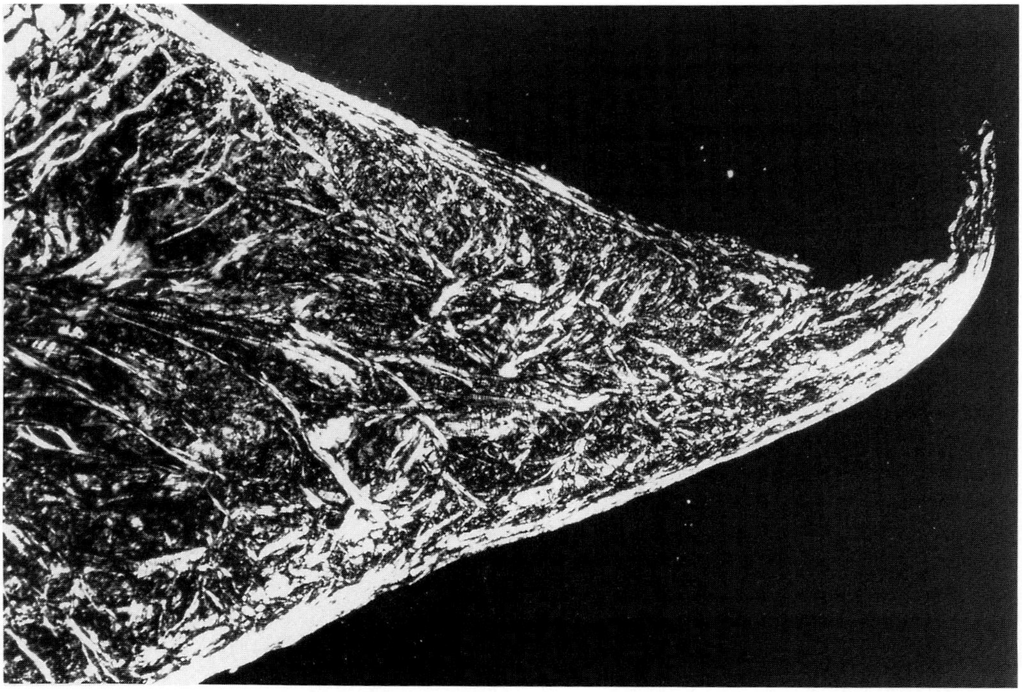

Fig. 6 *Photomicrograph of a section through the meniscus. Note the more prominent radial fibers of the tibial surface of the meniscus. (Reproduced with permission from Bullough PG, Munuera L, Murphy J, et al: The strength of the menisci of the knee as it relates to their fine structure.* J Bone Joint Surg *1970;52B:564–570.)*

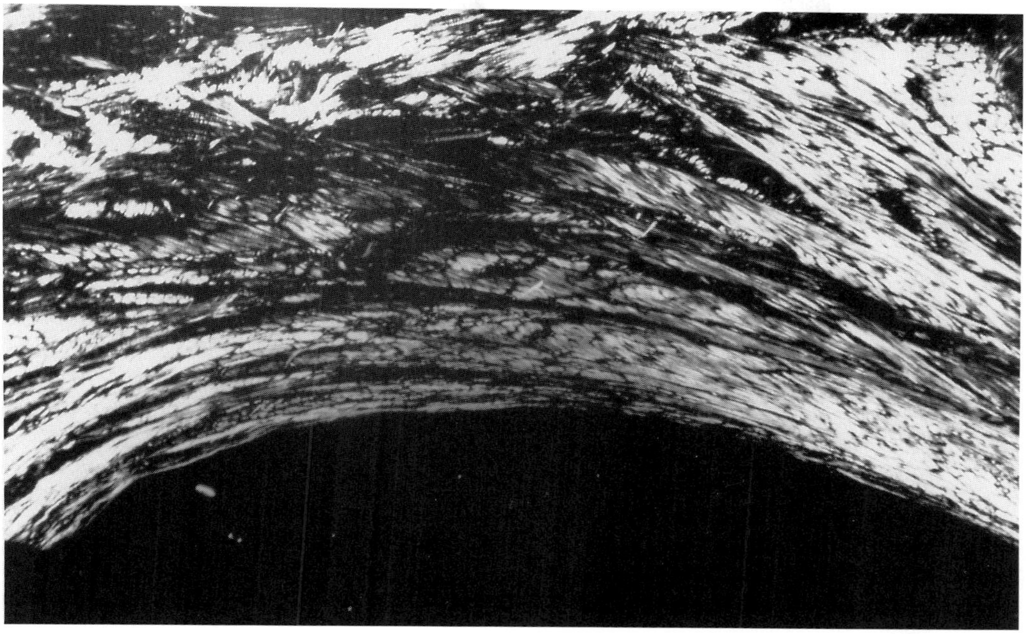

Fig. 7 *Longitudinal section of a medial meniscus viewed under polarized light illustrating the orientation of the coarse, deep circumferentially oriented collagen fibers. (Reproduced with permission from Arnoczky S, Adams M, DeHaven K, et al: Meniscus, in Woo SL-Y, Buckwalter JA (eds):* Injury and Repair of the Musculoskeletal Soft Tissues. *Park Ridge, Illinois, American Academy of Orthopaedic Surgeons, 1988, pp 483–537.)*

Meniscal Function

The meniscus is directly involved in loadbearing. At least 50% of the compressive load applied to the knee joint is transmitted through the meniscus when the knee is fully extended and 85% of the load is transmitted through the meniscus when the knee is flexed 90 degrees.[1] With load transmission, a net force acts radially, which is balanced by tensile stresses developed in the circumferential collagen fibers anchored by their tibial attachments at the anterior and posterior horns.

With loading and deformation of the meniscus, the interstitial fluid is forced to flow through a porous matrix of extremely low permeability; thus, the meniscus acts as an efficient shock absorber that attenuates the intermittent shock waves within the knee joint during various activities.

The menisci may also act as secondary stabilizers of the knee when the primary stabilizing structures are damaged. For example, Levy and associates[28] have shown the medial meniscus to be an important secondary restraint to anterior translation of the tibia in knees with deficient anterior cruciate ligaments.

Meniscal Injury

Meniscal injury can occur as an isolated lesion or in association with ligamentous injury. It is usually the result of compression and/or shear forces. The location of the lesion within the meniscus (vascular vs avascular zone), the tear configuration (radial vs peripheral), and the presence or absence of meniscal deformation are more pertinent to meniscal healing and repair than the age of the tear.[37] We recently successfully repaired a bucket-handle peripheral lateral meniscal tear that had been present for 12 years. A computed tomographic arthrogram taken three months after surgery was normal. We developed a simple classification scheme to categorize meniscal tears that accurately assesses types of tears amenable to repair on the basis of follow-up data (Fig. 8). Although some tears defy accurate description for coding, the system is easy to remember and facilitates proper evaluation of different types of meniscal repair techniques.

Biology of Meniscal Healing

After injury within the peripheral vascular zone, the meniscus can mount a reparative response similar to those of other vascular tissues—exudation, organization, vascularization, proliferation, and remodeling (Fig. 9).

The first phase of healing involves formation of a fibrin clot that is rich in inflammatory cells, an essential phase of any process of soft-tissue repair.[34] It provides a scaffold for matrix and is a chemotactic stimulus for the cellular elements involved in wound healing.[19,27,34] Vessels from the perimeniscal capillary plexus proliferate through this fibrin "scaffold," accompanied by the proliferation of undifferentiated mesenchymal cells (Fig. 10). Eventually, the lesion is filled with a cellular fibrovascular scar tissue that "glues" the wound edge together and appears continuous with the adjacent normal meniscal fibrocartilage. Vessels from the perimeniscal capillary plexus, as well as a proliferative vascular pannus, form the "synovial fringe," penetrating the fibrous scar to provide a marked inflammatory response (Fig. 11). Experimental studies in animals[5] have demonstrated that even complete radial lesions that extend to the periphery are completely healed with fibrovascular scarring by ten weeks (Fig. 12). Modulation of this scar tissue into normal-appearing fibrocartilage, however, requires several months. Clinical studies have supported this concept of meniscal healing and repair in the vascular zone, showing excellent results.[11,14,20,37,42] Surgical techniques have also been developed to improve the blood supply. For tears 1 or 2 mm more peripheral, the peripheral rim can be resected to a bleeding capsular bed, to which the meniscus can then be reattached.[11,15] Rasping of the perimeniscal synovium has also been advocated to stimulate the synovium and synovial cells to create an inflammatory response[21] in the region of repair.

Although the hematoma is a natural sequela of injury of vascularized tissue, it is absent from many wounds of the meniscus, which is avascular in its inner two-thirds. Experimental and clinical observations[5,25] have shown that these lesions are incapable of healing, thus providing the rationale for partial meniscectomy. However, more recent animal experiments[5,8] have successfully promoted healing in the avascular zone of the meniscus. In one study,[5] longitudinal lesions in the avascular portion of the meniscus in dogs were connected to the peripheral vasculature by a "vascular access channel" (Fig. 13). These lesions were then capable of healing through a process of fibrovascular scar proliferation. In this technique, a full-thickness vascular access channel was made at the midportion of the longitudinal lesion, connecting it with the vasculature of the perimeniscal capillary plexus.

A more recent animal study[8] demonstrated meniscal repair in the avascular zone by means of an exogenous fibrin clot. It had been theorized[39] that it is the absence of a hematoma and its associated factors, not the absence of a blood supply per se, that limits healing in the avascular portions of the meniscus. The basis for this theory is that meniscal cells in tissue culture media can proliferate and synthesize an extracellular matrix when they are exposed to factors normally present in the wound hematoma.[39] This clot seems to act as a scaffold for migration of cells, as a chemotactic stimulus, and as a stimulus for proliferation of cells and matrix synthesis.[19,27,34]

The chemotactic and mitogenic factors in the fibrin clot include platelet-derived growth factor and fibronectin, whose effects on the cellular component of the repair of wounds are well-known.[19,27,31,34,38,41] In 12 adult mongrel dogs, two full-thickness holes, 2 mm in diameter, were made in the avascular portion of the medial meniscus of each knee.[8] In one knee, the holes were filled with an exogenous fibrin clot (Fig. 14), taken from 10 ml of whole blood from the animal, agitated in a glass container, and washed free of excess erythrocytes. In the other knee, the defects were not filled and acted as controls. The defects filled with a fibrin clot healed through a proliferation of fibrous connective tissue that eventually was modulated into fibrocartilaginous tissue (Fig. 15). Control defects remained empty. The repair tissue was grossly and histologically different (Fig. 16) from the normal adjacent meniscal tissue, but it was morphologically similar to the tissue seen in repairs in the vascular area of the meniscus.

The origin of the reparative cells stimulated by the fibrin clot are unclear. Possibilities include fibroblasts from adjacent meniscal cells,[39,40] synovial cells,[3,6,26,35] and peripheral blood elements. An experimental study[2] demonstrated the ability of mononuclear blood cells to transform and proliferate in vitro as fibroblasts.

The defects filled with clot healed with an asymmetry in the previously circular defect, consistent with contraction of myofibroblasts within the edges of the wound. This is also seen in other areas of soft-tissue wound healing,[34] reducing the size of the defect.

Clinical trials with the use of an exogenous fibrin clot inserted into meniscal defects in conjunction with meniscus repair are currently under way (Fig. 17). Although the early results are promising, long-term biomechanical and biochemical evaluation of this reparative tissue is needed. Figure 18 demonstrates human meniscus repair in the avascular zone with insertion of a fibrin clot. A magnetic resonance imaging study performed three months after surgery was interpreted as showing a meniscal tear even though the meniscus appeared to be fully healed on an arthrogram. The question remains as to how this scar tissue will function in a young, active athlete who will stress the repair.

Other techniques currently under investigation include the use of synovial flaps sutured over meniscal tears[18] and methods involving a laser Doppler flowmeter and fluorometry to quantify the blood supply in relatively avascular portions of this meniscus; this would help to determine the amount of microcirculation necessary for meniscal healing.[16,29,32,36]

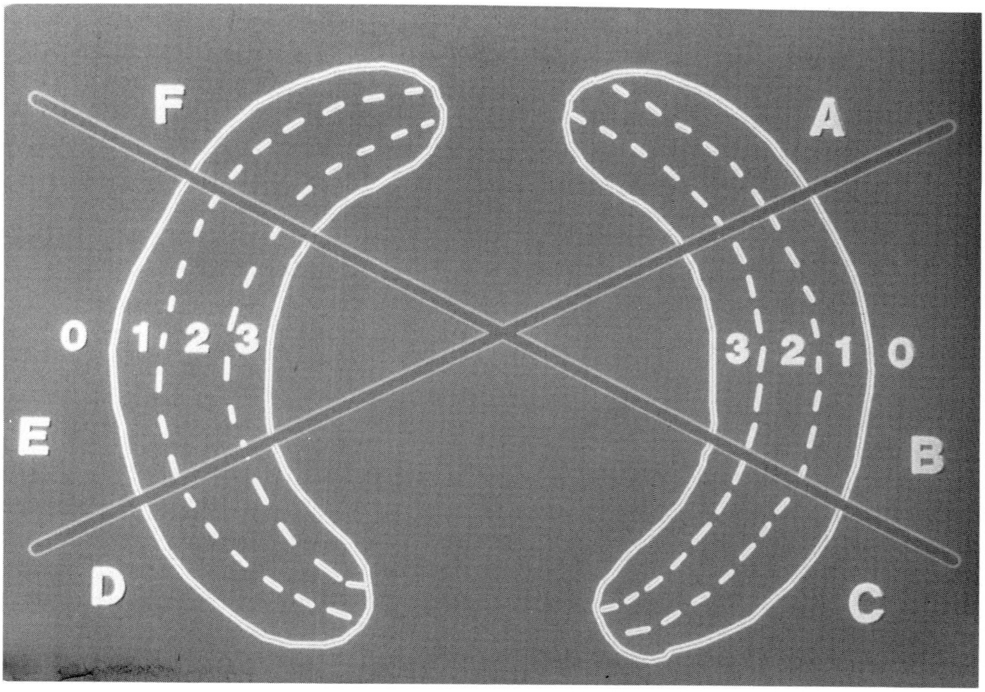

Fig. 8 *Classification scheme depicting types of meniscal tears. A, posteromedial; F, posterolateral; 0, synovial meniscal junction; 1, outer third of the meniscus; 2, middle third of the meniscus; and 3, inner third of the meniscus.*

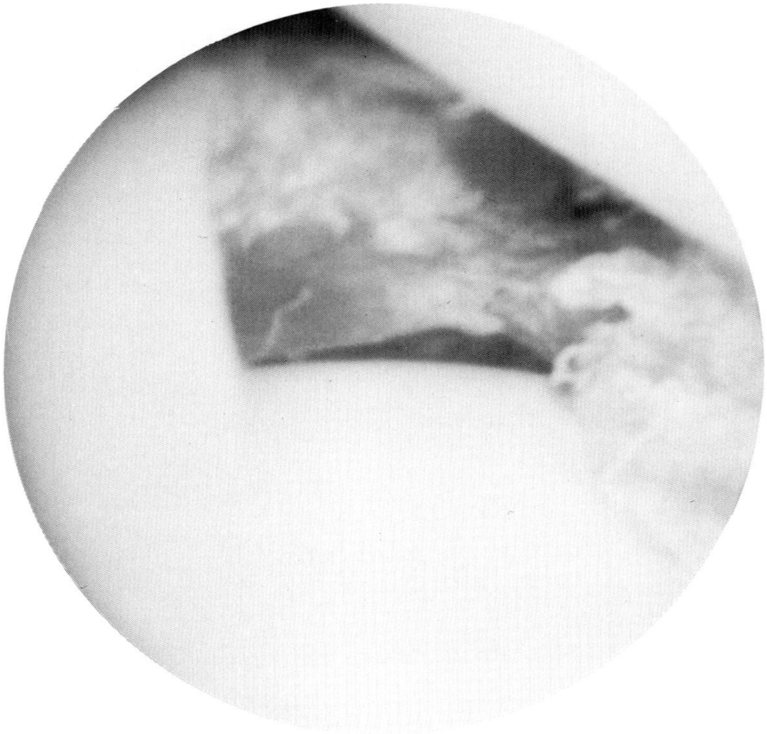

Fig. 9 *Arthroscopic view of medial meniscal tear in the vascular zone. Hemorrhage is seen on both sides of the meniscal tear.*

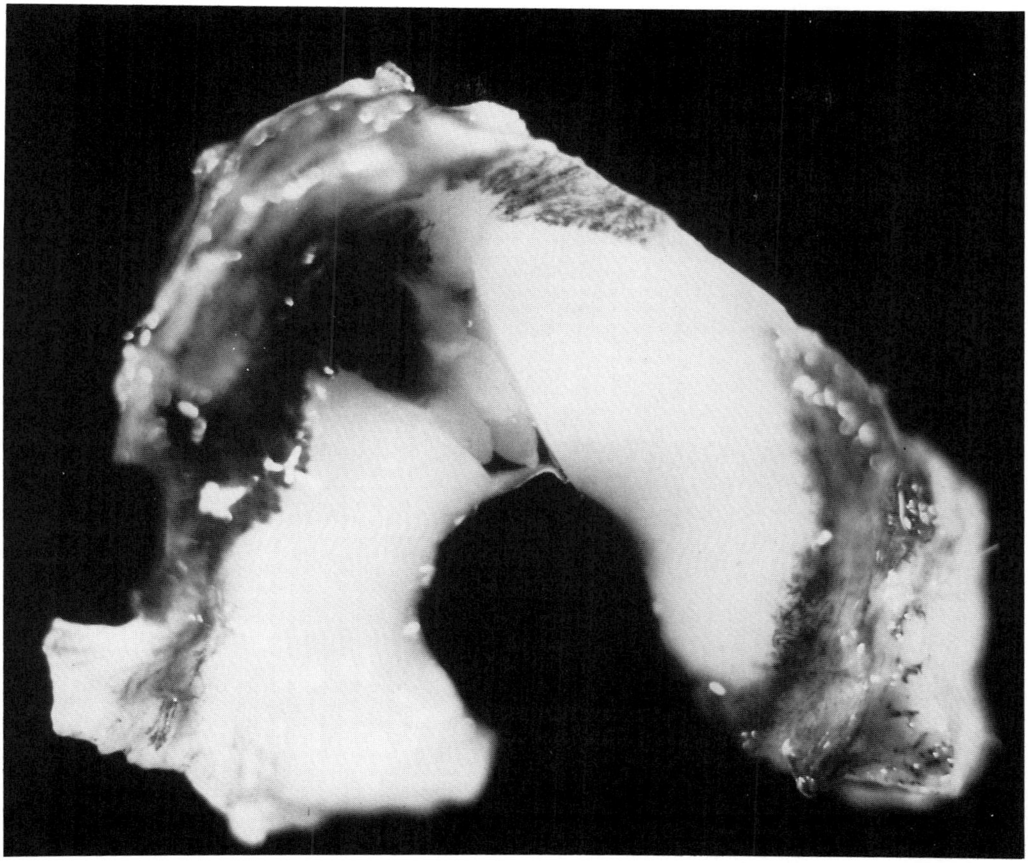

Fig. 10 *Canine medial meniscus perfused with india ink two weeks after complete radial transection. Note the proliferation of vessels from the perimeniscal capillary plexus into the fibrin clot. (Reproduced with permission from Arnoczky SP, Warren RF: The microvasculature of the meniscus and its response to injury: An experimental study in the dog.* Am J Sports Med *1983;11:131–141.)*

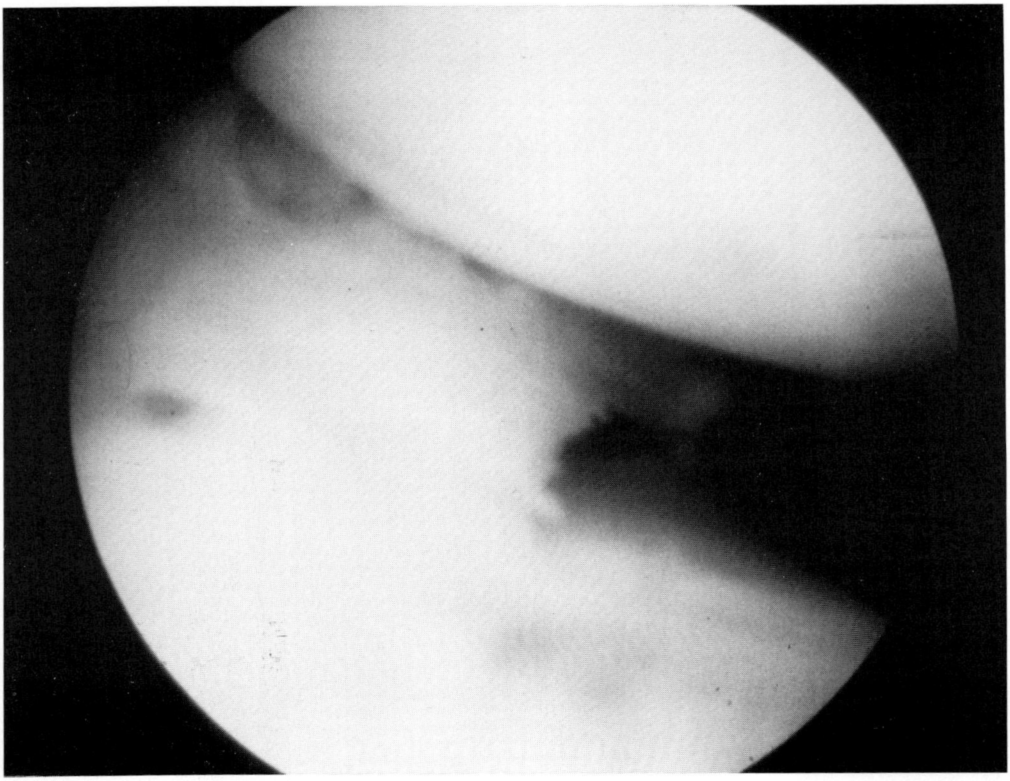

Fig. 11 *Arthroscopic view of medial meniscal repair shows complete healing seven weeks after surgery. Note that the synovial fringe anteriorly covers the meniscus.*

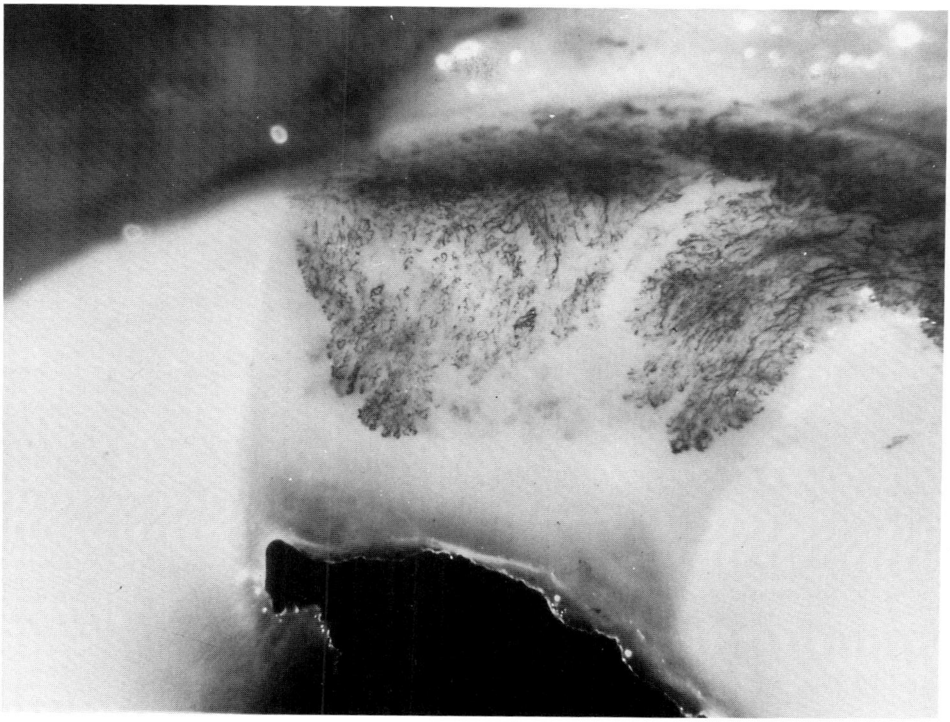

Fig. 12 *Specimen perfused with india ink shows the fibrovascular scar six weeks after complete transection of a canine medial meniscus. Note the proliferation of the vascular synovial tissue over the fibrovascular scar. (Reproduced with permission from Arnoczky SP, Warren RF: The microvasculature of the meniscus and its response to injury: An experimental study in the dog.* Am J Sports Med *1983:11:131–141.)*

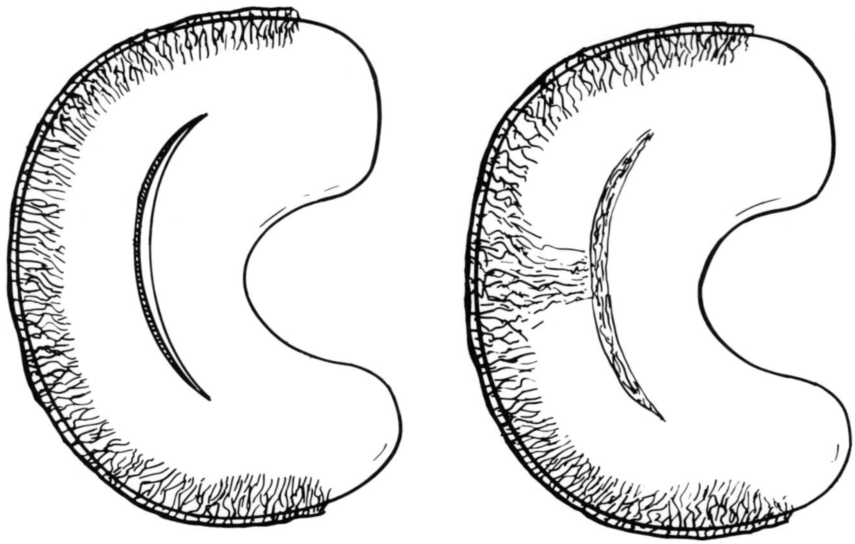

Fig. 13 ***Left,*** *Location and extent of the longitudinal lesion.* ***Right,*** *Location of the vascular access channel and the vascular response associated with it. (Reproduced with permission from Arnoczky S, Warren RF: The microvasculature of the meniscus and its response to injury: An experimental study in the dog.* Am J Sports Med *1983;11:131–141.)*

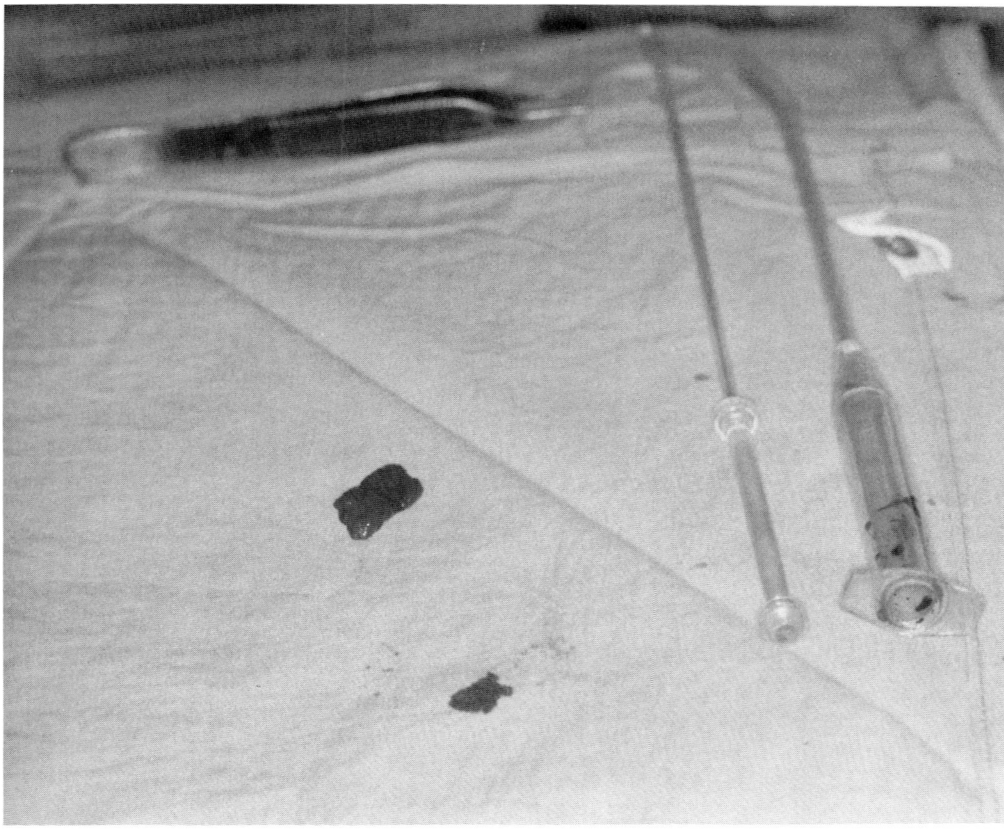

Fig. 14 *Exogenous fibrin clot. To the right of the clot is the fibrin clot inserter for arthroscopic use.*

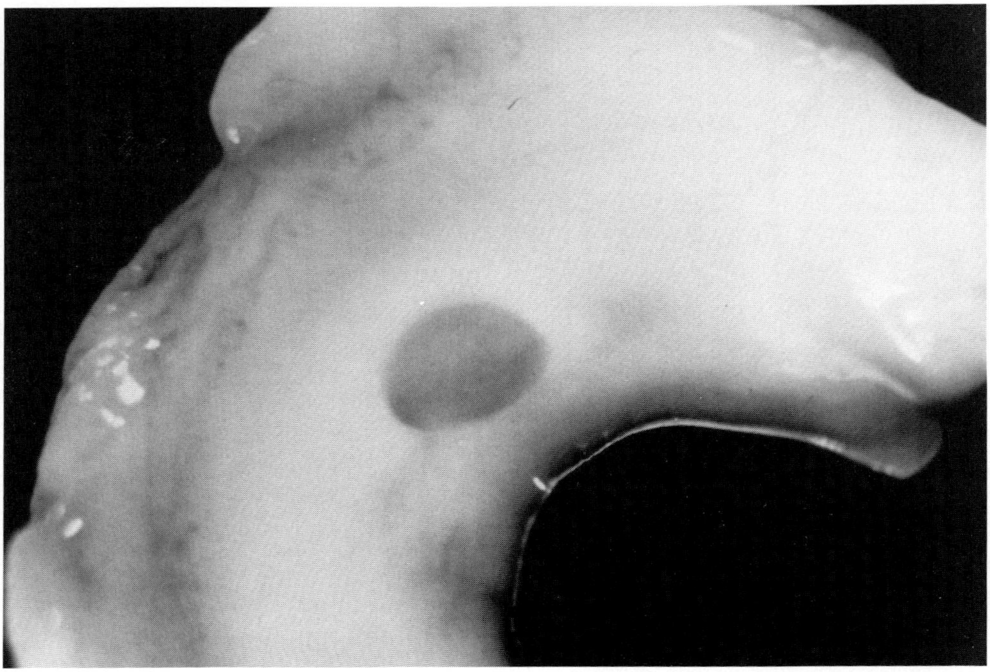

Fig. 15 *The gross appearance of the clot-filled defect six months after surgery. Although the tissue appears translucent, it fills the defect completely. Note the distorted shape of the circular defect after healing. (Reproduced with permission from Arnoczky SP, Warren RF, Spivak JM: Meniscal repair using an exogenous fibrin clot: An experimental study in dogs.* J Bone Joint Surg *1988;70A:1209–1217.)*

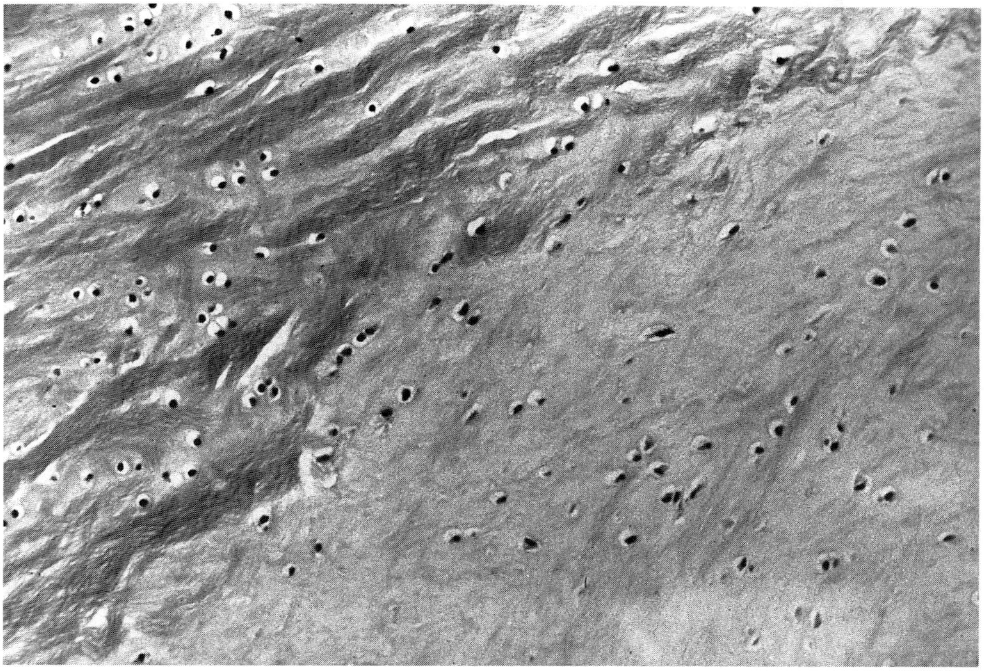

Fig. 16 *Photomicrograph showing the clot-filled defect with the meniscus at six months. The tissue in the defect has the histologic appearance of fibrocartilage but is still morphologically different from adjacent meniscal tissue. (Reproduced with permission from Arnoczky SP, Warren RF, Spivak JM: Meniscal repair using an exogenous fibrin clot: An experimental study in dogs.* J Bone Joint Surg *1988;70A:1209–1217.)*

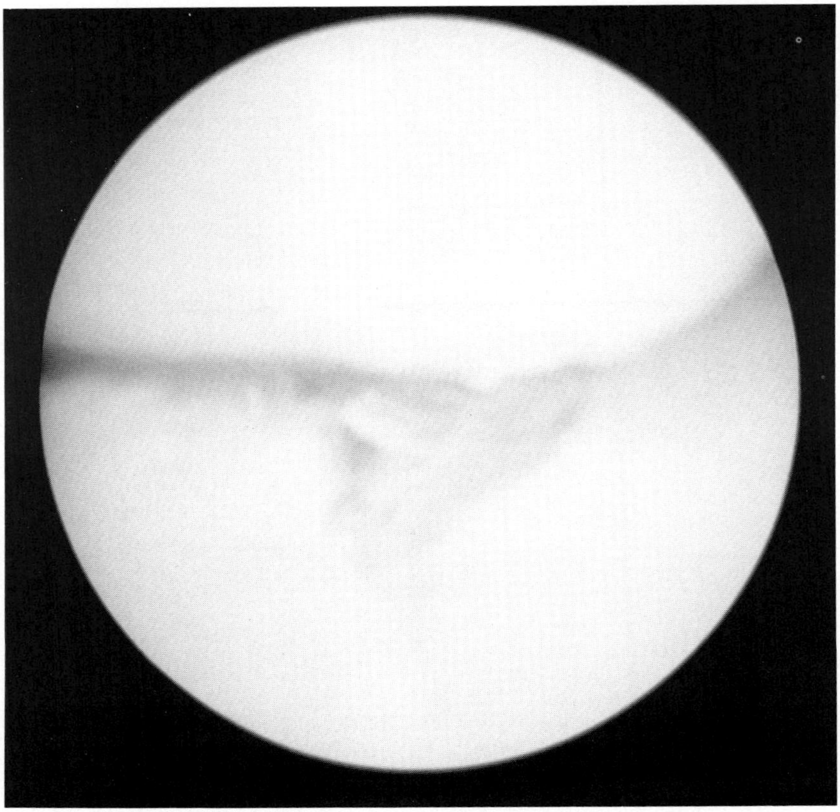

Fig. 17 *Arthroscopic view of exogenous fibrin clot inserted for meniscal repair.*

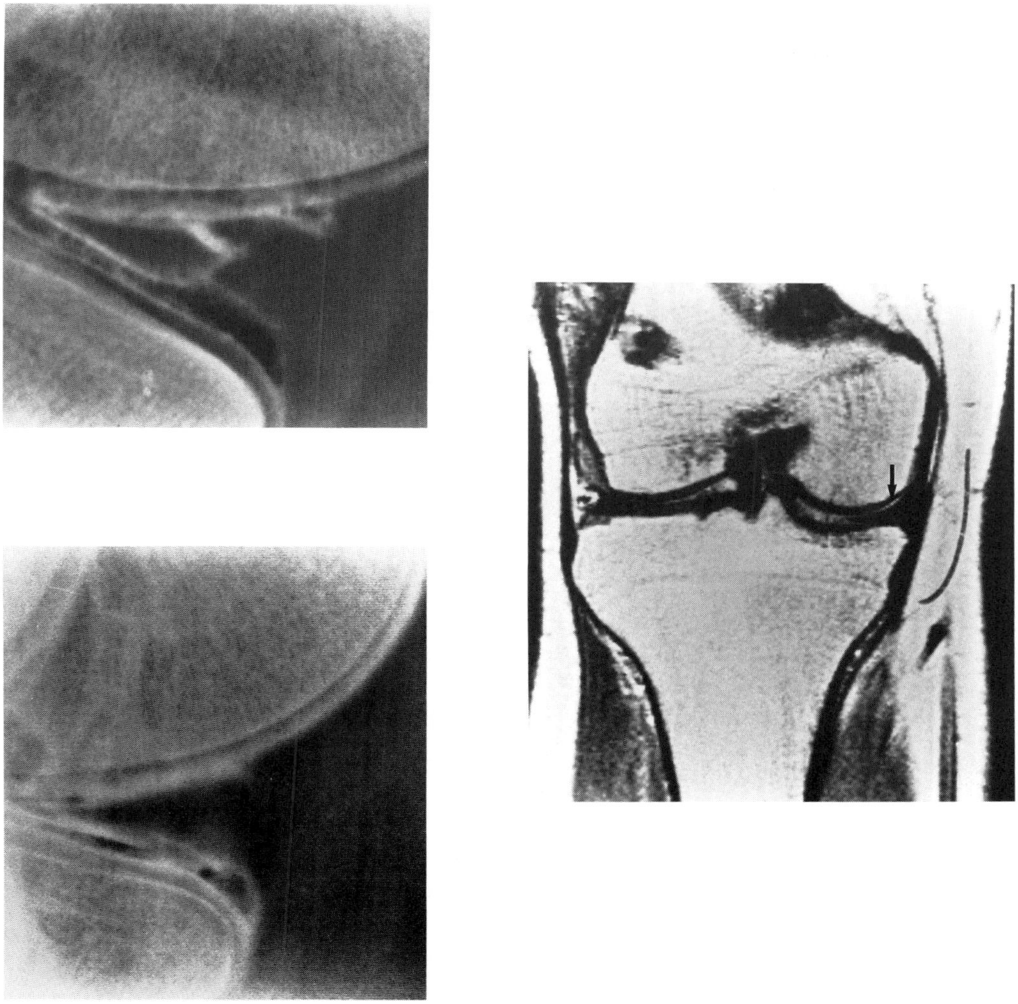

Fig. 18 *Medial meniscal tear in the avascular zone.* ***Top left,*** *Preoperative arthrogram.* ***Right,*** *Magnetic resonance imaging three months after meniscal repair shows apparent linear defect interpreted as a meniscal tear.* ***Bottom left,*** *Arthrogram three months after surgery shows complete healing of meniscal tear.*

Meniscal Regeneration

Controversy exists regarding the ability of a human meniscus to regenerate after meniscectomy. However, meniscal remodeling and regeneration have been documented in studies of rabbits and dogs.[7,13,24] After complete removal of the meniscus, it is thought, fibrocytes from the synovium and capsule migrate into the joint and are transformed into undifferentiated fibroblasts, which, in turn, form a loose fibrous connective tissue. In time, this tissue grossly resembles a meniscus and has the histologic appearance of fibrocartilage.

The importance of the peripheral synovial tissue in meniscal regeneration has been shown in experimental studies in rabbits.[24] In animals in which total meniscectomy was accompanied by synovectomy, there was no evidence of tissue regrowth at 12 weeks. However, total meniscectomy alone was followed by regrowth of a meniscus-like structure in 83% of the animals. A recent human clinical study evaluated 22 total meniscectomies ten years after resection. There was evidence of regeneration of at least one third of the normal meniscus in all cases[10] (Fig. 19).

Another recent experimental study of remodeling after partial meniscectomy in dogs demonstrated significant remodeling in approximately two thirds of the menisci[7] (Fig. 20). This was probably secondary to fibrin clots forming in the dead space created by the partial meniscectomy. The fibrocartilaginous tissue was grossly and histologically similar to the tissue seen in the study on fibrin clot.[22]

We recently studied the effects of various forms of surgical cutting tools on meniscal regeneration after partial meniscectomies in the avascular zone of the rabbit meniscus.[30,33] We compared the surgical scalpel, electrocautery, and a contact neodymium-YAG laser in 16 New Zealand white rabbits. The scalpel meniscectomies showed remodeling in 75% of the menisci, similar to our previous findings (Fig. 21).[7] In contrast, none of the electrosurgical meniscectomies (20 W) showed evidence of remodeling. In fact, a wide band of cellular necrosis was observed; this increased with time and was present in all specimens (Fig. 22).

The laser meniscectomies (20 W) showed an intermediate response. However, some menisci showed remodeling identical to that seen with the scalpel (Fig. 23). The carbonized tissue at the meniscal edge in some of these specimens, lacking the cooling effect of arthroscopic saline solution, was thought to prevent the fibrin clot from adhering. However, the damage did not increase with time—in fact, viable cells were present at the meniscal edge in specimens that did not show remodeling similar to the scalpel meniscectomies. It is believed that the contact neodymium-YAG laser, which can be used in saline solution, will eventually offer significant advantages over electrocautery and the scalpel.

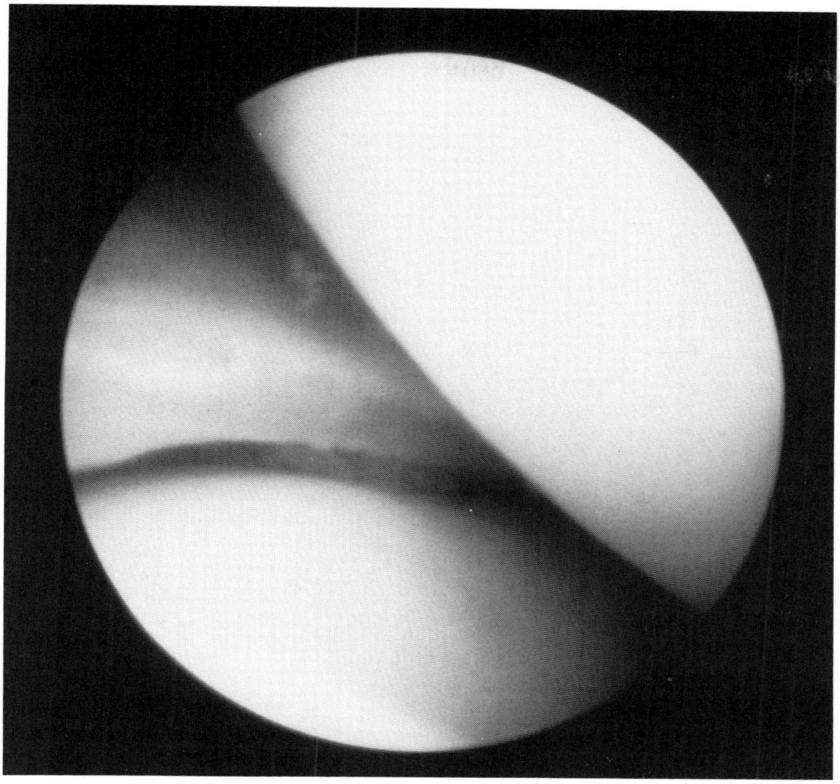

Fig. 19 *Arthroscopic view of human meniscus showing regeneration after complete medial meniscectomy.*

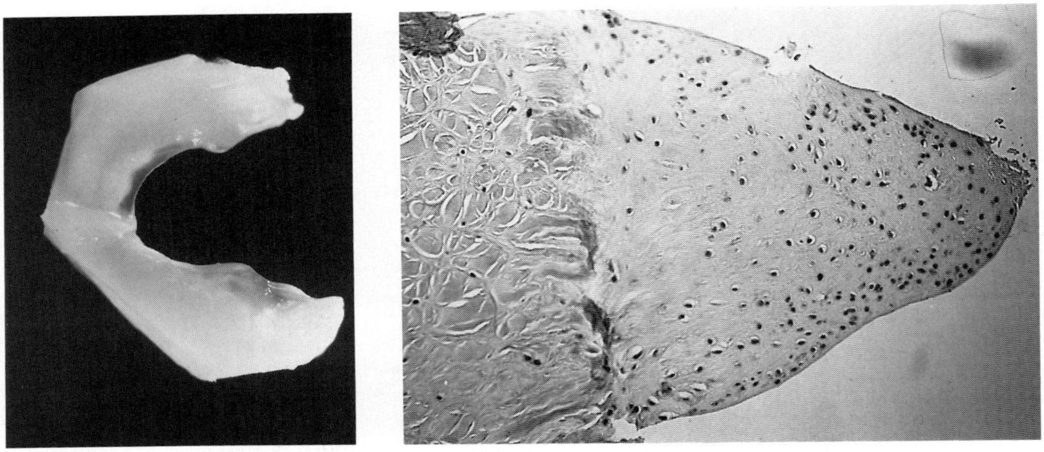

Fig. 20 *Meniscal remodeling in canine meniscus.* ***Left,*** *Note the translucent area of meniscal remodeling.* ***Right,*** *Histologic view. (Reproduced with permission from Arnoczky SP, Warren RF, Kaplan N: Meniscal remodeling following partial meniscectomy: An experimental study in the dog.* Arthroscopy *1985;1:247–252.)*

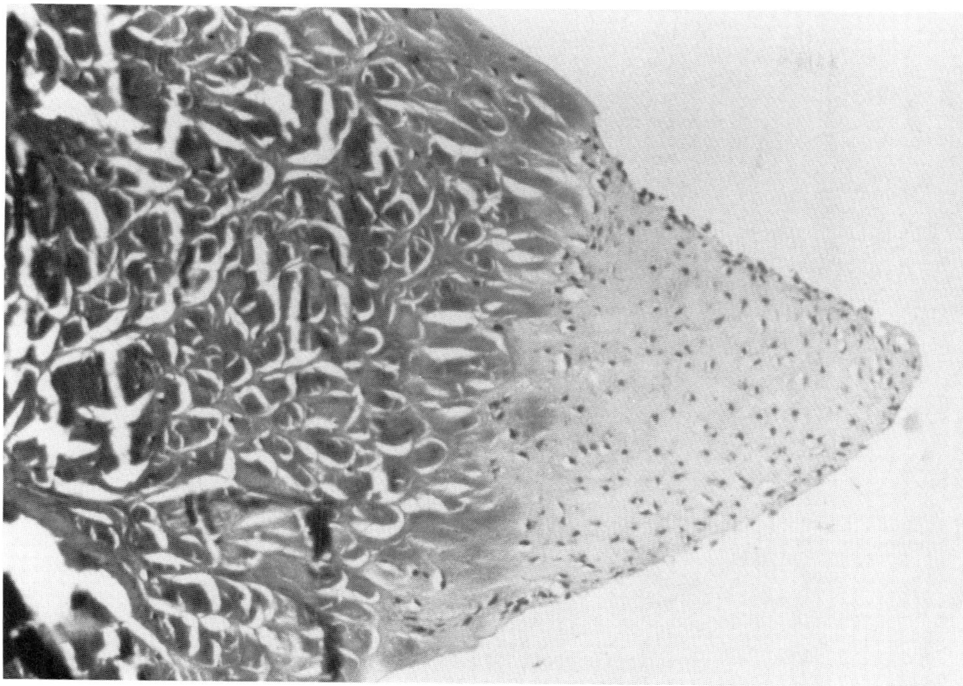

Fig. 21 *Meniscal remodeling in New Zealand white rabbits after scalpel meniscectomy in the avascular zone. (Reproduced with permission from Miller DV, O'Brien SJ, Arnoczky SP, et al: The use of the contact Nd-YAG laser in arthroscopic surgery: Effects on articular cartilage and meniscal tissue.* Arthroscopy *1989;5:245–253.)*

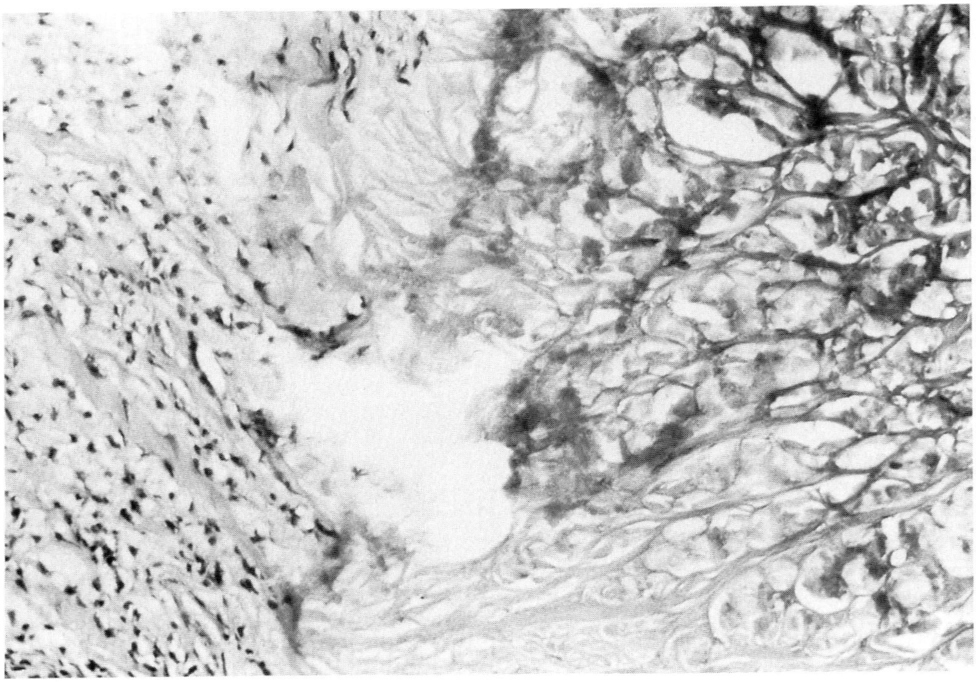

Fig. 22 *Safranin O stain of meniscal tissue after electrocautery meniscectomy in the avascular zone. Note the significant meniscal degeneration. The damage to the meniscus increased over time. (Reproduced with permission from Miller DV, O'Brien SJ, Arnoczky SP, et al: The use of the contact Nd-YAG laser in arthroscopic surgery: Effects on articular cartilage and meniscal tissue.* Arthroscopy *1989:5;245–253.)*

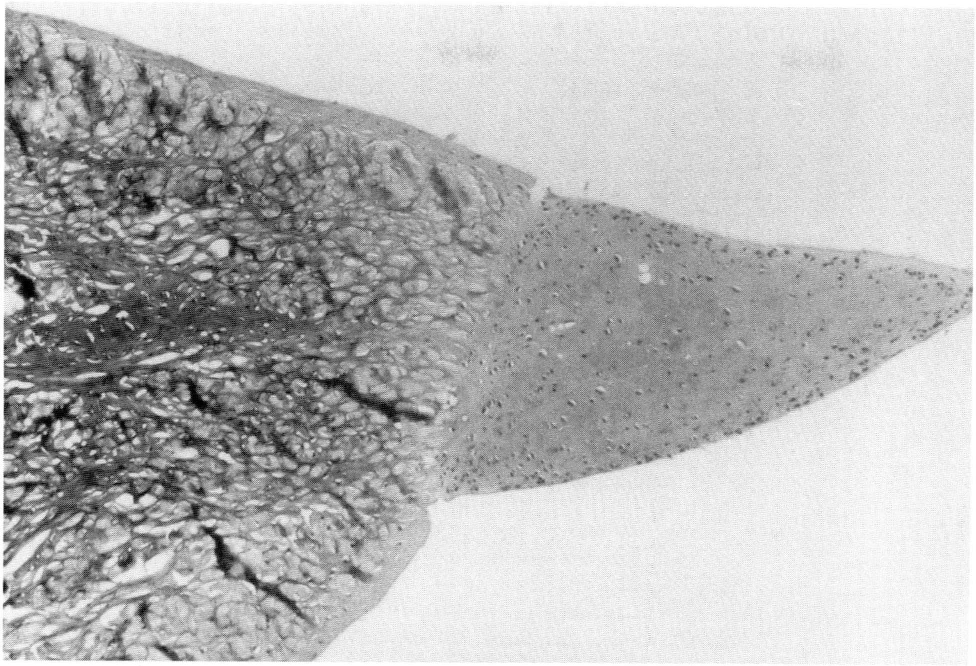

Fig. 23 *Section of meniscal tissue after partial meniscectomy with contact Nd:YAG laser in a vascular zone. The meniscal remodeling is similar to that in Figure 21. (Reproduced with permission from Miller DV, O'Brien SJ, Arnoczky SP, et al: The use of the contact Nd-YAG laser in arthroscopic surgery: Effects on articular cartilage and meniscal tissue.* Arthroscopy *1989;5:245–253.)*

References

1. Ahmad AM, Burke DL: *In vitro* measurement of static pressure distribution in synovial joints: Part I. Tibial surface of the knee. *J Biomed Eng* 1983;105:216–225.
2. Allgower M, Hulliger L: Origin of fibroblasts from mononuclear blood cells: A study on in vitro formation of the collagen precursor, hydroxyproline, in buffy coat culture. *Surgery* 1960;47:603–610.
3. Arnoczky SP, Cuzzell JZ, McDevitt CA, et al: Meniscal replacement using a cryopreserved allograft: An experimental study in the dog. *Trans Orthop Res Soc* 1984;9:220.
4. Arnoczky SP, Warren RF: Microvasculature of the human meniscus. *Am J Sports Med* 1982;10:90–95.
5. Arnoczky SP, Warren RF: The microvasculature of the meniscus and its response to injury: An experimental study in the dog. *Am J Sports Med* 1983;11:131–141.
6. Arnoczky SP, Warren RF, Ashlock MA: Replacement of the anterior cruciate ligament using a patellar tendon allograft: An experimental study. *J Bone Joint Surg* 1986;68A:376–385.
7. Arnoczky SP, Warren RF, Kaplan N: Meniscal remodeling following partial meniscectomy: An experimental study in the dog. *Arthroscopy* 1985;1:247–252.
8. Arnoczky SP, Warren RF, Spivak JM: Meniscal repair using an exogenous fibrin clot: An experimental study in dogs. *J Bone Joint Surg* 1988;70A:1209–1217.
9. Aspden RM, Yarker YE, Hukins DW: Collagen orientations in the meniscus of the knee joint. *J Anat* 1985;140:371–380.
10. Burr DB, Radin EL: Meniscal function and the importance of meniscal regeneration in preventing late medial compartment osteoarthrosis. *Clin Orthop* 1982;171:121–126.
11. Cassidy RE, Shaffer AJ: Repair of peripheral meniscus tears: A preliminary report. *Am J Sports Med* 1981;9:209–214.
12. Clark CR, Ogden JA: Development of the menisci of the human knee joint: Morphological changes and their potential role in childhood meniscal injury. *J Bone Joint Surg* 1983;65A:538–547.
13. Cox JS, Nye CE, Schaefer WW, et al: The degenerative effects of partial and total resection of the medial meniscus in dogs' knees. *Clin Orthop* 1975;109:178–183.
14. DeHaven KE: Peripheral meniscus repair: An alternative to meniscectomy. *Orthop Trans* 1981;5:399–400.
15. DeHaven KE, Hales W: Peripheral meniscal repair in a young athlete. *Orthop Consult* 1984;4:7–12.
16. Fanton GS, Andrish JT: Meniscofluoresis: An aid in determining prognosis of meniscal tears. *Cleve Clin Q* 1983;50:379–383.
17. Ghadially FN, Thomas I, Yong N, et al: Ultrastructure of rabbit semilunar cartilages. *J Anat* 1978;125:499–517.
18. Ghadially FN, Wedge JH, Lalonde JM: Experimental methods of repairing injured menisci. *J Bone Joint Surg* 1986;68B:106–110.
19. Giacometti L, Montagna W: Healing of skin wounds in primates, in Dunphy JE, Van Winkle W Jr (eds): *Repairs and Regeneration: The Scientific Basis for Surgical Practice.* New York, McGraw-Hill, 1969, pp 47–55.
20. Hamberg P, Gillquist J, Lysholm J: Suture of new and old peripheral meniscus tears. *J Bone Joint Surg* 1983;65A:193–197.
21. Henning CE, Lynch MA, Clark JR: Vascularity for healing of meniscus repairs. *Arthroscopy* 1987;3:13–18.

22. Jørgensen U, Sonne-Holm S, Lauridsen F, et al: Long-term follow-up of meniscectomy in athletes: A prospective longitudinal study. *J Bone Joint Surg* 1987;69B:80–83.
23. Kaplan EB: The embryology of the menisci of the knee. *Bull Hosp Joint Dis* 1955;16:111–124.
24. Kim JM, Moon MS: Effect of synovectomy upon regeneration of meniscus in rabbits. *Clin Orthop* 1987;224:64–70.
25. King D: The healing of semilunar cartilages. *J Bone Joint Surg* 1936;18:333–342.
26. Kleiner JB, Amiel D, Roux RD, et al: Origin of replacement cells for the anterior cruciate ligament autograft. *J Orthop Res* 1986;4:466–474.
27. Knighton DR, Hunt TK, Thakral KK, et al: Role of platelets and fibrin in the healing sequence: An in vivo study of angiogenesis and collagen synthesis. *Ann Surg* 1982;196:379–388.
28. Levy IM, Torzilli PA, Warren RF: The effect of medial meniscectomy on anterior-posterior motion of the knee. *J Bone Joint Surg* 1982;64A:883–888.
29. Limbird T, Swiontkowski MF, Schlehr F, et al: Direct in vivo measurement of meniscal blood flow. Presented at the Interim Meeting of the American Orthopaedic Society for Sports Medicine, San Francisco, Jan 21, 1987.
30. Miller DV, O'Brien SJ, Arnoczky SP, et al: The use of the contact Nd-YAG laser in arthroscopic surgery: Effects on articular cartilage and meniscal tissue. *Arthroscopy* 1989;5:245–253.
31. Mosesson MW, Amrani DL: The structure and biologic activities of plasma fibronectin. *Blood* 1980;56:145–158.
32. Nielsson GE, Terland T, Oberg P: Evaluation of a laser Doppler flowmeter for measurement of tissue blood flow. *IEEE Trans Biomed Eng* 1980;27:597–604.
33. O'Brien SJ, Miller DV: The contact Nd-YAG laser: A new approach to arthroscopic laser surgery. *Clin Orthop*, in press.
34. Peacock EE Jr: *Wound Repair*, ed 3. Philadelphia, WB Saunders, 1984.
35. Potenza AD, Herte MC: The synovial cavity as a "tissue culture in situ": Science or nonsense? *J Hand Surg* 1982;7:196–199.
36. Schlehr FJ, Limbird TA, Swiontkowski MF, et al: The use of laser Doppler flowmetry to evaluate anterior cruciate blood flow. *J Orthop Res* 1987;5:150–153.
37. Scott GA, Jolly BL, Henning CE: Combined posterior incision and arthroscopic intra-articular repair of the meniscus: An examination of factors affecting healing. *J Bone Joint Surg* 1986;68A:847–861.
38. Seppä HE, Yamada KM, Seppä ST, et al: The cell binding fragment of fibronectin is chemotactic for fibroblasts. *Cell Biol Int Rep* 1981;5:813–819.
39. Webber RJ, Harris MG, Hough AJ Jr: Cell culture of rabbit meniscal fibrochondrocytes: Proliferative and synthetic response to growth factors and ascorbate. *J Orthop Res* 1985;3:36–42.
40. Webber RJ, York L, Vander Schilden JL, et al: Fibrin clot invasion by rabbit meniscal fibrochondrocytes in organ culture. *Trans Orthop Res Soc* 1987;12:470.
41. Weiss RE, Reddi AH: Role of fibronectin in collagenous matrix-induced mesenchymal cell proliferation and differentiation in vivo. *Exp Cell Res* 1981;133:247–254.
42. Wirth CR: Meniscus repair. *Clin Orthop* 1981;157:153–160.
43. Yaseri K: Three-dimensional architecture of human normal menisci. *J Jpn Orthop Assoc* 1978;52:391–399.

Chapter 14

Sports-Induced Soft-Tissue Calcification

Gerald A. M. Finerman, MD
Matthew S. Shapiro, MD

Introduction

Pathologic calcification can be defined as deposits of calcium salts in abnormal locations. Calcific disease consists of a wide spectrum of orthopaedic and nonorthopaedic conditions and may be caused by systemic or local factors. Atherosclerosis, dental plaque, and calcification in tumors are all examples of pathologic calcification. Most soft-tissue calcification in otherwise healthy athletes is confined to calcification of the muscles, tendons, tendon sheaths, and ligaments.

Abnormal calcification typically occurs by one of three mechanisms.[10] Metastatic calcification occurs in otherwise normal tissues as a result of a derangement in calcium metabolism (hypercalcemia). Calcinosis causes widespread deposits of calcium salts in skin and other connective tissues despite normal calcium metabolism. Dystrophic calcification deposits calcium salts in damaged tissue. Most soft-tissue calcification in athletes is dystrophic.

Calcification is a normal bodily process, carefully controlled within rigorous limits. It is like other homeostatic processes such as coagulation or the immune reaction. When it is disrupted, disease results.[2] Although studies on the actual cellular mechanism of calcification are recent, much about it is understood. Extracellular fluid is undersaturated with inorganic calcium and phosphate in terms of crystal seeding, but metastable, or supersaturated, in terms of crystal growth. Serum does not precipitate calcium salts in vitro, but when a seed crystal of hydroxyapatite is added, crystal growth proceeds rapidly.[18]

Even abnormal calcium deposition is controlled. Mineral is always deposited into an organic matrix, usually by precipitation of calcium salts within collagen fibers. Plasma, urine, and joint fluid all contain potent natural inhibitors of calcium deposition such as pyrophosphate. Alkaline phosphatase destroys pyrophosphate, disabling the inhibitory effect. This may be one of the ways that this enzyme promotes calcium deposition. This mechanism also involves the functioning of diphosphonate medications that mimic the function of pyrophosphate.[18]

The molecular mechanism of normal calcification occurs in a two-

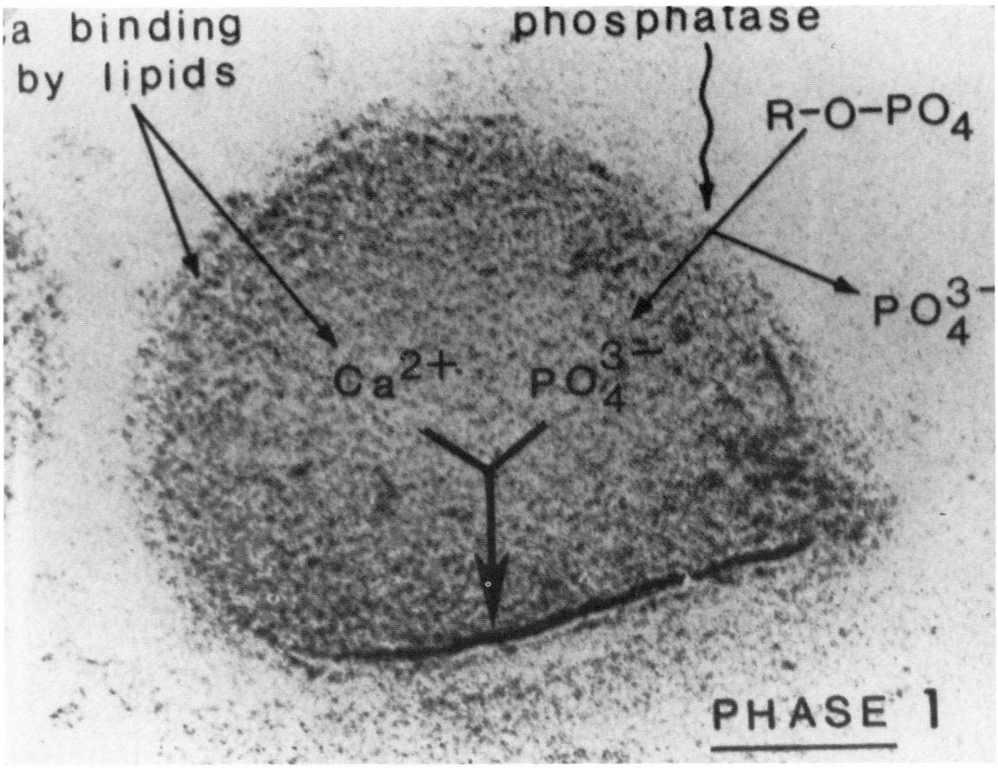

Fig. 1 *Negatively charged phospholipids contained within the matrix vesicle concentrate calcium. (Reproduced with permission from Anderson HC: Calcific diseases: A concept.* Arch Pathol Lab Med *1983;107:341–348.)*

stage process: initiation and crystal propagation. The membrane-bound matrix vesicle may be the initial site of extracellular calcification (Fig. 1). The negatively charged phospholipids within these vesicles concentrate calcium ions. The ions are then released into the extracellular matrix and deposited as calcium phosphate salts. Propagation of crystal formation (Fig. 2) then progresses automatically, as long as the normal inhibitory mechanisms are not activated. This process is enhanced by the presence of collagen, peptides such as osteonectin, and high calcium and phosphate levels in serum.[2]

Intracellular calcium levels are kept low through active transport pumps that remove calcium ions from the intracellular fluid. Both mitochondria and the matrix vesicles are active in this process. Calcium concentrations are 10,000 times higher in the mitochondria than in the intracellular fluid.[18] Both mechanisms protect the intracellular environment from accidental calcification. However, damage to cells

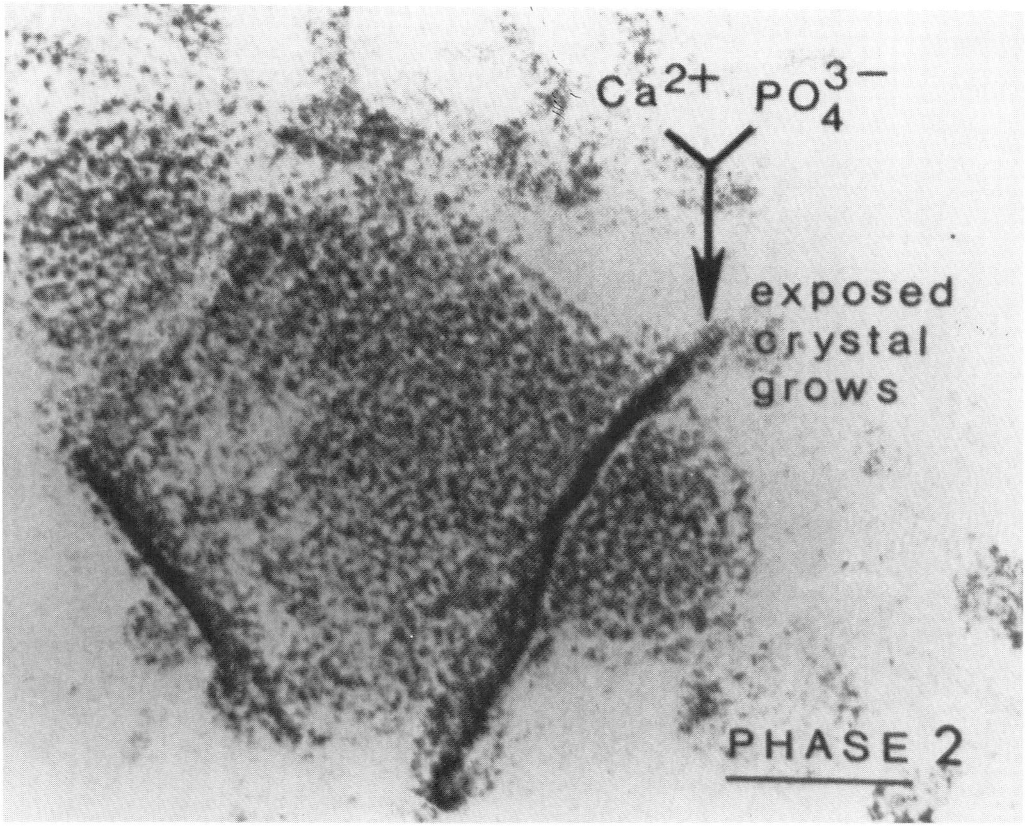

Fig. 2 *Crystal propagation continues automatically as the newly formed crystal is exposed to the supersaturated extracellular environment. (Reproduced with permission from Anderson HC: Calcific diseases: A concept.* Arch Pathol Lab Med *1983;107:341–348.)*

by external means releases stores of calcium into the extracellular tissues, promoting abnormal calcification. Electron micrographs have shown that the process of calcific tendinitis is mediated by membrane vesicles.[2] Dystrophic calcification in damaged tissue results because the normal calcification pathway exceeds the bounds of homeostatic control. Whatever the initiator, the actual deposition of crystalline calcium phosphate mineral represents a final common pathway. Thus, pathologic calcification can be considered normal calcification that occurs in an abnormal location.[9]

Heterotopic calcification must be differentiated from heterotopic ossification. Calcification is simply the deposition of inorganic calcium salts into an organic matrix. When these salts are subjected to the normal remodeling processes of bone, ossification occurs, creating

Outline 1 Differential diagnosis of calcification*

Muscle
- Calcinosis universalis
- Carbon monoxide poisoning (secondary to)
- Myositis ossificans
- Ochronosis
- Parasites, calcified
- Pyogenic myositis (secondary to)
- Scleroderma
- Synovial cell sacroma
- Volkmann's ischemic contracture

Tendon
- Calcinosis universalis
- Calcium pyrophosphate dihydrate
- de Quervain's disease
- Ganglia, calcified
- Multiple tendons, calcified
- Ochronosis
- Pelligrini-Stieda disease
- Peritendinous calcarea
- Posttraumatic
- Tendinitis, calcific

Ligament
- Ankylosing spondylitis
- Cooper's ligament
- Degenerative joint disease
- Fluorosis
- Idiopathic
- Posttraumatic
- Renal osteodystrophy

Bursa
- Bursal osteochondromatosis
- Bursitis, calcific
- Calcinosis
- Calcium pyrophosphate dihydrate
- Gout
- Hypervitaminosis
- Synovial cell sacroma

*Adapted from Greenfield GB: *Radiology of Bone Diseases*, ed 5. Philadelphia, JB Lippincott, 1990, pp 742–747.

bony structures containing trabeculae and cortex. Ossification begins at a focus of calcification; deposition of calcium salts is usually the inciting event in all soft-tissue calcifications.[10]

The nature of the calcium deposit has been studied extensively. Although the ossification in myositis ossificans resembles fracture callus, the appearance of the calcium in calcific tendinitis may range from a milky or cheese-like substance to a hard, dry, chalk-like material. Still, the crystal in all of these deposits is the same: hydroxyapatite. Variations in water content and organic matrix constituents account for the differences in appearance. The chemical nature of these crystals is very different from those in calcium pyrophosphate deposition disease.

Outline 1 lists the differential diagnoses for the radiologic appearance of calcifications in muscles, tendons, ligaments, and bursae. Although the list is extensive, most lesions in athletes fall into one of two categories: myositis ossificans or calcific tendinitis.

Calcification in Muscle

Perhaps the prototypical example of soft-tissue calcification is myositis ossificans. This disease has many names: heterotopic calcification, heterotopic ossification, heterotopic bone formation, myositis ossificans traumatica, myositis ossificans circumscripta, pseudomalignant myositis ossificans, pseudomalignant osseous tumor of soft tissue, traumatic periosteal proliferations, drill bone, rider's bone, ossifying hematoma, fibrodysplasia ossificans traumatica, and myo-osteosis. All these names have been used because the pathophysiology of the disorder is not clearly understood. The term "myositis ossificans" has been criticized because the suspected abnormality sometimes occurs without inflammatory changes in the muscle, and sometimes without involving the muscle at all. Even when it does occur in the muscle, it may not involve muscle tissue per se, but rather the nonmuscular connective tissue. Finally, the suspected inciting events do not always result in ossification. Despite these criticisms, the name myositis ossificans has the distinct advantages of common usage and general recognition.

Myositis ossificans was described as early as 1832 by Hasse. He described a group of Prussian soldiers who developed "drill bone," ossific deposits in the deltoids and pectoral muscles as a result of recurrent trauma from firing muskets.[17] Early orthopaedic surgeons were also familiar with "rider's bone," calcification in the adductor muscles of jockeys.[17]

Myositis ossificans may be classified into four broad groups: progressiva, traumatica (circumscripta), acquired, and pseudomalignant. Myositis ossificans progressiva is a rare hereditary dysplasia characterized by the relentless calcification of many muscles throughout the body. Myositis ossificans traumatica or circumscripta is the most usual form. Acquired myositis ossificans occurs in uninjured tissues in a wide spectrum of neurologic diseases, including 11% of patients with head injuries and 15% to 40% of patients with spinal cord injuries. It is also seen in tetanus, poliomyelitis, myelodysplasia, tabes dorsalis, syringomyelia, cerebral palsy, and stroke.[7] The exact mechanism is not known, but a systemic increase in the levels of bone morphogenic protein may be involved. Finally, pseudomalignant myositis ossificans, or a similar variant of this name, describes what appears to be traumatic myositis ossificans without any history of trauma. In most series, about one third of the patients with myositis ossificans have no history of trauma. These patients might, however, have suffered minor trauma, later forgotten, or repetitive microtrauma.

It is important to recognize pseudomalignant myositis ossificans. Among one group of patients with myositis ossificans but no known history of trauma, 20% underwent radical surgical procedures to eradicate what was mistakenly thought to be an osteogenic sarcoma. Osteogenic sarcoma and pseudomalignant myositis ossificans can be distinguished from each other on the basis of their natural courses and radiographic features, but an ossified mass without a history of trauma should receive careful attention.

Myositis ossificans is frequently considered to be synonymous with quadriceps contusion. Not every quadriceps contusion develops ossification, however, and not all muscle ossifications are secondary to trauma. In 1973 Jackson and Feagin[14] studied quadriceps contusions in 4,000 military cadets for a one-year period. There were 65 injuries, which they graded as mild (normal gait; normal deep knee bend; >90 degrees of flexion), moderate (swollen, tender thigh mass; <90 degrees of knee motion; limp; unable to perform a deep knee bend), or severe (<45 degrees of knee flexion; marked tenderness and swelling of the thigh).

It is almost impossible to classify these injuries early; the full nature of the injury does not become apparent for 24 to 48 hours. At this point, muscle contusions must be differentiated from other injuries such as ruptures or strains. This differentiation is based on the amount of muscle function preserved and the nature of the injury mechanism. The initial treatment consists of rest, ice, compression, and crutches. The goal of early treatment is to limit hemorrhage by avoiding early motion and any therapy that might be irritating, such as diathermy, ultrasound, massage, and heat. Once most of the pain is gone and there are no signs of inflammation, rehabilitation to restore motion begins. This is done with gentle active exercise. Once 90 degrees of motion is achieved, a functional rehabilitation program is instituted. This consists of progressive resistance exercises and agility drills, added in a gradual manner.

Of the 65 patients described by Jackson and Feagin,[14] 47 had mild injuries. These patients had an excellent prognosis, with only 6.5 days of disability. There were no cases of myositis ossificans. Seven patients had moderate injuries: their average disability lasted 56 days, and myositis ossificans developed in five of the seven, despite therapy. Eleven patients sustained severe injuries; myositis ossificans developed in eight of the 11. The average disability for this group was 72 days. Thus, for mild injuries without any functional deficit by 24 to 48 hours, symptomatic therapy is indicated and the risk of heterotopic ossification is low. For more severe injuries with limitation of motion, the risk of ossification is 70% to 75%. An important fact is that of the severely injured patients with an average disability of 66 days and a 70% incidence of myositis ossificans, none had any residual deficit at final follow-up.

Although the natural history of traumatic myositis has been described, debate about its pathophysiologic characteristics continues. Myositis ossificans has been produced experimentally in various ways. Heinen and associates[11] reported that others had produced heterotopic bone in the quadriceps muscle of rabbits by injecting alcoholic extracts of autologous bone or fracture callus, while similar preparations from connective tissue or muscle were ineffective. Those authors had concluded that there must be an osteogenic substance that stimulates the muscle to form bone. However, Heinen and associates produced similar ossifications by injecting alcohol or calcium chloride alone. Injections of blood itself did not cause bone formation. Thus, they argued that the muscle injury itself caused the ossification, and that the "osteogenic factor" was not important.

Several years later, Zaccalini and Urist[45] debated this concept. They developed an experiment with rabbits in which quadriceps muscles were injured by controlled blows. They were unable to produce ossifications in the muscle unless there was concomitant injury to the bone and/or periosteum. They suggested that some biologic factor from the bone induced ossification in injured muscle. In a later study, Urist and associates[41] found a biologic factor extracted from bone that could induce bone formation in rat muscle tissues. This diffusible polypeptide of approximately 400 daltons is known as bone morphogenic protein. They thought that normal muscle resists ossification, but various conditions involving both periosteum and muscle could predispose muscle to absorb bone morphogenic protein, thus inducing ossification.

Others agree that bony or periosteal injury is a prerequisite for muscle ossification. Many cases of myositis ossificans are accompanied by periosteal injury, and follow-up radiographs frequently show the ossific lesion tethered to the bone by a stalk. Other cases may be misdiagnosed instances of calcified subperiosteal hematoma. At least a portion of these lesions do not involve bone in any way. One report[31] suggested that a differentiating feature between myositis ossificans and parosteal osteosarcoma is that myositis always has a lucent zone between the ossific lesion and the bone. Zadek[46] reported a case of true ossifying hematoma that radiographically and pathologically had absolutely no contact with the bone. It appears, then, that although injury to bone or periosteum is involved in the production of some lesions of myositis ossificans, it is not an absolute prerequisite.

In one experiment, rabbit knees were immobilized in splints for one to two weeks.[26] After this period, immobilization was continued for eight to 12 weeks but the splints were removed daily for five minutes of forceful passive motion. Presumably, contractures developed in the muscle, and the forceful motion caused areas of necrosis and hemorrhage. During a period of two to three months, fibrous, cartilaginous, and bony tissue, resembling human myositis ossificans, developed in these areas (Fig. 3). The lesions were created without accompanying injury to the periosteum and bone, supporting the idea that these structures are not always participants in the ossification process. Other types of muscle trauma (incisions, thermal damage, blood) do not themselves produce ossification, and other models (alcohol, calcium chloride) produce it in only a small percentage of cases. This experiment suggested that a combination of muscle injury and resulting hematoma is required for calcium deposition to begin.

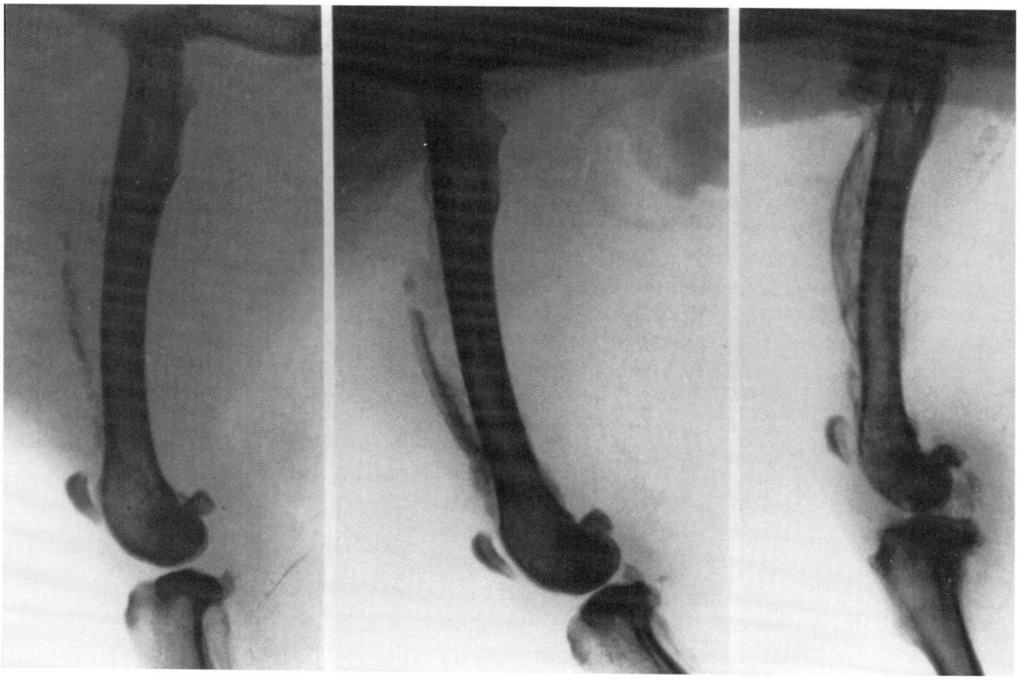

Fig. 3 *Experimental myositis ossificans produced in a rabbit model. (Reproduced with permission from Michelsson JE, Granroth G, Andersson LC: Myositis ossificans following forcible manipulation of the leg: A rabbit model for the study of heterotopic bone formation.* J Bone Joint Surg *1980;62A:811–815.)*

The actual event that triggers the deposition of calcium is unclear and many theories have been suggested. Possibly, some bone-producing substance causes hematogenous seeding of the traumatic intramuscular hematoma, but direct transmission of a bone-producing substance from bone or periosteum seems doubtful. Or, calcification may first occur at a site of necrosis, as part of a repair mechanism gone awry.[22] In the absence of normal inhibitors, this could stimulate increased calcification. A third theory involves lysosomal enzyme degradation resulting in localized pH changes and subsequent calcium salt precipitation.[47] Finally, it may result from a low-grade infection that induces a metaplasia of muscle and connective tissues into cartilage and bone.

Controlling calcification has received recent attention. As the number of total hip arthroplasties increases, heterotopic ossification is becoming a common problem. Several approaches have been used to minimize unwanted bone formation. Diphosphonates have been used,[38] but mineralization of osteoid occurs when treatment stops.

Irradiation in low doses has been successful in preventing ossification.[19] Nonsteroidal anti-inflammatory drugs (NSAIDs) also prevent heterotopic ossification.[34,35,37] This indicates the importance of inflammation (specifically the function of prostaglandins) in the calcification of soft tissues. The pathophysiologic sequence may be muscle trauma, inflammation, cellular proliferation, concentration of growth factors, induction of bone-forming cells, and, finally, ossification.

NSAIDs interrupt this mechanism at the inflammatory stage, and irradiation affects the proliferative stage, or the differentiation of bone-forming cells. Several theories on the cellular mechanisms have been proposed. Perhaps circulating bone morphogenic protein is concentrated in the hematoma, ultimately resulting in ossification. There may also be receptors for bone morphogenic protein that are activated or concentrated as a result of a particular type of muscle injury. Certain patients have a predisposition to form heterotopic bone, especially those with the DISH syndrome (disseminated idiopathic skeletal hyperostosis). These patients are likely to form bone after any type of musculoskeletal injury, perhaps because their bone morphogenic protein receptors are too numerous or too sensitive. Systemic growth factors (epidermal growth factor, fibroblast growth factor, platelet-derived growth factor, and somatomedin) may be released or concentrated by traumatized muscle. Another potential mechanism involves the deactivation of normal inhibitory mechanisms. Antibodies to bone morphogenic protein interfere with the ossification process in animal models, as does interleukin-1.[4,21] These factors may be inactivated in pathologic conditions. Calcification in ligaments and tendons probably occurs via a simpler mechanism.

The pathologic process of ossification begins with an initial injury to muscle and connective tissue associated with muscle fiber disruption and hemorrhage. Early in the process, a low-grade inflammatory reaction begins. The injured muscle fibers do not participate in the repair, but the intramuscular connective tissue proliferates through a process of cellular metaplasia and begins to form islands of cartilage and osteoid. Calcification begins and ossification progresses through both intramembranous and endochondral pathways. The histologic process is similar to normal callus formation, and indistinguishable from myositis ossificans progressiva. This suggests that myositis ossificans in either form is a normal physiologic mechanism that is out of homeostatic control. The resulting lesion was described by Ackerman[1] (Fig. 4). A central undifferentiated area of extreme cellularity exists, surrounded by a transitional zone of osteoid in a loose connective tissue stroma. The outer layer is mature lamellar bone. Normal muscle tissue is interspersed in all three layers. The central zone may contain areas of extreme pleomorphism and atypical mitoses that may alarm an unsuspecting pathologist if taken out of context. In this regard, the "zoning" phenomenon is important: if maturation occurs from the outside of the lesion in a centripetal manner, it is most probably benign. A lesion with a similar pathologic appearance that expands with the active cells peripherally is most probably malignant.

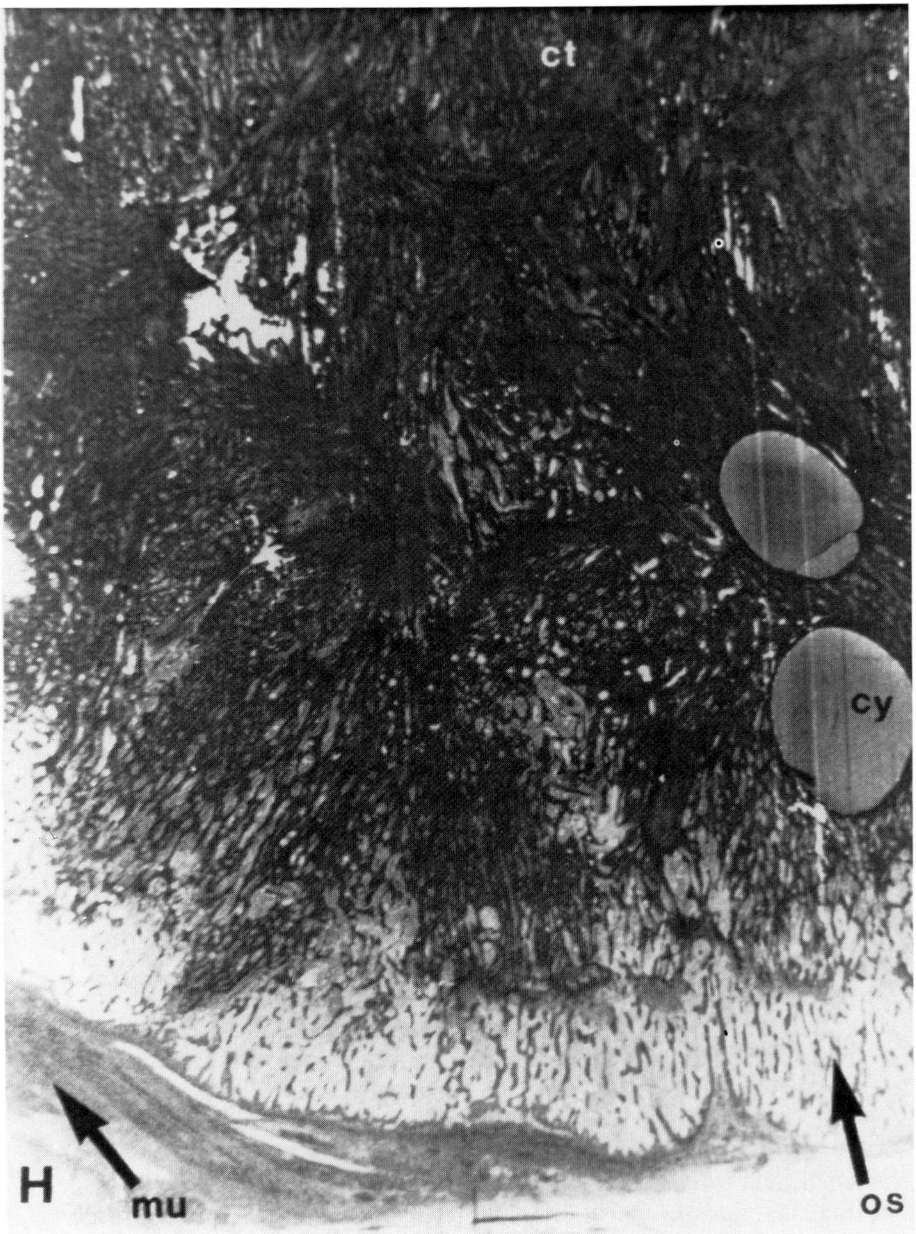

Fig. 4 *Histologic specimen of myositis ossificans: os, rim of cortical bone; mu, the muscle fibers in which the lesion began; cy, cysts that formed within the lesion; ct, hypercellular tissue at the center of the lesion. (Reproduced with permission from Hudson TM:* Radiologic-Pathologic Correlation of Musculoskeletal Lesions. *Baltimore, Williams & Wilkins, 1987.)*

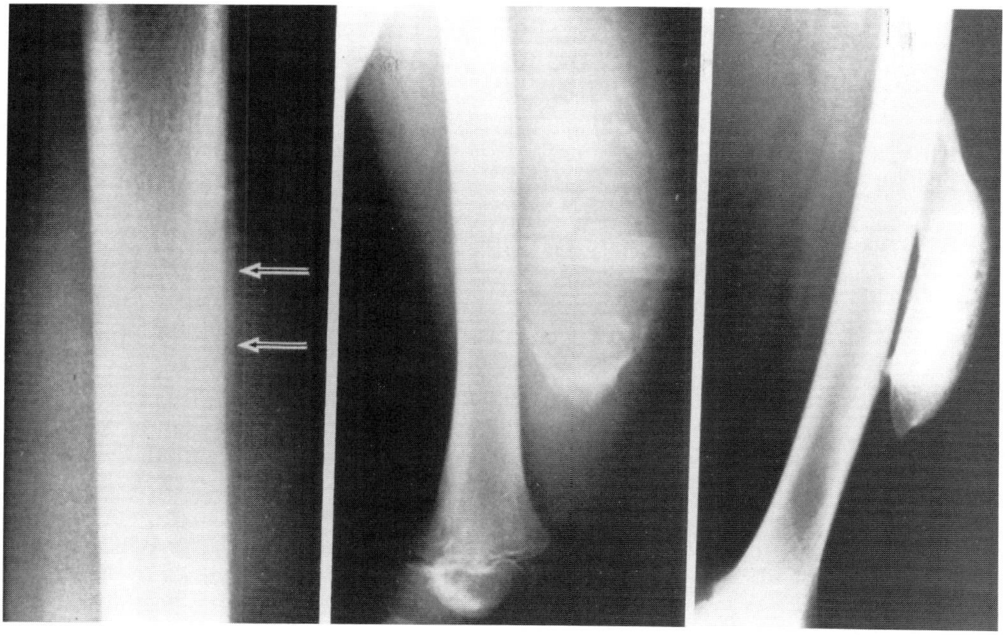

Fig. 5 *Radiographic progression of a typical myositis ossificans lesion in the thigh. (Reproduced with permission from Wilner D:* Radiology of Bone Tumors and Allied Disorders. *Philadelphia, WB Saunders, 1982.)*

The radiologic characteristics of the pathologic change has been also well described.[31] Soon after injury, a soft-tissue mass is visible (Fig. 5, *left*). After two to four weeks, flocculent calcific densities appear, and a periosteal reaction may also become visible. Six to eight weeks after injury, a lacy pattern of new bone is seen (Fig. 5, *center*). The periphery may be sharply circumscribed by a developing rim of cortical bone. At this time, the lesion may be confused with a malignancy, especially if it is an atraumatic lesion. In four cases studied, all the lesions had a lucent region between the outer rim and the underlying cortical bone. The existence of such a lucency may indicate that the lesion is not malignant, as osteosarcomas arise from bone. The absence of a lucency, however, does not prove that the lesion is malignant. Lesions of myositis ossificans develop rapidly, and become more organized over time, as opposed to malignancies. Usually, myositis ossificans reaches its maximum extent in ten to 12 weeks.

Computed tomography may help to clarify confusing cases. Computed tomography can usually detect the outer cortical rim of organizing bone, showing a clear boundary between ossified tissue and normal muscle.[48] Sarcomas do not show this organization, and there may be signs of infiltration of surrounding tissues. Sarcomas usually attach directly to bone, are more dense centrally than peripherally, and gradually enlarge over time. The myositis ossificans lesion matures in five to six months and then gradually begins to regress (Fig. 5, *right*).

The radiologic appearance can be used to characterize lesions as extraosseous, periosteal, or parosteal.[8] Parosteal lesions may be further divided into combined (extraosseous and periosteal lesions), secondary (a periosteal lesion that "leaks out" into the surrounding muscle tissue), or fascial-tendinous (lesions located near the insertion of tendons). These types of lesions are the least likely to resorb.[9]

Jackson and Feagin[14] developed the best clinical description of myositis ossificans. The four major risk factors for ossification are severe contusions, injuries near the musculotendinous junction, repeated injuries, and early exercise. Rest is the accepted treatment, and Hughston and associates[12] thought it would result "most frequently in incomplete resorption." Even minimal activity (walking) in the acute period may exacerbate the process of calcification. An additional risk factor is age. Although myositis ossificans is unusual in professional football players, it is common in college and high-school players. A mature periosteum-muscle interface or overall strength of the tissues may help prevent its development. Finally, poorly timed surgery (before the lesion matures) can exacerbate the condition and lead to early and more severe recurrences.

The most common site for myositis ossificans is the quadriceps femoris. This probably reflects the anatomic vulnerability of this muscle to contusion, rather than its predilection for ossification. Among patients with myositis ossificans, 50% to 75% have thigh lesions. About one third of the reported lesions occur in the arm, typically in the brachialis muscle (Fig. 6).[13] The natural histories of arm and thigh lesions are similar. Lesions have also been reported in the biceps, around the elbow and axilla,[5] and in the gastrocnemius, soleus, and hamstring muscles.[44]

The most common clinical finding is a soft-tissue mass. About one half of patients have a somewhat decreased range of motion. Pain is also common and occurs in about one third of patients, usually when the mass is accidentally compressed against the bone. Chronic inflammation is unusual. Most patients can return to their previous level of competition despite the persistence of the bony mass. Surgical excision is rarely required, unless the lesion is very large, located in an area particularly vulnerable to repetitive trauma, or remains painful or restricts motion.[5] Proper timing is important because surgery on "immature" lesions may result in early severe recurrence. It may be best to delay surgery until six months after injury. Myositis ossificans has been compared with the process of fracture healing.[13] Both have similar histologic features. Fractures may be actively remodeling 18 months or more after the injury. Each lesion should be evaluated individually, and bone scans used to determine cellular activity.

Alternative therapies are being developed. Molloy and McGuirk[27] treated a series of severe injuries by aspirating the hematoma and

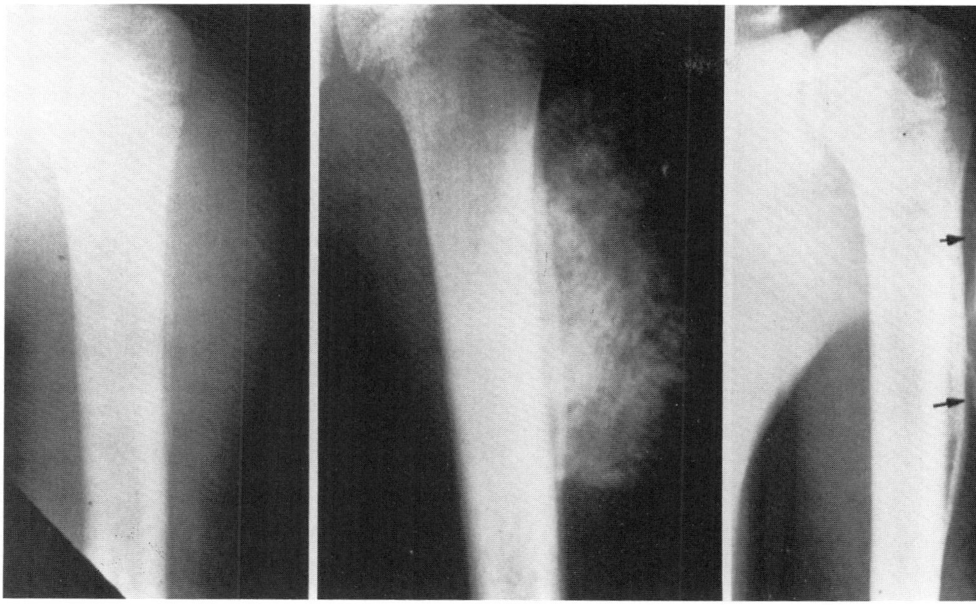

Fig. 6 *Myositis ossificans in the upper arm, a common location. (Reproduced with permission from Wilner D:* Radiology of Bone Tumors and Allied Disorders. *Philadelphia, WB Saunders, 1982.)*

instilling lidocaine, dexamethasone, and hyaluronidase. A small series showed good results, but evaluation with a controlled clinical series must be done before this treatment can be recommended.

The relationship of myositis ossificans to hemophilia should be mentioned. Areas of ectopic ossification are common in hemophilia; 15% of hemophiliacs in one series had such lesions. One third of these patients had multiple lesions. This provides some insight on the mechanism of ossification. Approximately 75% of hemophiliacs had intramuscular bleeding, but only a small fraction of these led to ossification. Yet, in some way, the presence of the hematoma remains linked to the production of the ossific deposit.[42] These and other observations may indicate that patients in whom myositis ossificans develops have an underlying diathesis that promotes the events that ultimately lead to ossification. One example is a football player who had recurrent episodes of subcutaneous ecchymosis and intramuscular hematomas, along with multiple areas of myositis ossificans.[15] An intensive examination revealed an unusual factor XI deficiency secondary to an incompletely recessive trait. Patients with these symptoms may be at increased risk for intracranial or intra-abdominal bleeding and should be advised against participating in contact sports.

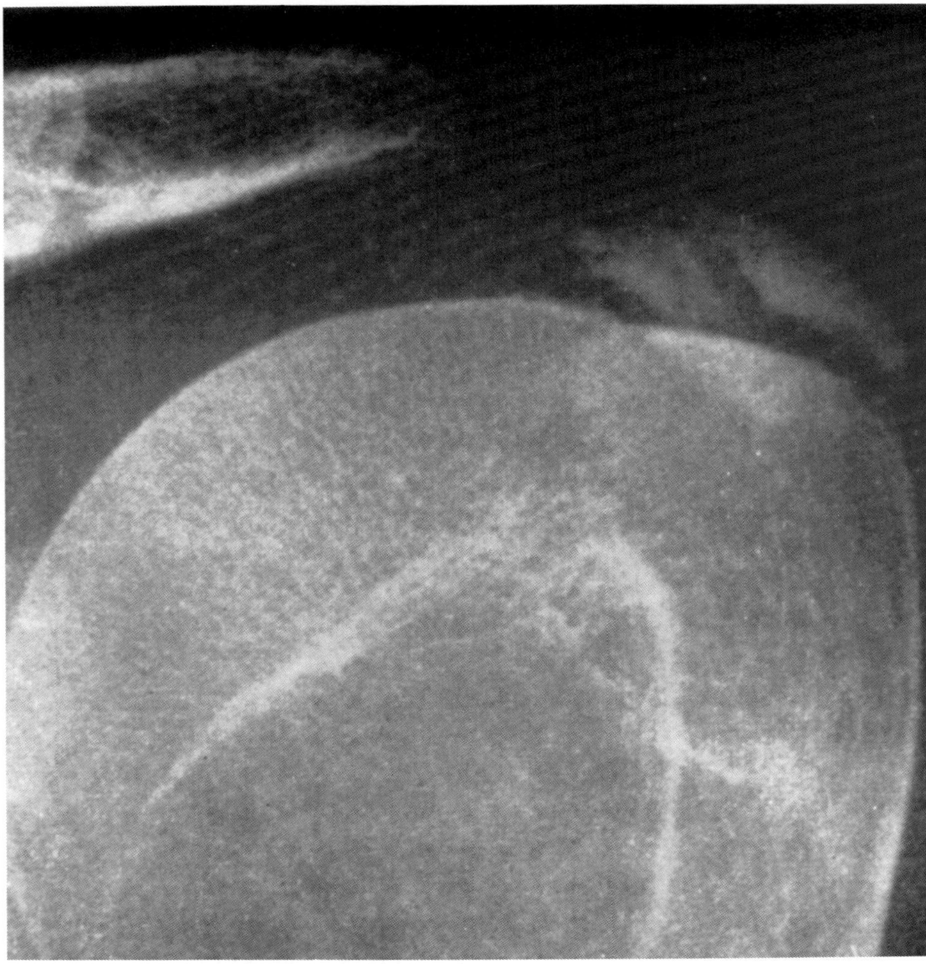

Fig. 7 *Calcific tendinitis of the shoulder. (Reproduced with permission from Murray RO, Jacobson HG:* The Radiology of Skeletal Disorders: Exercises in Diagnosis, *ed 2. Edinburgh, Churchill Livingstone, 1977.)*

Calcification in Tendon and Tendon Sheath

Athletes frequently have calcifications in the rotator cuff (Fig. 7). Calcific tendinitis may occur at many sites, but the symptoms of calcium in the rotator cuff are more severe and persistent, perhaps because the tendon rubs between two bony prominences.[25]

Calcium deposits in tendons are common but are usually asymptomatic, incidental findings. As many as 5.4% of normal hips may have calcification in or around the gluteus medius tendon.[16] Calcification is also present in 3% to 8% of all shoulders, often with multiple deposits. Perhaps only one third of these calcifications are symptomatic, usually among patients 40 to 59 years old.[25,36] McLaughlin[24] did not find a single case when examining more than 1,000 cadavers of elderly individuals, and there are no clear answers as to why only a fraction of these deposits become symptomatic.

In 1934, Codman[6] described several diseases of the rotator cuff, some involving calcium salt deposits. Later, Pedersen and Key[32] attributed the cause of calcareous tendinitis to the deposition of calcium in avascular, degenerated tendon. Symptoms occur only when the deposit is large enough to cause a mechanical dysfunction in the bursa. They pointed out that this condition exhibits minimal inflammation and is rarely accompanied by rotator cuff tears. There are apparently two clinical patterns associated with calcific tendinitis: an acute, inflammatory crisis, with marked pain and dysfunction; and a low-grade, chronic, often asymptomatic condition. Examples of both are common in the shoulder and have been described in detail. These conditions have also occurred in the gluteus maximus tendon,[16,43] in the elbow and wrist extensors and flexors,[9,30] and in the Achilles tendon.[20]

An acute inflammatory condition in the shoulder or other locations is often accompanied by transient calcifications in the soft tissues. The calcific deposits are self-limiting: when the symptoms abate, so does the calcification.[30] An acute condition may also occur in patients with chronic calcium deposits. In these cases, symptoms may occur only when the deposit enlarges and causes mechanical impingement of the cuff on the acromion. Another explanation may be that as the deposit enlarges and rises toward the surface of the tendon, it induces a reactive inflammatory condition in the bursa; this has been likened to a "calcium boil." Once the lesion ruptures into the bursa (or joint in the case of the hip), symptoms abate because the calcium is rapidly cleared away.[36] Or perhaps the rupture itself provokes the acute attack.[16] Whatever the actual mechanism, the acute period is usually self-limited and does not warrant surgical intervention. It is the prodromal period that frequently causes therapeutic difficulty.

Degenerating collagen fibers in the tendon tissue probably cause this initial lesion. This degeneration may occur in the avascular or hypervascular regions of the rotator cuff. Avascular lesions have also been found in the distal part of the supraspinatus tendon, where most cuff tears and calcific deposits are found.[33] In these areas, a low oxygen tension may stimulate the degenerated tendon tissue to undergo metaplasia into cartilage that subsequently calcifies.[40] This explanation has been questioned because the distal area is not really avascular at all; it is simply the junction of the muscular and osseous arterial networks.[29] Additionally, a vascular deficiency does not explain why other tendons undergo degeneration. Once necrotic tendon debris is produced, calcium salt deposition occurs.

Deposits associated with acute inflammation are typically milky or cheese-like in consistency, whereas chronic deposits appear as dry, gritty, chalk-like material. Both types are chemically identical hydroxyapatite.[23] Most cases can be treated symptomatically and will resolve.

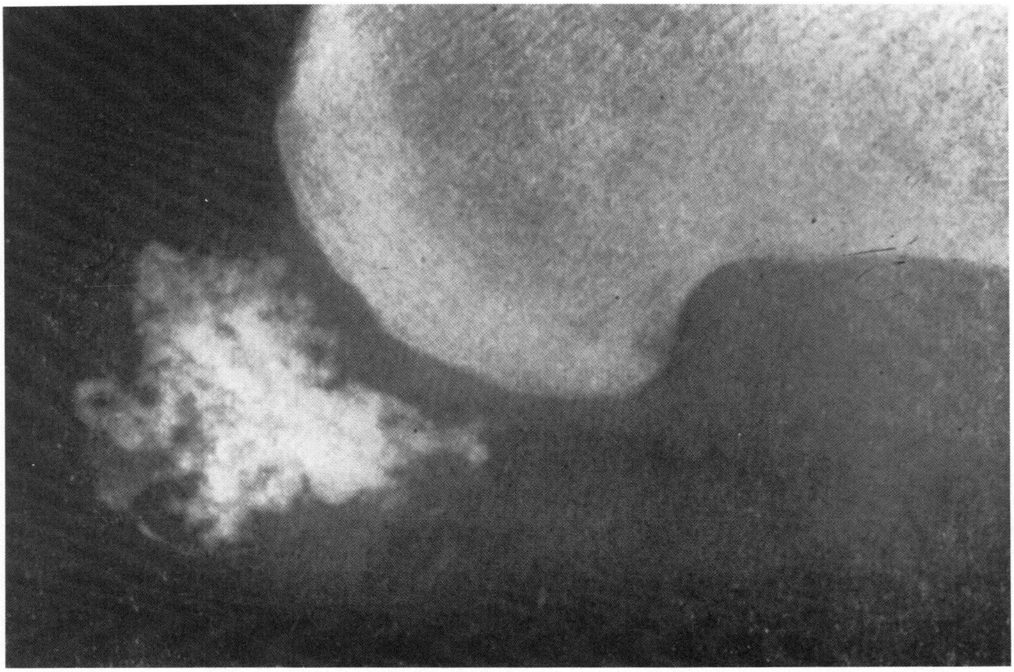

Fig. 8 *Calcific bursitis of the calcaneus. (Reproduced with permission from Murray RO, Jacobson HG:* The Radiology of Skeletal Disorders: Exercises in Diagnosis, *ed 2. Edinburgh, Churchill Livingstone, 1977.)*

Surgery should be reserved for chronic cases with long-standing symptoms that do not respond to conservative therapy. In these cases, simply evacuating the lesion produces a satisfactory outcome.[25]

Calcifications in Bursae and Ligaments and Around Joints

Calcific bursitis has been a common diagnosis in the past but is probably the same entity as calcific tendinitis. The transient calcifications of an acute inflammatory process occur within the substance of the tendons themselves, although there may be an accompanying bursal inflammation. This pattern occurs in the hip, shoulder, wrist, and elbow. It has specifically been reported as ischial, greater trochanteric, and calcaneal bursitis (Fig. 8). Persistent calcification in these areas is rare.[30]

Traumatic joint injuries often result in calcifications within the injured ligaments. In joints such as the ankle that are subject to repetitive injuries, ossicles often develop in and around the periarticular structures. The ossicles are usually asymptomatic. Severe joint injury also results in periarticular calcification of ligaments, joint capsule, and other connective tissues.[44] This often occurs in elbow injuries, especially dislocations and fracture-dislocations. Thompson and Garcia[39] reported a 3% incidence of myositis in elbow injuries and cited passive motion as a specific risk factor. Delaying surgical treatment beyond 24 hours also contributed to ossification.

Complete calcification of the acromioclavicular ligament has also been reported in the shoulder of a 37-year-old man.[28] In this particular patient, the calcified ligament caused an impingement syndrome. Calcified ligaments surrounding the hip joint of a professional soccer player were also reported. In this case, surgical excision was necessary.[3]

References

1. Ackerman LV: Extra-osseous localized non-neoplastic bone and cartilage formation (so-called myositis ossificans): Clinical and pathologic confusion with malignant neoplasms. *J Bone Joint Surg* 1958;49A:279–298.
2. Anderson HC: Calcific diseases: A concept. *Arch Pathol Lab Med* 1983;107:341–348.
3. Antao NA: Myositis of the hip in a professional soccer player: A case report. *Am J Sport Med* 1988;16:82–83.
4. Canalis E, Centrella M, Urist MR: Effect of partially purified bone morphogenetic protein on DNA synthesis and cell replication in calvarial and fibroblast cultures. *Clin Orthop* 1985;198:289–296.
5. Carlson WO, Klassen RA: Myositis ossificans of the upper extremity: A long-term follow-up. *J Pediatr Orthop* 1984;4:693–696.
6. Codman EA: *The Shoulder: Rupture of the Supraspinatus Tendon and Other Lesions in or About the Subacromial Bursa.* Boston, Thomas Todd, 1934.
7. Garland DE, Blum CE, Waters RL: Periarticular heterotopic ossification in head-injured adults: Incidence and locations. *J Bone Joint Surg* 1980;62A:1143–1146.
8. Gelmer WS, Anderson LD: Reactions of soft somatic tissue which may progress to bone formation. *South Med J* 1959;52:1432–1437.
9. Ghormley JW: Calcareous tendinitis. *Surg Clin North Am* 1961;41:1721–1728.
10. Greenfield GB: *Radiology of Bone Diseases*, ed 5. Philadelphia, JB Lippincott, 1990, pp 742–747.
11. Heinen JH Jr, Dabbs GH, Mason HA: The experimental production of ectopic cartilage and bone in the muscles of rabbits. *J Bone Joint Surg* 1949;31A:765–775.
12. Hughston JC, Whatley GS, Stone MM: Myositis ossificans traumatica (myo-osteosis). *South Med J* 1962;55:1167–1170.
13. Huss CD, Puhl JJ: Myositis ossificans of the upper arm. *Am J Sports Med* 1980;8:419–424.
14. Jackson DW, Feagin JA: Quadriceps contusions in young athletes: Relation of severity of injury to treatment and prognosis. *J Bone Joint Surg* 1973;55A:95–105.
15. Jokl P, Federico J: Myositis ossificans traumatica: Association with hemophilia (factor XI deficiency) in a football player. *JAMA* 1977;237:2215–2216.
16. Jones GB: Acute episodes with calcification around the hip joint. *J Bone Joint Surg* 1955;37B:448–452.

17. Kakulas BA, Adams RD: *Disease of Muscle*, ed 4. Philadelphia, Harper & Row, 1985.
18. Kim KM: Pathological calcification, in Trump BF, Srstila AV (eds): *Pathobiology of Cell Membranes*. New York, Academic Press, 1983.
19. Lo TC, Healy WL, Covall DJ, et al: Heterotopic bone formation after hip surgery: Prevention with single-dose postoperative hip irradiation. *Radiology* 1988;168:851–854.
20. Lotke PA: Ossification of the Achilles tendon: Report of seven cases. *J Bone Joint Surg* 1970;52A:157–160.
21. Mahy PR, Urist MR: Experimental heterotopic bone formation induced by bone morphogenetic protein and recombinant human interleukin-1B. *Clin Orthop* 1988;237:236–244.
22. Maki T, Suzuki N, Takahashi W, et al: The mechanism of calcification in necrotic foci and its biological significance. *Tohoku J Exp Med* 1972;107:57–71.
23. McCarty DJ Jr, Gatter RA: Recurrent acute inflammation associated with focal apatite crystal deposition. *Arthritis Rheum* 1966;9:804–819.
24. McLaughlin HL: Lesions of the musculotendinous cuff of the shoulder: III. Observations on the pathology, course and treatment of calcific deposits. *Ann Surg* 1946;124:354–362.
25. McLaughlin HL: The selection of calcium deposits for operation: The technique and results of operation. *Surg Clin North Am* 1963;43:1501–1504.
26. Michelsson JE, Granroth G, Andersson LC: Myositis ossificans following forcible manipulation of the leg: A rabbit model for the study of heterotopic bone formation. *J Bone Joint Surg* 1980;62A:811–815.
27. Molloy JC, McGuirk RA: Treatment of traumatic myositis ossificans circumscripta: Use of aspiration and steroids. *J Trauma* 1976;16:851–857.
28. Morimoto K, Mori E, Nakagawa Y: Calcification of the coracoacromial ligament: A case report of the shoulder impingement syndrome. *Am J Sports Med* 1988;16:80–81.
29. Moseley HF: The vascular supply of the rotator cuff. *Surg Clin North Am* 1963;43:1521–1522.
30. Murray RO, Jacobson HG: *The Radiology of Skeletal Disorders: Exercises in Diagnosis*, ed 2. Edinburgh, Churchill Livingstone, 1977.
31. Norman A, Dorfman HD: Juxtacortical circumscribed myositis ossificans: Evolution and radiographic features. *Radiology* 1970;96:301–306.
32. Pedersen HE, Key JA: Pathology of calcareous tendinitis and subdeltoid bursitis. *Arch Surg* 1951;62:50–63.
33. Rathbun JB, Mcnab I: The microvascular pattern of the rotator cuff. *J Bone Joint Surg* 1970;52B:540–553.
34. Ritter MA, Sieber JM: Prophylactic indomethacin for the prevention of heterotopic bone formation following total hip arthroplasty. *Clin Orthop* 1985;196:217–225.
35. Schmidt SA, Kjaersgaard-Andersen P, Pedersen NW, et al: The use of indomethacin to prevent the formation of heterotopic bone after total hip replacement: A randomized, double-blind clinical trial. *J Bone Joint Surg* 1988;70A:834–838.
36. Simon WH: Soft tissue disorders of the shoulder: Frozen shoulder, calcific tendinitis, and bicipital tendinitis. *Orthop Clin North Am* 1975;6:521–539.
37. Sodemann B, Persson PE, Nilsson OS: Prevention of heterotopic ossification by non-steroid antiinflammatory drugs after total hip arthroplasty. *Clin Orthop* 1988;237:158–163.
38. Thomas BJ, Amstutz HC: Results of the administration of diphosphonate for the prevention of heterotopic ossification after total hip arthroplasty. *J Bone Joint Surg* 1985;67A:400–403.

39. Thompson HC III, Garcia A: Myositis ossificans: Aftermath of elbow injuries. *Clin Orthop* 1967;50:129–134.
40. Uhthoff HK, Sarkar K, Maynard JA: Calcifying tendinitis: A new concept of its pathogenesis. *Clin Orthop* 1976;118:164–168.
41. Urist MR, Nakagawa M, Nakata N, et al: Experimental myositis ossificans: Cartilage and bone formation in muscle in response to a diffusible bone matrix-derived morphogen. *Arch Pathol Lab Med* 1978;102:312–316.
42. Vas W, Cockshott WP, Martin RF, et al: Myositis ossificans in hemophilia. *Skeletal Radiol* 1981;7:27–31.
43. Wepfer JF, Reed JG, Cullen GM, et al: Calcific tendinitis of the gluteus maximus tendon (gluteus maximus tendinitis). *Skeletal Radiol* 1983;9:198–200.
44. Wilner D: *Radiology of Bone Tumors and Allied Disorders.* Philadelphia, WB Saunders, 1982.
45. Zaccalini PS, Urist M: Traumatic periosteal proliferations in rabbits: The enigma of experimental myositis ossificans traumatica. *J Trauma* 1964;4:344–357.
46. Zadek I: Ossifying hematoma in the thigh: A case report. *J Bone Joint Surg* 1969;51A:386–390.
47. Zarins B, Ciullo JV: Acute muscle and tendon injuries in athletes. *Clin Sports Med* 1983;2:167–182.
48. Zeanah WR, Hudson TM: Myositis ossificans: Radiologic evaluation of two cases with diagnostic computed tomograms. *Clin Orthop* 1982;168:187–191.

Chapter 15

Inflammation and Tissue Repair

David J. Schurman, MD
Stuart B. Goodman, MD, FRCS(C)
R. Lane Smith, PhD

Introduction

Inflammation is a process that is typically perceived as an attempt to repair tissue injured by trauma, infection, or foreign antigens. For most of recorded history, inflammation was defined as a clinical entity consisting of local swelling, redness, heat, and pain. The advent of microscopy led to the association of specific cells—leukocytes—with inflammation. These cells were found to contain packets of enzymes that cleaned the wound of foreign invaders, or necrotic debris. In recent years, immunologic studies have indicated a high degree of specialization among the leukocytes, particularly lymphocytes. The macrophage plays a key role in directing traffic and communicating essential information to lymphocytes. Investigation of the methods of cell-to-cell communication has greatly expanded our understanding of inflammation, especially during the last two decades.

Wound Healing

One important natural form of inflammation that is an appealing basic model for a surgeon is wound healing. Under normal circumstances, the first few stages of wound healing constitute a physiologic, well-controlled, and integrated process of acute and then chronic inflammation. This unfolding process leads from granulation to epithelialization, repair, and scarring. An understanding of wound healing sets the stage for an appreciation of the potential of inflammation for both beneficial and harmful effects.

The healing of a simple wound entails three overlapping stages whose end point is the restoration of a functional barrier to mechanical, chemical, and thermal trauma:[7,10,22] (1) inflammation, (2) epithelialization, (3) scarring, wound contracture, and remodeling.

Inflammation

The inflammatory phase of wound healing begins immediately after injury. Transected blood vessels retract and constrict, resulting in local control of hemorrhage. Blood platelets and coagulation proteins mediate the formation of white and red thrombi, which further control bleeding.[13] In the area of injury the blood vessels dilate, and capillaries become more permeable to plasma proteins. Neutrophils and monocytes adhere to the walls of the capillaries and then exit into the perivascular space. The wound is filled with an inflammatory exudate composed of tissue fluid, plasma proteins, neutrophils, and monocytes. Clinically, the injured area is red, warm, and swollen.

Neutrophils and monocytes begin ingesting bacteria, foreign material, and tissue debris. During this process, some of these cells die and release their contents into the extracellular space. Intracellular enzymes such as the acid hydrolases and substances such as prostaglandins E_1 and E_2, kinins, and histamine enhance the inflammatory response and facilitate the digestion of necrotic debris.[11,22,42]

Platelet-derived growth factor causes the further migration of inflammatory cells and fibroblasts to the site of injury and repair.[13,20,33] The lymphatics are obstructed by tissue edema and by fibrinous deposits. A glycoprotein, fibronectin, aids in the localization of the reaction by causing an adherent network of fibroblasts, fibrin, and newly formed collagen to surround the area.

Epithelialization

Within about 24 hours of the injury, the second stage of wound healing, epithelialization, begins. Concurrent with the removal of necrotic debris, the epidermis begins to regenerate. Mitotic activity in the basal layer of the epidermis is followed by the migration of cells down the wound edge. Although the process is incompletely understood, fibrin strands and contact inhibition "guide" the newly formed basal cells that are adjacent to the wound edge into the defect.[27] Within about 48 hours, small wounds—those without extensive tissue loss—are covered by a thin layer of epithelium. This layer undergoes further mitotic activity and differentiation to reestablish a structured epithelial stratum.

Scarring

The third stage of wound repair, scarring and wound contracture, begins during the second or third day after the injury. Fibroblasts and other cells in the subcutaneous tissue migrate into the wound, probably originating from mesenchymal cells in the vicinity.[32] The fibroblasts use the fibrinous scaffolding in the wound and the phenomenon of contact inhibition to populate the wound space.[22] Fibroblasts begin secreting collagenous proteins and ground substance, reconstituting the subcutaneous layer. At the same time, new capillaries bud from existing vascular structures. During the next several weeks, as the inflammatory response dwindles, the subcutaneous layer matures further. This layer becomes less cellular, and collagenous bundles begin to dominate. At first, the collagen fibers are distributed randomly within a loose matrix of ground substance. However, concurrent collagen synthesis, deposition, and degradation provide a metabolic framework whereby thick bundles of collagen are formed. Within one or two weeks of injury, the wound begins to contract centripetally. This process is incompletely understood but is probably mediated by contractile fibroblasts called myofibroblasts.[23]

Wound healing may be inhibited by systemic or local factors.[7,22] Systemic factors include deficiency of essential vitamins and minerals (eg, vitamin C, copper, zinc, iron) or cytotic drugs, irradiation, corticosteroids, sepsis, anemia, poor oxygenation, and systemic diseases such as diabetes and renal failure. Local factors include poor local nutrition and oxygenation, hypovascularity, wound infection, and hematoma.

The final event in wound healing is remodeling of scar tissue, which can last as long as one year. Remodeling is not perceived to be linked with the inflammatory processes.

Tissue Healing

Inflammation and associated factors are part of normal wound healing and are prominent in abnormal wound healing. The deleterious effects of inflammation are most obvious during an infection in which the host's reaction to bacteria may actually be more harmful than the bacteria themselves. An imbalance of cytokines may lead to pathophysiologic fibrosis as well as destruction of connective tissue components. Rheumatoid arthritis, scleroderma, and even atherosclerosis are some conditions thought to be the result of malregulated cytokine influence.[3]

Historically, inflammation in soft tissues was studied histologically and defined by the types and numbers of particular cells present in various stages. Neutrophils predominate early and are replaced by macrophages and then by fibrocytes. It was later discovered that enzymes play an important role. Serine proteases trigger inflammatory cascades such as coagulation, kinin release, fibrinolysis, and complement activation.[6] These proteases are controlled by protease inhibitors. Genetically controlled deficiencies in protease inhibitors have been found to be responsible for a variety of soft-tissue diseases of the liver and lung. For example, the protease inhibitor antitrypsin can be inactivated by oxidation of stimulated neutrophils. A zone of oxidation around a stimulated neutrophil results from the release of oxygen radicals. This disarms the protease inhibitor, easing the localized breakdown of connective tissue.[6]

Knowledge of inflammatory mechanisms is growing. In addition to understanding the cell types and enzymes and antienzymes involved in inflammation, we have a better understanding of the cascades of enzymes, the interactions of those cascades, and a growing number of

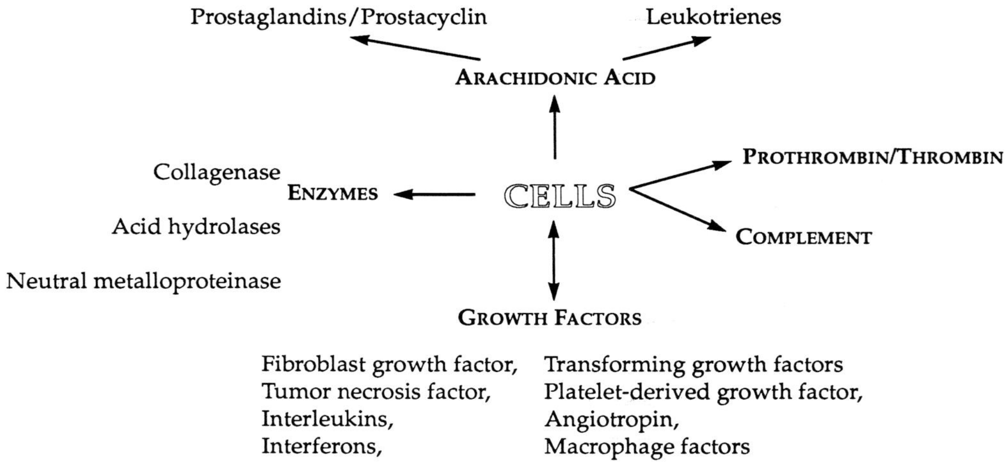

Fig. 1 *Modulators of inflammation and tissue repair.*

"traffic directors." We are learning more about the interaction of such factors as transforming growth factors alpha and beta,[4,24,25,30,31] interferons,[2,40] macrophage growth factors,[16–18,28,41] fibroblast growth factor,[12,19] platelet-derived growth factor,[25] tumor necrosis factor,[26] monocyte procoagulant-inducing factor,[15] epidermal growth factor,[4,5] and angiotropin[9,17] (Fig. 1).

No pharmacologic agent is known to stimulate healing, but growth factors may do just that. The identification, purification, and characterization of growth factors or cytokines may provide new insights into the mechanisms of inflammatory control and also offer exciting possibilities for therapeutic intervention. Conversely, we must not neglect some older, better-known controllers of inflammation. The arachidonic acid cascade is an important example. Stored as membrane-bound phospholipid, arachidonic acid is released by phospholipases and converted to biologically active forms principally through (1) cyclo-oxygenases, giving rise to the prostaglandins, prostacyclin, and thromboxanes, and (2) lipoxygenase, converting arachidonic acid to a variety of leukotrienes. Nonsteroidal anti-inflammatory drugs (NSAIDs) inhibit the cyclo-oxygenase pathways, and the corticosteroid drugs, by indirectly inhibiting phospholipases, prevent the release of the entire spectrum of activated arachidonic forms, including production of leukotrienes. There are now laboratory drugs that inhibit lipoxygenase pathways. Research is now being done to determine whether inhibiting either the cyclo-oxygenase or the lipoxygenase pathway separately might backfire by increasing arachidonic acid products on the unblocked side. Important therapeutic agents may soon result from this work.[14,21,34–37]

NSAIDs are extremely effective in preventing pain and in decreasing the destructive processes of a variety of clinical conditions (including trauma) in which inflammation is involved.[1,39] In at least one laboratory report on animals, NSAIDs compromised wound repair; that article included a single case report of impaired wound healing in a patient who ingested a high dose of perioperatively given ibuprofen.[29] Thus, inflammatory events themselves are neither beneficial nor harmful but play a physiologic role that can go awry if poorly regulated.

At each step of the inflammatory process, the pathway involved is likely to be physiologic and beneficial. Nevertheless, as with most physiologic events, the process itself can take a harmful turn. The inflammatory process consists of various events that under normal circumstances are advantageous, even required, for normal tissue healing. When such events are imbalanced, they can be harmful. The mesenchymal mitogenic effect of thrombin usually promotes cell division, stimulates cellular messengers, and is a chemoattractant for monocytes. When a clot is generated in an injury, the thrombin induces the release of plasminogen activator inhibitor, platelet-derived growth factor,[38] and interleukin-1.[39] All these substances are physiologically valuable. However, with the release of plasminogen activator inhibitor, intravascular clotting could lead to diffuse intravascular coagulation, a potentially lethal condition. Interleukin-1, an important cell-cell mediator responsible for many important physiologic events, including lymphocyte growth and regulation, has several deleterious effects if it is not properly regulated. Among these are osteoporosis, articular cartilage destruction, and fever.

Monocytes and macrophages are inflammatory cells that stimulate and react to other inflammatory events. Macrophages isolated from a wound site contain RNA for transforming, platelet-derived, and insulin-like growth factors.[30] Transforming growth factor is responsible for a wide variety of critical events in tissue healing, including the increase of wound strength,[4] by stimulating fibroblasts to produce collagen and fibronectin.[24,25] Either directly or indirectly, TGF-β can bring about all the complex events that lead to the formation of granulation tissue.[31] Although this cascade of events is critical for normal tissue function, healing, and embryogenesis, a recent report implicates overexpression of TGF-α as a possible major determinant in epidermal hyperplasia or psoriatic skin.[8]

Many metabolites of arachidonic acid are vital to the development of inflammation. The cyclo-oxygenase agents prostaglandin E_2 and prostacyclin are potent vasodilators. The leukotrienes increase vascular permeability, modulate interleukin-1, and cause cellular adhesion, chemotaxis of neutrophils, and degranulation of neutrophils.[14,21,34,36] Blocking the actions of prostaglandins or leukotrienes may reduce harmful inflammatory side effects. This can be useful if it is clear that the inflammatory process is no longer beneficial to healing, for example, in rheumatoid arthritis or in a postinflammatory synovitis. Leukotrienes are also believed to play an important role in allergic asthma and gout.[21] Thus, blocking the harmful effects of mediators when they serve no useful purpose is laudatory. In the normal course of events, prostaglandins and leukotrienes can play a critical role in the early stages of wound healing or in the presence of infection.

The stable prostaglandins, prostaglandins E_2 and I_2, have effects that are both inflammatory and anti-inflammatory. The anti-inflammatory effects include inhibition of the activation of neutrophils, platelets, and mononuclear phagocytes. For example, systemic treatment with prostaglandin E_2 in patients with Reiter's syndrome reduced swelling.[1]

References

1. Abramson SB, Weissmann G: The mechanisms of action of nonsteroidal antiinflammatory drugs. *Arthritis Rheum* 1989;32:1–9.
2. Adelmann-Grill BC, Hein R, Wach F, et al: Inhibition of fibroblast chemotaxis by recombinant human interferon gamma and interferon alpha. *J Cell Physiol* 1987;130:270–275.
3. Agelli M, Wahl SM: Cytokines and fibrosis. *Clin Exp Rheumatol* 1986;4:379–388.
4. Brown GL, Curtsinger LJ, White M, et al: Acceleration of tensile strength of incisions treated with EGF and TGF-β. *Ann Surg* 1988;208:788–794.
5. Buckley A, Davidson JM, Kamerath CD, et al: Epidermal growth factor increases granulation tissue formation dose dependently. *J Surg Res* 1987;43:322–328.
6. Carrell RW: Alpha$_1$-Antitrypsin: Molecular pathology, leukocytes, and tissue damage. *J Clin Invest* 1986;78:1427–1431.
7. Carrico TJ, Mehrhof AI Jr, Cohen IK: Biology of wound healing. *Surg Clin North Am* 1984;64:721–733.
8. Elder JT, Fisher GJ, Lindquist PB, et al: Overexpression of transforming growth factor α in psoriatic epidermis. *Science* 1989;243:811–814.
9. Folkman J, Ingber DE: Angiostatic steroids: Method of discovery and mechanism of action. *Ann Surg* 1987;206:374–383.
10. Forrest L: Current concepts in soft connective tissue wound healing. *Br J Surg* 1983;70:133–140.
11. Gorman RR: Prostaglandins, thromboxanes and prostacylin. *Int Rev Biochem* 1978;20:81.
12. Gospodarowicz D: Humoral control of cell proliferation: The role of fibroblast growth factor in regeneration, angiogenesis, wound healing, and neoplastic growth. *Prog Clin Biol Res* 1976;9:1–19.
13. Graham MF, Diegelmann RF, Lindblad WJ, et al: Effects of inflammation on wound healing: *In vitro* studies and *in vivo* studies, in Hunt TK, Heppenstall RB, Pines E, et al (eds): *Soft and Hard Tissue Repair: Biological and Clinical Aspects.* New York, Praeger, 1984, pp 361–379.
14. Greaves MW, Camp RD: Prostaglandins, leukotrienes, phospholipase, platelet activating factor, and cytokines: An integrated approach to inflammation of human skin. *Arch Dermatol Res* 1988;280(suppl):S33–S41.
15. Gregory SA, Kornbluth RS, Helin H, et al: Monocyte procoagulant inducing factor: A lymphokine involved in the T cell-instructed monocyte procoagulant response to antigen. *J Immunol* 1986;137:3231–3239.
16. Hibbs MS, Postlethwaite AE, Mainardi CL, et al: Alterations in collagen production in mixed mononuclear leukocyte-fibroblast cultures. *J Exp Med* 1983;157:47–59.
17. Höckel M, Jung W, Vaupel P, et al: Purified monocyte-derived angiogenic substance (angiotropin) induces controlled angiogenesis associated with regulated tissue proliferation in rabbit skin. *J Clin Invest* 1988;82:1075–1090.

18. Hunt TK, Knighton DR, Thakral KK, et al: Studies on inflammation and wound healing: Angiogenesis and collagen synthesis stimulated in vivo by resident and activated wound macrophages. *Surgery* 1984;96:48–54.
19. Joseph-Silverstein J, Rifkin DB: Endothelial cell growth factors and the vessel wall. *Semin Thromb Hemost* 1987;13:504–513.
20. Knighton DR, Hunt TK, Thakral KK, et al: Role of platelets and fibrin in the healing sequence: An in vivo study of angiogenesis and collagen synthesis. *Ann Surg* 1982;196:379–388.
21. König W, Bremm KD, Brom HJ, et al: The role of leukotriene-inducing and -metabolizing enzymes in inflammation. *Int Arch Allergy Appl Immunol* 1987;82:526–531.
22. Madden JW, Arem AJ: Wound healing: Biologic and clinical features, in Sabiston DC Jr (ed): *Textbook of Surgery: The Biological Basis of Modern Surgical Practice*, ed 13. Philadelphia, WB Saunders, 1986, vol 1, pp 193–213.
23. Majno G, Gabbiani G, Hirschel BJ, et al: Contraction of granulation tissue in vitro: Similarity to smooth muscle. *Science* 1971;173:548–550.
24. Marx JL: Cell growth control comes under scrutiny. *Science* 1988;239:1093–1094.
25. Mustoe TA, Pierce GF, Thomason A, et al: Accelerated healing of incisional wounds in rats induced by transforming growth factor-beta. *Science* 1987;237:1333–1336.
26. Nawroth PP, Bank I, Handley D, et al: Tumor necrosis factor/cachectin interacts with endothelial cell receptors to induce release of interleukin 1. *J Exp Med* 1986;163:1363–1375.
27. Odland G, Ross R: Human wound repair: I. Epidermal regeneration. *J Cell Biol* 1968;39:135–151.
28. Phan SH, McGarry BM, Loeffler KM, et al: Regulation of macrophage-derived fibroblast growth factor release by arachidonate metabolites. *J Leukocyte Biol* 1987;42:106–113.
29. Proper SA, Fenske NA, Burnett SM, et al: Compromised wound repair caused by perioperative use of ibuprofen. *J Am Acad Dermatol* 1988;18:1173–1179.
30. Rappolee DA, Mark D, Banda MJ, et al: Wound macrophages express TGF-alpha and other growth factors in vivo: Analysis by mRNA phenotyping. *Science* 1988;241:708–712.
31. Roberts AB, Sporn MB: Transforming growth factor-beta: Potential common mechanisms mediating its effects on embryogenesis, inflammation-repair, and carcinogenesis. *Int J Rad Appl Instrum [B]* 1987;14:435–439.
32. Ross R, Everett NB, Tyler R: Wound healing and collagen formation: VI. The origin of the wound fibroblast studied in parabiosis. *J Cell Biol* 1970;44:645–654.
33. Rutherford RB, Ross R: Platelet factors stimulate fibroblasts and smooth muscle cells quiescent in plasma serum to proliferate. *J Cell Biol* 1976;69:196–203.
34. Samuelsson B: An elucidation of the arachidonic acid cascade: Discovery of prostaglandins, thromboxane and leukotrienes. *Drugs* 1987;33(suppl 1):2–9.
35. Sinzinger H, Kaliman J, Mannheimer E: Effect of leukotrienes C4 and D4 on prostaglandin I2-liberation from human lymphatics. *Lymphology* 1986;19:79–81.
36. Sirois P, Borgeat P: Pharmacologie des leucotrienes [Pharmacology of the leukotrienes]. *J Pharmacol* 1984;15(suppl 1):53–68.
37. Tate GA, Mandell BF, Schumacher HR Jr, et al: Suppression of acute inflammation by 15 methyl prostaglandin E1. *Lab Invest* 1988;59:192–199.
38. Tracy PB: Regulation of thrombin generation at cell surfaces. *Semin Thromb Hemost* 1988;14:227–233.

39. Vane J: The evolution of non-steroidal anti-inflammatory drugs and their mechanisms of action. *Drugs* 1987;33(suppl 1):18–27.
40. Vogel SN, Douches SD, Kaufman EN, et al: Induction of colony stimulating factor in vivo by recombinant interleukin 1 alpha and recombinant tumor necrosis factor alpha 1. *J Immunol* 1987;138:2143–2148.
41. Wahl SM, Wahl LM: Regulation of macrophage collagenase, prostaglandin, and fibroblast-activating-factor production by anti-inflammatory agents: Different regulatory mechanisms for tissue injury and repair. *Cell Immunol* 1985;92:302–312.
42. Weeks JR: Prostaglandins. *Annu Rev Pharmacol* 1972;12:317–336.

Chapter 16

Inflammatory Mechanisms in Soft Tissues

A. Robin Poole, PhD, DSc

Collagens and proteoglycans are major extracellular components of many musculoskeletal tissues. Under some conditions, these proteins or fragments thereof may elicit an inflammatory immune response; thus, a sports injury may lead to disruption of collagens and proteoglycans, triggering an inflammatory process.

Immunology of Fibrillar Collagen Types I, II, and III and Cartilage Proteoglycans

Collagens

Collagen types I and III are confined to musculoskeletal tissues other than cartilage and have a wide distribution. Type I collagen is the major fibrillar collagen of most mature tissues (except cartilage), whereas type III collagen is synthesized in the same tissues as type I collagen but primarily during growth and development, in wound repair, and in inflammation; it is also one of the primary fibrillar collagens of the synovium. Type II collagen is restricted to cartilage and the vitreous of the eye. Normally, these collagens are not recognized by the immune system. When these three collagen types are degraded by collagenase, elastase, or cathepsin G,[79] they unwind at physiologic temperatures. This results in the exposure of epitopes on alpha chains, which are ordinarily masked within the triple helix of the molecule.[2,6,24,99,100] Therefore, when tissue is damaged, collagen is degraded and exposed in a denatured state to the immune system. Thus, the immune response is commonly directed primarily against denatured collagens. Moreover, because some epitopes are shared between different types of collagens,[100] cross-reactions may also occur.

There is also cross-reactivity between polyclonal anticollagen type II antibodies and the complement component C1q, once this collagen-like protein has been subjected to limited proteolysis by bacterial collagenase or by synovial fluid leukocytes from patients with rheumatoid arthritis.[50] Cross-reactivity is observed with C1q from synovial fluids of rheumatoid patients, but not with that from synovial fluids of patients with osteoarthritis and ankylosing spondylitis, unless it is exposed to leukocytes from rheumatoid patients. Also, cellular reactivity (and delayed hypersensitivity) to the collagen-like fragment of C1q is observed in vivo in guinea pigs immunized with native intact (containing the telopeptides) helical human type I collagen.[65] Antibodies are produced that recognize the collagen-like fragment of C1q and native type I collagen. These cross-reactions significantly expand the reactivities of immune cells and antibodies to type I collagen.

Aggregating Cartilage Proteoglycans

Normally these are located primarily in cartilage,[80] although aggregating proteoglycans with core proteins that are related immunologically are present in the sclera, aortic media, central and peripheral nervous system,[19,82] and tendons,[110] which contain aggregating molecules that resemble cartilage. There is no evidence in humans of cellular or humoral immune responses directed against intact or degraded glycosaminoglycan chains. Thus, the immune response is probably directed primarily against the core protein or core protein-associated epitopes, which may involve N- and O-linked oligosaccharides. The hyaluronic acid-binding region contains B-cell epitopes.[97] Putative T-cell epitopes are present throughout the core protein (P. Nyirkos, C. Webber, E. Buzas, and associates, unpublished data). Proteolytic fragments of these proteoglycans are recognized by T cells,[12-14] indicating that fragments of cartilage proteoglycan are immunoreactive when these molecules are degraded during tissue damage.

Immunology of Cartilage

Cartilage is an avascular tissue and, like the cornea, may escape normal immunologic surveillance. Immune-mediated destruction of cartilage allografts is often a slow process. There is evidence of circulating antibodies to chondrocytes in osteoarthritis.[72] Tissue-specific antigens have been recognized on articular chondrocytes.[35,36,38,61] These autoantigens, which may include cell-matrix components such as type II collagen and aggregating proteoglycans, can trigger immune responses if exposed or released as a result of trauma or inflammatory joint disease. Injection of minced rat articular cartilage into homologous rats leads to the development of delayed hypersensitivity.[118] A mixture of antibodies and sensitized cells isolated from these animals is cytotoxic for chondrocytes in vitro. Sera isolated from mice with cartilage proteoglycan-induced arthritis are also cytotoxic for mouse chondrocytes.[67]

Humoral Immune Responses to Collagens and Proteoglycans

Studies in Humans

Circulating antibodies to collagens have been detected in some healthy persons and in increased amounts in persons with rheumatic diseases. With antibodies to collagen types I, II, and III, the immune response is generally directed more to denatured collagens. An example of this was provided by the work of Collier and associates,[18] who observed increased antibodies to types I and II collagens in rheumatoid arthritis. Reactivity with denatured collagens is more pronounced both in normal subjects and in patient groups, particularly with respect to type II collagen. Increased reactivity with denatured collagen types I and II has also been reported by others.[69] Although this has not been reported for type IX collagen, reactivity with denatured collagen type XI was observed in patients with rheumatoid arthritis.

In patients with rheumatoid arthritis, osteoporosis, or Paget's disease (with and without osteoarthritis), and in those with osteoarthritis alone, antibodies to native collagen type II are more common than antibodies to native collagen type I.[15] Also, there is a high frequency of antibodies to cartilage collagen type IX in rheumatoid arthritis. Of all antibodies, those to type XI collagen were observed most often (in almost half of all patient groups). In studies of psoriatic patients with and without arthritis, antibodies to native and denatured collagen types I, II, and III were present in a high proportion of patients with arthritis but not in those without arthritis.[101] Antibodies to native collagen type II have been found in patients with ankylosing spondylitis with peripheral joint involvement.[16] These observations indicate an association of an immune response to cartilage collagens with arthritis involving the appendicular skeleton.

The site of origin of these antibodies in rheumatoid arthritis would appear to be the joint cavity, because antibody titers are higher in synovial fluid than in sera.[93]

These antibodies are usually associated with tissue destruction. In some cases they may precede disease, but antibodies to native collagen type II do not precede the clinical onset of rheumatoid arthritis.[70] They are associated with connective tissue disease that is less severe or of short duration.[15] Hence, these antibodies may ordinarily develop as a result of excessive exposure of collagen antigens to the immune system, particularly in the case of type II collagen, which is normally buried within cartilage. Antibodies to type II collagen develop in patients with otosclerosis and with Menière's disease.[117] These may develop as a result of damage to auditory cartilages and may contribute to the disease process.

It has been reported that there is no significant correlation between HLA-DR4, which is significantly associated with rheumatoid arthritis,[76,91] and the presence of the anticollagen antibodies.[18,114] Others, however, have found that patients positive for HLA-DR4 have significantly greater reactivity to denatured collagen type II than patients who are negative for HLA-DR4.[86] Yet, disease activity in rheumatoid arthritis is not correlated with the titer of anticollagen antibodies.[16,18,101] In other cases in which there is tissue damage, such as to type I collagen in thromboangiitis obliterans (Buerger's disease), antibodies develop to this molecule.[89] Therefore, with the exception of the immune response to cartilage collagen type II, which is correlated with damage to cartilage, humoral immune reactivity to collagens is apparently not specifically associated with any particular type of connective tissue damage in inflammatory and arthritic diseases.

Antibodies to cartilage proteoglycans (which aggregate with hyaluronic acid) have been detected only in patients with rheumatoid arthritis.[37] These findings have not, however, been confirmed, although several studies have been done (A.R. Poole, unpublished data).

Studies in Animals

The value of experimental studies in animals is the ability to investigate the roles of immunologic reactions in and their relationship to development of disease. In the case of antibodies to connective tissue macromolecules such as collagens and proteoglycans, few studies have been done. Purified antibodies to type II collagen can induce transient synovitis and loss of proteoglycan from cartilage.[57,112] Monoclonal mouse antibodies to cartilage proteoglycan can induce in vivo loss of cartilage proteoglycan (E. Dayer, L. Mathai, A.R. Poole, and associates, unpublished data).

Antibodies to homologous collagen types I and II have been found in the sera and the synovial fluids of dogs with spontaneous cruciate ligament rupture and osteoarthritis.[73] Antibodies were more common in dogs with arthritis a few weeks after ligament rupture. As in human studies,[15] these antibodies can develop early in the disease. Antibodies to type II collagen develop in mice with proteoglycan-induced arthritis as a consequence of cartilage damage.[67] Antibodies to homologous mouse cartilage proteoglycans (which aggregate with hyaluronic acid) appear in inflammatory arthritis in mice immunized with human proteoglycan[39,67] and antibodies to rabbit cartilage proteoglycans develop in rabbits immunized with immunoglobulin.[58,116]

Cellular Immune Response to Collagens and Proteoglycans

Studies in Humans

Collagens In studies of patients with rheumatic diseases, cellular immune responses to both helical (native) and denatured collagen types I, II, and III have been observed. As in the case of antibody studies, reactivity is usually much more pronounced against denatured collagen.[43,44,95] The reactions are quantitatively stronger and more common in patients with rheumatoid arthritis than in those with osteoarthritis, gout, or ankylosing spondylitis.[43,44,95] They are seen only occasionally in healthy persons.[43,44,95] Reactivity to type II collagen is again associated with inflammatory erosive arthritis. This also occurs in patients who have psoriasis with arthritis.[101] Selective reactivity to native human collagen type II is observed in osteoarticular disorders that include chondromalacia patellae, articular fracture, sprain, tendinitis, or tendon rupture, and in back pain.[34] Responses to types I and III collagen were not observed nor was an immune response detected in controls.

An immune response to type I collagen has been observed in diseases such as scleroderma in which there is evidence of increased collagen turnover[94] and in thromboangiitis obliterans,[1,89] which is an occlusive arterial disease affecting primarily smaller and medium-sized vessels. An immune response to type III collagen has also been observed.[1]

That a natural cellular immune reaction to these collagens may be genetically restricted is indicated by the observation that in healthy controls it is associated with the HLA antigen DR4, although this correlation was not observed in patients with osteoarticular syndromes.[34]

Proteoglycans A cellular immune response to cartilage proteoglycans has been detected in peripheral blood lymphocytes from patients with erosive joint diseases such as ankylosing spondylitis[44] and rheumatoid arthritis.[37,43,44] Proteoglycan-specific T-helper cells have been isolated as lines and a clone from patients with ankylosing spondylitis.[66] An immune response to proteoglycans may lead to cross-reactivity with proteoglycans in tissues such as the sclera of the eye, in arterial vessels, and in nerves of the central and peripheral nervous systems. Here shared B-cell epitopes have been demonstrated,[19,82] suggesting the presence of shared T-cell epitopes. Scleritis may develop in patients with rheumatoid arthritis as a result of such shared epitopes. A cellular immune response to cartilage proteoglycan is also found in relapsing polychondritis, an erosive disease affecting many cartilages.[51,83]

Studies in Animals

Collagens T-cell-dependent cellular immune responses to types I, II, and III collagens develop in animals with erosive inflammatory arthritis and osteoarthritis.[12–14] Again, the response is directed primarily against denatured collagens, particularly type III collagen, reactions against which are common in human rheumatoid arthritis. Immune responses to denatured collagen type III may be largely caused by the increased synthesis and turnover of this molecule that occurs in inflammation, with exposure of antigenic material in excessive amounts. Immune responses to type III collagen and, to a lesser extent, to type I collagen also develop as a result of surgery alone.[13] Studies have revealed that reactions to degraded rabbit collagen type III can be induced by direct immunization of rabbits. Hence, soft-tissue injury, with or without a significant inflammatory response, may induce an immune response.

Injection of type II collagen induces a cellular immune response with the development of arthritis in some strains of mice, rats, and primates.[81] This shows that the immune response to cartilage collagen type II observed in humans with erosive joint diseases such as rheumatoid arthritis can also produce such joint diseases. Transfer of type

II collagen-specific T-helper cells results in transfer of the chronic disease,[52] which cannot be transferred by means of antibodies to this molecule. Only a transient inflammation develops with antibody transfer. Hence, the importance of the cellular immune response to this molecule is well established in experimental animal studies.

Proteoglycans Experimental damage to articular cartilage caused by intra-articular inflammation[12,14] or joint instability[13] results in the development of a cellular immune response to homologous proteoglycan, which is not observed in healthy rabbits. A cellular reaction to mouse proteoglycan has also been observed in healthy BALB/c mice.[67] Immunization of these mice with heterologous human fetal proteoglycan leads to the development of erosive polyarthritis and spondylitis.[39,67] Thus, individuals with a preexisting reaction to cartilage proteoglycans may develop inflammatory arthritis. Ordinarily, this is not detectable in vivo. The immune response in healthy animals suggests that it may have developed as a result of a cross-reactive response to epitopes shared by bacteria or viruses with proteoglycans. There is one unconfirmed report of an arthritogenic T-lymphocyte clone with an immune response to both cartilage proteoglycan and mycobacterial antigen.[106]

Overview of the Immune Response to Collagen and Proteoglycans and Its Relationship to Disease

From these observations it is clear that an immune response to connective tissue components can be expressed in inflammation and arthritis and after traumatic tissue damage. Such reactions may occur naturally and be present before tissue damage, disease, or inflammation. Expression of such reactions, however, can be shown experimentally to result in diseases such as inflammatory erosive arthritis. Therefore, in soft-tissue injury the development and/or expression of such reactions may cause acute and chronic inflammation mediated primarily by neutrophils and by T-helper cells, respectively. These cellular immune reactions can then activate a number of effector pathways through the generation of cytokines from T lymphocytes and macrophages and monocytes responding to antigen.

Effector Pathways Mediating Inflammation and Tissue Turnover and Their Relationship to the Immune System

Immune responses to antigens and tissue damage caused by traumatic injury and inflammation are normally coordinated carefully and mediated by the actions of specific cells and chemical messengers (cytokines and growth factors) elaborated by them. These messengers are also produced by nonimmune cells, ie, cells other than B cells, monocytes, macrophages, and lymphocytes. Some of the interactions of these messengers and their effects on tissue physiology and turnover (synthesis and degradation) are as follows.

Responses of Tissues to Injury and Homing of Immune Effector Cells to Sites of Inflammation and Tissue Damage

The concentration of lymphocytes, neutrophils, monocytes, and macrophages at sites of tissue damage involves new blood vessel formation (angiogenesis), chemoattraction of cells, adherence to endothelial cells of vessels, and emigration into extravascular sites.

Angiogenesis

The growth of new capillary vessels is an essential part of the inflammatory response to wounding and wound repair. It provides a mechanism whereby cells that are concerned both with the expression of the immune response and with tissue repair can be brought to damaged or infected sites. It ensures the continuing nutrition of damaged tissue and effective repair.

Five structurally related peptides have been shown to be angiogenic, including fibroblast growth factors (acidic and basic),[96] angiogenin,[29] transforming growth factor alpha (TGF-α),[88] and transforming growth factor beta (TGF-β).[84] Tumor necrosis factor alpha (TNF-α)[31,60] is produced by activated macrophages. For a general review of angiogenic molecules, see Folkman and Klagsbrun.[30] Angiogenesis involves endothelial cell proliferation and migration and the secretion of proteinases by these cells. These include plasminogen activators[46,77] and latent collagenase,[46] which is activated by plasminogen activators. Procollagenase is also activated by a very small angiogenic factor.[113]

Homing of Neutrophils, Monocytes, and Lymphocytes and Adhesion to Endothelia

The regular trafficking of B and T lymphocytes is a normal feature of the expression of immunity. When tissues are damaged, signals are released that attract immune cells and stem cells to the tissues from which these signals originate. Interferon gamma, which is synthesized primarily by T cells in response to antigenic stimulation, promotes the adherence of T lymphocytes to endothelial cells.[119]

When synovial cells, fibroblasts, monocytes, and endothelial cells are activated by interleukin-1 and TNF-α they generate a 7-kd molecule (interleukin-8) that is a neutrophil chemotactic factor.[42,63,92] This molecule is also chemotactic for lymphocytes.[59] The chemoattractant activity of interleukin-1 appears to be the result of the activity of this molecule. As part of the response, the adhesion of monocytes,[7] lymphocytes,[11] and neutrophils[7,32] to endothelial cells is also increased by interleukin-1 and by TNF-α.[78] A monocyte-specific chemotactic factor of approximately 15 kd has also been identified.[62,85] TNF-α, also known as cachectin, induces the release of interleukin-1 by endothelial cells.[71] The adhesion of neutrophils to endothelial cells is inhibited by TGF-β; it also decreases the increased adhesion of neutrophils to endothelial cells induced by TNF-α.[33]

Effects of Cytokines and Growth Factors Produced in Injury and Inflammation on Connective Tissue Cells

Interleukin-1 Interleukin-1α and -1β are pivotal cytokines in the regulation of cellular activity. They are produced by a wide variety of cells, including neutrophils,[98] chondrocytes,[74] synovial cells,[22] and fibroblasts. They are also produced by monocytes, macrophages, and B cells as part of the immune recognition of antigen involving presentation of antigens by these cells to receptors on T lymphocytes. Interleukin-1 can dramatically influence the activities of a variety of cell types. It can stimulate the synthesis and secretion of the proteinases collagenase, stromelysin, and plasminogen activator by synovial cells, chondrocytes, and fibroblasts, and cause cartilage matrix destruction.[22,79,104] At the same time, it can arrest or down regulate the synthesis of cartilage collagens types II and IX[40,105] and proteoglycans.[103] Collagen synthesis by synovial cells is inhibited by interleukin-1,[64] affecting primarily type I, rather than type III, synthesis. Type I collagen (mRNA) is increased, indicating an effect on transcription. This inhibitory effect on synthesis is mediated by prostaglandin E_2. Also, interleukin-1 stimulates an increase in mRNA for the small dermatan sulfate proteoglycan made by skin fibroblasts[49] but without any detectable increase in secretion. Gingival fibroblasts synthesize increased amounts of sulfated proteoglycans in the presence of interleukin-1. Proliferation of these cells and skin fibroblasts is also stimulated.[5] Rates of proteoglycan degradation are unchanged. The synthesis of hyaluronic acid by synovial cells is also stimulated by interleukin-1.[47,115] Its synthesis by fetal tissue and its production in tissue repair are considered to be essential for the formation of new tissues.

Stimulation of plasminogen activator secretion in synovial cells also depends on prostaglandin E_2 synthesis.[68] The production of interleukin-1 by other cells can be induced by other mediators.

TNF-α TNF-α induces interleukin-1 production in vivo in rabbits, as does interferon gamma.[23] Their effects are synergistic. Interleukin-1 and prostaglandin E_2 production are stimulated by TNF-α in macrophages[4] and interleukin-1 production by endothelial cells is induced by TNF-α.[71]

Like interleukin-1, TNF-α can stimulate cartilage degradation mediated by chondrocytes,[87] and, also like interleukin-1, it inhibits proteoglycan synthesis. It stimulates an increased synthesis and secretion of collagenase and prostaglandin E_2 by synovial cells and dermal fibroblasts.[21] TNF-α inhibits the transcription and synthesis of type I collagen by fibroblasts[90] but stimulates fibroblastic proliferation.[109]

Interferon Gamma Interferon gamma enhances macrophage transcription of TNF-α, interleukin-1, and urokinase-like plasminogen activator genes[8,17,48] and blocks interleukin-1-induced prostaglandin release by monocytes.[8,10]

Interferon gamma stimulates synovial cell proliferation,[9] although inhibition of proliferation of dermal fibroblasts has been reported.[25]

Workers are agreed, however, that it dramatically inhibits types I and III collagen and fibronectin synthesis by synovial cells in vitro[3] and collagen synthesis in vivo.[45] It reduces types I and III collagen mRNA in dermal fibroblasts but in these cells it increases mRNA for fibronectin.[20] Transcriptional rates are unaffected for the collagens, but enhanced for fibronectin. Thus, the effects are at both posttranscriptional and transcriptional levels and vary among cells.

In scleroderma, collagen synthesis is excessive. Interferon gamma has a lasting inhibitory effect on collagen synthesis in normal fibroblasts and particularly in sclerodermal fibroblasts.[26] Hence, interferon gamma may be of use in the treatment of fibrosis. Type II collagen synthesis is also inhibited by interferon gamma with a suppression of transcription.[41] Angiogenesis is inhibited.[102] Interferon gamma induces the appearance of Ia antigens on synovial cells[3] and chondrocytes,[41,54] promoting immune responses. Hence, its increased production at sites of immune responses may inhibit tissue repair.

TGF-β This factor is produced by many cell types. In contrast to TNF, interleukin-1, and interferon gamma, TGF-β stimulates matrix synthesis, rapidly inducing fibrosis in vivo[84] through induction of collagen formation in fibroblasts, which can be detected in vitro.[84,107] It persistently increases production of types I and III collagen and fibronectin mRNAs.[53,108] This stimulation is associated with increased synthesis and secretion of the tissue inhibitor of the metalloproteinases (TIMP) but decreased production of the proenzymes collagenase and stromelysin.[27,75] Hence, it protects against tissue destruction. TGF-β also acts as a chemoattractant for monocytes, induces the production of a fibroblast growth factor,[111] and is a potent inhibitor of interleukin-1-induced B and T lymphocyte proliferation.[28,55,56] Thus, in contrast to interferon gamma, TGF-β appears to inhibit the immune response at the level of clonal expansion and to promote tissue repair.

References

1. Adar R, Papa MZ, Halpern Z, et al: Cellular sensitivity to collagen in thromboangiitis obliterans. *N Engl J Med* 1983;308:1113–1116.
2. Adelmann BC, Kirrane J: The structural basis of cell-mediated immunological reactions of collagen: The species specificity of the cutaneous delayed hypersensitivity reaction. *Immunology* 1973;25:123–130.
3. Amento EP, Bhan AK, McCullagh KG, et al: Influences of gamma interferon on synovial fibroblast-like cells: I. Induction and inhibition of collagen synthesis. *J Clin Invest* 1985;76:837–848.
4. Bachwich PR, Chensue SW, Larrick JW, et al: Tumor necrosis factor stimulates interleukin-1 and prostaglandin E_2 production in resting macrophages. *Biochem Biophys Res Commun* 1986;136:94–101.
5. Bartold PM: The effect of interleukin 1β on proteoglycans synthesized by human gingival fibroblasts *in vitro*. *Connect Tissue Res* 1988;17:287–304.
6. Beil W, Timpl R, Furthmayr H: Conformation dependence of antigenic determinants on the collagen molecule. *Immunology* 1973;24:13–24.

7. Bevilacqua MP, Pober JS, Wheeler ME, et al: Interleukin 1 acts on cultured human vascular endothelium to increase the adhesion of polymorphonuclear leukocytes, monocytes, and related leukocyte cell lines. *J Clin Invest* 1985;76:2003–2011.
8. Boraschi D, Censini S, Tagliabue A: Interferon-γ reduces macrophage-suppressive activity by inhibiting prostaglandin E_2 release and inducing interleukin 1 production. *J Immunol* 1984;133:764–768.
9. Brinckerhoff CE, Guyre PM: Increased proliferation of human synovial fibroblasts treated with recombinant immune interferon. *J Immunol* 1985;134:3142–3146.
10. Browning JL, Ribolini A: Interferon blocks interleukin 1-induced prostaglandin release from human peripheral monocytes. *J Immunol* 1987;138:2857–2863.
11. Cavender DE, Haskard DO, Joseph B, et al: Interleukin 1 increases the binding of human B and T lymphocytes to endothelial cell monolayers. *J Immunol* 1986;136:203–207.
12. Champion BR, Poole AR: Immunity to homologous cartilage proteoglycans in rabbits with chronic inflammatory arthritis. *Collagen Relat Res* 1981;1:453–473.
13. Champion BR, Poole AR: Immunity to homologous type III collagen after partial meniscectomy and sham surgery in rabbits. *Arthritis Rheum* 1982;25:274–287.
14. Champion BR, Sell S, Poole AR: Immunity to homologous collagens and cartilage proteoglycans in rabbits. *Immunology* 1983;48:605–616.
15. Charrière G, Hartmann DJ, Vignon E, et al: Antibodies to types I, II, IX, and XI collagen in the serum of patients with rheumatic diseases. *Arthritis Rheum* 1988;31:325–332.
16. Clague RB, Shaw MJ, Holt PJ: Incidence of serum antibodies to native type I and type II collagens in patients with inflammatory arthritis. *Ann Rheum Dis* 1980;39:201–206.
17. Collart MA, Belin D, Vassalli JD, et al: γ-Interferon enhances macrophage transcription of the tumor necrosis factor/cachectin, interleukin 1, and urokinase genes, which are controlled by short-lived repressors. *J Exp Med* 1986;164:2113–2118.
18. Collier DH, Kerwar SS, Garovoy MR, et al: Anticollagen antibodies and immune response gene products in rheumatoid arthritis. *Arthritis Rheum* 1984;27:1201–1209.
19. Cöster L, Rosenberg LC, van der Rest M, et al: The dermatan sulfate proteoglycans of bovine sclera and their relationship to those of articular cartilage: An immunological and biochemical study. *J Biol Chem* 1987;262:3809–3812.
20. Czaja MJ, Weiner FR, Eghbali M, et al: Differential effects of γ-interferon on collagen and fibronectin gene expression. *J Biol Chem* 1987;262:13348–13351.
21. Dayer JM, Beutler B, Cerami A: Cachectin/tumor necrosis factor stimulates collagenase and prostaglandin E_2 production by human synovial cells and dermal fibroblasts. *J Exp Med* 1985;162:2163–2168.
22. Dayer JM, Bréard J, Chess L, et al: Participation of monocyte-macrophages and lymphocytes in the production of a factor that stimulates collagenase and prostaglandin release by rheumatoid synovial cells. *J Clin Invest* 1979;64:1386–1392.
23. Dinarello CA, Cannon JG, Wolff SM, et al: Tumor necrosis factor (cachectin) is an endogenous pyrogen and induces production of interleukin 1. *J Exp Med* 1986;163:1433–1450.
24. Dodge GR, Poole AR: Immunohistochemical detection and immunochemical analysis of type II collagen degradation in human normal, rheumatoid and osteoarthritic articular cartilages and in explants of bovine articular cartilage cultured with interleukin-1. *J Clin Invest* 1989;83:647–661.

25. Duncan MR, Berman B: γ-Interferon is the lymphokine and β-interferon the monokine responsible for inhibition of fibroblast collagen production and late but not early fibroblast proliferation. *J Exp Med* 1985;162:516–527.
26. Duncan MR, Berman B: Persistence of a reduced collagen-producing phenotype in cultured scleroderma fibroblasts after short-term exposure to interferons. *J Clin Invest* 1987;79:1318–1324.
27. Edwards DR, Murphy G, Reynolds JJ, et al: Transforming growth factor beta modulates the expression of collagenase and metalloproteinase inhibitor. *EMBO J* 1987;6:1899–1904.
28. Ellingsworth LR, Nakayama D, Segarini P, et al: Transforming growth factor-βs are equipotent growth inhibitors of interleukin-1-induced thymocyte proliferation. *Cell Immunol* 1988;114:41–54.
29. Fett JW, Strydom DJ, Lobb RR, et al: Isolation and characterization of angiogenin, an angiogenic protein from human carcinoma cells. *Biochemistry* 1985;24:5480–5486.
30. Folkman J, Klagsbrun M: A family of angiogenic peptides. *Science* 1987;329:671–672.
31. Fràter-Schröder M, Risau W, Hallmann R, et al: Tumor necrosis factor type α, a potent inhibitor of endothelial cell growth in vitro, is angiogenic in vivo. *Proc Natl Acad Sci USA* 1987;84:5277–5281.
32. Gamble JR, Harlan JM, Klebanoff SJ, et al: Stimulation of the adherence of neutrophils to umbilical vein endothelium by human recombinant tumor necrosis factor. *Proc Natl Acad Sci USA* 1985;82:8667–8671.
33. Gamble JR, Vadas MA: Endothelial adhesiveness for blood neutrophils is inhibited by transforming growth factor-β. *Science* 1988;242:97–99.
34. Garbrecht FC, Ragsdale CG, Schultz JS, et al: Autoimmunity to articular collagen in patients with osteoarticular syndromes. *J Rheumatol* 1986;13:517–521.
35. Gertzbein SD, Lance EM: The stimulation of lymphocytes by chondrocytes in mixed cultures. *Clin Exp Immunol* 1976;24:102–109.
36. Gertzbein SD, Tait JH, Devlin SR, et al: The antigenicity of chondrocytes. *Immunology* 1977;33:141–145.
37. Glant T, Csongar J, Szücs T: Immunopathologic role of proteoglycan antigens in rheumatoid joint disease. *Scand J Rheumatol* 1980;11:247–252.
38. Glant T, Mikecz K: Antigenic profiles of human, bovine and canine articular chondrocytes. *Cell Tissue Res* 1986;244:359–369.
39. Glant TT, Mikecz K, Arzoumanian A, et al: Proteoglycan-induced arthritis in BALB/c mice: Clinical features and histopathology. *Arthritis Rheum* 1987;30:201–212.
40. Goldring MB, Birkhead J, Sandell LJ, et al: Interleukin-1 suppresses expression of cartilage-specific types II and IX collagens and increases types I and III collagens in human chondrocytes. *J Clin Invest* 1988;82:2026–2037.
41. Goldring MB, Sandell LJ, Stephenson ML, et al: Immune interferon suppresses levels of procollagen mRNA and type II collagen synthesis in cultured human articular and costal chondrocytes. *J Biol Chem* 1986;261:9049–9055.
42. Golds EE, Mason P, Nyirkos P: Inflammatory cytokines induce synthesis and secretion of *GRO* protein and a neutrophil chemotactic factor but not β2-microglobulin in human synovial cells and fibroblasts. *Biochem J* 1989;259:585–588.
43. Golds EE, Poole AR: Connective tissue antigens stimulate collagenase production in arthritic diseases. *Cell Immunol* 1984;86:190–205.
44. Golds EE, Stephen IB, Esdaile JM, et al: Lymphocyte transformation to connective tissue antigens in adult and juvenile rheumatoid arthritis, osteoarthritis, ankylosing spondylitis, systemic lupus erythematosus, and a nonarthritic control population. *Cell Immunol* 1983;82:196–209.

45. Granstein RD, Murphy GF, Margolis RJ, et al: Gamma-interferon inhibits collagen synthesis in vivo in the mouse. *J Clin Invest* 1987;79:1254–1258.

46. Gross JL, Moscatelli D, Rifkin DB: Increased capillary endothelial cell protease activity in response to angiogenic stimuli in vitro. *Proc Natl Acad Sci USA* 1983;80:2623–2627.

47. Hamerman D, Wood DD: Interleukin 1 enhances synovial cell hyaluronate synthesis. *Proc Soc Exp Biol Med* 1984;177:205–210.

48. Haq AU, Rinehart JJ, Maca RD: The effect of gamma interferon on IL-1 secretion of in vitro differentiated human macrophages. *J Leukocyte Biol* 1985;38:735–746.

49. Heino J, Kahari VM, Mauviel A, et al: Human recombinant interleukin 1 regulates cellular mRNA levels of dermatan sulphate proteoglycan core protein. *Biochem J* 1988;252:309–312.

50. Heinz HP, Brackertz D, Loos M: Enzymatic alteration of C1q, the collagen-like subcomponent of the first component of complement, leads to cross-reactivity with type II collagen. *FEBS Lett* 1988;228:332–336.

51. Herman JH, Dennis MV: Immunopathologic studies in relapsing polychondritis. *J Clin Invest* 1973;52:549–558.

52. Holmdahl R, Klareskog L, Rubin K, et al: T lymphocytes in collagen II-induced arthritis in mice: Characterization of arthritogenic collagen II-specific T-cell lines and clones. *Scand J Immunol* 1985;22:295–306.

53. Ignotz RA, Endo T, Massagué J: Regulation of fibronectin and type I collagen mRNA levels by transforming growth factor β. *J Biol Chem* 1987;262:6443–6446.

54. Jahn B, Burmester GR, Schmid H, et al: Changes in cell surface antigen expression on human articular chondrocytes induced by gamma-interferon: Induction of Ia antigens. *Arthritis Rheum* 1987;30:64–74.

55. Kehrl JH, Roberts AB, Wakefield LM, et al: Transforming growth factor β is an important immunomodulatory protein for human B lymphocytes. *J Immunol* 1986;137:3855–3860.

56. Kehrl JH, Wakefield LM, Roberts AB, et al: Production of transforming growth factor β by human T lymphocytes and its potential role in the regulation of T cell growth. *J Exp Med* 1986;163:1037–1050.

57. Kerwar SS, Englert ME, McReynolds RA, et al: Type II collagen-induced arthritis: Studies with purified anticollagen immunoglobulin. *Arthritis Rheum* 1983;26:1120–1131.

58. Kresina TF, Yoo JU, Goldberg VM: Evidence that a humoral immune response to autologous cartilage proteoglycan can participate in the induction of cartilage pathology. *Arthritis Rheum* 1988;31:248–257.

59. Larsen CG, Anderson AO, Appela E, et al: The neutrophil-activating protein (NAP-1) is also chemotactic for T lymphocytes. *Science* 1989;243:1464–1466.

60. Leibovich SJ, Polverini PJ, Shepard HM, et al: Macrophage-induced angiogenesis is mediated by tumour necrosis factor-α. *Nature* 1987;329:630–632.

61. Malseed ZM, Heyner S: Antigenic profile of the rat chondrocyte. *Arthritis Rheum* 1976;19:223–231.

62. Matsushima K, Larsen CG, DuBois CG, et al: Purification and characterization of a novel monocyte chemotactic and activating factor produced by a human myelomonocytic cell line. *J Exp Med* 1989;169:1485–1490.

63. Matsushima K, Morishita K, Yoshimura T, et al: Molecular cloning of a human monocyte-derived neutrophil chemotactic factor (MDNCF) and the induction of MDNCF mRNA by interleukin 1 and tumor necrosis factor. *J Exp Med* 1988;167:1883–1893.

64. Mauviel A, Teyton L, Bhatnagar R, et al: Interleukin-1α modulates collagen gene expression in cultured synovial cells. *Biochem J* 1988;252:247–255.
65. Menzel EJ, Smolen JS, Reid KB: Immunological cross-reactivity between the collagen-like fragment of human C1q and human type I collagen. *Mol Immunol* 1981;18:765–771.
66. Mikecz K, Glant TT, Baron M, et al: Isolation of proteoglycan-specific T lymphocytes from patients with ankylosing spondylitis. *Cell Immunol* 1988;112:55–63.
67. Mikecz K, Glant TT, Poole AR: Immunity to cartilage proteoglycans in BALB/c mice with progressive polyarthritis and ankylosing spondylitis induced by injection of human cartilage proteoglycan. *Arthritis Rheum* 1987;30:306-318.
68. Mochan E, Uhl J, Newton R: Evidence that interleukin-1 induction of synovial cell plasminogen activator is mediated via prostaglandin E_2 and cAMP. *Arthritis Rheum* 1986;29:1078–1084.
69. Morgan K, Clague RB, Collins I, et al: Incidence of antibodies to native and denatured cartilage collagens (types II, IX, and XI) and to type I collagen in rheumatoid arthritis. *Ann Rheum Dis* 1987;46:902–907.
70. Möttönen T, Hannonen P, Oka M, et al: Antibodies against native type II collagen do not precede the clinical onset of rheumatoid arthritis. *Arthritis Rheum* 1988;31:776–779.
71. Nawroth PP, Bank I, Handley D, et al: Tumor necrosis factor/cachectin interacts with endothelial cell receptors to induce release of interleukin 1. *J Exp Med* 1986;163:1363–1375.
72. Németh-Csóka M, Paroczai C, Mészáros T: The clinical diagnostic significance of serum antichondrocyte membrane antibodies in osteoarthritis. *Agents Actions* 1988;23:50–51.
73. Niebauer GW, Wolf B, Bashey RI, et al: Antibodies to canine collagen types I and II in dogs with spontaneous cruciate ligament rupture and osteoarthritis. *Arthritis Rheum* 1987;30:319–327.
74. Ollivierre F, Gubler U, Towle CA, et al: Expression of IL-1 genes in human and bovine chondrocytes: A mechanism for autocrine control of cartilage matrix degradation. *Biochem Biophys Res Commun* 1986;141:904–911.
75. Overall CM, Wrana JL, Sodek J: Independent regulation of collagenase, 72 KD progelatinase, and metalloproteinase inhibitor expression in human fibroblasts by transforming growth factor-β. *J Biol Chem* 1989;264:1860–1869.
76. Panayi GS, Wooley P, Batchelor JR: Genetic basis of rheumatoid disease: HLA antigens, disease manifestations, and toxic reactions to drugs. *Br Med J* 1978;2:1326–1328.
77. Pepper MS, Vassalli JD, Montesano R, et al: Urokinase-type plasminogen activator is induced in migrating capillary endothelial cells. *J Cell Biol* 1987;105:2535–2541.
78. Pober JS, Bevilacqua MP, Mendrick DL, et al: Two distinct monokines, interleukin 1 and tumor necrosis factor, each independently induce biosynthesis and transient expression of the same antigen on the surface of cultured human vascular endothelial cells. *J Immunol* 1986;136:1680–1687.
79. Poole AR: Changes in the collagen and proteoglycan of articular cartilage in arthritis. *Rheumatology* 1986;10:316–371.
80. Poole AR: Proteoglycans in health and disease: Structures and functions. *Biochem J* 1986;236:1–14.
81. Poole AR, Glant TT, Mikecz K: Autoimmunity to cartilage collagen and proteoglycan and the development of chronic inflammatory arthritis, in Glauert AM (ed): *The Control of Tissue Damage*. Amsterdam, Elsevier, 1988, pp 55–65.

82. Poole AR, Pidoux I, Reiner A, et al: Mammalian eyes and associated tissues contain molecules that are immunologically related to cartilage proteoglycan and link protein. *J Cell Biol* 1982;93:910–920.
83. Rajapakse D, Bywaters E: Cell-mediated immunity to cartilage proteoglycans in relapsing polychondritis. *Clin Exp Immunol* 1974;16:497–502.
84. Roberts AB, Sporn MB, Assoian RK, et al: Transforming growth factor type β: Rapid induction of fibrosis and angiogenesis in vivo and stimulation of collagen formation in vitro. *Proc Natl Acad Sci USA* 1986;83:4167–4171.
85. Robinson EA, Yoshimura T, Leonard EJ, et al: Complete amino acid sequence of a human monocyte chemoattractant, a putative mediator of cellular immunoreactions. *Proc Natl Acad Sci USA* 1989;86:1850–1854.
86. Rowley M, Tait B, Mackay IR, et al: Collagen antibodies in rheumatoid arthritis: Significance of antibodies to denatured collagen and their association with HLA-DR4. *Arthritis Rheum* 1986;29:174–184.
87. Saklatvala J: Tumour necrosis factor α stimulates resorption and inhibits synthesis of proteoglycan in cartilage. *Nature* 1986;322:547–549.
88. Schreiber AB, Winkler ME, Derynck R: Transforming growth factor-α: A more potent angiogenic mediator than epidermal growth factor. *Science* 1986;232:1250–1253.
89. Smolen JS, Youngchaiyud U, Weidinger P, et al: Autoimmunological aspects of thromboangiitis obliterans (Buerger's disease). *Clin Immunol Immunopathol* 1978;11:168–177.
90. Solis-Herruzo JA, Brenner DA, Chojkier M: Tumor necrosis factor-α inhibits collagen gene transcription and collagen synthesis in cultured human fibroblasts. *J Biol Chem* 1988;263:5841–5845.
91. Stastny P: Association of the B-cell alloantigen DRw4 with rheumatoid arthritis. *N Engl J Med* 1978;298:869–871.
92. Strieter RM, Kunkel SL, Showell HJ, et al: Endothelial cell gene expression of a neutrophil chemotactic factor by TNF-α, LPS, and IL-1β. *Science* 1989;243:1467–1469.
93. Stuart JM, Huffstutter EH, Townes AS, et al: Incidence and specificity of antibodies to types I, II, III, IV, and V collagen in rheumatoid arthritis and other rheumatic diseases as measured by ^{125}I-radioimmunoassay. *Arthritis Rheum* 1983;26:832–840.
94. Stuart JM, Postlethwaite AE, Kang AH: Evidence for cell-mediated immunity to collagen in progressive systemic sclerosis. *J Lab Clin Med* 1976;88:601–607.
95. Stuart JM, Postlethwaite AE, Townes AS, et al: Cell-mediated immunity to collagen and collagen α chains in rheumatoid arthritis and other rheumatic diseases. *Am J Med* 1980;69:13–18.
96. Thomas KA, Rios-Candelore M, Giménez-Gallego G, et al: Pure brain-derived acidic fibroblast growth factor is a potent angiogenic vascular endothelial cell mitogen with sequence homology to interleukin 1. *Proc Natl Acad Sci USA* 1985;82:6409–6413.
97. Thonar EJ, Kimura JH, Hascall VC, et al: Enzyme-linked immunosorbent assay analyses of the hyaluronate-binding region and the link protein of proteoglycan aggregate. *J Biol Chem* 1982;257:14173–14180.
98. Tiku K, Tiku ML, Skosey JC: Interleukin 1 production by human polymorphonuclear neutrophils. *J Immunol* 1986;136:3677–3685.
99. Timpl R: Immunological studies on collagen, in Ramachandran GN, Reddi AH (eds): *Biochemistry of Collagen*. New York, Plenum Press, 1976, pp 319–375.
100. Timpl R: Immunology of the collagens, in Piez KA, Reddi AH (eds): *Extracellular Matrix Biochemistry*. New York, Elsevier, 1984, pp 159–190.

101. Trentham DE, Kammer GM, McCune WJ, et al: Autoimmunity to collagen: A shared feature of psoriatic and rheumatoid arthritis. *Arthritis Rheum* 1981;24:1363–1369.
102. Tsuruoka N, Sugiyama M, Tawaragi Y, et al: Inhibition of in vitro angiogenesis by lymphotoxin and interferon-γ. *Biochem Biophys Res Commun* 1988;155:429–435.
103. Tyler JA: Articular cartilage cultured with catabolin (pig interleukin 1) synthesizes a decreased number of normal proteoglycan molecules. *Biochem J* 1985;227:869–878.
104. Tyler JA: Chondrocyte-mediated depletion of articular cartilage proteoglycans in vitro. *Biochem J* 1985;225:493–507.
105. Tyler JA, Benton HP: Synthesis of type II collagen is decreased in cartilage cultured with interleukin 1 while the rate of intracellular degradation remains unchanged. *Collagen Relat Res* 1988;8:393–405.
106. van Eden W, Holoshitz J, Nevo Z, et al: Arthritis induced by a T-lymphocyte clone that responds to *Mycobacterium tuberculosis* and to cartilage proteoglycans. *Proc Natl Acad Sci USA* 1985;82:5117–5120.
107. Varga J, Jimenez SA: Stimulation of normal human fibroblast collagen production and processing by transforming growth factor-β. *Biochem Biophys Res Commun* 1986;138:974–980.
108. Varga J, Rosenbloom J, Jimenez SA: Transforming growth factor-β (TGF-β) causes a persistent increase in steady-state amounts of type I and type III collagen and fibronectin mRNAs in normal human dermal fibroblasts. *Biochem J* 1987;247:597–604.
109. Vilček J, Palombella VJ, Henriksen-DeStefano D, et al: Fibroblast growth enhancing activity of tumor necrosis factor and its relationship to other polypeptide growth factors. *J Exp Med* 1986;163:632–643.
110. Vogel KG, Heinegård D: Characterization of proteoglycans from adult bovine tendon. *J Biol Chem* 1985;260:9298–9306.
111. Wahl SM, Hunt DA, Wakefield LM, et al: Transforming growth factor type β induces monocyte chemotaxis and growth factor production. *Proc Natl Acad Sci USA* 1987;84:5788–5792.
112. Watson WC, Brown PS, Pitcock JA, et al: Passive transfer studies with type II collagen antibody in B10.D2/old and new line and C57B1/6 normal and beige (Chediak-Higashi) strains: Evidence of important roles for C5 and multiple inflammatory cell types in the development of erosive arthritis. *Arthritis Rheum* 1987;30:460–465.
113. Weiss JB, Hill CR, Davis RJ, et al: Activation of a procollagenase by low-molecular-weight angiogenesis factor. *Biosci Rep* 1983;3:171–177.
114. Wooley PH, Luthra HS, O'Duffy JD, et al: Anti-type II collagen antibodies in rheumatoid arthritis: The influence of HLA phenotype. *Tissue Antigens* 1984;23:263–269.
115. Yaron I, Meyer FA, Dayer JM, et al: Human recombinant interleukin-1β stimulates glycosaminoglycan production in human synovial fibroblast cultures. *Arthritis Rheum* 1987;30:424–430.
116. Yoo JU, Kresina TF, Malemud CJ, et al: Epitopes of proteoglycans eliciting an anti-proteoglycan response in chronic immune synovitis. *Proc Natl Acad Sci USA* 1987;84:832–836.
117. Yoo TJ, Stuart JM, Kang AH, et al: Type II collagen autoimmunity in otosclerosis and Menière's disease. *Science* 1982;217:1153–1155.
118. Yoshioka Y, Tsuru S, Yokoyama M, et al: Experimental study on immunological reactions against the articular cartilage. *Int Arch Allergy Appl Immunol* 1982;68:152–156.
119. Yu CL, Haskard DO, Cavender D, et al: Human γ-interferon increases the binding of T lymphocytes to endothelial cells. *Clin Exp Immunol* 1985;62:554–560.

Chapter 17

Platelet-Derived Growth Factor and Transforming Growth Factor Beta in Wound Healing and Repair

Ronald L. Wilder, MD, PhD
Robert Lafyatis, MD
Elaine F. Remmers, PhD

Introduction

Although the cellular events involved in the healing and repair of musculoskeletal connective tissue injuries are reasonably well described, the molecular mechanisms regulating these responses are incompletely understood. New information, particularly on the roles of various cytokines and growth factors in inflammation and wound healing, however, is continually being published. This information may ultimately have far-reaching therapeutic implications.

We describe two polypeptide growth factors that appear to play important but apparently antagonistic roles in inflammatory and wound healing processes—platelet-derived growth factor (PDGF)[5,20,50,51] and transforming growth factor beta (TGF-β).[47,54] Other cytokines and growth factors are also involved in these biologic processes, but they are discussed only incidentally. They include, for example, interleukin-1, tumor necrosis factor, transforming growth factor alpha, epidermal growth factor, heparin-binding growth factors (fibroblast and endothelial cell growth factors), interferons, and insulin and insulin-like growth factors.

Platelet-Derived Growth Factor

Biochemistry

PDGF represents a family of related polypeptides that play a fundamental role in inflammation, neoplasia, and embryogenesis, as well as in wound healing.[5,20,50,51] It is likely that agents of this type affect the response of musculoskeletal tissues to sports-induced injury. It is now recognized that PDGF consists of two polypeptide chains with about 60% amino acid homology: A chains, which exist in two forms as a result of alternative splicing of RNA transcripts,[6,49,58] and B chains, which are 96% homologous to the transforming gene of simian sarcoma virus, v-*sis*. These chains form either homodimers or heterodimers.

Thus, at least three functional isoforms, AB, BB, and AA, exist. Although the isoforms are functionally similar, their potency and effects on various cell populations may differ. All have molecular weights of about 30,000.

Cell and Tissue Sources

PDGF was so named because it was originally isolated from human platelets. Human platelets contain predominantly the AB heterodimeric isoform, whereas porcine platelets contain predominantly the BB homodimeric isoform. PDGF production has since been demonstrated in endothelial cells, activated macrophages, and even fibroblasts, all of which participate in inflammation and wound healing. Other sources of PDGF include smooth muscle cells, megakaryocytes, embryonic blastocysts, and placental cytotrophoblasts. Many tumor cell lines also produce PDGF. Nonplatelet sources may produce isoforms of PDGF other than the AB heterodimer.[51]

Regulation of Production and Release

PDGF is stored in alpha-granules of platelets, and its release is stimulated by platelet aggregation, an early event during inflammation and wound healing. Its production and secretion by other cell types is initiated by a variety of stimuli,[51] many of which may be pertinent to wound healing processes. For example, in endothelial cells, thrombin increases steady state levels of A- and B-chain mRNA, increases B- but not A-chain transcription, and stimulates release of PDGF-like protein activity. Treatment of endothelial cells with phorbol esters, which activate protein kinase C, also stimulates production and release of PDGF in a similar manner. TGF-β stimulates A- and B-chain mRNA levels, increases both A and B transcription rates and stimulates release of PDGF-like activity. Interleukin-1 and tumor necrosis factor alpha both stimulate PDGF-like activity. In contrast to these stimulatory events, treatment of endothelial cells with forskolin or other agents that elevate intracellular cAMP blocks stimulation by all these agents except TGF-β. Similarly, acetyl low-density lipoproteins depress production of PDGF-like activity. Thus, both stimulatory and inhibitory pathways of PDGF production have been identified in endothelial cells.[8,9,15,17,24,56]

Several types of fibroblasts have been shown to produce A-chain mRNA and AA homodimeric PDGF when treated with endothelial growth factors, interleukin-1, and PDGF itself. Because fibroblasts, in contrast to endothelial cells, express PDGF receptors, this autocrine pathway for PDGF production is potentially important in the amplification of paracrine growth factor stimulation of fibroblasts.[41,45] Fibroblastoid cell PDGF B-chain production, to our knowledge, has been reported only for mouse embryo AKR-2B cells.[29]

The regulation of PDGF production by monocytes and macrophages is complex. Production of PDGF varies with the source of the macrophages, their differentiation state and type, and the nature of the stimulatory or differentiation signal. Much of the published work has been done on leukemic cell lines with monocytic characteristics,[1,34,40] which may not be relevant to wound macrophages. Nevertheless, it appears that controlling macrophage PDGF production is important for modulating the wound-healing process.

An important point of additional interest is that wound healing and embryogenesis have much in common. It is particularly pertinent that the production of PDGF-like activity appears to be developmentally regulated. For example, less B-chain mRNA and PDGF-like activity is released by aortic smooth muscle cells from adult rats than by smooth muscle cells from newborn rats. By contrast, A-chain mRNA expression is the same.[33] Thus, differential regulation of production of A- and B-chain PDGF probably has important physiologic functions.

Receptors

For PDGF to have an effect on a target cell, expression of high-affinity receptors, which specifically bind PDGF, is required. PDGF receptors have been identified on connective tissue cells throughout the body, including dermal, tendon, synovial, and other types of fibroblasts, vascular smooth muscle cells, glial cells, and chondrocytes. Endothelial cells lack PDGF receptors. At least two different receptors have been identified, initially on the basis of their differential ability to bind different isoforms of PDGF. Two genes were subsequently cloned. The type a PDGF receptor binds all three isoforms of PDGF, whereas the type b PDGF receptor binds only AB and BB isoforms. It is presumed that differential expression of the various isoforms of PDGF and their receptors provides wide latitude for modulating receptor-bearing target cell growth and function.[13,16-19,36,61,62]

The PDGF receptors are included in the *src* family of tyrosine kinase receptors, which also includes the colony-stimulating factor-1 receptor. In addition to the binding domain, these receptors contain a tyrosine kinase domain, which is required for receptor activity. The PDGF receptors are apparently associated with a separate phosphatidylinositol kinase molecule that seems to be important in inducing cell growth.[7] The study of PDGF receptors is progressing rapidly, and studies immediately relevant to inflammation and wound healing in connective tissues have begun to appear in the literature. For example, studies on rheumatoid arthritis have shown that expression of PDGF receptors is markedly increased in inflamed synovial tissues.[53] Similar upregulation of receptor expression is likely to be found in musculoskeletal injuries undergoing repair.

Effects of PDGF on Receptor-bearing Target Cells in Vitro

Many studies have examined the effects of PDGF on various target cells in vitro, particularly fibroblastoid cells.[5,20,50,51,61] Not all cells respond similarly, but many general features of the PDGF-induced response have been defined. These can be divided into immediate effects, which develop in one to five minutes and do not require gene transcription, early effects, which develop in 30 minutes to four hours and do require gene transcription, and late effects, which develop in four to 24 hours.

When stimulated by PDGF, the PDGF receptor expresses tyrosine kinase activity, which results within minutes in phosphorylation of itself and other proteins. Simultaneously, there is a decrease in the number of cell surface receptors secondary to internalization. Other immediate effects that have been described include the following: (1) stimulation of phospholipase C and A_2 activity, (2) increased phosphoinositol turnover, (3) increased diacylglycerol release, (4) increased intracellular Ca^{2+} release from internal stores, (5) increased release of free arachidonic acid, (6) increased cyclo-oxygenase, prostaglandins E and I_2 synthesis, (7) increased intracellular levels of cAMP, (8) increased NaH^+ exchange, (9) reorganization of actin filaments (membrane ruffling), and (10) modulation of endothelial growth factor receptors. From this list, it is clear that PDGF may potentially activate many pathways of intracellular second messengers. Various cell types may differ by using one pathway and not others. For example, recent data from our laboratory have shown that PDGF by itself does not stimulate prostaglandin E_2 production in synovial fibroblast-like cells from patients with rheumatoid arthritis (E.F. Remmers, R. Lafyatis, D.E. Yocum, and associates, and G.K. Kumkumian, R. Lafyatis, E.F. Remmers, and associates, unpublished data.)

Early effects of PDGF include increased RNA synthesis, increased protein synthesis, and acquisition of the "competent" state. Specific induction of the mRNAs for so-called competence genes c-*myc*, c-*fos*, JE, and KC has been a subject of considerable study. These genes appear to facilitate many of the downstream events in the functioning cell, such as responses to other polypeptide cytokines or to other mediators. For example, PDGF induces receptor expression of insulin-like growth factors, the low-density lipoprotein receptors. Other early events include stimulation of the amino acid "A" transport system, stimulation of synthesis of cholesterol and other lipids, stimulation of glycosaminoglycan synthesis, and stimulation of fluid endocytosis; PDGF also induces directed chemotaxis of smooth muscle cells, fibroblasts, and possibly monocytes, and, therefore, contributes to recruitment of cells to an injured tissue.

The most consistent late effect of PDGF stimulation of fibroblasts is cell division. In fact, PDGF is probably the most potent stimulator of fibroblastoid cell growth that has been identified. Other reported late effects of PDGF include induction of collagenase and collagen production in dermal fibroblasts, but collagenase gene expression is not induced in early-passage fibroblast-like cells from patients with rheumatoid arthritis (G.K. Kumkumian and associates, unpublished data). Thus, again, the data suggest that responses, even among "fibroblasts," can vary depending on the source, differentiation state, and presence of other growth factors or mediators.

Transforming Growth Factor Beta

Biochemistry

Initially TGF-β was isolated as a result of its ability to induce anchorage-independent growth in soft agar of NRK fibroblasts.[46] It is now known to consist of a multifunctional family of highly homologous cytokines that includes TGF-β1 (formerly known as TGF-β), TGF-β2, TGF-β3, TGF-β4, inhibins, activins, müllerian inhibiting substance, the decapentaplegic gene complex in *Drosophila*, and the putative V_g1 protein in *Xenopus*. The most extensively studied forms are TGF-β1 and TGF-β2, which appear to be functionally very similar. TGF-β1 is a homodimeric molecule, consisting of two polypeptide chains, each 12.5 kd, cross-linked by disulfide bonds. TGF-β2 is also a homodimer and is 71% homologous to TGF-β1. The peptides are strongly conserved. The mature TGF-β1 peptide is identical in humans, cows, pigs, and monkeys, and differs by only one amino acid in mice. The other forms of TGF-β similarly are strongly conserved structures across species, which suggests that they have important physiologic functions.[47,54]

Most of the TGF-β1 and TGF-β2 found in the body is biologically inactive, or "latent," and must be activated before they can modulate biologic function. In vitro, both TGF-β1 and TGF-β2 are activated by acidification. The mechanisms of activation in vivo remain incompletely defined, but plasmin and cathepsin D may play important roles. Activation may represent a physiologically critical mechanism for regulating the activity of these factors.[21,31,37,54]

Cell and Tissue Sources

The highest concentrations of TGF-β1 are found in platelets and bone,[47,48,54] but it is also readily demonstrable in tissues throughout the body, particularly in mesenchymally derived tissues, including chondrocytes and connective-tissue fibroblasts. Macrophages are also a source of TGF-β1.[2,14,57] Thus, many cell types that participate in the wound-healing process have the potential to produce and secrete TGF-β1. The tissue sources of TGF-β2 are not so well defined. TGF-β3 and TGF-β4 mRNAs have been identified in chondrocytes.[11,22,23]

Regulation of TGF-β Production and Release

Immunoreactive TGF-β1, as well as TGF-β1 mRNA, has been detected in many normal neonatal and adult murine tissues, but there is no correlation between relative mRNA abundance and specific protein abundance.[57] We have found that the abundance of TGF-β1 mRNA varies greatly in synovial tissues of patients with rheumatoid arthritis, but tends to be higher in rheumatoid than in osteoarthritic tissues. Tissue staining for TGF-β, however, tends to vary depending on the histologic abnormalities. For example, lymphocytic nodules tend not to stain with anti-TGF-β1 antibody, whereas fibrotic areas tend to stain intensely. Moreover, cultured rheumatoid synovial fibroblast-like cells spontaneously transcribe TGF-β1 mRNA and release TGF-β1 into the culture medium (R. Lafyatis, N.L. Thompson, E.F. Remmers and associates, unpublished data). In contrast, macrophages constitutively transcribe TGF-β1 mRNA, but cell activation with agents such as lipopolysaccharide is required to induce TGF-β protein synthesis and secretion.[2] These data suggest that the control of TGF-β synthesis and secretion is complex and may vary greatly according to tissue and cell type and differentiation state. Clearly, regulation of TGF-β1 mRNA transcription is not the primary step in regulating protein production. Regulation of the conversion of latent TGF-β to active protein may be more important in controlling its biologic effects than in controlling its synthesis and secretion.

Receptors

Three distinct receptors for TGF-β1 have been identified. A 280-kd, high-affinity receptor has been demonstrated on virtually all cells of the body, although the number per cell may vary. The receptor consists of a disulfide-linked glycosylated dimer. The receptor also has a high affinity for TGF-β2. In vitro studies have shown that it is distinct from other growth factor receptors, such as the PDGF receptors, in that it does not show ligand-induced clustering, does not downregulate, and does not autophosphorylate. Moreover, the number of receptors per cell does not change significantly over a wide range of conditions. It appears that modulation of the 280-kd receptor is not a primary control mechanism in the action of TGF-β.

Two additional high-affinity TGF-β1 receptors, one 65 kd and the other 85 kd, have been identified. The receptors bind TGF-β2 weakly. The differential affinity of TGF-β1 and TGF-β2 to these receptors may provide flexibility in regulation of tissue growth and cell differentiation by the TGF-β system.[4,60]

Effects of TGF-β on Receptor-Bearing Target Cells in Vitro

Although TGF-β1 was initially characterized by its ability to induce anchorage-independent growth of NRK cells, it has become clear that TGF-β1, as well as the other less extensively characterized forms of TGF-β, are pleiotropic, multifunctional growth factors.[35,47,54] Their biologic activities in vitro vary with the assay conditions (eg, anchorage-dependent vs anchorage-independent growth), the target cell type, its differentiation state, and the presence of other growth factors. For example, although TGF-β1 stimulates anchorage-independent growth of NRK and AKR-2B fibroblast cell lines, it does not stimulate anchorage-dependent growth of these cell lines.[46] In contrast, TGF-β1 inhibits both anchorage-dependent and anchorage-independent growth of early explant synovial fibroblast-like cell growth. These cells are strongly stimulated to grow by PDGF[27] (E.F. Remmers and associates, unpublished data). In fact, most studies on cells of fibroblast origin suggest that TGF-β slows or inhibits cell growth. This observation is consistent with data showing that TGF-β has important effects on the production of extracellular matrix and cell differentiation. It also stimulates fibroblast production of collagen and fibronectin and their incorporation into the extracellular matrix.[10,42,52] Moreover, in combination with basic fibroblast growth factor (a member of the heparin-binding growth factor family), it induces differentiation of mesenchymal tissue in *Xenopus* embryos.[26]

TGF-β1 also enhances the formation of extracellular matrix by its ability to inhibit the proteolytic degradation of newly formed matrix proteins. This occurs through two mechanisms: increased production of protease inhibitors, such as TIMP, the tissue inhibitor of metalloproteinases, and decreased production of proteases such as collagenase and stromelysin, which are key participants in the resorption of extracellular collagen and proteoglycan. These effects seem to result from direct modulation of mRNA transcription for these genes.[3,12,28,32] All of these observations suggest that TGF-β promotes differentiation of fibroblastoid cells.

TGF-β1 itself strongly inhibits the growth of capillary endothelial cells and stimulates the release of PDGF-like molecules.[9,24,47,56] It is chemotactic for monocytes at low concentrations and appears to stimulate release of various cytokines at higher concentrations.[47] The effects of TGF-β on macrophages are, however, complex, because TGF-β may also deactivate previously activated macrophages.[59]

TGF-β1 may also have inhibitory effects on other cells relevant to the healing of connective tissue injuries, particularly lymphoid cells and bone marrow hematopoietic precursor cells.[25,38,39] Thus, available data in vitro strongly suggest that the various forms of TGF-β play important roles in modulating various aspects of cell growth and differentiation, inflammation, and wound repair. Because of their multifunctional, multicellular effects, our understanding of their ultimate physiologic roles in vivo is still unclear.

The Effects of PDGF and TGF-β in Vivo

In vitro studies of the effects of PDGF and TGF-β on receptor-bearing target cells to a large extent address the direct effects of these cytokines. However, in vivo indirect effects are probably equally important. For example, although TGF-β1 inhibits endothelial cell proliferation, it may induce macrophages to release angiogenic peptides that indirectly induce angiogenesis. Similarly, although TGF-β1 and TGF-β2 directly inhibit the growth of most types of fibroblasts and induce extracellular matrix formation, macrophages and endothelial cells stimulated by TGF-β1 may produce cytokines, such as PDGF and interleukin-1, that may stimulate fibroblast growth and collagenase production. Because of the complicated cellular and molecular interactions, it is almost impossible to predict the in vivo effects of a given cytokine. Therefore, in vivo studies of cytokines are necessary and are beginning to appear in the literature.

Table 1 Basic data on platelet-derived growth factor and transforming growth factor beta

Data	PDGF	TGF-β
No. of isoforms	3	At least 4
Molecular weight	About 30,000	About 25,000
Major sources	Platelets, macrophages, endothelial cells, and fibroblasts	Platelets and bone (although almost all cells synthesize TGF-β)
Responding cells	Fibroblasts and smooth muscle cells	Almost all cells
Receptors	Two forms	Three forms
Major direct effect	Stimulation of target cell growth	Diverse effects depending on cell type, differentiation state, presence of other growth factors, and the like*

*On fibroblasts, for example, TGF-β inhibits growth and collagenase production and induces collagen and fibronectin production, promoting differentiation.

Three separate studies have been reported that demonstrate that PDGF, particularly in combination with insulin-like growth factor 1, accelerates in vivo wound healing, and increases tensile strength in incisional wounds in pigs and rats.[30,44,55] These data strongly suggest that PDGF, probably in combination with other cytokines, may be effective in modulating the wound-healing process.

Studies of TGF-β in vivo effects involved its direct injection into the skin of the newborn mouse. The investigators noted that TGF-β1 stimulated formation of a localized fibrous nodule with all the characteristics of granulation tissue.[47] These results indicate that TGF-β alone is sufficient to initiate the entire cascade of events resulting in the formation of granulation tissue. Subsequent studies have confirmed and extended these observations and suggest that TGF-β, like PDGF, may be useful for accelerating wound healing and repair.[43,55]

Conclusion

As reviewed above and summarized in Table 1, the various forms of PDGF and TGF-β almost certainly play fundamental but incompletely defined roles in the molecular regulation of healing and repair of musculoskeletal connective tissue injuries. Although these growth factors are produced by and affect many cell types, the clearest understanding of their effects is on molecular regulation of fibroblastoid cell growth and function. As summarized in Figures 1 and 2, the local wound paracrine sources of PDGF most likely to affect these cells are platelets, blood vessel endothelial cells, and macrophages, even though platelets and macrophages are the principal paracrine sources of TGF-β. Fibroblasts may themselves serve as autocrine sources of PDGF and TGF-β. These cytokines appear to have antagonistic effects on immature, quiescent fibroblasts. PDGF seems to stimulate accelerated growth of these cells directly and to perpetuate the immature fibroblast phenotype (the proliferative and extracellular matrix-degrading phase

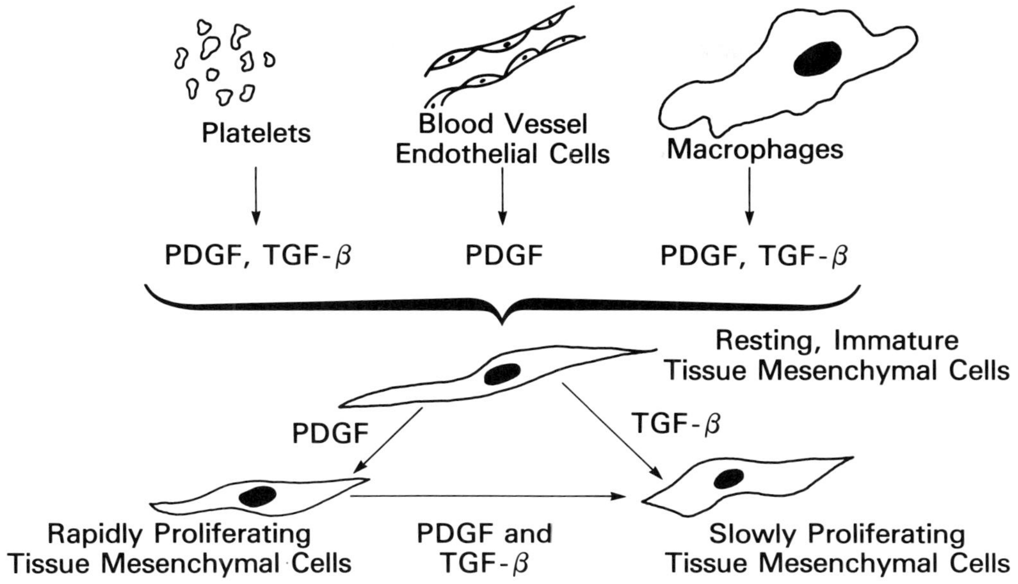

Fig. 1 *Paracrine control of wound mesenchymal cells by PDGF and TGF-β.*

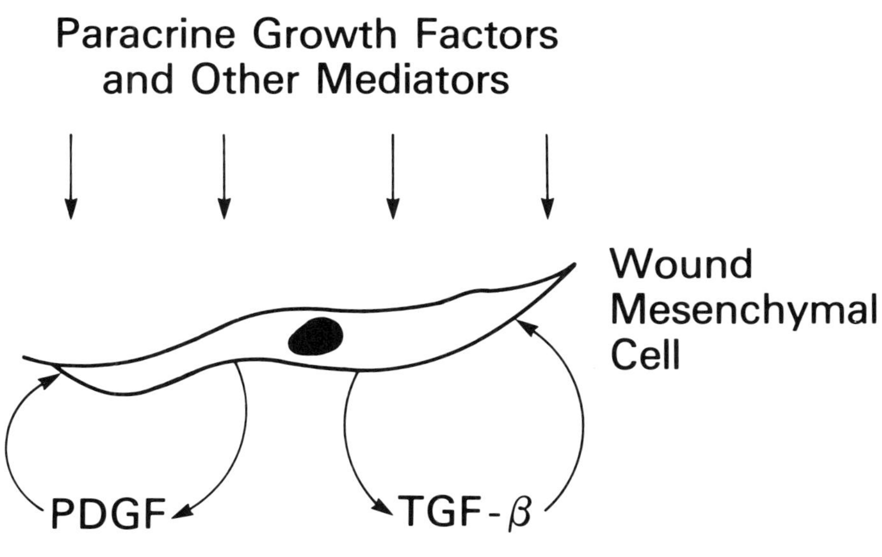

Fig. 2 *Autocrine control of wound mesenchymal cells by PDGF and TGF-β.*

of wound healing). On the other hand, TGF-β seems to stimulate the development of the mature fibroblast phenotype (slow cell growth with prominent extracellular matrix production, representing the fibrotic phase of wound healing). The degree to which the proliferative and resorptive phases predominate over the scarring and fibrotic phases in a wound probably depends on the site and type of the tissue injury (the differentiation state of the connective tissue fibroblasts) and on the extent and intensity of involvement of other cell types in the wound healing process (platelets, macrophages). If this conceptual model proves correct, it may ultimately be possible to modulate defective wound healing characterized by either insufficient or excess scar or extracellular matrix formation.

References

1. Alitalo R, Andersson LC, Betsholtz C, et al: Induction of platelet-derived growth factor gene expression during megakaryoblastic and monocytic differentiation of human leukemia cell lines. *EMBO J* 1987;62:1213–1218.
2. Assoian RK, Fleurdelys BE, Stevenson HC, et al: Expression and secretion of type beta transforming growth factor by activated human macrophages. *Proc Natl Acad Sci USA* 1987;84:6020–6024.
3. Chandrasekhar S, Harvey A: Transforming growth factor-beta is a potent inhibitor of Il-1 induced protease activity and cartilage proteoglycan degradation. *Biochem Biophys Res Commun* 1988;157:1352–1359.
4. Cheifetz S, Weatherbee JA, Tsang ML-S, et al: The transforming growth factor-beta system, a complex pattern of cross-reactive ligands and receptors. *Cell* 1987;48:409–415.
5. Cochran BH: The molecular action of platelet-derived growth factor. *Adv Cancer Res* 1985;45:183–216.
6. Collins T, Bonthron DT, Orkin SH: Alternative RNA splicing affects function of encoded platelet-derived growth factor A chain. *Nature* 1987;328:621–624.
7. Coughlin SR, Escobedo JA, Williams LT: Role of phosphatidylinositol kinase in PDGF receptor signal transduction. *Science* 1989;243:1191–1193.
8. Daniel TO, Gibbs VC, Milfay DF, et al: Agents that increase cAMP accumulation block endothelial c-sis induction by thrombin and transforming growth factor-beta. *J Biol Chem* 1987;262:11893–11896.
9. Daniel TO, Gibbs VC, Milfay DF, et al: Thrombin stimulates c-sis gene expression in microvascular endothelial cells. *J Biol Chem* 1986;261:9579–9582.
10. Dean DC, Newby RF, Bourgeois S: Regulation of fibronectin biosynthesis by dexamethasone, transforming growth factor beta, and cAMP in human cell lines. *J Cell Biol* 1988;106:2159–2170.
11. Duke PT, Hansen P, Iwata KK, et al: Identification of another member of the transforming growth factor type beta gene family. *Proc Natl Acad Sci USA* 1988;85:4715–4719.
12. Edwards DR, Murphy G, Reynolds JJ, et al: Transforming growth factor beta modulates the expression of collagenase and metalloproteinase inhibitor. *EMBO J* 1987;6:1899–1904.
13. Escobedo JA, Navankasatussas S, Cousens LS, et al: A common PDGF receptor is activated by homodimeric A and B forms of PDGF. *EMBO J* 1988;7:1387–1393.
14. Flanders KC, Thompson NL, Cissel DS, et al: Transforming growth factor-beta 1: Histochemical localization with antibodies to different epitopes. *J Cell Biol* 1989;108:653–660.

15. Fox PL, DiCorleto PE: Modified low density lipoproteins suppress production of a platelet-derived growth factor-like protein by cultured endothelial cells. *Proc Natl Acad Sci USA* 1986;83:4774–4778.
16. Gronwald RG, Grant FJ, Haldeman BA, et al: Cloning and expression of a cDNA coding for the human platelet-derived growth factor receptor: Evidence for more than one receptor class. *Proc Natl Acad Sci USA* 1988;85:3435–3439.
17. Hajjar KA, Hajjar DP, Silverstein RL, et al: Tumor necrosis factor-mediated release of platelet-derived growth factor from cultured endothelial cells. *J Exp Med* 1987;166:235–245.
18. Hart CE, Forstrom JW, Kelly JD, et al: Two classes of PDGF receptor recognize different isoforms of PDGF. *Science* 1988;240:1529–1531.
19. Heldin CH, Bäckström G, Ostman A, et al: Binding of different dimeric forms of PDGF to human fibroblasts: Evidence for two separate receptor types. *EMBO J* 1988;7:1387–1393.
20. Heldin CH, Wasteson A, Westermark B: Platelet-derived growth factor. *Mol Cell Endocrinol* 1985;39:169–187.
21. Huang SS, O'Grady P, Huang JS: Human transforming growth factor beta-alpha2-macroglobulin complex is a latent form of transforming growth factor beta. *J Biol Chem* 1988;263:1535–1541.
22. Jakowlew AB, Dillard PJ, Kondaiah P, et al: Complementary deoxyribonucleic acid cloning of a novel transforming growth factor-beta messenger ribonucleic acid from chick embryo chondrocytes. *Mol Endocrinol* 1988;2:747–755.
23. Jakowlew AB, Dillard PJ, Sporn MB, et al: Complementary deoxyribonucleic acid cloning of a messenger ribonucleic acid encoding transforming growth factor-beta 4 from chicken embryo chondrocytes. *Mol Endocrinol* 1988;2:1186–1195.
24. Kavanaugh WM, Harsh GR IV, Starksen NF, et al: Transcriptional regulation of the A and B chain genes of platelet-derived growth factor in microvascular endothelial cells. *J Biol Chem* 1988;263:8470–8472.
25. Kehrl JH, Wakefield LM, Roberts AB, et al: Production of transforming growth factor beta by human T lymphocytes and its potential role in the regulation of T cell growth. *J Exp Med* 1986;163:1037–1050.
26. Kimelman D, Kirschner M: Synergistic induction of mesoderm by FGF and TGF-beta and the identification of an mRNA coding for FGF in the early Xenopus embryo. *Cell* 1987;51:869–877.
27. Lafyatis R, Remmers EF, Roberts AB, et al: Anchorage-independent growth of synoviocytes from arthritic and normal joints: Stimulation by exogenous platelet-derived growth factor and inhibition by transforming growth factor-beta and retinoids. *J Clin Invest* 1989;83:1267–1276.
28. Laiho M, Saksela O, Andreasen PA, et al: Enhanced production and extracellular deposition of the endothelial-type plasminogen activator inhibitor in cultured human lung fibroblasts by transforming growth factor-beta. *J Cell Biol* 1986;103:2403–2410.
29. Leof EB, Proper JA, Goustin AS, et al: Induction of c-sis mRNA and activity similar to platelet-derived growth factor by transforming growth factor beta: A proposed model for indirect mitogenesis involving autocrine activity. *Proc Natl Acad Sci USA* 1986;83:2453–2457.
30. Lynch SE, Nixon JC, Colvin RB, et al: Role of platelet-derived growth factor in wound healing: Synergistic effects with other growth factors. *Proc Natl Acad Sci USA* 1987;84:7696–7700.
31. Lyons RM, Keski-Oja J, Moses HL: Proteolytic activation of latent transforming growth factor-beta from fibroblast-conditioned medium. *J Cell Biol* 1988;106:1659–1665.
32. Machida CM, Muldoon LL, Rodland KD, et al: Transcriptional modulation of transin gene expression by epidermal growth factor and transforming growth factor beta. *Mol Cell Biol* 1988;8:2479–2483.

33. Majesky MW, Benditt EP, Schwartz SM: Expression and developmental control of platelet-derived growth factor A-chain and B-chain/sis genes in rat aortic smooth muscle cells. *Proc Natl Acad Sci USA* 1988;85:1524–1528.
34. Mäkelä TP, Alitalo R, Paulsson Y, et al: Regulation of platelet-derived growth factor gene expression by transforming growth factor beta and phorbol ester in human leukemia cell lines. *Mol Cell Biol* 1987;7:3656–3662.
35. Marx JL: Cytokines are two-edged swords in disease. *Science* 1988;239:257–258.
36. Matsui T, Heidaran M, Miki M, et al: Isolation of a novel receptor cDNA establishes the existence of two PDGF receptor genes. *Science* 1989;243:800–803.
37. Miyazono K, Hellman U, Wernstedt C, et al: Latent high molecular weight complex of transforming growth factor beta 1: Purification from human platelets and structural characterization. *J Biol Chem* 1988;263:6409–6415.
38. Mulé JJ, Schwarz SL, Roberts AB, et al: Transforming growth factor-beta inhibits the in vitro generation of lymphokine-activated killer cells and cytotoxic T cells. *Cancer Immunol Immunother* 1988;26:95–100.
39. Ohta M, Greenberger JS, Anklesaria P, et al: Two forms of transforming growth factor-beta distinguished by multipotential haematopoietic progenitor cells. *Nature* 1987;329:539–541.
40. Pantazis P, Sariban E, Kufe D, et al: Induction of c-sis gene expression and synthesis of platelet-derived growth factor in human myeloid leukemia cells during monocytic differentiation. *Proc Natl Acad Sci USA* 1986;83:6455–6459.
41. Paulsson Y, Hammacher A, Heldin CH, et al: Possible positive autocrine feedback in the prereplicative phase of human fibroblasts. *Nature* 1987;328:715–717.
42. Penttinen RP, Kobayashi S, Bornstein P: Transforming growth factor beta increases mRNA for matrix proteins both in the presence and in the absence of changes in mRNA stability. *Proc Natl Acad Sci USA* 1988;85:1105–1108.
43. Pierce GF, Mustoe TA, Deuel TF: Transforming growth factor β induces increased directed cellular migration and tissue repair in rats, in Barbul A, Pines E, Caldwell M, et al (eds): *Growth Factors and Other Aspects of Wound Healing: Biological and Clinical Implications.* New York, Alan R Liss, 1988, pp 93–102.
44. Pierce GF, Mustoe TA, Senior RM, et al: In vivo incisional wound healing augmented by platelet-derived growth factor and recombinant c-sis gene homodimeric proteins. *J Exp Med* 1988;167:974–987.
45. Raines EW, Dower SK, Ross R: Interleukin-1 mitogenic activity for fibroblasts and smooth muscle cells is due to PDGF-AA. *Science* 1989;243:393–396.
46. Roberts AB, Anzano MA, Wakefield LM, et al: Type beta transforming growth factor: A bifunctional regulator of cellular growth. *Proc Natl Acad Sci USA* 1985;82:119–123.
47. Roberts AB, Thompson NL, Heine U, et al: Transforming growth factor-beta: Possible roles in carcinogenesis. *Br J Cancer* 1988;57:594–600.
48. Robey PG, Young MF, Flanders KC, et al: Osteoblasts synthesize and respond to transforming growth factor-type beta (TGF-beta) in vitro. *J Cell Biol* 1987;105:457–463.
49. Rorsman F, Bywater M, Knott TJ, et al: Structural characterization of the human platelet-derived growth factor A-chain cDNA and gene: Alternative exon usage predicts two different precursor proteins. *Mol Cell Biol* 1988;8:571–577.

50. Ross R, Bowen-Pope DF, Raines EW: Platelets, macrophages, endothelium, and growth factors: Their effects upon cells and their possible roles in atherogenesis. *Ann NY Acad Sci* 1985;454:254–260.
51. Ross R, Raines EW, Bowen-Pope DF: The biology of platelet derived growth factor. *Cell* 1986;46:155–169.
52. Rossi P, Karsenty G, Roberts AB, et al: A nuclear factor 1 binding site mediates the transcriptional activation of a type I collagen promoter by transforming growth factor-beta. *Cell* 1988;52:405–414.
53. Rubin K, Terracio L, Rönnstrand L, et al: Expression of platelet-derived growth factor receptors is induced on connective tissue cells during chronic synovial inflammation. *Scand J Immunol* 1988;27:285–294.
54. Sporn MB, Roberts AB, Wakefield LM, et al: Some recent advances in the chemistry and biology of transforming growth factor-beta. *J Cell Biol* 1987;105:1039–1045.
55. Sprugel KH, McPherson JM, Clowes AW, et al: The effects of different growth factors in subcutaneous wound chambers, in Barbul A, Pines E, Caldwell M, et al (eds): *Growth Factors and Other Aspects of Wound Healing: Biological and Clinical Implications.* New York, Alan R Liss, 1988, pp 77–91.
56. Starksen NF, Harsh GR IV, Gibbs VC, et al: Regulated expression of the platelet-derived growth factor A chain gene in microvascular endothelial cells. *J Biol Chem* 1987;262:14381–14384.
57. Thompson NL, Flanders KC, Smith JM, et al: Expression of transforming growth factor-beta 1 in specific cells and tissues of adult and neonatal mice. *J Cell Biol* 1989;108:661–669.
58. Tong BD, Auer DE, Jaye M, et al: cDNA clones reveal differences between human glial and endothelial cell platelet-derived growth factor A-chains. *Nature* 1987;328:619–621.
59. Tsunawaki S, Sporn M, Ding A, et al: Deactivation of macrophages by transforming growth factor-beta. *Nature* 1988;334:260–262.
60. Wakefield LM, Smith DM, Masui T, et al: Distribution and modulation of the cellular receptor for transforming growth factor-beta. *J Cell Biol* 1987;105:965–975.
61. Williams LT: Signal transduction by the platelet-derived growth factor receptor. *Science* 1989;243:1564–1570.
62. Yarden Y, Escobedo JA, Kuang WJ, et al: Structure of the receptor for platelet-derived growth factor helps define a family of closely related growth factor receptors. *Nature* 1986;323:226–232.

Chapter 18

Oxygen-Derived Free Radicals and Inflammation

Peter A. Ward, MD
Gerd O. Till, MD
Kent J. Johnson, MD

There is an increasing body of experimental and clinical evidence to suggest that oxygen-derived free radicals (oxyradicals) participate in the pathogenesis of acute inflammation. Evidence derived from experimental studies, both in vitro and in animal model systems, supports the concept that oxyradicals play an important role in the initiation and amplification as well as in the outcome of acute inflammatory reactions.

It is now increasingly recognized that oxyradicals are generated in a variety of conditions and that they play an important role in the inflammatory response. As indicated below, not only can their generation initiate or amplify an inflammatory reaction, but oxyradicals can also play a direct role in damage that often develops as a consequence of the acute inflammatory response. Although we can only speculate about the role played by oxyradicals in reactions to sports injuries, there is little doubt that when these injuries induce an acute inflammatory response, oxyradicals are generated and participate in the pathogenesis of the injury state.

The chemistry of oxyradicals within the context of the inflammatory response is relatively simple. An oxygen radical by definition is an unstable molecule in which oxygen has an unpaired electron in the outer orbit. The progressive reduction of molecular oxygen (O_2, dioxygen) by enzyme pathways listed below results in a family of products:

(1) O_2 + electron (e^-) $\rightarrow$ O_2^- (superoxide anion)
(2) $O_2^- + e^- \rightarrow H_2O_2$
(3) $H_2O_2 + e^- + Fe^{2+} \rightarrow HO^\bullet$ (hydroxyl radical) $+ OH^- + Fe^{3+}$
(4) $HO^\bullet + e^- \rightarrow H_2O$

This scheme indicates that two forms of oxyradicals exist: O_2^- and $HO^\bullet$, the former being moderately reactive while the latter is the most highly reactive of all oxygen radicals. This chemical scheme reveals two important conclusions: first, oxyradicals and the oxygen-reactive product H_2O_2 exist as a family of oxygen derivatives, the conclusion being that there is never a single and selective product; secondly, the reduction of H_2O_2 to $HO^\bullet$ is facilitated by the presence of the transition

Outline 1 Cellular sources of oxyradicals

Abundant formation
- Neutrophils
- Eosinophils
- Monocytes
- Macrophages

Little, if any, formation
- Lymphocytes
- Basophils
- Platelets

state of iron (Fe^{2+}); iron thus acts as a redox reagent cycling between Fe^{3+} and Fe^{2+}. The implication of this latter observation is that preventing the availability of iron with iron chelators, most of which only react with Fe^{3+}, effectively blocks the formation of $HO^{\cdot}$. There is now increasing evidence that O_2^- also plays an important role in bringing about the reduction of iron to its transition state:

(5) $O_2^- + Fe^{3+} \rightarrow Fe^{2+} + O_2$.

This points out another important feature of oxyradicals: they can act either as electron acceptors (ie, an oxidant) or as electron donors (ie, a reductant). Another important feature of the family of oxygen products is the ability of H_2O_2 to be converted in the presence of myeloperoxidase, which is derived chiefly from secretory granules of neutrophils.

Accordingly:

(6) $H_2O_2 + MPO + Cl^- \rightarrow HOCl$ (hypochlorous acid).

HOCl is a stable, powerful oxidant generated primarily from myeloperoxidase derived from neutrophils.[8] It is known that HOCl can bring about conversion of latent metalloproteinases (collagenase, gelatinase) of neutrophils to active enzymes and it may, therefore, be important in the hydrolysis of connective tissue matrix.[25]

Enzymes capable of generating oxyradicals in biologic systems are somewhat diverse, but perhaps the two most important are NADPH oxidase and xanthine oxidase. The former is found on the cell membrane and within membranes of intracellular granules in phagocytic cells (Outline 1), while the latter is found in some endothelial cells and appears to be present in rather high concentrations in the mucosa of the small bowel and within the liver.[6] There is also evidence that O_2^- may be generated by at least three other biologically relevant enzyme systems: cyclo-oxygenase, cytochrome P450 reductase, and enzymes of mitochondria,[3] although to what extent these pathways ordinarily generate sufficient amounts of O_2^- to be biologically meaningful is not clear at present.

Initiation of oxygen radical formation via NADPH oxidase of phagocytic cells occurs by a variety of mechanisms.[8] Engagement of cell membrane receptors by a variety of agonists initiates the signal transduction cascade[9] via the formation of inositol phosphates and diacylglycerol, the latter bringing about activation of protein kinase C, which, in turn, activates NADPH oxidase.[9] Receptor occupancy that results in this outcome includes receptors for Fc, formyl chemotactic peptides, C5a, CR3, (C3bi), leukotriene B, and platelet-activating factor, to name only a few examples. Circumstances leading to the activation of xanthine oxidase are less understood. Although it has been shown that ischemia leads to enzyme activation both in vitro (in endothelial cells) and in vivo,[6] the precise mechanisms have not been elucidated. One circumstance that has recently been associated with activation of xanthine oxidase in rat pulmonary endothelial cells is related to an interaction of these cells with phorbol ester-activated human neutrophils, which lack xanthine oxidase.[13] This interaction causes an activation of xanthine oxidase (ie, an irreversible conversion of xanthine dehydrogenase to xanthine oxidase) in a manner that does not require participation of oxygen products from the neutrophil. This activation process is presumably related to the release from the neutrophil of a granule constituent that brings about activation of xanthine oxidase in the endothelial cell, although this has not been proven.

Another important point to emphasize is that O_2^- can be found in the absence of available substrate whenever intracellular xanthine is activated. Because the substrates xanthine and hypoxanthine are not ordinarily present in measurable amounts within most normal cells, the activated enzyme is not effective in the absence of these purines. It is well known that ischemia breaks down adenosine triphosphate (ATP)[1] (Fig. 1), making available the substrate for xanthine oxidase. Another well-known example of ATP breakdown is exposure of cells to H_2O_2.[15] When a variety of cells are exposed to H_2O_2 (whether produced from activated phagocytic cells or generated from enzymes such as glucose oxidase), there is a rapid breakdown of ATP. Accordingly, therefore, several conditions that cause activation of xanthine oxidase also bring about the generation of its substrates.

Recently it has been reported that the well-known inflammatory mediator, histamine, released from tissue mast cells (physical, thermal, hypothermia), has the peculiar ability to enhance the catalytic activity of xanthine oxidase.[4] Optimal enhancement of the enzyme occurs at concentrations of histamine (1 μmol) known to be present in human plasma after traumatic or allergic episodes. Contact of xanthine oxidase with histamine results in a numerical lowering of the *K*m value of the enzyme, indicating more rapid hydrolysis of substrate. Not only does histamine have this effect on xanthine oxidase present in solution, incubation of endothelial cells with histamine also leads to enhanced intracellular xanthine oxidase activity, suggesting that histamine present either in interstitial fluids or in plasma can enhance both intracellular and extracellular xanthine oxidase. This is an example of how one product of the inflammatory system (histamine) can amplify the inflammatory response by a sequential effect on another important component (xanthine oxidase). It is important to note that the effect

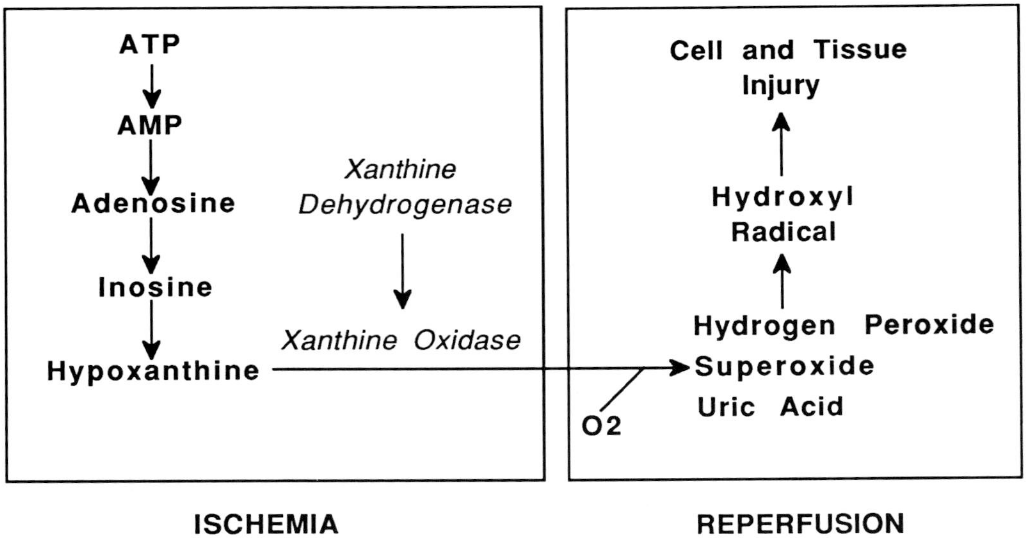

Fig. 1 *Proposed schema of events leading to cell and tissue injury following ischemia and perfusion.*

of histamine is selective: the activity of xanthine oxidase, but not of xanthine dehydrogenase, is enhanced (Fig. 2).

The biologic effects of oxygen radicals are diverse, as shown in Outline 2. The effect can be classified into two categories: direct biochemical alteration of cellular or noncellular constituents, such as connective tissue matrix and proteins, and indirect effects, which either amplify the inflammatory response or impair defenses against the inflammatory system. Among the former, there can be any number of biochemical modifications, including oxidation of cysteine residues, oxidation of glutathione, peroxidative changes, oxidative inactivation of enzymes of the glycolytic pathway, and even strand breaks in DNA.[14,16,24]

Compromise of protective anti-inflammatory factors also occurs. For instance, in patients with adult respiratory distress syndrome α_1-antiproteinase recovered from the lung by bronchoalveolar lavage has been reported to be oxidatively inactivated, resulting in a loss of the major protective shield against destructive proteinases derived from leukocytes.[10] Oxidants probably result in the loss of glutathione (through oxidation to generate oxidized glutathione), which is ordinarily present in large concentrations (millimoles) in the extracellular lung fluid in the alveolar compartment and would be expected to provide potent protection against oxidant damage. Another example of the indirect effects of oxygen radicals in accentuating tissue damage

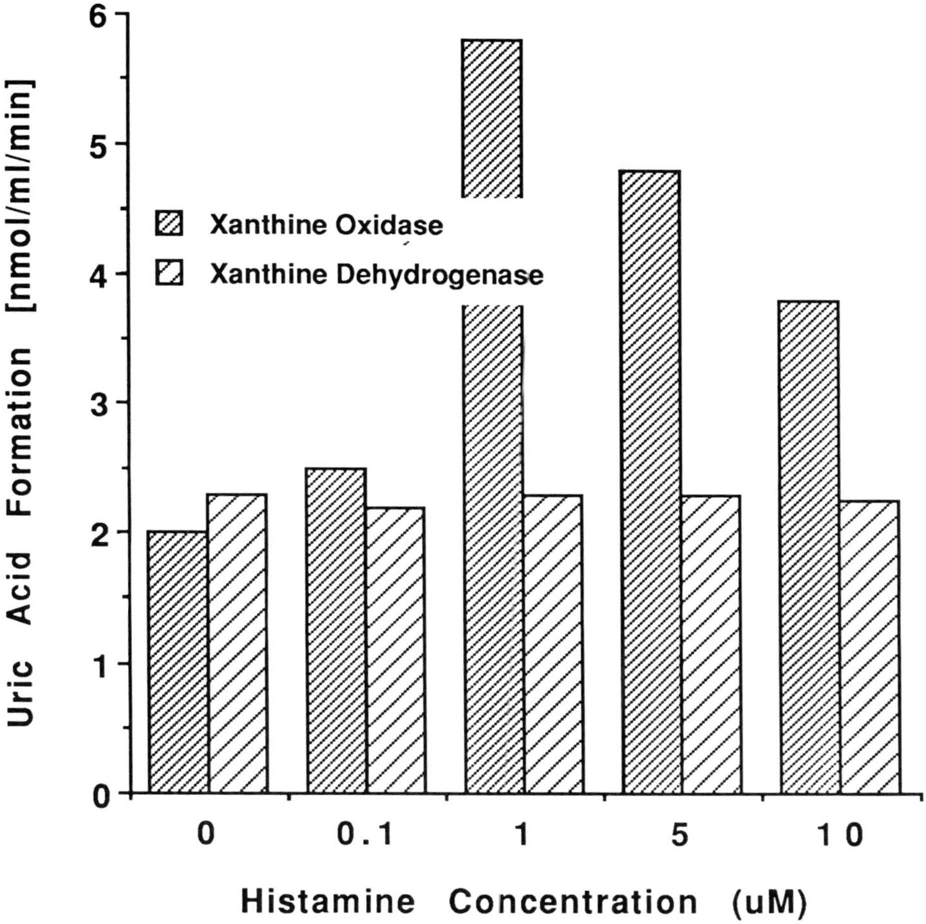

Fig. 2 *Dose-dependent enhancement by histamine of xanthine oxidase but not of dehydrogenase activity in rat plasma. The activity of both oxidases was determined by the rate of allopurinol-inhibitable uric acid production after the addition of xanthine (substrate) to rat plasma.*

Outline 2 Diverse mechanisms of damage mediated by oxyradicals

Biochemical changes
  Cross-linking of SH, peroxidative changes, DNA strand breaks, etc.

Loss of protective regulatory factors
  Inactivation of α_1-antiproteinase
  Reductions of GSH

Secondary activation of mediator pathways
  Complement activation
  Activation of latent enzymes (collagenase)

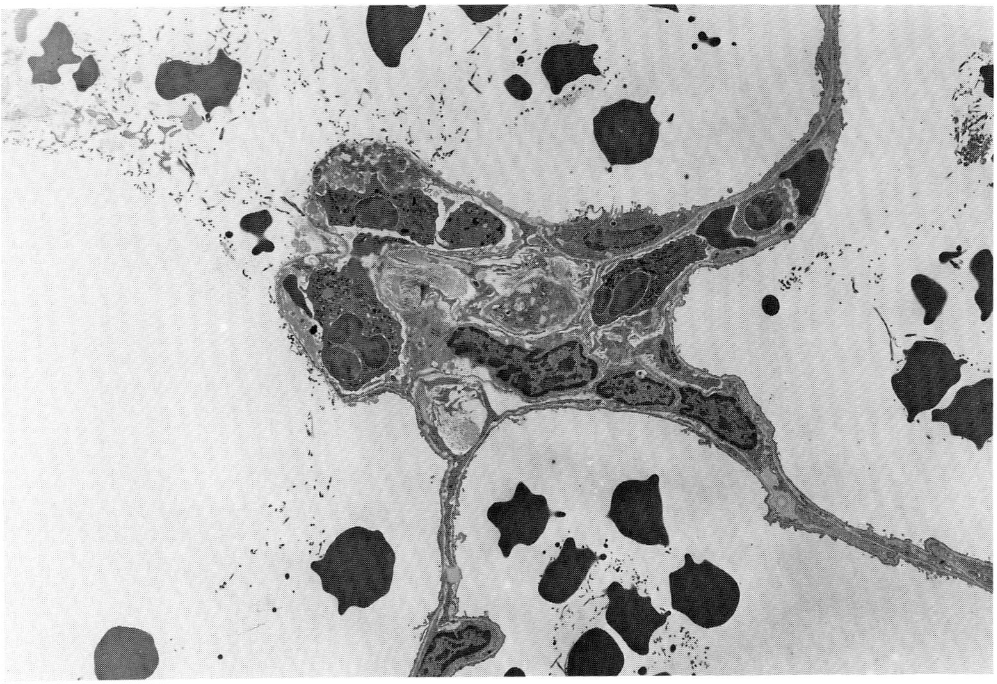

Fig. 3 *Transmission electron micrograph of rat lung after systemic complement activation. Aggregates of neutrophils are present within the interstitial capillaries of lung, along with destruction of endothelial cells and basement membrane, fibrin deposition, and intra-alveolar hemorrhage.*

can be found in the ability of O_2^- or its derivatives to result in the formation of chemotactic factors. There is evidence that chemotactic lipids as well as C5a can be generated as a result of O_2^- formation, perhaps ultimately via the formation of HO•.[11,12,21] In addition, it has been shown that a derivative of H_2O_2, presumably HOCl, can result in activation of latent metalloenzymes (collagenase, gelatinase) derived from phagocytic cells,[25] implying enhanced proteolysis of connective tissue matrices, including basement membrane, as a result of oxygen radical formation and protease secretion from phagocytic cells.

Stimulation of neutrophils within the vascular compartment by intravascular products of complement activation is not an innocuous event, as is shown by the morphologic changes. A transmission electron micrograph (Fig. 3) shows changes in the interstitial microvasculature of the lung obtained from an animal undergoing intravascular systemic activation of complement. Neutrophils have become sequestered within the interstitial capillaries where destruction of endothelial cells and basement membrane has occurred, associated with fibrin deposits, interstitial edema, and intra-alveolar hemorrhage. Interventional ma-

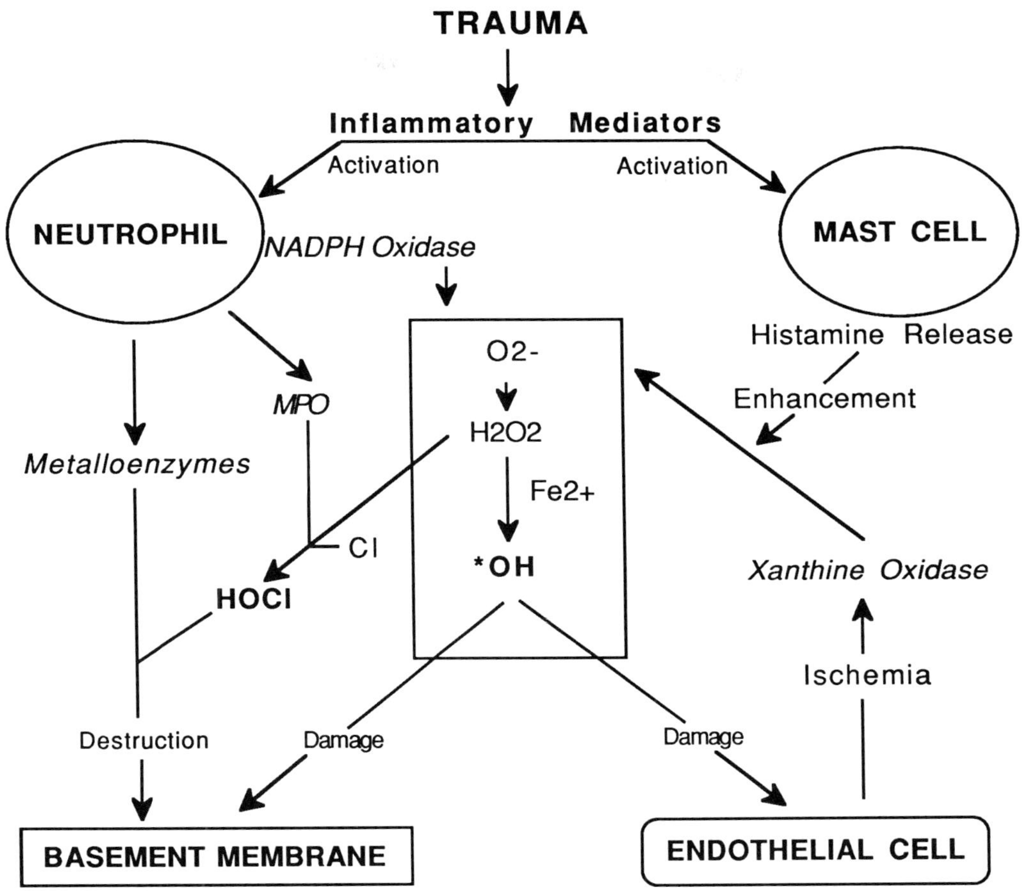

Fig. 4 *Proposed schema of events leading to oxyradical-mediated cell and tissue injury. Hydrogen peroxide (H_2O_2), superoxide anion (O_2^-), hydroxyl radical ($OH^\cdot$), hypochlorous acid (HOCl), chloride (Cl), myeloperoxidase (MPO).*

nipulations have shown that the vascular damage depends on the presence of neutrophils, the production of H_2O_2, and the availability of iron, suggesting that endothelial damage may be mediated by $HO^\cdot$. It is now probable that the vascular injury is initiated by the events depicted in Figure 4. The formation of O_2^- and H_2O_2 (by a combination of events involving oxygen products from both neutrophils and endothelial cells, as described above) leads initially to a breaching of the endothelial cell barrier, after which proteases from the neutrophil initiate hydrolysis of basement membrane[7] and other connective tissue matrices. Thus, tissue injury is in all likelihood the combined result of oxygen products and proteases derived from the phagocytic cells.

On the basis of this information, several interventions can be used

Outline 3 Protective interventions against oxyradicals

Naturally occurring antioxidant enzymes
- Superoxide dismutase
- Catalase
- Glutathione peroxidase-reductase

Scavengers
- Vitamins E, ceruloplasmin, dimethyl sulfoxide, dimethylthiourea

Iron chelators
- Deferoxamine

Inhibitors of xanthine oxidase
- Allopurinol

to intercept oxygen radicals in a manner that protects the tissue from injury after production of oxygen radicals. These are summarized in Outline 3. Naturally occurring enzymes include superoxide dismutase, catalase, and glutathione peroxidase, each of which removes toxic oxygen products. Superoxide dismutase causes rapid dismutation of O_2^- to H_2O_2, catalase destroys H_2O_2 (converting it to H_2O), and glutathione peroxidase catalyzes the oxidation of glutathione. Because of the rapid disappearance (within minutes) of these enzymes (which are ordinarily intracellular constituents) from the vascular compartment after their infusion, chemical alteration by the addition of carbohydrate groups (ficol, polyethylene glycol) to those enzymes greatly increases their duration in the circulation.[17,23] This has resulted in reagents that are particularly effective in protecting against formation of toxic oxygen products within the vascular compartment, but the extent to which these modified enzymes are able to gain entry to the intracellular compartment presently is not clear.

Other approaches include the use of scavengers of oxygen radicals. Such agents are vitamin E, ceruloplasmin, dimethyl sulfoxide, and dimethylthiourea. The last two agents are highly reactive with $HO^\cdot$ and appear to be effective scavengers of oxygen radicals in vitro and in experimental in vivo models of tissue injury related to products of the inflammatory system.[18,20,22]

Another approach to protecting tissues from injury is the use of compounds that chelate iron. Of special interest is the compound deferoxamine, which has the ability to chelate iron in its fully oxidized state, Fe^{3+}. This is the naturally occurring form of iron in ferritin; it also is speculated that there is a "mobile" pool of Fe^{3+}, presumably bound to a material chelate such as ATP to maintain the availability of the iron. Deferoxamine binds with accessible molecules of Fe^{3+}, making it unavailable for conversion to the transition state and formation of $HO^\cdot$ from H_2O_2.

Experimentally, treatment of animals undergoing acute vascular injury with deferoxamine affords a high degree of protection.[22,23] In this animal model system, the infusion of a potent activator of complement, the cobra venom factor, results in intravascular formation of

C5a, activation of blood neutrophils, generation of oxyradicals, and acute injury to endothelial cells. Pretreatment of animals with deferoxamine does not appear to alter the intracapillary accumulation of neutrophils within the lung interstitium, but a high degree of protection from injury is afforded, presumably because HO• cannot be formed in the absence of available Fe^{2+}. Although deferoxamine has considerable promise as a protective agent in these experimental animal model systems, the compound cannot readily be used in human clinical trials because of its toxicity in persons without iron overload, especially toxicity involving the central nervous system and the retina.[2]

As could be predicted from the preceding comments, inhibitors of xanthine oxidase can be expected to be useful in situations in which this enzyme contributes to the generation of oxyradicals. In the animal model previously described, treatment of animals with allopurinol or lodoxamide tromethamine attentuates the microvascular injury after infusion of the cobra venom factor.[19] These results are consistent with the earlier observation that, in the interaction of neutrophils and endothelial cells, a proportion of the endothelial cell injury appears to depend on products of xanthine oxidase contained within the endothelial cell.[13] As speculated earlier, it may be that the formation of O_2^- within the endothelial cell permits the reduction of Fe^{3+} to Fe^{2+}, which then can generate HO• after interaction with H_2O_2, which is diffusing from the neutrophil into the endothelial cell.[5] On the basis of this type of mechanism, it is not surprising that treatment with allopurinol only partially protects tissues from injury occurring during the inflammatory response.

One of the difficulties in generalizing this concept pertains to the fact that, in general, there is little evidence that human endothelial cells contain xanthine oxidase, at least according to the conventional methods of enzyme measurement. Whether, in humans, xanthine oxidase-derived toxic oxygen metabolites are involved in inflammatory cell and tissue injury remains to be seen; however, an increasing body of experimental and clinical evidence supports the concept that oxyradicals play a significant role in the pathogenesis of various traumatic and disease states.

References

1. Achterberg PW, Nieukoop AS, Schoutsen B, et al: Different ATP-catabolism in reperfused adult and newborn rat hearts. *Am J Physiol* 1988;254:H1091–H1098.
2. Davies SC, Marcus RE, Hungerford JL, et al: Ocular toxicity of high-dose intravenous desferrioxamine. *Lancet* 1983;2:181–184.
3. Fantone JC, Ward PA: Role of oxygen-derived free radicals and metabolites in leukocyte-dependent inflammatory reactions. *Am J Pathol* 1982;107:395–418.
4. Friedl HP, Till GO, Trentz O, et al: Roles of histamine, complement and xanthine oxidase in thermal injury of skin. *Am J Pathol* 1989;135:203–218.
5. Gannon DE, Varani J, Phan SH, et al: Source of iron in neutrophil-mediated killing of endothelial cells. *Lab Invest* 1987;57:37–44.

6. Granger DN: Role of xanthine oxidase and granulocytes in ischemia-reperfusion injury. *Am J Physiol* 1988;255:H1269–H1275.
7. Huber AR, Weiss SJ: Disruption of the subendothelial basement membrane during neutrophil diapedesis in an in vitro construct of a blood vessel wall. *J Clin Invest* 1989;83:1122–1136.
8. Klebanoff SJ, Clark RA: *The Neutrophil: Function and Clinical Disorders.* Amsterdam, North Holland Publishing Co, 1978, pp 410–434.
9. Lackie JM: The behavioural repertoire of neutrophils requires multiple signal transduction pathways. *J Cell Sci* 1988;89:449–452.
10. Merritt TA, Cochrane CG, Holcomb K, et al: Elastase and alpha-proteinase inhibitor activity in tracheal aspirated during respiratory distress syndrome: Role of inflammation in the pathogenesis of bronchopulmonary dysplasia. *J Clin Invest* 1983;72:656–666.
11. Perez HD, Weksler BB, Goldstein IM: Generation of a chemotactic lipid from an arachidonic acid by exposure to a superoxide-generating system. *Inflammation* 1980;4:313–328.
12. Petrone WF, English DK, Wong K, et al: Free radicals and inflammation: Superoxide-dependent activation of a neutrophil chemotactic factor in plasma. *Proc Natl Acad Sci USA* 1980;77:1159–1163.
13. Phan SH, Gannon DE, Varani J, et al: Xanthine oxidase activity in rat pulmonary artery endothelial cells and its alteration by activated neutrophils. *Am J Pathol* 1989;134:1201–1211.
14. Schraufstätter I, Hyslop PA, Jackson JH, et al: Oxidant-induced DNA damage of target cells. *J Clin Invest* 1988;82:1040–1050.
15. Spragg RG, Hinshaw DB, Hyslop PA, et al: Alterations in adenosine triphosphate and energy charge in cultured endothelial and P388D1 cells after oxidant injury. *J Clin Invest* 1985;76:1471–1476.
16. Taylor A, Davies KJ: Protein oxidation and loss of protease activity may lead to cataract formation in the aged lens. *Free Radic Biol Med* 1987;3:371–377.
17. Till GO, Beauchamp C, Menapace D, et al: Oxygen radical dependent lung damage following thermal injury of rat skin. *J Trauma* 1983;23:269-277.
18. Till GO, Hatherill JR, Tourtellotte WW, et al: Lipid peroxidation and acute lung injury after thermal trauma to skin: Evidence of a role for hydroxyl radical. *Am J Pathol* 1985;119:376–384.
19. Till GO, Morganroth ML, Grum CM, et al: Dual source of oxygen radicals in complement-mediated acute microvascular lung injury. *FASEB J* 1988;2:A1185.
20. Varani J, Fligiel SE, Till GO, et al: Pulmonary endothelial cell killing by human neutrophils: Possible involvement of hydroxyl radical. *Lab Invest* 1985;53:656–663.
21. Vogt W, von Zabern I, Hesse D, et al: Generation of an activated form of human C5 (C5b-like C5) by oxygen radicals. *Immunol Lett* 1987;14:209–215.
22. Ward PA, Till GO, Hatherill JR, et al: Systemic complement activation, lung injury, and products of lipid peroxidation. *J Clin Invest* 1985;76:517–527.
23. Ward PA, Till GO, Kunkel R, et al: Evidence for role of hydroxyl radical in complement and neutrophil-dependent tissue injury. *J Clin Invest* 1983;72:789–801.
24. Warren JS, Johnson KJ, Ward PA: Oxygen radicals in cell injury and cell death. *Pathol Immunopathol Res* 1987;6:301–315.
25. Weiss SJ, Peppin GJ: Collagenolytic metalloenzymes of the human neutrophil: Characteristics, regulation and potential function in vivo. *Biochem Pharmacol* 1986;35:3189–3197.

Chapter 19

Interleukin-1 and Endothelial Vascular Response in Inflammation

Walter Newman, PhD
Norma Graber, MA
Diane Wilson

Introduction

Endothelial cells are major participants in chronic and acute inflammation. They regulate the passage of cells and fluids between the bloodstream and the extravascular space. In addition, they respond to inflammatory stimuli by secreting soluble peptide hormones such as growth factors, colony-stimulating factors, and interleukins. These secretions affect hematopoiesis, chemotaxis, and wound healing.

There are eight defined interleukins, originally named for their ability to mediate signals between cells of the leukocytic lineage. For example, with appropriate stimulation, monocytes secrete a small-molecular-weight protein, named lymphocyte-activating factor.[5] Lymphocyte-activating factor is a potent co-stimulatory agent that causes rapid activation of the T-lymphocyte subclass of leukocytes. In 1978, scientists agreed to call lymphocyte-activating factor interleukin-1. Interleukin-1 has a wide range of effects on cells in vitro and is pyrogenic in vivo.[8]

In general, the remaining interleukins (interleukin-2 to interleukin-8) have either growth-promoting or cellular-differentiative effects on leukocytes and/or their bone marrow precursors. Interleukins may also affect nonhematopoeitic cell types. As a result, the more general name of cytokines is used for any soluble protein secreted by a cell that has proliferative or differentiative effects on similar cells or other cell types. Gallin and associates[4] examined many of these cytokines and their role in the inflammatory process, and Balkwill and Burke[1] developed a schematic overview of the known cytokines and their various properties.

Particular attention has been focused on the role of interleukin-1 in the inflammatory process. Interleukin-1 is secreted by a wide range of cell types in response to injury. Interleukin-1 is found at inflammation sites such as rheumatoid synovial fluid. When subcutaneously injected as a purified protein in experimental animals, interleukin-1 causes erythema and an influx of granulocytes from the bloodstream to the site of injection. Because it is present at very defined compartments of injury, interleukin-1 does not meet the classical definition of a hormone, which, to exert its effects, must circulate through the bloodstream. Neta and Oppenheim[7] reviewed the relevance of interleukin-1 for clinicians.

Endothelial cells respond rapidly to interleukin-1 consistent with their accessory nature in the inflammatory reaction. Procoagulant activity increases,[2] and there is a concomitant increase in adhesive capacity for granulocytes and monocytes.[3] This chapter describes a new endothelial cell surface antigen (a glycoprotein) that forms as a consequence of interleukin-1 treatment and that may play a role in the pro-inflammatory adhesive reaction. Several components of this response are resistant to dexamethasone. This suggests that there may be additional modes of intervention in the chronic inflammatory process that may lead to continued tissue destruction rather than healing. A key question is whether interleukin-1 actually participates in soft-tissue injuries.

An experiment using human cells in tissue-culture systems may suggest modes of intervention for the chronic steroid-resistant inflammatory process. Interleukin-1 quickly affects the endothelial lining of the blood vessel. Several laboratories have shown that the binding of leukocytes to the vascular wall is the first step in the emigration of the leukocytes into the tissue space. This process can be mimicked in vitro with interleukin-1 treatment of endothelial cells. Several aspects of this process may be related to the use of current anti-inflammatory agents of intervention.

A simple binding assay can monitor the effectiveness of any proposed anti-inflammatory agents. In constructing the assay, monolayer cultures of human endothelial cells are exposed for a short time to physiologic concentrations of interleukin-1. After the interleukin-1 is removed, leukocytes are added to the cultures and bind to the endothelial cells. Figure 1 shows this process. A human myelomonocytic tumor cell substitutes for normal human monocytes, because the adhesion process is the same. There is a dramatic increase in the number of cells bound to the endothelial cell monolayer treated with interleukin-1.

This assay can also be performed in a quantitative manner. The kind of data generated is shown in Table 1. To illustrate the generality of this event, other agents that induce the adhesive capacity in endothelial cells are also shown. Interleukin-1 induces a fivefold increase in the binding of tumor cells. Significant, although smaller, increases were seen with bacterial endotoxin and the protein tumor necrosis factor, another mediator of inflammation. Thrombin has been shown to stimulate endothelial cells to become adhesive for granulocytes or monocytes, in addition to its procoagulant effect. This has additional significance for the inflammatory process, but is not shown here. Hence, both inflammatory and thrombotic stimuli can lead to adhesion and emigration of leukocytes, an important early and presumably continuing process in chronic inflammation.

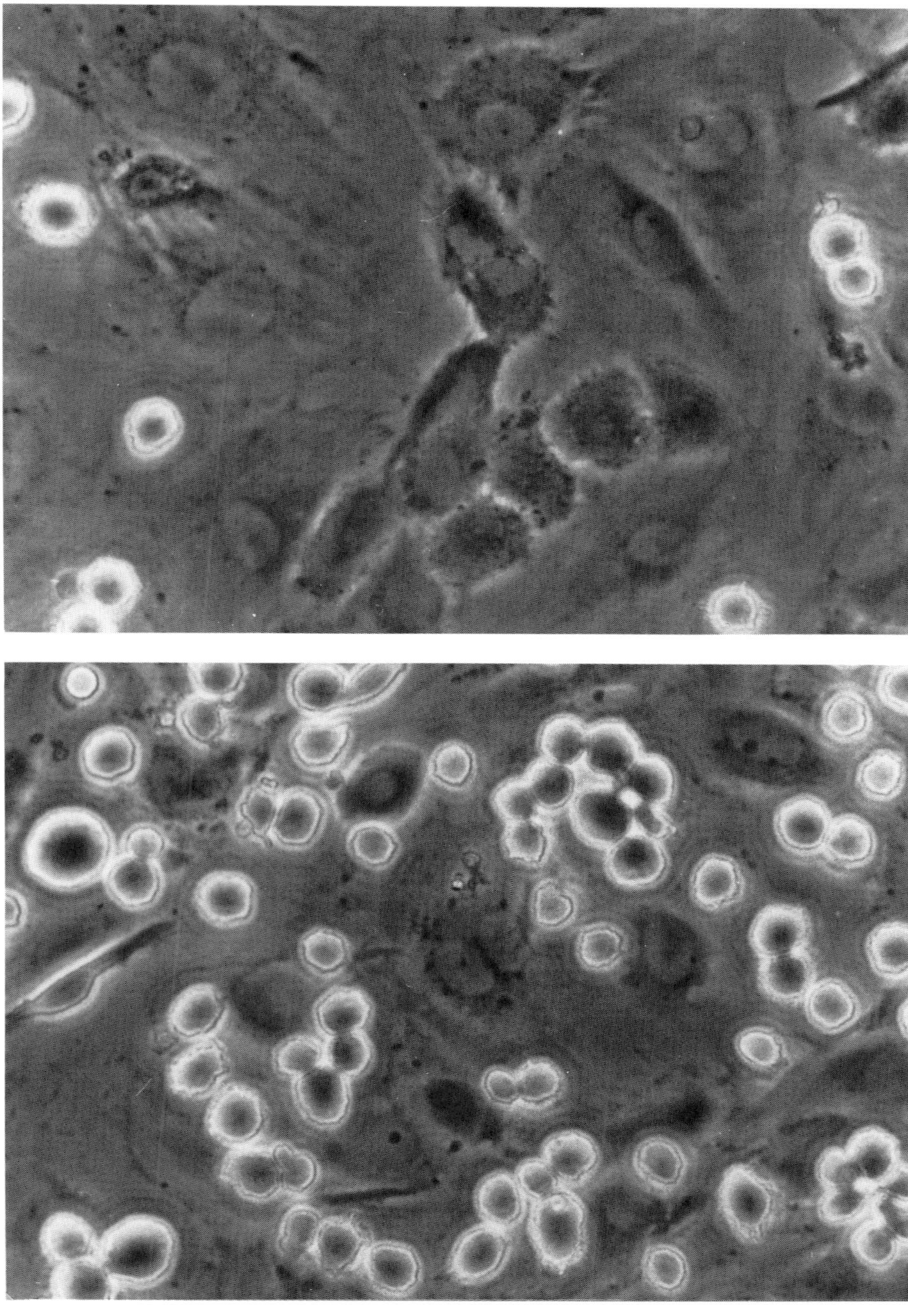

Fig. 1 ***Top,*** *Untreated endothelial cells essentially incapable of binding a monocyte-like cell line (THP-1).* ***Bottom,*** *Endothelial cells activated by interleukin-1 with many bound THP-1 cells.*

Table 1 Effect of inflammatory agents on the development of adhesiveness by cultured human endothelial cells*

Pretreatment of Endothelial Cells	Myelomonocytic Tumor Cell Bound (cpm)	Antibody Bound (cpm)
None	364	933
Interleukin-1	4,588	8,710
Endotoxin	1,178	4,204
Tumor necrosis factor	7,312	10,257

*Endothelial cells were exposed to 1 ng/ml of interleukin-1, 1μg/ml of *Escherichia coli* endotoxin, or 100 U/ml of recombinant tumor necrosis factor for four hours at 37 C; they were then rinsed to remove added inducers and overlaid with HL-60 tumor cells labeled with ^{51}Cr. After one hour for binding, the nonadherent cells were removed by gentle rinsing; the monolayers were solubilized in 1% Triton X-100 detergent and the supernatants counted in a gamma counter. In separate wells with the same regimen of pretreatments, endothelial cells were treated with 5 μg/ml of 1E7 for one hour, rinsed, and incubated with ^{125}I-goat antimouse antibody for an additional hour. The cell monolayers were rinsed, solubilized, and counted as above.

Monoclonal Antibody 1E7 Reacts Only With Activated Endothelial Cells

To establish a more precise biochemical definition of the activation process that endothelial cells undergo in response to interleukin-1, a murine monoclonal antibody called 1E7 was developed. It has the ability to react preferentially with endothelial cells pretreated with interleukin-1 for four hours, but it is essentially unreactive with untreated endothelial cells. Graber and associates[6] described this antibody in greater detail. Table 1 shows that activated endothelial cells bind a large amount of 1E7. A close correlation exists between the expression of the 1E7 antigen and the ability of activated endothelial cells to bind the myelomonocytic cell line. Additional experiments on the kinetics and dose-responsiveness of endothelial cells to interleukin-1 also show a close correlation between antigen expression and adhesiveness. This and other monoclonal antibodies, some of which block the adhesion of monocytes and granulocytes to "inflammatory" endothelial cells, are being tested for their in vivo anti-inflammatory properties. Those studying the mechanisms of sports-induced inflammation should test when possible for the presence of these pro-inflammatory adhesion proteins in the vasculature.

Effect of Dexamethasone on Endothelial Cell Activation by Interleukin-1

Glucocorticoids are widely used as anti-inflammatory agents in the treatment of chronic inflammation. Although their mechanism of action is not fully understood, in vitro experiments indicate that glucocorticoids can block the synthesis of inflammatory mediators such as interleukin-1. The effects of dexamethasone on the adhesion assay described have been investigated. One objective of the investigation was to determine whether the response of endothelial cells to interleukin-1, resulting in increased adhesive capacity for leukocytes, might

Table 2 Dexamethasone fails to block endothelial cell activation induced by interleukin-1*

Dexamethasone Concentration	Pretreatment Time (hr)	Endothelial Cell Pretreatment	Bound Cells (cpm)	Bound 1E7 Antibody (cpm)
None	24	None	230	ND
None	48	None	155	ND
None	24	Interleukin-1	4,629	47,558
None	48	Interleukin-1	4,422	51,567
10^{-6}	24	Interleukin-1	3,807	50,602
10^{-6}	48	Interleukin-1	4,959	55,797
10^{-7}	24	Interleukin-1	3,008	46,947
10^{-7}	48	Interleukin-1	4,737	49,257
10^{-8}	24	Interleukin-1	3,383	47,185
10^{-8}	48	Interleukin-1	3,298	52,279

*Endothelial cells were cultured for 24 or 48 hours before 1 ng/ml of interleuki-1 was added at the indicated concentrations of dexamethasone. Endothelial cells were cultured with drug during the pretreatment. Replicate plates were set up for either the adhesion assay or the antibody-binding experiment and processed as described in Table 1.

be another locus for the action of this anti-inflammatory agent. A second objective was to determine why certain patients do not respond to glucocorticoid therapy for chronic inflammation. Dexamethasone was tested at a range of concentrations and over a period of 24 to 48 hours preceding and including the interleukin-1 activation step to see whether it could block either the acquisition of adhesiveness or the expression of the 1E7 antigen. Table 2 shows the results of that experiment. Even at a concentration of 1 μmol, dexamethasone reduced neither adhesion nor antigen expression.

Conclusions

The prominent role played by endothelial cells in the inflammatory process means that a better understanding of that participation is necessary for the design of new methods of treating chronic inflammation. Improved understanding would also allow investigators to pose new questions about sports-induced trauma and inflammation. The adhesion of monocytes to the vessel wall is an important early step in the inflammatory process. Interleukin-1, tumor necrosis factor, or other as yet undiscovered pro-inflammatory cytokines may induce the adhesive capacity of endothelial cells for monocytes. This capacity can be studied with the described in vitro model system. Monitoring the acquisition of adhesiveness or the expression of the activation antigen 1E7 shows that the activation process is not blocked by the use of dexamethasone. This has two potential consequences. First, it may help explain why certain patients do not respond to treatment with glucocorticoids. Biopsy specimens from sites of chronic inflammation that express the IE7 antigen despite the administration of dexamethasone may help indicate why the treatment is unsuccessful. Second, the inability of glucocorticoids to block the endothelial cell activation process suggests that there may be an earlier phase of the inflammatory process that is amenable to intervention. It may be possible to devise strategies for interfering with the adhesion step in vivo that will lead to therapies that could be used alone or in conjunction with steroid application.

References

1. Balkwill FR, Burke F: The cytokine network. *Immunol Today* 1989;10:299–304.
2. Bevilacqua MP, Pober JS, Majeau GR, et al: Interleukin 1 (IL-1) induces biosynthesis and cell surface expression of procoagulant activity in human vascular endothelial cells. *J Exp Med* 1984;160:618–623.
3. Bevilacqua MP, Pober JS, Wheeler ME, et al: Interleukin 1 acts on cultured human vascular endothelium to increase the adhesion of polymorphonuclear leucocytes, monocytes, and related leukocyte cell lines. *J Clin Invest* 1985;76:2003–2011.
4. Gallin JI, Goldstein IM, Snyderman R (eds): *Inflammation: Basic Principles and Clinical Correlates.* New York, Raven Press, 1988, pp 195–264.
5. Gery I, Waksman BH: Potentiation of the T-lymphocyte response to mitogens: II. The cellular source of potentiating mediator(s). *J Exp Med* 1972;136:143–155.
6. Graber N, Gopal TV, Wilson D, et al: T-cells bind to cytokine activated endothelial cells via a novel, inducible sialoglycoprotein and ELAM-1. *J Immunol,* in press.
7. Neta R, Oppenheim JJ: Why should internists be interested in interleukin-1? *Ann Intern Med* 1988;109:1–3.
8. Oppenheim JJ, Kovacs EL, Matsushima K, et al: There is more than one interleukin 1. *Immunol Today* 1986;7:45–56.

Chapter 20

Mechanically Induced Synovitis

Mary L. Moran, MD
William J. Arnold, MD

Mechanically induced synovitis in joints, bursae, and tendon sheaths produces pain, swelling, and stiffness in a localized area. Warmth, erythema, and systemic features such as fever, anorexia, and weight loss are not as prominent in mechanically induced synovitis as they are in the systemic inflammatory arthritides such as rheumatoid and psoriatic arthritis. Specific examples of mechanically induced synovitis include Achilles tendinitis and plantar fasciitis in runners and rotator cuff impingement syndrome in competitive swimmers.

Few histopathologic studies of mechanically induced synovitis have been reported, because most of the overuse injuries causing this condition are treated conservatively.[1,4,11,13] Mechanically induced synovitis requiring surgical intervention has usually reached a chronic, fibrotic, and occasionally destructive stage that does not accurately depict the acute form.[1]

Mechanically induced synovitis in the joint, bursa, or tendon sheath has traditionally been ascribed to mechanisms of overuse, overload, or direct trauma. However, a complex array of environmental factors, such as the nature and type of sporting activity, also play a role in the initiation of mechanically induced synovitis. The training environment and schedule are also important in its pathogenesis. Most cases can be treated conservatively, by modifying the training environment and the individual characteristics of the athlete. The multidisciplinary treatment team must encourage the athlete to follow this approach and to avoid using combinations of analgesics and anti-inflammatory medications that allow continued abuse and create the potential for irreversible damage to mechanically inflamed synovial tissues.

As seen in Outline 1, the training environment can include extrinsic factors such as training error, preconditioning training, poor performance, poor technique, and inappropriate services.[8,10,11] Individual characteristics can include intrinsic factors such as leg-length discrepancy, pes planus, pes cavus, malalignment, scoliosis, and muscle imbalance. Most of these extrinsic and intrinsic factors can be modified to some degree to minimize the development of mechanically induced synovitis.

Outline 1 Etiologic factors in the development of mechanically induced synovitis

Training environment
- Poor preconditioning
- Poor technique
- Inappropriate equipment
- Training errors

Personal characteristics of athlete
- Leg-length discrepancy
- Scoliosis
- Pes planus; pes cavus
- Malalignment
- Excess weight
- Muscle imbalance

Sport
- Running (feet, ankles, knees, hips)
- Swimming (shoulders, neck)
- Tennis (shoulders, elbows)
- Rowing (spine, ischial region, sacroiliac joints)

Two sporting activities in which mechanically induced synovitis frequently occurs are running and swimming.

Mechanically Induced Synovitis in Runners

Runners have a high incidence of injury, especially to the foot, ankle, and knee.[3,6,14] The personal characteristics of runners commonly associated with mechanically induced synovitis are pes planus, pes cavus, leg-length discrepancy, femoral neck anteversion, quadriceps and hamstring insufficiency, excessive pronation (rearfoot valgus), muscular imbalance (sometimes a result of training techniques), lateral displacement of the patella, and a patellofemoral Q angle of more than 20 degrees.[11]

In a review of 1,650 runners by Clement and associates[4]; the most common anatomic features leading to mechanically induced synovitis included leg-length discrepancy, femoral neck anteversion, and quadriceps and hamstring insufficiency. These examples underscore the importance of evaluating the entire lower extremity in runners with mechanically induced synovitis. The physician should examine both lower extremities; observe body habitus, stance, and gait from the front and rear; measure leg length; evaluate hip (anteversion and retroversion), knee (varus, valgus, recurvatum), and tibial (internal and external torsion) alignment; and evaluate patellar and tibiotalar mechanics.[10,14] Finally, the examination should include a detailed study of the feet and the pattern of wear on the runner's shoes. This may give clear evidence of prolonged or excessive pronation or supination.[10,14] Muscle flexibility should be evaluated and attention given to the external rotators of the hip, the hamstrings, and the gastrocnemius and iliopsoas muscles.

In running, the training environment and extrinsic factors must also

Outline 2 Most prevalent causative factors in Achilles tendinitis*

Training errors
- Sudden increase in mileage
- Uphill training
- Single severe session
- Combination

Alignment factors
- Varus, with functional pronation
- Valgus, pes cavus foot

Other
- Gastrocnemius, soleus insufficiency
- Ineffective footwear

*Adapted with permission from Clement DB, Taunton JE, Smart GW: Achilles tendinitis and peritendinitis: Etiology and treatment. *Am J Sports Med* 1984;12:179-184.

be considered, particularly for athletes with Achilles tendinitis or plantar fasciitis. Many training errors lead to muscle imbalance, and training errors have been reported in 60% to 80% of running injuries. The most common mistakes in a runner's training program are excessive distance, sudden increases in mileage or intensity, and hill running. Specific guidelines[10] suggesting overuse in an athlete running more than 15 miles per week are an increase in mileage of more than 10% per month; a single run longer than three times the average daily mileage, speed training before achieving 25 miles per week for three months, frequent hill training, a return to previous mileage after a layoff, and continuous high mileage (more than 25 miles per week).

Running surfaces present an array of training problems that can lead to mechanically induced synovitis. Running on slippery, uneven surfaces, running in the same direction on a cambered surface, running on artificial turf, and hill running can all contribute to injury. Other extrinsic factors important for runners include stiff shoes and hard surfaces such as asphalt and cement.[14]

The clearest examples of the interaction among training environment, sport, and athlete in the initiation of mechanically induced synovitis are Achilles peritendinitis and plantar fasciitis.[7,8,10]

The pain in plantar fasciitis, or heel spur syndrome, is secondary to inflammation at the origin of the plantar fascia at the calcaneal tuberosity. These athletes complain of heel and arch pain. There is pain on palpation of the plantar fascia at its medial insertion on the calcaneus and pain on forced dorsiflexion of the toes. In most cases of plantar fasciitis, a pronated or pes cavus foot deformity is found.[3,10] Successful therapy begins with rest, ice, compression, and possibly anti-inflammatory medication, followed by a graduated exercise program and use of a well-designed orthotic. When fitted with the proper orthotic, most runners are able to continue running.[3,8,10] Other measures include reducing the distances run, stretching exercises, and using custom orthotics designed to dissipate stress on the heel and plantar fascia.

Achilles peritendinitis commonly causes gradual evolution of diffuse

Table 1 Prevalence of varus alignment in Achilles tendinitis*

Varus Alignment	No. of Cases
Unremarkable (0 to 2 degrees)	13
Mild (3 to 6 degrees)	35
Moderate (7 to 10 degrees)	49
Severe (more than 10 degrees)	12
Total	109

*Adapted with permission from Clement DB, Taunton JE, Smart GW: Achilles tendinitis and peritendinitis: Etiology and treatment. *Am J Sports Med* 1984;12:179–184.

heel pain with running. It is also associated with morning stiffness, tenderness, swelling, and, in the later stages, nodules and crepitus. An athlete susceptible to Achilles peritendinitis may exhibit tight gastrocnemius and iliopsoas muscles and pronation as a result of subtalar and forefoot varus. As shown in Outline 2, these characteristics lead to functional overpronation during weightbearing.[6] Normal subtalar varus of 3 degrees is optimal; increasing subtalar varus may play a role in the development of Achilles tendinitis (Table 1).

Mechanically Induced Synovitis in Swimmers

Mechanically induced synovitis in competitive swimmers also results from the combination of sport, the athlete's personal characteristics, and the training environment. The most common example is the rotator cuff impingement syndrome.[2,5,8,12,15] This syndrome of "mechanical impingement" of the rotator cuff (supraspinatus and biceps) on the coracoacromial arch occurs when the arm is fully abducted in freestyle, butterfly, backstroke, and synchronized swimming. This motion brings the rotator cuff against the anterior portion of the acromion. Repeated microtrauma to the bursa and rotator cuff tendons leads to inflammation, pain, and eventual thickening of the bursa.[5,9,15]

Swimmers force their shoulders through thousands of revolutions each day. The pain occurs at the junction of the recovery and pull-through phases of the stroke. There is tenderness anteriorly and superiorly in the shoulder, beneath and lateral to the coracoacromial arch. The pain can be reproduced during an examination when the arm is flexed and then internally rotated.

Common factors contributing to rotator cuff impingement syndrome in swimmers include training with hand paddles, anatomic variations, unilateral breathing, and competitive swimming for more than ten years. Certain anatomic features acquired by competitive swimmers predispose them to shoulder impingement syndrome. Competitive swimmers usually have relatively weak posterior shoulder musculature and poor upper-body posture with rounded shoulders. These factors probably increase their vulnerability to anterior shoulder problems. Exercise programs to strengthen the shoulder and scapular muscle groups are important because routine stroke work in the pool does not accomplish this.

Rotator cuff impingement in a swimmer's shoulder is reversible. Initial treatment includes ice and a reduction in the length and intensity of workouts. Other necessary measures include discontinuing the use of hand paddles and learning bilateral breathing techniques.[5,15]

Treatment of Mechanically Induced Synovitis

Mechanically induced synovitis responds well to conservative treatment. The universal approach in the acute stage is rest, ice, and, if possible, compression. In most cases, athletes should rest until the symptoms resolve. It is not appropriate to tell an athlete to give up the sport. If a runner must stop running for a period of time, participation in an alternative aerobic sport, such as swimming or bicycling, should be encouraged. When competitive swimmers are out of the water with rotator cuff impingement they should be encouraged to continue aerobic lower-extremity workouts in the water or on land to maintain cardiovascular fitness. [1,5,12]

It is appropriate and therapeutic to help the athlete understand the type of synovitis and the anatomic and environmental factors that may contribute to this problem. The athlete must understand the potential danger of using analgesics, nonsteroidal anti-inflammatory drugs, and corticosteroid injections. These treatments may give enough short-term relief for the athlete to continue intensive, improper training, an approach that can lead to irreversible fibrotic changes in the involved tissues. The use of nonsteroidal anti-inflammatory drugs, corticosteroid injections, and surgery should be reserved for chronic recalcitrant injuries that have not responded to conservative management and modifications in training and in individual characteristics.

Finally, overuse mechanically induced synovitis can be prevented in most cases by emphasizing preseason conditioning, muscle strengthening, and stretching before and after workouts.

References

1. Beck JL, Day RW: Overuse injuries. *Clin Sports Med* 1985;4:553–573.
2. Brunet ME, Haddad RJ Jr, Porche EB: Rotator cuff impingement syndrome in sports. *Phys Sportsmed* 1982;10:86–94.
3. Clement DB, Taunton JE, Smart GW: Achilles tendinitis and peritendinitis: Etiology and treatment. *Am J Sports Med* 1984;12:179–184.
4. Clement DB, Taunton JE, Smart GW, et al: A survey of overuse running injuries. *Phys Sportsmed* 1981;9:47–58.
5. Dominguez RH: Shoulder pain in swimmers. *Phys Sportsmed* 1980;8:37–42.
6. James SL, Bates BT, Osternig LR: Injuries to runners. *Am J Sports Med* 1978;6:40–50.
7. James SL, Brubaker CE: Biomechanics of running. *Orthop Clin North Am* 1973;4:604–615.
8. Lehman WL Jr: Overuse syndromes in runners. *Am Fam Physician* 1984;29:157–161.
9. Neer CS II: Anterior acromioplasty for the chronic impingement syndrome in the shoulder: A preliminary report. *J Bone Joint Surg* 1972;54A:41–50.

10. Paty JG Jr: Diagnosis and treatment of musculoskeletal running injuries. *Semin Arthritis Rheum* 1988;18:48–60.
11. Renström P, Johnson RJ: Overuse injuries in sports: A review. *Sports Med* 1985;2:316–333.
12. Richardson AB, Jobe FW, Collins HR: The shoulder in competitive swimming. *Am J Sports Med* 1980;8:159–163.
13. Seitz WH Jr, Froimson AI, Shapiro JD: Chronic impingement syndrome: The role of ultrasonography and arthroscopic anterior acromioplasty. *Orthop Rev* 1989;18:364–375.
14. Taunton JE, Clement DB, Smart GW, et al: Non-surgical management of overuse knee injuries in running. *Can J Sport Sci* 1987;12:11–18.
15. Weinberg, SK: Medical aspects of synchronized swimming. *Clin Sports Med* 1986;5:159–167.

Chapter 21

The Role of Joint Instability in Joint Inflammation and Cartilage Deterioration: A Study of the Glenohumeral Joint

Van C. Mow, PhD
Louis U. Bigliani, MD
Evan L. Flatow, MD
Roger G. Pollock, MD
May V. Parisien, MD
Louis J. Soslowsky, MS
Farshid Guilak, MS
Robert J. Pawluk, MS

Joint instability can significantly compromise the performance of the musculoskeletal system. Athletes with unstable joints commonly experience pain, giving way, and swelling that impair their ability to participate in sports activities. Prolonged vigorous use of an unstable joint frequently results in progressive deterioration of articular cartilage, increasing pain and producing further loss of joint function. Despite the importance of the relationship among joint instability, joint inflammation, and deterioration, the mechanisms of the effects of joint instability remain poorly understood. Although instability can adversely affect the function of any joint, instability of the shoulder and instability of the knee are the most common clinically significant problems. In this chapter, we examine the possible relationships between instability of the glenohumeral joint and joint deterioration.

Stability of the Glenohumeral Joint

In the short term, glenohumeral instability causes direct capsular damage and inflammation. The inflammatory response may result in contractures of the joint capsule, which may lead to altered subacromial mechanics, resulting in superimposed inflammation for secondary impingement. Over the longer term, it may lead to cartilage degeneration in the glenohumeral joint, perhaps by allowing abnormal motion that results in a shift in contact areas and pressures in the joint.

The glenohumeral joint has often been called a shallow "ball-and-socket" joint (Fig. 1). This simple geometric representation has been used to construct kinematic and biomechanical models of the shoulder and to design prostheses.[15,58] However, unlike the hip joint, which more truly resembles a ball and deep socket, the glenohumeral joint is a

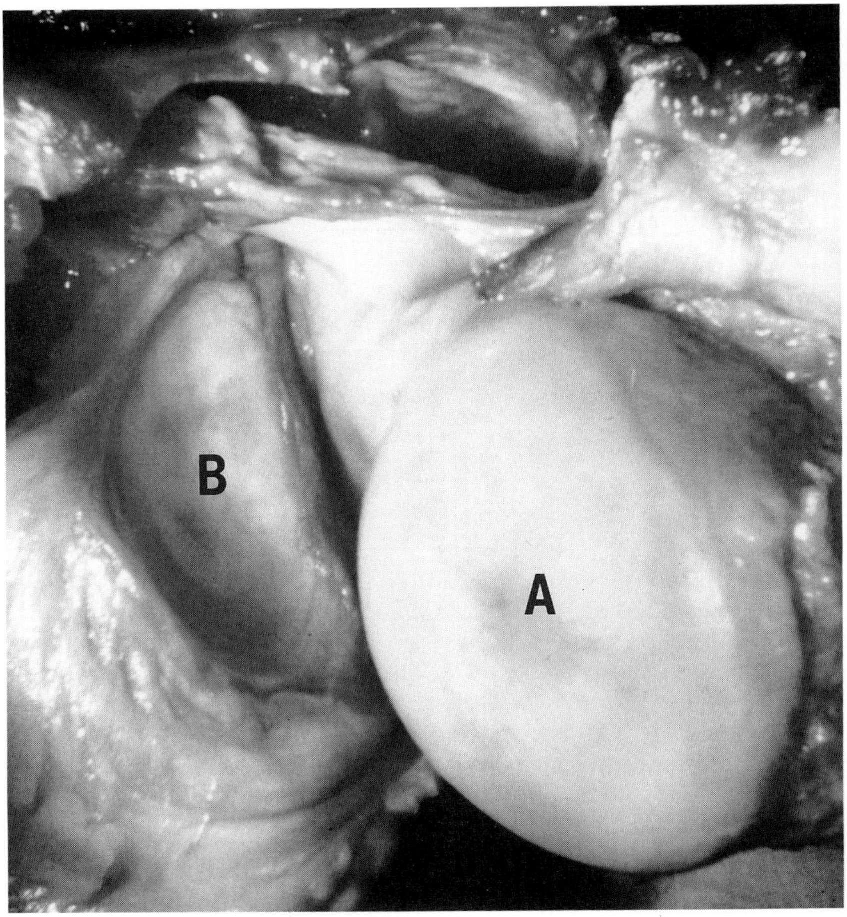

Fig. 1 *Photograph of the humeral head (A) and glenoid (B) showing the minimally constrained nature of the bony articulation.*

minimally constrained articulation. The surface area of the humeral head is three to four times that of the glenoid, and most of the articular surface of the head of the humerus is "out of the socket" because of the shallowness of the glenoid surface.[63] In addition, the transverse and vertical dimensions of the glenoid with respect to those of the humeral head (ie, glenohumeral indices), the amount of glenoid tilt, and the degree of humeral retrotorsion all provide stability for the glenohumeral joint. Most authors, however, emphasize the primacy of the surrounding soft-tissue structures in providing glenohumeral joint stability. These structures can be classified as either dynamic or static stabilizers.

Dynamic Stability

Dynamic stability is provided by the interaction of the rotator cuff muscles: the subscapularis, supraspinatus, infraspinatus, and teres minor. Magnuson[37] believed that the shoulder muscles were "the only structures which maintain the head of the humerus in contact with the glenoid and in proper position." Symeonides[69] discovered lesions of the subscapularis muscle in nearly all of his surgical cases and thought that subscapularis lengthening was the prime factor in producing instability of the shoulder. Electromyographic analyses of the shoulder during throwing have shown that, in normal shoulders, the activation of the subscapularis occurs in the late cocking stage, presumably to decelerate the external rotation of the shoulder. Moreover, in throwers with instability, there is a marked reduction in subscapularis activity, as well as in the activity of other internal rotators of the shoulder, suggesting a role for subtle differences in neuromuscular control in anterior instability.[17] The supraspinatus, infraspinatus, and teres minor were shown by Inman and associates[28] to be active continuously throughout both abduction and flexion, and also to play a role in depressing the humeral head as well as in compressing it against the glenoid. In this manner, the rotator cuff stabilizes the joint against the vertical (shearing) component of force exerted by the deltoid. More recently, Cain and associates[11] used a cadaver model to show that the posterior rotator cuff can reduce strain in the anterior structures of the glenohumeral joint by pulling the humeral head posteriorly during external rotation of the shoulder. Finally, Glousman and associates[17] have shown decreased electromyographic activity of the serratus anterior in throwers with anterior instability. They pointed out that decreased activity of this muscle diminishes protraction of the scapula at a time when the humerus is flexing forward and rotating externally. This results in further stress to the anterior supporting structures, perhaps contributing to further joint laxity.

Static Stability

The static restraints to anterior instability are the synovial joint lining, the joint capsule with its thickenings, known as the glenohumeral ligaments, and the glenoid labrum (Fig. 2). Most substantial of these tissues are the superior, middle, and inferior glenohumeral ligaments (SGHL, MGHL, and IGHL, respectively), which were first described by Schlemm in 1853.[44] The SGHL originates in the supraglenoid region and inserts onto the humerus adjacent to the anatomic neck near the tip of the lesser tuberosity. Because of its location, it is not a significant stabilizer against anterior displacement of the humeral head. The MGHL is a thick band originating from the anterosuperior quadrant of the glenoid and inserting onto the lesser tuberosity with the subscapularis tendon, to which it is adherent. The IGHL originates from the anteroinferior and posteroinferior quadrants of the glenoid and extends to the inferior region of the anatomic neck and the surgical

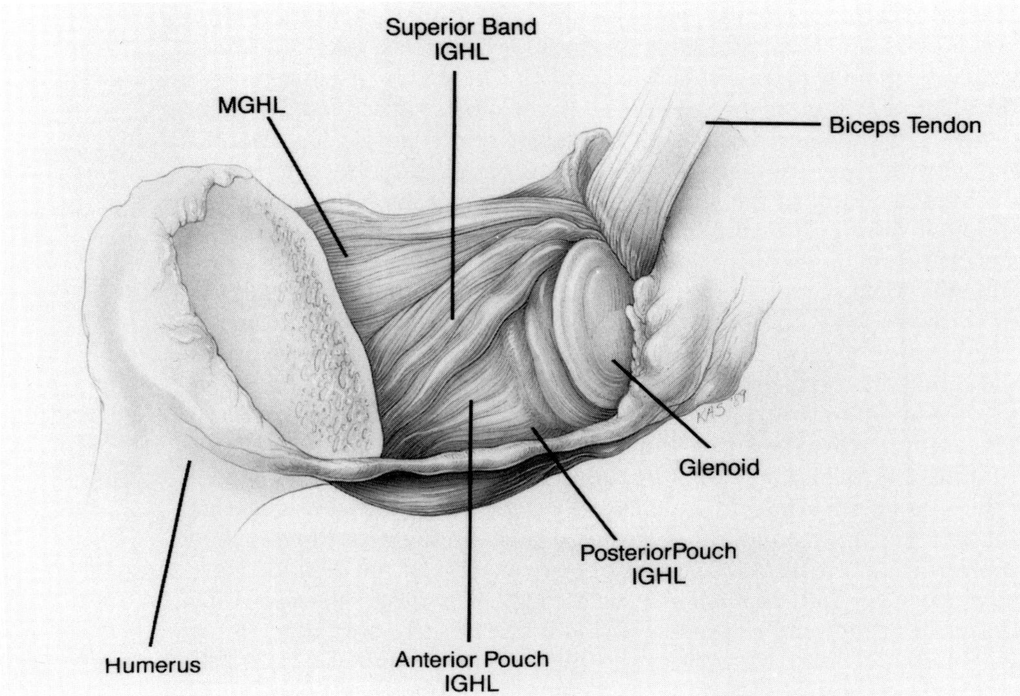

Fig. 2 *Schema of the glenohumeral ligaments, viewed with the joint capsule opened posteriorly. The IGHL demonstrates a prominent superior band as well as anterior and posterior axillary regions.*

neck of the humerus. Turkel and associates[73] subdivided this ligament into three regions: a superior band, which is most often the thickest portion of the capsule (in their dissections and in our own current series of approximately 20 fresh-frozen cadaver specimens); and an axillary pouch, which is subdivided into anterior and posterior regions. O'Brien and associates[53] provided a new nomenclature for the IGHL, as they described a posterior thickening comparable to the Turkel superior band—a "hammock-like" IGHL with anterior and posterior bands and a central axillary pouch.

The function of the anterior capsular structures has been a source of controversy. Bankart[7,8] stated that "the essential anatomical defect" causing recurrent anterior instability was the detachment of the fibrocartilaginous glenoid ligament (labrum) from the anterior margin of the glenoid (Fig. 2). Bost and Inman[9] expanded Bankart's emphasis on the labrum, referring to it as a ring of dense fibrocartilaginous tissue, which deepens the glenoid and enhances glenohumeral stability. Townley,[72] however, thought that the significance of the labrum as a mechanical stabilizer had been overstated. He demonstrated that in the abducted, externally rotated position, the labrum and the humeral head are not even in contact when the capsule is intact. In addition, with the labrum dissected away, stability of the joint is maintained as long as the remaining capsular insertion into the scapular neck is undisturbed. Townley introduced instead the concept of "the capsular mechanism," in which the entire capsule functions as an effective barrier against anterior instability. McLaughlin[43] suggested that the anterior glenoid labrum is merely an appendage of the IGHL and that separation of the IGHL from the glenoid rim is the significant lesion. Moseley and Overgaard[44] further clarified the nature of the capsular mechanism with a histologic study of the various anterior tissues, including the labrum. They observed that the labrum was not a consistent fibrocartilaginous disk like the meniscus of the knee; rather, it represented a redundant fold of fibrous capsular tissue with very little fibrocartilage.[44] Our dissections support the view that the labrum does not resemble the knee meniscus: it does not appear to deepen the glenoid or to bear load directly. Rather, it appears to represent a portion of the insertion of the IGHL into the glenoid.

Turkel and associates[73] performed a series of radiographic studies using radiopaque markers to demonstrate the position and tightness or laxity of the anterior structures (subscapularis muscle, MGHL, and IGHL) with varying positions of abduction and external rotation of the arm. These radiographic studies were then supplemented by sequential ligament-cutting experiments in cadavers. At 0 degrees of abduction, with the arm in neutral rotation, all structures were visibly lax (Fig. 3, *top left*). As external rotation increased, the subscapularis, the MGHL, and the superior band of the IGHL tightened, while the axillary pouch appeared redundant (Fig. 3, *top right*). At 45 degrees of abduction, in neutral rotation, the subscapularis and superior band of the IGHL became taut, while the axillary pouch remained relaxed (Fig. 3, *bottom left*). As external rotation increased in this position of abduction, the subscapularis became tighter, but it also began to rise with respect to the humeral head. The superior band of the IGHL also became taut and provided support at the inferior surface of the humeral head. Finally, at 90 degrees of abduction with neutral rotation, the subscapularis and superior band of the IGHL were again tight across the anterior aspect of the joint. As external rotation increased, the subscapularis came to lie superior to the humeral head, while the superior band of the IGHL was taut across the midportion of the anterior surface of the joint, and the axillary pouch was stretched across the inferior portion of the joint (Fig. 3, *bottom right*). Their ligament-sectioning studies verified these observations and again demonstrated that no single structure stabilized the glenohumeral joint in all positions. With abduction of the arm, the stabilizing function shifts from the superior to the inferior structures.[73]

The functional roles of different aspects of the IGHL are schematically summarized in Figure 3. Using sequential ligament-sectioning studies, Ovesen and Nielsen[54] obtained similar results. Further, Ham-

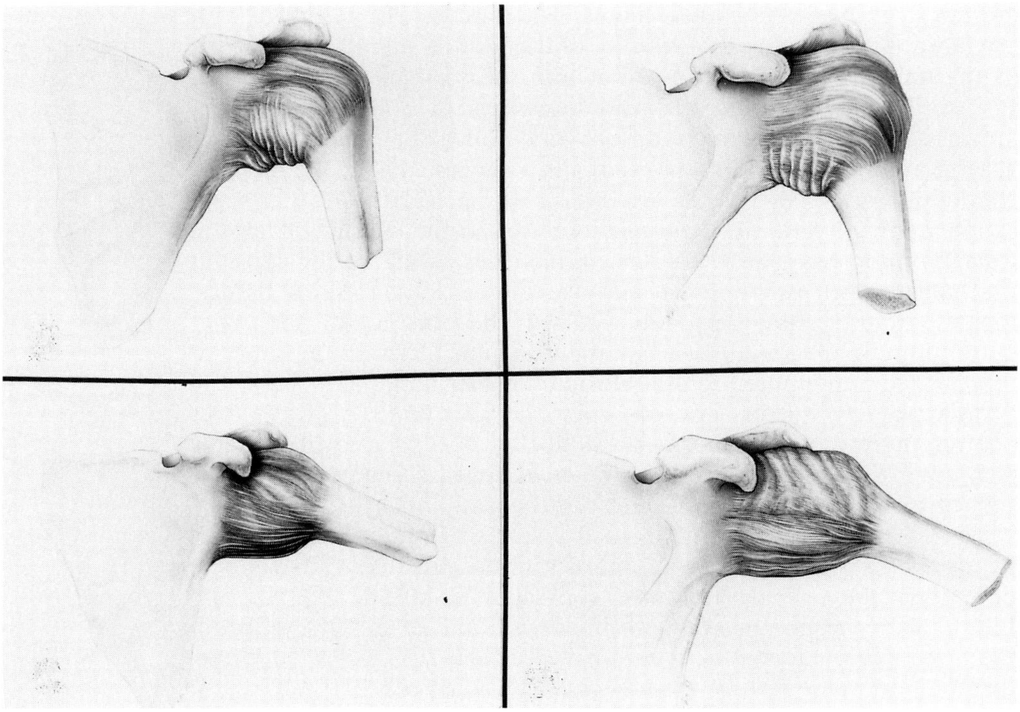

Fig. 3 *Schema of the capsular ligaments.* ***Top left,*** *With the arm in 0 degrees of abduction and 0 degrees of external rotation. The entire capsule is lax, and the inferior portions of the IGHL are redundant.* ***Top right,*** *With full external rotation, the MGHL and superior IGHL tighten, but the capsule remains lax inferiorly.* ***Bottom left,*** *The arm is in 90 degrees of abduction and O degrees of external rotation. The superior IGHL is now taut, and the axillary regions are no longer redundant.* ***Bottom right,*** *With increasing external rotation, the entire IGHL becomes taut, providing stability anteriorly and inferiorly.*

mon and associates[19] reported that different structures became primary restraints as the shoulder position changed, with the IGHL becoming primary for the "cocking position" during throwing—the combination of abduction, external rotation, and extension.

Articular Cartilage in the Shoulder

The shoulder experiences significant levels of compressive loading as the result of daily activities.[56] The magnitude of loading is expected to be high during competitive athletic activities, although no data exist to confirm this hypothesis. The pattern of load distribution on the glenohumeral joint surfaces depends on their anatomic shapes, their relative congruency, and the material properties of articular cartilage covering the joint surfaces. Excessive joint loading and abnormal patterns of loading at the joint surface, such as, for example, that associated with anterior instability, can lead to cartilage degeneration and osteoarthritis.[38] Although osteoarthritis of the shoulder is not as prevalent as that of the hip or knee, it is not an uncommon clinical problem.[52,65]

The specialized composition and ultrastructure of articular cartilage make it particularly suitable for withstanding the high stresses normally found within the joint.[45,50] Articular cartilage has two primary functions: (1) it distributes joint loading over a wide area, thus decreasing the stresses acting on the contacting articular surfaces; and (2) it allows relative movement of the opposing joint surfaces with minimal friction and wear.[3,46]

These functions of articular cartilage are determined by the physical properties of the tissue. In turn, these properties are controlled by tissue composition and the organization of the various components within the cartilaginous matrix. The extracellular matrix is composed of a dense network of fine collagen (type II) fibrils enmeshed in a concentrated solution of proteoglycans. The collagen and proteoglycan content of cartilage is approximately 20% and 5% by wet weight, respectively[50]; the remaining 75% is water, inorganic salts, and small amounts of other matrix proteins, glycoproteins, and lipids.[40,50,75] Collagen fibrils and proteoglycans are the main structural components of cartilage that support the joint and enable it to withstand the mechanical stresses developed within the tissue from loading.[1,32,45]

The collagen in articular cartilage has a high level of structural organization. It is inhomogeneously distributed, giving the tissue a layered character.[12,35,76] From light, transmission electron, and scanning electron microscopic studies, three separate structural zones for the collagen network have been identified (Fig. 4). In the superficial tangential zone (10% to 20% of the total tissue thickness), sheets of fine, densely packed fibers are randomly woven in planes parallel to the articular surface.[35,76] In the middle zone (40% to 60% of the total thickness), there are greater distances between the randomly oriented and homogeneously dispersed fibers. Below this, in the deep zone (about 30% of the total thickness), the fibers come together, forming larger, radially oriented fiber bundles, which then cross the tidemark inserting into the calcified cartilage. In the calcified cartilage these fiber bundles tend to form an interlocking "root" system, anchoring the cartilage to the underlying bone.[59]

The most important mechanical properties of collagen fibers are their tensile stiffness and strength. Because of the pronounced layering pattern of collagen fibril organization, articular cartilage's tensile properties vary with depth in a manner reflecting the fibrous organization.[32,61,77] The tissue also exhibits anisotropic properties in planes parallel to the articular surface.[32,61,77] The anisotropic tensile properties of the tissue may be related to the varying amount of collagen and cross-link density in different directions within planes parallel to the articular surface. To date, however, those aspects of collagen organization that

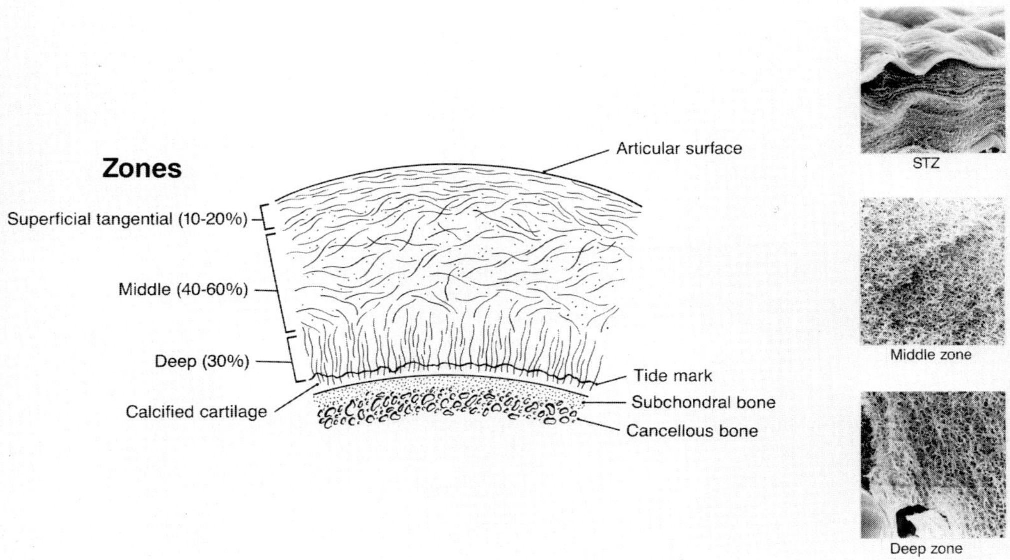

Fig. 4 *Schema and photomicrographs (× 3,000) of the ultrastructural arrangement of the collagen network throughout the depth of articular cartilage. (Reproduced with permission from Mow VC, Proctor CS, Kelly MA: Biomechanics of articular cartilage, in Nordin M, Frankel VH (eds):* Basic Biomechanics of the Musculoskeletal System. *Philadelphia, Lea & Febiger, 1989, p 34.)*

determine the pronounced anisotropic behavior of cartilage in tension are not known.[61,77]

Cartilage proteoglycans are large protein-polysaccharide molecules that exist in the tissue either as monomers or as aggregates.[20,22,50,60] A proteoglycan monomer consists of a long protein core to which approximately 150 glycosaminoglycan chains are covalently attached. Proteoglycan monomers may be visualized as having a bottle-brush-like structural arrangement, with the glycosaminoglycans attached to and radiating perpendicularly from the protein core (Fig. 5, *top*). In cartilage, most proteoglycan monomers associate with hyaluronate to form proteoglycan aggregates (Fig. 5, *bottom*). Recently it has been shown that proteoglycan aggregates and monomers can form elastic networks of considerable strength in solution, and the strength of the network formed by aggregates is significantly greater than that of monomers.[21,47] In cartilage, proteoglycans could also interact to form networks in the interfibrillar space, resulting in a stronger extracellular matrix. Moreover, many changes occurring in articular cartilage during maturation and degeneration result in alterations of the molecular structure of proteoglycans. These are, in turn, reflected in changes in

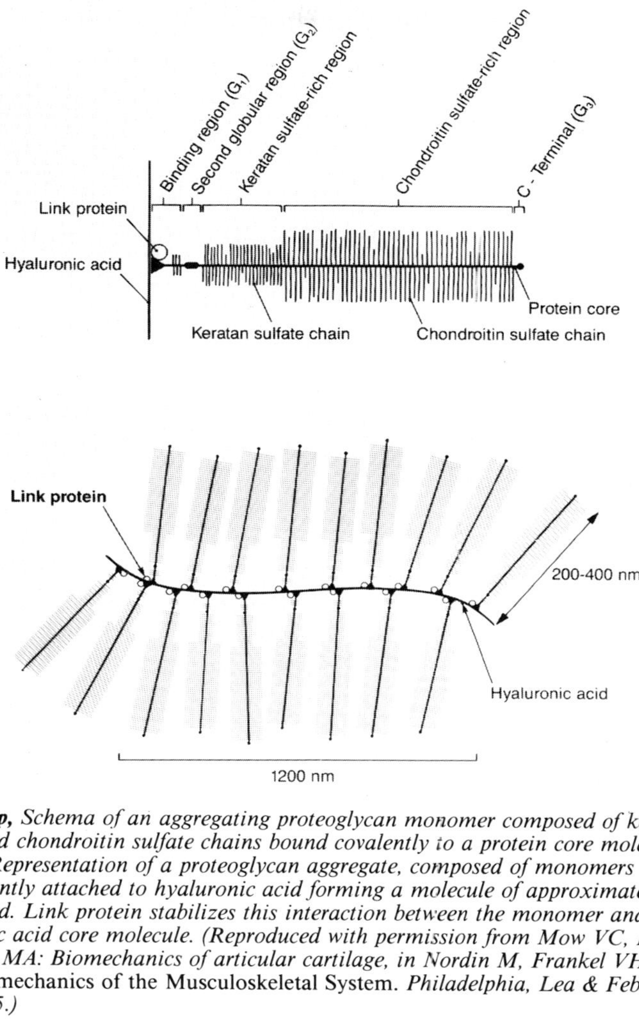

Fig. 5 ***Top,*** *Schema of an aggregating proteoglycan monomer composed of keratan sulfate and chondroitin sulfate chains bound covalently to a protein core molecule.* ***Bottom,*** *Representation of a proteoglycan aggregate, composed of monomers noncovalently attached to hyaluronic acid forming a molecule of approximately 200,000 kd. Link protein stabilizes this interaction between the monomer and the hyaluronic acid core molecule. (Reproduced with permission from Mow VC, Proctor CS, Kelly MA: Biomechanics of articular cartilage, in Nordin M, Frankel VH (eds):* Basic Biomechanics of the Musculoskeletal System. *Philadelphia, Lea & Febiger, 1989, p 35.)*

the physiochemical and biomechanical properties of cartilage, and thus its functional capacity in the joint.[3,40,45,46]

Water is the most abundant component of articular cartilage, constituting 70% to 80% of the tissue by weight.[36,40,45,71] A small percentage of this water is contained in the intracellular space, approximately 30% seems closely associated with the intrafibrillar space within collagen, and the remainder is contained in the molecular "pore" space of the extracellular matrix.[31,71] The water of articular cartilage plays important roles in organizing the extracellular matrix: (1) it is required for maintaining the proteoglycans of the extracellular matrix in solution; and

(2) together with proteoglycan, it modulates the diameter of the collagen fibrils.[31,45,49,50,71] Interstitial water may freely move under loading, and approximately 70% of the total water content may be forced out by compression.[13] Exudation of the interstitial fluid and the movement of this water through cartilage is the dominant mechanism controlling the compressibility of the tissue. Exudate from the tissue during compression contributes to the fluid film required for lubrication during diarthrodial joint function.[3,42,46] Interstitial fluid is also important in maintaining cartilage viability, because it permits the transport of the required nutrients and waste products between the chondrocytes in cartilage and the surrounding nutrient-rich synovial fluid.

The closely spaced (0.5 to 1.5 nm) negatively charged sulfate and carboxyl groups on the glycosaminoglycan chains of the proteoglycans create strong intramolecular and intermolecular charge-charge repulsive forces (Fig. 6). These forces tend to extend and stiffen the proteoglycans in the interfibrillar space formed by the collagen network. Mobile cations (eg, NA^{+} and Ca^{2+}) are attracted to the negatively charged groups of the proteoglycans within the extracellular matrix. These ions create a substantial osmotic swelling pressure (Donnan osmotic pressure) in cartilage. The magnitude of this swelling pressure is related to the density of the charged groups on the proteoglycans and the concentration of the counter-ions in the interstitial fluid.[40,41] When equilibrated in deionized water, the Donnan osmotic pressure of articular cartilage has been estimated to be 0.17 MPa.[40]

In the extracellular matrix, the swelling pressure is resisted and balanced by the tension developed in the collagen network surrounding the proteoglycan.[39] Consequently, this swelling pressure subjects the collagen network to a tensile stress even in the absence of external loads. Like collagen, cartilage proteoglycans are inhomogeneously distributed throughout the extracellular matrix—their concentration being highest in the middle zone and lowest in the superficial zone.[40,49] This non-uniform distribution causes an inhomogeneous swelling effect, which modulates the stress within the collagen network.

When an external stress is applied to the cartilage surface, the proteoglycan solution domain is decreased as the interstitial fluid flows out (Fig. 6). This results in an increase of the ion concentration in the interstitium, which, in turn, increases the Donnan osmotic swelling pressure and the charge-charge repulsive force. With compression, the bulk stress resisting the compression is also increased. Under load, equilibrium is achieved when the sum of these internal forces generated in the extracellular matrix is sufficient to balance the externally applied load on the tissue. In this manner, the physicochemical properties of the proteoglycans trapped in the extracellular matrix share the load carriage function of cartilage during compression. As indicated above, the Donnan osmotic pressure is 0.17 MPa at low compressive strains; at high compressive strains, this pressure may be as high as 0.5 MPa.[40] In physiologic solutions, the average elastic modulus of the extracellular matrix of human articular cartilage is approximately 0.78 MPa.[4] At high counter-ion concentrations (ie, without the Donnan osmotic

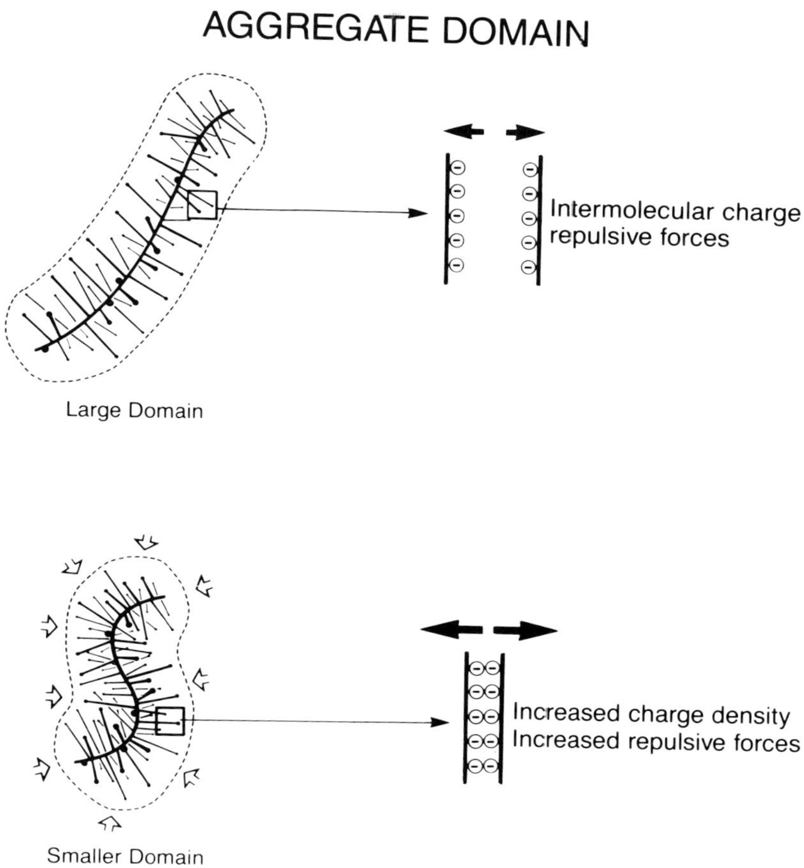

Fig. 6 *Proteoglycan aggregate domains.* ***Top,*** *Large domain and the repelling forces associated with the fixed negative charge groups on the glycosaminoglycans of a monomer.* ***Bottom,*** *Applied compressive stress decreases the aggregate solution domain, which in turn increases the charge density and thus the intermolecular charge repulsive forces. (Reproduced with permission from Mow VC, Proctor CS, Kelly MA: Biomechanics of articular cartilage, in Nordin M, Frankel VH (eds):* Basic Biomechanics of the Musculoskeletal System. *Philadelphia, Lea & Febiger, 1989, p 37.)*

pressure contribution), this modulus for bovine articular cartilage is approximately 0.45 MPa.[48] Thus, the Donnan osmotic pressure accounts for approximately 50% of the intrinsic compressive stiffness of articular cartilage.

Effects of Mechanical Environment on Articular Cartilage

Cartilage composition and properties vary with joint loading.[1,2] Some areas of the joint surface are habitually loaded (heavy weight-bearing areas).[1,2,29] Recently, several investigators have shown that alterations in the mechanical environment of the joint might alter the structure and composition of the cartilage.[29,55] Our hypothesis is that alteration of the joint-loading pattern resulting from primary anterior glenohumeral joint instability produces detrimental changes in articular cartilage that can lead to osteoarthritis.

In the 1960s, researchers began to characterize the histologic changes associated with abnormal stresses, generally involving immobilization and joint compression. Evans and associates[14] showed that early changes after immobilization include cartilage thinning, decreased chondrocyte size, and cleft formation. Salter and Field[64] noted late changes after immobilization with forced compression, similar to those changes documented by Evans and associates that were "limited to the area of the joint surfaces that had been in actual contact." Thaxter and associates[70] investigated the role of weightbearing, nonweightbearing, and rigidity of fixation on articular cartilage. They concluded that "pressures resulting from abnormal forced position are not necessary to produce degeneration of the immobilized joint," and that subjecting the joint to immobilization alone, without forced compression, was sufficient to induce these changes. From such early studies, it was postulated that such mechanically induced changes in articular cartilage were irreversible, could initiate arthritis, and were related to a decrease in the nutrient flow from the synovial fluid.

Recently, investigators began using in vivo animal models to evaluate how cartilage loading might modulate cartilage biochemistry. Kinzel and associates[33] demonstrated that the weightbearing region of the shoulders of dogs changed when they were made to ascend and descend a 21-cm step. In this model, lesions developed in the central caudal region, which is nonweightbearing during normal gait on level surfaces. This model directly evaluates the effects on cartilage of increased mechanical forces generated from weightbearing in regions not normally in contact. Hillberry and associates[24] also used an in vivo canine model to investigate the effects of increased mechanical loading on articular cartilage. Using an instrumented spatial linkage to measure the relative motion of the scapula and humerus in vivo, they developed a three-dimensional geometric representation of the surfaces of the joints. Moreover, using data from instrumented spatial linkages, they determined the relative position of the two surfaces and the corresponding contact areas between them. In a related study, Van Sickle and Hillberry[74] used this model to evaluate the effect of increased mechanical forces on the modulation of articular cartilage biochemistry in the central caudal region of the humeral head. They found that the increased mechanical forces increased the chondroitin sulfate content in the extracellular matrix of articular cartilage. Other investigators have also noted increased matrix proteoglycan content in canine articular cartilage after moderately increased mechanical loading. Further, moderately increased mechanical loading has been shown to increase the thickness of the articular cartilage. These experimental results indicate that increased mechanical loading promotes the metabolic activity of the chondrocytes, which results in an increase in the proteoglycan content of the matrix. This increase in the proteoglycan content may then augment the ability of articular cartilage to resist compressive loading.

All of these studies provide basic scientific support for our hypothesis that primary anterior glenohumeral joint instability can lead to secondary osteoarthritis. That is, secondary glenohumeral joint osteoarthritis results from failure of glenohumeral joint cartilage to respond to altered joint loading and contact stress patterns at the articulating surfaces.

Determinations of Glenohumeral Geometry and Contact Areas

Recently, several authors[6,27,67] have used analytic stereophotogrammetry to provide precise quantification of joint surface anatomy of the patellofemoral joint and the glenohumeral joint. For the glenohumeral joint, Soslowsky and associates[67] reported that the normal humeral head and glenoid surfaces may be approximated by spheres with radii of 23.5 mm and 24.3 mm, respectively, with standard deviations of less than 1% of the radius. Moreover, the radius of the glenoid tends to be slightly greater than that of the humeral head. This degree of joint conformity renders the glenohumeral joint ideal for fluid film lubrication.[3,46]

In the past, investigators have attempted to determine the contact areas and pressures in joints by using circulating dyes, silicone rubber casting, ultrasonic transducers, miniature piezoresistive transducers, and pressure film.[10,18,26,34,62] Major drawbacks to these techniques are that they require the placement of (1) a relatively thick (0.3-mm) plastic film into a generally congruent joint space; (2) relatively stiff electronic transducers at discrete locations; or (3) viscous dyes and rubber castings. These devices or substances alter the contact areas and contact stresses at the joint surfaces and thus alter physiologic values. In addition, the pressure film technique generally requires several minutes to make an imprint, and the miniature piezoresistive transducer provides information only at discrete points.

To eliminate these problems, we have developed a method for estimating joint contact areas using precise information about joint geometry obtained from stereophotogrammetry in conjunction with joint compression studies in our laboratory. This technique has already been applied to the patellofemoral and thumb carpometacarpal joints and will be used for the glenohumeral joint.[5,68]

Briefly, this technique involves mounting the application of loads through appropriate tendons to produce joint motion and contact in a range of anatomic positions. At specified times, a pair of stereophotographs is obtained to evaluate the three-dimensional coordinates of optical targets fixed to the opposing bones in this configuration. The joint capsule is then opened without disturbing the relationship of the joint surfaces to the optical targets, and these exposed surfaces are

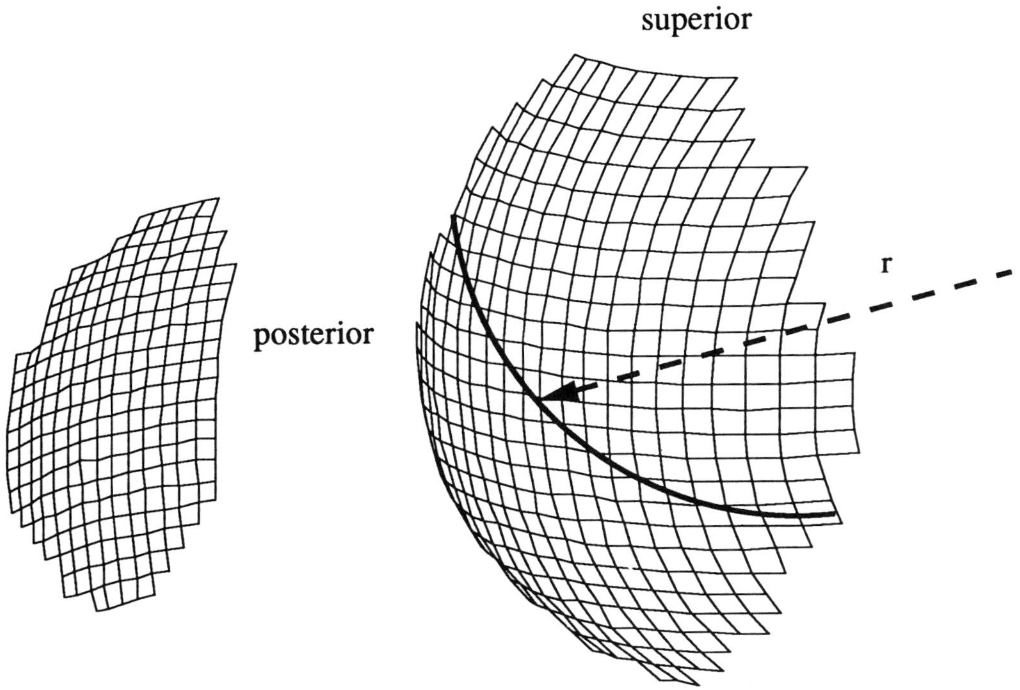

Fig. 7 *Computer graphics representation of the glenoid* ***(left)*** *and humeral head* ***(right)*** *articular surfaces, as obtained using stereophotogrammetry.*

analyzed using stereophotogrammetry. The data are used to create a three-dimensional computer-graphics representation of each joint surface.[66] These geometric models are then rotated and translated in space to assume the relative position of the actual surfaces in the intact joint while in a loaded state. In this manner, information about the contact areas in the joint may be obtained without interposing any material that would interfere with these measurements. Figure 7 shows a computer-graphics representation of the glenohumeral joint surfaces. These surfaces can be manipulated to simulate joint contact at various joint positions.

Glenohumeral Joint Deterioration From Altered Biomechanics in Unstable Shoulders

Inman and associates[28] in 1944 provided a biomechanical analysis of shoulder motion, noting that elevation of the extremity depends on motion at both the glenohumeral and the scapulothoracic joints. They found that the ratio of this motion throughout the arc of abduction is

2:1, glenohumeral to scapulothoracic. Other investigators found this ratio to be 3:2 or 5:4 after the first 30 degrees of abduction.[16,57] Poppen and Walker[57] found the center of rotation of the glenohumeral joint for abduction in the scapular plane to be within 6 mm of the geometric center of the humeral head in normal shoulders. However, in patients with shoulder disorders, including rotator cuff tears and instability, the centers of rotation could be found as far as 13 mm from the geometric center, more than twice the normal value. Moreover, in normal shoulders, the average vertical excursion of the humeral head on the glenoid was only 1.5 mm for each 30 degrees of forward elevation. In two of the three patients with previous anterior dislocations, this excursion was double the normal value.[57] More recently, Howell and associates[25] reported on glenohumeral joint mechanics in the horizontal plane. In their control group of patients with normal shoulders, the humeral head was precisely centered with respect to the glenoid in the horizontal plane for all positions except the position of maximum extension and external rotation, the cocking position of throwing. In that position, the humeral head was translated 4 mm posteriorly. In seven of 12 patients with recurrent anterior instability, the humeral head was translated 3.5 mm anteriorly in extension and external rotation. The normal posterior translation, observed in normal shoulders in the cocking position, was absent in the unstable shoulders, presumably as the result of failure of the anterior capsular mechanism.[25]

Alterations in joint contact areas and stresses were shown to cause changes in articular cartilage in a canine model.[24,33] Similarly, the abnormal motion described in patients with anterior instability of the shoulder results in abnormal contact stresses and may be a factor in the development of degenerative joint disease. Samilson and Prieto[65] reported on a series of 70 patients with glenohumeral arthritis and a history of shoulder dislocation. This group included patients who had undergone surgical repair of the unstable shoulder as well as those treated nonsurgically. The authors concluded that the incidence of glenohumeral arthrosis after shoulder dislocations is not known but is probably higher than previously suspected.[65] Neer and Foster[51] reported that a major reason for the failure of instability repairs was not recognizing that instability is multidirectional in some patients.[30] Only the anterior component of the instability had been repaired, as in the Putti-Platt or Magnuson repairs. This created excessive tightness anteriorly on a hypermobile joint, causing subluxation or dislocation of the humeral head posteriorly, which the authors believed led to arthritis. Neer and associates[52] described 25 patients with "arthritis of recurrent dislocation." Most had undergone previous surgery for instability and had fixed subluxation in the direction opposite to that of the initial dislocation. These patients typically were younger than most patients in the shoulder replacement series (average age of 45 years, compared with 60 years for osteoarthritic patients) and had severe erosion of the posterior glenoid. Hawkins and Hawkins[23] recently reported similar findings in patients who had repairs that excessively tightened the shoulder anteriorly and who subsequently developed glenohumeral arthritis.

References

1. Akizuki S, Mow VC, Müller F, et al: Tensile properties of human knee joint cartilage: I. Influence of ionic conditions, weight bearing, and fibrillation on the tensile modulus. *J Orthop Res* 1986;4:379–392.
2. Akizuki S, Mow VC, Müller F, et al: Tensile properties of human knee joint cartilage: II: Correlations between weight bearing and tissue pathology and the kinetics of swelling. *J Orthop Res* 1987;5:173–186.
3. Armstrong CG, Mow VC: Friction, lubrication and wear of synovial joints, in Owen R, Goodfellow J, Bullough P (eds): *Scientific Foundations of Orthopaedics and Traumatology*. London, William Heinemann Medical Books, 1980, pp 223–232.
4. Armstrong CG, Mow VC: Variations in the intrinsic mechanical properties of human articular cartilage with age, degeneration, and water content. *J Bone Joint Surg* 1982;64A:88–94.
5. Ateshian GA, Soslowsky LJ, Froimson M, et al: Determination of patellofemoral contact areas from stereophotogrammetric models of joint surfaces. *Biomech Symp* 1989;98:105–108.
6. Ateshian GA, Soslowsky LJ, Froimson M, et al: Stereophotogrammetric determinations of patellar cartilage thickness and surface geometry. *Adv Bioeng* 1988;14:167–170.
7. Bankart ASB: Recurrent or habitual dislocation of the shoulder joint. *Br Med J* 1923;2:1132–1133.
8. Bankart ASB: The pathology and treatment of recurrent dislocation of the shoulder joint. *Br J Surg* 1938;26:23–29.
9. Bost FC, Inman VT: The pathological changes in recurrent dislocation of the shoulder: Report of Bankart's operative procedure. *J Bone Joint Surg* 1942;24:595–613.
10. Brown TD, Shaw DT: In vitro contact stress distribution on the femoral condyles. *J Orthop Res* 1984;2:190–199.
11. Cain PR, Mutschler TA, Fu FH, et al: Anterior stability of the glenohumeral joint: A dynamic model. *Am J Sports Med* 1987;15:144–148.
12. Clarke IC: Articular cartilage: A review and scanning electron microscope study: 1. The interterritorial fibrillar architecture. *J Bone Joint Surg* 1971;53B:732–750.
13. Edwards J: Physical characteristics of articular cartilage. *Proc Inst Mech Eng* 1967;181:16–24.
14. Evans EB, Eggers GWN, Butler JK, et al: Experimental immobilization and remobilization of rat knee joint. *J Bone Joint Surg* 1960;42A:737–758.
15. Fenlin JM Jr: Total glenohumeral joint replacement. *Orthop Clin North Am* 1975;6:565–583.
16. Freedman L, Munro RR: Abduction of the arm in the scapular plane: Scapular and glenohumeral movements. A roentgenographic study. *J Bone Joint Surg* 1966;48A:1503–1510.
17. Glousman R, Jobe F, Tibone J, et al: Dynamic electromyographic analysis of the throwing shoulder with glenohumeral instability. *J Bone Joint Surg* 1988;70A:220–226.
18. Greenwald AS, Haynes DW: Weight-bearing areas in the human hip joint. *J Bone Joint Surg* 1972;54B:157–163.
19. Hammon DJ, France EP, Terry GC: Stabilizing function of passive shoulder restraints. *Trans Orthop Res Soc* 1987;12:77.
20. Hardingham TE: Proteoglycans: Their structure, interactions and molecular organization in cartilage. *Biochem Soc Trans* 1981;9:489–497.

21. Hardingham T, Muir H, Kwan MK, et al: Viscoelastic properties of proteoglycan solutions with varying proportions present as aggregates. *J Orthop Res* 1987;5:36–46.
22. Hascall VC: Interactions of cartilage proteoglycans with hyaluronic acid. *J Supramol Struc* 1977;7:101–120.
23. Hawkins RH, Hawkins RJ: Failed anterior reconstruction for shoulder instability. *Orthop Trans* 1984;8:404–405.
24. Hillberry BM, Van Sickle DC, Maturo CJ, et al: A model for studying the influence of mechanical usage on articular cartilage. Presented at the 15th Symposium of the European Society of Osteoarthrology, Kuopio, Finland, June 25–27, 1986.
25. Howell SM, Galinat BJ, Renzi AJ, et al: Normal and abnormal mechanics of the glenohumeral joint in the horizontal plane. *J Bone Joint Surg* 1988;70A:227–232.
26. Huberti HH, Hayes WC: Contact pressures in chondromalacia patellae and the effects of capsular reconstructive procedures. *J Orthop Res* 1988;6:499–508.
27. Huiskes R, Kremers J, de Lange A, et al: Analytical stereophotogrammetric determination of three-dimensional knee-joint geometry. *J Biomech* 1985;18:559–570.
28. Inman VT, Saunders JB deCM, Abbott LC: Observations on the function of the shoulder joint. *J Bone Joint Surg* 1944;26:1–30.
29. Jurvelin J, Kiviranta I, Tammi M, et al: Effect of physical exercise on indentation stiffness of articular cartilage in the canine knee. *Int J Sports Med* 1986;7:106–110.
30. Kaltsas DS: Comparative study of the properties of the shoulder joint capsule with those of other joint capsules. *Clin Orthop* 1983;173:20–26.
31. Katz EP, Wachtel EJ, Maroudas A: Extrafibrillar proteoglycans osmotically regulate the molecular packing of collagen in cartilage. *Biochim Biophys Acta* 1986;882:136–139.
32. Kempson GE: Mechanical properties of articular cartilage, in Freeman MAR (ed): *Adult Articular Cartilage.* Tunbridge Wells, England, Pitman Medical, 1979, pp 333–414.
33. Kinzel GL, Hall AS Jr, Hillberry BM: Measurement of the total motion between two body segments: I. Analytical development. *J Biochem* 1972;5:93–105.
34. Kurosawa H, Fukubayashi T, Nakajima H: Load-bearing mode of the knee joint: Physical behavior of the knee joint with or without menisci. *Clin Orthop* 1980;149:283–290.
35. Lane JM, Weiss C: Review of articular cartilage collagen research. *Arthritis Rheum* 1975;18:553–562.
36. Lipshitz H, Ethredge R III, Glimcher MJ: Changes in the hexosamine content and swelling ratio of articular cartilage as functions of depth from the surface. *J Bone Joint Surg* 1976;58A:1149–1153.
37. Magnuson PB: Treatment of recurrent dislocation of the shoulder. *Surg Clin North Am* 1945;25:14–20.
38. Mankin HJ, Brandt KD, Shulman LE: Workshop on Etiopathogenesis of Osteoarthritis: Proceedings and recommendations. *J Rheumatol* 1986;13:1130–1160.
39. Maroudas AI: Balance between swelling pressure and collagen tension in normal and degenerate cartilage. *Nature* 1976;260:808–809.
40. Maroudas AI: Physicochemical properties of articular cartilage, in Freeman MAR (ed): *Adult Articular Cartilage*, ed 2. Tunbridge Wells, England, Pitman Medical, 1979, pp 215–290.
41. Maroudas AI, Muir H, Wingham J: The correlation of fixed negative charge with glycosaminoglycan content of human articular cartilage. *Biochim Biophys Acta* 1969;177:492–500.

42. McCutchen CW: The frictional properties of animal joints. *Wear* 1962;5:1–17.
43. McLaughlin HL: Recurrent anterior dislocation of the shoulder: I. Morbid anatomy. *Am J Surg* 1960;99:628–632.
44. Moseley HF, Overgaard B: The anterior capsular mechanism in recurrent anterior dislocation of the shoulder: Morphological and clinical studies with special references to the glenoid labrum and the gleno-humeral ligaments. *J Bone Joint Surg* 1962;44B:913–927.
45. Mow VC, Holmes MH, Lai WM: Fluid transport and mechanical properties of articular cartilage: A review. *J Biomech* 1984;17:377–394.
46. Mow VC, Lai WM: Recent developments in synovial joint biomechanics. *Siam Rev* 1980;22:275–317.
47. Mow VC, Mak AF, Lai WM, et al: Viscoelastic properties of proteoglycan subunits and aggregates in varying solution concentrations. *J Biomech* 1984;17:325–338.
48. Mow VC, Schoonbeck JM: Contribution of Donnan osmotic pressure towards the biphasic compressive modulus of articular cartilage. *Trans Orthop Res Soc* 1984;9:262.
49. Muir H: Proteoglycans as organizers of the intercellular matrix. *Biochem Soc Trans* 1983;11:613–622.
50. Muir H: The chemistry of the ground substance of joint cartilage, in Sokoloff L (ed): *The Joint and Synovial Fluid*. New York, Academic Press, 1980, vol 2, pp 27–94.
51. Neer CS II, Foster CR: Inferior capsular shift for involuntary inferior and multidirectional instability of the shoulder: A preliminary report. *J Bone Joint Surg* 1980;62A:897–908.
52. Neer CS II, Watson KC, Stanton FJ: Recent experience in total shoulder replacement. *J Bone Joint Surg* 1982;64A:319–337.
53. O'Brien SJ, Neves M, Rozbruch R, et al: Anatomy and histology of the inferior glenohumeral ligament complex. Presented at the Fifth Open Meeting of the American Shoulder and Elbow Surgeons, Las Vegas, February 1989.
54. Ovesen J, Nielsen S: Stability of the shoulder joint: Cadaver study of stabilizing structures. *Acta Orthop Scand* 1985;56:149–151.
55. Palmoski M, Perricone E, Brandt KD: Development and reversal of a proteoglycan aggregation defect in normal canine knee cartilage after immobilization. *Arthritis Rheum* 1979;22:508–517.
56. Poppen NK, Walker PS: Forces at the glenohumeral joint in abduction. *Clin Orthop* 1978;135:165–170.
57. Poppen NK, Walker PS: Normal and abnormal motion of the shoulder. *J Bone Joint Surg* 1976;58A:195–201.
58. Post M, Haskell SS, Jablon M: Total shoulder replacement with a constrained prosthesis. *J Bone Joint Surg* 1980;62A:327–335.
59. Redler I, Mow VC, Zimny ML, et al: The ultrastructure and biomechanical significance of the tidemark of articular cartilage. *Clin Orthop* 1975;112:357–362.
60. Rosenberg L, Hellmann W, Kleinschmidt AK: Electron microscopic studies of proteoglycan aggregates from bovine articular cartilage. *J Biol Chem* 1975;250:1877–1883.
61. Roth V, Mow VC: The intrinsic tensile behavior of the matrix of bovine articular cartilage and its variation with age. *J Bone Joint Surg* 1980;62A:1102–1117.
62. Rushfeldt PD, Mann RW, Harris WH: Improved techniques for measuring in vitro the geometry and pressure distribution in the human acetabulum: I. Ultrasonic measurement of acetabular surfaces, sphericity and cartilage thickness. *J Biomech* 1981;14:253–260.

63. Saha AK: Dynamic stability of the glenohumeral joint. *Acta Orthop Scand* 1971;42:491–505.
64. Salter RB, Field P: The effects of continuous compression on living articular cartilage: An experimental investigation. *J Bone Joint Surg* 1960;42A:31–49.
65. Samilson RL, Prieto V: Dislocation arthropathy of the shoulder. *J Bone Joint Surg* 1983;65A:456–460.
66. Scherrer PK, Hillberry BM: Piecewise mathematical representation of articular surfaces. *J Biomech* 1979;12:301–311.
67. Soslowsky LJ, Ateshian GA, Bigliani LU, et al: Sphericity of glenohumeral joint articulating surfaces. *Trans Orthop Res Soc* 1989;14:228.
68. Soslowsky LJ, Ateshian GA, Pollock RG, et al: An in situ method to determine diarthrodial joint contact areas using stereophotogrammetry. *Adv Bioeng* 1989;15:129–130.
69. Symeonides PP: The significance of the subscapularis muscle in the pathogenesis of recurrent anterior dislocation of the shoulder. *J Bone Joint Surg* 1972;54B:476–483.
70. Thaxter TH, Mann RA, Anderson CE: Degeneration of immobilized knee joints in rats: Histological and autoradiographic study. *J Bone Joint Surg* 1965;47A:567–585.
71. Torzilli PA: Influence of cartilage conformation of its equilibrium water partition. *J Orthop Res* 1985;3:473–483.
72. Townley CO: The capsular mechanism in recurrent dislocation of the shoulder. *J Bone Joint Surg* 1950;32A:370–380.
73. Turkel SJ, Panio MW, Marshall JL, et al: Stabilizing mechanisms preventing anterior dislocation of the glenohumeral joint. *J Bone Joint Surg* 1981;63A:1208–1217.
74. Van Sickle DC, Hillberry BM: In vivo biomechanical modulation of adult articular cartilage. Presented at the 15th Symposium of the European Society of Osteoarthrology, Kuopio, Finland, June 25–27, 1986.
75. Venn MF: Variation of chemical composition with age in human femoral head cartilage. *Ann Rheum Dis* 1978;37:168–174.
76. Weiss C, Rosenberg L, Helfet AJ: An ultrastructural study of normal young adult human articular cartilage. *J Bone Joint Surg* 1968;50A:663–674.
77. Woo SLY, Akeson WH, Jemmott GF: Measurements of nonhomogeneous directional mechanical properties of articular cartilage in tension. *J Biomech* 1976;9:785–791.

Chapter 22

Induction of Synovial Inflammation by Matrix Molecules, Implant Particles, and Chemical Agents

Mark W. Rodosky, MD
Freddie H. Fu, MD

Each component of the musculoskeletal system must perform its essential function with a high level of efficiency for an athlete to excel in sports. Synovium is no exception, playing a vital role in the normal motion of joints.[97] Inflammation of this layer with a concomitant effusion can interfere with the function of the articulating joint and may create an environment hostile to articular cartilage.[33,35,37,38,44] Synovitis has been shown to result from a variety of stimuli, including artificial-ligament wear particles.[7,59,74,91,101,113] This chapter summarizes current knowledge pertinent to sports medicine about the synovial tissue response to matrix molecules, implant wear particles, and chemical agents.

Synovium

Composition and Structure

The synovial membrane is the connective tissue lining of the joint cavity and is therefore a type of mesothelium (Fig. 1). It covers all intra-articular structures except the central portion of the menisci and the articular cartilage.[26,27,48] The synovial membrane comprises a layer of lining cells and matrix molecules immediately adjacent to the joint space, called the synovial intima, and a supporting layer of subintimal tissue that merges at its external surface with the fibrous capsule of the joint (Fig. 2).[50] The embryologic origin of the synovial membrane is the mesenchyme of the original skeletal blastema[8]; for this reason, it is similar to other connective tissues in the body. In fact, synovium is seen to arise from ordinary connective tissue in a variety of situations, such as in pseudarthrosis,[26] in experimental animals when air-inflated cavities are created,[32] and in regeneration of synovium after synovectomy.[81]

The synovial intima is composed of synovial intimal cells, which form a compact layer one to three cells deep set in a matrix.[10,120] This compact layer is not a continuous layer of cells as would exist in a

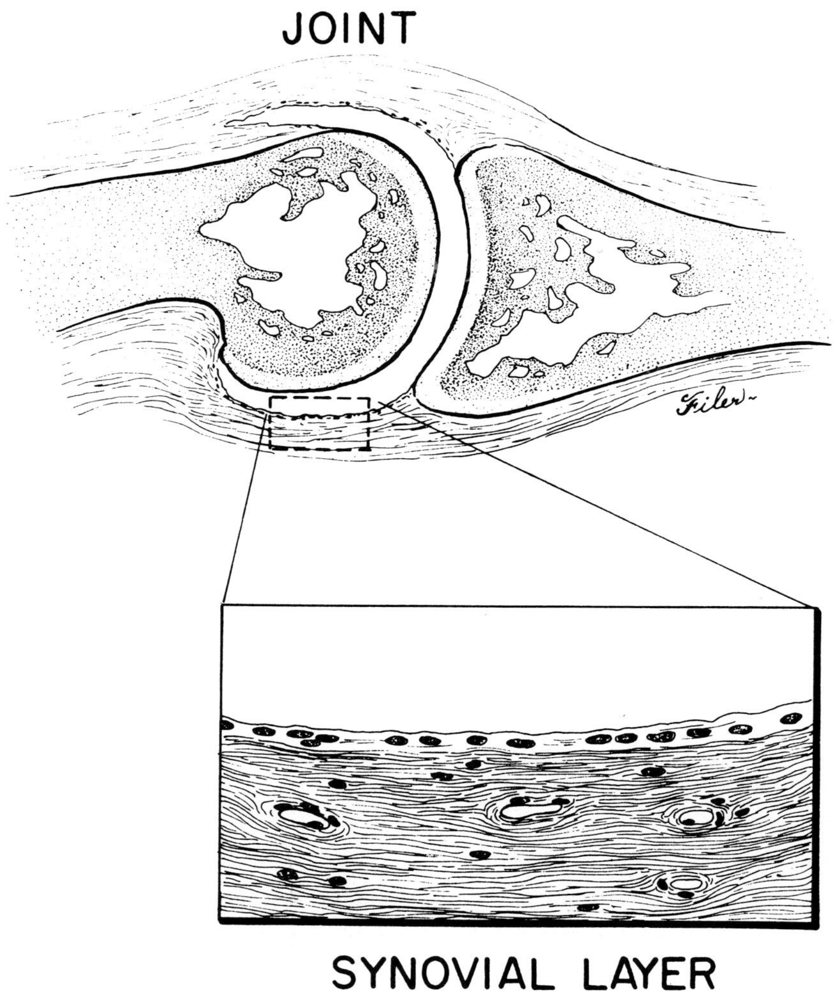

Fig. 1 *Schema of joint showing location of synovium.*

true epithelium. Instead, gaps filled by matrix substances exist between many of the cells (Fig. 2). This allows both the synovial cells and the matrix to come into contact with joint fluids.[50] The intimal matrix between synovial cells contains organized structures of banded collagen fibrils, unbanded fibrils, and electron-dense amorphous material including hyaluronate.[56,57] Mitotic intimal cells are never seen and it seems that the synovial membrane sheds cells and matrix with replacement from subintimal tissue.[10,50]

Intimal cells may be divided into two main cell types, A and B.

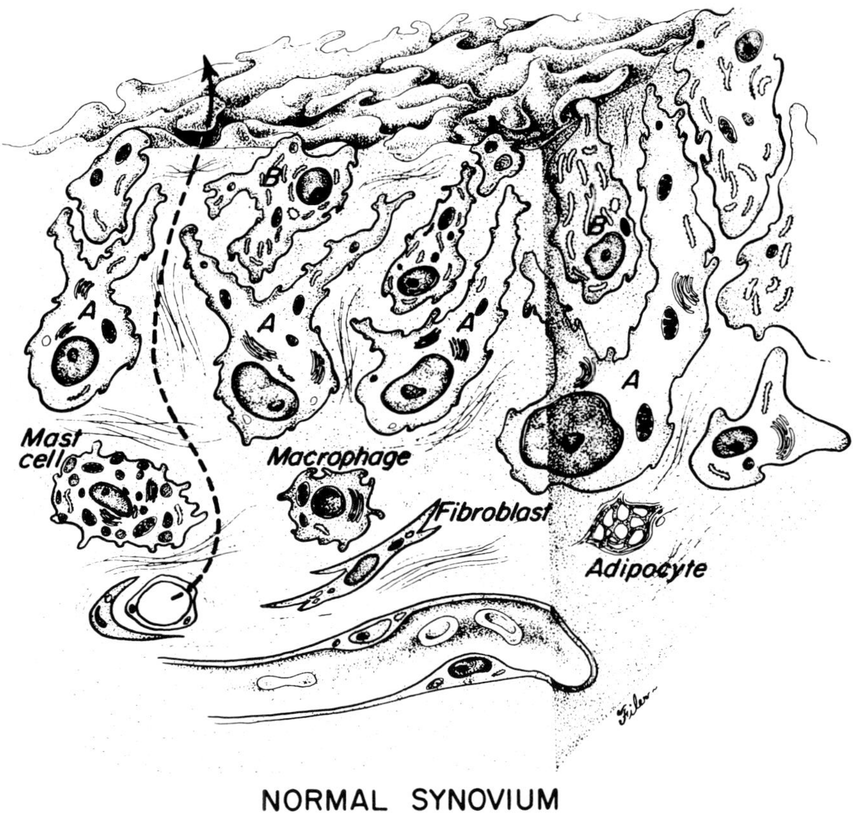

Fig. 2 *Normal synovium. The intimal layer consists of types A and B cells. The subintimal layer shows the vascular structures and the various cell types seen normally. The arrow indicates the path taken by synovial fluid as it filters through the subintimal capillary and extracellular matrix on its way to the interior of the joint.*

Most authors believe that the two cell types do not represent distinct or different types of cells but interconvertible variants with morphologic characteristics that depend on functional activity.[50] Cells with features of both are referred to as type AB and are quite common. The type A cell (Fig. 3, *left*) contains a prominent Golgi complex, many vesicles and vacuoles, small amounts of rough endoplasmic reticulum, and many filopodia; the type B cell is essentially the converse.[10,50] The predominant cell in normal human joints is type A.[10,80] It is thought to be the secretor of the hyaluronic acid that serves as a synovial lubricating factor.[58,97] Type A cells are also thought to be phagocytic with remarkable capacity for endocytosis.[51,55] Their lysosomes have

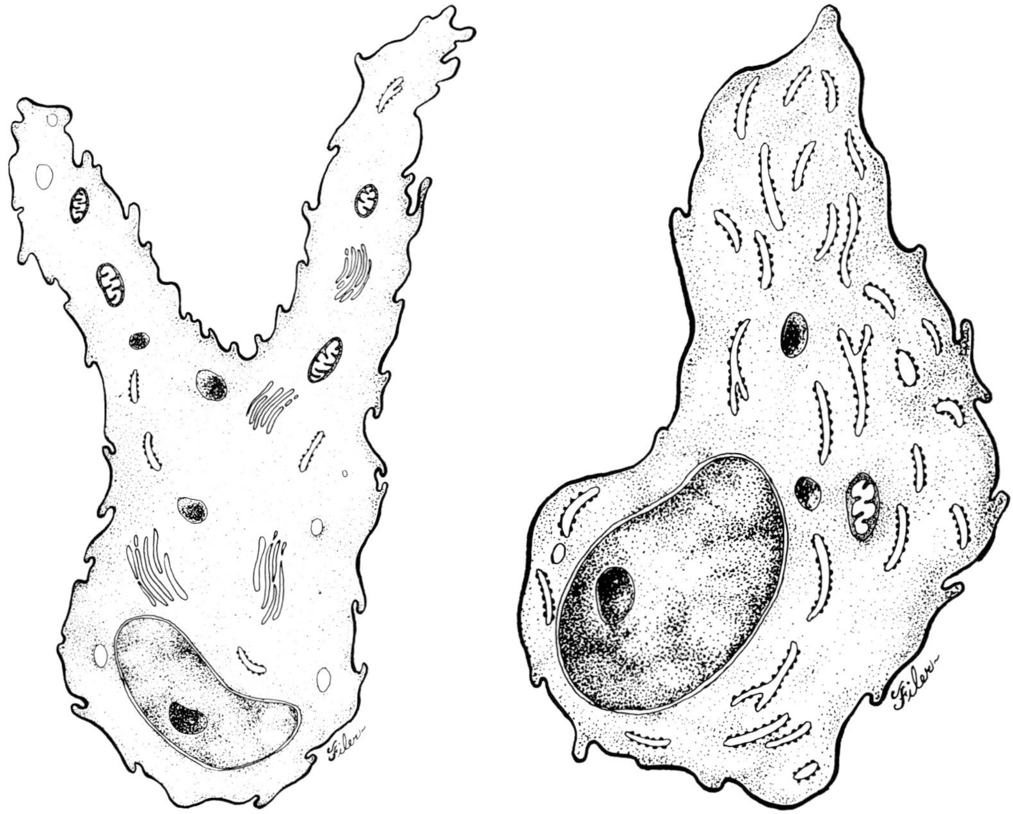

Fig. 3 *Cells of synovial intima.* ***Left,*** *Type A cell showing its prominent Golgi complex, vesicles, vacuoles, small amount of rough endoplasmic reticulum, and filopodia.* ***Right,*** *Type B cell showing its well-endowed rough endoplasmic reticulum.*

been shown to take up a variety of materials placed intra-articularly.[50] The B cells with their well-endowed rough endoplasmic reticulum are believed to be responsible for polypeptide secretion (Fig. 3, *right*). These cells, as will be discussed later, have the capacity to secrete enzymes that can degrade cartilage.[18,23,33,38,64,67] The type B cell predominates in abnormal joints, including those in people with meniscal and ligamentous disease.[50,120]

The subintimal tissue (Fig. 2) lies below the intima, without separation by any type of basal laminae.[50] The cell types encountered in subintimal tissue include fibroblasts, adipocytes, macrophages, and mast cells.[106] An abundant supply of blood vessels and lymphatics is located in this layer. Free nerve endings do not exist in the subintimal tissue, but many autonomic fibers are present in the adventitia of blood vessels.[61] Pacinian corpuscles can be found at the border of capsule and synovial membrane. The precise way in which pain is sensed from the synovium has not yet been elucidated.[50]

Synovial Function

The absence of a basal lamina and the presence of matrix-filled gaps between synovial cells allows a free passageway between synovial fluid and blood vessels.[63] In the normal joint, synovial fluid is formed by a filtration process through subintimal capillaries and extracellular matrices on its way to the interior of the joint (Fig. 2). Plasma proteins are filtered by size and charge, with the large ones such as α_2-macroglobulin, fibrinogen, and IgM present in small amounts in noninflammatory synovium. The electrolyte concentration of synovial fluid is similar to that of plasma.[50,63] As previously mentioned, the synovial cells contribute hyaluronate to the joint fluid. The hyaluronate is thought to be responsible for the lubrication of synovial-synovial and synovial-cartilage interfaces, which play a major role in the resistance to joint motion.[77,97] Because abnormal joints have shown a preponderance of type B cells and it is the type A cell that is thought to secrete hyaluronate, inflammation of the synovium may lead to a decrease in synovial lubrication. This may result in increased mechanical load to the synovial membrane and further inflammation.

The synovial membrane has an absorptive function that works in balance with its secretory role. It serves as a clearing device whose purpose is to remove substances that might otherwise accumulate within the joint cavity. The absorption of fluid from the joint space by synovial intimal cells is evidenced by the many micropinocytotic vesicles and pinocytotic vacuoles found in these cells.[10,50,120] Large molecules such as IgM and albumin may leave the joint cavity via the matrix-filled channels between cells to the numerous subintimal lymphatic channels.[19] The phagocytic capabilities of synovial cells enable them to phagocytize debris present at the synovial fluid-cell interface. This has been proven by numerous experiments with intra-articular injections of various substances, including colloidal gold,[52] platinum uracil-blue,[54] colloidal carbon,[3] ferritin,[89] and iron dextran.[9] Synovium has also been shown to absorb substances placed intravascularly, including carbon particles,[103] iron dextran,[17] and graphite dust.[12] The above-mentioned substances were found in both the synovial intimal cells and subintimal macrophages.

After absorption, the materials have a tendency to persist in the synovial membrane.[50] Gold deposits have been found in rheumatoid arthritis patients more than 20 years after chrysotherapy.[115] In a study on the long-term effects of sodium aurothiomalate, Ghadially and associates[53] found aurosomes in synovial intimal cells and subintimal macrophages two years after intra-articular injections. As will be discussed later, artificial ligaments shed wear particles, which are taken up by synovial cells and may cause these cells to secrete substances harmful to articular cartilage. Once these materials are deposited in synovium they may persist indefinitely.

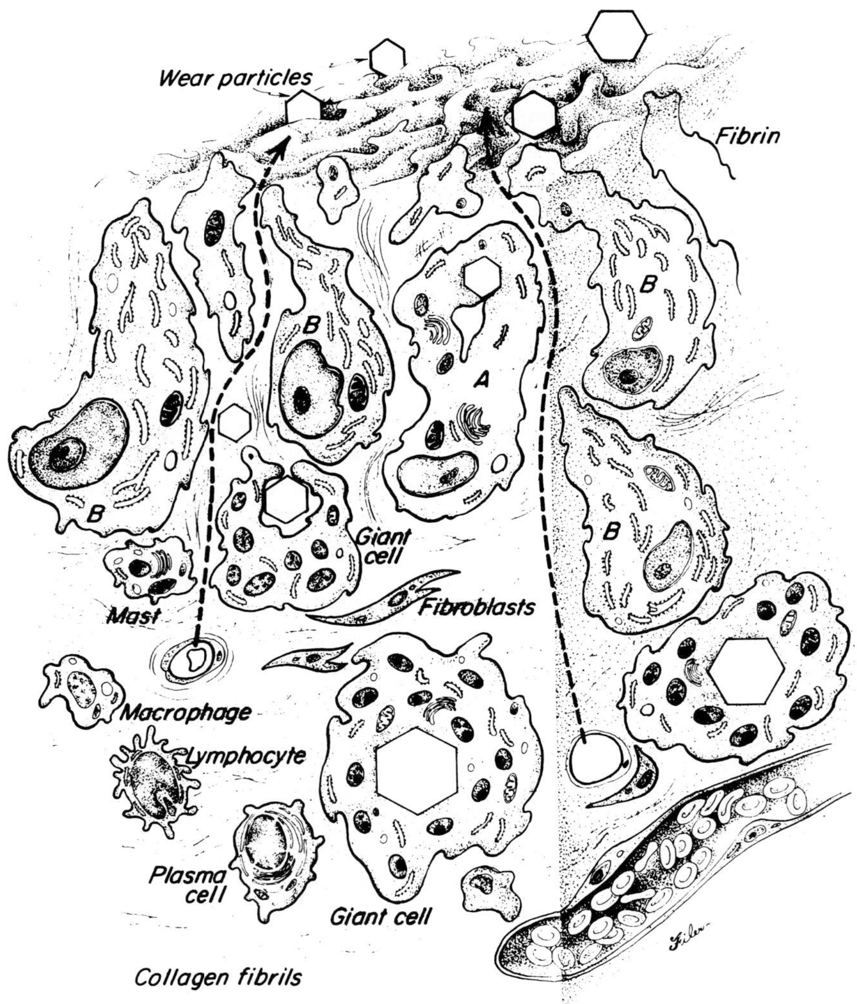

CHRONICALLY INFLAMED SYNOVIUM

Fig. 4 *Chronically inflamed synovium showing congestion of blood vessels, hypertrophy of intimal cell layer, increase in type B cells, fibrinous exudate at surface of intimal cell layer, fibrosis, and wear particles taken up by intimal cells and giant cells. The arrows represent the path of synovial fluid, which is commonly increased in synovitis.*

Synovial Inflammation

The inflammatory response is mediated by a highly regulated complex system of cells, proteins, and molecular mediators. It provides the organism with the ability to defend itself against local injurious stimuli. However, as evidenced in the inflammatory synovium of rheumatoid arthritis patients, the inflammatory process may be potentially harmful to the joint.

Synovial inflammation may be induced by two types of stimuli: trauma or substances foreign to the synovial membrane. Traumatically induced inflammation is not addressed further in this chapter. Substances foreign to the joint are those not normally found there. This can mean anything from large amounts of hemosiderin and immune complexes to particulate debris formed from the breakdown of articular cartilage or artificial ligaments. While the rheumatologist wonders about the former, the sports medicine physician is concerned about the latter. In this category we include matrix molecules, implant wear particles, and chemical agents.

Synovial inflammation produced by these stimuli includes stages along the continuum of inflammation. The synovial membrane is a richly vascularized tissue with many blood vessels and lymphatics in its subintimal layer. In acute inflammation, the blood vessels become congested and dilated. Granulocytes and mononuclear cells infiltrate the edematous subintimal tissue layer.[50,62,71]

The most common synovial response encountered in response to matrix molecules, implant particles, and chemical agents is chronic inflammation.[1,42,82,91,101,119] In addition to the above vascular changes, the chronically inflamed synovium shows several characteristic features (Fig. 4). Villi that are seen normally become more numerous and larger.[101] The intimal cell layer hypertrophies, with an increase both in matrix and in cell size and number.[50] The usual morphology of the synovial cell changes, which may be related to its state of activation.[4,117] (The amount of neutral proteinases produced by synoviocytes has been shown to correlate with a change in cell morphology. Agents that change synoviocyte morphology increase neutral proteinase production. Particle uptake changes both synoviocyte morphology and neutral proteinase production. It has been hypothesized that the change in cell morphology is related to the synoviocyte's state of activation in terms of enzyme production.[4,117]) A fibrinous exudate can be seen on the surface of the intimal cells adjacent to the joint cavity.[42] The inflammatory inducer, whether it be cartilage fragments or implant particles, can be found adhering to the intimal cells, phagocytosed by intimal cells, or in the subintimal tissue. Increased numbers of macrophages are found in the congested subintima adjacent to or already having engulfed the foreign agent. Foreign-body giant cell formation also is seen in this layer, as well as a few lymphocytes and plasma cells.[91] Fibroblastic proliferation and increased fibrosis of the synovium occur.[42,71,82,91,119]

The synovitis described above is often associated with a joint effusion. The vascular changes allow increased egress of fluids, cells, and large macromolecules into and through the extracellular matrix and into the joint cavity.[79] Large plasma proteins such as fibrinogen, the source of fibrinous exudates, and α_2-macroglobulin, a proteinase inhibitor, can now be found in the joint cavity. Fluid pressure within

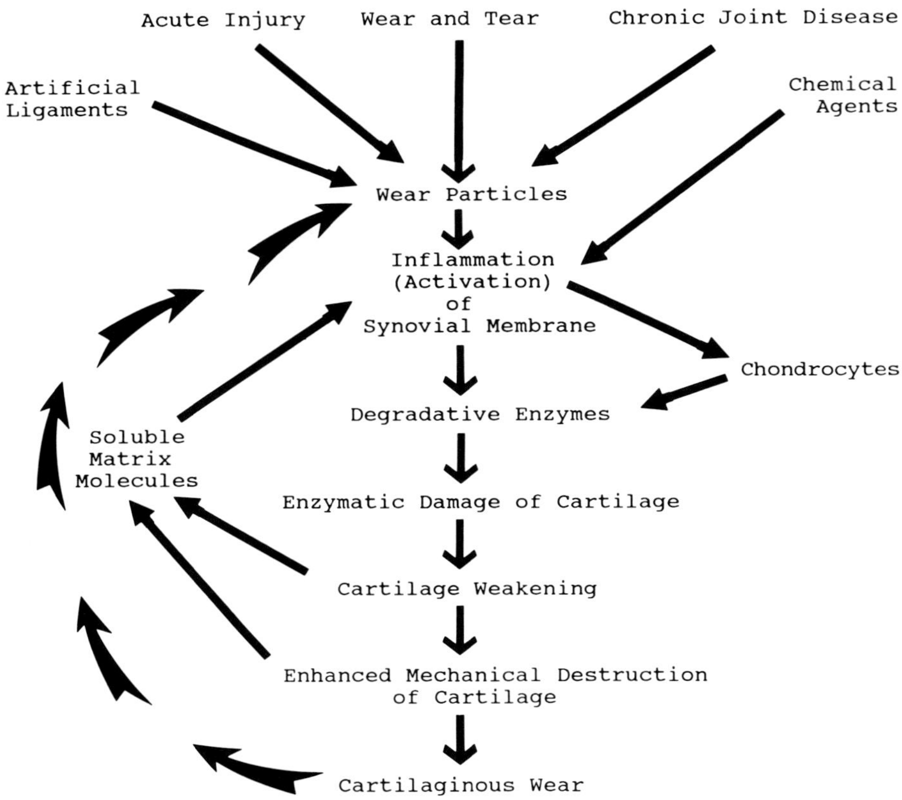

Fig. 5 *Proposed biomechanical-biochemical cause of osteoarthritis.*

the joint may reach a point at which synovial blood flow is diminished.[63] Synovial cells and the infiltrating inflammatory cells release enzymes and inflammatory mediators within the joint.[38] The accumulation of proteinases within the joint may saturate the entire population of proteinase inhibitors, allowing the enzymes to act negatively on joint soft tissues, including cartilage.[2,65] The inflammatory mediators, such as interleukin-1 and prostaglandin E_2, may enhance the destructive effect and lead to feedback mechanisms that encourage continued damage to the joint's soft tissues.[31,44,102] We know of these events through recent study of the effect of cartilaginous wear particles and matrix molecules in relation to osteoarthritis.

Synovial Response to Matrix Molecules

Osteoarthritis has traditionally been thought of as a disease of "wear and tear" leading to mechanical destruction of the joint, but recent

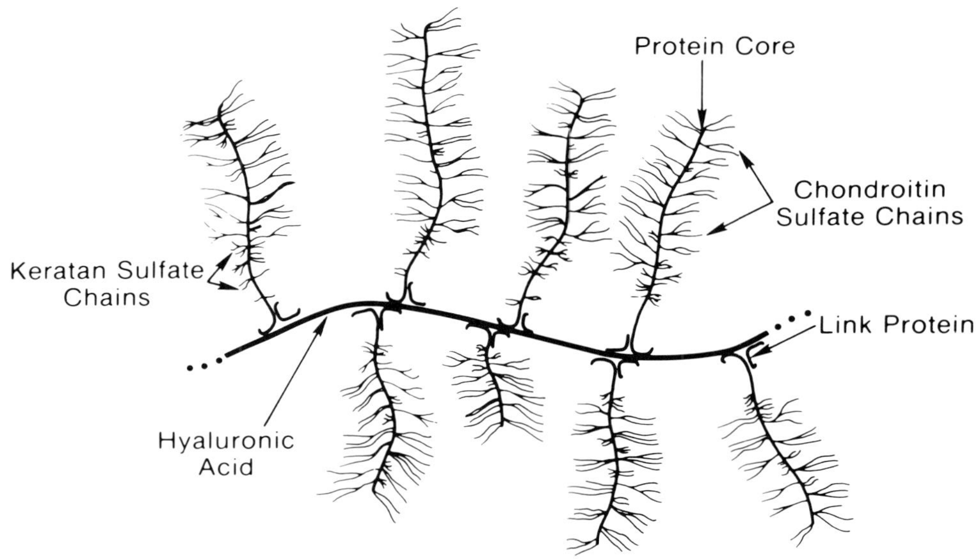

Fig. 6 *Structure of proteoglycan aggregate. (Reproduced with permission from Buckwalter JA: The fine structure of human intervertebral disc, in White AA III, Gordon SL (eds): American Academy of Orthopaedic Surgeons* Symposium on Idiopathic Low Back Pain. *St. Louis, CV Mosby, 1982, pp 108–143.)*

findings suggest biochemical and cellular contributions to osteoarthritis.[33,70] These findings are directly related to the induction of synovial inflammation by cartilage particles and matrix molecules (Fig. 5).

Physicians have known for many years that particles of cartilage and various other articular tissues tend to accumulate in the synovial fluid of osteoarthritic joints and that these "wear particles" incite a synovial reaction.[24,69,73,82] In recent years, a magnetic separation technique originally used to analyze wear particles in the lubricating oil of machines was adapted by Evans and associates to the study of wear particles in human synovial fluids.[36,39–41,105] They found an increased number of wear particles not only in osteoarthritic joints but also in knees with torn menisci, anterior cruciate ligament disruption, and chondromalacia patellae. The wear particles consisted of cartilaginous debris as well as collagenous fibers. Animal studies in which cartilaginous particles were injected in the knees of rabbits have shown that the synovium absorbs the particles and becomes chronically inflamed. The rabbits also exhibit articular cartilage damage, as revealed by friability, pitting, and loss of metachromasia.[37] A review by Ehrlich and associates[33] stated that the cause of such articular cartilage damage is the action of neutral proteolytic enzymes. This etiology can be linked to inflamed synovium. In order to understand this linkage, one must have a basic understanding of the composition and structure of articular cartilage.

Articular cartilage consists of chondrocytes surrounded by an extracellular matrix. The matrix is composed of type II collagen, several minor collagens, proteoglycan aggregates, and various noncollagenous proteins. The proteoglycan aggregates are formed largely of keratan sulfate and chondroitin sulfate. These sulfated proteoglycan chains attach to a protein core, which is then linked to a hyaluronic acid chain via a link protein (Fig. 6). Type II collagen becomes interspersed with the proteoglycan aggregates, interacting to give articular cartilage its lubricating and shock-absorbing features.[20] The type II collagen molecules help stabilize the viscoelastic proteoglycan molecules within the cartilage.[21]

Synoviocytes are known to synthesize and release at least three important neutral proteinases that have the capacity to degrade cartilage: collagenase, gelatinase, and stromelysin.[18,23,29,38,46,64,66,67,98,117] Collagenase is able to digest the collagenous lattice within the articular matrix. Gelatinase acts to digest partially degraded collagen and stromelysin digests proteoglycan.[11,23] Although the loss of proteoglycan molecules appears repairable, breakdown and removal of type II collagen from cartilage may be irreversible.[30] In addition to neutral proteases, synoviocytes have been shown to secrete interleukin-1 and prostaglandin E_2.[31,44,102] The inflammatory mediator interleukin-1, previously called catabolin by cartilage researchers, can cause chondrocytes to decrease matrix synthesis as well as to resorb their surrounding matrix.[44] It is well known that synoviocytes from normal joints secrete neglible quantities of these enzymes and mediators. The inflamed synovium of diseased joints is somehow triggered to release these chondrolytic factors.[33,37,39] Evans and associates[39] postulated that joints with some initial type of mechanical damage shed cartilaginous wear particles into synovial fluid. The wear particles are then taken up by the synovial membrane, resulting in activation of the synoviocytes. The inflamed and activated synovium secretes neutral proteinases and cytokines such as interleukin-1, which in turn can lead to further articular weakening and mechanical damage (Fig. 5).

Evidence to support the above hypothesis comes from in vitro and in vivo studies. Working with cultured rabbit synovial cells, Werb and Reynolds[117] showed that synoviocytes can be activated through the process of endocytosing particles. The synoviocytes phagocytosed 1-μ latex beads and carbon particles, resulting in a change in cell shape and the production of neutral proteinases.[117] Evans and associates[38] took this work one step further by growing normal human synoviocytes in monolayer culture via standard techniques and co-cultivating them with wear particles recovered from human osteoarthritic synovial fluids. The synovial cells released large quantities of latent collagenase and other proteinases. When cartilage wear particles are injected in rabbit knees, the synovium is seen to phagocytose the particles and

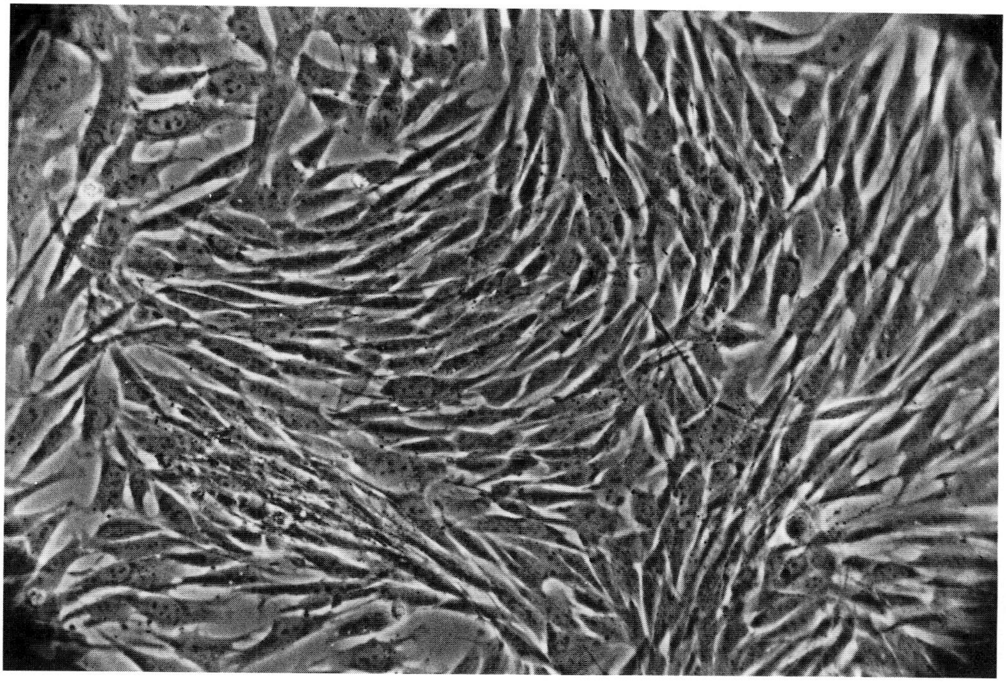

Fig. 7 *Lapine synovial cell seen as grown in culture (×100).*

display a state of chronic inflammation.[37] Organ cultures of such synovia produced as much as five times the normal amount of collagenase.

Proteoglycans released from enzymatically digested cartilage may also serve to activate synovial cells. The proteoglycan content of human synovial fluid increases during transient synovitis in children and in osteoarthritic joints.[60,83] Cartilage particles are better activators of synovial cells than latex beads of the same size.[35] Proteoglycans released from cartilage after proteolytic cleavage of core proteins can diffuse passively from cartilaginous wear particles.[95] Cartilage proteoglycans consist primarily (95%) of large, highly sulfated glycosaminoglycan polysaccharides.[20] Large sulfated polysaccharides such as carrageenan and dextran sulfate produce severe arthritis after injection in rabbit knees.[1,47] Furthermore, intra-articular injections of either partially purified soluble extracts of lapine articular cartilage or highly purified proteoglycan monomers from bovine nasal cartilage provoked synovial changes in rabbit knees.[14] Synoviocytes recovered from their knees exhibited activation and produced increased quantities of collagenases.

Another matrix molecule that has been implicated in joint synovitis is hydroxyapatite, seen in bone matrices. McCarty and associates[84]

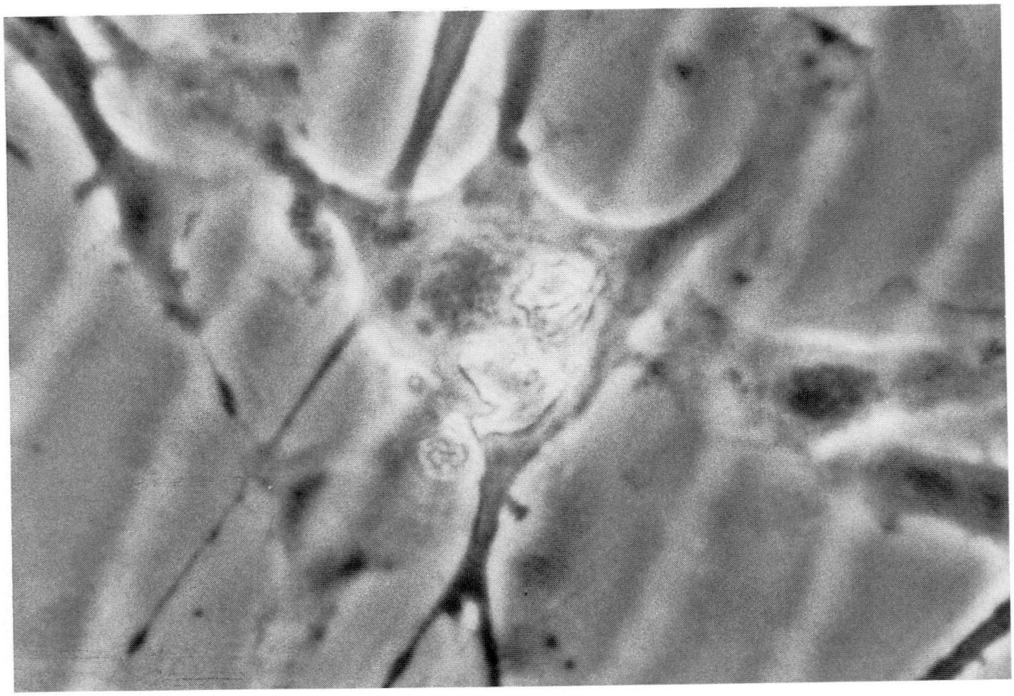

Fig. 8 *Photomicrograph of synoviocyte having phagocytosed an artificial-ligament wear particle (phase contrast ×1,000). (Reproduced with permission from Olson EJ, Kang JD, Fu FH, et al: The biochemical and histological effects of artificial ligament wear particles: In vitro and in vivo studies.* Am J Sports Med *1988;16:558–570.)*

looked at the synovial fluid and tissue from a group of patients with glenohumeral osteoarthritis and bilateral rotator cuff defects, joint stiffness, and instability. Their synovial fluid contained hydroxyapatite crystals in clumps, active synovial collagenase, and collagen types I, II, and III in an almost acellular synovial fluid. The synovial tissue was chronically inflamed and hypertrophied. Menkes and associates[87] reported a similar arthropathy characterized by mineral deposition, chronic proliferative synovitis, cartilage degeneration, and tendon erosion. Whether the hydroxyapatite is a cause or a result of this inflammatory condition is uncertain; however, Schumacher and associates[104] have shown that hydroxyapatite can lead to synovitis when injected into canine joints.

Synovial Response to Implant Particles

Artificial Ligaments

The literature contains several reports relating a high incidence of meniscal tears, early traumatic arthritis, and functional instability to

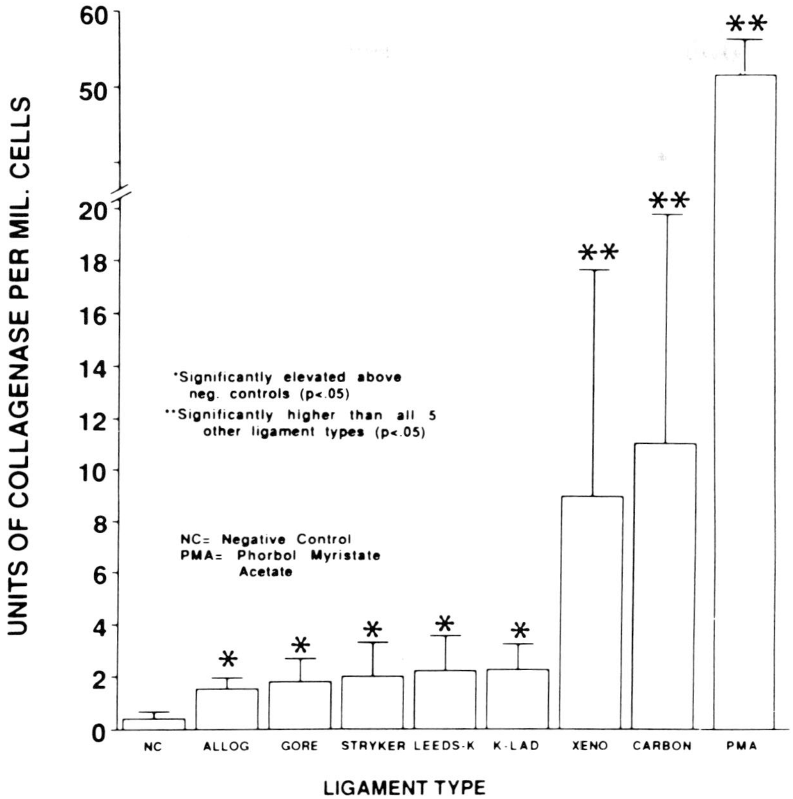

Fig. 9 *Collagenase production by synovial cells in response to 2 mg/ml of artificial-ligament wear particles. (Reproduced with permission from Olson EJ, Kang JD, Fu FH, et al: The biochemical and histological effects of artificial ligament wear particles: In vitro and in vivo studies.* Am J Sports Med *1988;16:558–570.)*

deficiency of the anterior cruciate ligament.[25,28,34,43,75] As a result, sports medicine specialists increasingly have turned to the use of artificial ligaments to treat patients with symptomatic knees with deficient anterior cruciate ligaments.[5,6,13,76,85,86,90,92] These artificial ligaments are subject to many loading cycles because the knee flexes and extends 2 million to 4 million times per year in the average person, and as many as 8 million times per year in athletes. Biomechanical studies have shown that the implanted ligaments are subjected to tensioning, bending, and abrasion against bony structures, as well as to interfiber friction.[107,108] This can result in ligament wear, fiber failure, and the generation of artificial-ligament wear particles.[59,74,101] In an attempt to prevent bony abrasion and to contain any wear debris that may form, some surgeons have wrapped the synthetic ligaments in soft tissues

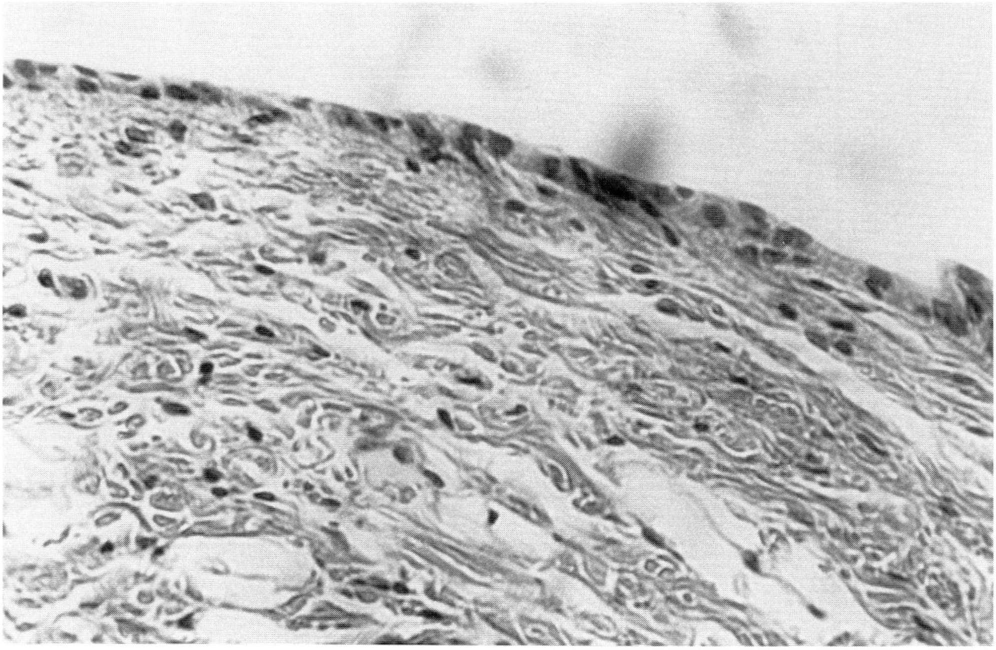

Fig. 10 *Normal synovium from a rabbit (×200).*

before implantation. This approach has been unsuccessful, however, because the release of artificial-ligament wear particles was not eliminated.[85]

Although it is recognized that these devices shed wear particles intra-articularly, the long-term effect of the debris is not yet known. Artificial ligaments are typically placed in young people and it is anticipated that they may remain in place for as long as 50 years. Will these artificial ligament wear particles act similarly to cartilaginous wear particles and have the same ability to induce synovial inflammation and activation leading to chondrolytic enzyme production?

Olson and associates[91] examined this question by studying the synovial response to artificial-ligament wear debris. They carried out both in vitro and in vivo biochemical and histologic studies in a rabbit model. Wear particles closely matching the size of particles recovered in animal and clinical studies were produced from a number of artificial ligaments.

In Vitro Studies

A line of lapine synovial cells (HIG-82) previously established by Georgescu and associates[49] was used for in vitro study. The HIG-82 cell line was established by spontaneous transformation from an aging

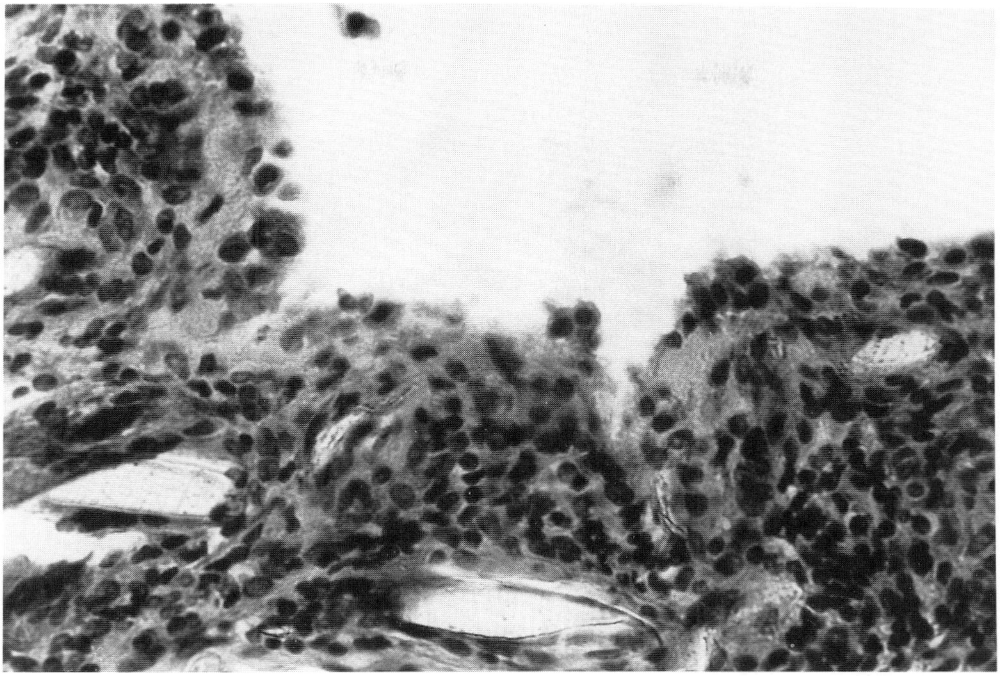

Fig. 11 *Chronically inflamed rabbit synovium after in vivo exposure to artificial-ligament wear particles. The synovium is hypertrophied with deposits of wear particles seen in the subintimal layer (×200).*

primary synovial cell culture and has the morphologic appearance of type B synovial cells (Fig. 7). The HIG-82 cell line has advantages over primary cultures in that the cells are identical to one another and do not undergo senescent changes onsubculturing. The karyotype of the HIG-82 cell line is extremely similar to that of a healthy female rabbit and has retained many of the properties of primary synovial cells, including phagocytic abilities.

The artificial-ligament wear debris was co-cultured with the HIG-82 synovial cells. Wear particles as large as 40 μ were occasionally internalized, whereas particles of less than 15 μ were phagocytosed readily (Fig. 8). The synovial cells that enveloped ligament debris subsequently underwent changes in cell shape consistent with cell activation. There was a significant increase in synovial cell production of neutral proteinases, including collagenase, gelatinase, and stromelysin (Fig. 9). In addition, there was indirect evidence for increased interleukin-1 production in response to the wear particles.

These results were consistent with the work of Evans,[35] Werb and Reynolds,[117] and Werb and associates,[116] suggesting that production of neutral proteinases by synoviocytes is a result of activation via phag-

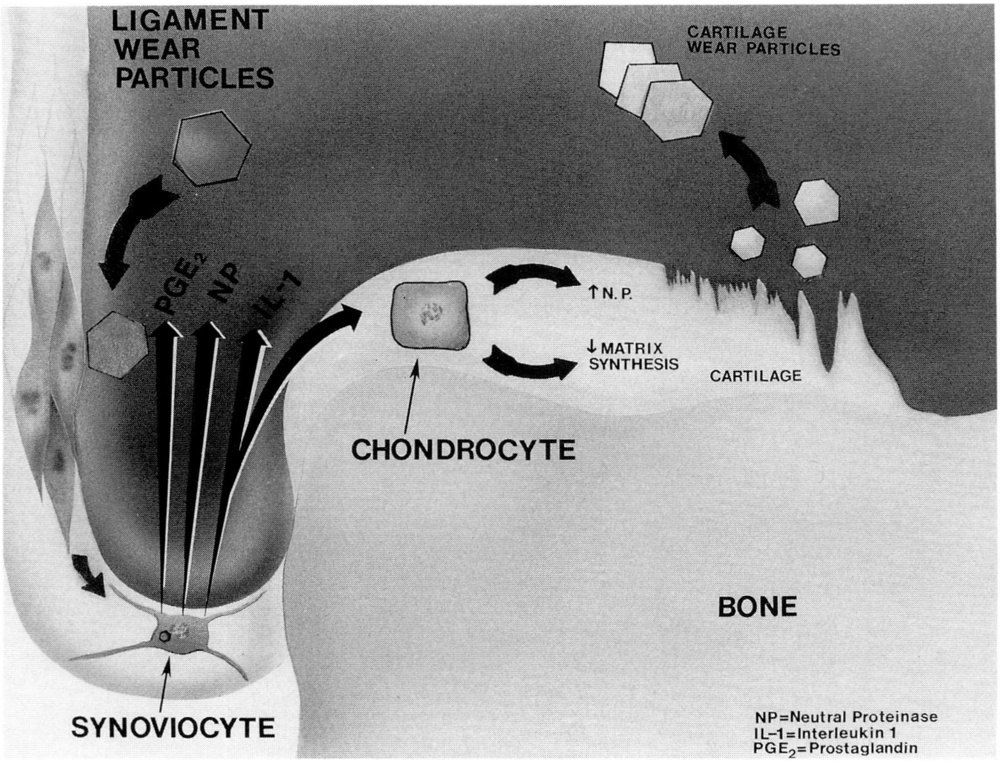

Fig. 12 *Hypothetical model of wear particles, including arthritic changes in articular cartilage. (Reproduced with permission from Olson EJ, Kang JD, Fu FH, et al: The biochemical and histological effects of artificial ligament wear particles: In vitro and in vivo studies.* Am J Sports Med *1988;16:558–570.)*

ocytosis. Whether extracellular binding by synovial cells to wear particles that are too large for phagocytosis may also activate synovial cells is not yet known; however, macrophages are known to produce enzymes after binding to, but not internalizing, wear particles.[35] As stated previously, neutral proteinases and interleukin-1 are harmful to articular cartilage.

In Vivo Studies

The in vivo aspect of the work of Olson and associates[91] consisted of injecting the artificial-ligament wear particles into rabbit knees. The amount of wear particles injected was consistent with the estimated amount of particles that would be formed from artificial ligament rupture. After 14 weeks, the rabbits were killed and histologic studies were undertaken. The wear particles were scattered throughout the knee in both the synovial intimal and subintimal layers. The highest concentration of particles was noted in the retrotibial and retrofemoral synovial folds. The synovium was found to be chronically inflamed, as evidenced by hypertrophy and a vigorous foreign-body response with dense macrophage and foreign-body giant cells seen around subintimal wear particles (Figs. 10 and 11).

Clinical Relevance

Olson and associates demonstrated that artificial-ligament wear particles can induce synovial inflammation and subsequent production of chondrolytic enzymes (Fig. 12). Short-term follow-up studies of prosthetic cruciate replacements have corroborated their findings. Indelicato and associates[74] reported satisfactory results in 34 of 39 patients with polytetrafluoroethylene cruciate replacements; however, 23% of these patients had sterile effusions, which may have been related to synovial inflammation. Several of these patients had polytetrafluoroethylene particles in synovial biopsy specimens. Glousman and associates[59] reported that four of 82 polytetrafluoroethylene cruciate replacements ruptured, with evidence of polytetrafluoroethylene wear particles in inflamed synovium. Rushton and associates[101] reported that ten of 39 patients who underwent anterior cruciate ligament replacement with a carbon-fiber device had persistent pain and effusions. Five of these patients were found to have chronic synovial inflammation and carbon-fiber wear debris within the synovium. All these clinical follow-up reports were made approximately two years postoperatively and should be interpreted with caution. The reported cases of synovitis may have resulted from poor surgical technique that led to large quantities of wear debris. On the other hand, in the patients with good results in the short term, small quantities of wear particles may continue to be released over many years. As pointed previously, synovial tissue tends to accumulate nondegradable substances. If small quantities accumulate over time, one could postulate that synovial activation might eventually occur, leading to chondrolytic enzyme release. Because one of the long-term goals of ligament reconstruction is to prevent osteoarthritis through restoration of joint stability, these findings may be important.

Experiences with joint replacement also substantiate the work of Olson and associates. Metals have been shown to cause synovitis and to stimulate production of collagenase and chondrolytic activating factors.[45,71] Polyethylene, silicone, and polymethylmethacrylate have all been found to be related to synovitis and subsequent bony resorption adjacent to implants.[22,72,88,110,118]

Synovial Response to Chemical Agents

The sports medicine specialist should be aware of two chemical agents that may induce synovial inflammation in surgical patients: glutaraldehyde and ethylene oxide.

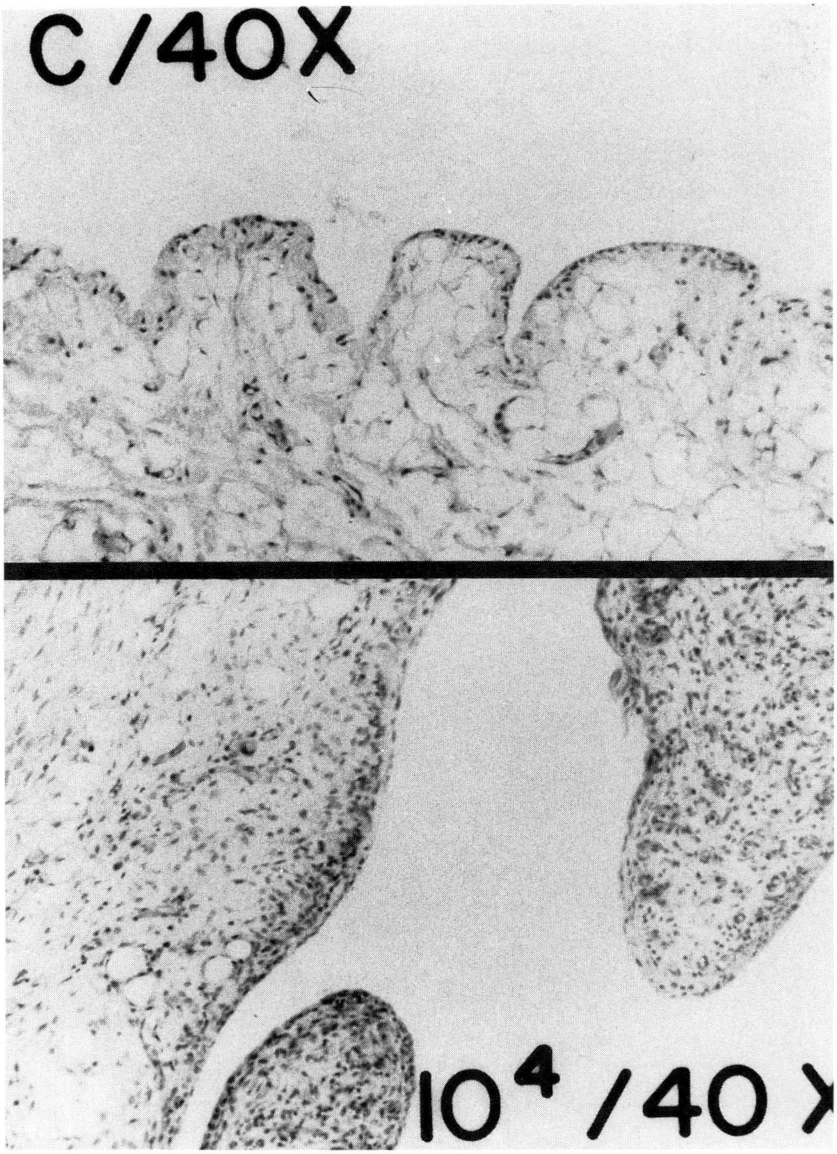

Fig. 13 ***Top,*** *Normal synovium from rabbit.* ***Bottom,*** *Inflamed rabbit synovium after exposure to 50% glutaraldehyde showing subintimal edema, vascular congestion, and proliferation of intimal cell layer (×40). (Reproduced with permission from Harner CD, Fu FH, Mason GC, et al: Cidex-induced synovitis.* Am J Sports Med *1989;17:96–102).*

Glutaraldehyde

Glutaraldehyde in a 2% concentration is used in the commercially available disinfectant Cidex. Cidex was developed in the early 1960s as a safe, rapidly acting (ten minutes) chemical solution for disinfection of medical, dental, and hospital instruments.[15,16,63,94,99,100,109,111] Clinical studies, including a large retrospective study of 12,505 cases by Johnson and associates,[78] showed Cidex to be an effective, practical, safe, and economical means of preparing instruments. However, until the recent studies by Harner and associates,[62] the potentially toxic effect of this substance on the intra-articular tissues had never been examined. They studied the effects of Cidex by injecting it into rabbit knees at concentrations ranging from 0 to 10,000 ppm (50% solution). At concentrations of 100 ppm (0.5% solution), synovial inflammation was evidenced by subsynovial edema, vascular congestion, mononuclear cell infiltrates, and proliferation of the synovial intimal cell layer (Fig. 13). In addition to their rabbit study, they examined the intraoperative levels of Cidex in rinse solutions of several hospitals. They found that the concentration of Cidex in the rinse solutions of the arthroscopic instruments was often between 100 and 300 ppm. If these instruments are placed intra-articularly without adequate irrigation, synovial toxicity could result.

Glutaraldehyde also has been encountered in anterior cruciate ligament reconstruction using a tendon bioprosthesis. This device is a bovine tendon that is preserved in glutaraldehyde to allow heteroplastic transplantation. Teitge[112] and van Steensel and associates[114] have reported that this ligament replacement was associated with a high incidence of chronic synovitis presumed to be related to the glutaraldehyde.

Ethylene Oxide

Ethylene oxide is a chemical used in the technique of gas sterilization. Paulos and associates[93] reported their experience with 200 cases of anterior cruciate ligament reconstructions using allografts; the majority of these allografts were freeze-dried, ethylene oxide-sterilized patellar tendon-bone preparations. They stated that 15% of their patients developed intense synovitis with a foreign-body giant cell reaction. This manifested clinically with effusion and pain approximately five to 18 months after surgery. Ethylene oxide levels in the allografts were assayed and found to be low. However, high levels of ethylene glycol residues were found. Ethylene glycol and ethylene chlorhydrin are known to form when ethylene oxide is exposed to water or chloride.[96] Paulos and associates[93] reasoned that the ethylene glycol residues were the most probable cause of the induction of synovial inflammation in their patients.

References

1. Aaron RK, Sledge CB, Shortkroff S: Experimental arthritis induced by polysaccharide macromolecules. *Arthritis Rheum* 1987;30:679–688.
2. Abe S, Nagai Y: Evidence for the presence of a complex of collagenase with alpha$_2$-macroglobulin in human rheumatoid synovial fluid: A possible

regulatory mechanism of collagenase activity in vivo. *J Biochem* 1973;73:897–900.
3. Adam WS: Fine structure of synovial membrane: Phagocytosis of colloidal carbon from the joint cavity. *Lab Invest* 1966;15:680–691.
4. Aggeler J, Frisch SM, Werb Z: Changes in cell shape correlate with collagenase gene expression in rabbit synovial fibroblasts. *J Cell Biol* 1984;98:1662–1671.
5. Allen PR, Amis AA, Jones MM, et al: Evaluation of preserved bovine tendon xenografts: A histological, biomechanical and clinical study. *Biomaterials* 1987;8:146–152.
6. Amis AA, Campbell JR, Kempson SA, et al: Comparison of the structure of neotendons induced by implantation of carbon or polyester fibres. *J Bone Joint Surg* 1984;66B:131–139.
7. Amis AA, Kempson SA, Campbell JR, et al: Anterior cruciate ligament replacement: Biocompatibility and biomechanics of polyester and carbon fibre in rabbits. *J Bone Joint Surg* 1988;70B:628–634.
8. Andersen H: Development, morphology and histochemistry of the early synovial tissue in human foetuses. *Acta Anat* 1964;58:90–115.
9. Ball J, Chapman JA, Muirden KD: The uptake of iron in rabbit synovial tissue following intra-articular injection of iron dextran: A light and electron microscope study. *J Cell Biol* 1964;22:351–364.
10. Barland P, Novikoff AB, Hamerman D: Electron microscopy of the human synovial membrane. *J Cell Biol* 1962;14:207–220.
11. Barrett AJ, Saklatvala J: Proteinases in joint disease, in Kelly WN, Harris ED Jr, Ruddy S, et al (eds): *Textbook of Rheumatology*. Philadelphia, WB Saunders, 1982, pp 195–209.
12. Bellamy R, Wood TP: Graphite localization in the synovial membrane of the knee: Case report. *J Bone Joint Surg* 1978;60A:1149–1151.
13. Bolton CW, Bruchman WC: The GORE-TEX expanded polytetrafluoroethylene prosthetic ligament: An in vitro and in vivo evaluation. *Clin Orthop* 1985;196:202–213.
14. Boniface RJ, Cain PR, Evans CH: Articular responses to purified cartilage proteoglycans. *Arthritis Rheum* 1988;31:258–266.
15. Borick PM: Antimicrobial agents as liquid chemosterilizers. *Biotechnol Bioeng* 1965;7:435–443.
16. Borick PM, Dondershine FH, Chandler VL: Alkalinized glutaraldehyde, a new antimicrobial agent. *J Pharm Sci* 1964;53:1273–1275.
17. Brighton CT, Bigley EC Jr, Smolenski BI: Iron-induced arthritis in immature rabbits. *Arthritis Rheum* 1970;13:849–857.
18. Brinckerhoff CE, McMillan RM, Fahey JV, et al: Collagenase production by synovial fibroblasts treated with phorbol myristate acetate. *Arthritis Rheum* 1979;22:1109–1116.
19. Brown DL, Cooper AG, Bluestone R: Exchange of IgM and albumin between plasma and synovial fluid in rheumatoid arthritis. *Ann Rheum Dis* 1969;28:644–651.
20. Buckwalter JA, Cooper RR: The cells and matrices of skeletal connective tissues, in Albright JA, Brand RA, (eds): *The Scientific Basis of Orthopaedics*, ed 2. Norwalk, Appleton & Lange, 1987, pp 1–29.
21. Buckwalter J, Hunziker E, Rosenberg L, et al: Articular cartilage: Composition and structure, Woo SL-Y, Buckwalter JA (eds): *Injury and Repair of the Musculoskeletal Soft Tissues*. Park Ridge, Illinois, American Academy of Orthopaedic Surgeons, 1988, pp 405–425.
22. Charosky CB, Bullough PG, Wilson PD Jr: Total hip replacement failures: A histological evaluation. *J Bone Joint Surg* 1973;55A:49–58.
23. Chin JR, Murphy G, Werb Z: Stromelysin, a connective tissue-degrading metalloendopeptidase secreted by stimulated rabbit synovial fibroblasts in

parallel with collagenase: Biosynthesis, isolation, characterization, and substrates. *J Biol Chem* 1985;260:12367–12376.

24. Chrisman OD, Fessel JM, Southwick WO: Experimental production of synovitis and marginal articular exostoses in the knee joints of dogs. *Yale J Biol Med* 1965;37:409–412.
25. Clancy WG Jr, Nelson DA, Reider B, et al: Anterior cruciate ligament reconstruction using one-third of the patellar ligament, augmented by extra-articular tendon transfers. *J Bone Joint Surg* 1982;64A:352–359.
26. Collins DH: *The Pathology of Articular and Spinal Diseases.* London, Edward Arnold, 1949.
27. Davies DV: The biology of joints, in Copeman WSC (ed): *Textbook of the Rheumatic Diseases*, ed 4. Edinburgh, E & S Livingstone, 1969, pp 40–86.
28. DeHaven KE: Diagnosis of acute knee injuries with hemarthrosis. *Am J Sports Med* 1980;8:9–14.
29. Deshmukh-Phadke K, Nanda S, Lee K: Macrophage factor that induces neutral protease secretion by normal rabbit chondrocytes: Studies of some properties and effects on metabolism of chondrocytes. *Eur J Biochem* 1980;104:175–180.
30. Dingle JT: Heberden Oration 1978: Recent studies on the control of joint damage. The contribution of the Strangeways Research Laboratory. *Ann Rheum Dis* 1979;38:201–214.
31. Dingle JT, Saklatvala J, Hembry R, et al: A cartilage catabolic factor from synovium. *Biochem J* 1979;184:177–180.
32. Edwards JC, Sedgwick AD, Willoughby DA: The formation of a structure with the features of synovial lining by subcutaneous injection of air: An in vivo tissue culture system. *J Pathol* 1981;134:147–156.
33. Ehrlich MG, Armstrong AL, Treadwell BV, et al: Degradative enzyme systems in cartilage. *Clin Orthop* 1986;213:62–68.
34. Ericksson E: Sports injuries of the knee ligaments: Their diagnosis, treatment, rehabilitation and prevention. *Med Sci Sports* 1976;8:133–144.
35. Evans CH: Cellular mechanisms of hydrolytic enzyme release in osteoarthritis. *Semin Arthritis Rheum* 1982;11(suppl 1):93–95.
36. Evans CH, Bowen ER, Bowen J, et al: Synovial fluid analysis by ferrography. *J Biochem Biophys Meth* 1980;2:11–18.
37. Evans CH, Mazzocchi RA, Nelson DD, et al: Experimental arthritis induced by intraarticular injection of allogenic cartilaginous particles into rabbit knees. *Arthritis Rheum* 1984;27:200–207.
38. Evans CH, Mears DC, Cosgrove JL: Release of neutral proteinases from mononuclear phagocytes and synovial cells in response to cartilaginous wear particles in vitro. *Biochim Biophys Acta* 1981;677:287–294.
39. Evans CH, Mears DC, McKnight JL: A preliminary ferrographic survey of the wear particles in human synovial fluid. *Arthritis Rheum* 1981;24:912–918.
40. Evans CH, Mears DC, Stanitski CL: Ferrographic analysis of wear in human joints: Evaluation by comparison with arthroscopic examination of symptomatic knees. *J Bone Joint Surg* 1982;64B:572–578.
41. Evans CH, Tew WP: Isolation of biological materials by use of erbium: III. Induced magnetic susceptibilities. *Science* 1981;213:653–654.
42. Ewald FC, Sledge CB, Corson JM, et al: Giant cell synovitis associated with failed polyethylene patellar replacements. *Clin Orthop* 1976;115:213–219.
43. Feagin JA Jr, Curl WW: Isolated tear of the anterior cruciate ligament: 5-year follow-up study. *Am J Sports Med* 1976;4:95–100.
44. Fell HB, Jubb RW: The effect of synovial tissue on the breakdown of articular cartilage in organ culture. *Arthritis Rheum* 1977;20:1359–1371.
45. Ferguson GM, Watanabe S, Georgescu HI, et al: The synovial production

of collagenase and chondrocyte activating factors in response to cobalt. *J Orthop Res* 1988;6:525–530.
46. Frisch SM, Clark EJ, Werb Z: Coordinate regulation of stromelysin and collagenase genes determined with cDNA probes. *Proc Natl Acad Sci USA* 1987;84:2600–2604.
47. Gardner DL: Production of arthritis in the rabbit by the local injection of the mucopolysaccharide caragheenin. *Ann Rheum Dis* 1960;19:369–376.
48. Gardner E: The structure and function of joints, in Hollander JL, McCarty DJ Jr (eds): *Arthritis and Allied Conditions: A Textbook of Rheumatology*, ed 8. Philadelphia, Lea & Febiger, 1972, pp 32–50.
49. Georgescu HI, Mendelow D, Evans CH: HIG-82 an established cell line from rabbit periarticular soft tissue, which retains the activatable phenotype. *In Vitro Cell Dev Biol* 1988;24:1015–1022.
50. Ghadially FN: *Fine Structure of Synovial Joints: A Text and Atlas of the Ultrastructure of Normal and Pathological Articular Tissues.* London, Butterworths, 1983.
51. Ghadially FN: Overview article: The articular territory of the reticuloendothelial system. *Ultrastruct Pathol* 1980;1:249–264.
52. Ghadially FN, Lalonde JM: Electron-probe x-ray analysis of granules and particles found in aurosomes produced by colloidal gold. *Virchows Arch [Cell Pathol]* 1980;32:185–189.
53. Ghadially FN, Lalonde JM, Thomas I, et al: Long-term effects of myochrysine on the synovial membrane and aurosomes. *J Pathol* 1978;125:219–224.
54. Ghadially FN, Lock CJ, Lalonde JM, et al: Platinosomes produced in synovial membrane by platinum coordination complexes. *Virchows Arch [Cell Pathol]* 1981;35:123–131.
55. Ghadially FN, Roy S: Phagocytosis by synovial cells. *Nature* 1967;213:1041.
56. Ghadially FN, Roy S: Ultrastructural changes in the synovial membrane in lipohaemarthrosis. *Ann Rheum Dis* 1969;28:529–536.
57. Ghadially FN, Roy S: Ultrastructure of rabbit synovial membrane. *Ann Rheum Dis* 1966;25:318–326.
58. Ghadially FN, Roy S: *Ultrastructure of Synovial Joints in Health and Disease.* New York, Appleton-Century-Crofts, 1969.
59. Glousman R, Shields C Jr, Kerlan R, et al: Gore-Tex prosthetic ligament in arterior cruciate deficient knees. *Am J Sports Med* 1988;16:321–326.
60. Gysen P, Adams A, Meyner G, et al: Proteoglycans, N-terminal procollagen type III peptide and kinogens in synovial fluid, in Franchimont P (ed): *Articular Synovium.* Basel, S Karger, 1982, pp 129–141.
61. Halata Z, Groth HP: Innervation of the synovial membrane of the cat's joint capsule. *Cell Tissue Res* 1976;169:415–418.
62. Harner CD, Fu FH, Mason GC, et al: Cidex-induced synovitis. *Am J Sports Med* 1989;17:96–102.
63. Harris ED Jr: Biology of the joint, in Kelly WN, Harris ED Jr, Ruddy S, et al (eds): *Textbook of Rheumatology*, ed 2. Philadelphia, WB Saunders, 1985, vol 1, pp 254–271.
64. Harris ED Jr: Role of Collagenases in joint destruction, in Sokoloff L (ed): *The Joints and Synovial Fluid.* New York, Academic Press,1978, vol 1, pp 243–272.
65. Harris ED Jr, Faulkner CS II, Brown FE: Collagenolytic systems in rheumatoid arthritis. *Clin Orthop* 1975;110:303–316.
66. Harris ED Jr, Krane SM: An endopeptidase from rheumatoid synovial tissue culture. *Biochim Biophys Acta* 1972;258:566–576.
67. Harris ED Jr, Krane SM: Collagenases: Part 1. *N Engl J Med*

1974;291:557–563; Part 2. *N Engl J Med* 1974;291:605–609; Part 3. *N Engl J Med* 1974;291:652–661.

68. Haselhuhn DH, Brason FW, Borick PM: "In use" study of buffered glutaraldehyde for cold sterilization of anesthesia equipment. *Anesth Analg* 1967;46:468–474.
69. Horwitz T: Bone and cartilage debris in the synovial membrane: Its significance in the early diagnosis of neuro-arthropathy. *J Bone Joint Surg* 1948;30A:579–588.
70. Howell DS, Sapolsky AI, Pita JC, et al: The pathogenesis of osteoarthritis. *Semin Arthritis Rheum* 1976;4:365–383.
71. Howie DW, Vernon-Roberts B: The synovial response to intraarticular cobalt-chrome wear particles. *Clin Orthop* 1988;232:244–254.
72. Howie DW, Vernon-Roberts B, Oakeshott R, et al: A rat model of resorption of bone at the cement-bone interface in the presence of polyethylene wear particles. *J Bone Joint Surg* 1988;70A:257–263.
73. Hulten O, Gellerstedt N: Über Abnutzungsprodukte in Gelenken und ihre Resorption unter dem Bilde einer Synovitis detritica. *Acta Chir Scand* 1940;84:1–29.
74. Indelicato PA, Pascale MS, Huegel MO: Early experience with the GORE-TEX polytetrafluoroethylene anterior cruciate ligament prosthesis. *Am J Sports Med* 1989;17:55–62.
75. Jacobsen K: Osteoarthrosis following insufficiency of the cruciate ligaments in man: A clinical study. *Acta Orthop Scand* 1977;48:520–526.
76. Jenkins DH, McKibbin B: The role of flexible carbon-fibre implants as tendon and ligament substitutes in clinical practice: A preliminary report. *J Bone Joint Surg* 1980;62B:497–499.
77. Johns RJ, Wright V: Relative importance of various tissues in joint stiffness. *J Appl Physiol* 1962;17:824–828.
78. Johnson LL, Shneider DA, Austin MD, et al: Two per cent glutaraldehyde: A disinfectant in arthroscopy and arthroscopic surgery. *J Bone Joint Surg* 1982;64A:237–239.
79. Kushner I, Somerville JA: Permeability of human synovial membrane to plasma proteins: Relationship to molecular size and inflammation. *Arthritis Rheum* 1971;14:560–570.
80. Leonardelli J, Catanzariti L: La synoviale normale: Données morphologiques et histophysiologiques. *Lille Med* 1971;16:277–284.
81. Levene A: The response to injury of rat synovial membrane. *J Pathol Bacteriol* 1957;73:87–90.
82. Lloyd-Roberts GC: The role of capsular changes in osteoarthritis of the hip joint. *J Bone Joint Surg* 1953;35B:627–642.
83. Lohmander LS, Wingstrand H, Heinegård D: Transient synovitis of the hip in the child: Increased levels of proteoglycan fragments in joint fluid. *Trans Orthop Res Soc* 1986;11:485.
84. McCarty DJ, Halverson PB, Carrera GF, et al: "Milwaukee shoulder": Association of microspheroids containing hydroxyapatite crystals, active collagenase, and neutral protease with rotator cuff defects. I. Clinical aspects. *Arthritis Rheum* 1981;24:464–473.
85. McPherson GK, Mendenhall HV, Gibbons DF, et al: Experimental mechanical and histologic evaluation of the Kennedy ligament augmentation device. *Clin Orthop* 1985;196:186–195.
86. Mendes DG, Angel D, Grishkan A, et al: Histological response to carbon fibre. *J Bone Joint Surg* 1985;67B:645–649.
87. Menkes CJ, Simon F, Delrieu F, et al: Destructive arthropathy in chondrocalcinosis articularis. *Arthritis Rheum* 1976;19(suppl 3):329–348.
88. Mirra JM, Marder RA, Amstutz HC: The pathology of failed total joint arthroplasty. *Clin Orthop* 1982;170:175–183.

89. Muirden KD: An electron microscope study of the uptake of ferritin by the synovial membrane, abstract. *Arthritis Rheum* 1963;6:289.
90. Nikolaou PK, Seaber AV, Glisson RR, et al: Anterior cruciate ligament allograft transplantation: Long-term function, histology, revascularization, and operative technique. *Am J Sports Med* 1986;14:348–360.
91. Olson EJ, Kang JD, Fu FH, et al: The biochemical and histological effects of artificial ligament wear particles: In vitro and in vivo studies. *Am J Sports Med* 1988;16:558–570.
92. Park JP, Grana WA, Chitwood JS: A high-strength Dacron augmentation for cruciate ligament reconstruction: A two-year canine study. *Clin Orthop* 1985;196:175–185.
93. Paulos LE, Rosenberg TD, Gurley WD: Anterior cruciate ligament allografts, in Friedman MJ, Ferkel RD (eds): *Prosthetic Ligament Reconstruction of the Knee.* Philadelphia, WB Saunders, 1988, pp 186–192.
94. Pepper RE, Chandler VL: Sporicidal activity of alkaline alcoholic saturated dialdehyde solutions. *Appl Microbiol* 1963;11:385–388.
95. Pottenger LA, Lyon NB, Hecht JD, et al: Influence of cartilage particle size and proteoglycan aggregation on immobilization of proteoglycans. *J Biol Chem* 1982;257:11479–11485.
96. Prolo DJ, Oklund SA: Sterilization of bone by chemicals, in Friedlaender GE, Mankin HJ, Sell KW (eds): *Osteochondral Allografts: Biology, Banking, and Clinical Applications.* Boston, Little, Brown, 1981, pp 233–238.
97. Radin EL, Paul IL, Swann DA, et al: Lubrication of synovial membrane. *Ann Rheum Dis* 1971;30:322–325.
98. Ridge SC, Oronsky AL, Kerwar SS: Induction of the synthesis of latent collagenase and latent neutral protease in chondrocytes by a factor synthesized by activated macrophages. *Arthritis Rheum* 1980;23:448–454.
99. Rittenbury MS, Hench ME: Preliminary evaluation of an activated glutaraldehyde solution for cold sterilization. *Ann Surg* 1965;161:127–130.
100. Rubbo SD, Gardner JF, Webb RL: Biocidal activities of glutaraldehyde and related compounds. *J Appl Bacteriol* 1967;30:78–87.
101. Rushton N, Dandy DJ, Naylor CP: The clinical arthroscopic and histological findings after replacement of the anterior cruciate ligament with carbon-fibre. *J Bone Joint Surg* 1983;65B:308–309.
102. Saklatvala J, Pilsworth LM, Sarsfield SJ, et al: Pig catabolin is a form of interleukin 1: Cartilage and bone resorb, fibroblasts make prostaglandin and collagenase, and thymocyte proliferation is augmented in response to one protein. *Biochem J* 1984;224:461–466.
103. Schumacher HR: Fate of particulate material arriving at the synovium via the circulation: An ultrastructural study. *Ann Rheum Dis* 1973;32:212–218.
104. Schumacher HR, Smolyo AP, Tse RL, et al: Arthritis associated with apatite crystals. *Ann Intern Med* 1977;87:411–416.
105. Seifert WW, Westcott VC: A method for the study of wear particles in lubricating oil. *Wear* 1972;21:27–42.
106. Shaw NE, Martin BF: Histological and histochemical studies on mammalian knee-joint tissues. *J Anat* 1962;96:359–373.
107. Sidles JA, Garbini JL, Larson RV, et al: Fiber-fiber interactions within finite ligament grafts. *Trans Orthop Res Soc* 1988;13:189.
108. Sidles JA, Larson RV, Garbini JL, et al: Can the peripheral portion of an anterior cruciate ligament graft be nearly isometric? *Trans Orthop Res Soc* 1988;13:198.
109. Snyder RW, Cheatle EL: Alkaline glutaraldehyde: An effective disinfectant. *Am J Hosp Pharm* 1965;22:321–327.
110. Stinson NE: Tissue reaction induced in guinea-pigs by particulate polymethylmethacrylate, polythene and nylon of the same size range. *Br J Exp Pathol* 1965;46:135–146.

111. Stonehill AA, Krop S, Borick PM: Buffered glutaraldehyde: A new chemical sterilizing solution. *Am J Hosp Pharm* 1963;20:458–465.
112. Teitge RA: Bovine xenograft reconstruction of the ACL, in Feagin JA (ed): *The Crucial Ligaments.* New York, Churchill Livingstone, 1988, pp 529–534.
113. Thomas NP, Turner IG, Jones CB: Prosthetic anterior cruciate ligaments in the rabbit: A comparison of four types of replacement. *J Bone Joint Surg* 1987;69B:312–316.
114. van Steensel CJ, Schreuder O, van den Bosch BF, et al: Failure of anterior cruciate-ligament reconstruction using tendon xenograft. *J Bone Joint Surg* 1987;69A:860–864.
115. Vernon-Roberts B, Doré JL, Jessop JD, et al: Selective concentration and localization of gold in macrophages of synovial and other tissues during and after chrysotherapy in rheumatoid patients. *Ann Rheum Dis* 1976;35:477–486.
116. Werb Z, Hembry RM, Murphy G, et al: Commitment to expression of the metalloendopeptidases, collagenase and stromelysin: Relationship of inducing events to changes in cytoskeletal architecture. *J Cell Biol* 1986;102:697–702.
117. Werb Z, Reynolds JJ: Stimulation by endocytosis of the secretion of collagenase and neutral proteinase from rabbit synovial fibroblasts. *J Exp Med* 1974;140:1482–1497.
118. Willert H-G, Semlitsch M: Reactions of the articular capsule to wear products of artificial joint prostheses. *J Biomed Mater Res* 1977;11:157–164.
119. Worsing RA Jr, Engber WD, Lange TA: Reactive synovitis from particulate Silastic. *J Bone Joint Surg* 1982;64A:581–585.
120. Wynne-Roberts CR, Anderson C: Light- and electron-microscopic studies of normal juvenile human synovium. *Semin Arthritis Rheum* 1978;7:279–286.

Chapter 23

Mechanisms of Pain Sensation Resulting From Inflammation

Kenneth M. Hargreaves, DDS, PhD

Introduction

Sports-related injuries often give rise to the classic signs of inflammation—pain, edema, hyperthermia, erythema, and loss of function. Pain caused by inflammation produces a distinct perception that differs from that produced by transient, painful stimuli such as a venipuncture. Inflammatory pain is often a spontaneous, prolonged aching sensation produced in response to even innocuous stimuli. This chapter reviews the physiologic basis for pain sensation, how this neural system is activated and altered during inflammation, and how this system may contribute to the development of inflammation.

Anatomic and Physiologic Basis of Pain and Perception

The perception of pain is thought to signal the occurrence of tissue damage or the potential for damage.[20] Noxious stimuli, such as exercise-induced tissue damage, are detected by the terminal endings of two major classes of nociceptive (pain-detecting) afferent nerve fibers: the C fibers and the A-δ fibers. Analysis of the fiber population in the human sural nerve indicates that there are approximately three to five times more C fibers than A fibers. However, it is presumed that not all of these fibers are nociceptors.[38] Nociceptive fibers are distributed throughout the skin, periosteum, muscles, and joints.[9,53] Although most knowledge on the detection of pain comes from studies on A-δ and C fibers in skin, pain caused by sports-induced injuries arises primarily from nociceptors located in muscle and joints. While the properties of cutaneous and deep nociceptors are thought to be generally similar, there are some differences.

The finely myelinated, relatively fast-conducting nociceptive fibers in skin are termed A-δ fibers. These fibers respond primarily to noxious mechanical stimuli, but some respond to chemical or thermal stimuli. They have been proposed to mediate the initial (or "first") sensation of pain, which has a sharp or "bright" perceptual quality.[9,53] Joints and muscles are innervated by similar finely myelinated A-δ fibers (also called group III fibers). A-δ fibers located in joints are distributed throughout the ligaments and periosteum. These fibers can be classified according to their responsiveness to passive movement and to noxious stimulation.[46] Under normal conditions, 30% of joint A-δ fibers respond only to noxious stimuli, and an additional 24% of these fibers do not respond to movement at all. These fibers are activated by chemicals such as the prostaglandins as well as by noxious joint movements. In muscle, A-δ fibers are thought to be distributed throughout muscle fibers, connective tissue, tendons, and endothelial walls.[48] These fibers are activated by muscle contraction, but also respond to hypertonic saline solution, bradykinin, and potassium.[34] Current evidence suggests that muscle A-δ fibers are probably important for perceptions of joint pain; their role in mediating muscle pain may be only secondary.[46,53]

The second group of nociceptive fibers are unmyelinated, slowly conducting nerve fibers. In skin, these nerves are termed polymodal C fibers, because they respond to several forms of stimulus, including thermal, mechanical, and chemical. The C polymodal nociceptors are responsive to bradykinin, potassium, acetylcholine, leukotrienes, and prostaglandins.[33,53] The C fibers probably mediate secondary pain. Secondary pain occurs after the initial "sharp, pricking" pain and is generally described as having a dull, aching, or burning quality.[9,53] Joints and muscle are innervated by similar unmyelinated C nociceptors (or group IV fibers), which have polymodal response properties.[24] In normal joints, 34% of C fibers are activated by noxious stimuli, while an additional 36% do not respond to movement at all.[46] Like the A-δ fibers located in joints, C fibers are activated by chemicals, such as prostaglandins, as well as noxious joint movements.[46] The sensation of pain arising from muscle is thought to be mediated primarily by C polymodal nociceptors.[53] In muscle, the C fiber afferents show little response to contraction but vigorously respond to ischemia, potassium, bradykinin, and prostaglandins.[34,53] Activation of muscle C fibers differs from stimulation of cutaneous C fibers by a prolonged alteration in spinal cord activity (ie, an increase in the receptive field size of dorsal horn neurons) and flexion reflexes.[7,51] Accordingly, injury to muscle may produce more extensive central nervous system changes than an equivalent amount of cutaneous injury.

Primary afferent nerves fan out as they enter their cutaneous receptive fields. Compared with C fibers, A-δ fibers innervating spinal dermatomes generally have more receptive field spots spread out over a greater surface area.[4] Although free nerve terminals lack morphologic specialization compared with other forms of cutaneous receptor types (eg, pacinian corpuscles), they are believed to possess some degree of biochemical specialization in terms of membrane receptors and stored neuropeptide substances. Ultrastructural studies have demonstrated that free nerve endings contain granular vesicles,[1,5,19,49] which may release neuropeptides such as substance P or calcitonin gene-related peptide (CGRP); these substances may be of importance in the modulation of inflammatory responses to tissue damage.

In addition to the A-δ and C fiber nociceptors, evidence indicates that the sympathetic nervous system may also contribute to the sensation of pain by any of several proposed mechanisms. First, visceral afferents appear to travel with sympathetic efferents and to encode for visceral pain.[21] Second, sympathetic efferents may alter the responses of certain low-threshold mechanoreceptors thought to be involved with chronic pain conditions such as causalgia.[44] Third, stimulation of sympathetic nerve fibers may alter the responses of some A-δ nociceptors that have terminal endings in inflamed tissue.[43] These findings suggest that the sympathetic nervous system may augment or modify the information obtained by the A-δ and C fiber afferent nociceptors for the perception of pain.

The spinal dorsal horn contains four major components related to the processing of noxious stimuli.[9,53] The first component, primary nociceptive afferents (eg, A-δ and C fibers), enter the spinal dorsal horn in Lissauer's tract. A-δ and C fibers terminate primarily in laminae I, IIa, and V of the dorsal horn. The primary nociceptive afferents are thought to transmit information by the synaptic release of neuropeptides such as substance P and CGRP or amino acids such as glutamate.

The second component of the dorsal horn is the local circuit neuron. Local circuit neurons are thought to modulate and perhaps to transfer nociceptive signals from the primary afferents to the projection neurons.[9,53]

The third component of the dorsal horn is the projection neuron. Projection neurons and local circuit neurons can be divided into two major classes, wide-dynamic-range (WDR) and nociceptive-specific (NS) neurons. The WDR neurons are activated by weak mechanical stimuli (eg, hair movement) but respond maximally to intense, potentially tissue-damaging stimuli. In contrast, the NS neurons respond only to noxious forms of mechanical, thermal, or chemical stimuli. The major projection, or output, system of pain is the spinothalamic tract. This tract is composed of axonal projections of WDR and NS neurons. These axons cross to the contralateral side of the spinal cord and ascend rostrally to the thalamus. From the thalamus, additional neurons convey this information to the cerebral cortex. The projection neurons encode information about the location, intensity, duration, and stimulus type of the noxious input.

The fourth component in the dorsal horn is the terminal endings of descending neurons. These neurons form an important component of the endogenous pain-suppression system. This system is activated under conditions of pain or stress and acts to inhibit the transmission of nociceptive information.[2,9,18]

Development of Sensitization and Hyperalgesia Caused by Tissue Damage

In general, inflammatory mediators have two main effects on the peripheral nociceptive nerve ending. Mediators excite and sensitize the peripheral nerve ending, and they also evoke peripheral release of neuropeptides such as substance P.[9,53] In response to mediators released during tissue injury, peripheral nerves become sensitized. Sensitized cutaneous fibers have spontaneous activity, a decreased threshold, and prolonged responses (afterdischarges) to suprathreshold stimuli. Although both polymodal C fibers and A-δ fibers can be sensitized, their susceptibilities seem to differ. Studies on human and monkey skin indicate that C fibers become sensitized at less intense noxious temperatures, whereas A-δ fibers become sensitized at higher or more intense temperatures.[6,35] Fibers that innervate joints can also become sensitized; during inflammation in joints, the spontaneous activity of C and A-δ fibers more than doubles, and their responses to joint movements that are not noxious increase twofold to sevenfold.[46] The biochemical substances that mediate sensitization are unknown, although some inflammatory mediators such as prostaglandins can mimic most of the attributes of sensitization.[33,34]

These electrophysiologic changes in the response properties of nociceptors, together with changes in the central nervous system,[6,54] result in the perceptual state of hyperalgesia. Hyperalgesia is characterized by spontaneous pain, a decreased pain threshold, and an increased magnitude of perceived pain for any given stimulus.[9,53] In many clinical models of inflammation it is a common finding and its presence differentiates pain caused by inflammation from that caused by transient stimuli. The presence of hyperalgesia after exercise-induced tissue damage explains why the injured athlete reports pain even after such a mild stimulus as stretching.

Relationship Between Mediator Release and Pain Recognition

In contrast to a transient pain-producing stimulus (eg, venipuncture), pain from inflammation is associated with prolonged hyperalgesia that is the result of the sustained actions of peripheral inflammatory mediators, which are thought to interact in the development of a local positive-feedback cycle (Fig. 1) and to central nervous system changes.[6,54] Tissue trauma, such as that found in sports-induced injuries, can activate the synthesis of prostaglandins and the release of bradykinin from its blood-borne precursor, kininogen. Because prostaglandins, bradykinin, and histamine all increase either the permeability or the vasodilation of local blood vessels,[36] they act synergistically to increase plasma extravasation. It is this accumulation of extravasated fluid into tissue spaces that produces the clinical sign of edema. In addition, plasma extravasation replenishes these short-lived local mediators by providing a fresh supply of kininogen, prostaglandins (released by bradykinin), histamine, and other mediators. Their continued synthesis or release explains the prolonged course of inflammation, which far exceeds the duration of the athletic endeavor (Fig. 1).

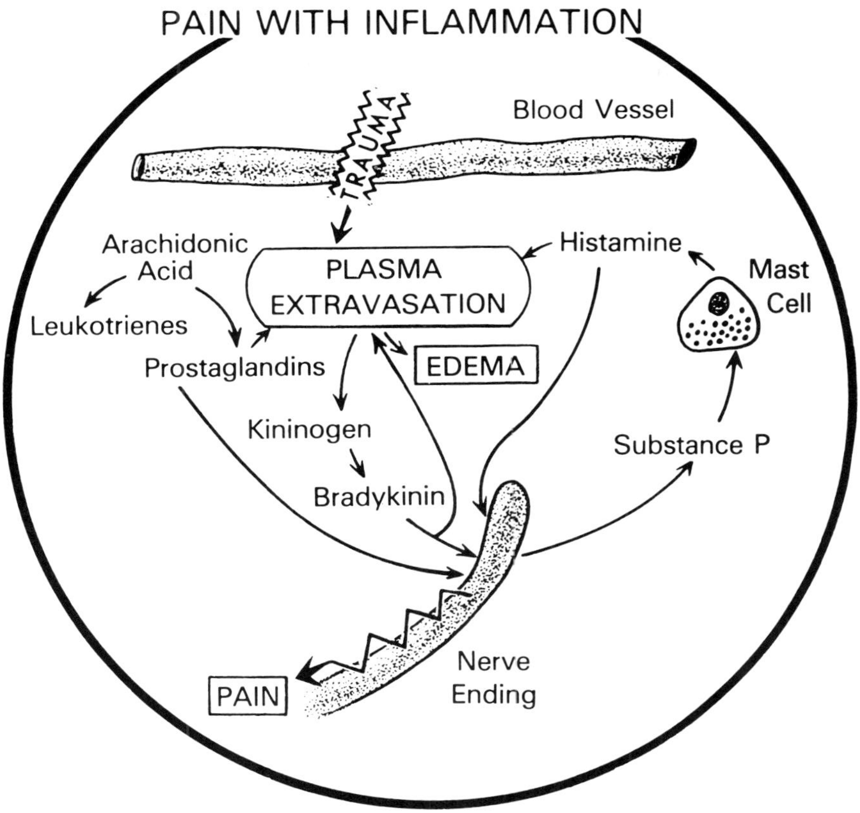

Fig. 1 *Schema of the positive-feedback relationship that develops during the course of inflammation secondary to sports-related injuries. (Reproduced with permission from Hargreaves KM, Troullos ES, Dionne RA: Pharmacologic rationale for the treatment of acute pain.* Dent Clin North Am *1987;31:675–694.)*

Many studies have evaluated the effects of inflammatory mediators on some dependent measure related to nociception. For example, prostaglandins, leukotrienes, bradykinin, histamine, serotonin, acetylcholine, and potassium all activate primary afferents located in skin, muscle, or joints.[33,34,46,53] In addition, pretreatment with prostaglandin E_2 potentiates the stimulating effects of a subsequent application of bradykinin.[34] In studies measuring a behavioral endpoint, such as flexion reflex or pain report, prostaglandins, leukotrienes, bradykinin, potassium, and dihydroxyeicosatetraenoic acids (diHETES) are active when administered into peripheral tissue.[23,27,29,42,50,52] However, these studies merely document the ability of mediators, usually administered at supraphysiologic doses, to stimulate processes related to nociception. Little is known about the actual tissue concentration of these mediators during inflammation and to what extent they are involved in mediating pain caused by different types of tissue injury (thermal vs chemical vs overexercise). An additional complicating factor is that stress or pain can activate endogenous pain-suppression systems in some[12,15] but not all[13] conditions. Accordingly, pain caused by inflammation is not related solely to peripheral release of inflammatory mediators, but represents an integration of peripheral and central processes.

Interactions Between Peripheral Nerves and Inflammatory Mediators

In addition to sensation, another effect of inflammatory mediators is to modulate the release of neuropeptides stored in the peripheral nociceptive nerve ending (Fig. 1). The cell body of the primary afferent nerve fiber synthesizes the neuropeptides substance P and CGRP, as well as other substances, that are transported to both the central nervous system and the periphery.[45] These neuropeptides are highly concentrated in peripheral tissue such as joints, and the electrical or chemical stimulation of peripheral nerves releases immunoreactive substance P.[39,55] These peptides have pro-inflammatory effects: administration of substance P and CGRP induces plasma extravasation in skin and exacerbates ongoing joint inflammation.[25,26] These findings suggest that peripheral nerves may be able to modulate the development of inflammation.

Whether peripheral nerves alter inflammation has been directly tested in several experiments. Generally, either nerve transection or application of neurotoxins reduces the magnitude of inflammation.[8,10,22] Consistent with this observation, electrical or chemical stimulation of peripheral nerves can evoke plasma extravasation in both cutaneous beds and in joints.[25,36] Polymodal C fibers have been implicated in several of these studies, because many of the effects of nerve stimulation can be blocked by administration of substance P antagonists or capsaicin, a neurotoxin that inactivates C fibers.[25,36] Thus, the peripheral nerve not only detects and signals the occurrence of tissue damage, it also participates in the development of tissue inflammation (Fig. 1). However, the sympathetic nervous system may also contribute to the development of inflammation, since sympatholytic agents such as reserpine reduce inflammatory changes in joints.[28] Moreover, β_2-antagonists such as albuterol or butoxamine significantly reduce joint injury caused by chronic inflammation.[28]

Peripheral nerves can also modulate inflammation by altering the release or metabolism of inflammatory mediators. Neuropeptides from primary afferents, such as substance P, act synergistically with other inflammatory mediators to stimulate histamine release from mast cells.[25,27] Administration of substance P to synoviocytes obtained from human joints stimulates these cells to secrete prostaglandin E_2 and collagenase and to proliferate in culture.[30] In addition, substance P stimulates monocytes to release substances such as interleukin-1, interleukin-6, and tumor necrosis factor.[31] Activation of the sympathetic nervous system or administration of norepinephrine stimulates the synthesis and release of prostaglandins from vascular tissue.[3,32,56] In addition, peripheral nerves are capable of synthesizing prostaglandins.[11] Another potential target for catecholamines are leukocytes, which have adrenergic receptors[40] and are responsive to administration of adrenergic agents.[14,37] The basis for the modulation of inflammation by peripheral nerves might be their ability to regulate the synthesis or release of inflammatory mediators.

Relationship Between the Magnitude of Tissue Injury and the Report of Pain

On first consideration, it might be assumed that there is a close relationship between the magnitude of tissue injury and the patient's report of pain. Indeed, studies on animals indicate that there is a linear relationship between the dose of an inflammatory agent and the magnitude of nociceptive responses.[17] Similarly, humans reported dose-related increases in pain when bradykinin or potassium was applied in an experimental model of inflamed skin.[52]

The relationship between the injury and the pain reported, however, seems more complex when examined in a clinical setting. In outpatients undergoing a highly standardized surgical procedure, only 23% of the variability of postoperative pain was associated with variations in indices of tissue damage.[47] Factors that probably complicate this relationship include psychological health, personality traits, expectations, cognitive assessments of pain,[41] and intersubject differences in activation of endogenous analgesic systems. In patients with different types of injuries—joint vs soft tissue—and in different stages of inflammation or repair (acute vs chronic), the relationship between the magnitude of the initial trauma and the level of pain reported becomes even more obscure.

References

1. Arwill T, Edwall L, Lilja J, et al: Ultrastructure of nerves in the dentinal-pulp border zone after sensory and autonomic nerve transection in the cat. *Acta Odontol Scand* 1973;31:273–281.
2. Basbaum AI, Fields HL: Endogenous pain control systems: Brainstem spinal pathways and endorphin circuitry. *Annu Rev Neurosci* 1984;7:309–338.
3. Boeynaems JM, Demolle D, Galand N: Adrenergic stimulation of vascular prostacyclin: Role of alpha$_1$ receptors in smooth muscle cells. *Eur J Pharmacol* 1987;144:193–200.
4. Burgess PR, Perl ER: Cutaneous mechanoreceptors and nociceptors, in Iggo A (ed): *Handbook of Sensory Physiology: Volume II. Somatosensory System.* Berlin, Springer-Verlag, 1973, pp 29–78.
5. Byers MR: Dental sensory receptors. *Int Rev Neurobiol* 1984;25:39–94.
6. Coderre TJ, Melzack R: Cutaneous hyperalgesia: Contributions of the peripheral and central nervous systems to the increase in pain sensitivity after injury. *Brain Res* 1987;404:95–106.

7. Cook AJ, Woolf CJ, Wall PD, et al: Dynamic receptive field plasticity in rat spinal cord dorsal horn following C-primary afferent input. *Nature* 1987;325:151–153.
8. Courtright LJ, Kuzell WC: Sparing effect of neurological deficit and trauma on the course of adjuvant arthritis in the rat. *Ann Rheum Dis* 1965;24:360–368.
9. Dubner R, Bennett GJ: Spinal and trigeminal mechanisms of nociception. *Annu Rev Neurosci* 1983;6:381–418.
10. Gamse R, Holzer P, Lembeck F: Decrease of substance P in primary afferent neurones and impairment of neurogenic plasma extravasation by capsaicin. *Br J Pharmacol* 1980;68:207–213.
11. Goswami SK, Gould RM: Prostanoid synthesis in peripheral nerve. *Biochim Biophys Acta* 1985;834:263–266.
12. Gracely RH, Dubner R, Wolskee PJ, et al: Placebo and naloxone can alter post-surgical pain by separate mechanisms. *Nature* 1983;306:264–265.
13. Grevert P, Goldstein A: Endorphins: Naloxone fails to alter experimental pain or mood in humans. *Science* 1978;199:1093–1095.
14. Hammerschmidt DE, Jeanneret C, Husak M, et al: Lymphocyte aggregation in response to adrenergic stimulation. *Blood* 1988;71:1470–1474.
15. Hargreaves KM, Dionne RA, Mueller GP, et al: Naloxone, fentanyl, and diazepam modify plasma beta-endorphin levels during surgery. *Clin Pharmacol Ther* 1986;40:165–171.
16. Hargreaves KM, Dubner R: Mechanisms of pain and analgesia, in Dionne R, Phero J (eds): *Management of Pain and Anxiety*. New York, Elsevier Press, in press.
17. Hargreaves KM, Dubner R, Brown F, et al: A new and sensitive method for measuring thermal nociception in cutaneous hyperalgesia. *Pain* 1988;32:77–88.
18. Hargreaves KM, Troullos ES, Dionne RA: Pharmacologic rationale for the treatment of acute pain. *Dent Clin North Am* 1987;31:675–694.
19. Hoyes AD, Barber P: Ultrastructure of the corneal nerves in the rat. *Cell Tissue Res* 1976;172:133–144.
20. IASP Subcommittee on Taxonomy: Pain terms: A list with definitions and notes on usage. *Pain* 1979;6:249–252.
21. Jänig W, Kollmann W: The involvement of the sympathetic nervous system in pain: Possible neuronal mechanisms. *Arzneim Forsch* 1984;34:1066–1073.
22. Joris J, Hargreaves K: Involvement of the peripheral nerve system in the development of carrageenan-induced inflammation, abstract. *Soc Neurosci* 1987;13:1017.
23. Katori M, Hori Y, Uchida Y, et al: Different modes of interaction of bradykinin with prostaglandins in pain and acute inflammation. *Adv Exp Med Biol* 1986;198:393–398.
24. Kumazawa T, Mizumura K: Thin-fibre receptors responding to mechanical, chemical, and thermal stimulation in the skeletal muscle of the dog. *J Physiol* 1977;273:179–194.
25. Lembeck F, Holzer P: Substance P as a neurogenic mediator of antidromic vasodilation and neurogenic plasma extravasation. *Naunyn Schmiedebergs Arch Pharmacol* 1979;310:175–183.
26. Levine JD, Coderre TJ, Helms C, et al: Beta$_2$-adrenergic mechanisms in experimental arthritis. *Proc Natl Acad Sci USA* 1988;85:4553–4556.
27. Levine JD, Lam D, Taiwo YO, et al: Hyperalgesic properties of 15-lipoxygenase products of arachidonic acid. *Proc Natl Acad Sci USA* 1986;83;5331–5334.

28. Levine JD, Lau W, Kwiat G, et al: Leukotriene B4 produces hyperalgesia that is dependent on polymorphonuclear leukocytes. *Science* 1984;225:743–745.
29. Levine JD, Moskowitz MA, Basbaum AI: The contribution of neurogenic inflammation in experimental arthritis. *J Immunol* 1985;135(suppl):843s–847s.
30. Lotz M, Carson DA, Vaughan JH: Substance P activation of rheumatoid synoviocytes: Neural pathway in pathogenesis of arthritis. *Science* 1987;235:893–895.
31. Lotz M, Vaughan JH, Carson DA: Effect of neuropeptides on production of inflammatory cytokines by human monocytes. *Science* 1988;241:1218–1221.
32. Malik KU: Interaction of arachidonic acid metabolites and adrenergic nervous system. *Am J Med Sci* 1988;295:280–286.
33. Martin HA, Basbaum AI, Kwiat GC, et al: Leukotriene and prostaglandin sensitization of cutaneous high-threshold C- and A-delta mechanoreceptors in the hairy skin of rat hindlimbs. *Neuroscience* 1987;22:651–659.
34. Mense S: Nervous outflow from skeletal muscle following chemical noxious stimulation. *J Neurophysiol* 1977;267:75–88.
35. Meyer RA, Campbell JN: Myelinated nociceptive afferents account for the hyperalgesia that follows a burn to the hand. *Science* 1981;213:1527–1529.
36. Morton CR, Chahl LA: Pharmacology of the neurogenic oedema response to electrical stimulation of the saphenous nerve in the rat. *Naunyn Schmiedebergs Arch Pharmacol* 1980;314:271–276.
37. Nielson CP: Beta-adrenergic modulation of the polymorphonuclear leukocyte respiratory burst is dependent upon the mechanism of cell activation. *J Immunol* 1987;139:2392–2397.
38. Ochoa J, Mair WGP: The normal sural nerve in man: I. Ultrastructure and numbers of fibres and cells. *Acta Neuropathol* 1969;13:197–216.
39. Olgart L, Gazelius B, Brodin E, et al: Release of substance P-like immunoreactivity from the dental pulp. *Acta Physiol Scand* 1977;101:510–512.
40. Panosaian JO, Marinetti GV: Alpha$_2$-adrenergic receptors in human polymorphonuclear leukocyte membranes. *Biochem Pharmacol* 1983;32:2243–2247.
41. Price DD, Harkins SW, Baker C: Sensory-affective relationships among different types of clinical and experimental pain. *Pain* 1987;28:297–307.
42. Rackham A, Ford-Hutchinson AW: Inflammation and pain sensitivity: Effects of leukotrienes D4, B4 and prostaglandin E1 in the rat paw. *Prostaglandins* 1983;25:193–203.
43. Roberts WJ, Elardo SM: Sympathetic activation of A-delta nociceptors. *Somatosen Res* 1985;3:33–44.
44. Roberts WJ, Foglesong ME: Identification of afferents contributing to sympathetically evoked activity in wide-dynamic-range neurons. *Pain* 1988;34:305–314.
45. Rosenfeld MG, Mermod JJ, Amara SG, et al: Production of a novel neuropeptide encoded by the calcitonin gene via tissue-specific RNA processing. *Nature* 1983;304:129–135.
46. Schaible HG, Schmidt RF: Discharge characteristics of receptors with fine afferents from normal and inflamed joints: Influence of analgesics and prostaglandins. *Agents Actions* 1986;19(suppl):99–117.
47. Schmidt EA, Hargreaves KM, Dionne RA: Surgical trauma and duration as predictors of post-operative pain, abstract. *J Dent Res* 1988;67:212.
48. Stacey MJ: Free nerve endings in skeletal muscle of the cat. *J Anat* 1969;105:231–254.
49. Tervo T, Palkama A: Innervation of the rabbit cornea: A histochemical and electron-microscopic study. *Acta Anat* 1978;102:164–175.

50. Tyers MB, Haywood H: Effects of prostaglandins on peripheral nociceptors in acute inflammation; in Rainsford KD, Ford-Hutchinson AW (eds): *Prostaglandins and Inflammation.* Basel, Birkhauser Verlag, 1979, pp 65–78.
51. Wall PD, Woolf CJ: Muscle but not cutaneous C-afferent input produces prolonged increases in the excitability of the flexion reflex in the rat. *J Physiol* 1984;356:443–458.
52. Whalley ET, Clegg S, Stewart JM, et al: The effect of kinin agonists and antagonists on the pain response of the human blister base. *Naunyn Schmiedebergs Arch Pharmacol* 1987;336:652–655.
53. Willis WD Jr: *The Pain System: The Neural Basis of Nociceptive Transmission in the Mammalian Nervous System.* Basel, S Karger, 1985.
54. Woolf CJ: Evidence for a central component of post-injury pain hypersensitivity. *Nature* 1983;306:686–688.
55. Yaksh TL: Substance P release from knee joint afferent terminals: Modulation by opioids. *Brain Res* 1988;458:319–324.
56. Yousufzai SY, Gracy RA, Aboul-Khair HS, et al: In vivo electrical stimulation of the sympathetic nerve of the eye increases inositol phosphate production and prostaglandin release in the rabbit iris muscle. *J Neurochem* 1988;50:752–758.

Future Directions

Sports-induced soft-tissue inflammation is a common cause of pain and impaired performance in recreational and competitive athletes. In some patients, sports-induced inflammation results from a single acute load that exceeds the strength of the tissue. In others, it results from repetitive loading that exceeds the adaptive capacity of the tissue. Despite the frequency and importance of the problem, the pathophysiology of sports-induced soft-tissue inflammation, especially inflammation resulting from repetitive loading, remains poorly understood. Diagnostic criteria are not well established, the incidence and prevalence of the common sports-induced inflammation syndrome have not been defined, and the mechanisms remain unknown.

Extensive knowledge and well-developed research methods that can be used to define the pathophysiology of sports-induced inflammation exist in three areas. These are (1) studies of the structure, composition, and material properties of soft tissues, (2) clinical experience with and studies of the diagnosis and treatment of sports-induced inflammation syndromes, and (3) investigations of the basic inflammatory mechanisms. Thus far, the research methods and knowledge derived from these three areas have not been combined effectively to study the problems of sports-induced soft-tissue inflammation. The following recommendations draw on these three areas and suggest approaches that may advance understanding of the pathophysiology of sports-induced soft-tissue inflammation.

Develop Clinical Diagnostic Criteria

Lack of consistent diagnostic criteria compromises treatment and investigation of sports-induced soft-tissue inflammation. In particular, the lack of reliable, well-accepted diagnostic criteria impedes treatment comparisons, epidemiologic studies, clinical research, basic research, natural history studies, development of new diagnostic methods, and refinement of current diagnostic methods.

Diagnostic criteria could be developed and refined through several methods. One possibility would be to establish a consensus group of clinical experts. With the assistance of basic scientists, this group could develop diagnostic criteria similar to those developed for selected rheumatologic conditions. This approach is more likely to be successful if it includes a wide range of individuals and if the criteria developed are clinically applicable to large-scale use. The criteria could then be verified through clinical trials by many physicians. This project might consider such sports-related soft-tissue inflammation syndromes as muscle strains, patellofemoral joint pain, and specific forms of tendinitis.

Barriers to implementing this approach include difficulties in organizing the consensus group, in achieving consensus, and in obtaining financial support for such a large-scale project.

Study Specific Syndromes

One of the limitations of further study of sports-induced soft-tissue inflammation, including the development and study of animal models, is the lack of well-defined, carefully studied examples of human soft-tissue inflammation syndromes. If specific clinical diagnostic criteria could be developed, selected groups of patients could be studied to determine the relationships between the clinical presentation (the history, physical findings, pain measurements, and performance deficit) and the clinically defined mechanisms of injury. Imaging studies, laboratory studies, and tissue and fluid samples, where appropriate, could be part of this study. Although routine use of imaging studies, laboratory studies, and tissue and fluid samples might not be appropriate, they could help define selected clinical syndromes. Here, too, however, there would be organizational, consensual, and financial barriers to implementation.

Investigate Epidemiology

The incidence and prevalence of common sports-induced soft-tissue inflammation syndromes remain unknown. Studies based on the clinical diagnostic criteria developed under the first recommendation could determine the incidence and prevalence of sports-induced soft-tissue inflammation syndromes and identify associations between specific syndromes and age, sex, activity type, and activity intensity. These studies could be performed simultaneously by several institutions. However, this recommendation cannot be implemented until reliable, valid, and widely accepted clinical diagnostic criteria are developed.

Develop Animal Models

Well-defined animal models of soft-tissue inflammation caused by mechanical loading do not currently exist. As a result, it is difficult to design controlled experimental studies of the mechanisms, treatments, and methods of prevention of sports-induced soft-tissue inflammation. Potentially useful experimental studies include efforts to produce inflammation by acute and repetitive loading of tendons, ligaments, joint capsules, tendon and ligament insertions into bone, myotendinous junctions, and skeletal muscle. Different loading mechanisms should be explored to identify those that predictably cause soft-tissue inflammation resembling sports-induced soft-tissue inflammation in humans. This necessitates a definition of sports-induced inflammation syndromes as previously outlined. Experimental models of mechanically induced tendinitis, synovitis, and inflammation of muscle, myotendinous junctions, and tendon and ligament insertions would be particularly helpful. Another approach would be to study tendinitis and other mechanically induced soft-tissue inflammation syndromes that occur spontaneously in such animals as greyhounds and racehorses.

However, experimental models have important potential limitations. These include the difficulty of studying the relationship between inflammation and pain, the difficulty of studying the relationship between inflammation and performance deficit, and the uncertainty of the relationship between an animal model and similar human conditions. In addition, attempts to develop experimental models of mechanically induced soft-tissue inflammation may show that the relationship between repetitive loading and soft-tissue inflammation varies considerably among individuals and among tissues.

Develop Mechanical and Mathematical Computer Models of Soft-Tissue Responses to Loading

Developing mechanical and mathematical computer models of human soft tissues would make it possible to study loading effects in complex synovial joints and soft tissues. Models based on specific human joints and tissues could examine the effects of alterations in loading on many specific tissues. For example, a model of the glenohumeral joint could be used to study the effects of displacement of the humeral head relative to the glenoid and the effects on surrounding soft tissues such as the joint capsule, surrounding ligaments, the labrum and adjacent muscles, and their insertions.

Explore Possible Immune System Mechanisms

Although a relationship between sports-induced soft-tissue inflammation and immune system activation has not been demonstrated, some forms of chronic, mechanically induced inflammation may have an immune system component. Studying animal models or examining human tissue with histochemical methods are ways of exploring this issue. Difficulty in obtaining human tissue samples and lack of animal models as well as the problems outlined under the first two recommendations are the primary barriers to implementing this recommendation.

Explore the Possible Existence of Urine, Serum, or Tissue Markers for Inflammation

Sports-induced soft-tissue inflammation may be associated with the release of inflammatory mediators. Examination of aspirates, biopsy specimens, urine, or serum from humans with sports-induced soft-tissue inflammation might identify increased levels of these inflammatory mediators. Animal models might be useful in demonstrating the relationship between the severity or mechanism of soft-tissue inflammation and the marker levels. If such markers can be identified and measured, a series of clinical studies on the diagnosis and treatment of sports-induced soft-tissue inflammation could be initiated.

However, there is no strong evidence to suggest that such an exploration would be productive. At present, it is not clear which inflammatory mediators should be studied, or if increased levels of any inflammatory mediators can be identified in patients with mechanically induced soft-tissue inflammation. Even if such inflammatory mediators were identified, the information might not be useful in diagnosing and assessing the severity of mechanically induced soft-tissue inflammation.

Investigate Possible Urine, Serum, or Tissue Markers for Increased Soft-Tissue Turnover

Increased turnover of matrix molecules may be associated with the adaptation of soft tissues to increased loading and many sports-induced soft-tissue inflammation syndromes. Release of these molecules or one of their degradation products might be detected by analyzing tissue, serum, or urine. Investigative approaches include examining human tissue, serum, and urine from patients with sports-induced soft-tissue inflammation or similar studies in animal models. However, specific serum and tissue markers reflecting increased soft-tissue turnover may not exist, or they may be so variable or difficult to measure that they would be of little value.

Measure Strain Load and Deformation in Vivo for Normal and Inflamed Soft Tissues

Although the mechanical (or material) properties as represented by the stress-strain curve of many soft tissues have been well described using standard engineering techniques, the load (or stress) and deformation (or strain) of these tissues in vivo have not been extensively studied. Investigations in this area will depend on the development of new methods to measure these quantities. Possible approaches include the use of in vivo strain gauges to measure tissue elongation under controlled loading conditions, or other kinematic methods to determine the elongation of these tissues. Once the strains are known, then the corresponding stress can be determined by in vitro techniques. Once the levels of stress and strain in vivo are known, appropriate animal models of sports-induced soft-tissue inflammation can be developed. Particularly, the level and frequency of stresses and strains that cause soft tissue to be inflamed can be evaluated. Barriers to implementation of this recommendation include limitations of methods for studying the levels of in vivo stress and strain as well as the lack of animal models.

Investigate in Vivo Cellular and Matrix Responses of Soft Tissues to Single and Repetitive Loads

Although it is generally accepted that persistent increased loading of soft tissues tends to increase their strength, especially in young individuals, the mechanism is unknown and the quantitative features of the response are not well defined. A series of experiments with animal models demonstrating changes in cell function and in matrix composition and organization in response to loading would be useful. The cellular functions studied should include proliferation and synthetic activity. Matrix studies should include measures of composition and organization. At present, there is no method of applying controlled in vivo loading.

Investigate the in Vivo Cellular and Matrix Responses to Soft-Tissue Inflammation

Mechanically induced inflammation may alter the cells and matrices of soft tissues, but this has not been proven. An animal model of sports-induced soft-tissue inflammation would make it possible to demonstrate the morphologic, biochemical, and cellular responses to inflammation. Methods similar to those outlined above could be used to study the tissues once an animal model of mechanically induced soft-tissue inflammation has been developed.

Explore the Possible Relationships Between Training-Induced Changes in Muscle Function and the Development of Sports-Induced Soft-Tissue Inflammation

Despite the effects of training on tissues, even highly conditioned athletes may develop sports-induced soft-tissue inflammation. Why this occurs is not clear. One possible explanation is that muscles that normally absorb loads by decelerating limb motion become less active with prolonged training. This would then increase the load on musculoskeletal soft tissues. Specifically, as prolonged training increases the efficiency of sport-specific movements, the passive musculoskeletal soft tissues may absorb more load—and muscle contraction less—during deceleration of joints. Another explanation might be that some conditioning programs include patterns of muscle action that increase loading of soft tissues in ways that cause inflammation.

These possibilities could be investigated by comparing the patterns of muscle action and muscle strength in selected groups of highly trained athletes and in control groups. Another approach would be to measure in vivo soft-tissue loading in trained and untrained animals during activity. It might then be possible to associate changes in patterns of muscle action and soft-tissue loading with sports-induced soft-tissue inflammation syndromes. If these patterns could be identified, new training methods might be devised. However, it would be difficult to assess patterns of muscle action and soft-tissue loading with current methods.

Investigate the Use of Imaging Studies

The value of most imaging studies in the assessment of sports-induced soft-tissue inflammation is unclear. However, experiments could be designed to correlate imaging studies with clinical syndromes and with the degree of severity. The imaging techniques that have the most promise are magnetic resonance imaging, magnetic resonance imaging spectroscopy, radioactive isotope scanning, and positron emission tomography. The difficulty lies in the lack of well-defined clinical diagnostic categories of sports-induced soft-tissue inflammation.

Investigate Age-Related Changes

Aging may alter the response of soft tissues to repetitive loading and the incidence, prevalence, clinical mechanism, duration, and intensity of sports-induced soft-tissue inflammation. If clinical diagnostic criteria can be developed, the relationship between sports-induced inflammation and aging should be investigated. If acceptable animal models can be developed, age-related changes in the tissue response to mechanically induced inflammation might be found. Implemention of this recommendation must await the development of clinical diagnostic criteria and suitable animal models.

Investigate the Mechanism and Treatment of Sports-Induced Soft-Tissue Calcification

Occasionally, sports-induced soft-tissue inflammation results in calcification of such tissues as muscle, tendon, ligament, and joint capsule. Although the clinical presentation is well-described and the risk factors are known, the mechanism remains unclear. Our understanding of this problem can be increased through basic investigations of soft-tissue calcification and the development of experimental models of sports-induced inflammation that result in soft-tissue calcification. At present, no satisfactory experimental model has been developed.

Section Three

Modifiers of Inflammation

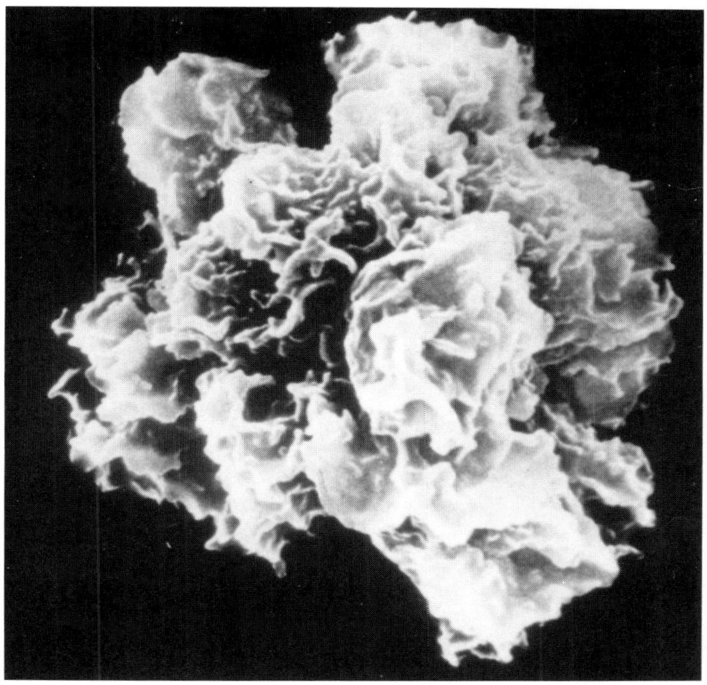

Group Leaders

Wayne Leadbetter, MD
William Quillen, PhD, PT, SCS

Group Participants

Steven Abramson, MD
Jeffrey Basford, MD, PhD
W. Watson Buchanan, MD, FRCP (Edin, Glasg, and C)
Jesse DeLee, MD
Cyril Frank, MD, FRCS (C)
James Goodwin, MD
Herbert Haupt, MD
Kenneth Knight, PhD, ATC
Terry Malone, EdD, PT, ATC
Fred Nelson, MD
Edward Percy, MD, FRCS (C)
Ethan Saliba, MEd, ATC, PT

Overview

Changing the inflammatory process in connective tissue requires inciting a cellular and/or matrix tissue response. In clinical medicine, such attempts are common and involve the prescription of a modifier. Potential modifiers include anti–inflammatory medications (which may be oral, injectable, or topical) and physical techniques such as thermotherapy, cryotherapy, electrical-field induction, and rehabilitative exercise.

Modifiers of sports-induced inflammation have been employed to decrease the pain of inflammation to allow compliance with rehabilitation and to avoid pain-induced disuse atrophy, neurologic discoordination, and altered muscle function after injury. In such cases, a modifier may be employed as part of the total rehabilitative therapy program to minimize the ill effects of immobilization, soft-tissue atrophy, adhesions, joint stiffness, or articular cartilage degeneration. Modifiers are also used to decrease inflammation in freshly healed, relatively vascular tissues during the period of retraining and reconditioning after injury, to control symptoms of inflammation in "overuse" injuries, especially chronic symptoms in the older athlete stemming from the degenerative sequelae of previous injury, and to stem the acute "inflammatory overshoot" occurring in response to acute trauma, thereby limiting the zone of soft-tissue necrosis or damage and dysfunctional behavior caused by pain.

In the broadest sense, modification of inflammation is intended to reduce the zone of secondary tissue damage and necrosis resulting from the aftermath of traumatic cellular and matrix events, to promote healing leading to more rapid return of structural integrity through the formation of scar, and, ultimately, to permit an earlier safe return to sports performance. Because inflammation is the immediate sequela of wounding and the precursor of repair, modification of inflammation implies an attempt either to diminish scar formation (eg, tendinitis, fibrobursitis, capsular contracture) or to augment scar formation (eg, ligament repair, healing of intratendinous degeneration).

Once thought to be metabolically inactive, the mesenchymally derived connective tissues are now seen as capable of a wide variety of biochemical and cellular responses to overload and overuse. Thus, there is also the possibility of response to an imposed modifier. However, the understanding of such responses and their treatment has not been as well documented because many initial soft-tissue sports-injury complaints are not treated surgically. Indeed, the paradox of "the absence of inflammation" in some tendinitic conditions may be the result of the timing of the observation during the cycle of inflammatory repair. In addition, more attention must be given to the potentially significant sports-induced matrix changes that may be a prelude to classic inflammation. Further, although an animal model for synovitic inflammation is available, a reliable tendon model for overuse injuries has proven to be more elusive.

Statistically, the chronic inflammatory conditions of synovial structures and tendon constitute the majority of sports injuries. These injuries are typified by unwanted responses such as friction-induced bursitis or overuse tendinitis and the more poorly understood tendinosis phenomenon in which no classic inflammatory response is noted but there is pain. Pain, however, does not indicate that inflammation is definitely present. Mechanical stress or strain, such as occurs with distension or isolated excessive pressure can stimulate nerve endings and create pain without classic inflammation. Inflammation may be structurally insignificant, self-healing, and nonserious with treatment centered on the symptoms of pain or structurally significant with treatment based on strength return, residual instability, and preexisting degenerative disease, in addition to pain. In this second category of injury, there is a demand for progressive rehabilitation or surgery.

As previously noted, not all pain is inflammatory, and pain is not always proportional to the severity of injury because of changing thresholds of perception in the athlete. When this is coupled with the limited ability to quantify soft-tissue injury, "inflammation" can be a catch-all term covering an imprecise clinical diagnosis.

Because it is difficult to define the injury and to identify the presence of true inflammation, the assessment of improvement after modifier use if often based on comparisons with an undefined starting point. There is less disagreement regarding the need to control pain that interferes in any way with function, and there is agreement that rehabilitation should be initiated during this period of observation and treatment.

Assuming that structural injury is associated with inflammation, it is not certain that optimum healing occurs under "normal" circumstances or conditions of rest. The sports clinician tends to seek treatment that is complete and effective, that is, that relieves inflammatory symptoms and at the same time produces a genuine healing response. However, in practice the present choices of therapeutic modifiers of soft-tissue inflammation range among those that seem to offer complete tissue restoration (for example, electrical-field induction, therapeutic exercise), those that claim to alter the course of the inflammatory repair cycle (for example, physical techniques such as thermotherapy and cryotherapy, nonsteroidal anti-inflammatory drugs, corticosteroids), and those that appear to affect symptoms for which a beneficial cellular response is either disputed or not well documented (for example, anabolic steroids, dimethyl sulfoxide). In addition, modification of inflammatory mediators may actually accentuate damage. Salicylates and NSAIDs have been shown to unmask mediators and change the function of the arachidonic acid cascade. However, the inflammatory process within the body represents an open system with several hundred chemical mediators; a full understanding of this system may not be needed to justify the use of a modifier in the treatment of the disability. Because of the short duration of some inflammatory patterns, a modifier may not affect loss of function by decreasing classic chemical reactions, but is more likely to affect the secondary responses of inflammation such as muscle spasm and neuroreflexic pain.

The Role of Specific Modifiers

The section on modifiers of inflammation provides a broad overview of potentially useful measures that range from commonly used techniques such as thermotherapy, cryotherapy, NSAIDs, and corticosteroid injections to those with unproven clinical effectiveness such as electrical-field induction and laser therapy.

NSAIDs

The role of oral anti-inflammatory medication in the treatment of sports trauma appears to be governed by the old adage, "First, do no harm." This is underscored by the potential suppression of normal wound healing response and the diverse adverse side effects of oral corticosteroids that currently limit their indications in acute and chronic injuries. In contrast, NSAIDs have several indications and fewer potential side effects because of their different site of action in the arachidonic acid cycle. Both ligand and inflammatory cell reactions and chemical mediator release secondary to mechanically induced cell death represent common sources of chronic inflammation. A classic model is the crystal-driven types of inflammation such as gout or pseudogout. Excitation of polymorphonuclear cells can be stimulated by fibronectin and other breakdown products of injured collagen structures, favoring further mediator release and neutrophil activation. NSAIDs enter into this cycle in a variety of ways to stabilize cell membranes and dampen the effects of the arachidonic acid cascade. Paradoxically, the resultant decrease in prostaglandin synthesis has been shown to unmask other mediators and, in a complex fashion, to result in potentially increased damage from inflammation. Although concern regarding retardation of wound healing by NSAIDs can be tempered by their lack of adverse effect on the function of fibroblasts and tissue macrophages, NSAIDs have not been proven to speed wound healing. The efficacy of NSAIDs may be less when there is no continuing trigger for cell hyperactivity with which NSAIDs interfere, thus explaining their relative lack of efficacy in inflammation caused by acute injury compared with that caused by chronic injury.

Salicylates are in the same position as the other NSAIDs. Acetylsalicylic acid and other analgesic and anti–inflammatory agents may be only one component in a therapeutic regimen in specific conditions, but may aggravate initial hematoma formation and be counterproductive in some situations. Decreasing the disability produced by painful, reflexively controlled muscle spasm may be the primary value of these agents.

Anabolic Steroids—DMSO

Both dimethyl sulfoxide and anabolic steroids have been advocated for the treatment of athletic injuries. Yet neither of these potential modifiers can be therapeutically justified on the basis of our present understanding of the balance between their cellular and metabolic effects. Although the inhibition of the oxidative function of stimulated neutrophils by dimethyl sulfoxide may suggest a role for in vivo anti–inflammatory activity, well-controlled studies have not substantiated its efficacy in relieving symptoms or demonstrated a posttreatment healing response. Similarly, evidence of dysplastic collagen fibril development resulting from anabolic steroid treatment and the statistical association of pathologic tendon rupture with increased lysosomal activity argue against its use.

Corticosteroids

As oral corticosteroids act earliest in the anti–inflammatory cascade, blocking the release of arachidonic acid, these medications have great effect on many different biologic systems and have a greater risk-benefit ratio. Corticosteroids decrease collagen synthesis by fibroblasts as well as inhibit cytokine release from mononuclear cells. There is no support in the literature for the use of oral corticosteroids in the treatment of sports trauma. Major design flaws in all reported drug studies have left many questions open to further study with respect to both NSAIDs and oral corticosteroids.

Corticosteroid injection therapy continues to be widely employed although the mechanism of its alleged therapeutic effect has not been documented. The potential adverse structural effects on ligament and tendon tissues must be weighed against the potential therapeutic benefit of this powerful pharmacologic agent. The best indication for local corticosteroids seems to be inflammatory processes in which suppression of neutrophils and higher levels of chemical mediators may prevent further tissue injury. They are contraindicated in acute macrotrauma because of their catabolic effects. The healing induced by injection therapy has not been conclusively documented but has been implied in some animal models. No controlled clinical studies have been done and clinical response remains anecdotal. Because a reliable animal model is lacking, present research depends on injecting normal tendon structures. Thus, any extrapolation of conclusions to diseased or injured structures is questionable. A best, such therapy remains adjunctive.

Physical Modalities

There is much debate about the various physical techniques' indications, efficacy, and potential to modify the inflammation-repair cycle. However, clinical experience suggests that they have a role.

Thermotherapy or heat application relieves the secondary symptoms of inflammation such as spasm. Local effects on enzymes have been documented. Its greatest effect is to facilitate exercise. Cryotherapy may reduce local tissue temperature and local blood flow to an injured area, thereby influencing the secondary necrotic effects of the initial trauma. Although such processes have been readily documented in acute injury by decreased edema and pain, cellular responses continue to be conjectural. In chronic overuse injuries, the effects of cold on inflammation have not been investigated.

Studies suggest that ice massage, ultrasound, iontophoresis, and phonophoresis are equally efficacious. Animal modeling may affect the conclusions drawn about treatment-induced cellular effects in inflammation. Although one study found electromicroscopic evidence of healing in the Achilles tendon of rats with partial rupture treated with ultrasound, another found no anti–inflammatory effect on inflammation induced by subcutaneous implants of polyurethene foam impregnated with dead tubercle bacilli. Research on high-voltage galvanic electrical stimulation suggests that edema, secondary hypoxia, and microvascular leakage are decreased in several animal models, but no conclusive studies have been done on human subjects.

Both low-energy laser therapy and bioelectrical-field induction therapy remain investigational in the treatment of soft-tissue injury. Laser stimulation initiates many cellular metabolic and proliferative processes, including DNA synthesis, protein metabolism, enzyme production, and respiratory function. This is reflected in increased collagen synthesis along with increased phagocytosis and changes in prostaglandin concentration, bacterial binding by lymphocytes, and lymph and blood flow, suggesting a potential role for this therapy. Similarly, cells subjected to electrical fields in vitro show increased protein synthesis and sulfate uptake, reflecting possible glycosaminoglycan synthesis.

Therapeutic Exercise

Tissue remodeling and responses to therapeutic exercise have been theorized to follow a pattern of a specific adaptation to an imposed level of demand. Such a response to therapeutic exercise has been termed "Wolf's law of soft tissue." Cellular and biomechanical responses to exercise are documented in tendon, ligament, and muscle, and include changes in collagen fibril size, strength, and stiffness. Exercise, particularly to the point of fatigue, can damage the ultrastructure of a tendon unit and, it is suggested, this combined with motion stimulates repair of the tendon by triggering a healing response. To what degree a true inflammatory reaction is generated or participates in this process is not clear. Studies demonstrate that cells in muscle, tendon, ligament, skin, and cartilage generally respond to "windows" of increased loading by increasing matrix synthesis, metabolic activity, and replication rates and by modifying the production of matrix components. An important concept is that pathologic loading effects (excessive loads or no load) outside these "windows" can reduce cell synthesis, increase degradative activity, or increase or decrease both. Present interest centers on how loading stimulates or signals the cell for specific matrix production. Whether these tissue changes are cell-driven or the indirect effect of various exercise-induced agents (such as hormones, changes in nutrition, or release of biochemical mediators, and growth factors) is being debated. It seems likely that a multifactorial pathway will be defined as the data accumulate.

Chapter 24

Oral Corticosteroids

Timothy W. Behrens, MD
James S. Goodwin, MD

History of Corticosteroids

Corticosteroids are the most powerful and the most toxic drugs available for treating inflammatory diseases. Their discovery was a major advance in the treatment of inflammatory diseases. The toxicities resulting from the high dosages prescribed in the early 1950s, however, led to the realization that corticosteroids must be administered cautiously.

In the 1920s, Hench observed that the symptoms of patients with rheumatoid arthritis were similar to those of patients with adrenal insufficiency. This stimulated investigation of the role of adrenal cortical hormones in inflammatory diseases. In the 1930s Mason and associates[46] had isolated cortisone (compound E) from adrenal tissue and tried to synthesize it and other adrenal cortical hormones. By 1948 the quantity of synthesized cortisone was sufficient for clinical trials to begin.[39] Hench and Kendall received the Nobel Prize in 1950 for their work on the use of cortisone in treating rheumatic diseases.

Pharmacology and Physiology

Glucocorticoids are 21-carbon steroid hormones synthesized from cholesterol. The term "glucocorticoid" refers to the ability of these agents to stimulate hepatic glycogen deposition and gluconeogenesis. Figure 1 shows the structures of the commonly used synthetic glucocorticoids. The activity of glucocorticoids depends on the presence of a hydroxyl group on carbon 11 of the steroid backbone. Two of the most commonly used glucocorticoids, cortisone and prednisone, are inactive until converted in vivo to the corresponding 11-hydroxyl compounds, cortisol and prednisolone.

The clinical potency of the various synthetic steroids depends on the rate of absorption, the concentration at target tissues, and the rate of metabolism and subsequent clearance. These factors must be considered when glucocorticoids are used. Table 1 presents the half-life

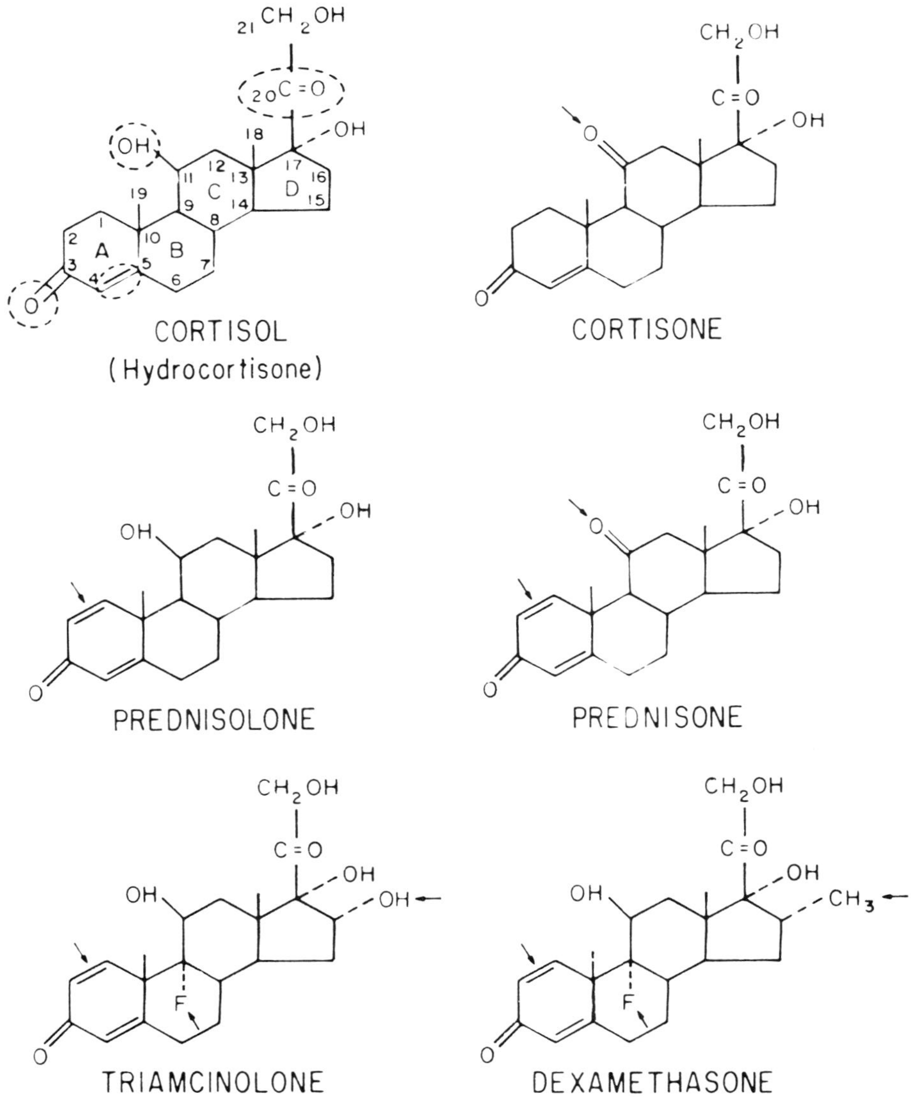

Fig. 1 *Structures of the commonly used synthetic glucocorticoids. (Reproduced with permission from Behrens TW, Goodwin JS: Glucocorticosteroids, in McCarty DJ (ed):* Arthritis and Allied Conditions: A Textbook of Rheumatology, *ed 11. Philadelphia, Lea & Febiger, 1989, pp 604–621.)*

and relative potency of the commonly used glucocorticoid preparations.[4,36,59] The relative potencies are estimates based on studies that measured hypothalamic-pituitary-adrenal axis suppression, glycogen

Table 1 Biologic activity of commonly used glucocorticoids*

Synthetic Glucocorticoids	Plasma Half-Life (min)	Relative Potency		Approximate Equivalent Dose (mg)
		Glucocorticoid	Mineralocorticoid	
Cortisol	80 to 120	1.0	1.0	20
Cortisone	80 to 120	0.8	0.8	25
Prednisone	200 to 210	3.5 to 4.0	0.8	5
Prednisolone	120 to 300	4.0	0.8	5
Triamcinolone	180 to 240	5.0	0	4
Dexamethasone	150 to 270	30 to 150	0	0.75

*Reproduced with permission from Behrens TW, Goodwin JS: Glucocorticoids, in McCarty DJ (ed): *Arthritis and Allied Conditions: A Textbook of Rheumatology,* ed 11. Philadelphia, Lea & Febiger, 1989, pp 604–621.

deposition, and other parameters that may or may not correlate with the desired clinical effect. Although Table 1 may be useful as an approximate guide, the clinician should exercise caution when calculating dose equivalents for an individual patient.[48]

Most glucocorticoids are readily absorbed after oral administration, and food intake does not influence absorption. Approximately 90% of endogenous circulating cortisol binds with high affinity to the plasma protein corticosteroid-binding globulin. Another 5% to 8% binds to albumin, a high-capacity, low-affinity reservoir for steroids. Only the 2% to 5% of unbound circulating glucocorticoids are free to exert a biologic action. Those associated with proteins are inactive and protected from metabolic degradation.[6] Most synthetic steroids, with the exception of prednisolone, have a low affinity for corticosteroid-binding globulin and bind predominantly to albumin.[6] The volume of distribution and levels of protein binding of synthetic steroids may influence the frequency of adverse reactions. Lewis[44] reported that, of patients receiving glucocorticoid therapy, those with a serum albumin level of less than 2.5 mg/dl were twice as likely to have cushingoid side effects as the control group with normal albumin levels. The increased potency of dexamethasone may in part be related to its lesser degree of plasma binding relative to other synthetic steroids.[59]

The glucocorticoids are metabolized by enzymatic modifications in the liver. Hydroxylation of the 4,5 double bond and ketone groups and subsequent conjugation with glucuronide or sulfate groups render steroids inactive and water-soluble. The kidney excretes 95% of the conjugated metabolites, and the remainder are lost in the gut. The rates of metabolic degradation and clearance of steroids from the circulation are important determinants of potency. The plasma half-life is a commonly used index of the rate of clearance of glucocorticoids. However, both the distribution and the clearance of different glucocorticoids vary considerably among individuals. Thus, the half-life often underestimates true clearance times.

The decreased clearance rates of prednisolone and dexamethasone relative to cortisol accounts for much of their enhanced potency (Table 1). Modifications of the steroid molecule around the A ring (Fig. 1) decrease the rate of metabolism by the liver and delay clearance.[6] The differences in the half-life of synthetic steroids mean that patients with prolonged clearance rates for prednisolone[42] or dexamethasone[47] are more likely to experience side effects.

Clearance rates of glucocorticoids are also affected by a variety of drugs and disease states. Phenytoin, phenobarbital, and rifampin can increase steroid clearance by inducing hepatic enzyme activity. Estrogen therapy and estrogen-containing oral contraceptives decrease clearance and may decrease the amount of steroid required.[59] Liver disease does not alter the metabolism of glucocorticoids significantly, and dosage adjustments are not necessary.[59] Dosage adjustments are also generally not recommended for patients with kidney disease. During pregnancy, the clearance rate of cortisol is reduced whereas corticosteroid-binding globulin levels increase.[59] Glucocorticoids can decrease plasma salicylate levels by enhancing renal clearance of salicylates. Patients on fixed-dose salicylate therapy may develop rapid increases in serum salicylate levels, possibly to toxic levels, if glucocorticoids are withdrawn or gradually decreased.[41]

Cortisol and the Hypothalamic-Pituitary-Adrenal Axis

Cortisol accounts for 90% of the total hormonal output of the adrenal cortex. Secretion rates for cortisol vary from 8 to 25 mg/day in healthy humans, with an average plasma concentration of 86 mg/ml for females and 116 mg/ml for males.[6] The production of cortisol in the body is regulated by a neuroendocrine axis formed by the hypothalamus, the pituitary gland, and the adrenal glands. The hypothalamus releases a peptide, corticotropin-releasing factor, that stimulates the secretion of this hormone by the anterior pituitary. Corticotropin stimulates the release of cortisol and other steroids from the adrenal cortex. Several mechanisms control the rate of cortisol release. Endogenous rhythms in the brain make the release of corticotropin and cortisol pulsatile. Release is more frequent in the late evening and early morning hours, resulting in a circadian rhythm of plasma cortisol levels. Most endogenous cortisol is released during the last four hours of sleep and the first five hours after awakening.[6] By late afternoon, cortisol levels may be undetectable. Emotions and physical factors, including hormones and neural input, influence cortisol release and may increase plasma cortisol levels above normal.

The most important means of controlling cortisol release is feedback inhibition of corticotropin-releasing factor, and thus corticotropin release, by glucocorticoids, including all the synthetic glucocorticoids. This feedback inhibition is rapid and normally regulates cortisol levels in the physiologic range. However, in the patient treated with glucocorticoids, the axis may be progressively suppressed with continued exposure. A prolonged (weeks to months) period of high-dose steroid therapy may make the axis totally unresponsive. The length of time necessary for recovery of the axis after glucocorticoids are discontinued

Outline 1 Metabolic effects of glucocorticoids*

Carbohydrate metabolism
- Impaired glucose uptake and utilization by peripheral tissues
- Increased gluconeogenesis and glycogen deposition in liver
- Glucose intolerance in susceptible patients

Lipid metabolism
- Stimulation of lipolysis and increased free fatty acid levels (countered by increased insulin release and gluconeogenesis)
- Increased fat deposition in truncal and facial areas

Protein metabolism
- Inhibition of synthesis and enhanced breakdown of proteins in peripheral tissues
- Increased plasma levels of free amino acids
- Stimulation of negative nitrogen balance

Nucleic acid metabolism
- RNA synthesis stimulated in liver and inhibited in other tissues
- DNA synthesis inhibited in most peripheral tissues.

Fluid and electrolyte metabolism
- Increased sodium retention and potassium loss independent of mineralocorticoid action
- Increased glomerular filtration rate

Bone and calcium metabolism
- Partially blocked intestinal absorption of calcium
- Decreased renal reabsorption of calcium and phosphate, resulting in hypercalciuria
- Inhibited osteoblast function

*Modified with permission from Baxter JD, Tyrrell JB: The adrenal cortex, in Felig P, Baxter JD, Broadus AE, et al (eds): *Endocrinology and Metabolism*, ed 2. New York, McGraw-Hill, 1987, pp 511–650.

varies widely among individuals, but generally correlates with dose and duration of treatment.[30]

Metabolic Effects of Glucocorticoids

Like other hormones, glucocorticoids affect many different tissues and organ systems. At normal levels, these various metabolic effects help maintain homeostasis. However, when steroids are present in high levels because of endogenous overproduction or exogenous administration, these metabolic effects are accentuated and may lead to the toxicity associated with corticosteroid administration and Cushing's syndrome.

The metabolic effects of glucocorticoids are summarized in Outline 1. In general, steroids are catabolic promoters. They block glucose uptake by tissues, enhance protein breakdown, and decrease new protein synthesis in muscle, skin, bone, connective tissue, fat, and lymphoid tissue.[14,59] DNA synthesis and cell proliferation are inhibited in fibroblasts, lymphocytes, and adipocytes.[14,59] Organisms exposed for long periods to supraphysiologic levels of corticosteroids have a type of wasting disease: they lose bone, connective tissue, and muscle and gain water and fat.

Mechanism of Action

All steroid hormones (vitamin D, glucocorticoids, sex hormones, mineralocorticoids) act by binding to high-affinity receptors found in

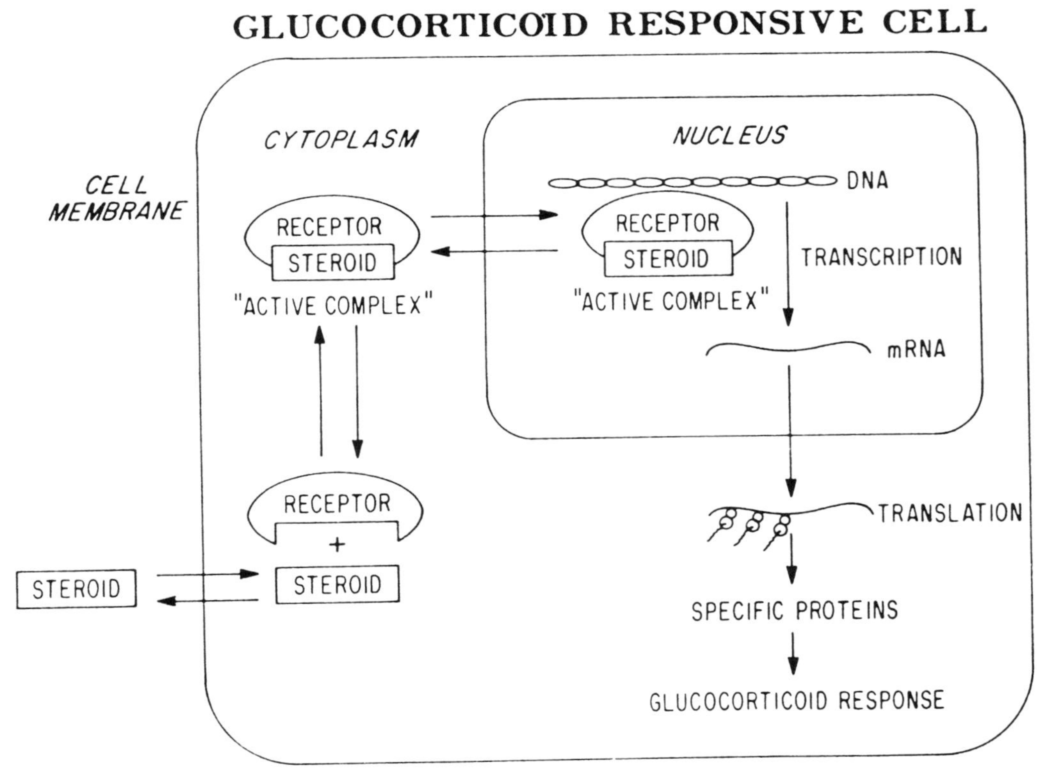

Fig. 2 *Model of the molecular basis of glucocorticoid action. (Reproduced with permission from Behrens TW, Goodwin JS: Glucocorticosteroids, in McCarty DJ (ed):* Arthritis and Allied Conditions: A Textbook of Rheumatology, *ed 11. Philadelphia, Lea & Febiger, 1989, pp 604–621.)*

relatively low numbers (2 to 6 × 10^4 per cell) in the cytoplasm[8] (Fig. 2). The steroid-receptor complex in turn has a high affinity for nuclear interphase chromosomes and thus binds to chromosomal DNA.[51] This triggers DNA transcription and the formation of messenger RNA, leading to new protein synthesis. The specific genes transcribed and proteins produced after exposure to steroid hormones depend on the steroid hormone used and the type of target cell. Specificity of cell response is provided for in at least two ways. First, the steroid-receptor complex binds to specific regulatory sequences, which in turn leads to transcription of the particular gene containing that sequence. Second, only the part of the genome contained in an accessible portion of chromatin sensitive to digestion with deoxyribonuclease is susceptible to induction by steroid hormones. This accessible portion differs depending on cell type.[51]

All well-defined physiologic and pharmacologic effects of steroid hormones are mediated by this process. This implies that pharmacologic and/or physiologic effects are separated in time from drug administration. For example, the clinical response to glucocorticoids in short-term therapy occurs several hours after the drug is given. Thus, in many ways glucocorticoid action is less direct than the action of other drugs because it depends on the synthesis of other compounds.

Gryglewski and associates[31] observed that prior infusion of glucocorticoids inhibited the production of prostaglandins in isolated perfused rabbit mesentery. This inhibition could be overcome by the infusion of arachidonic acid. They concluded that glucocorticoids inhibit prostaglandin production by blocking the release of the precursor arachidonic acid from cellular stores. They also proposed that the anti-inflammatory properties of glucocorticoids were secondary to this effect on arachidonic acid.

This hypothesis was difficult for most investigators to accept. Nonsteroidal anti-inflammatory drugs (NSAIDs) were known to work by inhibiting arachidonic acid metabolism,[60] and the anti-inflammatory effects of glucocorticoids were clearly different and more powerful than those of NSAIDs. If arachidonic acid metabolism were a straight-line pathway from membrane phospholipid to arachidonic acid to "prostaglandins," glucocorticoids and NSAIDs would be expected to have very similar actions, even if they cause inhibition at different points. This problem was clarified when Samuelsson[55] identified the lipoxygenase metabolic pathways for arachidonic acid (Fig. 3). With this more complex schema, it is possible for both NSAIDs and glucocorticoids to inhibit arachidonic acid release from membrane phospholipid, while having different effects. The glucocorticoids inhibit both cyclo-oxygenase and lipoxygenase products, whereas NSAIDs inhibit only cyclo-oxygenase products.

The evidence supporting this concept has increased considerably. Danon and Assouline[19] showed that synthesis of both RNA and protein is required for steroids to inhibit prostaglandin production. In 1979 and 1980, Blackwell and Flower,[11,25] Hirata and associates,[37] and Axelrod[4] identified a phospholipase A_2-inhibitory glycoprotein. Called lipocortin, it is synthesized and released by cells exposed to glucocorticoids. However, several investigators have failed to inhibit the endogenous production of arachidonic acid metabolites in vitro[15] and in vivo[49] with glucocorticoids, perhaps because arachidonic acid can be released from membrane phospholipid by at least two pathways, and lipocortin can inhibit only one of them. Lipocortin appears to be a family of molecules; one of these molecules has been cloned and found to have potent anti-inflammatory actions.[64] Davidson and associates[21] suggested that lipocortins are identical to calpactins, ubiquitous intracellular proteins that bind calcium and phospholipid. If this is the case, then inhibition of arachidonic acid release by lipocortin (and by glucocorticoids) may be caused by a masking of the substrate for phospholipase A_2—the membrane phospholipids—rather than inhibition of the enzyme per se.[21]

As the physiologic and pathophysiologic roles of various lipoxygen-

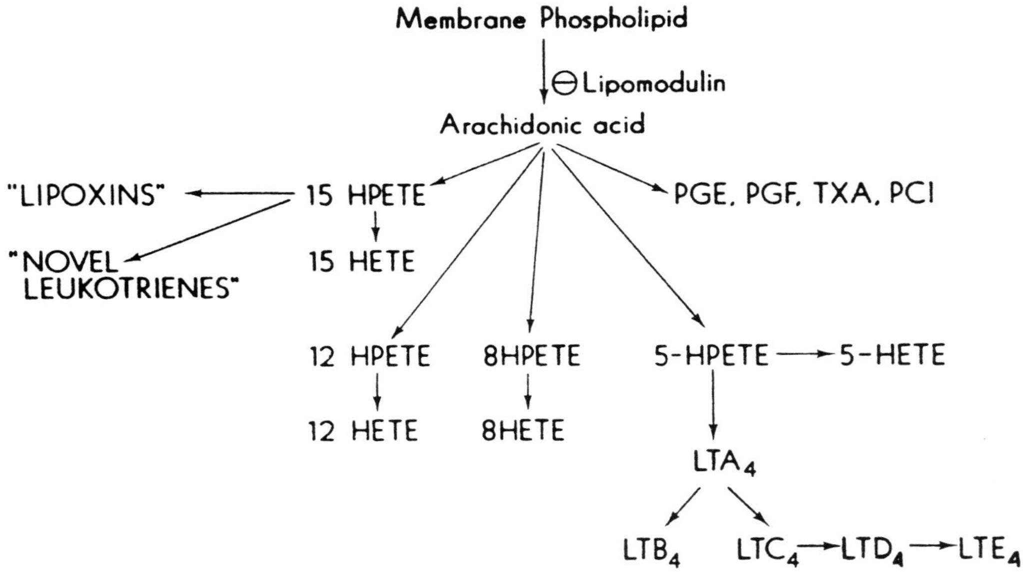

Fig. 3 *Current schema of arachidonic acid metabolism. (Reproduced with permission from Behrens TW, Goodwin JS: Glucocorticosteroids, in McCarty DJ (ed):* Arthritis and Allied Conditions: A Textbook of Rheumatology, *ed 11. Philadelphia, Lea & Febiger, 1989, pp 604–621.)*

ase metabolites of arachidonic acid, particularly the leukotrienes, are clarified, they help explain how glucocorticoids inhibit arachidonic acid metabolism and result in anti-inflammatory and other therapeutic actions. Leukotrienes C_4 and D_4 are slow-reacting substances of anaphylaxis (SRS-A). Their suppression might explain the therapeutic efficacy of glucocorticoids in the treatment of asthma.[55] Leukotriene B_4 appears to play a major role in the inflammatory response. Very small concentrations can cause margination, chemotaxis, and aggregation of neutrophils and stimulate pain receptors.[26,29] The pharmaceutical industry is now searching for specific inhibitors of the synthesis of leukotrienes and also leukotriene receptor antagonists. Such drugs might have a relatively specific therapeutic anti-inflammatory or antiasthmatic action while lacking the whole spectrum of therapeutic actions or the array of toxic effects of the glucocorticoids.

Anti-inflammatory Effects

The glucocorticoids are the most powerful anti-inflammatory agents available to the clinician. The administration of glucocorticoids results in a complex series of changes in the actions of cells involved in inflammatory reactions.[53] After a single dose of glucocorticoids in humans, the number of circulating neutrophils increases, peaking four to six hours later.[17] This increase and the increase in the half-life of neutrophils in the circulation are accompanied by and secondary to a decrease in the margination, migration, and accumulation of neutrophils at the site of inflammation. The four cardinal signs of inflammation—heat, redness, swelling, and pain—decrease. Glucocorticoids also reduce the numbers of monocytes migrating to and accumulating in inflammation sites, thus preventing the signs of acute inflammation and interfering with delayed hypersensitivity reactions.[67]

Glucocorticoids also directly suppress the action of cells involved in the inflammatory response. They inhibit the production of phagocytosis by neutrophils and monocytes, the release of degradative enzymes such as collagenase and plasminogen activator by neutrophils and synovial lining cells, and the production of inflammatory lymphokines and monokines such as interleukin–1.[22,61,66] Glucocorticoids clearly have in vivo and in vitro effects on migration and accumulation of granulocytes and monocytes. However, which other actions of glucocorticoids on inflammatory cell function actually contribute to the anti-inflammatory effect is unknown because most data were obtained from in vitro models and isolated cell populations. It is reasonable to assume, however, that the "lysosomal stabilizing" effects and the decreased release of inflammatory mediators and degradative enzymes probably do play roles in glucocorticoid action.[22,65]

Immunosuppressive Effects

The immunosuppressive properties of corticosteroids were recognized quickly.[9] In general, T lymphocytes are more sensitive to the in vivo immunosuppressive effects of corticosteroids than are B lymphocytes. Fauci and associates[24] emphasized the importance of the redistribution of lymphocytes and monocytes in mediating corticosteroid action in humans. A single dose of corticosteroids results in a 70% decline in circulating lymphocytes and a 90% decline in circulating monocytes. Corticosteroids also deplete T lymphocytes, especially helper T cells, from the circulation to a greater extent than they do B lymphocytes. This occurs within four to six hours and reverts to normal by 24 hours.[24] A similar phenomenon occurs daily during long-term steroid administration. The lymphocytopenia appears to be the result of redistribution of circulating lymphocytes to other lymphoid compartments, particularly the bone marrow, and not of cell lysis or death.

B lymphocytes are relatively resistant to the in vivo immunosuppressive effects of corticosteroids. Specific antibody synthesis after inoculation with pneumococcal capsular polysaccharide, pertussis vaccine diphtheria toxoid, and streptococcal-O-antigens is not affected by glucocorticoid therapy.[20] However, serum IgG, IgA, and IgM levels are suppressed after a brief course of daily high-dose methylprednisolone. Maximal suppression occurs two to four weeks after treatment. In vivo, steroids may augment immunoglobulin levels in certain clinical situations such as adult combined immunodeficiency by inhibiting suppressor cell function.[63]

Cell-mediated immune reactions are generally inhibited by in vivo corticosteroid effects. Patients taking steroids are often anergic, reflecting an inability to express cutaneous delayed hypersensitivity despite previous sensitization. Bovornkitti and associates[12] showed that in 68 of 70 patients treated with 40 mg of prednisone per day a tuberculin test converted from positive to negative within two weeks. The skin test reaction reconverted to positive six days after the prednisone therapy was stopped. Steroids may suppress graft rejection by inhibiting the proliferation of alloreactive T lymphocytes and the generation of cytotoxic T lymphocytes.[9,40] Corticosteroids suppress most in vitro T lymphocyte proliferative responses, and they appear to interfere with early activation events.[9]

Natural killer (NK) cells and antibody-dependent cellular cytotoxicity effector cells are important in vivo in tumor surveillance, acute graft rejection, and lysis of virally infected cells. Parrillo and Fauci[52] found that 12 mg of dexamethasone suppressed NK-cell activity in vivo at 24 and 48 hours, but activity returned to normal by 96 hours.

Many of the suppressive effects of glucocorticoids would appear to be secondary to inhibition of the production and action of a variety of lymphokines and monokines. These peptides communicate between cells of the immune system, carrying messages that stimulate cells to proliferate, differentiate, or perform specific functions. Interleukin–1 is produced by monocytes and in turn can enhance T cell production of interleukin–2, colony stimulating factor, interferon gamma, and other lymphokines. Glucocorticoids are one of the few classes of agents that can inhibit the production of interleukin–1.[56] They also profoundly inhibit interleukin–2 production.[10] The observation that exogenous interleukin–2 restores proliferation of glucocorticoid-treated lymphocytes suggests that steroids do not affect the initial activation events of lymphocytes but that rather they prevent the cell from passing through an early cell cycle phase.[10] Glucocorticoids also block the production of interferon gamma by T lymphocytes, at the level of DNA transcription.[2]

Side Effects

The toxic effects of prolonged glucocorticoid therapy are many and limit the use of these agents (Outline 2). The most prominent adverse side effect is impaired wound healing. Steroids effectively abolish collagen synthesis in granulation tissue and inhibit many fibroblastic functions in cell culture. Steroids interfere with the formation of a fibrous scar and suppress the secondary control "inflammation" necessary to promote proper wound healing.[5] Peacock and VanWinkel[54] noted,

> It would appear that most commonly used corticosteroids whose effect on wound healing has been reported tend to inhibit wound healing in the dosage used in laboratory animals. There are insufficient data to allow one to transfer these results to human surgical patients, however. In most instances the dosages used in animals were consid-

Outline 2 Side effects of glucocorticoid therapy*

- Very common (should be anticipated in all patients)
  - Osteoporosis
  - Increased appetite
  - Obesity
  - Impaired wound healing
  - Psychiatric disorders, particularly euphoria
  - Glucose intolerance
  - Increased risk of infection
  - Suppression of hypothalamic-pituitary-adrenal axis
  - Growth arrest in children
- Frequent
  - Myopathy
  - Osteonecrosis
  - Hypertension
  - Plethora
  - Thin, fragile skin, striae, purpura
  - Edema secondary to sodium and water retention
  - Hyperlipidemia
- Uncommon, but early recognition important
  - Posterior subcapsular cataracts
  - Glaucoma
  - Benign intracranial hypertension
  - "Silent" intestinal perforation
  - Peptic ulcer disease (often gastric)
  - Hypokalemic alkalosis
  - Hyperosmolar nonketotic coma
- Rare
  - Pancreatitis
  - Hirsutism
  - Panniculitis
  - Gastric hemorrhage
  - Secondary amenorrhea
  - Impotence
  - Epidural lipomatosis
  - Allergy to synthetic steroids

*Reproduced with permission from Behrens TW, Goodwin JS: Glucocorticoids, in McCarty DJ (ed): *Arthritis and Allied Conditions: A Textbook of Rheumatology*, ed 11. Philadelphia, Lea & Febiger, 1989, pp 604–621.

erably higher than those normally administered to patients. . . . There appears to be a marked species variation in response to a given dose of any one of the corticosteroids.

Other side effects include osteoporosis,[7,13,28,34] myopathy,[3,38,62] psychiatric complications,[45] susceptibility to infections,[18,24,27] ocular complications,[23,43] suppression of the hypothalamic-pituitary-adrenal axis,[50,57] and bone osteonecrosis.[1,68]

One of the most puzzling aspects of glucocorticoid therapy is the wide range of susceptibility to the side effects. Some patients receiving prolonged, high-dose therapy tolerate glucocorticoids without adverse effects, whereas others treated with small doses for brief intervals develop devastating side effects. This differential sensitivity depends in part on individual differences in plasma protein binding. Hypoalbuminemic patients are especially at risk. It also depends in part on variations in metabolism and clearance of synthetic steroids. Sensitivity to glucocorticoids in mice is closely linked to the H2 histocompatibility region,[33] and there is some evidence of analogous linkages in humans. Differences in glucocorticoid sensitivity among different mouse strains have been associated with differences in glucocorticoid receptor content[33] and in stimulation of lipocortin synthesis.[32]

Therapeutic Use of Steroids in Sports Trauma

The prescription of oral steroids in the treatment of sports trauma is not common. In the last ten years, not a single peer-reviewed study evaluating the therapeutic use of oral corticosteroids in sports injuries has appeared. A survey of practicing orthopaedic surgeons in the Milwaukee area found that not one used oral corticosteroids to treat sports injuries. In an extensive review of the use of steroids in treating sprain and strain injuries, Cox[16] noted that prolonged systemic administration of corticosteroids is rarely used for athletic injuries, but that some individuals use systemic steroids in limited doses. This treatment is reserved for chronic conditions such as tennis elbow or tendinitis of the shoulder and is used when all other therapeutic measures have failed.

A short, high-dose treatment regimen of oral dexamethasone has been used to reduce pain and neurologic compromise in lumbar radiculopathy caused by disk prolapse.[58] However, in 1985 Haimovic and Beresford[35] concluded a placebo-controlled, double-blind study of 33 hospitalized patients treated with dexamethasone. The treatment provided short-term pain relief in five of 21 patients. Long-term follow-up failed to show that dexamethasone was more effective in sustaining pain relief.

Therefore, the use of oral corticosteroids for the routine treatment of sports-related injuries cannot be recommended. Those physicians who do use oral steroids to treat the inflammation and edema associated with acute injuries should exercise extreme caution.

References

1. Anderton JM, Helm R: Multiple joint osteonecrosis following short-term steroid therapy: Case report. *J Bone Joint Surg* 1982;64A:139–141.
2. Arya SK, Wong-Staal F, Gallo RC: Dexamethasone-mediated inhibition of human T cell growth factor and gamma-interferon messenger RNA. *J Immunol* 1984;133:273–276.
3. Askari A, Vignos PJ Jr, Moskowitz RW: Steroid myopathy in connective tissue disease. *Am J Med* 1976;61:485–492.
4. Axelrod L: Glucocorticoid therapy. *Medicine* 1976;55:39–65.
5. Baxter JD, Forsham PH: Tissue effects of glucocorticoids. *Am J Med* 1972;53:573–589.
6. Baxter JD, Tyrrell JB: The adrenal cortex, in Felig P, Baxter JD, Broadus AE, et al (eds): *Endocrinology and Metabolism*, ed 2. New York, McGraw-Hill, 1987, pp 511–650.
7. Baylink DJ: Glucocorticoid-induced osteoporosis. *N Engl J Med* 1983;309:306–308.
8. Behrens TW, Goodwin JS: Glucocorticoids, in McCarty DJ (ed): *Arthritis and Allied Conditions: A Textbook of Rheumatology*, ed 11. Philadelphia, Lea & Febiger, 1989, pp 604–621.

9. Behrens TW, Goodwin JS: Glucocorticosteroids, in Bray M, Morley J (eds): *The Pharmacology of Lymphocytes.* New York, Springer-Verlag, 1988.
10. Bettens F, Kristensen F, Walker C, et al: Lymphokine regulation of activated (G1) lymphocytes: II. Glucocorticoid and anti-Tac-induced inhibition of human T lymphocyte proliferation. *J Immunol* 1984;132:261–265.
11. Blackwell GJ, Carnuccio R, Di Rosa M, et al: Macrocortin: A polypeptide causing the anti-phospholipase effect of glucocorticoids. *Nature* 1980;287:147–149.
12. Bovornkitti S, Kangsadal P, Sathirapat P, et al: Reversion and reconversion rate of tuberculin skin reactions in connection with the use of prednisone. *Dis Chest* 1960;38:51–55.
13. Bressot C, Meunier PJ, Chapuy MC, e al: Histomorphometric profile, pathophysiology and reversibility of corticosteroid-induced osteoporosis. *Metab Bone Dis Relat Res* 1979;1:303–311.
14. Canalis E: Effect of glucocorticoids on type I collagen synthesis, alkaline phosphatase activity, and deoxyribonucleic acid content in cultured rat calvariae. *Endocrinology* 1983;112:931–939.
15. Chandrabose KA, LaPetina EG, Schmitges CJ, et al: Action of corticosteroids in regulation of prostaglandin biosynthesis in cultured fibroblasts. *Proc Natl Acad Sci USA* 1978;75:214–217.
16. Cox JS: Current concepts in the role of steroids in the treatment of sprains and strains. *Med Sci Sports Exerc* 1984;16:216–218.
17. Dale DC, Fauci AS, Guerry D IV, et al: Comparisons of agents producing a neutrophilic leukocytosis in man: Hydrocortisone, prednisone, endotoxin, and etiocholanolone. *J Clin Invest* 1975;56:808–813.
18. Dale DC, Petersdorf RG: Corticosteroids and infectious diseases. *Med Clin North Am* 1973;57:1277–1287.
19. Danon A, Assouline G: Inhibition of prostaglandin biosynthesis by corticosteroids requires RNA and protein synthesis. *Nature* 1978;273:552–554.
20. David DS, Grieco H, Cushman P Jr: Adrenal glucocorticoids after twenty years: A review of their clinically relevant consequences. *J Chronic Dis* 1970;22:637–711.
21. Davidson FF, Dennis EA, Powell M, et al: Inhibition of phospholipase A2 by "lipocortins" and calpactins: An effect of binding to substrate phospholipids. *J Biol Chem* 1987;262:1698–1705.
22. Dinarello CA: Interleukin-1. *Rev Infect Dis* 1984;6:51–95.
23. Dujovne CA, Azarnoff DL: Clinical complications of corticosteroid therapy: A selected review, in Azarnoff DL (ed): *Steroid Therapy.* Philadelphia, WB Saunders, 1975, pp 27–41.
24. Fauci AS, Dale DC, Balow JE: Glucocorticosteroid therapy: Mechanisms of action and clinical considerations. *Ann Intern Med* 1976;84:304–315.
25. Flower RJ, Blackwell GJ: Anti-inflammatory steroids induce biosynthesis of a phospholipase A2 inhibitor which prevents prostaglandin generation. *Nature* 1979;278:456–459.
26. Ford-Hutchinson AW, Bray MA, Doig MV, et al: Leukotriene B, a potent chemokinetic and aggregating substance released from polymorphonuclear leukocytes. *Nature* 1980;286:264–265.
27. Ginzler E, Diamond M, Kaplan D, et al: Computer analysis of factors influencing frequency of infection in systemic lupus erythematosus. *Arthritis Rheum* 1978;21:37–44.
28. Gluck OS, Murphy WA, Hahn TJ, et al: Bone loss in adults receiving alternate day glucocorticoid therapy: A comparison with daily therapy. *Arthritis Rheum* 1981;24:892–898.

29. Goetzl EJ, Brindley LL, Goldman DW: Enhancement of human neutrophil adherence by synthetic leukotriene constituents of the slow-reacting substance of anaphylaxis. *Immunology* 1983;50:35–41.
30. Graber AL, Ney RL, Nicholson WE, et al: Natural history of pituitary-adrenal recovery following long-term suppression with corticosteroids. *J Clin Endocrinol* 1965;25:11–16.
31. Gryglewski RJ, Panczenko B, Korbut R, et al: Corticosteroids inhibit prostaglandin release from perfused mesenteric blood vessels of rabbits and from perfused lungs of sensitized guinea pig. *Prostaglandins* 1975;10:343–355.
32. Gupta C, Goldman AS: Dexamethasone-induced phospholipase A2-inhibitory proteins (PLIP) influenced by the H–2 histocompatibility region. *Proc Soc Exp Biol Med* 1985;178:29–35.
33. Gupta C, Goldman AS: H–2 histocompatibility region: Influence on the murine glucocorticoid receptor and its response. *Science* 1982;216:994–996.
34. Hahn TJ: Corticosteroid-induced osteopenia. *Arch Intern Med* 178;138:882–885.
35. Haimovic IC, Beresford HR: Treatment of lumbosacral radicular pain with dexamethasone: A controlled study, abstract. *Neurology* 1985;35(suppl 1):252.
36. Haynes RC Jr, Murad F: Adrenocorticotropic hormone: Adrenocortical steroids and their synthetic analogs; inhibitors of adrenocortical steroid biosynthesis, in Gilman AG, Goodman LS, Rall TW, et al (eds): *Goodman and Gilman's The Pharmacologic Basis of Therapeutics*, ed 7. New York, Macmillan, 1985, pp 1459–1489.
37. Hirata F, Schiffmann E, Venkatasubramanian K, et al: A phospholipase A2 inhibitory protein in rabbit neutrophils induced by glucocorticoids. *Proc Natl Acad Sci USA* 1980;77:2533–2536.
38. Horber FF, Scheidegger JR, Grünig BE, et al: Evidence that prednisone-induced myopathy is reversed by physical training. *J Clin Endocrinol Metab* 1985;61:83–88.
39. Kendall EC: Some observations on the hormone of the adrenal cortex designated compound E. *Mayo Clin Proc* 1949;24:298–301.
40. Keown PA, Stiller CR: Control of rejection of transplanted organs. *Adv Intern Med* 1986;31:17–46.
41. Klinenberg JR, Miller F: Effect of corticosteroids on blood salicylate concentration. *JAMA* 1965;194:601–604.
42. Kozower M, Veatch L, Kaplan MM: Decreased clearance of prednisolone, a factor in the development of corticosteroid side effects. *J Clin Endocrinol Metab* 1974;38:407–412.
43. Levine SB, Leopold IH: Advances in ocular corticosteroid therapy, in Azarnoff DL (ed): *Steroid Therapy*. Philadelphia, WB Saunders, 1975, pp 62–77.
44. Lewis GP, Jusko WJ, Graves L, et al: Prednisone side-effects and serum-protein levels: A collaborative study. *Lancet* 1971;2:778–781.
45. Ling MH, Perry PJ, Tsuang MT: Side effects of corticosteroid therapy: Psychiatric aspects. *Arch Gen Psychiatry* 1981;38:471–477.
46. Mason HL, Myers CS, Kendall EC: Chemical studies of the suprarenal cortex: Identification of the substance which possesses the qualitative action of cortin; its conversion into diketone closely related to androstenedione. *J Biol Chem* 1936;116:267–276.
47. Meikle AW, Clarke DH, Tyler FH: Cushing syndrome from low doses of dexamethasone: A result of slow plasma clearance. *JAMA* 1976;235:1592–1593.
48. Meikle AW, Tyler FH: Potency and duration of action of glucocorticoids: Effects of hydrocortisone, prednisone and dexamethasone on human pituitary-adrenal function. *Am J Med* 1977;63:200–207.

49. Náray-Fejes-Tóth A, Fejes-Tóth G, Fischer C, et al: Effect of dexamethasone on in vivo prostanoid production in the rabbit. *J Clin Invest* 1984;74;120–123.
50. Nichols T, Nugent CA, Tyler FH: Diurnal variation in suppression of adrenal function by glucocorticoids. *J Clin Endocrinol* 1965;25:343–349.
51. O'Malley BW: Steroid hormone action in eucaryotic cells. *J Clin Invest* 1984;74:307–312.
52. Parrillo JE, Fauci S: Comparison of the effector cells in human spontaneous cellular cytotoxicity and antibody-dependent cellular cytotoxicity: Differential sensitivity of effector cells to in vivo and in vitro corticosteroids. *Scand J Immunol* 1978;8:99–107.
53. Parrillo JE, Fauci AS: Mechanisms of glucocorticoid action on immune processes. *Annu Rev Pharmacol Toxicol* 1979;19:179–201.
54. Peacock EE Jr, VanWinkel W Jr: *Surgery and Biology of Wound Repair.* Philadelphia, WB Saunders, 1979, p 128.
55. Samuelsson B: Leukotrienes: Mediators of immediate hypersensitivity reactions and inflammation. *Science* 1983;220:568–575.
56. Snyder DS, Unanue ER: Corticosteroids inhibit murine macrophage Ia expression and interleukin-1 production. *J Immunol* 1982;129:1803–1805.
57. Streck WF, Lockwood DH: Pituitary adrenal recovery following short-term suppression with corticosteroids. *Am J Med* 1979;66:910–914.
58. Tsairis P: Corticosteroid therapy in the management of lumbar radiculopathy. *Contemp Orthop* 1988;17:53–57.
59. Tyrrell JB, Baxter JD: Glucocorticoid therapy, in Felig P, Baxter JD, Broadus AE, et al (eds): *Endocrinology and Metabolism*, ed 2. New York, McGraw-Hill, 1987, pp 788–817.
60. Vane JR: Inhibition of prostaglandin synthesis as a mechanism of action for aspirin-like drugs. *Nature* 1971;232:231–235.
61. Vane J, Botting R: Inflammation and the mechanism of action of anti-inflammatory drugs. *FASEB J* 1987;1:89–96.
62. Van Marle W, Woods KL: Acute hydrocortisone myopathy. *Br Med J* 1980;281:271–272.
63. Waldmann TA, Blaese RM, Broder S, et al: Disorders of suppressor immunoregulatory cells in the pathogenesis of immunodeficiency and autoimmunity. *Ann Intern Med* 1978;88:226–238.
64. Wallner BP, Mattaliano RJ, Hession C, et al: Cloning and expression of human lipocortin, a phospholipase A_2 inhibitor with potential anti-inflammatory activity. *Nature* 1986;320:77–81.
65. Weissmann G, Thomas L: Studies on lysosomes: II. The effect of cortisone on the release of acid hydrolases from a large granule fraction of rabbit liver induced by an excess of vitamin A. *J Clin Invest* 1963;42:661–669.
66. Werb Z, Mainardi CL, Vater CA, et al: Endogenous activation of latent collagenase by rheumatoid synovial cells: Evidence for a role of plasminogen activator. *N Engl J Med* 1977;296:1017–1023.
67. Weston WL, Mandel MJ, Yeckley JA, et al: Mechanism of cortisol inhibition of adoptive transfer of tuberculin sensitivity. *J Lab Clin Med* 1973;82:366–371.
68. Zizic TM, Marcoux C, Hungerford DS, et al: Corticosteroid therapy associated with ischemic necrosis of bone in systemic lupus erythematosus. *Am J Med* 1985;79:596–604.

Chapter 25

Nonsteroidal Anti-inflammatory Drugs: Mechanisms of Action and Therapeutic Considerations

Steven B. Abramson, MD

Introduction

Nonsteroidal anti-inflammatory drugs (NSAIDs) have anti-inflammatory, analgesic, and antipyretic properties. These drugs have been postulated to act by inhibiting the synthesis of prostaglandins. However, increasing evidence indicates that this hypothesis may not account for all the effects of NSAIDs at all dosages. For example, suppressing inflammation requires higher doses than does simply inhibiting prostaglandin synthesis. Also, sodium salicylate is an ineffective inhibitor of cyclo-oxygenase at concentrations used clinically. Thus, these aspirin-like drugs may have important pharmacologic actions in addition to their anti-inflammatory effects. This chapter examines the evidence for diverse mechanisms of action of NSAIDs and their use in sports injuries.

Physicochemical Characteristics and Pharmacokinetics

As a class, NSAIDs are weakly acidic benzoic acid derivatives with diverse chemical structures. The most commonly used NSAIDs are the salicylates, originally derived from extracts of willow bark. The active ingredient of willow bark, salicin, is converted to salicylic acid in vivo. Like salicin, aspirin (acetylsalicylic acid) rapidly hydrolyzes to salicylate after it is absorbed.[7] Salicylic acid is also the active agent at the inflammatory site. When aspirin or salicylic acid was administered orally to dogs with carrageenan-induced edema, the principal compound recovered from the inflammatory exudate was salicylic acid.[1]

Most NSAIDs have a pKA between 3 and 5. Therefore, at lower pH levels, the percentage of the drug in a non-ionized state increases. This affects the tissue distribution of drug, causing NSAIDs to accumulate in areas of greater acidity, such as an inflamed joint, the stomach, and the renal medulla.[4] NSAIDs are also lipophilic compounds. At acid pH levels, lipophilicity increases[10] and promotes the association of

NSAIDs with the lipid bilayers of inflammatory cells.[16] Acetaminophen has antipyretic and analgesic properties but not anti-inflammatory properties. This neutral compound may not concentrate at inflammatory sites or within inflammatory cells.[4]

Raghoebar and associates[16] studied the association between radioisotope-labeled aspirin and salicylic acid and various cell types. Both drugs have a dose-dependent association with monocytes and neutrophils but little association with lymphocytes. The degree of association between the neutrophils significantly increases at lower pH levels, consistent with the prediction that the un-ionized species accumulates more readily in the lipid bilayer of the plasma membrane. The effect of pH levels and the different reactions with cell types indicate that the association of NSAIDs with inflammatory cells is a diffusion-limited process determined by the physicochemical properties of the drug, the conditions of the local environment, and the nature of the cell membrane.[16]

The actions of NSAIDs, with the exception of aspirin, are reversible, although there is little evidence that plasma levels correlate with clinical response. One study found an increasing clinical response to naproxen as the dose increased: 76% of the patients improved when plasma concentrations exceeded 50 mg/L.[7] NSAIDs bind strongly to plasma proteins and have the potential to displace other drugs. Although this property is not usually clinically significant, caution must be exercised in prescribing NSAIDs when warfarin anticoagulants, methotrexate, and phenytoin are also being taken.[7] High-dosage NSAIDs such as salicylate are of special concern. Because the pathways of metabolism of salicylate are saturable, steady-state plasma concentrations increase to a greater extent than would be predicted by an increase in dosage. Disproportionate increases in the concentration of unbound drug in plasma occur because the binding of salicylate to plasma proteins is also saturable.

Mechanisms of Action

Prostaglandin-Dependent Effects

In 1971, Sir John Vane proposed that local production of prostaglandins was necessary to the inflammatory process,[19] and his hypothesis has been largely substantiated. The potential pro-inflammatory effects of prostaglandins are not confined to their ability to induce signs of inflammation. For example, prostaglandins synthesized by rheumatoid synovium stimulate bone resorption by mouse calvaria in vitro[17] and may contribute to the periarticular osteoporosis of rheumatoid disease.

Klaushofer and associates[9] demonstrated that NSAIDs inhibit thrombin-induced bone resorption in mouse calvaria. Interestingly, this study found that the potency of NSAIDs as prostaglandin inhibitors differed from their potency in other model systems, indicating tissue variability. Thus, the potency of an NSAID in a whole-tissue preparation such as cultured bone may be influenced by tissue penetration as well as by other local factors.

Prostaglandins also affect humoral and cell-mediated immunity. Macrophages and circulating monocytes produce significant amounts of prostaglandin E_2 when exposed to various stimuli. If added to mononuclear or T-cell cultures at concentrations detectable at inflammation sites, prostaglandin E_2 suppresses antigen responsiveness, cytokine production, clonal proliferation, and monocyte cytotoxic activity. Thus, by suppressing prostaglandin synthesis, NSAIDs may enhance cellular responsiveness. For example, indomethacin enhances delayed hypersensitivity reactions and short-term allograft survival in experimental animals. Goodwin[6] found that indomethacin restores the delayed hypersensitivity reaction in selected anergic human subjects.

Humoral immune responses may also be affected by prostaglandins. Goodwin also showed that NSAIDs could suppress immunoglobulin production in peripheral blood mononuclear cells stimulated with pokeweed mitogen. Adding prostaglandin E_2 to the cultures stimulated immunoglobulin production again. Subsequent studies indicated that prostaglandin E_2 exerts a preferential inhibitory effect on the suppressor T-cells that inhibit immunoglobulin production by B cells.[6] Because NSAIDs suppress prostaglandins, the suppressor T-cells are able to inhibit immunoglobulin production.

Prostaglandin-Independent Effects of NSAIDs

Problems With the Prostaglandin Hypothesis That NSAIDs can inhibit prostaglandin synthesis is clearly important in understanding their effects. However, the Vane hypothesis cannot be applied to all products of the arachidonic acid cascade or to all NSAIDs at all dosages. The three major antipyretic and analgesic drugs have diverse effects on prostaglandin biosynthesis. For example, aspirin has antipyretic, anti-inflammatory, and analgesic effects when used in dosages of 4 to 6 g/day. It inhibits prostaglandin synthesis in disrupted cell preparations. At lower dosages (650 every four to six hours), aspirin has antipyretic and analgesic but not anti-inflammatory effects. The plasma salicylate levels of persons taking lower doses, however, are sufficient to inhibit prostaglandin biosynthesis in vivo by the kidneys, platelets, and vascular endothelium. Higher plasma concentrations (18 to 30 mg/dl) are required to achieve an anti-inflammatory effect. These observations suggest two possibilities: either the cyclo-oxygenase of cells at inflammatory sites is relatively insensitive to aspirin, or aspirin has a mode of action distinct from its capacity to inhibit prostaglandin biosynthesis.

Evidence that aspirin-like drugs exert significant clinical effects independent of prostaglandins is seen in the action of sodium salicylate. Sodium salicylate was the first NSAID used to treat rheumatic diseases and shares many of the properties of aspirin. But it does not inhibit prostaglandin biosynthesis in disrupted cell preparations at plasma

Outline 1 Diverse cellular processes inhibited by nonsteroidal anti-inflammatory drugs

Membrane-associated enzymatic activities
  NADPH oxidase (neutrophil)
  Phospholipase C (macrophage)
  12-Hydroperoxyeicosatetraenoic acid peroxidase (platelet)
Uptake of precursor arachidonate and its insertion into macrophage membranes
Transmembrane anion transport (erythrocytes, renal tubules)
Oxidative phosphorylation and calcium translocation in mitochondria
Release of histamine from mast cells in response to fibrinogen degradation products

concentrations of less than 5 to 10 mmol.[2] Nonacetylated salicylates do not inhibit human platelet function in vitro or ex vivo, nor do they prolong bleeding time.[5] Because aspirin and salicylic acid are clinically equivalent anti-inflammatory agents and aspirin is rapidly hydrolyzed to salicylic acid in vivo, it is doubtful that the only action of NSAIDs is to inhibit the synthesis of prostaglandin. Vane used an animal model to show that salicylate salicylic acid reduces prostaglandin concentration in inflammatory exudates,[1] but whether this reduction resulted from a direct effect on prostaglandin synthesis or reflected a global decrease in the inflammatory response by other mechanisms was unclear.

The prostaglandin hypothesis is further complicated by the fact that the stable prostaglandins (prostaglandin E_2, prostaglandin I_2) possess both pro-inflammatory and anti-inflammatory effects. The pro-inflammatory effects include the production of vasodilation, synergistic action with the complement component C5a or leukotriene B_4, the mediation of fever and myalgia in response to interleukin-1, synergistic action with bradykinin to provoke pain, and inhibition of T-suppressor cells. Zurier and Ballas[22] showed that high doses of stable prostaglandins inhibit inflammation in animal models of arthritis, and lower doses inhibit local inflammation induced by carrageenan-like agents. More importantly, it is clear that prostaglandin I_2 and stable prostaglandins of the E-type inhibit the activation of neutrophils, platelets, and mononuclear phagocytes. This effect results, at least in part, from an increase in cyclic adenosine monophosphate. Thus, the anti-inflammatory effects of NSAIDs may not derive entirely from inhibition of prostaglandin synthesis.

Effects on Diverse Cells and Their Membranes NSAIDS exert effects on inflammatory cells separate from their ability to inhibit prostaglandin synthesis (Outline 1). The broad spectrum of effects results from the physicochemical properties of NSAIDs that favor their association with the plasma membrane of certain cells.[1,16] This association may alter the fluidity of the membrane and disrupt the molecular interactions required for normal signal transduction across the lipid bilayer.[1] Some NSAIDs can inhibit a variety of membrane-associated processes, including superoxide anion generation by a cell-free NADPH oxidase system of neutrophils, mononuclear cell phospholipase C activity, and the 12-hydroperoxyeicosatetraenoic acid per-

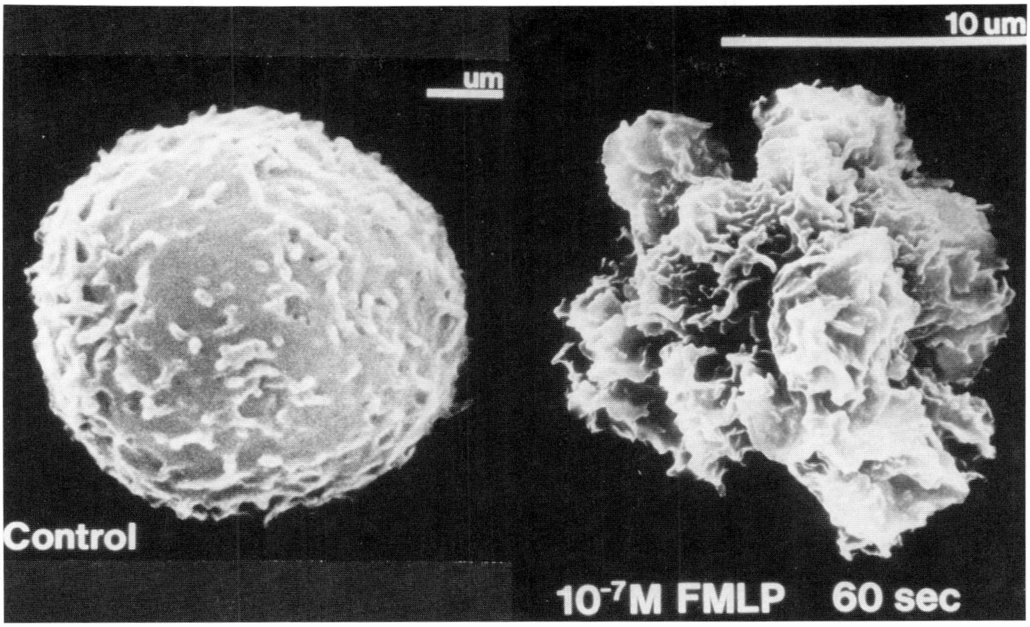

Fig. 1 *Effect of the chemoattractant formyl-methionyleucylphenylalanine on the surface characteristics and adhesiveness of human neutrophils. The scanning electron micrograph on the left shows a single neutrophil suspended in buffer. On the right is an aggregate of neutrophils fixed 60 seconds after the addition of 10^{-7}M of f-MLP. The increased adhesiveness of these cells is associated with an increase in surface area as reflected by the marked ruffling of the plasma membrane. Neutrophil aggregation is effectively inhibited by NSAIDs.*

oxidase of the lipoxygenase pathway in platelets.[1,4] Aspirin-like drugs inhibit calcium movement across the mitochondrial membrane where they uncouple oxidative phosphorylation.[11] Aspirin (but not acetaminophen) also alters the uptake of precursor arachidonate and its insertion into the membrane of monocytes and macrophages in human cultures.[1] Salicylates (but not acetaminophen) inhibit anion transport across a variety of cell membranes, including human erythrocyte, rabbit choroid plexus, and human renal tubular epithelium.[1] Finally, certain NSAIDs can inhibit the release of histamine by mast cells exposed to fibrinogen degradation products.[20]

NSAIDs also exert significant effects on the metabolism of cartilage and bone (in vitro and in vivo) that probably do not depend on the inhibition of cyclooxygenase.[14] Studies have also shown that some classes of NSAIDs such as the salicylates inhibit glycosaminoglycan synthesis by articular cartilage.

Effects on the Neutrophil The ability of NSAIDs to inhibit the release of lysosomal enzymes and the chemotactic response of neu-

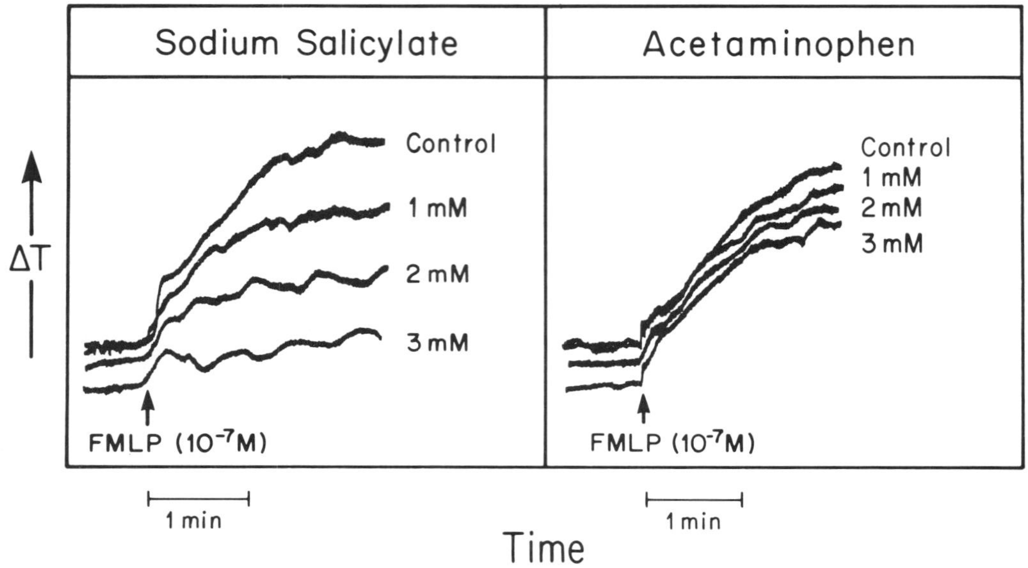

Fig. 2 *The effect of sodium salicylate and acetaminophen on f-MLP-induced neutrophil aggregation. Neutrophils were preincubated with buffer or drug before exposure to the chemoattractant f-MLP. Changes in light transmission, recorded over time, are represented by curves similar to those generated in the measurement of platelet aggregation. Sodium salicylate is a poor inhibitor of prostaglandin synthesis (and does not inhibit platelet aggregation), but is as effective as other NSAIDs in its capacity to inhibit neutrophil aggregation. Acetaminophen, structurally related to salicylate but without anti-inflammatory properties, does not effectively inhibit aggregation.*

trophils was demonstrated even before Vane showed that NSAIDs inhibited cyclo-oxygenase. The concentrations needed for inhibition and neutrophil activation were comparable to anti-inflammatory rather than analgesic doses. However, because these concentrations were substantially higher than the expected unbound plasma concentrations in vivo, the clinical importance of these observations was questioned. Recently, studies have found that the effect of NSAIDs observed in vitro can be reproduced in neutrophils harvested from the blood and synovial fluid of subjects taking NSAIDs in conventional doses.[13] Thus, the predicted unbound concentration of drug in an aqueous medium such as plasma may be an unreliable indicator of actual tissue accumulation for lipophilic NSAIDs.

The inhibition of neutrophil function by NSAIDs is not related to its ability to inhibit prostaglandin synthesis. Sodium salicylate, an ineffective cyclo-oxygenase inhibitor, is as effective as aspirin in inhibiting neutrophil functions.[1] Furthermore, there are differences among the cyclo-oxygenase inhibitors. All NSAIDs inhibit cell-cell aggregation (Figs. 1 and 2), but they exert diverse effects on other neutrophil func-

Outline 2 Effects of NSAIDs on neutrophil functions*

Effects common to all classes of NSAIDs
- Inhibition of aggregation
- Formyl-methionyleucylphenylalanine binding
- Intracellular cyclic AMP increased after stimulation†

Effects that differ among NSAIDs
- Inhibition of superoxide anion by intact cells and cell-free NADPH oxidase
- Alteration of membrane viscosity (increased by piroxicam and indomethacin; decreased by salicylates

*NSAID classes examined include oxicams, salicylates, propionic acid derivatives, indole acetic acids, and fenamates.
†Fenamates not tested.

tions (Outline 2). For example, piroxicam inhibits the generation of superoxide anion from neutrophils exposed to concanavalin A or phorbol myristate acetate.[8] Ibuprofen does not. Minta and Williams[12] demonstrated that piroxicam and indomethacin (but not meclofenamate, salicylate, or ibuprofen) inhibit the production of superoxide anion by a cell-free, membrane preparation of NADPH oxidase. They also corroborated previous observations that NSAIDs can inhibit the binding of the chemoattractant formyl-methionyleucylphenylalanine (f-MLP) to neutrophils. Purified neutrophil membrane preparations can be used to show that sodium salicylate and piroxicam inhibit f-MLP binding at dosages that prevent neutrophil activation.[1] Acetaminophen does not inhibit ligand binding at concentrations as high as 3 mmol/L (unpublished observation).

However, these isolated effects of NSAIDs on f-MLP binding cannot explain their effects on the neutrophil. NSAIDS also inhibit activation in response to other ligands, such as C5a, platelet-activating factor, and leukotriene B_4, as well as to other stimuli such as phorbol myristate acetate. Furthermore, Perez and associates[15] showed that meclofenamate inhibits C5a-induced neutrophil functions, but does not inhibit the binding of radioisotope-labeled C5a. NSAIDs must therefore exert other actions that may pertain to nonspecific disruptive effects on signaling within the plasmalemma (Fig. 3).

Application to Sports-Induced Injuries

NSAIDs are commonly used in sports medicine to help heal the inflammatory process and provide simple analgesia. NSAIDs and acetaminophen (a chemically related compound that is not anti-inflammatory) all have analgesic properties. However, the toxicity of NSAIDs is related to their capacity to inhibit prostaglandins, a property not shared by acetaminophen. Thus, for sports-related injuries and other disorders such as osteoarthritis that require both analgesia and anti-inflammation, the risk-benefit ratio for NSAID use depends on the need for anti-inflammatory action rather than for pain relief alone.

Unfortunately, there are no clear guidelines. There are few controlled

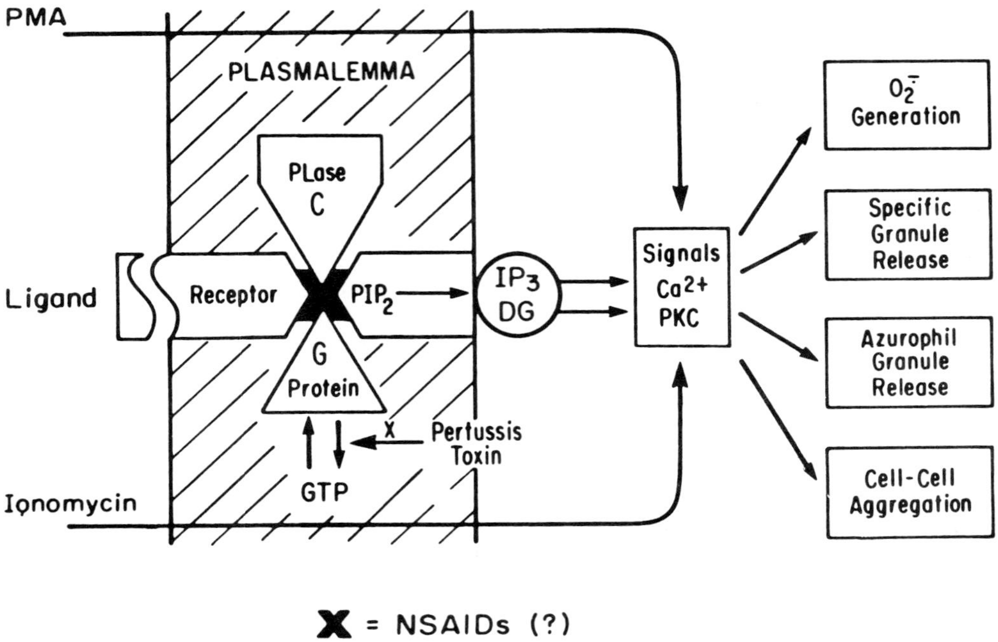

Fig. 3 *Stimulus-response coupling in the neutrophil. X represents the insertion into the lipid bilayer and the uncoupling of protein-protein interactions by NSAIDs. PMA, phorbol myristate acetate; PLase C, phospholipase C; PIP_2, phosphatidylinositol 4,5 bisphosphate; IP_3, inositol 1,4,5-trisphosphate; DG, diacylglycerol; PKC, protein kinase C; GTP, guanosine triphosphate.*

studies that compare simple analgesics with NSAIDs for their effects on sports injuries. One problem is that sports injuries take various forms, which makes it impossible to identify a single pathophysiologic mechanism or to generalize about the effects of NSAIDs on the basis of their use in one type of injury. Few studies have analyzed the biochemical and histopathologic characteristics of specific sports-injury syndromes. For example, little is known about the key inflammatory mediators that are released after mechanical trauma and that perpetuate an inflammatory process. There are no adequate studies of the evolution and influx of inflammatory cells, some of which destroy tissue whereas others affect the normal reparative processes. Perhaps anti-inflammatory therapy retards the normal healing process, but there seems to be no clinical evidence to support this concern. In theory, this is not surprising. The essential cells for normal healing of injured tissue are fibroblasts and tissue macrophages. Cell functioning (with the obvious exception of prostaglandin synthesis) appears to be unimpaired by NSAIDs. Corticosteroids, on the other hand, decrease collagen synthesis by fibroblasts and inhibit the release of cytokines from mononuclear cells.

Another problem in analyzing the efficacy of NSAIDs in sports injuries is the inadequacy of study designs. Weiler and associates[20] found only three studies of highly competitive athletes that included a placebo control. Blazina[3] compared oxyphenbutazone (600 mg/day for two days and 200 mg/day for three days) with a placebo in a double-blind trial in 46 college football players. Both groups received physical therapy. Although the patients treated with oxyphenbutazone were more likely to have an "excellent" response, the differences were not statistically significant, and there was no analgesic treatment group for comparison. One group compared indomethacin (150 mg/day) with a placebo in 30 professional football players in England who had sprains, strains, and direct trauma.[20] Rapid improvement occurred in both groups and the indomethacin group did not fare significantly better. In a study of acute minor injuries in professional athletes,[18] low or analgesic doses of ibuprofen or placebo were less effective than piroxicam (20 mg/day) in reducing pain and passive functional disability. Neither of the NSAIDs reduced the time necessary for recovery.

Although differences favoring NSAIDs were found in two of these controlled studies, the differences were not striking. Other studies on acute injuries compared two NSAIDs without a placebo group. The differences between the drugs were nonexistent or small. Most athletes improved in seven days.[20] None of the studies showed that NSAIDs delayed recovery. Most adverse reactions to these short courses of drug therapy were mild.

Similar studies have been performed on the recreational athlete. Weiler and associates[20] reviewed these studies and concluded that "none of these studies is useful in evaluating the use of NSAIDs in sports medicine because they contained major flaws."

A similar conclusion can be drawn regarding studies on NSAID therapy in various other sports medicine settings. Patients tend to do well with NSAIDs, but differences between the drugs and a placebo are small or nonexistent.

References

1. Abramson SB, Weiseman G: The mechanisms of action of nonsteroidal antiinflammatory drugs. *Arthritis Rheum* 1989;32:1–9.
2. Atkinson DC, Collier HOJ: Salicylates: Molecular mechanism of therapeutic action. *Adv Pharmacol Chemother* 1980;17:233–288.
3. Blazina ME: Oxyphenbutazone as an adjunct to the conventional treatment of athletic injuries. *Clin Med* 1969;76:19.
4. Day RO: Modes of action of non-steroidal anti-inflammatory drugs. *Med J Aust* 1988;148:195–199.
5. Estes D, Kaplan K: Lack of platelet effect with the aspirin analog, salsalate. *Arthritis Rheum* 1980;23:1303–1307.
6. Goodwin JS: Immunologic effects of nonsteroidal antiinflammatory drugs. *Am J Med* 1984;77:7.
7. Graham GC: Pharmacokinetics and metabolism of non-steroidal anti-inflammatory dugs. *Med J Aust* 1987;147:597–602.

8. Kaplan H, Edelson M, Korchak H, et al: Effects of nonsteroidal antiinflammatory agents on human neutrophil functions in vitro and in vivo. *Biochem Pharmacol* 1984;33:371–378.
9. Klaushofer K, Hoffman O, Czerwenka E, et al: Comparison of the inhibitory effect of nonsteroidal antiinflammatory drugs on bone prostaglandin synthesis and resorption. *J Rheumatol* 1987;15:486–491.
10. Lombardino J, Otterness I, Wiseman E: Acidic antiinflammatory agents. *Arzneim Forschung* 1975;25:1629–1634.
11. McDougal P, Markham A, Cameron I, et al: Action of the nonsteroidal antiinflammatory agent, flufenamic acid, on calcium movements in isolated mitochondria. *Pharmacology* 1988;37:1327–1330.
12. Minta J, Williams MJ: Some nonsteroidal antiinflammatory drugs inhibit the generation of superoxide anions by activated polymorphs by blocking ligand-receptor interactions. *Rheumatology* 1985;12:751–757.
13. Montecucco C, Mazzone A, Pasotti D, et al: Effect of piroxicam therapy on granulocyte function elastase concentration in peripheral blood and synovial fluid in rheumatoid arthritis patients. *Inflammation*, in press.
14. Palmoski MJ, Brandt KD: Effect of salicylate on proteoglycan metabolism in normal canine articular cartilage in vitro. *Arthritis Rheum* 1980;23:1010–1020.
15. Perez HD, Elfman F, Marder S: Meclofenamate sodium monohydrate inhibits chemotactic factor-induced human polymorphonuclear leukocyte function: A possible explanation for its antiinflammatory effect. *Arthritis Rheum* 1987;30:1023–1031.
16. Raghoebar MR, Van Den Berg WB, Van Ginneken CAM: Mechanisms of cell association of some non-steroidal antiinflammatory drugs with isolated leukocytes. *Biochem Pharmacol* 1988;37:1247–1250.
17. Robinson DR, Tashjian AH Jr, Levine L: Prostaglandin-stimulated bone resorption by rheumatoid synovia: A possible mechanism for bone destruction in rheumatoid arthritis. *J Clin Invest* 1975;56:1181–1188.
18. Santilli G, Tuccimei V, Cannistia FM: Comparative study with piroxicam and ibuprofen versus placebo in the supportive treatment of minor sports injuries. *JIMR* 1980;8:265.
19. Vane JR: Inhibition of prostaglandin synthesis as a mechanism of action for aspirin-like drugs. *Nature* 1971;231:232–235.
20. Weiler JM, Albright JP, Buckwalter JA: Nonsteroidal antiinflammatory drugs, in Lewis AJ, Furst DE (eds): *Antiinflammatory Agents in Sports Medicine*. New York, Marcel Dekker, 1987, pp 71–78.
21. Wojtecka-Lukasis E, Stanchurska J, Kopec M, et al: Anti-inflammatory drugs modulate histamine release from mast cells induced by fibrinogen degradation products. *Ann Rheum Dis* 1988;47:328–332.
22. Zurier RB, Ballas M: Prostaglandin E suppression of adjuvant arthritis: Histopathology. *Arthritis Rheum* 1973;16:251–258.

Chapter 26

Aspirin and Nonacetylated Salicylates: Use in Inflammatory Injuries Incurred During Sporting Activities

W. Watson Buchanan, MD, FRCP (Edin, Glasg, and C)
K.D. Rainsford, PhD, MRCPath, FRSC

One of the most commonly self-administered and prescribed anti-inflammatory and analgesic drugs is aspirin (acetylsalicylic acid). Studies have examined its use in treating both acute and chronic sports-induced injuries.[1,9,17,43,70] This chapter discusses the pharmacokinetic disposition and pharmacodynamic effects of aspirin and related salicylates and the rationale for their use in treating sports injuries.

Pharmacokinetics and Biodisposition

Absorption

Palatability, ease of consumption, and ready availability often make simply formulated or buffered aspirin the pain-reliever of choice for injured athletes. Both are more rapidly absorbed by the body than slow-release, enteric-coated preparations.[50]

Salicylic acid and its derivatives are rapidly absorbed by passive diffusion of undissociated molecules in the stomach and, to a lesser extent, in the small intestine.[50] The rate of absorption is largely determined by the physical characteristics of the formulation[50] and its state (liquid, soluble or insoluble tablet, or enteric-coated capsule). Enteric-coated capsules are absorbed more in the small intestine because the time needed before the drug is released exceeds the rate of gastric emptying. The large surface area of the intestinal tract compensates for the alkaline pH that would otherwise delay absorption. Absorption of aspirin and salicylic acid is, in general, enhanced in the acidic environment of the stomach, where the pH is less than the p*K*a of the drug. Although aspirin hydrolyzes spontaneously in aqueous solutions, this is a slow process and little or no free salicylate exists in the lumen of the stomach or intestine. Thus, the drug is principally absorbed as aspirin and not as salicylic acid.[50]

Solutions, "plain" tablets, and capsules of aspirin or other salicylic acids are generally well absorbed in relatively short times (one to three hours). Effervescent soluble tablets[67] and some of the strongly "buffered" preparations are absorbed most rapidly.[39] Absorption is influenced by a number of factors, including the rate of gastric emptying, the ingestion of food with the drug, the volume of food ingested, intake of concurrent medications (especially those such as metaclopramide that affect the rate of gastric emptying), posture during intake, and exercise.[12,50] The effect of food on total bioavailability is minimal; food may delay the rate of absorption, but does not affect the kinetics of drug absorption.[74] Some types of antacids may have a marked influence on salicylate absorption, especially if they are taken in large doses.[50]

Athletes often use topical ointments containing methyl salicylate to control pain and swelling. Percutaneous absorption is rapid, but toxic reactions may occur if the applied dose exceeds 10 g.[74] Rapid absorption occurs over a wide range of pH values so it is not possible to modulate the rate of absorption by altering the acidity of the preparation.[74]

Biotransformation

When aspirin is taken, esterase enzymes in gastrointestinal mucosa, plasma, erythrocytes, and liver rapidly hydrolyze the parent compound to salicylate and acetate. The acetylsalicylate or salicylate concentrations in the blood or other body fluids can be determined by various calorimetric, chromatographic, and fluorometric methods.[50] However, the reliability of these methods for measuring acetylsalicylate varies markedly.[50]

Aspirin has a half-life of only 15 to 20 minutes, so only small amounts are detectable in the blood after ingestion.[58] The acetyl component may be chemically acetylated into gastric cell biomolecules or it may be excreted as carbon dioxide after passing through the Krebs cycle.[52]

In its ionized form, salicylic acid is partly excreted in an unchanged form and partly biotransformed into four metabolites.[37] Gentisuric acid may be formed either from salicylic acid by hepatic microsomal oxidative enzymes, or from gentisic acid by glycine conjugation.[73] The biotransformations of salicylic acid to salicyluric acid or to salicyl phenolic glucuronide follow Michaelis-Menten kinetics, while the other two pathways exhibit first-order or linear kinetics.[12] As a result, the plasma half-life of salicylate increases nonlinearly as the dosage increases. Consequently, the increased concentration in the blood is disproportionate to the increase in the dose of salicylate.[35,47]

Levy[35] showed that when the dose of aspirin is increased from 250 mg to 1.0 g, the plasma half-life increases from three to 20 hours. This has important clinical applications. If anti-inflammatory doses of aspirin prescribed are equal to a total of 3 g/day or more, twice-daily administration will maintain adequate therapeutic blood concentrations because of the long plasma half-life.[8] Because of the existence of the potentially saturable metabolic pathways, there is a sudden increase in plasma salicylate concentrations when dosage is increased even slightly. The timing of this also influences the pattern of plasma salicylate levels.

Salicylic acid induces its own biotransformation to salicyluric acid.[10,18,59] Müller and associates[44] compared steady-state plasma concentrations after one week and after three weeks of salicylate therapy and found that levels decreased approximately 50%. Hence, patients treated with salicylate therapy for several weeks may find that the therapeutic effects diminish. This phenomenon, however, would not affect athletes whose injuries seldom require such prolonged anti-inflammatory, analgesic therapy.

Methyl salicylate metabolizes to salicylate quite slowly. Early studies compared the excretion rates for methyl salicylate with those for salicylate,[19,71] but there is practically no research on the quantitative aspects of the metabolic pathways of this widely used drug. The methyl portion may hydrolyze to salicylic acid and methanol.

Methanol is subsequently oxidized by the metabolic pathways to acetaldehyde,[71] which is known to be associated with ocular and other toxic reactions. Long-term use of high doses of methyl salicylate should thus be avoided.

Biodisposition

Once absorbed, salicylate is distributed extensively in body fluids. The volume of distribution ranges from 9.6 to 12.7 L or 0.14 to 0.18 L/kg for an adult weighing 70 kg and approximately 0.12 to 0.14 L/kg in a child.[72] Both acetylsalicylate and salicylate are bound to serum albumin at two primary sites (diazepam and warfarin) and at a number of secondary, low-affinity sites.[64] Acetylsalicylate binds less than salicylate, and binding may accompany acetylation of albumin and esterase-like deacetylation by this protein. At therapeutic serum concentrations (that is, 100 mg/ml), approximately 80% to 90% of acetylsalicylate is protein-bound. At higher concentrations, however, only 70% to 75% is bound. Thus, protein-binding is nonlinear.[18,68] As the serum concentration increases, more free or unbound acetylsalicylate is available for distribution into the tissues.

The pH of the plasma has a profound effect on protein-binding. In rats, a decrease in the plasma pH level from 7.4 to 7.2 causes the amount of unbound acetylsalicylate to double.[12] A decrease in serum albumin concentration, such as occurs in patients with inflammatory joint disease, also increases the concentration of unbound acetylsalicylate. If the serum albumin concentration decreases from 5 g/100 ml to 2 g/100 ml, the amount of unbound acetylsalicylate increases from 10% to 50%.[75] Inflammatory synovial fluid has significantly lower concentrations of acetylsalicylate and salicylate than plasma because of its lower albumin concentration.[69] Salicylates readily cross the placenta and also enter breast milk.[50]

Excretion

In the kidneys, the salicylic acids are passively reabsorbed by the distal tubules; this is profoundly affected by changes in the pH of the urine. Administering sodium bicarbonate or other alkalis with aspirin causes the plasma concentration of salicylate to decrease significantly.[36] This is clinically important because antacids are frequently prescribed to reduce dyspepsia in patients taking salicylates.

Monitoring Therapy

The therapeutic plasma concentration of salicylate is normally considered to range from 15 to 30 mg/100 ml or 1 to 2 mmol/L. However, there is at least a fivefold variation in serum concentrations of salicylate among patients given the same dose.[50] Boardman and Hart[5] found that a daily 3-g dose of aspirin was needed to produce an anti-inflammatory effect (meaured by the reduction in joint circumference) in patients with rheumatoid arthritis.[5] They did not attempt to correlate this measure with therapeutic serum concentrations. It has not been possible to demonstrate an anti-inflammatory effect with salicylate therapy in a dose-response manner.[33] Pushing salicylate therapy to the limits of tolerance and then "backing off"[33] is no longer regarded as sound clinical practice, especially in elderly subjects with preexisting hearing loss, because of the risk of ototoxicity and gastrointestinal side effects.

Mechanisms of Action

Inhibition of cyclo-oxygenase, first described by Vane,[66] is widely cited as the major mechanism of action of nonsteroidal anti-inflammatory analgesics. However, this is not the only major mechanism of anti-inflammatory action.[49,50]

Inhibition of cyclo-oxygenase may represent only part of the mechanism of many of the toxic effects these drugs have on the stomach, kidneys, skin, and lungs.[50,53,54] For example, the analgesic and anti-inflammatory effects of sodium salicylate and choline magnesium salicylate in equimolar dosage are equal to those of aspirin in the treatment of rheumatoid arthritis.[31,48] The salicylate dimer, salsalate (salicylsalicylic acid as diplosal) hydrolyzes after oral absorption to two molecules of salicylate. It is as effective as aspirin in relieving the pain of osteoarthritis of the knee if the dosages achieve comparable plasma salicylate levels.[38] Nonacetylated salicylates are also effective in treating chronic inflammatory states despite the fact that they are weaker prostaglandin inhibitors.[50] Rosenkranz and associates[56] have shown that effective therapeutic doses of salicylate for treatment of rheumatoid diseases do not affect urinary excretion of prostaglandin E_2. Aspirin, however, does cause a significant reduction.

Aspirin has long been considered a more potent analgesic than the nonacetylated metabolite, salicylate.[30] However, no definitive study in humans with different inflammatory diseases has proven this. Although the analgesic response to aspirin is dose-dependent, it does not appear to correlate with serum concentrations.[34] There is, however, substantial evidence that aspirin is more effective than salicylate as an antipyretic.[60]

Most laboratory studies on the effects of aspirin and nonacetylated salicylates on the biochemical pharmacology of inflammation use acute rather than chronic models. These models may have direct relevance to certain acute sports injuries. Thus, aspirin may surpass salicylate or salicylic acid in controlling soft-tissue injuries and relieving pain. Although the effects of aspirin and salicylate may be similar in chronic inflammations such as occur in rheumatoid arthritis, they may be different in an acute injury. Properly controlled therapeutic trials must therefore be conducted, especially for sport injuries. If salicylates are as effective as aspirin in treating acute inflammatory states, then these drugs should be used because they cause less gastric irritation and do not cause bronchial asthma or allergic reactions.[50,74]

Salicylates have other mechanisms of action relevant to the control of inflammation. These include uncoupling of oxidative phosphorylation, inhibiting lysosomal enzyme release and free-radical generation, and inhibition of neutrophils, lymphocytes ,and monocytes.[49–51,53] Inhibition of the generation of radicals may be linked to salicylate's ability to scavenge superoxide or hydroxyl radicals to form gentisate.[50]

Analgesia

Aspirin, salicylate, and their congeners are classically considered peripherally acting analgesics.[50] One interpretation of a series of elegant crossover perfusion experiments performed by Lim and associates in 1969 supports this hypothesis.[50] Linked with this hypothesis is the recognition that controlling inflammation is an integral part of the peripheral analgesia elicited by the salicylates.[50] Other studies on rabbits confirmed these earlier observations.[55] Now, detailed investigation of the mechanisms of analgesic action in the spine have shown that aspirin and salicylate act directly on both the central and the peripheral nervous systems. Studies on laboratory animals[7,27,63] indicate that salicylates act on components of the spinothalamic tracts, including those mediated by substance P.[27] Table 1 summarizes the mechanisms of spinothalamic actions of salicylate compared with those of the opiates and acetaminophen.

Recent studies have also distinguished between the antinociceptive and the anti-inflammatory actions of aspirin and salicylate.[24,26] These investigations also showed that the drugs have analgesic actions on central as well as peripheral nerves.

Many clinical studies have measured the analgesic effects of apirin in specific models of human pain.[4,16,29,32,62,65] The results indicate that in some instances acetylsalicylate can provide analgesia at certain sites in the central nervous system comparable to opiates. Further, the degree of analgesia from ingested aspirin correlates with plasma salicylate levels but not with those of the parent drug.[16]

Analgesia and the other anti-inflammatory effects of methyl salicylate have received little attention. Methyl salicylate may act by a "counterirritant" mechanism,[74] although the basis for this nebulous description is unclear.

Table 1 Central vs peripheral actions of analgesics

Actions	Acetylsalicylic Acid	Salicylic Acid	Acetaminophen	Morphine
At spinal/central level				
Thalamic nerve stimulation	Decreased	Not established	Decreased	Decreased
Pre-optic/hypothalamic nerve activities	Decreased	Not established	Not established	Decreased
Ascending axons	No action	Not established	No action	Decreased
Postsynaptic substance P production	Decreased	Not established	Decreased	Decreased
5-Hydroxytryptamine turnover	Increased	Increased	Not established	Increased
Prostaglandins E_2 and I_2 production	Not established	Decreased	Decreased	Not established
At peripheral level				
Prostaglandins E_2 and I_2 production	Decreased	No action	Variable decrease*	No action
Nerve membrane conductance	Decreased	Decreased	Not established	Not established
ATP production	Decreased†	Decreased	Not established	No action

*Variable decrease depending on the system being investigated.
†From a salicylate derived by metabolism.

Antithrombotic Actions

Most nonsteroidal anti-inflammatory drugs (NSAIDs) with analgesic action impair platelet aggregation by inhibiting synthesis of thromboxane A_2. Unlike aspirin, most NSAIDs do not covalently bind to the active site of cyclo-oxygenase, and synthesis is resumed when the drug is withdrawn. In contrast, aspirin irreversibly acetylates platelet cyclo-oxygenase; the effect persists for the life of the platelet (about five days).[6,57] Nonacetylated salicylates, including diflunisal and salsalate, do not affect platelet aggregation or thromboxane formation.[13,56] In normal subjects, aspirin may prolong bleeding time slightly and high doses of salicylates may cause hypoprothrombinemia, but these findings become significant only in patients with bleeding disorders.[40]

The most serious potential adverse effect of aspirin is hemorrhage into acutely inflamed and traumatized tissues. A high incidence of postoperative bleeding after dental extraction has been reported in cases in which aspirin was administered before surgery.[23] If the drug is given two hours after the operation, when hemostasis is well established, no significant bleeding occurs.[61]

If aspirin is taken concomitantly with ethanol, there may be a synergistic effect, causing gastric bleeding.[11,14,20,45,46]

Therapeutic Application in Sports Injuries

NSAIDs are frequently prescribed to reduce inflammation and facilitate return to full function. However, properly designed, placebo-controlled therapeutic trials have not been performed to confirm their effectiveness in sports injuries. Many reports include assumptions rather than facts.[9]

Muckle's[42,43] controlled trials showed that aspirin was as effective as ibuprofen in the treatment of soft-tissue injuries to the lower limbs of British football players. Other NSAIDs such as naproxen and indomethacin showed gastric side effects and several participants in these controlled trials withdrew from therapy.[70] Other reports are noticeably deficient in recording adverse effects.

Andersen and Gøtzsche[1] compared aspirin with naproxen in 79 patients with injuries of less than 14 days' duration. Both drugs were associated with improvement in pain symptoms, but their effects were not statistically different. Heere[22] described a multicenter, double-blind, parallel study of piroxicam, indomethacin, naproxen, and aspirin in 1,290 patients with acute sprains and tendinitis. Improvement in pain symptoms occurred with all four drugs in 80% of patients, with piroxicam being the most effective drug. Neither of these studies included placebo-treated or an untreated groups. Because acute sports injuries tend to improve spontaneously, the results may be expressed as drug A = drug B = drug C = drug D = 0.

Of the available NSAIDs, aspirin is both inexpensive and relatively safe for occasional use.[21,50] It is best prescribed as a soluble tablet because this form provides a more rapid onset and longer duration of analgesia than conventional forms, and may also be better tolerated in the upper gastrointestinal tract.[25,62] If there is risk of associated local hemorrhage (that is, hematomas), as in knee injuries,[3] aspirin should be avoided. It may also be dangerous if taken in full therapeutic doses during physical exertion in the heat.[17] Further, dehydration with exercise may make renal dysfunction caused by aspirin more likely.[50] Elderly patients may suffer cognitive dysfunction, and they, as well as others, may be susceptible to salicylate intoxication.[2] It is not known whether aspirin in therapeutic doses impairs an athlete's reaction time.

Sports injuries vary considerably and such a global term conceals the complexity of this heterogeneous group of injuries. Depending on the situation and the injury, aspirin and other analgesic and anti-inflammatory agents may be only one component of the therapeutic regimen, may have limited efficacy, or may be contraindicated, as in a head or knee injury in which associated "concealed" bleeding would be exacerbated by these drugs' tendency to promote bleeding.

The complexities of neuromuscular "cycling" in muscle sprains are obvious indications for muscle relaxants. The combination of these drugs with aspirin has not been tested in different types of injuries. The relative ineffectiveness of aspirin and other NSAIDs in the treatment of certain soft-tissue injuries may be related to the need for a muscle relaxant or a mild antidepressant to control the cycle of associated muscle spasms. Such combination therapies have yet to be examined in properly conducted double-blind studies. In addition, the safety of nonacetylated salicylates in acute sports injuries requires full and intense study because of their lack of effect on thrombotic reactions and their propensity for producing gastrointestinal side effects.

References

1. Andersen LA, Gøtzsche PC: Naproxen and aspirin in acute musculoskeletal disorders: A double-blind, parallel study in patients with sports injuries. *Pharmatherapeutica* 1984;3:531–537.
2. Anderson RJ, Potts DE, Gabow PA, et al: Unrecognized adult salicylate intoxication. *Ann Intern Med* 1976;85:745–748.
3. Beall S, Gardner J, Coxley D: Anterolateral compartment syndrome related to drug-induced bleeding: A case report. *Am J Sports Med* 1983;11:454–455.
4. Blendinger I, Eberlein HJ: Comparison of intravenous acetylsalicylic acid and dipyrone in postoperative pain: An interim report. *Br J Clin Pharmacol* 1980;10(suppl 2):339S–341S.
5. Boardman PL, Hart FD: Clinical measurements of the anti-inflammatory effects of salicylates in rheumatoid arthritis. *Br Med J* 1967;4:264–268.
6. Burch JW, Stanford N, Majerus PW: Inhibition of platelet prostaglandin synthetase by oral aspirin. *J Clin Invest* 1978;61:314–319.
7. Carlsson KH, Monzel W, Jurna I: Depression by morphine and the non-opioid analgesic agents, metamizol (dipyrone), lysine acetylsalicylate, and paracetamol, of activity in rat thalamus neurones evoked by electrical stimulation of nociceptive afferents. *Pain* 1988;32:313–326.
8. Cassell S, Furst D, Dromgoole S, et al: Steady-state serum salicylate levels in hospitalized patients with rheumatoid arthritis: Comparison of two dosage schedules of choline magnesium trisalicylate. *Arthritis Rheum* 1979;22:384–388.
9. Cody KA, Gaska JA: A primer on sports-related injuries. *Am Drugs* 1985;189:89–95.
10. Day RO, Shen DD, Azarnoff DL: Induction of salicyluric acid formation in rheumatoid arthritis patients treated with salicylates. *Clin Pharmacokinet* 1983;8:263–271.
11. DeSchepper PJ, Tjandramaga TB, De Roo M, et al: Gastrointestinal blood loss after diflunisal and after aspirin: Effect of ethanol. *Clin Pharmacol Ther* 1978;23:669–676.
12. Dromgoole SH, Furst DE, Paulus HE: Rational approaches to the use of salicylates in the treatment of rheumatoid arthritis. *Semin Arthritis Rheum* 1981;11:257–283.
13. Estes D, Kaplan K: Lack of platelet effect with the aspirin analog, salsalate. *Arthritis Rheum* 1980;23:1303–1307.
14. Falaye JM, Odutola TA: The economic potential and the role of aspirin and alcohol ingestion in relation to haematemesis and melaena. *Niger Med J* 1978;8:526–530.
15. Findlay SW, DeAngelis RL, Kearney MF, et al: Analgesic drugs in breast milk and plasma. *Clin Pharmacol Ther* 1981;29:625–633.
16. Forster C, Anton F, Reeh PW, et al: Measurement of the analgesic effects of aspirin with a new experimental algesimetric procedure. *Pain* 1988;32:215–222.
17. Fred HL: Reflections on a 100-mile run: Effects of aspirin therapy. *Med Sci Sports Exerc* 1980;12:212–215.
18. Furst D, Tozer TN, Melmon KL: Salicylate clearance, the resultant of protein binding and metabolism. *Clin Pharmacol Ther* 1979;26:380–389.
19. Gross M, Greenberg LA: *The Salicylates: A Critical Bibliographic Review.* New Haven, Hillhouse Press, 1948.
20. Goulston K, Cooke AR: Alcohol, aspirin, and gastro-intestinal bleeding. *Br Med J* 1978;4:664–665.
21. Hadler NM: The argument for aspirin as the NSAID of choice in the management of rheumatoid arthritis. *Drug Intell Clin Pharmacol* 1984;18:34–38.

22. Heere LP: Piroxicam in acute musculoskeletal disorders and sports injuries. *Eur J Rheumatol Inflamm* 1987;9:60–64.
23. Hepso HU, Lokken P, Bjornson J, et al: Double-blind crossover study of the effect of acetylsalicylic acid on bleeding and post-operative course after bilateral oral surgery. *Eur J Clin Pharmacol* 1976;10:217–225.
24. Higeuchi S, Tanaka N, Shiori Y, et al: Two modes of analgesic action of aspirin, and the site of analgesic action of salicylic acid. *Int J Tissue React* 1986;8:327–331.
25. Holland IS, Seymour RA, Ward-Booth RP, et al: An evaluation of different doses of soluble aspirin and aspirin tablets in postoperative dental pain. *Br J Clin Pharmacol* 1988;26:463–468.
26. Hunskaar S, Berge OG, Hole K: Dissociation between antinociceptive and anti-inflammatory effects of acetylsalicylic acid and indomethacin in the formalin test. *Pain* 1986;25:125–132.
27. Hunskaar S, Fasmer OB, Hole K: Acetylsalicylic acid, paracetamol and morphine inhibit behavioral responses to intrathecally administered substance P or capsaicin. *Life Sci* 1985;37:1835–1841.
28. Koch PA, Schultz CA, Wills RJ, et al: Influence of food and fluid ingestion on aspirin bioavailability. *J Pharm Sci* 1978;67:1533–1535.
29. Korttila K, Pentti OM, Auvinen J: Comparison of i.m. lysine acetylsalicylate and oxycodone in the treatment of pain after operation. *Br J Anaesth* 1980;52:613–617.
30. Lasagna L: Analgesic drugs. *Am J Med Sci* 1961;242:620–627.
31. Lecher BJ, Blechman WJ: Double-blind comparison—trilisate tablets vs. aspirin. *Fla Fam Phys* 1978;28:50–56.
32. Lee MH, Zaretsky HH, Ernst M, et al: The analgesic effects of aspirin and placebo on experimentally induced tooth pulp pain. *J Med* 1986;16:417–428.
33. Levy G: Clinical pharmacokinetics of aspirin. *Pediatrics* 1978;62:867–872.
34. Levy G: Clinical pharmacokinetics of salicylates: A re-assessment. *Br J Clin Pharmacol* 1980;10(suppl 2):285S–290S.
35. Levy G: Pharmacokinetics of salicylate elimination in man. *J Pharm Sci* 1965;54:959–967.
36. Levy G, Leonards JR: Urine pH and salicylate therapy. *JAMA* 1971;217:81.
37. Levy G, Tsuchiya T: Salicylate accumulation kinetics in man. *N Engl J Med* 1987;287:430–432.
38. Liyange SP, Tambar PK: Comparative study of salsalate and aspirin in osteoarthrosis of the hip or knee. *Curr Med Res Opin* 1978;5:450–453.
39. Mason WD, Winer N: Kinetics of aspirin, salicylic acid, and salicyluric acid following oral administration of aspirin as a tablet and two buffered solutions. *J Pharm Sci* 1981;70:262–265.
40. Mielke CH Jr: Comparative effects of aspirin and acetaminophen on hemostasis. *Arch Intern Med* 1981;141:305–310.
41. Mongan E, Kelly P, Nies K, et al: Tinnitus as an indication of therapeutic serum salicylate levels. *JAMA* 1973;226:142–145.
42. Muckle DS: Comparative study of ibuprofen and aspirin in soft-tissue injuries. *Rheumatol Rehabil* 1974;13:141–147.
43. Muckle DS: A double blind trial of ibuprofen and aspirin in the treatment of soft tissue injuries sustained in professional football. *Br J Sports Med* 1974;14:46–47.
44. Müller FO, Hundt HKL, de Kock AC: Decreased steady-state salicylic acid plasma levels associated with chronic aspirin ingestion. *Curr Med Res Opin* 1975;3:417–422.
45. Murray HS, Strottman MP, Cooke AR: Effect of several drugs on gastric potential differences in man. *Br Med J* 1974;1:19–21.

46. Needham CD, Kyle J, Jones PF, et al: Aspirin and alcohol in gastrointestinal haemorrhage. *Gut* 1971;12:819–821.
47. Paulus HE, Siegel M, Mongan E, et al: Variations of serum concentrations and half-life of salicylate in patients with rheumatoid arthritis. *Arthritis Rheum* 1971;14:527–532.
48. Preston SJ, Arnold MH, Beller EM, et al: Comparative analgesic and anti-inflammatory properties of sodium salicylate and acetylsalicylic acid (aspirin) in rheumatoid arthritis. *Br J Clin Pharmacol*, in press.
49. Rainsford KD (ed): *Anti-Inflammatory and Anti-Rheumatic Drugs*. Boca Raton, CRC Press, 1985, vol 1.
50. Rainsford KD: *Aspirin and the Salicylates*. London, Butterworths, 1984.
51. Rainsford KD: Biochemical effects of anti-inflammatory drugs in inflammatory diseases, in Williamson WRN (ed): *Anti-Inflammatory Compounds*. New York, Marcel Dekker, 1987, pp 123–152.
52. Rainsford KD, Schweitzer A, Brune K: Distribution of the acetyl compared with the salicyl moiety of acetylsalicylic acid: Acetylation of macromolecules in organs wherein side-effects are manifest. *Biochem Pharmacol* 1983;32:1301–1308.
53. Rainsford KD, Velo GP (eds): *New Developments in Anti-Rheumatic Therapy*. Lancaster, Kluwer Academic, 1989.
54. Rainsford KD, Velo GP (eds): *Side Effects of Anti-Inflammatory Drugs*. Lancaster, MTP Press, 1987.
55. Rohdewald P, Derendorf H, Drehsen G, et al: Changes in cortical evoked potentials as correlates of the efficacy of weak analgesics. *Pain* 1982;12:329–341.
56. Rosenkranz B, Fischer C, Meese CO, et al: Effects of salicylic and acetylsalicylic acid alone and in combination on platelet aggregation and prostanoid synthesis in man. *Br J Clin Pharmacol* 1986;21:309–317.
57. Roth GJ, Stanford N, Majerus PW: Acetylation of prostaglandin synthase by aspirin. *Proc Natl Acad Sci USA* 1975;72:3073–3076.
58. Rowland M, Riegelman S: Pharmacokinetics of acetylsalicylic acid and salicylic acid after intravenous administration in man. *J Pharm Sci* 1968;57:1313–1319.
59. Rumble RH, Brooks PM, Roberts MS: Metabolism of salicylate during chronic aspirin therapy. *Br J Clin Pharmacol* 1980;9:41–45.
60. Seed JC: A clinical comparison of the antipyretic potency of aspirin and sodium salicylate. *Clin Pharmacol Ther* 1965;6:354–358.
61. Seymour RA, Rawlins MD: Efficacy and pharmacokinetics of aspirin in post-operative dental pain. *Br J Clin Pharmacol* 1982;13:807–810.
62. Seymour RA, Williams FM, Luyk NM, et al: Comparative efficacy of soluble aspirin and aspirin tablets in postoperative dental pain. *Eur J Clin Pharmacol* 1986;30:495–498.
63. Shyu KW, Lin MT: Hypothalamic monoaminergic mechanisms of aspirin-induced analgesia in monkeys. *J Neural Transm* 1985;62:285–293.
64. Sjoholm I, Kober A: Binding of drugs to human serum albumin with special reference to the binding of some anti-rheumatic agents. *Br J Clin Pract* 1980;6(suppl):6–9.
65. Skjelbred P: The effects of acetylsalicylic acid on swelling, pain and other events after surgery. *Br J Clin Pharmacol* 1984;17:379–384.
66. Vane JR: Inhibition of prostaglandin synthesis as a mechanism of action for aspirin-like drugs. *Nature* 1971;231:232–235.
67. Volans GN: Effects of food and exercise on the absorption of effervescent aspirin. *Br J Clin Pharmacol* 1974;1:137–141.
68. Wanwimolruk S, Birkett DJ, Brooks PM: Protein binding of some non-steroidal anti-inflammatory drugs in rheumatoid arthritis. *Clin Pharmacokinet* 1982;7:85–92.

69. Wanwimolruk S, Brooks PM, Birkett DJ: Protein binding of non-steroidal anti-inflammatory drugs in plasma and synovial fluid of arthritic patients. *Br J Clin Pharmacol* 1983;15:91–94.
70. Williams JGP, Engler C: A double-blind comparative trial naproxen and indomethacin in sports injuries. *Eur J Rheumatol Inflamm* 1979;12:51–55.
71. Williams RT: *Detoxication Mechanisms*, ed 2. New York, Wiley, 1959.
72. Wilson JT, Brown RD, Bocchini JA Jr, et al: Efficacy, disposition and pharmacodynamics of aspirin, acetaminophen and choline salicylate in young febril children. *Ther Drug Monit* 1982;4:147–180.
73. Wilson JT, Howell RL, Holladay MW, et al: Gentisuric acid: Metabolic formation in animals and identification as a metabolite of aspirin in man. *Clin Pharmacol Ther* 1978;23:635–643.
74. Woodbury DM: Analgesic-antipyretics, anti-inflammatory agents, and inhibitors of uric acid synthesis: Salicylates and congeners, phenacetin and congeners, antipyrine and congeners, indomethacin, colchicine, allopurinol, in Goodman LS, Gilman A (eds): *The Pharmacological Basis of Therapeutics*, ed 4. London, MacMillan, 1970, pp 314–347.
75. Wosilait WD: Theoretical analysis of the binding of salicylate by human serum albumin: The relationship between free and bound drug and therapeutic levels. *Eur J Clin Pharmacol* 1976;9:285–290.

Chapter 27

Dimethyl Sulfoxide: Its Role as an Anti-inflammatory Agent in Athletic Injuries

Edward C. Percy, MD, FRCS(C)

Introduction

Topical therapy with dimethyl sulfoxide (DMSO) has been advocated for the resolution of sports-induced local inflammatory conditions involving muscles and tendons. More recent research and experience suggest that this is inappropriate. The following discussion describes the historical background, the pharmacologic action, and the present reputable medical uses of this drug. It is not thought at this time that DMSO should play a significant role in the treatment of athletic injury.

The remarkable and yet controversial chemical compound DMSO was reportedly first prepared by Alexander Saylzeff in 1866.[11] It was not, however, until the 1950s that this substance found commercial use as a powerful solvent and as a medium for chemical reactions. The chemical can be manufactured easily from lignin, the noncellulosic constituent of wood. In 1960 the lignin-bearing spent liquor derived from the digestion of the pulp was reacted with sulfur to form dimethyl sulfide. DMSO was then produced from the partial oxidation of that substance. Dimethyl sulfide is used as an odorant for natural and artificial gases.[16]

DMSO is a most unusual solvent that, like alcohol, mixes in all proportions with water. It lowers the freezing points of biologic fluids, a quality useful for preserving animal and human tissues and cells. In animal studies, it has been reported to protect against radiation.[2] Because of its ability to penetrate intact normal skin easily, it can be used as a carrier of other substances. This characteristic has practical applications in agriculture because various chemicals can be transported into a plant simply by applying a solution to the bark or spraying it on the leaves.[12]

DMSO also functions as an endocellular cryophylactic agent, protecting against freezing damage rather than preventing freezing. With the exception of spermatozoa, human mammalian cells are largely destroyed during slow freeezing and thawing; hence, this chemical, with its ability to penetrate cells and replace their water content, is able to prevent freezing damage. Thus, it has an important role in the preservation of erythrocytes, platelets, and bone marrow elements.[5]

In 1962, researchers handling the chemical noted a peculiar taste in their mouths and a garlic-like odor on their breaths. This discovery led to the finding that DMSO penetrated the intact skin. Further investigation suggested that it might act as an anti-inflammatory agent. Jacob and associates[7] described its use in the treatment of inflammatory musculoskeletal disorders. A number of investigative reports followed rapidly. DMSO was claimed to be an excellent local analgesic agent, a bacteriostatic agent, a diuretic, and a potentiator of other compounds. Those involved in the animal sciences were quick to realize the potential properties of the chemical and it was soon widely used in both large and small animals.[10]

A 1964 article in *Life* claimed that "if DMSO lives up to scientists' expectations, it will come closer to being the legendary panacea than any drug in all medical history."[9] The value of DMSO seemed more creditable when a professional hockey player who had sustained a painful shoulder separation was able to return to the Stanley Cup playoffs two days after a local application of DMSO. As a result of this report, I carried out a double-blind study with DMSO in 1965, but a report by the FDA describing the formation of cataracts in experimental animals exposed to this drug led to the termination of this clinical trial. FDA restrictions on DMSO investigations were withdrawn in 1969; in 1973 further studies were begun.

Chemical Formulation and Pharmacologic Properties

DMSO is a clear, colorless, and essentially odorless liquid that mixes with water and most organic solvents. It does readily penetrate intact, usually impermeable, skin. Ramler and Zaffaroni[14] suggested that the rapid movement of the DMSO molecule through the intact skin depends on a reversible configurational change of the protein that occurs when DMSO substitutes for water. Substances with low molecular weights can be transported through the intact skin by this means. Even in concentrations as low as 5%, a mushroom-like flavor is rapidly detected in the mouth and a garlic-like odor appears on the breath within minutes of its application on the skin. It is metabolized in humans by oxidation to dimethyl sulfone or by reduction to dimethyl sulfide. DMSO and dimethyl sulfone are excreted in the urine and feces and dimethyl sulfide is eliminated through the lungs along with methyl sulfinic acid; this leads to the malodorous breath.

DMSO produces degranulation of the mass cells. Liberation of histamine leads to a local reaction that can result in burning, itching, prickling pain, congestion, edema, urticaria, and dermatitis. It is also reported to cause dehydration and vacuolization of the upper epidermal cells, making the skin slightly scaly and dry. Although lens opacities and changes in the refractive index have occurred in monkeys, dogs, and rabbits given high doses of DMSO, such changes have not been reported in humans.[17] Iwasa and associates[6] reported decreased levels of albumin and α-fetoprotein and increased levels of haptoglobin. Beilke and associates[3] reported that neutrophil viability was not reduced by either DMSO or dimethyl sulfone, but the inhibition of the oxidative function of stimulated neutrophils by DMSO may provide an alternative explanation for the effects of the compound on the microbicidal activity of neutrophils and as an in vivo anti-inflammatory agent. DMSO can also produce nerve blockade by lowering the conduction velocity of the nerve impulses. Jacob and Herschler[8] reported on DMSO's wide range of primary pharmacologic actions in laboratory studies. Included in this list, in addition to those already noted above, are enhanced reduction of the effectiveness of other drugs, cholinesterase inhibition, nonspecific enhancement of resistance to infection, vasodilation, muscle relaxation, enhancement of cell differentiation and function, anatagonism to platelet aggregation, and an influence on serum cholesterol in experimental hypercholesterolemia.

The teratogenic action of DMSO has ben confirmed in the Rhode Island chick embryo. This action has also been demonstrated in mammals but only after relatively high and repeated doses.[4]

The ability of DMSO to penetrate the intact skin has not escaped the attention of the lay public. In two recent "whodunits," *Trial Run* by Dick Francis and *Sudden Death* by William X. Kienzle, the authors selected DMSO as a murder weapon because of this ability.

Clinical Applications of DMSO

The initial interest in and use of this chemical for musculoskeletal lesions have waned considerably since the first enthusiastic reports. A number of the earliest reports were not true double-blind studies and thus had questionable scientific validity. One of the main problems encountered in doing a double-blind study is to find a satisfactory control substance. Percy and Carson[13] reported on the use of DMSO in tennis elbow and rotator cuff tendinitis. It was thought that a 5% solution, one too weak to allow the patients to identify the drug by its taste and the garlic-like odor on the breath, was too weak to have a definite clinical anti-inflammatory effect. A 70% solution was used as the control. It was our belief that DMSO in itself was not effective in the treatment of these two conditions.

DMSO has a number of unpleasant side effects, usually related to the site of its local application. Local rash, burn, blisters, itchiness, hives, and scaling and dryness of the skin were noted in our series. There were no major complications.

Albrechtsen and Harvey[1] studied the biomechanical effect of topical DMSO on the Achilles tendons of mice. They applied 100 ml of a 70% solution in 30% sterile water for 12 intervals over 28 days. The model identified an initial area of decreasing mean separation force (at zero to seven days), an area of increasing mean separation force (at seven to 22 days), and a subsequent area of decreasing mean separation force (at 22 to 28 days). The maximum decrease in group mean separation force was 20.2% in the seven-day treatment group. Tendon weakening suggests that vigorous activity should be avoided during any DMSO use.

It must be remembered that DMSO is a powerful solvent that can leach out materials from the container in which it is placed, and it can carry undesirable substances through the skin into the body should the solution contain impurities.

Present Uses of DMSO

From a review of the literature it appears that the role of DMSO as an anti-inflammatory agent in the treatment of musculoskeletal injuries remains in limbo. Personal communication with a number of veterinary surgeons suggests that it is no longer widely used in the treatment of large or small animals. The drug apparently has a local analgesic effect at its site of application. It is still widely used in the treatment of interstitial cystitis. In such cases it is injected directly into the bladder.[18] It is used extensively in blood banking for the preservation of platelets, bone marrow elements, and erythrocytes. Indeed, because of its cryoprotective actions, it may well be used in the future to protect against ischemic injuries caused by such cold trauma.[16]

A number of investigators have reported successful treatment of gastrointestinal amyloidosis.[20] DMSO apparently still has a role in the treatment of the dermatologic manifestations of scleroderma. Although it has been reported to reduce cerebral edema, its use has been abandoned because of reported morbidity.[22] Its role in the treatment of rheumatoid arthritis and osteoarthritis remains unknown.[21]

There is an interesting report by Reinstein and associates[15] of a patient who developed mixed sensorimotor peripheral neuropathy while taking Sulindac and who applied 90% DMSO to his upper and lower extremities. Fortunately, he did eventually make a full recovery. An article by Swanson and associates[19] added credence to the initial report.

References

1. Albrechtsen SJ, Harvey JS Jr: Dimethyl sulfoxide: Biomechanical effects on tendons. *Am J Sports Med* 1982;10:177–179.
2. Ashwood-Smith MJ: Radioprotective and cryoprotective properties of dimethyl sulfoxide in cellular systems. *Ann NY Acad Sci* 1967;141:45–62.
3. Beilke MA, Collins-Lech C, Sohnle PG: Effects of dimethyl sulfoxide on the oxidative function of human neutrophils. *J Lab Clin Med* 1987;110:91–96.
4. Caujolle FM, Caujolle DH, Cros SB, et al: Limits of toxic and teratogenic tolerance of dimethyl sulfoxide. *Ann NY Acad Sci* 1967;141:110–126.
5. Huggins CE: Frozen blood: Principles of practical preservation. *Monogr Surg Sci* 1966;140:3.
6. Iwasa F, Galbraith RA, Sassa S: Effects of dimethyl sulphoxide on the synthesis of plasma proteins in the human hepatoma Hep G2: Induction of an acute-phase-like reaction. *Biochem J* 1988;253:927–930.

7. Jacob SW, Bischel M, Hirschler RJ: DMSO: A new concept in pharmacotherapy. *Curr Ther Res* 1964;6:134–135.
8. Jacob SW, Herschler R: Pharmacology of DMSO. *Cryobiology* 1986;23:14–27.
9. Kerr A: DMSO. *Life Magazine* 1964;57:1–2.
10. Knowles RP: Clinical experience with DMSO in small animal practice. *Ann NY Acad Sci* 1967;141:478–483.
11. Leake CD: Introductory remarks. *Ann NY Acad Sci* 1967;141:1–2.
12. Leonard CD: Use of dimethyl sulfoxide as a carrier for iron in nutritional foliar sprays applied to citrus. *Ann NY Acad Sci* 1967;141:148–158.
13. Percy EC, Carson JD: The use of DMSO in tennis elbow and rotator cuff tendonitis: A double-blind study. *Med Sci Sports Exerc* 1981;13:215–219.
14. Ramler DH, Zaffaroni A: Biological implications of DMSO based on a review of its chemical properties. *Ann NY Acad Sci* 1967;141:13–23.
15. Reinstein L, Mahon R Jr, Russo GL: Peripheral neuropathy after concomitant dimethyl sulfoxide use and Sulindac therapy. *Arch Phys Med Rehabil* 1982;63:581–584.
16. Robbins MD: Pulp plant wrings profit from lignin. *Chem Eng* 1961;269:100–102.
17. Rubin LF, Barnett KC: Ocular effects of oral and dermal application of dimethyl sulfoxide in animals. *Ann NY Acad Sci* 1967;141:333–345.
18. Stewart BH: Intravesical DMSO in the treatment of chronic interstitial cystitis. *AUA Update Ser* 1983;2:5–6.
19. Swanson BN, Boppana VK, Vlasses PH, et al: Dimethyl sulfoxide inhibits bioactivation of Sulindac. *J Lab Clin Med* 1983;102:95–101.
20. Takahashi A, Matsumoto J, Nishimura S, et al: Improvement of endoscopic and histologic findings of AA-type gastrointestinal amyloidosis by treatment with dimethyl sulfoxide and prednisolone. *Gastroenterol Jpn* 1985;20:143–147.
21. Trice JM, Pinals RS: Dimethyl sulfoxide: A review of its use in rheumatic disorders. *Semin Arthritis Rheum* 1985;15:45–60.
22. Yellowlees P, Greenfield C, McIntyre N: Dimethylsulphoxide-induced toxicity. *Lancet* 1980;2:1004–1006.

Chapter 28

The Role of Anabolic Steroids as Modifiers of Sports-Induced Inflammation

Herbert A. Haupt, MD

Abuse of anabolic steroids by athletes is nearly epidemic. They are used by both competitive athletes and young body builders in local health clubs who want the cosmetic effects of increased size and strength. Some athletes report a more rapid recovery from injury while taking anabolic steroids: others report an increased incidence of injuries. This chapter reviews the available research on the effect of anabolic steroids on injury and inflammation in sports.

Pharmacology

Anabolic steroids are derivatives of testosterone and closely resemble it. They are generally grouped in two categories, the alpha alkyl derivatives and the norderivatives. The alpha alkyl derivatives have an alkyl group added to the 17th carbon atom (C17) in the testosterone nucleus. They are active orally and produce cholestatic jaundice. The length of the alkyl group at C17 influences the rate at which the drug is metabolized and the length of time it is active.[14] The second group, the norderivatives, have an absent methyl group at the 19th carbon (C19) on the basic testosterone nucleus. Removing this methyl group reduces the androgenic properties of the steroid nucleus.

Anabolic steroids can be ranked according to their relative anabolic and androgenic properties. The anabolic-androgenic ratio is determined in animals treated with anabolic steroids by comparing the weight of the levator ani muscles (an index of anabolic activity) to the weight of the seminal vesicles on the ventral prostrate gland (an index of androgenic activity).[14,19] Testosterone propionate has an anabolic-androgenic ratio of 1:1. Methandienone (dianabol) also has an anabolic/androgenic ratio of 1:1. Stanozolol has a ratio of 100:1 because its effect is much more anabolic than androgenic.[14]

The mechanism of action of anabolic steroids is unclear and complicated. They affect athletes on many different levels, from the cellular to the psychological.

Receptors for anabolic steroids exist on muscle cells. Through these receptors, the steroids stimulate protein synthesis. Steroids also cause a shift to a positive nitrogen balance—resulting in growth of all organ systems, not just muscles.[16,19,23,25] Steroid use can also increase endogenous growth hormone release, enhancing the anabolic effects.[4] Finally, anabolic steroids have significant motivational and placebo effects. Athletes taking anabolic steroids become more aggressive in all activities, including training. They intensify their training sessions and report that feelings of fatigue decrease. Even athletes who are given placebos but believe they are taking anabolic steroids demonstrate significant increases in strength.[5]

Previous studies have shown that anabolic steroids are effective only when given to athletes who have had previous resistance training and who continue such training while using the steroids.[16] When given to athletes without previous resistance training, anabolic steroids have little effect. There is a relationship between overtraining and the athlete's testosterone-cortisol ratio. Several studies verify that the serum testosterone-cortisol ratio increases as the athlete gains strength during training.[1,15,20,21] As training intensifies, levels of cortisol become higher in response to stress.[7] The increased cortisol has catabolic effects on the skeletal muscle, creating the negative calcium and nitrogen balances that characterize the overtrained state and lower the serum testosterone-cortisol ratio. In fact, overtraining may be defined as a decrease in the free testosterone-cortisol ratio by more than 30%.[1]

Exogenous anabolic steroid supplementation increases the testosterone-cortisol ratio and reverses the catabolic effects of the glucocorticosteroids.[2] The anticatabolic effect of testosterone is mediated by its ability to displace cortisol from the glucocorticosteroid receptors on muscles and other organ systems.[15,20,28] Anabolic steroids reverse the negative nitrogen balance, loss of body weight, and muscle wasting associated with excess cortisol production in overtraining. They are best classified as anticatabolic for this reason.

Anabolic steroids, therefore, have both anabolic and catabolic effects. The anabolic effects result from their ability to attach to the androgenic muscle receptors, their ability to induce a positive nitrogen balance, the associated increase in endogeneous growth hormone release, and their motivational and placebo effects. The anticatabolic effects include reversal of the catabolic effects of increased endogeneous cortisol release during intense training. Anabolic steroids may also be able to reverse an inflammation-induced catabolic state resulting from increased cortisol release.

Connective Tissue Effects

Some athletes report increased injury to musculotendinous structures while using anabolic steroids. Three reports (two on triceps tendon tears and one on a spontaneous rupture of the extensor pollicus longus tendon) suggest that extended use of anabolic steroids may weaken tendinous structures.[6,18,22] A pathologic examination of the ruptured extensor pollicus tendon found that the fibers had degenerated and spots of calcification had formed. This suggests that the rupture was secondary to inflammation and degeneration of the tendon itself.

Several animal studies[26,27,32] have investigated the effects of steroids on tendons. Michna and Stang-Voss[27] combined anabolic steroid use with an endurance running program in mice. The steroids activated cellular metabolism in the tendon. Extracellular lysosomes appeared and induced degenerative changes in the fine structure of the myotendinous junction. Calcification occurred in the area of cell degeneration. The collagen fibers dissociated into subfibrils and ruptured. They also showed marked variations in diameter, contour irregularities, and disorganized internal packing.

Michna[26] also demonstrated that the duration of anabolic steroid treatment affected the number of dysplastic collagen fibrils. During the first week of steroid treatment, the extracellular accumulation of collagen increased, suggesting increased synthesis. The number of collagen fibrils and their volume density also increased. This could be an adaptation by the tendons to the increased muscular strength resulting from the steroid treatment. However, after ten weeks of treatment, the number of thick fibrils decreased and the number of thin fibrils increased significantly. Volume density decreased because of the predominance of thinner fibrils. The increase in thin fibrils and the decreased density and cross-sectional area of the tendon fibrils suggest that the tendon strength decreased. In addition, the number of dysplastic collagen fibrils increased dramatically, especially in the animals treated with both anabolic steroids and exercise. The degree of dysplasia also depended on the duration of the treatment and was more pronounced at ten weeks than at one week.

Another study on rat tendons by Wood and associates[32] also suggests that tendons weaken with anabolic steroid use. They measured the crimp angle and crimp length in the rat tendon. The crimp angle significantly increased and crimp length significantly decreased during treatment with anabolic steroids, especially when treatment was combined with exercise. Their findings suggest that the tendon must elongate more, requiring increased muscular contraction to produce a given stress. The increased elongation of the tendon at a given stress could theoretically lower the amount of stress necessary for breakage. The treated group also had a lower modulus of elasticity. As the strength of the tendon is directly proportional to its modulus of elasticity, the tendons in the rats treated with anabolic steroids and exercise were less efficient, had theoretically lower breaking strains, and were weaker than the control tendons.

These studies suggest that the use of anabolic steroids, especially when coupled with exercise, predisposes tendons to rupture. This is supported by the experiences of athletes. Additional study is necessary to determine how quickly these tendons heal after rupture and whether the tendency to rupture can be reversed if steroid use is discontinued.

Immunologic Effects

Anabolic steroids affect the user's immunologic status. A recent study showed that anabolic steroids decreased IgG, IgM, and, especially, IgA.[30] The use of the anabolic steroid ethyl estrenol can decrease the development of autoimmune disease in mice and C19 nortestosterone derivatives can favorably modify the immune system in mice, as well as in persons with systemic lupus erythematosus.[17,31]

Studies show a relationship between low adrenal androgenic-anabolic metabolites and the occurrence of rheumatoid arthritis. They suggest a sexual predisposition for rheumatoid arthritis resulting from an imbalance of sex hormones.[24] Other studies found an improvement in the erythrocyte sedimentation rate, morning stiffness, pain, and fibrin deposition in patients with rheumatoid arthritis who were treated with anabolic steroids.[8] These improvements may be secondary to the fibrinolytic effect of the steroids. Anabolic steroids also promote fibrinolysis in both healthy persons and in those with atherosclerotic disease.[14] Other studies show no significant improvement in the clinical manifestations of rheumatoid arthritis after treatment with anabolic steroids.[9]

Although anabolic steroids do attach to the glucocorticoid receptors, they do not appear to have any significant effect on basal plasma cortisol production or adrenal gland response to corticotropin.[28]

Training usually increases glucose tolerance and decreases insulin resistance. This condition helps prevent coronary artery disease. Anabolic steroid use, however, induces a diabetic state characterized by decreased glucose tolerance and increased insulin resistance.[3] The diabetic state is transient and reverses when steroid use is discontinued. No one has investigated whether steroid use can induce a permanent diabetic state.[11]

Anabolic steroids can affect the inflammatory response in soft tissues. They affect the immune system, cause fibrinolytic changes, and alter glucose homeostasis.

Anabolic steroids may be used to counter bone demineralization. Even NASA is considering their use by astronauts during space flights.[20]

One of the original therapeutic uses of anabolic steroids was in the treatment of anemia.[14] They have been effective in aplastic anemia, anemia secondary to whole-body irradiation, and hemophilia B-Leyden.[9,10,12,13] Their effectiveness results from their ability to increase megakaryocytopoiesis and the hematopoietic-inductive microenvironment.

Conclusion

Although much is known about the effects of anabolic steroids on both animals and humans, additional research is needed to clarify their mechanisms of actions and other physiologic effects. Their role in modifying soft-tissue inflammation needs further investigation. Extrapolating from current research provides some insight, but whether anabolic steroid use is beneficial or not remains unclear. Steroids may be able to improve an athlete's psychological state and diminish immunologic and perhaps inflammatory responses. However, they may also have adverse effects on tendinous structures. Many athletes experience an increased injury rate with anabolic steroids, yet others report improved performance and response to injury. As anabolic steroid abuse continues, athletes need credible information on potential beneficial and adverse effects. Therapeutic prescription of these drugs is not indicated because of the potential damage to tendinous structures and connective tissues and the lack of any controlled therapeutic studies proving their usefulness in the recovery from specific structural injury.

References

1. Adlercreutz H, Härkonen M, Kuoppasalmi K, et al: Effect of training on plasma anabolic and catabolic steroid hormones and their response during physical exercise. *Int J Sports Med* 1986;7(suppl 1):27–28.
2. Alén M, Häkkinen K: Androgenic steroid effects on serum hormones and on maximal force development in strength athletes. *J Sports Med Phys Fitness* 1987;27:38–46.
3. Alén M, Häkkinen K, Komi PV: Changes in neuromuscular performance and muscle fiber characteristics of elite power athletes self-administering androgenic and anabolic steroids. *Acta Physiol Scand* 1984;122:535–544.
4. Alén M, Rahkila P, Reinilä M, et al: Androgenic-anabolic steroid effects on serum thyroid, pituitary and steroid hormones in athletes. *Am J Sports Med* 1987;15:357–361.
5. Ariel G, Saville W: Anabolic steroids: The physiological effects of placebos. *Med Sci Sports* 1972;4:124–126.
6. Bach BR Jr, Warren RF, Wickiewicz TL: Triceps rupture: A case report and literature review. *Am J Sports Med* 1987;15:285–289.
7. Barron JL, Noakes TD, Levy W, et al: Hypothalamic dysfunction in overtrained athletes. *J Clin Endocrinol Metab* 1985;60:803–806.
8. Belch JJF, Madhok R, McArdle B, et al: Stanozolol as a treatment for rheumatoid arthritis, abstract. *Br J Rheumatol* 1985;24:102–103.
9. Bird HA, Burkinshaw L, Pearson D, et al: A controlled trial of nandrolone decanoate in the treatment of rheumatoid arthritis in postmenopausal women. *Ann Rheum Dis* 1987;46:237–243.
10. Briët E, Wijnands MC, Veltkamp JJ: The prophylactic treatment of hemophilia B Leyden with anabolic steroids. *Ann Intern Med* 1985;103:225–226.
11. Cohen JC, Hickman R: Insulin resistance and diminished glucose tolerance in powerlifters ingesting anabolic steroids. *J Clin Endocrinol Metab* 1987;64:960–963.
12. Gallicchio VS, Chen MG, Watts TD: Regeneration of murine megakaryocytopoiesis and the hematopoietic inductive microenvironment after sublethal whole body irradiation by treatment with an anabolic steroid. *Acta Haematol* 1985;73:80–85.
13. Gardner FH: Anabolic steroids in aplastic anemia. *Acta Endocrinol* 1985;271(suppl):87–96.
14. Gribbin HR, Matts SG: Mode of action and use of anabolic steroids. *Br J Clin Pract* 1976;30:3–5.

15. Häkkinen K, Pakarinen A, Alén M, et al: Serum hormones during prolonged training of neuromuscular performance. *Eur J Appl Physiol* 1985;53:287–293.
16. Haupt HA, Rovere GD: Anabolic steroids: A review of the literature. *Am J Sports Med* 1984;12:469–484.
17. Hazelton RA, McCruden A, Stimson WH, et al: The effects of 19-nortestosterone treatment on clinical and laboratory parameters in patients with systemic lupus erythematosus, abstract. *Ann Rheum Dis* 1981;40:626.
18. Herrick R, Herrick S: Ruptured triceps in a powerlifter presenting as cubital tunnel syndrome: A case report. *Am J Sports Med* 1987;15:514–516.
19. Kopera H: The history of anabolic steroids and a review of clinical experience with anabolic steroids. *Acta Endocrinol* 1985;271(suppl):11–18.
20. Kraemer WJ: Endocrine responses to resistance exercise. *Med Sci Sports Exerc* 1988;20(suppl):S152-S157.
21. Kraemer WJ, Deschenes MR, Fleck SJ: Physiological adaptations to resistance exercise: Implications for athletic conditioning. *Sports Med* 1988;6:246–256.
22. Kramhøft M, Solgaard S: Spontaneous rupture of the extensor pollicis longus tendon after anabolic steroids. *J Hand Surg* 1986;11B:87.
23. Martinez JA, Buttery PJ, Pearson JT: The mode of action of anabolic agents: The effect of testosterone on muscle protein metabolism in the female rat. *Br J Nutr* 1984;52:515–521.
24. Masi AT, Josipovic DB, Jefferson WE: Low adrenal androgenic-anabolic steroids in women with rheumatoid arthritis (RA): Gas-liquid chromatographic studies of RA patients and matched normal control women indicating decreased 11-deoxy-17-ketosteroid excretion. *Semin Arthritis Rheum* 1984;14:1–23.
25. Michelsen CB, Askanazi J, Kinney JM, et al: Effect of an anabolic steroid on nitrogen balance and amino acid patterns after total hip replacement. *J Trauma* 1982;22:410–413.
26. Michna H: Organization of collagen fibrils in tendon: Changes induced by an anabolic steroid. II. A morphometric and stereologic analysis. *Int J Sports Med* 1983;4:59.
27. Michna H, Stang-Voss C: The predisposition to tendon rupture after doping with anabolic steroids, abstract. *Int J Sport Med* 1983;4:59.
28. Morris DD, Garcia MC: Effects of phenylbutazone and anabolic steroids on adrenal and thyroid gland function tests in healthy horses. *Am J Vet Res* 1985;46:359–364.
29. Stepaniak PC, Furst JJ, Woodard D: Anabolic steroids as a countermeasure against bone demineralization during space flight. *Aviat Space Environ Med* 1986;57:174–178.
30. Study: Steroids lower immunity, lipids. *Phys Sportsmed* 1988;16:56–60.
31. Verheul HA, Schot LP, Deckers GH, et al: Effects of tibolone, lynestrenol, ethylestrenol, and desogestrel on autoimmune disorders in NZB/W mice. *Clin Immunol Immunopathol* 1986;38:198–208.
32. Wood TO, Cooke PH, Goodship AE: The effect of exercise and anabolic steroids on the mechanical properties and crimp morphology of the rat tendon. *Am J Sports Med* 1988;16:153–158.

Chapter 29
Thermotherapy

William E. Prentice, PhD, PT, ATC
Terry R. Malone, EdD, PT, ATC

Introduction

Thermotherapy uses a heating agent to increase tissue temperature in a general or specific (local) fashion. This transfer can require direct physical contact or involve passage through the air. Infrared sources are most commonly used, including hot packs, hydrotherapy, paraffin baths, contrast baths, fluidotherapy, and luminous or nonluminous lamps. Diathermy uses high-frequency currents to provide selective heating. (Ultrasound is discussed elsewhere in this volume.) The physiologic effects of thermotherapy include vasodilation, altered pain sensation, enhanced nutrition and metabolism, increased collagen extensibility, and decreased sensitivity to muscle stretch.

Thermotherapy

The use of various techniques to increase tissue temperature is called thermotherapy.[1,16,17] Thermotherapy is usually used in the later stages of a rehabilitation program. Cryotherapy, the use of cold to reduce tissue temperature, is most effective in the early stages of healing, soon after injury. Cold applications can be continued into the reconditioning stage of injury management.

Electromagnetic Radiation

Radiation is a process by which energy in various forms travels through space. The sun emits radiant energy as a result of high-intensity reactions. Other objects also produce radiant energy.[18,36,40]

All matter produces energy that radiates in the form of heat. When a chemical or electrical force of sufficient intensity is applied to any object, various forms of radiant energy are produced by movement of electrons. Many therapeutic techniques, including infrared sources and the diathermy, produce radiant energy. Radiant energy that produces heat and lies beyond the visible red portion of the light spectrum is called infrared radiation. Radiant energy that produces chemical changes and is located beyond the violet end of the visible spectrum is called ultraviolet radiation. As the temperature increases in a particular substance, molecular vibrations increase electron activity. This movement of electrons produces electromagnetic waves. The higher the temperature, the greater the frequency of the electromagnetic waves produced. Heat-produced electromagnetic waves are usually absorbed but have little penetration.[37]

Beyond the infrared portion of the spectrum are several large regions of radiation termed diathermic. These include radio, television, and nerve- and muscle-stimulating frequencies. Beyond the ultraviolet end of the spectrum is the high-frequency ionizing and penetrating radiation region that includes X-rays and alpha, beta, and gamma rays.[38]

When electromagnetic radiations strike or come into contact with various objects, some rays are reflected, others are transmitted through the tissues and refracted, and still others penetrate to deeper layers and are absorbed. Generally, radiation with the longest wavelength has the greatest penetration.

If the therapeutic energy is not absorbed by the tissues, then it must be transmitted to deeper layers according to the law of Grotthus-Draper. As the amount of energy absorbed increases, the amount that is transmitted decreases, resulting in less penetration.[31] The transmitted energy travels in a straight line until it comes into contact with a tissue that reflects or turns it away, or until its angle of transmission is changed or refracted within the tissue.

All sources of electromagnetic radiation are subject to the relationship between the absorption and the transmission of energy. The sources that emit radiations with relatively longer wavelengths can transmit energy through the superficial tissue layers, thus penetrating to the deeper tissues where it is absorbed.

Mechanisms of Heat Transfer

The therapist transfers energy in the form of heat from the source to the patient to achieve specific physiologic responses. The laws of thermodynamics govern the transformation of energy.[28] Heat is transmitted through one of four mechanisms: conduction, convection, radiation, or conversion. Evaporation, another way of dissipating heat, does not apply to heat transfer by therapeutic techniques.[28]

Conduction and radiation transfer energy entirely as a result of temperature differences. Convection depends on both temperature difference and mass transport. All three mechanisms use infrared sources to produce a heat exchange. Tissue can gain or lose heat through any of these three mechanisms.[1,5]

Conduction involves the exchange of thermal energy through direct contact. Energy flows from the warmer object to the cooler object or from the higher-energy molecules to the lower-energy molecules, thus equalizing the temperatures of the objects. For example, applying a hot pack to the body rapidly increases the temperature of the cutaneous tissue. Increased temperatures in the deeper tissues depend to some extent on the thickness of the insulating subcutaneous fat. Thus, heat transfer through conduction is primarily superficial.

Convection transfers heat through direct contact of a surface with another medium and the movement of that medium over the surface. For example, density gradients created by temperature differences or some external force can cause fluids to move over a surface. In the case of a warm whirlpool, a turbine moves warm water across a cooler skin surface, thus adding heat to the skin.

In radiation, electromagnetic energy is emitted from a specific source, such as an infrared baker or heating lamp, to heat the surface of the body. The human body itself produces radiant heat. Unlike conduction and convection, radiant energy exchange does not require a transport medium. However, there is usually some medium, such as air, that separates the two surfaces and minimally affects the energy exchange.[28]

Conversion is the transformation of one form of energy, usually nonthermal, into thermal energy, resulting in the production of heat in the tissues. The diathermic frequencies, such as shortwave and ultrasound, are generally considered to be deep-heating, producing heat by converting electrical or soundwave energy into thermal energy as it penetrates the tissues.[35]

Thermotherapy is generally regarded as beneficial for patients with chronic conditions. However, few researchers have reported on the use of thermotherapy in inflammatory conditions. The general consensus is that such use may aggravate the inflammation and it is thus contraindicated.[26]

Although activity generally increases with temperature, recent studies indicate that heating articular tissue to 42 C may inhibit the articular enzymes responsible for the inflammatory cycle.[9,34] The intra-articular temperature is normally lower than that of the surrounding tissues even when inflammatory arthritides exist.[23–25,32] Local hyperthermia in joints may help activate anti-inflammatory medications and inhibit articular enzymes.[6,34,39] The temperature needed for these proposed beneficial effects is approximately 42 C. The selective heating required to achieve this is a key issue that must be addressed in determining the appropriate use of thermotherapy techniques.[43]

Application of Infrared Sources

Perhaps the greatest confusion about the relationship between electromagnetic radiations and therapeutic techniques is associated with the infrared region. Infrared modalities are not limited to luminous and nonluminous infrared bakers or lamps. Most sources emit radiations with wavelengths and frequencies that fall within the infrared region. Cold packs,[10] hot packs,[11] whirlpools, paraffin baths,[3,10] contrast baths, and fluidotherapy[7] are all infrared sources.[20,36]

Infrared sources are used to produce local or generalized heating or cooling of the superficial tissues. Infrared wavelengths are temperature-dependent. Sources with lower temperatures have longer wavelengths. This means that an ice pack has a longer wavelength and thus a greater depth of penetration than a hot pack. Temperatures in infrared sources range from 0 C with ice to more than 3,000 C with infrared lamps. The wavelengths for these temperatures range from 1,000 to 10,500 nm, with corresponding frequencies ranging between 2×10^{12} and 4×10^{13} Hz.

Regardless of the mechanisms of heat transfer, the physiologic effects of heat are rarely the result of direct absorption of infrared energy. Infrared energy is not capable of penetrating the tissues to a depth greater than 2 cm.[2,30] Thus, infrared sources have primarily superficial effects that involve the cutaneous blood vessels and nerve receptors.

Absorption of infrared energy cutaneously can both increase and decrease subcutaneous circulation in muscle and fat layers.[4,19,21,44] If energy is absorbed cutaneously long enough to raise the temperature of the circulating blood, the hypothalamus reflexly increases blood flow to the underlying tissue. If the primary treatment goal is to increase tissue temperature and blood flow to the deeper tissues, a technique such as diathermy or ultrasound is recommended, because they produce energy that can penetrate the cutaneous tissues and be absorbed directly by the deep tissues. If the primary treatment goal is to reduce tissue temperature and decrease blood flow to an injured area, superficial application of ice or cold is the only appropriate technique.

The most effective use of infrared is as an analgesic to reduce pain associated with injury.[27,33] Infrared sources selectively stimulate cutaneous nerve receptors.[12,13] In an aggressive program of rehabilitation, reducing pain is a means of facilitating therapeutic exercise.[22,36]

The physiologic effects of thermotherapy include vascular changes that result in vasodilation, increased nutrition, and enzymatic activities. Increased blood flow and altered pain sensation interrupt the pain-spasm cycle.[29] Tissue extensibility and metabolism are enhanced.[41,42] Muscle spasm is decreased by the inhibition of the gamma fibers of the muscle spindle, thus decreasing sensitivity to muscle stretch.[14]

Treatments for the hands, muscles, and ankles, and for conditions that manifest themselves relatively near the surface of the skin can use superficial heating to achieve appreciably higher body temperatures.[8] Because the superficial techniques treat a larger area of the body than do ultrasound or microwave sources, the total amount of heat absorbed is much higher. Fluidotherapy, hydrotherapy, and paraffin baths create nearly the same temperature increase.[15]

Diathermy

The diathermic high-frequency currents have more than 1 million cycles per second. When such short-duration impulses come into contact with human tissue, there is not sufficient time for ion movement to take place. Consequently, there is no stimulation of either motor or sensory nerves. However, the energy of such a rapidly vibrating electrical current produces heat as it passes through tissue cells, resulting in a temperature increase.

Electrotherapeutic shortwave and microwave devices have preset frequencies and wavelengths that cannot be altered. Shortwave diathermy units are set either at 13.56 MHz, with a corresponding wavelength of 22 m, or at 27.12 MHz, with a wavelength of 11 m.[36]

Microwave units have shorter wavelengths than shortwave diathermy units. Microwave units are set at wavelengths of 33 cm or 12 cm with respective frequencies of 915 MHz and 2,450 MHz. Microwaves penetrate a bit more deeply than shortwaves because the energy used is concentrated in one spot rather than being spread out over a large area.[36]

Although its general physiologic actions are known, much information is needed about the effects of thermotherapy at the tissue and cellular levels. In vivo studies on normal and injured populations are needed. Researchers must determine if selective actions are possible with the various techniques, but few have examined these problems in either animal models or clinical populations.

References

1. Abraham WM: Heat vs cold therapy for the treatment of muscle injuries. *Athlet Train* 1974;9:177.
2. Abramson DI, Mitchell RE, Tuck S Jr, et al: Changes in blood flow, oxygen uptake and tissue temperatures produced by the topical application of wet heat. *Arch Phys Med Rehabil* 1961;42:305–318.
3. Abramson DI, Tuck S Jr, Chu LSW, et al: Effect of paraffin bath and hot fomentations on local tissue temperatures. *Arch Phys Med Rehabil* 1964;45:87–94.
4. Abramson DI, Tuck S Jr, Chu LSW, et al: Indirect vasodilatation in thermotherapy. *Arch Phys Med Rehabil* 1965;46:412–420.
5. Abramson DI, Tuck S Jr, Lee SW, et al: Comparison of wet and dry heat in raising temperature of tissues. *Arch Phys Med Rehabil* 1967;48:654–661.
6. Benz R, Beckers F, Zimmermann U: Reversible electrical breakdown of lipid bilayer membranes: A charge-pulse relaxation study. *J Membrane Biol* 1979;48:181–204.
7. Borrell RM, Henley EJ, Ho P, et al: Fluidotherapy: Evaluation of a new heat modality. *Arch Phys Med Rehabil* 1977;58:69–71.
8. Borrell RM, Parker R, Henley EJ, et al: Comparison of in vivo temperatures produced by hydrotherapy, paraffin wax treatment, and fluidotherapy. *Phys Ther* 1980;60:1273–1276.
9. Castor CW, Yaron M: Connective tissue activation: VIII. The effects of temperature studied in vitro. *Arch Phys Med Rehabil* 1976;57:5–9.
10. Chambers R: Clinical uses of cryotherapy. *Phys Ther* 1969;49:245–249.
11. Cordray YM, Krusen EM Jr: Use of hydrocollator packs in the treatment of neck and shoulder pains. *Arch Phys Med Rehabil* 1959;40:105–108.
12. Crockford GW, Hellon RF: Vascular responses of human skin to infra-red radiation. *J Physiol* 1959;149:424–432.
13. Crockford GW, Hellon RF, Parkhouse J: Thermal vasomotor responses in human skin mediated by local mechanisms. *J Physiol* 1962;161:10–20.

14. Currier DP, Kramer JF: Sensory nerve conduction: Heating effects of ultrasound and infrared. *Physiother Can* 1982;34:241–246.
15. Downer AH: *Physical Therapy Procedures: Selected Techniques*, ed 3. Springfield, Charles C Thomas, 1978.
16. Downey JA: Physiological effects of heat and cold. *J Am Phys Ther Assoc* 1964;44:713–717.
17. Fischer E, Solomon S: Physiological responses to heat and cold, in Licht S, Kanenetz HL (eds): *Therapeutic Heat and Cold*, ed 2. Baltimore, Waverly Press, 1965, pp 126–169.
18. Goldman L: *Introduction to Modern Phototherapy*. Springfield, Charles C Thomas, 1978.
19. Greenberg RS: The effects of hot packs and exercise on local blood flow. *Phys Ther* 1972;52:273–278.
20. Griffin JE, Karselis TC: *Physical Agents for Physical Therapists*. Springfield, Charles C Thomas, 1978.
21. Hendler E, Crosbie R, Hardy JD: Measurement of heating of the skin during exposure to infrared radiation. *J Appl Physiol* 1958;12:177–185.
22. Henricson AS, Fredricksson K, Persson I, et al: The effect of heat and stretching on the range of hip motion. *J Orthop Sports Phys Ther* 1984;6:110–115.
23. Hollander JL, Horvath SM: The influence of physical therapy procedures on the intra-articular temperature of normal and arthritic subjects. *Am J Med Sci* 1949;218:543–548.
24. Hollander JL, Stoner EK, Brown EM Jr, et al: Joint temperature measurement in the evaluation of anti-arthritic agents. *J Clin Invest* 1951;30:701–706.
25. Horvath SM, Hollander JL: Intra-articular temperature as a measure of joint reaction. *J Clin Invest* 1949;28:469–473.
26. Krusen EM Jr, Wakim KG, Leden UM, et al: Effects of hot packs on peripheral circulation. *Arch Phys Med* 1950;31:145–150.
27. Lehmann JF, Brunner GD, Stow RW: Pain threshold measurements after therapeutic application of ultrasound, microwaves and infrared. *Arch Phys Med Rehabil* 1958;39:560–565.
28. Lehmann JF, de Lateur BJ: Therapeutic heat, in Lehmann JF (ed): *Therapeutic Heat and Cold*, ed 3. Baltimore, Williams & Wilkins, 1982, pp 404–562.
29. Lehmann JF, Masock AJ, Warren CG, et al: Effect of therapeutic temperatures on tendon extensibility. *Arch Phys Med Rehabil* 1970;51:481–487.
30. Lehmann JF, Silverman DR, Baum BA, et al: Temperature distributions in the human thigh, produced by infrared, hot pack and microwave applications. *Arch Phys Med Rehabil* 1966;47:291–299.
31. Licht S (ed): *Therapeutic Electricity and Ultraviolet Radiation*. New Haven, Elizabeth Licht, 1959.
32. Mainardi CL, Walter JM, Spiegel PK, et al: Rheumatoid arthritis: Failure of daily heat therapy to affect its progression. *Arch Phys Med Rehabil* 1979;60:390–393.
33. McCray RE, Patton NJ: Pain relief at trigger points: A comparison of moist heat and shortwave diathermy. *J Orthop Sports Phys Ther* 1984;5:175–178.
34. McGhie JB, Wold E, Pettersen EO, et al: Combined electron radiation and hyperthermia: Repair of DNA strand breaks in NHIK 3025 cells irradiated and incubated at 37, 42.5, or 45° C. *Radiat Res* 1983;96:31–40.
35. Michlovitz S (ed): *Thermal Agents in Rehabilitation*. Philadelphia, FA Davis, 1986.
36. Prentice WE: *Therapeutic Modalities in Sports Medicine*. St. Louis, Times/Mirror Mosby College Publishing, 1986.

37. Schriber W: *A Manual of Electrotherapy*. Philadelphia, Lea & Febiger, 1975.
38. Sears FW, Zemansky MW, Young HD: *University Physics*, ed 5. Reading, Addison-Wesley, 1976.
39. Song CW: Effect of hyperthermia on vascular functions of normal tissues and experimental tumors: Brief communication. *J Natl Cancer Inst* 1978;60:711–713.
40. Stillwell GK: Therapeutic heat and cold, in Krusen FH, Kottke FJ, Ellwood PM Jr (eds): *Handbook of Physical Medicine and Rehabilitation*, ed 2. Philadelphia, WB Saunders, 1971, pp 259–272.
41. Warren CG: The use of heat and cold in the treatment of common musculoskeletal disorders, in Kessler RM, Hertling D (eds): *Management of Common Musculoskeletal Disorders: Physical Therapy Principles and Methods*. Philadelphia, Harper & Row, 1983, pp 115–127.
42. Warren CG, Lehmann JF, Koblanski JN: Heat and stretch procedures: An evaluation using rat tail tendon. *Arch Phys Med Rehabil* 1976;57:122–126.
43. Weinberger A, Fadilah R, Lev A, et al: Deep heat in the treatment of inflammatory joint disease. *Med Hypoth* 1988;25:231–233.
44. Wyper DJ, McNiven DR: Effects of some physiotherapeutic agents on skeletal muscle blood flow. *Physiotherapy* 1976;62:83–85.

Chapter 30

Cold as a Modifier of Sports-Induced Inflammation

Kenneth L. Knight, PhD, ATC

Cold has been used since the 1950s for the immediate care of sports injuries. In the mid-1960s, physicians also began to use cold as part of rehabilitation treatment. Cryotherapy—the therapeutic use of cold—is said to cause vasoconstriction and decrease hemorrhaging during immediate care, and to cause cold-induced vasodilation during rehabilitation. These statements are contradictory, vague, and inadequate. In both situations, cold may decrease many phases of the inflammatory response, but a definitive statement is not possible because so little research has been done on the topic. The main benefits of cryotherapy may stem from factors other than the way it modifies the inflammatory response.

Indirect evidence suggests that the primary reason to use immediate cryotherapy is to slow metabolism and limit secondary hypoxic injury. Great strides have been made in using cold to preserve tissues during abdominal and cardiac surgery, because cold reduces the metabolic rate to the point that the tissue does not undergo hypoxic injury during the period of anoxia. In sports trauma, the primary injury may include direct ultrastructural changes that cannot be helped by cryotherapy. Cold applications can, however, limit the extent of secondary hypoxic injury. Because of vascular damage and vascular alterations during the inflammatory response, the area may become hypoxic. Tissues within the injury site that escaped primary injury and those on the periphery of the injury may suffer secondary hypoxic injury. By decreasing the metabolic rate, cold applications reduce the total tissue damage and consequently, the extent of healing required.

During rehabilitation, cold decreases pain and allows earlier pain-free active exercise. It is the earlier exercise that stimulates repair. Cold applications without exercise probably hinder repair.

Using cold to modify sports-induced inflammation is a relatively new, complex, and misunderstood concept. Cold is used regularly, but the bounds of its use, the explanations for its use, and the mechanisms by which it works continue to be debated. As a result, practitioners may use cold improperly.

Part of the confusion stems from the fact that cold is used both in immediate care and during rehabilitation. Although these two phases of injury management have different objectives, cold is an effective technique.[69]

Historical Perspective

Cold compresses were a recognized adjunct to surgery as early as 1881[24] but they were not used for sports injuries until much later. In the 1930s, the common treatment for acute sports injuries was hot compresses or soaks combined with soapsuds or Epsom salts.[91] Sports medicine texts in the 1940s advocated cold treatments for acute injuries, but only for 30 to 60 minutes and only if applied within the first 30 minutes after injury.[14,15] For injuries more than 30 minutes old, whether or not ice had been used initially, hot soaks or compresses were recommended. During the 1950s, the time for using cold was extended to the first 24 to 72 hours after injury.[13,32,100,118] By the early 1970s, cold was used almost universally by sports medicine practitioners for immediate care[11,30,107] but its use had not been adopted by the entire medical community.[11,117] The common rationale for using cold was that it decreased blood flow and hemorrhaging.

Cold as an adjunct to rehabilitation of acute musculoskeletal injuries was introduced in 1965 by an army physician[43] and a physical therapist.[51] More than 6,000 patients with sprains, strains, and contusions suffered during basic training were treated with a technique called cryokinetics in which cold applications alternated with active exercise. More than 80% of the patients returned to active duty after one to three treatments. This report stimulated others to try the procedure[12,66,90,124] and to speculate about its mechanism.[2,12,26,39,124] The most prevalent speculation was that cold-induced vasodilation increased blood flow to the tissue. Few recognized that this contradicted the theory that immediate applications of cold resulted in vasoconstriction. Although there is little doubt about the efficacy of cold during both immediate care and rehabilitation, little research has substantiated its use or explained its mechanisms of action. Because of the lack of direct research, there is no definitive explanation of the effects of cold on sports-induced soft-tissue inflammation. Nonetheless, peripheral research provides a basis for the working hypotheses that this chapter examines.

Tissue Response to Cold Applications

The most important local physiologic effects of cold applications are decreases in temperature, inflammation, metabolic rate, circulation, and muscle spasm; an increase in tissue stiffness; and a transient increase, followed by a decrease, in pain. All other responses appear to be temperature-dependent. Metabolic rate and circulation also have a great impact on inflammation. A detailed review of each of the effects of cryotherapy can be found in my text.[69]

Temperature Changes

Cold applications cause a logarithmic decrease in local surface temperature. Surface temperature plateaus within a few minutes at a few degrees above the temperature of the cold pack (or other means of application).[72–74] Depending on the heat-storage capacity of the cooling device, tissue temperature remains fairly constant throughout the application or begins a gradual increase.[3,69]

Deep temperatures decrease later and less rapidly than surface temperatures, and they continue to decrease for a period after the cooling device is removed.[50,120,121] The magnitude of decrease depends on the depth of the measurement, the cooling device, and the time of exposure.[87] For example, a decrease of 12 C was reported at 3 cm after ten minutes of ice-pack application.[16]

When the body part is removed from an ice-water bath or a cold pack is removed from the skin, the surface temperature begins to increase, but more slowly than it decreased.[72,74,120,121] The rate of rewarming may be related to the amount of heat lost, which in turn is influenced by the body part involved, the body surface area exposed, the type of cooling device, and the length of application.[69,87] After 30 to 40 minutes of immersion in 1 C water, a finger rewarms to the contralateral temperature within 20 minutes, but an ankle or a forearm requires more than 150 minutes to rewarm.[72,74]

Contralateral limb temperature does not respond to cold applied to the other limb. Although contralateral temperatures decrease during experiments that require subjects to lie still for hours,[72,74] this is caused by inactivity and/or environmental temperature—not by the cold-pack application.[69,72,74]

Decreased Inflammation

The effects of cold on trauma-induced inflammation have not been investigated. Most research has concentrated on the healing of surgically induced wounds or on the inflammation resulting from the injection of various substances into surgical wounds. Depending on the substance used, local hypothermia can decrease, increase, or delay inflammation.[110]

Cold applied to wounds injected with turpentine or *Staphylococcus* organisms delayed development of the inflammatory response but did not alter it.[1,23,114,115] There was an associated decrease in movement of leukocytes to the wound area.

In a review of work on this topic, Schmidt and associates[110] concluded that cold aggravates prostaglandin-mediated inflammation and inhibits formol-induced inflammation. Because the later is an acute necrotizing inflammation that acts similarly to traumatically induced inflammation, this confirms clinical experience that cold applications are effective in treating trauma.

Cold decreases the effects of histamine on the vascular membrane,[21,102] neutrophil activation,[89] synovial collagenase,[36,49] and synovial fluid leukocytes,[36] and enhances the effects of antibiotics.[17] However, more research is needed to determine the effect of cold on the various phases of trauma-induced inflammation.

Decreased Metabolic Rate

Much tissue degeneration associated with trauma and surgery is hypoxic in nature and secondary to profound vascular alterations.[2] Cold applications decrease the tissue's metabolic activity, thus improving the chances for survival during the period of anoxia caused by insufficient blood flow.[22,94,104,105] Hypothermia reduces the energy needs of the cell,[18,38,59,93,116] thus conserving the limited supplies of oxygen.

Anoxic hearts,[9,35,108] lungs,[48,83] muscles,[58,125] and other organs[46,68,78,94,97,104] survive longer with local hypothermia than with normothermia. In one study, anoxic hearts remained viable for less than 35 minutes at 37 C, but for 230 minutes at 15 C.[9]

As an organism is cooled more deeply, the depression of metabolism becomes more profound.[27,53,88,97,98] Whole-body[27] and forearm[3] oxygen consumption decrease almost linearly with temperature decreases down to 15 C to 17 C, with a forearm oxygen consumption Q_{10} of 2.5.[4] Hearts maintained with hypothermia during ischemic arrest have significantly higher levels of adenosine triphosphate, creatine phosphate, and glycogen, and less histologic disturbance than those maintained at normal temperatures.[27,99,116] Cold applications also decrease upper-extremity muscle injury caused by tourniquet ischemia.[58]

Morbidity also decreases in experimental animals treated with hypothermia after crush wounds,[19] lethal burns,[95] and spinal cord trauma.[5,6,22] A decreased metabolic rate has been credited with this beneficial effect.

Cooling burned tissue below 10 C may be detrimental,[41] and delaying the application by even two minutes negates its beneficial effect.[34] Cooling decreases the magnitude of the injury, that is, it decreases the amount of necrotic tissue.[41,123] Cold applications may even decrease the nonthermal cell death that results from local ischemia and that occurs long after the initial injury.[123]

Although laboratory research has shown that hypothermia slows metabolism, the specific mechanisms of action and the clinical applications of this information are still being debated.

Decreased Circulation

There is much confusion about the circulatory response to cryotherapy. Reports indicate that cold applications both increase and decrease blood flow, that cold applied immediately after an acute injury decreases blood flow and helps control swelling, and that cold applied during rehabilitation (24 to 48 hours after the injury) increases blood flow and promotes healing.[69] It seems absurd that cold applications decrease circulation one day and increase it the next simply because the clinical objective has changed. This confusion stems from various attempts to explain cold-induced vasodilation.

The literature states that cold-induced vasodilation occurs during a cold application or afterwards, contains conflicting statements on how long it lasts (from one to 30 minutes),[12,26,40,55] and makes no direct statement about its magnitude.[69] Despite this confusion, cold-induced vasodilation is generally accepted in sports medicine.[2,11,39,67,86,87,124]

The term cold-induced vasodilation was coined by Lewis[82] to explain temperature fluctuations during and after immersion of the finger in ice water. Lewis assumed a direct relationship between blood flow and temperature that was later proven to be invalid.[40] Also, the increase in temperature above pre-immersion levels that Lewis reported occurs only in fingers that have been cooled to approximately 20 C before immersion.[72,74,82]

Blood flow decreases during cold-pack application and during immersion in ice water at temperatures ranging from 1 C to 15 C for as long as 192 minutes.[4,73,75] Blood flow remains depressed for as long as 45 minutes after cold-pack application.[69,75] Both research and review studies[70] lead to the conclusion that cold-induced vasodilation does not increase blood flow during therapeutic applications of cold, and that the therapeutic value of cold during immediate care and rehabilitation is unrelated to the effects of cold on circulation.

Cold and Wound Healing

Hypothermia depresses wound healing by slowing metabolism and circulation.[78,84,87] A sharp reduction in endogenous respiration of the regenerating lip mucosa of rats occurs during hypothermia and leads to depressed carbohydrate and protein metabolism.[1] Lowering the environmental temperature from 20 C to 12 C for five days decreases the tensile strength of healing incisions in rabbits. Because vasoconstriction requires intact innervation, however, this effect does not occur if the skin is denervated before the wounds are inflicted.[78] Both these examples involve extended periods of whole-body hypothermia. The effect of 20 to 40 minutes of cold applications during wound healing is unknown. Many users of cryotherapy during rehabilitation combine it with exercise,[39,55,75,90] and believe that the sooner exercise can be initiated, the quicker rehabilitation will be. Clinical research substantiates this; patients with ankle sprains[56] and total knee arthroplasty[52] recover more quickly when treated with cold and exercise than when treated with heat and exercise. Combining cold and exercise increases blood flow substantially more than heat applications do.[75]

Theoretical Basis for the Use of Cryotherapy

The immediate care and the rehabilitation of sports injuries have different objectives. During immediate care, the goals are to remove the cause of the injury and to limit the negative results of the injury (secondary hypoxic injury, swelling, pain, spasm).[69] During rehabilita-

Table 1 Use of cryotherapy and thermotherapy*

Physiologic Effects	Efficacy in Immediate Care of Acute Injury	Efficacy in Rehabilitation	
		Acute Injury	Chronic Injury
Cold			
Decreases circulation	0	–	–
Decreases metabolism	+ + +†	–	–
Decreases inflammation	–	–	–
Decreases pain (anesthesia)	+	+ + +‡	+
Decreases muscle spasm	+	+	0
Increases tissue stiffness	0	–	–
Overall effect	+	+	?
Heat			
Increases circulation	0	+	+
Increases metabolism	–§	+	+
Increases inflammation	+	+	–
Decreases pain (analgesia)	+	0‖	+
Decreases muscle spasm	+	+	0
Decreases tissue stiffness	0	0	+
Overall effect	–	–	+

*Adapted with permission from Knight KL: *Cryotherapy: Theory, Technique, and Physiology.* Chattanooga, Chattanooga Corp, 1985.

†Inhibits secondary hypoxic injury.

‡Allows or requires active exercise.

§Promotes secondary hypoxic injury.

‖Often does not facilitate active exercise.

tion, the goal is to return the athlete to previous conditioning levels.[71] Because these objectives are so different, the reasons for using cryotherapy during these two phases of sports-injury management also differ (Table 1).

Cryotherapy During Immediate Care

Decreased circulation has long been seen as the major beneficial effect of ice applications during immediate care.[14,15,30,32,100,118] The traditional theory contends that slowed circulation lessens swelling by decreasing extravascular hemorrhaging. However, the clotting mechanism generally seals torn vessels within three to five minutes.[92,111,122] Because removing the athlete from the playing field or court, evaluating the injury, and applying the ice pack takes longer than this, the beneficial effects cannot be attributed to decreased extravascular hemorrhaging.

Slowed metabolism provides a logical explanation for the beneficial effects of ice.[70] When the metabolic rate of cells on the periphery of the injury is decreased, they require less oxygen and are more resistant to the period of hypoxia brought on by damage to the local vascular system and inflammatory vascular response (Fig. 1). This results in less secondary hypoxic injury, less total tissue damage, less tissue debris, and less edema. This theory has been widely accepted,[8,10,20,106] but has no direct proof.

How quickly cold must be applied to limit secondary hypoxic injury

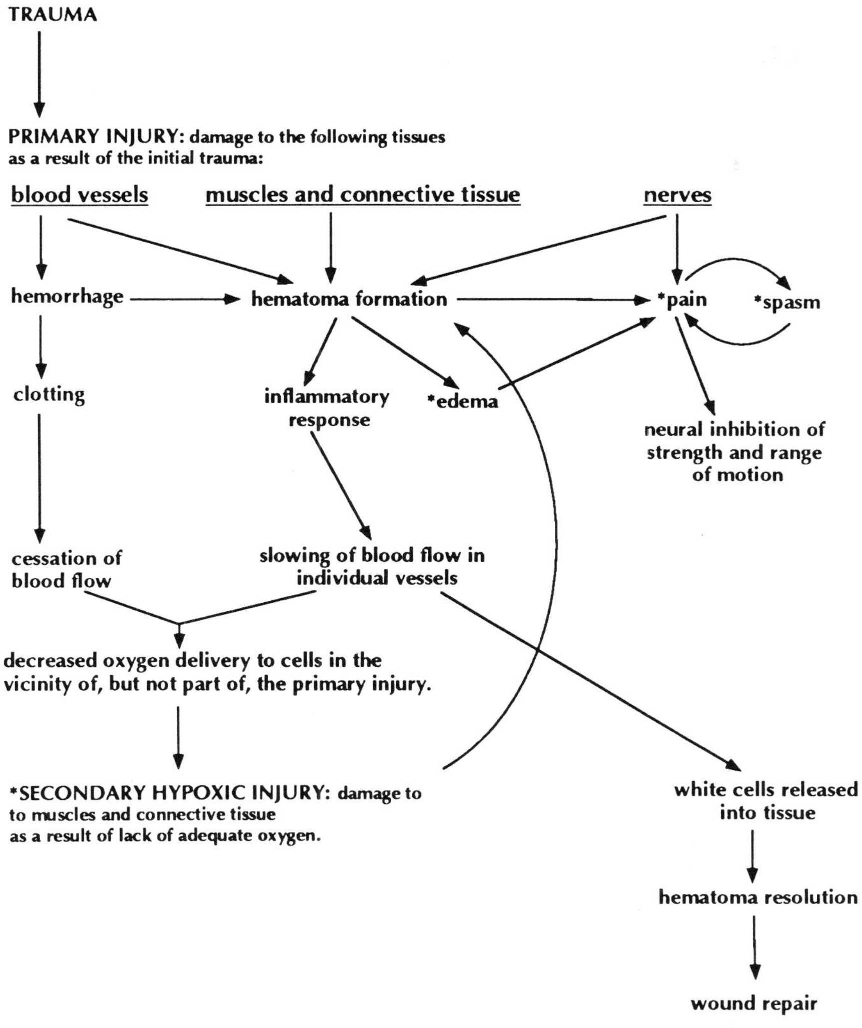

Fig. 1 *Summary of the response of the inflammatory system to acute trauma. The phases that respond to intervention by cold applications to the injury site are labeled with asterisks. (Reproduced with permission from Knight KL:* Cryotherapy: Theory, Technique, and Physiology. *Chattanooga, Chattanooga Corporation, 1985.)*

effectively is unknown. Neurons in the brain suffer irreversible damage after three to five minutes of ischemia, whereas it takes one to two hours of ischemia to produce irreversible damage to liver cells.[103] Jennings and associates[63,64] reported irreversible injury in the myocardium after 20 to 60 minutes of total ischemia. Vogt and Farber[119] reported no renal cell death after 20 minutes of total ischemia, but widespread death after 30 minutes.

Heat applications during this period have the opposite effect (Table 1). Heat speeds up the metabolic rate and, therefore, the tissue's oxygen consumption. This causes more secondary hypoxic injury on the periphery, resulting in increased tissue debris and more edema.

Cold applications to decrease pain and muscle spasm can be beneficial or detrimental. They may make the injured athlete more comfortable and minimize inhibition, thus allowing the athlete to begin therapeutic exercise sooner. However, they may also be detrimental if the athlete returns to the sport too quickly or too vigorously.

Decreasing circulation and inflammation during the immediate care of acute injuries has a negative impact on healing. Decreased circulation contributes to secondary hypoxic injury, and the inflammatory process is a necessary prerequisite to resolution and subsequent wound healing (Fig. 1).

Thus, the primary reason for using cryotherapy during the immediate care of acute musculoskeletal injury and as an adjunct to surgery is to decrease the metabolic rate.[18,69,97]

Cryotherapy During Rehabilitation

The decreases in circulation, metabolic rate, and inflammation and the increase in tissue stiffness resulting from cold applications are detrimental to rehabilitation[1,85]; at this time, increased circulation and metabolism are needed (Table 1). Cold, however, has some desirable effects, such as decreased pain and decreased spasm.

The exercise component of cryokinetics, however, offers benefits that more than compensate for the decreases in circulation and metabolism caused by cold.[47,75,76] Exercise-induced vasodilation during cryokinetics is much greater than that resulting from heat applications.[75] In addition, exercise retards the development of adhesions, reverses neural inhibition,[33,66,79] and activates the lymphatic system[25] to remove much of the tissue debris.[65]

In rats, immediate mobilization after standardized experimentally induced contusions led to a more pronounced macrophage reaction,[77] faster hematoma resolution,[60] increased vascular ingrowth,[62] quicker regeneration of muscle and scar tissue,[60] and increased tensile strength of the healed muscle.[61] Immobilization for two to five days delayed contraction and maturation of the scar as measured 42 days later.[60]

Because pain prevents active exercise for many days after even minor joint sprains,[33,76] cold-induced pain relief allows active exercise much earlier than would otherwise be possible.[47,76] Increased tissue stiffness hinders active exercise, and so exerts a negative effect during rehabilitation.

Cryokinetics can also begin much earlier than thermal therapy.[29,47,81] Thermotherapy must be delayed until the vascular system is repaired and oxygen delivery is normal, a period of 48 to 72 hours, or additional secondary hypoxic injury will occur. Cryokinetics can begin one to 24 hours after injury.[12]

Heat applications are not as effective as cold applications as an adjunct to exercise during rehabilitation. Although both decrease pain, cold is a better facilitator of active exercise.[80] Exercising after heat applications often causes a recurrence of pain and muscle spasm.

Chronic Injuries

The use of cold applications for chronic injuries differs from their use in acute injuries for two reasons: (1) The major problem with chronic injuries is not a primary injury, but a chronic inflammatory response. Secondary hypoxic injury should not occur in a chronic injury. The primary goal, therefore, is to decrease the inflammatory process. (2) Muscle spasm usually does not occur in chronic injuries.

There are no consistent guidelines for the use of heat or cold in treating chronic inflammation. Some investigators advocate the use of ice applications as long as pain persists.[45] Others recommend heat before and cold after activity.[57] Some even advocate a choice of heat or cold, without providing guidelines for the use of either.[54]

Cryotherapy Before and After Surgery

Preoperative local hypothermia has been used to produce surgical anesthesia before amputation of gangrenous limbs,[7,31,112] to lower the elevated body temperature caused by some neurologic diseases,[111] to preserve tissue during abdominal and thoracic surgery, to suspend the spread of infection and toxic absorption in gangrenous patients in whom amputation was delayed,[44] and to decrease muscle injury from tourniquet ischemia.[58]

The use of cold after orthopaedic surgery is controversial. A small, insignificant decrease in forearm temperatures when cold applications were placed on plaster casts and bulky compression dressings led Omer and Brobeck[96] to conclude that the cold applications had no value. Although the patients consistently felt more comfortable when treated with ice packs after surgery, Omer and Brobeck thought this response was totally subjective. The results of Schaubel's[109] review of 800 consecutive surgical cases indicate otherwise.

Of the 800 patients, 345 were treated with ice caps over their casts or dressings for 48 hours.[109] In the 72-hour period after surgery, the group treated with cold applications had fewer split casts; lower temperature, pulse, and respiration rates; nearly normal leukocyte counts; lower doses of narcotic per patient; and fewer postoperative complications. Other studies also reported a decrease in drug use,[113] postoperative draining, and hospitalization[17] in patients treated with cold immediately after surgery. Even cold sitz baths result in decreased postpartum perineal pain and swelling, and a quicker return to normal activities.[37]

Research involving questionable application techniques has caused people to question the use of cold in controlling swelling. In rabbit legs with femoral fractures treated for 24 hours with circulating water at temperature of 5 C to 15 C, swelling increased, but in limbs cooled with water at 20 C to 25 C for 24 hours or at 10 C for six hours there was no increase.[85] Rheumatoid hands treated with two four-minute immersions in 10 C water beginning 48 hours after surgery demonstrated no decrease in swelling.[101] For swelling control to be effective, cold treatments must begin within 30 minutes of surgery, last 30 to 60 minutes, and be repeated every two hours for the first 24 hours or more after surgery. Crushed rat paws placed between two rubber tubes filled with water at 11.5 C to 12.5 C for two to ten hours showed no significant differences from a control group. Farry and associates[42] found increased subcutaneous tissue swelling in both injured and uninjured pig forelegs treated with crushed ice packs for two 20-minute periods one hour apart.

Interpretation of these results must be tempered. Continuous application for several hours is probably too long, whereas a few minutes is too short.[70] Cold applications should be combined with compression and elevation.[43] In those cases in which the location of the swelling was investigated, researchers found that the swelling occurred in the soft tissue overlying the injured ligament, rather than in the ligament itself,[43,85] indicating that the increased swelling resulted from additional injury caused by excessive cold applications.

References

1. Abakumova EA: Vliianie gipotermii na zazhivlenie ran [Effect of hypothermia on inflammation]. *Stomatologia* 1978;57:19–21.
2. Abraham WM: Heat vs. cold therapy for the treatment of muscle injuries. *Athlet Train* 1974;18:144–147.
3. Abramson DI, Chu LS, Tuck S Jr, et al: Effect of tissue temperatures and blood flow on motor nerve conduction velocity. *JAMA* 1966;198:1082–1088.
4. Abramson DI, Kahn A, Tuck S, et al: Relationship between a range of tissue temperature and local oxygen consumption in the resting forearm. *Lab Clin Med* 1957;50:789.
5. Albin MS, White RJ, Acosta-Rua G, et al: Study of functional recovery produced by delayed localized cooling after spinal cord injury in primates. *J Neurosurg* 1968;29:113–120.
6. Albin MS, White RJ, Locke GS, et al: Localized spinal cord hypothermia: Anesthetic effects and application to spinal cord injury. *Anesth Analg* 1967;46:8–16.
7. Allen FM: Reduced temperatures in surgery: I. Surgery of limbs. *Am J Surg* 1941;52:225–237.
8. American Academy of Orthopaedic Surgeons: *Athletic Training and Sports Medicine.* Park Ridge, American Academy of Orthopaedic Surgeons, 1984.
9. Angell WW, Rikkers L, Dong E, et al: Organ viability with hypothermia. *J Thorac Cardiovasc Surg* 1969;58:619–624.
10. Arnheim DD: *Modern Principles of Athletic Training: The Science of Sports Medicine. Injury Prevention, Causation, and Management*, ed 6. St. Louis, Times Mirror/Mosby, 1985.
11. Barnes L: Cryotherapy: Putting injury on ice. *Phys Sportsmed* 1979;7:130–136.
12. Behnke RS: Cold therapy. *Athlet Train* 1974;9:178–179.
13. Bennett D: Water at 67° to 69° Fahrenheit to control hemorrhage and swelling encountered in athletic injuries. *J Natl Athlet Train Assoc*, Winter 1961, pp 12–14.

14. Bevan R: *The Athletic Trainer's Handbook*. Englewood Cliffs, Prentice-Hall, 1956, pp 63–75.
15. Bilik SE: *The Trainer's Bible*, ed 8. New York, TJ Reed & Co, 1946, pp 257–263.
16. Bing HI, Carlsten A, Christiansen S: The effect on muscular temperature produced by cooling normal and ultraviolet radiated skin. *Acta Med Scand* 1945;121:577–591.
17. Bingham R: The therapeutic effect of cold in bone and joint infection. *Am J Orthop Surg* 1968;10:186–189.
18. Blair E: *Clinical Hypothermia*. New York, McGraw-Hill, 1964, pp 22–30.
19. Blalock A: A comparison of the effects of the local application of heat and of cold in the prevention and treatment of experimental traumatic shock. *Surgery* 1942;11:356–359.
20. Booher JM, Thibodeau GA: *Athletic Injury Assessment*. St. Louis, Times Mirror/Mosby, 1985.
21. Boykin JV Jr, Crute SL: Mechanisms of burn shock protection after severe scald injury by cold-water treatment. *J Trauma* 1982;22:859–866.
22. Bricolo A, Ore GD, Da Pian R, et al: Local cooling in spinal cord injury. *Surg Neurol* 1976;6:101–106.
23. Brooks B, Duncan G: The influence of temperature on wounds. *Ann Surg* 1941;114:1069–1075.
24. Bryant T: *A Manual for the Practice of Surgery*, ed 3. Philadelphia, Henry C Lea's Son, 1881, pp 121 and 961.
25. Casley-Smith JR: An electron microscopic study of injured and abnormally permeable lymphatics. *Ann NY Acad Sci* 1964;116:803–830.
26. Chu DA, Lutt CJ: The rationale of ice therapy. *J Nat Athlet Train Assoc* 1969;4:8–9.
27. Civalero LA, Moreno JR, Senning Å: Temperature conditions and oxygen consumption during deep hypothermia. *Acta Chir Scand* 1962;123:179–188.
28. Cohn LH, Collins JJ Jr: Local cardiac hypothermia for myocardial protection. *Ann Thorac Surg* 1974;17:135–140.
29. Condit RE: Wound repair, letter. *Am Fam Phys* 1976;13:28–30.
30. Craig TT (ed): *Comments in Sports Medicine*. Chicago, American Medical Association, 1973, p 171.
31. Crossman LW, Ruggiero WF, Hurley V, et al: Reduced temperatures in surgery: II. Amputations for peripheral vascular disease. *Arch Surg* 1942;44:139–156.
32. Dayton OW: *Athletic Training and Conditioning*. New York, Ronald Press, 1960, pp 126–127.
33. Dehne E, Torp RP: Treatment of joint injuries by immediate mobilization: Based upon the spinal adaptation concept. *Clin Orthop* 1971;177:218–232.
34. Demling RH, Mazess RB, Wolberg W: The effect of immediate and delayed cold immersion on burn edema formation and resorption. *J Trauma* 1979;19:56–60.
35. Dillard DH: Congenital heart disease: Definitive surgery during infancy. *Surg Rounds* 1981;4:24–31.
36. Dorwart BB, Hansell JR, Schumacher HR: Effects of heat, cold and mechanical agitation on crystal-induced arthritis in the dog, abstract. *Arthritis Rheum* 1973;16:540–556.
37. Droegemuller W: Cold sitz baths for relief of perineal pain. *Clin Obstet Gynecol* 1980;23:1039–1043.
38. Drucker WR: Rationale for hypothermia in therpy of hypovolemia, in Mills LC, Moyer JH (eds): *Shock and Hypotension: Pathogenesis and Treatment*. New York, Grune & Stratton, 1965, pp 670–677.

39. Edwards AG: Increasing circulation with cold. *J Natl Athlet Train Assoc* 1973;6:15–16.
40. Edwards M, Burton AC: Correlation of heat output and blood flow in the finger, especially in cold-induced vasodilation. *J Appl Physiol* 1960;15:201–208.
41. Epstein MF, Crawford JD: Cooling in the emergency treatment of burns. *Pediatrics* 1973;52:430–432.
42. Farry PJ, Prentice NG, Hunter AC, et al: Ice treatment of injured ligaments: An experimental model. *NZ Med J* 1980;91:12–14.
43. Grant AE: Massage with ice (cryokinetics) in the treatment of painful conditions of the musculoskeletal system. *Arch Phys Med* 1964;45:233–238.
44. Gibbel MI, Atkins RA, Burns A: The use of dry ice refrigeration when delaying an inevitable amputation. *Am J Surg* 1960;99:326–329.
45. Gieck JH, Saliba EN: Application of modalities in overuse syndromes. *Clin Sports Med* 1987;6:427–466.
46. Hägerdal M, Harp J, Nilsson L, et al: The effect of induced hypothermia upon oxygen consumption in the rat brain. *J Neurochem* 1975;24:311–316.
47. Handling KA: Rehabilitating athletic injuries with cryotherapy. *J Phys Educ Recreat Dance* 1982;53:338–340.
48. Harjula A, Baldwin JC, Shumway NE: Donor deep hypothermia or donor pretreatment with prostaglandin E_1 and single pulmonary artery flush for heart-lung graft preservation: An experimental primate study. *Ann Thorac Surg* 1988;46:553–555.
49. Harris ED Jr, McCroskery PA: The influence of temperature and fibril stability on degradation of cartilage collagen by rheumatoid synovial collagenase. *N Engl J Med* 1974;290:1–6.
50. Hartviksen K: Ice therapy in spasticity. *Acta Neurol Scand* 1962;38(suppl 3):79–84.
51. Hayden CA: Cryokinetics in an early treatment program. *J Am Phys Ther Assoc* 1964;44:990–993.
52. Hecht PJ, Bachmann S, Booth RE Jr, et al: Effects of thermal therapy on rehabilitation after total knee arthroplasty: A prospective randomized study. *Clin Orthop* 1983;178:198–201.
53. Hegnauer AH, D'Amato HE: Oxygen consumption and cardiac output in the hypothermic dog. *Am J Physiol* 1954;178:138–142.
54. Herring SA, Nilson KL: Introduction to overuse injuries. *Clin Sports Med* 1987;6:225–240.
55. Hocutt JE Jr: Cryotherapy. *Am Fam Phys* 1981;23:141–144.
56. Hocutt JE Jr, Jaffe R, Ryland CR, et al: Cryotherapy in ankle sprains. *Am J Sports Med* 1982;10:316–319.
57. Hunter SC, Poole RM: The chronically inflamed tendon. *Clin Sports Med* 1987;6:371–388.
58. Ikemoto Y, Kobayashi H, Usui M, et al: Changes in serum myoglobin levels caused by tourniquet ischemia under normothermic and hypothermic conditions. *Clin Orthop* 1988;234:296–302.
59. Iung OS, Wade FV: The treatment of burns with ice water, pHisoHex, and partial hypothermia. *Industr Med Surg* 1963;32:365–370.
60. Järvinen M: Healing of a crush injury in rat striated muscle: 2. A histological study of the effect of early mobilization and immobilization on the repair processes. *Acta Pathol Microbiol Scand* 1975;83:269–282.
61. Järvinen M: Healing of a crush injury in rat striated muscle: 3. A micro-angiographical study of the effect of early mobilization and immobilization on capillary ingrowth. *Acta Pathol Microbiol Scand* 1976;84:85–94.
62. Järvinen M: Healing of a crush injury in rat striated muscle: 4. Effect of early mobilization and immobilization on the tensile properties of gastrocnemius muscle. *Acta Chir Scand* 1976;142:47–56.

63. Jennings RB, Ganote CE, Reimer KA: Ischemic tissue injury. *Am J Pathol* 1975;81:179–198.
64. Jennings RB, Hawkins HK, Lowe JE, et al: Relation between high energy phosphate and lethal injury in myocardial ischemia in the dog. *Am J Pathol* 1978;92:187–214.
65. Johnston MG: Potential role of the lymphatic vessel in regulating inflammatory events. *Surv Synth Pathol Res* 1983;1:111–119.
66. Juvenal JP: Cryokinetics, a new concept in the treatment of injuries. *Scholastic Coach* 1966;35:40–42.
67. Kalenak A, Medlar CE, Fleagle SB, et al: Athletic injuries: Heat vs. cold. *Am Fam Phys* 1975;12:131–134.
68. Kelly MJ, Wheatley R, Smith JH, et al: Cooling prevents ischaemic testicular damage after spermatic cord clamping in rats. *Int J Androl* 1987;10:721–726.
69. Knight KL: *Cryotherapy: Theory, Technique, and Physiology.* Chattanooga, Chattanooga Corp, 1985, pp 15–31 and 73–155.
70. Knight KL: Effects of hypothermia on inflammation and swelling. *Athlet Train* 1976;11:7–10.
71. Knight KL: Guidelines for rehabilitation of sports injuries. *Clin Sports Med* 1985;4:405–416.
72. Knight KL, Aquino J, Johannes SM, et al: A reexamination of Lewis' cold-induced vasodilation—in the finger and the ankle. *Athlet Train* 1980;15:24–27.
73. Knight KL, Bryant KS, Halvorsen J: Circulatory changes in the forearm in 1, 5, 10, and 15°C water, abstract. *Int J Sports Med* 1981;4:281.
74. Knight KL, Elam JF: Rewarming of the ankle, finger, and forearm after cryotherapy: Further investigation of Lewis' cold-induced vasodilation. *J Can Athlet Ther Assoc* 1981;8:17–18.
75. Knight KL, Londeree BR: Comparison of blood flow in the ankle of uninjured subjects during therapeutic applications of heat, cold, and exercise. *Med Sci Sports Exerc* 1980;12:76–80.
76. Kraus H: Prevention and treatment of skiing injuries. *J Trauma* 1961;1:457–463.
77. Kvist H, Järvinen M, Sorvari T: Effect of mobilization and immobilization on the healing of contusion injury in muscle: A preliminary report of a histological study in rats. *Scand J Rehabil Med* 1974;6:134–140.
78. Kvitsinskayia EA, Krivulis DB, Sorokin IA: Vliianie gipotermii na metabolizm v pecheni pri ee koservatii [Effect of hypothermia on metabolism in the liver during preservation]. *Biull Eksp Biol Med* 1978;86:179–182.
79. Lee JM, Warren MP: *Cold Therapy in Rehabilitation.* London, Bell & Hyman, 1978, pp 69–81.
80. Lehmann JF, De Lateur BJ: Cryotherapy, in Lehmann JF (ed): *Therapeutic Heat and Cold*, ed 3. Baltimore, Williams & Wilkins, 1982, pp 563–602.
81. Lehmann JF, De Lateur BJ: Therapeutic heat, in Lehmann JF (ed): *Therapeutic Heat and Cold*, ed 3. Baltimore, Williams & Wilkins, 1982.
82. Lewis T: Observations upon the reactions of the vessels of the human skin to cold. *Heart* 1930;15:177–208.
83. Locke TJ, Hooper TL, Flecknell PA, et al: Preservation of the lung: Comparison of topical cooling and cold crystalloid pulmonary perfusion. *J Thorac Cardiovasc Surg* 1988;96:789–795.
84. Lundgren C, Muren A, Zederfeldt B: Effect of cold-vasoconstriction on wound healing in the rabbit. *Acta Chir Scand* 1959;118:1–4.
85. Matsen FA III, Questad K, Matsen AL: The effect of local cooling on postfracture swelling: A controlled study. *Clin Orthop* 1975;109:201–206.

86. McDonald WD, Guthrie JD Jr: Cryotherapy in the postoperative setting. *J Foot Surg* 1985;24:438–441.
87. Meeusen R, Lievens P: The use of cryotherapy in sports injuries. *Sports Med* 1986;3:398–414.
88. Michenfelder JD, Theye RA: Hypothermia: effect on canine brain and whole-body metabolism. *Anesthesiology* 1968;29:1107–1112.
89. Moore FD Jr, Warner KG, Assousa S, et al: The effects of complement activation during cardiopulmonary bypass: Attenuation by hypothermia, heparin, and hemodilution. *Ann Surg* 1988;208:95–103.
90. Moore RJ, Nicolette RL, Behnke RS: The therapeutic use of cold (cryotherapy) in the care of athletic injuries. *J Natl Athlet Train Assoc* 1967;2:6–13.
91. Morehead JJ: *Traumatotherapy: The Treatment of the Injured.* Philadelphia, WB Saunders, 1931, pp 17–18.
92. Mustard JF, Packham MA: The reaction of the blood to injury, in Movat HZ (ed): *Inflammation, Immunology, and Hypersensitivity*, ed 2. Hagerstown, Harper & Row, 1979, pp 557–664.
93. Nordström CH, Rehncrona S: Reduction of cerebral blood flow and oxygen consumption with a combination of barbiturate anaesthesia and induced hypothermia in the rat. *Acta Anaesthesiol Scand* 1978;22:7–12.
94. O'Connor JV, Wilding T, Farmer P, et al: The protective effect of profound hypothermia on the canine central nervous system during one hour of circulatory arrest. *Ann Thorac Surg* 1986;41:255–259.
95. Ofeigsson OJ, Mitchell R, Patrick RS: Observations on the cold water treatment of cutaneous burns. *J Pathol* 1972;108:145–150.
96. Omer GE Jr, Brobeck AG: An evaluation of ice application with postoperative dressings. *Clin Orthop* 1971;81:117–121.
97. Popovic V, Popovic P: *Hypothermia in Biology and Medicine.* New York, Grune & Stratton, 1974, pp 79–115.
98. Race D, Cooper E, Rosebaum M: Hemorrhagic shock: The effect of prolonged low flow on the regional distribution of blood and its modification by hypothermia. *Ann Surg* 1968;167:454–466.
99. Rao KS, Schutz RW, Feinberg H, et al: Metabolic evidence that regional hypothermia induced by cold saline protects the heart during ischemic arrest. *J Surg Res* 1976;20:421–425.
100. Rawlinson K: *Modern Athletic Training.* Englewood Cliffs, Prentice-Hall, 1961, pp 48–54.
101. Rembe EC: Use of cryotherapy on the postsurgical rheumatoid hand. *Phys Ther* 1970;50:19–23.
102. Rippe B, Grega GJ: Effects of isoprenaline and cooling on histamine induced changes of capillary permeability in the rat hindquarter vascular bed. *Acta Physiol Scand* 1978;103:252–262.
103. Robbins SL, Cotran RS: *Pathologic Basis of Disease*, ed 2. Philadephia, WB Saunders, 1979, pp 12–90.
104. Robertson CS, Foltz R, Grossman RG, et al: Protection against experimental ischemic spinal cord injury. *J Neurosurg* 1986;64:633–642.
105. Rosenfeldt FL: Myocardial preservation 1987: What is the state of the art? *Aust NZ J Surg* 1987;57:349–353.
106. Roy S, Irvin R: *Sports Medicine: Prevention, Evaluation, Management, and Rehabilitation.* Englewood Cliffs, Prentice-Hall, 1983.
107. Ryan AJ: Technological advances in sports medicine and in the reduction of sports injuries. *Exerc Sports Sci Rev* 1973;1:285–312.
108. Sapsford RN, Blackstone EH, Kirklin JW, et al: Coronary perfusion versus cold ischemic arrest during aortic valve surgery: A randomized study. *Circulation* 1974;49:1190–1199.

109. Schaubel HJ: The local use of ice after orthopedic procedures. *Am J Surg* 1946;72:711–714.
110. Schmidt KL, Ott VR, Röcher G, et al: Heat, cold and inflammation. *Z Rheumatol* 1979;38:391–404.
111. Schwartz SI, Troup SB: Hemostasis, surgical bleeding, and transfusion, in Schwartz SI, Lillehei RC, Shires GT, et al (eds): *Principles of Surgery*, ed 2. New York, McGraw-Hill, 1974, pp 97–132.
112. Shafer K: *Shafer's Medical-Surgical Nursing*, ed 7. St. Louis, CV Mosby, 1980, pp 231–232.
113. Smith MP: Reduction of postoperative pain. *Northwest Med* 1964;63:698–701.
114. Svanes K: Studies in hypothermia I: The influence of deep hypothermia on the formation of cellular exudate in acute inflammation in mice. *Acta Anaesthesiol Scand* 1964;8:143–156.
115. Svanes K: Studies in hypothermia: II. The influence of deep hypothermia on the formation of fluid exudate in acute inflammation in mice. *Acta Anaesthesiol Scand* 1964;8:157–166.
116. Takami H, Matsuda H, Hirose H, et al: Myocardial energy metabolism in preserved heart: Comparison of simple storage and hypothermic perfusion. *J Heart Transplant* 1988;7:205–212.
117. Temperman PS, Devlin M: Therapeutic heat and cold: A practitioner's guide. *Postgrad Med* 1983;73:69–76.
118. Thorndike A: Frequency and nature of sports injuries. *Am J Surg* 1959;98:316–324.
119. Vogt MT, Farber E: On the molecular pathology of ischemic renal cell death: Reversible and irreversible cellular and mitochondrial metabolic alterations. *Am J Pathol* 1968;53:1–26.
120. Walton M, Roestenburg M, Hallwright S, et al: Effects of ice packs on tissue temperatures at various depths before and after quadriceps hematoma: Studies using sheep. *J Orthop Sports Phys Ther* 1986;8:294–300.
121. Waylonis GW: The physiologic effects of ice massage. *Arch Phys Med* 1967;48:37–42.
122. Weatherall DJ, Bunch C, Sharp AA: The blood and blood-forming organs, in Smith LH Jr, Thier SO (eds): *Pathophysiology: The Biological Principles of Disease*. Philadelphia, WB Saunders 1981, pp 326–478.
123. Wiedeman MP, Brigham MP: The effects of cooling on the microvasculature after thermal injury. *Microvasc Res* 1971;3:154–161.
124. Wise DD: Ice and the athlete. *Physiother Can* 1973;25:213–217.
125. Wright JG, Kerr JC, Valeri CR, et al: Regional hypothermia protects against ischemia-reperfusion injury in isolated canine gracilis muscle. *J Trauma* 1988;28:1026–1031.

Chapter 31

Therapeutic Ultrasound: Influence on Inflammation and Healing

Joe H. Gieck, EdD, ATC, PT
Ethan Saliba, MEd, ATC, PT

Ultrasound is acoustical energy that causes molecular motion as it travels through matter. Ultrasound of varying intensities and frequencies has several medical uses, including diagnostic imaging and surgical and therapeutic applications. This chapter deals principally with therapeutic ultrasound. Therapeutic ultrasound has been recommended for some time as a deep-heating agent for such conditions as tendinitis, bursitis, and arthritis. Recently, this treatment has also gained recognition for its role in soft-tissue healing.

Historical Perspectives

Ultrasound has been used for medical purposes for the past 50 years. The discovery that high-frequency acoustical energy affected biologic tissues was made during World War I. At that time, ultrasound energy was used in the newly developed underwater detection devices. The reaction of small fish passing through the sonated fields led to the discovery that marine life is adversely affected by ultrasound. This discovery prompted biologic experimentation with high-frequency acoustical energy. The first medical reports of therapeutic ultrasound date from the late 1930s in Germany. In 1955, the Council on Physical Medicine and Rehabilitation of the American Medical Association recommended ultrasound as an adjunctive therapy for pain and for soft-tissue and joint dysfunction.

Despite the large number of studies on ultrasound, there is some question about which responses are consistently attainable. Most early studies used animal models, and the ultrasound dosages administered exceeded recommended therapeutic ranges. Dosimetry was often vaguely described, and instrument calibration was not precise enough to confirm exactly what energy levels were being delivered. Many professionals currently consider ultrasound to be a safe treatment when properly applied. Its principal therapeutic benefit may be derived from the closeness it requires between clinician and patient, that is, the way it provides an opportunity to "touch."

Physical Principles

The audible ranges of sound are between 16 and 20,000 Hz. Frequencies beyond 20,000 Hz are, therefore, considered ultrasound. Therapeutic ultrasound operates at frequencies between 0.75 and 3.3 MHz, and most devices in the United States operate at a 1-MHz frequency. European units have optional frequencies, including 0.75, 1.5, and 3.0 MHz. Therapeutic ultrasound units currently marketed can diversify treatment applications by using interchangable sound heads that have crystals of different sizes and different operating frequencies.

Ultrasound is created by a reverse piezoelectric effect in which high-frequency electrical currents are converted into mechanical energy as they pass over a crystal contained in the transducer or sound head. The mechanical energy is transmitted to organic molecules in longitudinal waves, producing thermal and nonthermal responses. Energy is transferred to a patient by the use of a coupling medium. Because ultrasound travels easily through solids and liquids but is readily reflected or absorbed by atmospheric gases, it requires the use of a conductive medium at the air-transducer interface. Ultrasound energy is delivered in a continuous or pulsed mode at intensities from 0.1 to 3.0 W/cm^2. The continuous-wave mode and higher intensities are generally used to elicit thermal responses; the pulsed mode at lower intensities is used principally for nonthermal effects. The pulsed mode incorporates a duty cycle, which lowers the average power delivered to the tissues. Low-intensity, pulsed ultrasound, makes it possible to produce nonthermal responses without appreciable heat generation.

Ultrasound is probably best known for its ability to generate heat deep within a muscle or joint capsule while minimizing heat production in superficial tissues, such as skin and fat. This characteristic allows clinicians to direct heat of an appropriate temperature to the target tissue. It is believed that other, nonthermal cellular responses also occur along with the thermal actions and that, by reducing inflammation and promoting wound healing, these responses are of benefit in treating sports injuries.

The depth of penetration of ultrasound is inversely related to its frequency. Higher-frequency ultrasound has less beam divergence, but a higher absorption rate in superficial tissues; therefore, less energy is available to be transmitted to deeper tissues. Therapeutic responses have been reported to be diminished by as much as 50% (termed half-value thickness or 50% energy attenuation) at 5 cm with a frequency of 1 MHz and at 2 cm with a frequency of 3.3 MHz. Clinically, higher frequencies are used to treat cutaneous lesions or bony areas, such as the wrist, hand, or temporomandibular joint, that have minimal superficial tissue covering. Lower-frequency ultrasound is used to treat areas with thicker soft tissue, such as over muscle bellies.

Therapeutic Responses

Energy applied to a system is absorbed, transmitted, or deflected. Heat production in tissues is proportional to the intensity of ultrasound delivered and to the absorption coefficient of the tissues. Intensity—the rate at which energy is delivered per unit area—is expressed in watts per square centimeter (W/cm^2). It is measured by dividing the total power output in watts by the surface area (effective radiating surface) of the crystal in square centimeters. Tissues with a high protein content absorb ultrasound more readily than do other tissues. Nerve and muscle, therefore, absorb the greatest amount of ultrasound energy. Deflection (reflection and refraction) of ultrasound energy is greatest at heterogeneous tissue interfaces, especially at the bone-muscle interface. This deflection creates standing waves, causing an increased thermal response.

Thermal Responses

A thermal response of between 40 C and 45 C for at least five minutes is required to obtain a therapeutic effect.[15] Therapeutic effects of heat application include increased blood flow, increased extensibility of tissues (when combined with stretching), decreased pain, and decreased muscle spasms. These temperatures are easily obtainable with ultrasound within the recommended ranges. The intensity of ultrasound is determined by the degree of thermal response desired and by the thickness of the overlying soft tissue. Tissues that are actively inflamed should not be subjected to increased heat because this can exacerbate the inflammation.

The amount of heating at various depths and tissue types has been studied by Lehmann and de Lateur.[34] They stated that to create vigorous heat in deep structures, such as the hip, as much as 4 W/cm^2 (total output, 40 W) was necessary. For moderate heating, 2 W/cm^2 (total output, 10 to 20 W) was needed. Mild heating was attained in superficial structures with 0.1 to 1.0 W/cm^2 (total output, 1 to 10 W). Lehmann and de Lateur thought that to obtain the appropriate dosage for vigorous heating, the intensity should be increased until discomfort is elicited, at which point the output is decreased slightly. Ultrasound units marketed today generally do not allow outputs above 20 to 25 W. With improved instrumentation, high outputs are not needed to provide comparable energy levels.

When determining the dosimetry of ultrasound, factors to be considered include the total wattage output, the duration of application, and the size of the treatment area.[34] Along with the wattage requirements, a period of five minutes per 5 sq in of treatment area has been recommended to elicit the desired response. If the surface area treated is too large, the energy absorbed is insufficient to create a therapeutic response.

Nonthermal Responses

Along with the thermal responses, the nonthermal effects of ultrasound for promoting wound healing are gaining wider use. During ultrasound treatment, both thermal and nonthermal effects are present, although the thermal responses often cloud nonthermal effects. Pulsed ultrasound with temporal average intensities of 0.1 to 0.2 W/cm^2 is used to elicit nonthermal effects while eliminating or minimizing thermal responses.[15] Proposed mechanisms for nonthermal effects include cavitation and acoustical microstreaming.

Cavitation is the formation of tiny oscillating cavities or gas bubbles in the medium being insonated. Molecular oscillation that occurs when ultrasound is applied can cause pressure fluctuations within the region, causing gases to flow from regions of high pressure into areas of lower pressure. Gas bubbles can fluctuate significantly in both size and degree of oscillation.

Cavitation can be either stable or transient. Stable cavitation is considered to have relatively low pressure amplitudes and is a term used to describe the oscillation of tiny gas bubbles already present within the ultrasound field. This oscillation, called acoustical microstreaming, results in the movement of fluid in the vicinity of the bubble.

Acoustical microstreaming increases the flow of ions and metabolites over cellular membranes and intracellular structures in addition to altering membrane permeability. This increases diffusion of ions and metabolites across cell membranes, facilitating cellular metabolism. Changes in the permeability of calcium have been demonstrated and are associated with enhancing the progression of the reparative processes. Alterations in sodium ion permeability may change the electrical activity of nerves and are a proposed mechanism of pain reduction.

Transient or collapsible cavitation, which occurs at relatively high pressures, can be extremely damaging. Transient cavitation, which involves the expansion and sudden collapse of cavities, results in focal high pressures and temperatures in the tissues and can cause local tissue damage and free radical production.[15]

Inflammatory Responses

Ultrasound has long been used to treat inflammatory conditions although experimental studies have not verified its benefits or the mechanisms involved. Ultrasound has not been shown to decrease the inflammatory response of acute soft-tissue injury, although low-intensity, pulsed ultrasound has been found to hasten the inflammatory response in some studies and to provide primarily a placebo effect in others[15] Several studies have reported that ultrasound, when compared with sham ultrasound treatment, has no significant anti–inflammatory effect.

Goddard and associates[25] induced an inflammatory response in rat and monitored inflammatory cell infiltration into subcutaneously implanted sponges. The effects that ultrasound, sham ultrasound, and the administration of a nonsteroidal anti–inflammatory drug (NSAID had on the cell infiltration were then compared. The investigators concluded that ultrasound had no anti–inflammatory effect, because the amount of protein present in the sponges was similar in the u trasound and sham ultrasound groups, and significantly higher in both groups than in the rats who received the NSAID. This inflammatory model had been used previously and was believed to offer a highly reproducible method of measuring both fluid exudation and cellular infiltration associated with inflammation.

Snow and Johnson[47] concluded that ultrasound did not significantly affect acute inflammation in human soft tissues. Inflammation was induced in two cutaneous regions of the abdomens of the subjects by exposure to ultraviolet light. One site was treated with ultrasound and the other received sham ultrasound (double-blind method). Ultrasound was applied for five minutes (20% duty cycle at 1.0 W/cm^2). Monitoring the magnitude of temperature differences between the inflamed area and the surrounding normal skin showed that the ultrasound-treated area did not differ significantly from the sham ultrasound site.

Several studies have shown that ultrasound has an effect on the inflammatory process, although the mechanisms are still being investigated. Many of the changes noted after ultrasound application are attributed to changes in cellular permeability, especially of calcium ions.

Dyson,[15] McDiarmid and Burns,[37] and Patrick[39] all advocated the use of pulsed ultrasound within the first 24 hours after injury. This was to minimize the development of organized edema and to reduce pain and muscle spasm, shortening the rehabilitation times for soft-tissue injuries. Patrick advocated this through case studies and did not attempt to explain the mechanisms for such action.

When ultrasound is used so soon after injury, it is best to wait until active bleeding has ceased, to ensure that the mechanical nonthermal energy does not disrupt the clotting mechanism. The pulsed average intensity delivered during the acute phase should be low to minimize a thermal response, which is contraindicated.

Dyson[15] described the effect of ultrasound on the three stages of wound healing: acute inflammatory (early and late), proliferative, and remodeling. In acute inflammation, ultrasound is thought to enhance the natural occurrence of degranulation of mast cells by increasing transport of calcium ions across cell membranes. This process is responsible for releasing chemotactic agents that draw the cellular components of inflammation (neutrophils and monocytes) to the injured site.

Macrophages are also associated with the late stage of acute inflammation and may be affected by insonation. Along with the phagocytic function, these cells release chemotactic agents and growth factors that are thought to be essential for the development of connective tissue. Because these cells are drawn to the injury site sooner by chemotactic influence, the entire inflammatory process may be hastened so that the repair phase begins earlier.

Dyson[15] thought that ultrasound is less efficacious in chronic inflammation and generally does not interrupt the process beneficially unless the irritative stimulus is removed.

The proliferative phase of inflammation, which normally begins three to four days after injury, provides the framework for connective tissue reconstruction and replacement. Ultrasound may affect the speed and effectiveness of this phase by increasing the entry of calcium into fibroblasts and endothelial cells. Calcium carries a message to these cells, which respond by enhancing their "metabolic machinery" to a reparative mode. Ultrasound during this phase of tissue repair is believed to enhance the tensile strength of the wound by increasing collagen production, to promote wound contraction by augmenting the myofibroblasts, and to enhance angiogenesis by influencing endothelial cell activity. McDiarmid and associates[38] reported that ultrasound stimulates fibroblast motility and influences the ultrastructure of these connective tissue precursor cells by increasing their total protein content. Collagen synthesis is increased, which increases the tensile strength of the newly formed scar.

Attempts to influence the mechanical properties of scar tissue with ultrasound have been made during the remodelling phase. With increased collagen production and the possible effects on fiber patterning, the strength and elasticity of the scar may be enhanced.[15]

Cellular Responses

The cellular responses gained from ultrasound have been attributed to both thermal and nonthermal microstreaming effects. These responses include an increase in the diffusion rate of ions across membranes and repolarization of nerve and muscle membranes. The effect on the diffusion rate in turn affects the ion concentration gradients and intracellular metabolism. Thermal effects have also been credited with the increase in active transport processes.

The rate of protein synthesis can be increased or decreased by exposure to ultrasound. Higher intensities using a continuous wave (1.0 W/cm^2 for five minutes) inhibited protein synthesis. Continuous wave at lower intensities (0.5 W/cm^2 average intensity) enhanced protein synthesis by 20%. Lower intensities in a pulsed mode at 0.1 W/cm^2 increased protein synthesis by 30%.[28]

Circulation

Again, conflicting results have been found regarding the effect of ultrasound on blood flow. Investigators using the stationary application technique observed blood stasis in chick embryo, frog mesentery, and mammalian vessels. Damage to endothelial cells lining the embryonic vessels was also observed.[18,50] With short exposure times (five minutes) damage was considered reversible, but longer exposures (15 minutes) resulted in more permanent injury. Blood stasis was attributed to the production of standing waves and did not occur if the recommended moving sound head technique was used.

Mixed results were found in limb perfusion after ultrasound therapy. Although several investigators noted significant increases in blood flow,[1,33] others found inconsistent and insignificant changes.[30,40]

Immune Response

The effect of ultrasound on immunologic response was also investigated. Ultrastructural changes on the cell's surface after insonation are thought to be important in immune reactions and may result in the cell becoming more or less susceptible to detection by the immune system. Several researchers reported ultrastructural changes and decreased phagocytic activity in experimental animals after insonation.[2,46] However, Bekhome[7] reported that ultrasound therapy to the tonsilar regions appeared to stimulate immunologic reactivity in patients with subcompensated tonsillitis.[7]

Skeletal System

Low-intensity ultrasound used during bone repair can accelerate healing.[14,16] Higher intensities over bone have shown many deleterious effects, including reduced skeletal growth in dogs (exposures of 3 to 4 W/cm^2), periosteal loss (0.5 to 1.0 W/cm^2 with continuous-wave and a stationary technique), bleeding in the bone marrow of canine femurs (0.5 W/cm^2), a 5 C temperature increase in bone marrow temperatures (2.5 W/cm^2) that resulted in increased peripheral blood clotting time and marrow damage, and reduced calcium metabolism after insonation of rat knees.[6,31,42]

Central Nervous System

Although ultrasound has an analgesic effect, the mechanism responsible for this is not currently known.[34] The analgesic properties of ultrasound reportedly stem from various influences, including thermal effects, effects on nerve conduction, counterirritant responses, presynaptic inhibition by A-β fiber stimulation, autonomic nerve responses, and increased cortisol levels.

Studies of the effect of ultrasound on nerve conduction are inconclusive, as conduction has been found to be increased in some studies and decreased in others.[10,22,25] Low-intensity ultrasound was found to increase nerve conduction, whereas higher intensities decreased neural activity.[27] Antich[4] reported that ultrasound caused a superficial sensory nerve irritation, ultimately decreasing the transmission of pain. Herrick[29] reported an interruption in nerve conduction with the application of 0.8 MHz at 1.0 W/cm^2. This response was attributed to a thermal effect.

Several reports indicated that nerves are selectively heated to a much higher degree than surrounding soft tissues.[3,48] This selective heating results from reflection of energy at the heterogeneous soft tissue-nerve interface and the enhanced absorption of ultrasound by nerves because of their high protein content. Evidence that this occurs includes reports that sciatic nerves in dogs were destroyed, whereas surrounding muscles were not affected.[29] Alterations in such neural activities as action potentials, reflex discharge, and brain waves were dissimilar to those produced by heat; therefore, nonthermal influences as well as those caused by thermal effects were suspected.[49]

Clinical Applications

Joint Contractures

Ultrasound generates a thermal response in targeted joint structures, such as muscle, tendon, or joint capsule. The heat increases the extensibility of collagen fibers by altering the properties of the viscoelastic components of the connective tissue matrix. The tissues elongate and range of motion increases when the involved tissues are heated during stretching exercises. In this manner, ultrasound, in combination with appropriate exercise, is effective in treating joint contractures.[35]

Scar Tissue

The effects of ultrasound on scar tissue have been attributed to both thermal and nonthermal responses. Loss of joint mobility caused by fibrotic muscle and adhesion formation has been effectively treated with ultrasound. This benefit was attributed to the thermal response that occurs with the selective absorption of ultrasound by connective tissue. Another proposed effect of ultrasound on scar tissue is a reduction in the cement substance between the collagen fibrils.[8] This loosens the bonds between the individual macromolecules, enhancing the extensibility of the tissue and softened scar tissue. To optimize the benefit of increased mobility after ultrasound treatment, stretching exercises should be incorporated. The combination of stretching and ultrasound has been found to enhance residual elongation of connective tissue.[35] Another potential benefit from ultrasound treatment of scar tissue is the analgesic effect of decreasing C fiber activity.

Muscle Spasm Reduction

The ability of ultrasound to reduce muscle spasms is believed to derive from a direct alteration in the skeletal muscle contractile process, reduction in muscle spindle activity, reduction of pain, and increased blood flow to the involved musculature. Although many clinical reports have noted the effectiveness of ultrasound in reducing muscle spasms, few physiologic processes were described to account for this response. Lehmann and Guy[35] reported that second afferent and gamma activity decreased when heat was applied. This relieves the spasms by decreasing neural firing to the muscle.

Tissue Healing

Studies have shown that ultrasound can both increase and decrease tissue regeneration. A 32% increase in the rate of wound healing has been reported with the application of low-intensity, pulsed ultrasound. Dyson and associates[17] examined the effect of nine different dosages of ultrasound on the rate of regeneration in superficial wounds made in rabbit ears. Significant increases in healing rate were found with 0.25 to 1.0 W/cm² pulsed at 20% and with 0.1 W/cm² continuous-wave ultrasound. Pulsed ultrasound at an average intensity of 0.1 W/cm² and a maximal intensity of 0.5 W/cm² (20% duty cycle) resulted in the greatest rate of tissue regeneration. Maximal intensities above some unestablished level were also thought to inhibit regeneration even when the average intensity was low.

Varicose ulcers treated with low-intensity ultrasound were 27% smaller in area than were the controls. The mechanism of tissue regeneration was attributed to nonthermal responses with the lower intensities. Higher intensities inhibited protein synthesis.

Variations of the animal studies in clinical trials produced less dramatic but still positive results when ultrasound was applied over pressure ulcers. McDiarmid and associates,[38] using parameters similar to those used by Dyson and Suckling,[19] found that clean wounds showed no significant increase in healing rate. Infected sores, although they still healed more slowly than clean wounds, had better healing rates with ultrasound than did their sham-treatment counterparts.[38]

Roche and West,[44] in a study of the effectiveness of ultrasound on venous ulcers, found that the treated wound healed significantly faster and showed the greatest reduction in size at 14 days. They also noticed that larger wounds healed faster than smaller wounds. Other reports confirmed that ultrasound used in conjunction with traditional therapy produce a faster rate of healing and that the wounds have a healthier, cleaner appearance when treated with low-intensity, pulsed ultrasound three times a week.[19,41]

Roberts and associates[43] found that pulsed ultrasound applied to repaired rat tendons (0.8 W/cm², five days a week for six weeks) decreased tensile strength when compared with sham treatment. It has been recommended that ultrasound treatments begin approximately two weeks after the injury, during the proliferative phase of tissue healing. Earlier application increased wound edema and delayed healing time.[52]

Most studies that examine the effects of ultrasound on wound healing treat open skin lesions because the size and progress of such wounds can be measured. Other wounds, such as soft-tissue contusions, sprains, and strains, are probably affected by ultrasound in a similar manner, but the effectiveness of such a treatment is more difficult to measure. Frieder and associates[24] treated partially ruptured rat Achilles tendons with 1.5 W/cm^2 continuous-wave ultrasound for three minutes. Electron microscopy showed that tissues insonated for three weeks had ultrastructural changes indicating a more advanced stage of healing than was seen in untreated tissues.

Tissue healing is thought to occur principally through nonthermal cellular mechanisms such as acoustical streaming. The recommended parameters are intensities between 0.5 and 1.0 W/cm^2 pulsed at 20% for both skin and other soft-tissue wounds. A lower frequency should be used when deeper penetration is desired. Skin lesions and ulcers are generally treated with frequencies of 3.0 MHz or above.

Tendinitis and Bursitis

The benefits attained from using ultrasound to treat tendinitis and bursitis are believed to result from the reduction of pain and edema and are attributed to the thermal effects of ultrasound application. Increased shoulder range of motion has been demonstrated after ultrasound treatments for subacromial bursitis,[20] although these results have been challenged in a controlled study by Downing and Weinstein.[13] Because ultrasound has not proven to be an effective anti–inflammatory technique, its benefits in treating tendinitis and bursitis may be questioned.

Calcium Deposits

The effect ultrasound has on calcium deposits is poorly substantiated by controlled clinical studies. Several reports claim a reduction in the size of calcific deposits after insonation.

There have been reports of resorption of calcific deposits in the supraspinatus tendons and in the stump ends of amputated limbs.[9,45] It is uncertain whether the resorption is caused by thermal responses, which increase local blood flow, or by a change in calcium metabolism. Calcium ion permeability through cell membranes has been shown to be increased after the application of pulsed ultrasound.[15] This mechanism may influence the resorption of intercellular calcium deposits, although this has not been shown experimentally or radiologically. Flax[23] reported that calcium deposits resolved as often in the control groups as in the treatment groups.

Phonophoresis

Phonophoresis, a technique that uses mechanical energy to drive whole molecules of medication into the tissues, is commonly used to administer anti–inflammatory agents, such as cortisol, dexamethasone, and salicylates. The treatment is painless and delivers the drug molecules into the subcutaneous tissue without injections. Davick and associates[11] investigated the distribution and deposition of various dosages of corticosteroids administered by phonophoresis. The study was conducted on dogs whose tissue was histologically examined with light microscopy to obtain counts of tritiated cortisol cream. When compared with ultrasound alone, 10% cortisol with ultrasound showed the greatest penetration, although this was only into the deep epidermal layers of the skin.

Griffin and associates[26] conducted a double-blind study to compare the clinical effectiveness of ultrasound used alone and used with hydrocortisone cream. When patients with various degenerative joint diseases were treated, 68% of those receiving phonophoresis had relief from pain and improved range of motion. Only 28% of the patients treated with the ultrasound alone had these improvements.

Most clinical trials have used continuous-wave ultrasound. The higher heat may increase tissue permeability to topically applied medicine, allowing it to be absorbed more easily. However, the driving force of phonophoresis more probably results from the mechanical pressure wave. Current studies have failed to reproduce the penetrative capabilities previously claimed.[11]

Stress Fracture Assessment

In 1986, Lowdon[36] reported a 92% accuracy rate in detecting stress fractures from soft-tissue lesions. Continuous-wave ultrasound at a frequency of 0.75 MHz was used at 0 to 2.0 W/cm^2. The intensity was increased gradually until the patient experienced a sensation. A positive sensation was described as a sharp needle or pinprick or pressure, bruising, or aching. The ultrasound results were compared with those for radiography and bone scintigraphy.

Precautions and Contraindications

Ultrasound is generally considered to be safe. Many of the deleterious effects associated with ultrasound were reported in studies that administered dosages beyond therapeutic ranges.[3,31,32] A stationary treatment technique, which is not recommended in clinical applications, was also frequently used.

Ultrasound is known to have potentially harmful effects. Because this potential harm exceeds any benefit that it might provide, ultrasound use is precluded over the uterus during pregnancy, over the eyes because of possible cataract formation, in thrombophlebitic conditions, and in peripheral vascular disease and hypesthesia, in which the thermal responses would not disperse or harmful intensities be apparent.

Also, ultrasound should not be used on immature epiphyses. There have been conflicting reports on the effects of ultrasound on unclosed epiphyses. Vaughen and Bender[51] concluded that ultrasound had no effect on the integrity or closure time of epiphyses in rabbits. Elmer and Fleischer[21] found no statistically significant increase in growth of in vitro mouse tibias after three ultrasound treatments at 1.8 W/cm^2 for five minutes each. There was an increased uptake of marked proline into the protein of cartilaginous epiphyses. However, De Forest and associates[12] reported increased chondroblast activity that resulted in widening, slipping, and fracturing of upper tibial epiphyses in rabbits after insonation. He used 5 to 10 W of ultrasound although the exact dosage was difficult to ascertain.

Ultrasound should not be used on bony prominences. Because of the high absorption of ultrasound in bone and the tissue interface with impedance differences, a significant heating effect occurs in superficial bone and the periosteum. There are reports of periosteal damage, marrow destruction, and cortical necrosis with higher dosages in the therapeutic range.[32] Dosages in excess of 1.5 W/cm^2 over superficial bone require caution. The stationary technique of ultrasound application should not be used because blood stasis from blood cell aggregation has been reported with this technique.[5,6] If circulation and sensation are adequate and safe therapeutic dosages are administered, the thermal increases should be dissipated.

Ultrasound over the brain and spine, especially after laminectomy, should be avoided. Histologic changes were found in the spinal cords of rats after ultrasound, although no functional compromise resulted.[3] Other concerns with insonation over the central nervous system include the increased possibility of cavitation over fluid-filled cavities and the risk of vascular compromise of the cord or meninges.[29]

Ultrasound should not be used over reproductive organs, the heart, or pacemakers; over the stellate ganglion or vagus nerve in advanced heart disease; in acute infections; or over malignancies because of the increased risk of metastases.

References

1. Abramson DI, Burnett C, Bell Y, et al: Changes in blood flow, oxygen uptake and tissue temperatures produced by therapeutic physical agents: I. Effects of ultrasound. *Am J Phys Med* 1960;39:51–62.
2. Anderson DW, Barrett JT: Ultrasound: A new immunosuppressant. *Clin Immunol Immunopathol* 1979;14:18–29.
3. Anderson TP, Wakim KG, Herrick JF, et al: An experimental study of the effects of ultrasonic energy on the lower part of the spinal cord and peripheral nerves. *Arch Phys Med Rehabil* 1951;32:71–83.
4. Antich TJ: Phonophoresis: The principles of the ultrasonic driving force and efficiency in the treatment of common orthopaedic diagnoses. *J Orthop Sports Phys Ther* 1982;4:99–102.
5. Ardan NI Jr, Janes JM, Herrick JF: Ultrasonic energy and surgically produced defects in bone. *J Bone Joint Surg* 1957;39A:394–402.
6. Barth G, Wachsmann F: Biological basis for ultrasonic therapy, in Pohlman R (ed): *Ultrasound Therapy*. Stuttgart, Georg Thieme Verlag, 1949, p 162.
7. Bekhome AK: Reaktsiia leĭkergii u bol'nykh khronicheskim tonzillitom do i posle ul'trazvukovoĭ terapiio [Leukergia reaction in patients suffering from chronic tonsillitis before and after ultrasound therapy]. *Vestn Otorinolaringol* 1977;4:62–65.
8. Bierman W: Ultrasound in the treatment of scars. *Arch Phys Med Rehabil* 1954;35:209–214.
9. Carstensen EL: Mechanism of absorption of ultrasound in biologic materials. *IRE Trans Med Electrol* 1960;7:158–165.
10. Currier DP, Greathouse D, Swift T: Sensory nerve conduction: Effect of ultrasound. *Arch Phys Med Rehabil* 1978;59:181–185.

11. Davick JP, Martin RK, Albright JP: Distribution and deposition of tritiated cortisol using phonophoresis. *Phys Ther* 1988;68:1672–1675.
12. De Forest RE, Herrick JF, Janes JM, et al: Effects of ultrasound on growing bone: An experimental study. *Arch Phys Med Rehabil* 1953;34:21–30.
13. Downing D, Weinstein A: Ultrasound therapy of subacromial bursitis: A double-blind study, abstract. *Arthritis Rheum* 1983;26(suppl):S87.
14. Duarte LR: The stimulation of bone growth by ultrasound. *Arch Orthop Trauma Surg* 1983;101:151–159.
15. Dyson M: Mechanisms involved in therapeutic ultrasound. *Physiotherapy* 1987;73:116–120.
16. Dyson M, Brookes M: Stimulation of bone repair by ultrasound, in Lerski RA, Morley P (eds): *Proceedings of the Third Meeting of the World Federation of Ultrasound in Medicine and Biology.* Oxford, Pergamon Press, 1983, pp 61–66.
17. Dyson M, Pond JB, Joseph J, et al: The stimulation of tissue regeneration by means of ultrasound. *Clin Sci* 1968;35:273–285.
18. Dyson M, Pond JB, Woodward B, et al: The production of blood cell stasis and endothelial damage in the blood vessels of chick embryos treated with ultrasound in a stationary wave field. *Ultrasound Med Biol* 1974;1:133–148.
19. Dyson M, Suckling J: Stimulation of tissue repair by ultrasound: A survey of the mechanisms involved. *Physiotherapy* 1978;64:105–108.
20. Echternach JL: Ultrasound: An adjunct treatment for shoulder disabilities. *Phys Ther* 1965;45:865–869.
21. Elmer WA, Fleischer AC: Enhancement of DNA synthesis in neonatal mouse tibia after exposure to ultrasound. *J Clin Ultrasound* 1975;2:191–195.
22. Farmer WC: Effect of intensity of ultrasound on conduction of motor axons. *Phys Ther* 1968;48:1233–1237.
23. Flax HJ: Ultrasound treatment of peritendinitis calcarea of the shoulder. *Am J Phys Med* 1964;43:117–124.
24. Frieder S, Weisberg J, Fleming B, et al: A pilot study: The therapeutic effect of ultrasound following partial rupture of the Achilles tendons in male rats. *J Orthop Sports Phys Ther* 1988;10:39–46.
25. Goddard DH, Revell PA, Cason J, et al: Ultrasound has no anti-inflammatory effect. *Ann Rheum Dis* 1983;42:582–584.
26. Griffin JE, Echternach JL, Price RE, et al: Patients treated with ultrasonic driven hydrocortisone and with ultrasound alone. *Phys Ther* 1967;47:594–601.
27. Halle JS, Scoville CR, Greathouse DG: Ultrasound's effect on the conduction latency of the superficial radial nerve in man. *Phys Ther* 1981;61:345–350.
28. Harvey W, Dyson M, Pond JB, et al: The in vitro stimulation of protein synthesis in human fibroblasts by therapeutic levels of ultrasound, in de Vlieger M, Kazner E, Muller HR, et al (eds): *Proceedings of the Second European Congress on Ultrasonics in Medicine.* Amsterdam, Excerpta Medica, 1975, pp 10–21.
29. Herrick JF: Temperatures produced in tissue by ultrasound: Experimental study using various technics. *J Acoust Soc Am* 1953;25:12–16.
30. Hogan RD, Franklin TD, Avery KS, et al: Microvascular responses to ultrasound in normal, ischemic and denervated skeletal muscle. Presented at the 26th Annual Convention of the American Institute of Ultrasound Medicine, Las Vegas, March 1981.
31. Kolář J, Babický A, Káclová J, et al: Influence of ultrasound on bone mineral metabolism. *Nature* 1964;202:411–412.

32. Kolář J, Babický A, Káclová J, et al: The effect of ultrasound on the mineral metabolism in bones. *Orthop Traumatol Protez* 1965;26:43–51.
33. Lehmann JF: Ultrasound and therapy, in Licht S, Kamenetz HL (eds): *Therapeutic Heat and Cold*, ed 2. Baltimore, Waverley Press, 1965, pp 321–386.
34. Lehmann JF, de Lateur BJ: Diathermy and superficial heat and cold therapy, in Kottke FJ, Stillwell GK, Lehmann JF (eds): *Krusen's Handbook of Physical Medicine and Rehabilitation*, ed 3. Philadelphia, WB Saunders, 1982, pp 275–350.
35. Lehmann JF, Guy AW: Ultrasonic therapy, in Reid JM, Silov MR (eds): *Interaction of Ultrasound and Biological Tissues*. DHE Publication (FDA) BRH/DBE, 1972.
36. Lowdon A: Application of ultrasound to assess stress fractures. *Physiotherapy* 1986;72:160–161.
37. McDiarmid T, Burns PN: Clinical applications of therapeutic ultrasound. *Physiotherapy* 1987;73:155–162.
38. McDiarmid T, Burns PN, Lewith T, et al: Ultrasound and the treatment of pressure sores. *Physiotherapy* 1985;71:66–70.
39. Patrick MK: Applications of therapeutic pulsed ultrasound. *Physiotherapy* 1978;64:103–104.
40. Patrick MK: Ultrasonic therapy: Has it a place in the 70s? *Physiotherapy* 1973;59:282–283.
41. Paul BJ, Lafratta CW, Dawson AR, et al: Use of ultrasound in the treatment of pressure sores in patients with spinal cord injury. *Arch Phys Med* 1960;41:438–440.
42. Payton OD, Lamb RL, Kasey ME: Effects of therapeutic ultrasound on bone marrow in dogs. *Phys Ther* 1975;55:20–27.
43. Roberts M, Rutherford JH, Harris D: The effect of ultrasound on flexor tendon repairs in the rabbit. *Hand* 1982;14:17–20.
44. Roche C, West J: A controlled trial investigating the effect of ultrasound on venous ulcers referred from general practitioners. *Physiotherapy* 1984;70:475–477.
45. Rubin D, Kuitert JH: Use of ultrasonic vibration in the treatment of pain arising from phantom limbs, scars and neuromas: A preliminary report. *Arch Phys Med Rehabil* 1955;36:445–452.
46. Saad AH, Williams AR: Effects of therapeutic ultrasound on clearance rate of blood borne colloidal particles in vivo. *Br J Cancer* 1982;45(suppl):202–205.
47. Snow CJ, Johnson KA: Effect of therapeutic ultrasound on acute inflammation. *Physiotherapy Can* 1988;40:162–167.
48. Stuhlfauth K: Neural effects of ultrasonic waves. *Br J Phys Med* 1952;15:10–14.
49. Takagi SF, Higashino S, Shibuya T, et al: The actions of ultrasound on the myelinated nerve, the spinal cord and the brain. *Jap J Physiol* 1960;10:183–193.
50. ter Haar G, Wyard SJ: Blood cell banding in ultrasonic standing wave fields: A physical analysis. *Ultrasound Med Biol* 1978;4:111–123.
51. Vaughen JL, Bender LF: Effects of ultrasound on growing bone. *Arch Phys Med Rehabil* 1959;40:158–160.
52. Ziskin MC, Michlovitz SL: Therapeutic ultrasound, in Michlovitz SL (ed): *Thermal Agents in Rehabilitation*. Philadelphia, FA Davis, 1986, pp 161–162.

Chapter 32

High-Voltage Pulsed Galvanic Stimulation as a Modifier of Sports-Induced Inflammation

William S. Quillen, PhD, PT, SCS
Thomas M. Mohr, PhD, PT
Brian V. Reed, PhD, PT

Introduction

Electrical stimulation has been promoted and used in sports medicine to treat both acute and chronic musculoskeletal injuries and related symptoms. There is considerable anecdotal and empiric support for the use of stimulation to modify inflammation. There are, however, few relevant scientific studies demonstrating phenomenologic relationships or causative mechanisms.

The effects of electrical stimulation on the inflammatory cascade may result from either direct or reflexive effects on pain sensation or transmission, blood flow (macrocirculation and microcirculation), or fluid dynamics. A scientifically supportable mechanism has yet to be identified.

Thus, although high-voltage, pulsed galvanic stimulators (HVPGSs) are commonly used in sports medicine, their mechanism of action as a modifier of sports-induced inflammation remains at best speculative. Further research using validated physiologic models is necessary.

Historical Overview

Electricity has been used in medicine since Roman times. The physician Scribonius Largus used electric eels, rays, and torpedo fish to treat headache and gout.[8] By 1768, both the voltaic pile (battery) and the hand-cranked faradic generator had been developed.[8] This freed medical practitioners from reliance on naturally occurring sources of electricity. Physicians then attempted to use electricity to treat a variety of ailments, including acute and chronic musculoskeletal dysfunctions.

Electrotherapy flourished in the late 19th and early 20th centuries. Gottschalk,[9] expressing the conventional wisdom at the time, noted "there is probably no one agent at the physician's command by which so much good can be accomplished as by a skillfully handled static machine."[9] Nonetheless, the general lack of scientific evidence supporting the therapeutic benefits of electrotherapy and the aura of charlatanism that surrounded some practitioners[8] led to a general decline in its use after the turn of the century. New interest has been aroused in the last 15 years. Electrical stimulation devices of various types are now standard in most sports medicine clinics in the United States.

Traditional "medical galvanism" was associated for more than a century with the treatment of denervated muscle and the performance of iontophoresis. The low-voltage, direct-current generator (LVDCG) used produced a long-duration (>300 ms), rectangular waveform with a high average current flow. HVPGSs developed as an offshoot of research conducted at the Bell Telephone Laboratories in the late 1940s.[15] HVPGSs have been in clinical use for more than 35 years, and their popularity peaked in the last decade. Whether these units should be called "galvanic" is problematic. Although they produce a monophasic pulsatile current, the HVPGS waveform is radically different (primarily in duration) and produces distinctly different physiologic responses and potential effects.

This chapter focuses on HVPGSs because of their widespread popularity and use in sports medicine facilities. Indeed, special sections on HVPGSs have been added to several standard electrotherapy textbooks,[15,22] and at least one text[2] on their use has been published.

HVPGSs are electrical stimulation units with an output of more than 100 to 150 V, and a pulsatile, monophasic waveform (often twin-peaked) that is 5 to 100 μs in duration. The short pulse and the high voltage dramatically reduce skin resistance to current flow, thus allowing a potentially unlimited depth of penetration. Most HVPGSs incorporate a long interpulse interval into the microsecond pulse duration and allow frequency modulation of the current generated.

The FDA has a list of "approved" applications for all electrotherapy equipment. HVPGSs can be used for temporarily relaxing muscle spasms, preventing or retarding disuse atrophy, increasing local blood circulation, reeducating muscles atrophied from disuse, preventing postsurgical phlebothrombosis through stimulation of calf muscles, and maintaining or increasing range of motion.

Other popular uses of HVPGSs, as suggested by Alon and DeDomenico,[2] include reducing edema and enhancing wound healing. Until recently, these uses were based primarily on anecdotal case studies or empiric observations of small clinical series. However, a small number of phenomenological studies[13,14,18] and well-controlled clinical trials[7] are now available.

Biologic Effects of Electrotherapeutic Currents

An electrical current passing through biologic tissues may produce thermal, chemical, or physical effects. These may be directly mediated or initiate a reflexive response. These effects occur at a cellular level, although under certain conditions they may directly affect tissue structures. To effect these responses, sufficient, but not excessive, pulse charge energy must be delivered to the cell or tissue as described by the Arndt-Schultz principle.[10]

An HVPGS, with its short pulse and low average current flow, produces negligible electrical to thermal conversion[2] under Joule's law ($H = 0.24\ I^2\ Rt$, where H is the amount of heat production, I is the total current intensity, R is the resistance, and T is the duration of current flow).

Electrochemical effects occur at both cellular and tissue levels. The unidirectional flow of an LVDCG redistributes sodium ions beneath the anode and chloride ions beneath the cathode of a circuit. This results in an alkali accumulation beneath the negative pole and the formation of an acidic reaction under the positive pole. Unlike traditional LVDCG, the HVPGS causes no measurable changes in tissue pH.[16] The most important cellular electrochemical changes involve enhancement enzyme activity. Cheng and associates[4] demonstrated enhanced formation of adenosine triphosphate from mitochondrial-membrane-bound H^+ adenosine triphosphatase and adenosine diphosphate. The external energy of appropriately configured electrotherapy currents may augment the energy replenishment process for cellular metabolism.

Electrophysical effects do not change the molecular configuration of ions. Rather, the electrical pulse charge may cause ions or other nondissociated molecules such as proteins or lipoproteins to move.[2,10] The excitation of a peripheral nerve is a classic example. An adequate electrical current moves sodium and potassium ions across membranes, producing an action potential and subsequent indirect effects. The movement of other ions, free amino acids, and proteins in the presence of current flow is termed cataphoresis and may further alter concentration gradients to trigger local and remote responses.[2]

The exact physiologic mechanisms by which an HVPGS directly or reflexively affects the inflammatory cascade have not been conclusively identified in a controlled in vivo model. There is little evidence to indicate that HVPGSs affect biologic tissues in any unique or special way.

Theoretically, the presence of even the smallest pulse charges from an electrical current can attract or repel charged ions, proteins, or other cellular debris in the interstitium during the inflammatory cascade. Indirect activation of segmental and systemic mechanisms, such as local chemical mediators or the autonomic nervous system, may alter permeability, circulation, and reabsorption of edema and effusions. Therefore, the extrapolation of thermal, chemical, and physical mechanisms identified in vitro to in vivo models remains speculative.

Scientific Studies

Studies using electrical stimulation to alter blood flow in human subjects are few. Wakim and associates[21] reported that percutaneous stimulation increased mean blood flow more than 80% in normal individuals. Currier[5] reported significant increases in blood flow at the popliteal artery after intermittent stimulation of the gastrocnemius muscle. Dooley and Kasprak[6] found that transcutaneous or implanted electrode stimulation of the spinal cord or selected nerve roots resulted in peripheral vasodilation.

Edema and effusion secondary to tissue trauma may result from direct microvessel trauma or increased permeability to plasma proteins induced by the chemical mediators histamine and bradykinin. The HVPGS, either alone or in conjunction with cryotherapy, has been advocated for treatment of acute edema.[3,12,17,20] No well-controlled scientific evidence supported these claims until Reed's study was published in 1988.[18]

Reed postulated that HVPGSs reduced microvessel permeability to plasma proteins, thus limiting the further development of preexisting edema. Using the microvasculature of the hamster cheek pouch, he simulated an acute in vivo inflammatory response with a histamine superfusion.

Intravenous fluorescein-labeled dextran (150 kd) served as a tracer of plasma proteins under fluorescence microscopy. Protein leaks from the microvessels were quantified every five minutes for a 25-minute baseline period and again after a five-minute superfusion with histamine (10^{-5} mol/L). The HVPGS was applied to the vascular bed of the animals in a standard clinical fashion in doses of 0, 10, 30, or 50 V at the time of the histamine superfusion. Histamine increased microvessel leakiness in all four groups. However, animals that received either a 30-V or a 50-V dose had significantly fewer leaks than the other two groups. No alterations in microvessel blood flow were observed.

Reed could not identify a specific mechanism responsible for the reduced permeability. The fluorescein-dextran efflux used in the study was electrically neutral, so the results could not be explained by charge repulsion. Altered lymphatic activity could not explain the results because the cheek pouch has no lymphatic network.[11] Athough no alterations in microvessel blood flow were observed, leakiness may have been indirectly affected by this factor. Tyml and associates[19] observed transient flow stasis in the capillaries of frog skin in response to an applied electrical current. Possibly the HVPGS constricts arterioles and terminal arterioles, thus decreasing microvessel flow and reducing leakiness. Decreased microvessel pore size could also have restricted the efflux of proteins and fluorescein-dextran. This model investigated the potential effects of the HVPGS on one mechanism of edema, but the actual physiologic mediators are still undetermined.

Mohr and associates[13,14] studied the effect of the HVPGS on edema reduction and blood flow in rat paws. Paw volumes were measured before trauma and at 24, 48, 72, and 96 hours after the trauma. In the treatment group, paw volumes were also measured before and after treatment. A standard dose of 40 V was applied for 20 minutes. Animals in both groups had significantly decreased paw volume over time, but there was no significant difference between the two groups in the amount of edema reduction. The treatment group did have lower mean paw volumes than the control group during the treatment period.

Mohr and associates[14] also assessed the effect of the HVPGS on blood flow velocity in the rat hind limb in response to four different pulse rates (2, 20, 80, and 120 pulses per second). Flow was also measured in the unstimulated limb. All four pulse rates increased blood flow (measured at the femoral artery), with the most significant increases occurring at 20 pulses per second. The increase began within the first minute of stimulation and persisted for as long as 14 minutes. Blood flow velocity also increased as voltage intensity increased. This response was local rather than systemic because the velocity in the unstimulated hind limb did not change.

HVPGSs used to ameliorate edema from the inflammatory cascade reduce fluid loss to the interstitium and increase lymphatic flow and circulation after capillary bed repair. Theoretically, the mechanisms demonstrated by Reed[18] and Mohr and associates[13,14] should facilitate resolution of edema. The correct timing of the intervention and the threshold dose necessary to evoke an appropriate response remain to be determined.

References

1. Alon G: *High Voltage Stimulation.* Chattanooga, Chattonooga Corp, 1984.
2. Alon G, DeDomenico G: *High Voltage Stimulation: An Integrated Approach to Clinical Electrotherapy.* Chattanooga, Chattanooga Corp, 1987.
3. Brown S: Ankle edema and galvanic muscle stimulation. *Phys Sportsmed* 1981;9:137.
4. Cheng N, Van Hoof H, Bockx E, et al: The effects of electric currents on ATP generation, protein synthesis, and membrane transport of rat skin. *Clin Orthop* 1982;171:264–272.
5. Currier DP: Electrical stimulation effect on localized blood flow, abstract. *Phys Ther* 1983;63:761.
6. Dooley DM, Kasprak M: Modification of blood flow to the extremities by electrical stimulation of the nervous system. *South Med J* 1976;69:1309–1311.
7. Feedar JA, Kloth LC: Acceleration of wound healing with high voltage pulsating direct current, abstract. *Phys Ther* 1985;65:741.
8. Geddes LA: A short history of the electrical stimulation of excitable tissue including electrotherapeutic applications. *Physiologist* 1984;27(suppl):S15–S47.
9. Gottschalk FB: *Static Electricity, Xray and Electrovibration.* Chicago, T Eisele, 1903.
10. Griffin JE, Karselis TC: *Physical Agents for Physical Therapists.* Springfield, Charles C Thomas, 1978.
11. Ladd MP, Kottke FJ, Blanchard RS: Studies of the effect of massage on the flow of lymph from the foreleg of the dog. *Arch Phys Med* 1952;33:604–612.
12. Lamboni P, Harris B: The use of ice, airsplints and high voltage galvanic stimulation in effusion reduction. *Athlet Train* 1983;18:23.
13. Mohr TM, Akers TK, Landry RG: Effect of high voltage stimulation on edema reduction in the rat hind limb. *Phys Ther* 1987;67:1703–1707.
14. Mohr TM, Akers TK, Wessman HC: Effect of high voltage stimulation on blood flow in the rat hind limb. *Phys Ther* 1987;67:526–533.

15. Nelson RM, Currier DP (eds): *Clinical Electrotherapy*. Norwalk, Appleton & Lange, 1987.
16. Newton RA, Karselis TC: Skin pH following high voltage pulsed galvanic stimulation. *Phys Ther* 1983;63:1593–1596.
17. Ralston DJ: High voltage galvanic stimulation: Can there be a state of the art? *Athlet Train* 1985;20:291–293.
18. Reed BV: Effect of high voltage pulsed electrical stimulation on microvascular permeability to plasma proteins: A possible mechanism in minimizing edema. *Phys Ther* 1988;68:491–495.
19. Tyml K, Weigelt H, Schäfer D: Are endothelial cells rich in filaments involved in the phenomenon of electrically induced stoppages of flow in frog capillaries? *Int J Microcirc Clin Exp* 1985;4:121–130.
20. Voight ML: Reduction of post traumatic ankle edema with high voltage pulsed galvanic stimulation. *Athlet Train* 1984;19:278–311.
21. Wakim KG, Terrier JC, Elkins EC, et al: Effects of percutaneous stimulation of the circulation in normal and in paralyzed lower extremities. *Am J Physiol* 1948;153:183–189.
22. Wolf SL (ed): *Electrotherapy*. New York, Churchill Livingstone, 1981.

Chapter 33

Low-Energy Laser Therapy

Jeffrey R. Basford, MD, PhD

Introduction

Low-energy laser therapy may be a safe and effective treatment for a variety of soft-tissue, neurologic, and musculoskeletal conditions. It has been accepted in many parts of the world, but has not yet been approved by the Food and Drug Administration for clinical use. This chapter reviews the scientific basis and potential importance of this treatment.

Interest in laser radiation as a stimulative agent, rather than merely as a destructive one, began in the 1960s when alterations in cell function and wound healing after irradiation were reported. Additional work confirmed these findings, and research continues. Although there is still some controversy, many published studies report that laser radiation (as well as monochromatic radiation from noncoherent sources) can stimulate the metabolic and proliferative processes of cells. Investigations in animals and humans are more difficult to interpret but also often support stimulative effects.

Studies dealing specifically with inflammation and soft-tissue injury (other than wounds) are rare. However, cell studies and clinical trials suggest potential tissue-repair and anti-inflammatory effects. Although there may be important clinical applications of low-energy laser therapy, its usefulness for treating soft-tissue injury and inflammation remains unclear.

Background

Light has been a part of medical treatment for thousands of years. The ancient Greeks used sunlight to treat arthritis, jaundice, malnutrition, and parasites.[39] In Italy during the Middle Ages, sunlight was part of the quarantine process for the plague. In the 18th and 19th centuries, sunlight and its components, such as ultraviolet light, were used to treat rickets and tuberculosis.[39] Today, although little emphasized in medicine, light is still used in treating psoriasis and neonatal hyperbilirubinemia.

Table 1 Reported cellular effects after low-energy laser irradiation*

Phenomenon	Change	Model	Laser
Adenosine triphosphate synthesis[37,54]	Increase	Rat liver mitochondria	Helium-neon
Bacterial phage growth[67]	Increase	*Escherichia coli*	Helium-neon
Bacterial proliferation[13]	Increase	*E coli*	Argon
	Decrease	*Staphylococcus aureus*	Argon
Cell binding affinities[37,55]	Increase	Human lymphocytes and fibroblasts	Helium-neon
Cell granule release[68]	Increase	Mouse mast cells	Helium-neon
Cell motility[60]	Increase	Human sperm	Krypton
Collagen and protein synthesis[4,19,28,43,49,63]	Increase	Human fibroblasts	Helium-neon
	Increase	Rabbit skin	Helium-neon plus gallium-arsenide
	Decrease	Human synovium	Neodymium-PO_4 glass
	Decrease	Bovine cartilage	Neodymium-YAG
Intercellular matrix[73]	Increase	Mouse retina	Helium-neon
Mammalian cell proliferation[1,26,34]	Increase	Mouse fibroblasts	Ruby
	Decrease	Human lymphocytes	Helium-neon
Membrane potential[37,53,54]	Increase	Rat liver mitochondria	Helium-neon
	Increase	Human fibroblasts	Helium-neon
Neurotransmitter release[69]	Increase	Acetylcholine (guinea pigs)	Ruby
Oxyhemoglobin dissociation[30]	Increase	——	——
Phagocytosis[48]	Increase	Human lymphocytes	Ruby
Prostaglandin synthesis[49]	Increase	Rat skin	Helium-neon
RNA synthesis[19]	Increase	Mouse skin	Helium-neon

* Adapted from Basford[5]

The nondestructive, stimulative effect of laser irradiation was first described in the 1960s by investigators who found alterations in cell function and wound healing that could not be explained on the basis of heating. These first reports were often sketchily presented in obscure European and Russian journals—a situation that resulted in heightened skepticism and delayed knowledge of this work in the West. Later results, however, encouraged further investigation. Laser therapy has gained increasing acceptance and is now readily available in many parts of the world.

Laser therapy in the United States is restricted by the FDA's insistence that low-energy lasers are new therapeutic "devices" that must be reviewed before being approved as "safe and effective" for human use. One laser was presented to an FDA panel as an adjunctive treatment for rheumatoid arthritis. The presentation was unsuccessful, but additional trials are planned or under way. Even if these new trials are successful, however, it is unlikely that any device will gain approval in the next two or three years.

Nevertheless, there is considerable interest in low-energy lasers, supported by reports from the United States and overseas (Table 1 and Outline 1). Although lasers have FDA sanction for human treatment only as part of an investigational protocol, some people are using lasers to treat themselves or others for various athletic, dance, and musculoskeletal injuries.

Outline 1 Conditions in which low-energy laser therapy is reportedly effective

Ankylosing spondylitis
Dental disease
Edema
Musculoskeletal pain
Neuropathy
Osteoarthritis
Peyronie's disease
Radiculopathy
Rheumatoid arthritis
Sjögren's syndrome
Tendinitis
Trigeminal neuralgia
Vascular headaches
Wound healing

This chapter examines the current and potential significance of laser irradiation for treating soft-tissue injury and inflammation.

Scientific Basis of Laser Therapy

Two obvious questions about laser stimulation must be addressed. First, can sufficient radiation penetrate to the depths necessary for clinical effectiveness? Second, if penetration does occur, what is the mechanism of action? The first question can be answered by examining the optical properties of the soft-tissues. The second question is more difficult to answer, but some information is available.

The transmission of light through tissue is a complex function of tissue structure, wavelength, and pigmentation. Several definite facts are known. There is an optical "window" of sorts for skin and many soft tissues. This window admits light in the portion of the spectrum from about 0.6 to 1.0 or 1.3 μ,[14,25] a region that includes most of the low-energy lasers in use (Outline 2). In addition, longer wavelengths tend to penetrate soft tissue more easily than shorter wavelengths, although results vary depending on the specific tissue being examined.[14,25] Thus, for example, a 0.7-μ beam loses about 37% (1/e) of its initial intensity at a depth of 0.75 mm, whereas a longer 1.2-μ wavelength beam penetrates about 2.2 mm before decreasing to the same amount.[2,35] Although these decreases are precipitous, many of the effects outlined in Table 1 are reported at intensities as low as 1 mW/cm^2 and energy densities as low as 1 mJ/cm^2.[34] Typical treatments have probe-tip intensities of 50 mW/cm^2 or more and energy densities of 1 to 4 J/cm^2. This is sufficient energy to produce effects at depths of 0.5 to 2.0 cm. For example, 1% of a beam in the 0.6- to 0.85-μ portion of the spectrum can penetrate the chest wall[2] and a 1-mW helium-neon laser can transilluminate a finger. Thus, if low-energy laser does have any effects, they should occur in tissues within a centimeter or two of the skin's surface. Treatment effectiveness at greater depths seems progressively more problematic.

The central tenet of low-energy laser therapy is that stimulation is

Outline 2 Common characteristics of low-energy lasers*

Laser types
- Argon (0.476 to 0.514 μ)
- Gallium-aluminum arsenide (0.904 μ)
- Gallium-arsenide (0.840 μ)
- Helium-neon (0.633 μ)
- Krypton (0.476 to 0.647 μ)
- Ruby (0.694 μ)

Modes of operation
- Continuous wave
- Pulsed (typically 10 to 5,000 pulses per second)
- Q-switched (nanosecond pulses)

Techniques
- Acupuncture
- Irradiation of multiple points in a grid pattern
- Irradiation of nerves proximal to treated area
- Scanning over treated area

* Power, <1 to 50 mW.

produced by nonthermal photobiologic reactions and occurs in the absence of significant temperature increases. This means that laser powers and treatment energies are restricted to ranges of 50 mW or less and 1 to 4 J or less where both measurements[10,21,42,69] and simple calculations confirm that temperature increases after treatment are routinely 0.5 C or less. (By comparison, therapeutic ultrasound and shortwave diathermy easily increase tissue temperatures 4 C or 5 C.[38])

It must be remembered that there are other physical agents that do not depend on thermal effects. For example, electrical stimulation has a nonthermal basis, and natural processes such as photosynthesis, vision, and plant growth have photobiologic origins.

Mechanism of Action

Initially, potential mechanisms of action for laser therapy were based on the specific properties of laser radiation—coherency, collimation, and monochromaticity. Although there is still interest in mechanisms based on coherency,[22] experiments with noncoherent sources[34] and the realization that coherency is rapidly lost in tissue have lessened the emphasis on this explanation. Collimation is difficult to accept as a mechanism because successful laser stimulation has been reported in experiments that used lenses to expand laser beams over broad areas. Monochromaticity, at specific biologically active frequencies, has strong support.[34] Thus, lasers may serve as intense, but not unique, sources of stimulating energy.

The location of laser-induced stimulation in a cell is not known; it may be that different reactions occur in different cells at different wavelengths. However, work with bacteria, yeast, human cells,[34,67] and cell organelles such as mitochrondria[54] implicates the respiratory chain as a point of action. Respiratory chain components and flavoproteins may be absorbers that interact resonantly with light at specific frequencies.[67] This mechanism is attractive because it may explain why lasers of different wavelengths differ in effectiveness. For example, absorption and penetration values that depend on wavelength (frequency) provide some support for a widely held belief that visible irradiation (eg, helium-neon) may be more effective for wound healing, whereas infrared radiation may be more effective for inflammation modification.

Research Findings

Research evaluation is complicated by the multitude of experimental models, lasers, dosages, and treatment schedules reported (Table 1 and Outline 2). In addition, research quality has been variable and, until recently, well-designed, controlled studies have been relatively rare. Fortunately, the situation has improved, and evaluation should become easier in the next few years. For now, stimulation effects seem best established on the cellular level. Findings are harder to replicate and controversy is magnified as more complex tissue, animal, and human models are studied.

Cell Studies

Changes in cellular processes such as proliferation, DNA synthesis, protein metabolism, enzyme production, and respiratory function are routinely reported after irradiation with laser and nonlaser monochromatic light (Table 1). Even though the evidence seems almost overwhelming, not all investigators have found effects.[18,24,50] This dichotomy cannot be attributed merely to error; much of the confusion may result from the use of different techniques and models.

Tissue, Animal, and Human Studies

Tissue, animal, and human studies are more difficult to interpret than cellular investigations. Nevertheless, a variety of neurologic, pain, musculoskeletal, and wound-healing effects have been reported.

Neurologic Function Although reports are not unanimous, a number of morphologic and physiologic changes have been reported after low-energy irradiation of both intact and injured nervous tissue. For example, low-power ($<$20-mW) helium-neon laser irradiation is reported to speed healing and preserve action potentials in the peripheral (sciatic nerve) and central (optic nerve) nervous system tissue of experimentally injured rats and dogs.[41,57–59,61] Research on humans is more restricted, but some investigators have found that irradiation slows conduction, produces action potentials, has possible effects on the sympathetic nervous system, and inhibits clonus.[9,64,70,71] Other investigations have found no effects.[21,72]

Pain Studies of nocioception, pain, and analgesia have also had mixed results. Large, frequently uncontrolled studies involving as many as 2,500 subjects have found improvement in 60% to more than 80% of those treated for neuropathy, osteoarthritis, and headache.[27,36,62] Other studies, often smaller but better controlled, found little or no benefit in treating lateral epicondylitis,[42] osteoarthritis of the thumb[7] or knees,[46] and carpal tunnel syndrome.[74]

Soft-Tissue Injury Wound healing was one of the first areas of investigation[16,47] and is still an active area of study. Experimental evaluation remains hampered by the different lasers, techniques, and models studied. Accelerated wound healing (particularly in the early phases) is frequently reported in rabbits and rodents after irradiation with coherent or noncoherent monochromatic light.[23,33,56,63] Experiments on pigs, whose skin is similar to that of humans, appear less encouraging and show lesser or no benefits from treatment.[6,29,32,66]

Even when an increase in the healing rate or strength of a wound is found, it may have limited significance in the overall healing process because it often occurs only in the earliest stages of healing. Species effects may also be important. Small, loose-skinned animals, such as rabbits and rodents, may be more responsive to laser stimulation than swine or humans. Health may also be important. Irradiation may do little to accelerate healing in a healthy animal, but may be beneficial in a metabolically impaired situation.

The clinical usefulness of laser therapy for wound healing is unsettled. Nevertheless, studies and laboratory findings suggest increased procollagen production[19] and increased wound strength. Irradiation may also shift the hemoglobin-oxygen dissociation curve so that oxygen is released more easily in ischemic tissue.[30] Laser stimulation may also stimulate lymphatic vessel growth,[40] lessen edema, and accelerate healing.

Inflammation Few studies have directly investigated the effect of low-energy laser irradiation on inflammation. Nevertheless, inferences can be drawn from cell, animal, and human investigations, even though these studies may not have addressesd this problem directly. For example, prostaglandins are reported to increase in wounds after irradiation.[47] Changes in bacterial binding by lymphocytes,[53] increased phagocytosis,[19] and altered lymph[40] and blood flow have been reported. Changes reported in collagen synthesis after low-energy laser irradiation[1,19] also suggest that laser treatment may alter the course of inflammatory processes and soft-tissue healing.

Much attention and several controlled, clinical trials have focused on rheumatoid arthritis, in which inflammation and immune effects play important parts. Most of the studies report (alone or in some combination), diminished joint warmth, lessened joint circumferences, improved range of motion, and less need for medication after treatment with various visible and infrared lasers.[8,11,20,44,52,65] Additional studies of Sjögren's syndrome[15] and ankylosing spondylitis[17] show similarly encouraging results. However, these findings, even if statistically significant, may not be marked enough to justify laser use for rheumatoid disease, or for inflammation in general.

These investigations also attempted to isolate blood-borne inflammatory and immune-related products. Alterations in C-reactive protein, serum immune complexes, erythrocyte sedimentation rate, and leukocyte counts have been reported.[11,20,52] However, the alterations were not consistent[8] and may not be significant.

Safety Issues

Thermal injury is not an issue with low-power lasers, and safety concerns center on protecting the eye because of the sensitivity of the retina and the focusing ability of the cornea. Even a brief glance into a 1-mW helium-neon beam can cause a headache, and attenuating goggles should be worn by both the patient and the therapist during treatment. While infrared beams are not visible, they present the same risks and require the same precautions.

The issue of carcinogenicity has also been raised. Most, but not all, cell studies found limited or no neoplasm stimulation or mutagenesis.[3,12,31,45,51] Lasers are widely used in surgery and in everyday life (for example, as pointers and bar code scanners) with almost no adverse side effects.

References

1. Abergel RP, Dwyer RM, Neeker CA, et al: Laser treatment of keloids: A clinical trial and an in vitro study with Nd:YAG laser. *Lasers Surg Med* 1984;4:292.
2. Anderson RR, Parrish JA: The optics of humans skin. *J Invest Dermatol* 1981;77:13–19.
3. Apfelberg DB, Chadi B, Maser MR, et al: Study of carcinogenic effects of in vitro argon laser exposure of fibroblasts. *Plast Reconstr Surg* 1983;71:92–97.
4. Barabás K, Bakos J, Szábo DL, et al: "In vitro" effect of neodymium phosphate glass laser irradiation on the rheumatoid synovial membrane, abstract. *Lasers Surg Med* 1988;8:176.
5. Basford JR: Low-energy laser therapy: Controversies and new research findings. *Lasers Surg Med* 1989;9:1–5.
6. Basford JR, Hallman HO, Sheffield CG, et al: Comparison of cold-quartz ultraviolet, low-energy laser, and occlusion in wound healing in a swine model. *Arch Phys Med Rehabil* 1986;67:151–154.
7. Basford JR, Sheffield CG, Mair SD, et al: Low energy helium neon laser treatment of thumb osteoarthritis. *Arch Phys Med Rehabil* 1987;68:794–797.
8. Bliddal H, Hellesen C, Ditlevsen P, et al: Soft-laser therapy of rheumatoid arthritis. *Scand J Rheumatol* 1987;16:225–228.
9. Bork CE, Snyder-Mackler L: Effect of helium-neon laser irradiation on peripheral sensory nerve latency. *J Am Phys Ther Assoc* 1988;68:223.
10. Brunner R, Haina D, Landthaler M, et al: Application of laser light of low power density: Experimental and clinical investigations. *Curr Probl Dermatol* 1986;15:111–116.
11. Colov HC, Palmgren N, Jensen GF, et al: Convincing clinical improvement of rheumatoid arthritis by soft laser therapy, abstract. *Lasers Surg Med* 1987;7:77.

12. Dasdia T, Melloni E, Marchesini R, et al: A study to evaluate whether low watt laser irradiation can affect colony formation capability of human tumor cells in vitro, abstract. *Lasers Surg Med* 1988;8:177.
13. Dzinic M, Nanusevic O: Effects of low dose laser radiation on bacterial growth, in Waidelich W, Waidelich R (eds): *Laser Optoelectronics in Medicine.* Berlin, Springer-Verlag, 1988, pp 681–684.
14. Eichler J, Knof J, Lenz H: Measurements on the depth of penetration of light (0.35-1.0 microgram) in tissue. *Radiat Environm Biophys* 1977;14:239–242.
15. Frucuoso FJG, Moset JM: Estudio a doble ciego randomizado sobre los efectos bioestimulantes del laser de baja potencia (904 NM DE AS-GA, Biondo) en la irradiacion de glandula parotida en pacientes afectos de sindrome de Sjögren. *Bol Cent Doc Laser* 1987;13:4.
16. Gamaleja NF: Laser biomedical research in the USSR, in Wolbarsht ML (ed): *Laser Applications in Medicine and Biology.* New York, Plenum Press, 1977, p 1.
17. Gartner C, Becker M: Laser treatment of back pain and enthesiopathy in ankylosing spondylarthritis, in Waidelich W, Waidelich R (eds): *Laser Optoelectronics in Medicine.* Berlin, Springer-Verlag, 1988, pp 742–746.
18. Gfrorer A, Spahn J, Wagner WD, et al: Studies of laser-induced cell growth with yeast in continuous culture, in Waidelich W, Waidelich R (eds): *Laser Optoelectronics in Medicine.* Berlin, Springer-Verlag, 1988, pp 694–698.
19. Glassberg E, Lask GP, Uitto J: Biological effects of low energy laser irradiation, abstract. *Lasers Surg Med* 1988;8:186.
20. Goldman JA, Chiapella J, Casey H, et al: Laser therapy of rheumatoid arthritis. *Lasers Surg Med* 1980;1:93–101.
21. Greathouse DG, Currier DP, Gilmore RL: Effects of clinical infrared laser on superficial radial nerve conduction. *Phys Ther* 1985;65:1184–1187.
22. Greguss P: The concept of "biologon" and the influence of laser light on vital activities, in Waidelich W, Waidelich R (eds): *Laser Optoelectronics in Medicine.* Berlin, Springer-Verlag, 1988, pp 699–702.
23. Haina D, Brunner R, Lanthaler M, et al: Animal experiments in light-induced wound healing. *Laser Basic Biomed Res* 1982;22:1.
24. Hallman HO, Basford JR, O'Brien JF, et al: Does low-energy helium-neon laser irradiation alter "in vitro" replication of human fibroblasts? *Lasers Surg Med* 1988;8:125–129.
25. Hardy JD, Hammel HT, Murgatroyd D: Spectral transmittance and reflectance of excised human skin. *J Appl Physiol* 1956;9:257–264.
26. Hardy LB, Hardy FS, Fine S, et al: Effect of ruby laser radiation on mouse fibroblast culture, abstract. *Fed Proc* 1967;26:668.
27. Hasan P, Rijado A, Purnomo S, et al: Clinical experience of the Mix HeNe and IR low energy laser: A review of 404 cases, in Waidelich W, Waidelich R (eds): *Laser Optoelectronics in Medicine.* Berlin, Springer-Verlag, 1988, pp 736–741.
28. Herman JH, Khosla RC: *In vitro* effects of Nd:YAG laser radiation on cartilage metabolism. *J Rheumatol* 1988;15:1818–1826.
29. Hunter J, Leonard L, Wilson R, et al: Effects of low energy laser on wound healing in a porcine model. *Lasers Surg Med* 1984;3:285–290.
30. Itzkan I, Tang S, Bourgelais D: Laser wound healing can be explained by the photodissociation of oxyhemoglobin, abstract. *Lasers Surg Med* 1988;8:175.
31. Jamieson CW, Litwin MS, Longo SE, et al: Enhancement of melanoma cell culture growth rate by ruby laser radiation. *Life Sci* 1969;8:101–106.
32. Jongsma FHM, Bogaard AEJM, van Gemert MJC, et al: Is closure of open skin wound in rats accelerated by argon laser exposure? *Lasers Surg Med* 1983;3:75–80.

33. Kana JS, Hutschenreiter G, Haina D, et al: Effect of low-power density laser radiation on healing of open skin wounds in rats. *Arch Surg* 1981;116:293–296.
34. Karu TI: Photobiological fundamentals of low-power laser therapy. *IEEE J Quant Elect* 1987;QE-23:1703.
35. Kolari PJ: Penetration of unfocused laser light into the skin. *Arch Dermatol Res* 1985;277:342–344.
36. Kroetlinger M: On the use of the laser in acupuncture. *Int J Acupuncture Electrother Res* 1980;5:297–311.
37. Kubasova T, Kovács L, Somosy Z, et al: Biological effect of He-Ne laser: Investigations on functional and micromorphological alterations of cell membranes, in vitro. *Lasers Surg Med* 1984;4:381–388.
38. Lehmann JF, De Lateur BJ: Diathermy and superficial heat and cold therapy, in Kottke FJ, Stillwell GK, Lehmann JF (eds): *Krusen's Handbook of Physical Medicine and Rehabilitation.* Philadelphia, WB Saunders, 1982, pp 275–350.
39. Licht SH: History of ultraviolet therapy, in Licht SH (ed): *Therapeutic Electricity and Ultraviolet Radiation,* ed 4. Baltimore, Waverly Press, 1987, pp 191–211.
40. Lievens PC: The influence of laser on the lymphatic system, abstract. *Lasers Surg Med* 1988;8:175–176.
41. Lubart R, Rochkind S, Nissan M, et al: Investigations on different laser wavelengths and power in peripheral and central nervous systems, in Waidelich W, Waidelich R (eds): *Laser Optoelectronics in Medicine.* Berlin, Springer-Verlag, 1988, pp 763–765.
42. Lundeberg T, Haker E, Thomas M: Effect of laser versus placebo in tennis elbow. *Scand J Rehabil Med* 1987;19:135–138.
43. Lyons RF, Abergel RP, White RA, et al: Biostimulation of wound healing in vivo by a helium-neon laser. *Ann Plast Surg* 1987;18:47–50.
44. Mach ES, Tsurko VV, Lebedeva OI, et al: Kliniko-instrumental'naia otsenka lazernoĭ terapii revmatoidnogo artrita [Clinical and instrumental evaluation of the effect of laser therapy in patients with rheumatoid arthritis]. *Revmatologiia* 1983;3:36–39.
45. Marchesini R, Dasdia T, Melloni E, et al: Effect of low-energy laser irradiation on colony formation capability in different human tumor cells in vitro. *Lasers Surg Med* 1989;9:59–62.
46. McAuley R, Ysla R: Soft laser: A treatment for osteoarthritis of the knee? *Arch Phys Med Rehabil* 1985;66:553.
47. Mester A, Mester AF: Data for laser biostimulation in wound-healing, in Waidelich W, Waidelich R (eds): *Laser Optoelectronics in Medicine.* Berlin, Springer-Verlag, 1988, pp 731–735.
48. Mester E, Mester AF, Mester A: The biomedical effect of laser application. *Lasers Surg Med* 1985;5:31–39.
49. Mester E, Toth N, Mester A: The biostimulative effect of laserbeam. *Laser Basic Biomed Res* 1982;22:4.
50. Meyers AD, Joyce J, Cohen JJ: Effects of low-watt helium neon laser radiation on human lymphoctye cultures. *Lasers Surg Med* 1987;6:540–542.
51. Ming-Chien KAO, Jui-Chang TSAI, Teh-Cheng JOU, et al: Biological effects of low power laser irradiation on cultured C-6 glioma cells, abstract. *Lasers Surg Med* 1988;8:176.
52. Oyamada Y, Izu S: Application of low energy laser in chronic rheumatic arthritis and related rheumatoid diseases. Presented at the meeting of the International Society for Lasers in Surgery and Medicine, Tel Aviv, 1985.
53. Passarella S: The effect of helium-neon laser irradiation on structure and function of isolated mitochrondria in vitro. Presented at the First Omega Low Power Laser Seminar, London, April 1988.

54. Passarella S, Casamassima E, Molinari S, et al: Increase of proton electrochemical potential and ATP synthesis in rat liver mitochondria irradiated in vitro by helium-neon laser. *FEBS Lett* 1984;175:95–99.
55. Passarella S, Casamassima E, Quagliariello E, et al: Quantitative analysis of lymphocyte-Salmonella interaction and effect of lymphocyte irradiation by helium-neon laser. *Biochem Biophys Res Commun* 1985;130:546–552.
56. Ribari O: The stimulating effect of low power laser rays: Experimental examinations in otorhinolaryngology. *Rev Laryngol Otol Rhinol* 1981;102:531–533.
57. Rochkind S, Barrnea L, Razon N, et al: Stimulatory effect of He-Ne low dose laser on injured sciatic nerves of rats. *Neurosurgery* 1987;20:843–847.
58. Rochkind S, Nissan M, Barr-Nea L, et al: Treatment of peripheral and central nervous systems after injury using low energy laser irradiation: Experimental results, in Waidelich W, Waidelich R (eds): *Laser Optoelectronics in Medicine*. Berlin, Springer-Verlag, 1988, pp 760–762.
59. Rosner M, Belkin M, Erlich M, et al: Low energy laser irradiation prevents the early morphological and electrophysiological effects of optic nerve injury, in Waidelich W, Waidelich R (eds): *Laser Optoelectronics in Medicine*. Berlin, Springer-Verlag, 1988, pp 703–705.
60. Sato H, Landthaler M, Haina D, et al: The effect of laser light on sperm motility and velocity in vitro. *Andrologia* 1984;16:23–25.
61. Schwartz M, Doron A, Erlich M, et al: Effects of low-energy He-Ne laser irradiation of posttraumatic degeneration of adult rabbit optic nerve. *Lasers Surg Med* 1987;7:51–55.
62. Shiroto C, Ono K, Ohshiro T: Laser stimulation therapy using a diode laser, in Waidelich W, Waidelich R (eds): *Laser Optoelectronics in Medicine*. Berlin, Springer-Verlag, 1988, pp 755–759.
63. Simunovic Z, Ivankovich AD: Low-energy He-Ne + I.R. laser effects on wound healing in animals and human body, abstract. *Lasers Surg Med* 1988;8:175.
64. Snyder-Mackler L, Bork C, Bourbon B, et al: Effect of helium-neon laser on musculoskeletal trigger points. *Phys Ther* 1986:66:1087–1090.
65. Soto JJM, Moller I: La lasertherapia como coadyuvante en el tratemiento de la A.R. (artritis reumatoidea). *Bol Cent Doc Laser* 1987;14:4.
66. Surinchak JS, Alago ML, Bellamy RF, et al: Effects of low-level energy lasers on the healing of full-thickness skin defects. *Lasers Surg Med* 1983;2:267–274.
67. Tiphlova O, Karu T: Role of primary photoacceptors in low-power laser effects: Action of He-Ne laser radiation on bacteriophage T4-Escherichia coli interaction. *Lasers Surg Med* 1989;9:67–69.
68. Trelles MA, Mayayo E, Miro L, et al: Are mast cells implicated in the interaction of low-power-laser and tissue?, abstract. *Lasers Surg Med* 1988;8:174.
69. Vizi ES, Mester E, Tisza S, et al: Acetylcholine releasing effect of laser irradiation on Auerbach's plexus in guinea-pig ileum. *J Neural Transm* 1977;40:305–308.
70. Walker JB: Temporary suppression of clonus in humans by brief photostimulation. *Brain Res* 1985;340:109–113.
71. Walker JB, Akhanjee LK: Laser-induced somatosensory evoked potentials: Evidence of photosensitive in peripheral nerves. *Brain Res* 1985;344:281–285.
72. Wu WH, Ponnudurai R, Katz J, et al: Failure to confirm report of light-evoked response of peripheral nerve to low power helium-neon laser light stimulus. *Brain Res* 1987;401:407–408.
73. Yew DT, Ling Wong SL, Chan Y: Stimulating effect of the low dose laser: A new hypothesis. *Acta Anat* 1982;112:131–136.
74. Ysla R, McAuley R: Effects of low power infra-red laser stimulation on carpal tunnel syndrome: A double-blind study. *Arch Phys Med Rehabil* 1985;66:577.

Chapter 34

Bioelectrical Events and Intervention in Soft-Tissue Injury and Repair

Fred Nelson, MD

Introduction

Scientific interest in electrical-field stimulation of soft-tissue regeneration began when electrical field effects on bone during deformation were observed. After much research, electrical currents and specific magnetic fields were later applied in the treatment of fracture nonunions. Mechanically produced electrical polarization of biologic systems results from deformation of crystalline biopolymers such as collagen. Deformation in cartilage exposed to cyclic loading generates an intrinsic electrical field produced in part by streaming ionic fluids.

Membrane potentials, nerve conduction, and the electrical mechanism of a heartbeat are familiar biologic functions associated with electricity and electrical fields. All biochemical events are driven by changes in electrical charge and fields. Influences from neighboring electrical fields affect the cell in homeostasis or during stress.

An increasing body of research evidence shows the links between mechanical and electrical coupling in living organisms. Cells and other matrix components become polarized, altering ion fluxes and cell membrane functions. These alterations have important implications for the initiation and termination of biologic responses vital to growth, repair, and remodeling of tissues.[35]

Naturally Occurring Electrical Fields

Electrical fields in the body occur naturally and are important for growth, remodeling, and repair. A better understanding of their role in repair may provide the best opportunity for intervention in injury. However, the role of electrical fields in growth and remodeling must first be understood.

The Hodgkin-Huxley model describes the familiar sequence in nerve conduction depending on Na^+ and K^+.[53] The system has a threshold of potential energy that, when applied, causes an excitation that results in a chain sequence that initiates the nerve-conduction pattern.

Table 1 Spectrum of normal functional electrical potentials

Event	Tissue Gradient
Membrane potential	10^5 V/cm
Synaptic potential	10^3 V/cm
Electroencephalogram	10^{-1} V/cm
Circadian rhythm (human)	10^{-7} V/cm

The potential difference of 90 mV has an excitement threshold within one order of magnitude of the resting-membrane potential. Although important in nerve conduction, this membrane model is different from the typical cell membrane.

All cells have a membrane potential of about 100 mV. Most cell membranes can be influenced by electrical fields that are six or seven orders of magnitude less than those required to initiate nerve conduction.[62] For example, the 15-Hz magnetic fields used in stimulation of bone nonunions deliver a potential gradient of 3 mV/cm and current densities of 10^{-6}A/cm^2. Most cells have a membrane potential difference of 100 mV and a membrane thickness of 4 nm, resulting in a gradient of 10^5 V/cm across the membrane. The magnetic field is only 3 mV/cm. An electroencephalogram measures the potential difference across a given cell as 10^{-1} V/cm. Thus, the naturally occurring electrical signal is six orders of magnitude less than the membrane potential. The mechanisms involved in maintaining this Ca^{2+} based membrane model are discussed more fully in the section on mechanisms of field stimulation.

The surface of the cell has an electrical bilayer. Negatively charged ions cover the positive ends of the glycoprotein receptors, their sialic acid terminals, and other molecular components. These repelling forces facilitate the movement of blood cells through the endothelium by allowing the cells to slither between the layers. Disturbances in the movements of this bilayer lead to changes in cell receptivity.

The spectrum of normal functional electrical potentials ranges from 10^5 to 10^{-7} V/cm, as shown in Table 1.

Normal electrical fields for cellular activity are far below those necessary for nerve transmission and are within the range of imposed external electrical fields.

The stress-generated potentials[81] are also sources of natural electrical energy. Early research on bone stimulation and repair focused on the piezoelectric effect,[98] one of the stress-generated potentials. The piezoelectric effect is the accumulation of an electric charge on the surface of a solid material as a result of the deformation of that material. The rate of deformation is important.[13] The deformation that occurs in bone and tendon with weightbearing takes place in the first millisecond.[6] Stress-generated potentials also arise from the flow of ionic fluids and are called streaming potentials.[77] At the osteonal level, streaming potentials develop when wet bone tissue is bent.[84] The electrical gradient produced is similar to that induced by artificially applied electrical fields in nonunion stimulation. Mechanically stressed wet bone has a gradient range of 20 mV/cm for bone in general and of 200 to 500 mV/cm for bone next to a haversian canal.[54,89,90]

Streaming potentials occur in bone and in soft tissues such as cartilage[42,43,49] and ligaments.[7,8,97] Their production changes under certain tissue conditions. For example, normal bone and osteoporotic bone show differences in their electrical double layers (the relatively charged layer at the molecular surface of collagen and the oppositely charged neighboring ionic layer of bone).[83] Hence, mechanical forces are naturally converted into electrical fields and currents.

There is another steady-state potential in bone that responds to injury.[27] The growing epiphyseal area of bone is electronegative whereas the diaphysis is positive. If the diaphysis is fractured, it becomes electronegative even before the initial metabolic response to the injury.[44]

A SQUID magnetometer can detect small electrical currents within a limb.[48] The SQUID magnetometer is a noninvasive instrument that eliminates the effects of ambient fields such as the earth's gravity and detects the electrical field patterns in the limb. A human leg has up-and-down current flows of as much as 12 μA. The currents are similar from one person to another and are reproducible from day to day for each individual. Exercise affects these currents because of the bone stress aroused by muscular activity, not because of changes in blood flow or oxygen tension. The electrical currents themselves are not from the bone but rather from the electrical flow through soft tissue.

Fields in Repair and Growth

The way that salamanders and newts regenerate their tails has intrigued biologists for years.[28,29] Borgens[28] stated that the "flow of electrical current into an injury to a single cell, or out of the damaged region of an animal's integument, may be one of the earliest evolutionary response—and signal—to wounding" [*sic*]. In these amphibians the current is directed out the stump at a density of about 10 μA/cm^2.[29] The current appears to arise from the skin and flow through the core of the severed limb (Fig. 1). If the current is retarded by skin coverage, chemical intervention, or some other process, limb regeneration is retarded or stopped entirely. Artificially produced currents in frogs create some regeneration. Even mammals show current gradients from skin wounds.

Embryonic development as well as morphogenesis in plants appears to be under the control of electrical fields.[16] The low-frequency fluctuation of the earth's magnetic field may have had a strong influence on evolution. Malignancies appear to have a relatively high electronegative force, perhaps resulting from local vascular interstitial closed circuits.[75]

Cell-to-Cell Communication

The gap junctions between cells, which are similar in construction to cell membrane channels, enable chemical and electrical coupling to occur.[61] Maintaining these junctions is important for normal cell ho-

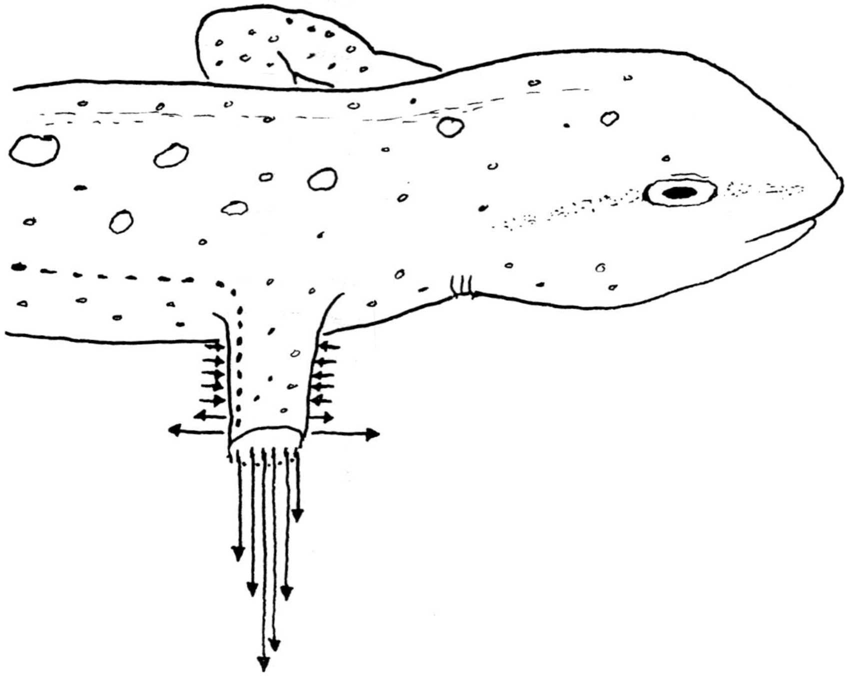

Fig. 1 *Current densities in an amputated limb after 20 hours. (Adapted with permission from Borgens RB, Vanable JW Jr, Jaffe LF: Bioelectricity and regeneration.* Bioscience *1979;29:468–474.)*

meostasis and resistance to tumor modification.[100] They can break down if both protein kinase C and phorbol esters are activated, decreasing intercellular communication and promoting growth.[92] There is little research on the function of these gap junctions in the repair process. Because they are affected by low-energy fields, however, they must be considered in any study of the mechanism by which electrical fields produce their effects.[4]

Artificially Produced Tissue Fields

Considerable research on clinical electrical stimulation followed investigation of naturally produced currents.[10,11,13,15,17,27] The relaxation time for electrochemical coupling was estimated to be in the range of 1 ms, resulting in the development of a magnetic pulse now in clinical use.[79] These electrical fields were then tested extensively to prove that tissue damage or other undesired effects did not occur. Since the FDA approved clinical application of electrical stimulation in 1979, the mechanism of the effect of these fields has been closely scrutinized.

Researchers are concerned that the electromagnetic contamination of the environment may have an adverse effect on human life.[10]

In soft-tissue stimulation, the tissue gradients for current and voltage must be carefully defined. The total current used and voltage delivered are quite different from those that individual tissues absorb. Current density means the amperes of current per square centimeter of base. Current density can be calculated or actually measured in tissues. Clinically used currents are about 1 to 20 $\mu A/cm^2$. The voltage gradient is considered in steps per centimeter of tissue. The voltage gradient in most clinically used currents is 1 to 3 mV/cm. Black[21] developed an excellent guide to the terminology and physics of the electrical fields used in clinical applications.

In a freshly amputated newt tail, the electrical field averages 5 mV/cm.[66] In vitro, the effective potential of cells is approximately 1 mV/cm. Clinical current flows are approximately 10 $\mu A/cm^2$.

Mechanisms of Electromagnetic Field Effects

Most investigations of electrical field stimulation involve bone. The three major clinical applications are direct current applied to the bone surface,[31] magnetic stimulation,[1,10–12,23,55,64,65,70,78–80] and capacitive coupling stimulation.[23]

Cell Membrane Components

The cell membrane is one of the primary targets of electromagnetic stimulation.[74] The important components of the cell membrane are the lipid-protein bilayer, the cell channels, the cell gap junctions or cell-to-cell channels, and the cell receptors. The cell membrane is modulated by some electromagnetic fields.[2,3,5,10] The primary effect of electromagnetic fields is on the surface of the cell membrane and not on the membrane potential. The surface charge alters ligand binding,[36] the primary basis for changes in receptor response. The response to these signals may be primarily at the receptor, channel, or some other membrane or nonmembrane locus. The channel responds to low-frequency, low-intensity fields ($<$500 Hz) because of the Lorentz force, the force that a magnetic field has on a charged moving particle. Higher-frequency fields ($>$500 Hz) are more likely to have an effect on the ion-binding sites of the cell membrane.[79] Further, the delivery system used[55] and tissue distortion[51] also play major roles in cellular responses. Additional potentially important harmonics are produced by these fields.[55]

Cell Receptors

Cell receptors are glycoproteins with sialic acid terminals. On the cell membrane, multiple receptors produce a dense polyanionic surface. These receptors are specific for hormone, antibodies, and neurotransmitters (Fig. 2). The receptors may then stimulate an internal cytoskeleton, part of which has an actin-like periodicity.

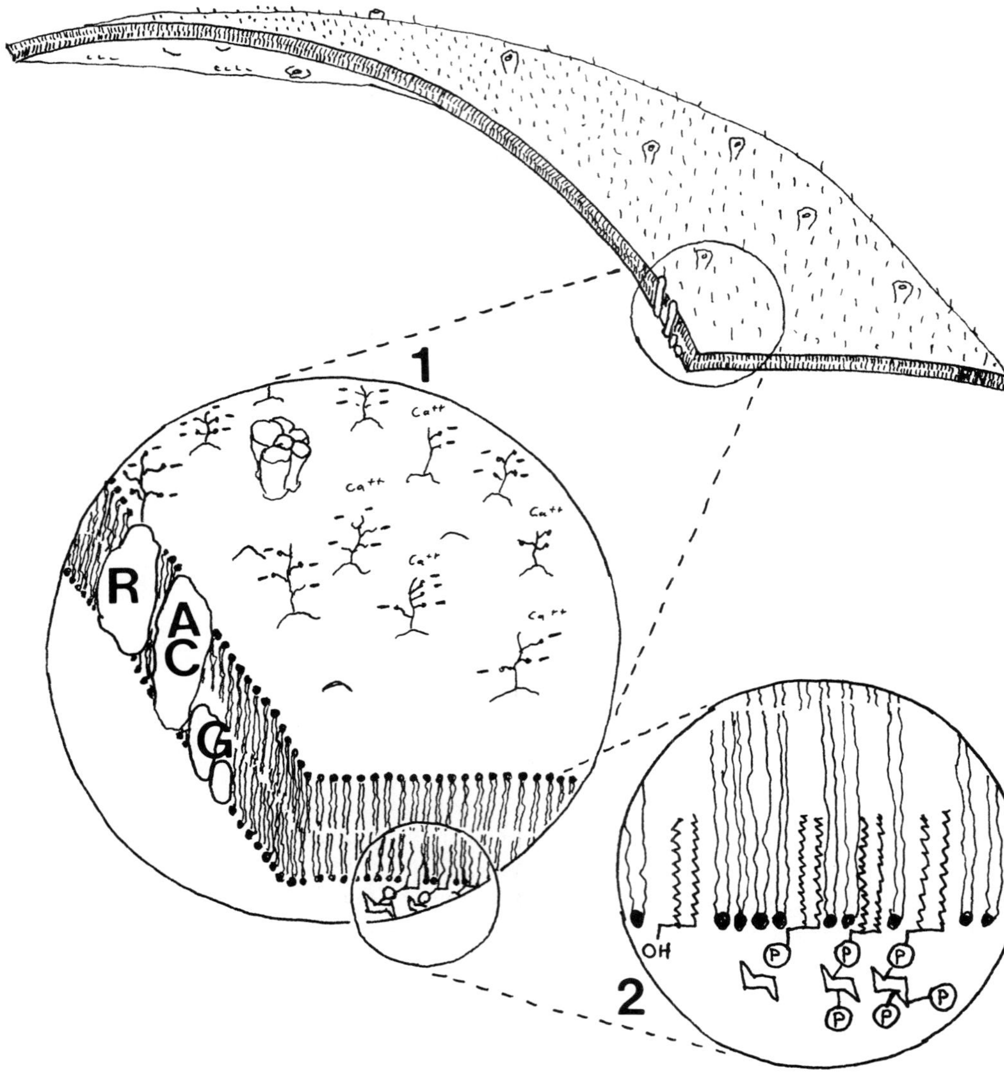

Fig. 2 *Slice of cell membrane showing fluid mosaic model. The first magnification (1) shows the negatively charged channel and receptor surface, which is opposed by a cationic field that includes calcium. Receptors (R) contain negatively charged glycoprotein extensions. Adenyl cyclase (AC) occupies an intramembranous location near the guanine nucleotide proteins (G). The second magnification (2) shows the inositol lipids involved in protein kinase C activation and intracellular calcium release.*

Three groups of intracellular enzymes respond to signals initiated at the cell membrane when exposed to an electromagnetic field[2,5]: (1) Protein kinase activated by membrane-bound adenylate conversion of adenosine triphosphate to cyclic AMP; (2) protein kinase that is cAMP-independent and performs messenger functions; and (3) ornithine decarboxylase involved in polyamine synthesis, required for DNA synthesis and cell growth.

Protein kinase C functions as a receptor and an enzyme. It is calcium-dependent and activated by diacylglycerol. Diacylglycerol is formed from inositol phospholipids that are transformed in response to cell surface stimuli. Activating a single diacylglycerol-receptor creates a spreading wave effect of receptors on the surface of the cell membrane. A synergism seems to exist between electromagnetic fields and the chemical environments. This is important for cancer research examining the effect of phorbol esters (which have a stimulatory effect similar to that of diacylglycerol) and electromagnetic fields (such as the 50- to 60-Hz fields created by power lines).

The parathyroid hormone receptor transmits to adenylate cyclase on the internal surface of the cell membrane. Its receptivity can be diminished by an external field of only 1 to 3 mV/cm, or eight orders of magnitude less than the membrane potential. Part of the effectiveness of the weak electrical signals used on tissue stimulation may result from nonlinear vibration modes in the protein. Stimulating the receptor causes the amount of free cytoplasmic calcium to double or even quadruple within 30 to 60 seconds.

Ornithine decarboxylase can change rapidly in response to external electromagnetic fields. It may be a useful marker for recording the cellular membrane response to manipulation of external fields.[33,34] The enzyme sequence is influenced by a number of growth factors and hormones active on the cell surface. Its additional sensitivity to external fields increases its usefulness in the study of electrical stimulation.

The response of glycoprotein cell receptors is important. When stimulated, the entire glycoprotein cell receptor complex may be incorporated into the cell by pinocytosis, creating a self-limited reaction to the specific stimulator. However, not all receptors respond in this way.

The burst pattern was originally selected as a electromagnetic pulse to help couple electrochemical processes with relaxation times of milliseconds. However, a single repetitive pulse is as effective as the 21-pulse signal now in use. Pulses of much narrower main and opposite polarity widths may promote more efficient electrochemical coupling.[79] In the presence of a proper DC magnetic field, ion binding may be influenced by AC magnetic fields of lower frequencies than was previously recognized.

Channels

Channels are protein-based petal-shaped openings in the cell membrane. They are usually specific for various ions, and can be influenced by certain electromagnetic fields. The disaggregation of the protein that constitutes the components of the channnel may be a mechanism for the effect of the electrical environment.[24,25] The channels can be ligand-

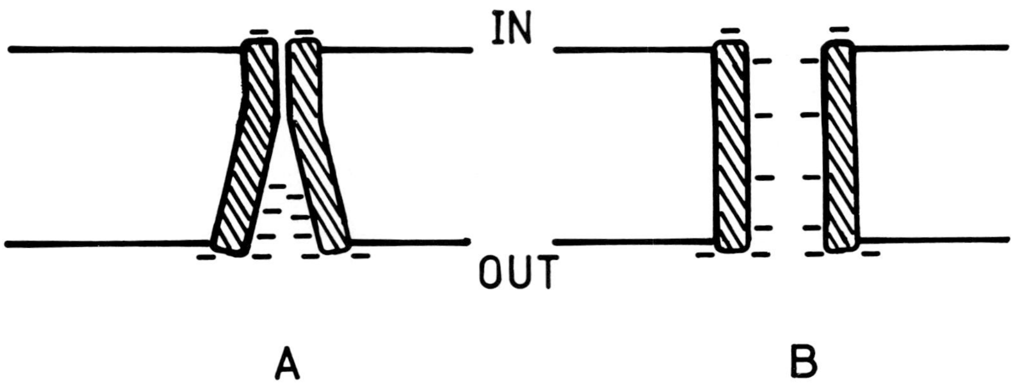

Fig. 3 *Voltage gated channel. With depolarization, the charge density shifts, causing the inner region to dissociate and open. (Reproduced with permission from Blank M: The surface compartment model (SCM): Role of surface charge in membrane permeability.* Bioelectrochem Bioenerg *1982;9:615–624.)*

gated (charge responds to the attachment of a specific molecule) or voltage-gated (charge movements are associated with enzymatic reactions), or affected by movement of gating charges in an electrical field.[26] The changes in the electrical double layer of these protein channels components results in a change in the gating for sodium, potassium, and calcium channels (Fig. 3). This process quickly reaches equilibrium, so there is a potential difference in effect if different frequency and/or pulses of fields are used.[67]

Cyclotron Resonance

"Cyclotron resonance" refers to the oscillating pattern that an ion takes as it traverses an electromagnetic field, particularly when that pattern matches or is a harmonic of the oscillation experienced by the molecule as it passes through a helical channel. Some cell channels may be helical, causing the passing ion to take on a specific oscillation. Energy is transferred to the channel by an electromagnetic field when the time-varying field is in proper resonance.[59] There are specific resonance harmonics[68] based on the proposed 16 turns of the helix of the calcium channel. These resonances differ for different ions. For example, in a specific, fixed direct magnetic field the resonance frequency for Ca^{2+} is 16 Hz; for Mg^{2+} it is 24.6 Hz.[99]

The cyclotron resonance theory is simply another explanation for the effect of electromagnetic fields on cell membranes and intracellular events in which the level of calcium is important. However, some biophysical characteristics of fluid media and dynamic friction may prevent this model from occurring.[50] Researchers are also investigating the effects of the Lorentz field on a charged messenger and resonance-like effects for appropriately selected fields.[36]

Gap Junctions

Although gap junctions are affected mostly by tumor-producing agents such as phorbol esters, certain electromagnetic fields can enhance this effect.[40] A 450-MHz field modulated at 16 Hz impairs cell-gap function. The 450-MHz signal alone has no effect. Although there is no specific research on the role of cell gaps in tissue repair, they are probably important for cell-to-cell (paracrine) functioning.

Cytoskeleton

Cells are supported by an infrastructure called the cytoskeleton. Some of the fibers of this cytoskeleton are actin fibers. The importance of the cytoskeleton in cell orientation and cell migration is not clear. Cytoskeletal stress-fiber orientation is disrupted by electrically induced intracellular calcium.[74] However, the electrical field effect on cell motility does not appear to depend on the cytoskeleton.[38]

Calmodulin

Calmodulin is a multifunctional calcium-dependent protein. It associates with ribosomes, nuclear membranes, mitochondria, endoplasmic reticulum, enzymes, and the cell membrane. Stimulating the cell with a 2.45-GHz field may have an effect on the calmodulin regulation of the calcium pump in certain neurons,[9] changing their conducting power. The calmodulin complex can also have a direct effect on the calcium-dependent K^+ channel. The mitogenic effect of calmodulin, as well as its membrane effect, may be influenced by a 16-Hz electromagnetic field.[39]

Cell Migration and Alignment

Cells migrate along the path of an electric current, toward the cathode.[38] The motion depends on the calcium channel and specifically involves the cytoskeleton. A primary mechanism of this movement appears to be a total cell-potential difference of 1 to 2 mV between the anodal and cathodal sides of the cell.[76] This difference in potential may selectively increase the channel opening on the cathodal side and cause cellular motion to that side.[74] Fibroblast cells break off from a confluent cell culture mass and migrate away on a perpendicular line under the influence of a 0.14 $\mu A/cm^2$ current driven by a 1-kHz sinusoidal magnetic current.[57]

Cell orientation may be influenced by electrical fields in vitro. The most effective electrical potentials and currents are still under investigation.[85] Electromagnetic fields have no documented effect on cell orientation in living ligament or tendon.

Chemotaxis

Various chemicals are involved in chemotaxis, including the kinins. Electrical stimulation produces a vascular ingrowth.[86] However, the electrochemical mechanism of the vascular ingrowth is not understood. A 60-kHz sine capacitively coupled current produces vascular ingrowth in an implanted sponge. The clinically used, 72-Hz magnetic signal is associated with improved vascularity in avascular necrotic bone,[1] but the mechanism of this effect is not known.

Streaming Potentials

Although the fluid steam produced by external electrical fields has not been measured, studies suggest that the effects of clinically useful electrical fields match those produced by steaming potentials developed with normal activity.[69] The orientation of a 1-Hz direct electrical current used as a stimulus to prevent joint contracture in rats is important.[91] The intensity and frequency developed are similar to those from normal activity. The clinical complement of this action is the reduced incidence of joint contracture seen with early mobilization.

Other Cell Components

The mechanisms of electrical and magnetic fields change DNA and other cellular chemical functions, including protein production. There is a direct effect on RNA and DNA.[26] In cells exposed to 220-Hz sine waves, mRNA is lower in molecular weight than in cells exposed to 72 Hz.[47] Other research reveals reduced synthesis in molecular polypeptides with molecular weights of 50,000 to 90,000 and increased production of peptides with molecular weights of 20,000 to 50,000.[46] This demonstrates the effects of electromagnetic field on electrochemical entities within the cell.

Matrix Production

The essential function of electrical stimulation is matrix production. Direct currents produce matrix changes that are not seen in magnetic stimulation. Brighton and McCluskey[32] presented the research in excellent graphic form, recording the type of currents used and their biochemical effects in nearly 100 studies.

Current Research on Soft Tissues and Sports Injuries

Field and Currents

The electrical fields used in soft-tissue research are direct current, capacitive coupling, and electromagnetic fields. The direct currents are usually faradic with a continuous electrical current. Some direct currents have been delivered sinusoidally at various low frequencies. The most useful reports on electrical stimulation indicate the current or signal delivered to the tissue in voltage gradients (mV/cm) and current densities (μA/cm^2) and the actual tissue response. Unfortunately, this is not often done. Another useful concept is the duty cycle, or the actual percentage of time that a pulse or current is delivered per unit of time. For example, a high-frequency wave may be delivered for the first 100 ms of a second, for a 10% duty cycle. Duty cycles may be used with larger units of time as well.

Stimulation of Fresh Wounds

Epithelialization is one index of wound healing. Direct stimulation of fresh skin lesions with a 15-Hz pulsed electromagnetic field and both longitudinal and perpendicular orientation did not stimulate early healing.[45] However, epithelialization increased significantly at days 3, 4, and 6 after the injury with rectangularly pulsed electrical stimulation at 128 pulses/sec to a 30-mA peak, 140-ms pulse.[71] Another index of wound healing is wound strength. An 80-Hz pulsed field increased tissue strength after three weeks.[60]

It is difficult to determine the delivered current to the involved tissues. One experiment stimulated both sham and actual wounds. The sham wounds produced more fibrous tissue,[72] but this might have been a byproduct of the lower-intensity electrical fields felt there. Other studies on wound healing and collagen formation have had mixed results with faradic stimulation.[22]

Healing of Chronic Wounds

Direct-current stimulation of chronic ulcers caused by neurologic injury has been studied. A 50-mA current (40-Hz pulse, 250 μ in width) applied to leg ulcers stimulated the rate of healing.[90,95] Similar results were obtained over four weeks of treatment with a 64 pulse/sec (pulse width, 140 μs) electrical current.[82] A 75-Hz pulsed magnetic field is effective in the treatment of ulcers of venous origin[56] because it stimulates granulation. These studies imply that different fields use different mechanisms to produce their effects.

Tendon

A constant 20-μA direct current applied to tendon has improved tendon repair strength in dogs.[88] In an uncontrolled study of the over-the-top iliotibial band reconstruction procedure for anterior cruciate replacement, a similar current produced a strong repair.[87] In a study involving rabbit patellar tendon, an 8.5-μA direct-current stimulation of the severed tendon increased the healing tensile strength at six weeks but a 15-μA current had no significant effect.[30] A direct-current experiment on tendons in vitro found that a 7-μA current increased incorporation of proline and conversion to hydroxyproline and enhanced intrinsic tenoplastic repair.[73] Reporting current densities in these studies would make them more helpful.

A 15-Hz electromagnetic field used in rabbit tendon healing affected hydroxyproline production but made no significant difference in tensile strength.[93] Patients with chronic rotator cuff tendinitis benefitted from treatment with a 75-Hz pulsed magnetic field, probably because of improved blood supply.[20] A 1.5-Hz magnetic field with a 90-μs repeating pulse pattern (20 ms positive, 4 μs negative) had no stimulatory effect on severed equine digital flexor tendons.[96]

Capacitive coupling has been used in horses to reduce the incidence of tendinitis, suspensory and check ligament desmitis, carpal tunnel syndrome, and bursitis.[94] How the field produces its preventive effect is not known.

Ligament

A square-wave, 100-μA, 1-Hz alternating current reduces joint contractures in rats if the stimulation is transverse rather than longitudinal.[90,91] The same type of current improves transected ligament healing if it parallels the ligament.[58]

A 1-Hz square-wave direct magnetic field increases collagen content and histologic maturity at six weeks in rabbit ligaments.[41] An experiment that stimulated fibroblasts from chick tendon found that a 0.35-$\mu A/cm^2$ current with parallel orientation at 1 Hz was most effective in stimulating proliferation.[37]

Skin Flap

Electromagnetic fields pulsed at 20, 72, and 500 Hz were used on skin flaps for four days. The flaps were evaluated at eight days.[52] The 20-Hz field produced a positive effect, but the 72-Hz field was most effective. The 500-Hz fields had no statistically significant effect. A 15-Hz field was used to show that exposure times (six vs 18 hours per day) made no significant difference in the stimulatory effects of that field.[63]

Effects on Other Tissues

An electrical field can produce tissue heating, as can some of the electromagnetic fields, particularly the high-frequency fields. The effect of a 26-MHz field may result from heating.[21] However, a 26-MHz carrier frequency for a 900-Hz modulated signal produces more rapid healing in facial plastic procedures.[18] Other high-frequency fields have been used as carriers for various frequencies to reduce edema in initial soft-tissue healing.[19] The thermal effects do not play a role in this healing effect, but minimal heating can have a direct effect on cell activity. The heating effect has been investigated as a clinical tool in treating cancer to kill specific cells. Microwave frequencies such as 2.45 GHz (2.45 billion cycles per second) are used for this purpose.

References

1. Aaron RK, Lennox D, Bunce GE, et al: The conservative treatment of osteonecrosis of the femoral head: A comparison of core decompression and pulsing electromagnetic fields. *Trans Orthop Res Soc* 1989;14:78.
2. Adey WR: Cell membranes: The electromagnetic environment and cancer promotion. *Neurochem Res* 1988;13:671–677.
3. Adey WR: Cell membranes: The electromagnetic environment and cancer promotion, in Monnier A (ed): *Melanges de neurophysiologie.* Paris, 1988, pp 7–34.

4. Adey WR: Evidence for tissue interactions with microwave and other nonionizing electromagnetic fields in cancer promotion, in Fiala J, Pokorny J (eds): *Biophysiological Aspects of Cancer.* Prague, Charles University Press, 1987, p 141.
5. Adey WR: The cellular microenvironment and signaling through cell membranes, in O'Connor ME, Lovely RH (eds): *Electromagnetic Fields and Neurobehavioral Function.* New York, Alan R Liss, 1988, pp 81–106.
6. Anderson JC, Eriksson C: Electrical properties of wet collagen. *Nature* 1968;218:166–168.
7. Anderson JC, Eriksson C: Piezoelectric properties of dry and wet bone. *Nature* 1970;227:491–492.
8. Arber SL: A model of cell electromagnetic susceptibility associated with the membrane electric field. *Physiol Chem Phys Med NMR* 1986;18:49–51.
9. Arber SL: Microwave enhancement of membrane conductance: Calmodulin hypothesis. *Physiol Chem Phys Med NMR* 1985;17:227–233.
10. Bassett CA: Fundamental and practical aspects of therapeutic uses of pulsed elecromagnetic fields (PEMF's). *CRC Crit Rev Bioeng,* in press.
11. Bassett CA: Low energy pulsing electromagnetic fields modify biomedical processes. *Bioessays* 1987;6:36–42.
12. Bassett CA: The development and application of pulsed electromagnetic fields (PEMFs) for ununited fractures and arthrodeses. *Orthop Clin North Am* 1984;15:61–87.
13. Bassett CA, Becker RO: Generation of electric potentials by bone in response to mechanical stress. *Science* 1962;137:1063–1064.
14. Bassett CR, Mitchell SN, Schink MM: Treatment of therapeutically resistant non-unions with bone grafts and pulsing electromagnetic fields. *J Bone Joint Surg* 1982;64A:1214–1220.
15. Bassett CA, Pawluk RJ, Pilla AA: Acceleration of fracture repair by electromagnetic fields: A surgically noninvasive method. *Ann NY Acad Sci* 1974;238:242–262.
16. Becker RO: Electromagnetic controls over biological growth processes. *J Bioelect* 1984;3:105–118.
17. Becker RO: The bioelectric factors in amphibian-limb regeneration. *J Bone Joint Surg* 1961;43A:643–656.
18. Bentall RHG: An interdisciplinary approach to low level biological effects of induced current, in Allen MJ, Underwood PNR (eds): *Charged and Field Effects on Biosystems.* United Kingdom, Abucus Press, 1984, pp 331–345.
19. Bentall RHG: Low-level pulsed radiofrequency fields and the treatment of soft-tissue injuries. *Bioelectrochem Bioenerg* 1986;16:531–548.
20. Binder A, Parr G, Hazleman B, et al: Pulsed electromagnetic field therapy of persistent rotator cuff tendinitis: A double-blind controlled assessment. *Lancet* 1984;1:695–698.
21. Black J: *Electrical Stimulation: Its Role in Growth, Repair and Remodeling of the Musculoskeletal System.* New York, Praeger, 1986.
22. Black J: Electrical stimulation of hard and soft tissues in animal models. *Clin Plast Surg* 1985;12:243–257.
23. Black J: Tissue response to exogenous electromagnetic signals. *Orthop Clin North Am* 1984;15:15–31.
24. Blank M: Biological switches. *Chemtech* 1988;18:434–438.
25. Blank M: The surface compartment model: A theory of ion transport focused on ionic processes in the electrical double layers at membrane protein surfaces. *Biochem Biophys Acta* 1987;906:277–294.
26. Blank M, Goodman R: An electrochemical model for the stimulation of biosynthesis by external electric fields. *Bioelectrochem Bioenerg* 1988;19:569–580.

27. Borgens RB: Endogenous ionic currents traverse intact and damaged bone. *Science* 1984;225:478–482.
28. Borgens RB: What is the role of naturally produced electric current in vertebrate regeneration and healing. *Int Rev Cytol* 1982;76:245–298.
29. Borgens RB, Vanable JW Jr, Jaffe LF: Bioelectricity and regeneration. *Bioscience* 1979;29:468–474.
30. Bose K, Ang EJ, Loo WM, et al: Effects of electrical stimulation in rabbit patellar tendon healing. *Trans BRAGS* 1988;8:50.
31. Brighton CT, Black J, Friedenberg ZB, et al: A multicenter study of the treatment of non-union with constant direct current. *J Bone Joint Surg* 1981;63A:2–13.
32. Brighton CT, McCluskey WP: Cellular response and mechanism of action of electrically induced osteogenesis. *Bone Mineral Res* 1986;4:213–254.
33. Byus CV, Kartun K, Pieper S, et al: Increased ornithine decarboxylase activity in cultured cells exposed to low energy modulated microwave fields and phorbol ester tumor promoters. *Cancer Res* 1988;48:4222–4226.
34. Byus CV, Pieper SE, Adey WR: The effects of low-energy 60-Hz environmental electromagnetic fields upon the growth-related enzyme ornithine decarboxylase. *Carcinogenesis* 1987;8:1385–1389.
35. Castor CW: Regulation of connective tissue metabolism, in McCarty DJ (ed): *Arthritis and Allied Conditions: A Textbook of Rheumatology*, ed 11. Philadelphia, Lea & Febiger, 1989, pp 256–272.
36. Chiabrera A, Bianco B: The role of the magnetic field in the EM interaction with ligand binding, in Blank M, Findl E (eds): *Mechanistic Approaches to Interactions of Electric and Electromagnetic Fields With Living Systems*. New York, Plenum Press, 1987, pp 79–95.
37. Cleary SF, Liu LM, Graham R, et al: Modulation of tendon fibroplasia by exogenous electric currents. *Bioelectromagnetics* 1988;9:183–194.
38. Cooper MS, Schliwa M: Motility of cultured fish epidermal cells in the presence and absence of direct current electric fields. *J Cell Biol* 1986;102:1384–1399.
39. Fitzsimmons RJ, Farley JR, Adey WR, et al: Evidence that calcium/calmodulin-dependent release of mitogen(s) mediate electric field (EF) stimulated bone cell proliferation in vitro, abstract. *Clin Res* 1987;35:149A.
40. Fletcher WH, Shiu WW, Haviland DA, et al: A modulated-microwave field and tumor promoters similarly enhance the action of alpha-lymphotoxins (αLT). *Trans Bioelectromag Soc* 1986;8:12.
41. Frank C, Schachar N, Dittrich D, et al: Electromagnetic stimulation of ligament healing in rabbits. *Clin Orthop* 1983;175:263–272.
42. Frank EH, Grodzinsky AJ: Cartilage electromechanics: I. Electrokinetic transduction and the effect of electrolyte pH and ionic strength *J Biomech* 1987;20:615–627.
43. Frank H, Grodzinsky AJ: Cartilage electromechanics: II. A continuum model of cartilage electrokinetics and correlation with experiments. *J Biomech* 1987;20:629–639.
44. Friedenberg ZB, Brighton CT: Bioelectric potentials in bone. *J Bone Joint Surg* 1966;48A:915–923.
45. Glassman LS, McGrath MH, Bassett CAL: Effect of external pulsing electromagnetic fields on the healing of soft tissue. *Ann Plast Surg* 1986;16:287–295.
46. Goodman R, Henderson AS: Patterns of transcription and translation in cells exposed to EM fields: A review, in Blank M, Findl E (eds): *Mechanistic Approaches to Interactions of Electric and Electromagnetic Fields With Living Systems*. New York, Plenum Press, 1987, pp 217–230.
47. Goodman R, Henderson AS: Some biological effects of electromagnetic fields. *Bioelectrochem Bioenergy* 1986;15:39.

48. Grimes DI, Lennard RF, Swithenby SJ: Macroscopic ionic currents within the human leg. *Phys Med Biol* 1985;30:1101–1112.
49. Grodzinsky AJ: Electromechanical and physicochemical properties of connective tissue. *CRC Crit Rev Biomed Eng* 1983;9:133–199.
50. Halle B: On the cyclotron resonance mechanism for magnetic field effects on transmembrane ion conductivity. *Bioelectromagnetics* 1988;9:381–385.
51. Hart FX: Pulse shape distortion by tissue. *J Bioelect* 1987;6:93–107.
52. Herbst E, Bryant GC, Sisken BF: Increased skin flap survival in rats subjected to low frequency electromagnetic fields. *Trans BRAGS* 1987;7:72.
53. Hodgkin AL, Huxley AF: A quantitative description of membrane current and its application to conduction and excitation in nerve. *J Physiol* 1952;117:500–544.
54. Iannacone W, Korostoff E, Pollack SR: Microelectrode study of stress-generated potentials obtained from uniform and nonuniform compression of human bone. *J Biomed Mater Res* 1979;13:753–763.
55. Jackson SF: Biophysical studies of pulsed magnetic field interaction with biological systems: Part I. Biophysical interactions, in Chiabrera A, Nicolini C, Schwan HP (eds): *Interactions Between Electromagnetic Fields and Cells.* New York, Plenum Press, 1985, pp 537–545.
56. Jeran M, Bagnacani M, Zaffuto S, et al: Effect of low frequency electromagnetic fields on the healing of skin lesions of venous origin: A double blind study. *Trans BRAGS* 1987;7:81.
57. Joshi R, Ross SM, Carter P, et al: Responses of rabbit ligament fibroblasts to sinusoidal electric currents. *Trans BRAGS* 1987;7:52.
58. Kenney TG, Dahners LE: The effect of electrical stimulation on ligament healing in a rat model. *Trans Orthop Res Soc* 1988;13:107.
59. Liboff AR: Geomagnetic cyclotron resonance in living cells. *J Biol Phys* 1985;13:99–102.
60. Liburdy RP, Vanek PF Jr, Kemski MH, et al: Influence of pulsed electromagnetic fields on soft tissue wound healing: In vivo and in vitro studies. *Trans BRAGS* 1988;8:49.
61. Loewenstein WR: Junctional intercellular communication: The cell-to-cell membrane channel. *Physiol Rev* 1981;61:829–913.
62. Luben RA, Cain CD, Chen MC-Y, et al: Effects of electromagnetic stimuli on bone and bone cells in vitro: Inhibition of responses to parathyroid hormone by low-energy low-frequency fields. *Proc Natl Acad Sci USA* 1982;79:4180–4184.
63. Luce EA, Bryant GC: Dose-response of electromagnetic field current in rat skin flap survival. *Trans BRAGS* 1986;6:72.
64. MacGinitie LA, Grodzinsky AJ, Frank EH, et al: Frequency and amplitude dependence of electric field interactions: Electrokinetics and biosynthesis, in Blank M, Findl E (eds): *Mechanistic Approaches to Interactions of Electric and Electromagnetic Fields With Living Systems.* New York, Plenum Press, 1987, pp 133–149.
65. Marsland TP: Biophysical studies of pulsed magnetic field interaction with biological systems: Part II. Physical aspects, in Chiabrera A, Nicolini C, Schwan HP (eds): *Interactions Between Electromagnetic Fields and Cells.* New York, Plenum Press, 1985, pp 546–555.
66. McGinnis ME, Vanable JW Jr: Electric fields in newt stumps. *Trans BRAGS* 1985;5:9.
67. McLeod BR, Liboff AR: An estimation of the damping factor for biological ions in low frequency EM fields. *Trans Bioelectromag Soc* 1986;8:11.
68. McLeod BR, Liboff AR, Smith S, et al: The calcium ion cyclotron resonance: Exploring the cell response to harmonics. *Trans BRAGS* 1987;7:25.

69. McLeod KJ, Rubin CT: Dose dependent response of bone remodeling to the magnitude of induced electric fields. *Trans Orthop Res Soc* 1989;14:309.
70. McLeod KJ, Rubin CT: The role of electric field intensity in the regulation of bone remodeling activity in-vivo. *Trans BRAGS* 1988;8:18.
71. Mertz PM, Davis SC, Eaglstein WH: Pulsed electromagnetic stimulation increases the rate of epithelialization in partial thickness wounds. *Trans BRAGS* 1988;8:48.
72. Mikulics MH, Esterhai JL, Black J, et al: Faradic stimulation produces an increase in ultimate tensile strength in surgically induced full thickness skin incisions. *Trans BRAGS* 1986;6:73.
73. Nessler JP, Mass DP: Direct-current electrical stimulation of tendon healing in vitro. *Clin Orthop* 1987;217:303–312.
74. Neumann E: Membranes and electromagnetic fields. *Trans Bioelectromag Soc* 1986;8:1.
75. Nordenstrom B: Biologically closed electric circuits: Activation of vascular interstitial closed electric circuits for treatment of inoperable cancers. *J Bioelect* 1984;3:137–153.
76. Onuma EK, Hui SW: Electric field-directed cell shape changes, displacement and cytoskeletal reorganization are calcium dependent. *J Cell Biol* 1988;106:2067–2075.
77. Pienkowski D, Pollack SR: The origin of stress-generated potentials in fluid-saturated bone. *J Orthop Res* 1983;1:30–41.
78. Pienkowski D, Pollack SR, Brighton CT: Electromagnetic stimulation of osteotomized rabbit fibulae: Comparison of asymmetrical and symmetrical signal waveforms. *Trans BRAGS* 1988;8:19.
79. Pilla AA, Kaufman JJ, Ryaby JT: Electrochemical kinetics at the cell membrane: A physicochemical link for electromagnetic bioeffects, in Blank M, Findl E (eds): *Mechanistic Approaches to Interactions of Electric and Electromagnetic Fields With Living Systems.* New York, Plenum Press, 1987, pp 39–62.
80. Pilla AA, Wener F, Costa F, et al: In vivo dosimetry of electromagnetic stimulation for optimal fracture repair. *Trans Orthop Res Soc* 1988;13:306.
81. Pollack SR: Bioelectrical properties of bone: Endogenous electrical signals. *Orthop Clin North Am* 1984;15:3–14.
82. Pollack SV: Effect of pulsed electrical stimulation on failing skin flaps in Yorkshire pigs. *Trans BRAGS* 1989;9:37.
83. Pollack SR, Berretta D, Steinberg ME, et al: Osteoporosis and the electrical double layer in bone. *Trans BRAGS* 1989;9:37.
84. Pollack SR, Korostoff E, Starkebaum W, et al: Microelectrode studies of stress generated potentials in bone, in Brighton CT, Black J, Pollack SR (eds): *Electrical Properties of Bone and Cartilage: Experimental Effects and Clinical Applications.* New York, Grune & Stratton, 1979, pp 69–81.
85. Ross SM, Frank CB: Effects of uniform applied electric currents on behavior of ligament fibroblasts. *Trans BRAGS* 1987;7:53.
86. Sisken BF, Barr E, Kotwick J: Use of the Ivalon sponge model for studying the effects of electrical stimulation on wound healing. *Trans BRAGS* 1989;9:37.
87. Stanish WD: The effect of electrical stimulation on soft tissue healing. *Trans BRAGS* 1986;6:69.
88. Stanish WD, Rubinovich M, Kozey J, et al: The use of electricity in ligament and tendon repair. *Phys Sportsmed* 1985;13:109–116.
89. Starkebaum W, Pollack SR, Korostoff E: Microelectrode studies of stress-generated potentials in four-point bending of bone. *J Biomed Mater Res* 1979;13:729–751.
90. Stefanovska A, Vodonik L, Benko H, et al: Exogenous electrical currents: Influence on wound healing. *Trans BRAGS* 1987;7:22.

91. Tart RP, Dahners LE: The effect of electrical stimulation on joint contracture in a rabbit model. *Trans Orthop Res Soc* 1989;14:195.
92. Trosko JE: Mechanisms of tumor promotion: Possible role of inhibited intercellular communication. *Eur J Cancer Clin Oncol* 1987;23:599–601.
93. VanZuiden LJ: Pulse electromagnetic stimulation of tendon healing. *Trans BRAGS* 1986;6:70.
94. Vasko KA, Lockhart KA: The use of bioelectricity for the treatment of soft tissue injuries in equine sports medicine. *Trans BRAGS* 1986;6:71.
95. Vodonik L, Stefanovska A, Benko H, et al: Soft tissue healing with low frequency pulsed currents. *Trans BRAGS* 1986;6:74.
96. Watkins JP, Auer JA, Morgan SJ, et al: Healing of surgically created defects in the equine superficial digital flexor tendon: Effects of pulsing electromagnetic field therapy on collagen-type transformation and tissue morphologic reorganization. *Am J Vet Res* 1985;46:2097–2103.
97. Williams WS, Breger L: Piezoelectricity in tendon and bone. *J Biomech* 1975;8:407–413.
98. Williams WS, Johnson M, Gross D: Piezoelectric description of strain-related potentials from whole bone and single osteons, in Brighton CT, Black J, Pollack SR (eds): *Electrical Properties of Bone and Cartilage: Experimental Effects and Clinical Applications.* New York, Grune & Stratton, 1979, pp 83–93.
99. Winters WD, Darnell B, Liboff AR, et al: Inhibition of normal fibroblast cell contraction by exposure to magnetic fields. *Trans Bioelectromag Soc* 1988;10:71.
100. Yamasaki H: The role of cell-to-cell communication in tumor promotion, in Buttorworth BE, Slaga TJ (eds): *Banbury Report 25: Nongenotoxic Mechanisms in Carcinogenesis.* Cold Spring Harbor, 1987, pp 297–309.

Chapter 35

Corticosteroid Injection Therapy in Sports Injuries

Wayne B. Leadbetter, MD

Since 1951, when Hollander and associates[40] popularized corticosteroid intra-articular injection therapy in rheumatoid arthritis, the injection of long-acting microcrystalline corticosteroid esters has gained wide use in the treatment of sports injury, although its therapeutic benefits remain controversial.[22,55] Despite impressions that the development of nonsteroidal anti-inflammatory drugs (NSAIDs) has decreased the indications for injection of corticosteroids,[22] injection therapy is repeatedly advised by experts in the field. This is particularly perplexing, because neither the cause of the persistent symptoms of inflammation nor the mechanism of action of corticosteroids is entirely known.

Background

Hydrocortisone acetate crystal suspension became available for clinical trials in 1951 after the successful synthesis of compound E (cortisone) by Hench and associates.[34] The first widespread clinical use of intra-articular injection therapy was initiated when Hollander[39] reported his experience with 7,353 injections into bursae and tendons, as well as joints, using 25 mg of hydrocortisone acetate. Hollander and associates[40] noted that, in the inflamed rheumatoid knee, the joint temperature decreased to normal within 24 hours and local tenderness, pain, and effusion lessened in almost all cases. Such local therapy was soon advocated for a broad spectrum of soft-tissue inflammations[77] (Outline 1). This led to a rapid spread in application to athletic injury, a practice that recent surveys show is still prevalent.[15]

Available Parenteral Corticosteroids

The adrenal corticosteroid hormones (or their semisynthetic or synthetic analogs) are employed as replacement or adjuvant therapeutic agents in treating an enormous variety of diseases. Biologic activity is

Outline 1 Common inflammatory indications for injection therapy*

- Bursitis
  - Calcareous bursitis
  - Olecranon
  - Prepatellar
  - Subdeltoid
  - Other bursae
- Fibrositis
  - Localized
    - Dupuytren's contracture, fasciitis, myalgia and myositis, scapulocostal syndrome, tender point and "trigger" point syndromes
  - Systemic
    - Arthralgia, fibromyalgic syndrome (muscular rheumatism), myalgia, myopathies, neuralgia, polymyalgia rheumatica, vasomotor instability
- Ganglion
- Neuritis
  - Neuralgia
  - Neuropathy
  - Carpal tunnel syndrome
- Periarthritis and arthritis
  - Adhesive capsulitis
  - Frozen shoulder
  - Scapulohumeral capsulitis
  - Synovitis
- Reflex neurovascular dystrophy
  - Causalgia
  - Posttraumatic dystrophy
  - Shoulder-hand syndrome
  - Sudeck's atrophy
- Tendinitis
  - Epicondylitis (tennis elbow)
- Tenosynovitis
  - Bicipital
  - de Quervain's syndrome
  - Tenovaginitis ("trigger" finger)

*Adapted from Steinbrocker and Neustadt.[77]

related directly to the chemical structure and is characterized by two types: (1) mineralocorticoids, which affect the excretion of sodium, potassium, and the like, and (2) glucocorticoids, which affect carbohydrate metabolism, particularly glucogenesis.

Glucocorticoid and the anti-inflammatory activities of cortisol have been found to be closely related. The evolution of synthetic parenteral corticosteroids was advanced when Hollander and associates[41] showed that hydrocortisone esterified with a branch chain compound (hydrocortisone tertiary butyl acetate) was rapidly hydrolized by joint enzymes and thus could double the duration of the local anti-inflammatory effect. The newer molecules represent attempts to prolong a desirable local effect by increasing solubility. Relatively insoluble medications include methylprednisolone acetate, triamcinolone acetonide, triamcinolone diacetate, triamcinolone hexacetonide, and dexamethasone acetate. More soluble preparations include cortisone acetate, hydrocortisone acetate, and prednisolone derivatives. Most soluble is betamethasone sodium phosphate. In an attempt to achieve broader clinical efficacy, soluble and insoluble derivatives of the same molecule are combined. Structural modifications found to enhance glucocorticoid activity include fluorination at C9 and at C6, dehydrogenation (double bond) at C1-C2 and at C6-C7, methylation at C2, C6, C16, and C21, hydroxylation at C16, and deoxygenation at C21.

All parenteral corticosteroids include a significant number of inactive ingredients. Among these are polysorbate, sorbitol solution, sterile water, methylparaben, benzol alcohol, sodium chloride, creatine, edetate disodium, sodium bisulfite, sodium hydroxide, carboxymethylcellulose, and benzalkonium chloride. Although exact formulations vary from manufacturer to manufacturer, it is important to recognize the potential for significant damage to soft tissues, especially tendon, that can be produced by these coincident chemicals.

As yet, the role that the pH of the carrier solution plays in local tissue biology is unknown. The reported pH of betamethasone sodium phosphate and acetate mixture ranges from 6.8 to 7.2. Attention should be given to pH when a given agent is chosen on the assumption that this will affect tissue tolerance.

Mode of Action and Effects

Both orally and parenterally administered corticosteroids appear to enter into the inflammatory cycle at a point between membrane phospholipid breakdown and the production of arachidonic acid by inhibition of phospholipidase A enzyme.[25,30] Aspirin and nonsteroidal medications affect the arachidonic acid cycle chain after arachidonic acid production. Because of their earlier action in the inflammatory cascade, steroids are unique in their potential suppressive effects on inflammation, which is why they are used in a wide variety of diseases. However, because this step precedes the cycle of inflammation and repair, corticosteroids have the potential to inhibit the harmful side effects of the inflammatory reaction caused by lysosomal release. They can also suppress and retard the onset of wound repair.[25] Using an experimental model for allergic inflammation of the air-pouch type in rats, Kurihara and associates[52] demonstrated that local administration of either dexamethasone or indomethacin inhibited leukocyte infiltration, but that only dexamethasone reduced the chemotactic activity of the exudate. This suggested that anti-inflammatory steroids manifest their inhibitory effect on leukocytic infiltration by inhibiting the generation of chemotactic factors at the inflammatory site.[52] However, the effects of locally administered steroids on arachidonic acid metabolites in the inflammatory reaction can vary. Lundberg and Gerdin,[58] investigating the response of granulation tissue in a cutaneous wound model in the rat by employing challenging doses of prostaglandin E_2 and leukotriene B_4, found that methylprednisolone decreased local blood flow and albumin extravasation by 29% and 31% respectively without influencing neutrophil infiltration.

Bjork and associates[8] found that systemic injection with methylprednisolone in a hamster model of immune-complex-induced inflammatory reaction produced microvascular leakage only on the venular side of the microcirculation in immunized animals exposed to antigen. The leakage was largely inhibited by treatment with methylprednisolone. They proposed a central effect with possible suppression of agonist receptor function or modulation of a final common effector mechanism of the endothelial cell after interaction with the agonist receptor. The rationale for local injection includes stabilization of cellular membrane integrity, primarily through the inhibition of phospholipase A_2, which stabilizes lysosomal enzymes, decreases cellular swelling and edema, and decreases the number of neutrophils.[36]

Cortisone and hydrocortisone are cleared rapidly from joint cavities. The half-life of drug samples tagged with carbon 14 varies from 60 to 107 minutes. The acetate derivatives of these compounds are less soluble in aqueous solutions, but are removed even more rapidly—85% within one hour and 98% by three hours.[32] After entering the blood, corticosteroids are metabolized in the liver and excreted by the kidney. That intra-articular steroids exert a systemic effect is shown by joint improvement remote from the injection site and by suppression of the hypothalamic-pituitary-adrenal axis. Gray and associates,[32] in an exhaustive review of parenteral corticosteroid treatment in rheumatic disorders, noted the following potential modes of action: (1) enhancement of hyaluronate concentration and polymerization in synovial fluid; (2) increased viscosity of synovial fluid; (3) fewer leukocytes in the synovial fluid; (4) decreased synthesis of collagenase and prostaglandins; (5) production of a peptide factor that may depress neutrophil migration, as well as that of monocytes and macrophages (this peptide may inhibit the assembly of cytoplasmic microtubules within leukocytes, an effect similar to that of colchicine, and may be mediated indirectly by enhanced intracellular cyclic adenosine triphosphatase; (6) suppression of cellular immunity in rheumatoid synovium by suppression of T lymphocytes; (7) inhibition of lymphocyte-mediated activities, including lymphokine production, T-suppressor cell function, and antibody-dependent cell cytotoxicity; and, finally, (8) decreasing antibody production, including alterations in immunoglobulin synthesis and complement level. The significance of all these mechanisms of action requires further research. Further, it has been found that the dose of corticosteroid ester used intra-articularly is not proportional to the effective oral dose. Because any excess of corticosteroid over the amount that synovial membrane retains is absorbed into the systemic circulation, the optimal amount for local injection is the maximal amount that can be held locally. Crystalline suspensions are apparently taken up by synovial lining cells. These form a depot or repository for the medication, which is later inactivated by hydrolysis.[38]

In regard to the adverse effects of parenteral corticosteroids on tissue, concerns center on the intra-articular suppression of articular cartilage metabolism and deleterious effects on tendon and ligament structures. Mankin and Conger[59] noted that corticosteroids administered intra-articularly in the knee temporarily reduced the synthesis of matrix of articular cartilage in rabbits. This effect was dose-related. Roach and associates,[74] comparing the effects of steroids, aspirin, and sodium salicylates on articular cartilage in the rabbit knee, noted that the salicylates had beneficial effects and that the steroids accelerated cartilage generation. Chandler and associates[18] described an elderly woman with progressive hip osteoarthritis in whom a Charcot-like arthropathy developed after 18 monthly intra-articular injections of 50 mg of hydrocortisone acetate. Articular damage was ascribed to excessive joint mobility and accumulated trauma resulting from steroid-related pain relief. Chandler and Wright[19] described rapid radiographic deterioration in 15 of 25 knees after intra-articular steroid therapy. Despite such reports, evidence for steroid arthropathy remains anecdotal, with scattered case reports, and confused by variables such as antecedent trauma or gross ligamentous instability.[6,35] Many reports do not support the idea that this adverse effect is common. Balch and associates,[5] in a study of 65 knees with rheumatoid arthritis or osteoarthritis, found that gross deterioration did not correlate with the number of injections but rather with the activity and underlying disease process. In their own series of 80,000 injections over a period of 20 years, the incidence of rapid joint damage was less than 1%. Hollander and associates[42] noted instability associated with osteonecrosis in 79 injected hip and knee joints of 62 patients. This represented less than 0.8% of more than 8,000 individuals given multiple intra-articular injections over many years. Pathologic evidence for cortisone- or steroid-induced arthropathy is notably lacking. Existing studies show bone fragmentation, cartilage metaplasia in synovium, soft-tissue calcareous debris (resembling the changes of Charcot arthropathy[6]), chronic hypertrophic synovitis, and paravascular lymphoid and plasma cell invasion, referred to as "lymphoplasmocytic inflammatory infiltrate."[35] These changes appear to be indistinguishable from progressive osteoarthritic degeneration secondary to peak loading, excessive ligamentous laxity, and joint instability with acceleration of joint damage, possibly aggravated by deprivation of normal protective proprioceptive sensations. However, no controlled studies proving the causal relationship of injection to joint degeneration exists. Nonetheless, as Gray and associates[32] pointed out, "It is eminently possible that repetitive intra-articular injections given at short intervals (less than monthly) may exert a deleterious effect on joint structures."

Research regarding the potentially harmful or healing effects of steroid injection into ligament or tendon is greatly hampered by the lack of an appropriate animal model of overuse injuries. To date, studies have used injections into normal tendon or ligament tissue; therefore, it should be noted, whether the following studies are directly applicable to injection into diseased or injured tendons has not been proved, but only implied.

Noyes and associates[69] and Butler and associates[16] provided authoritative reviews of the local effect of methylprednisolone acetate injection into the anterior cruciate ligaments of rhesus monkeys. The two protocols called for an intercollagenous injection or two intra-articular injections in the knees. They found that alterations in ligament behavior depended on the dosage and the time after injection. A 20-mg (large-dose) group was studied at six and 15 weeks and a 4-mg (small-dose) group was studied at 15 and 52 weeks. The large-dose group showed significantly decreased maximum load (21% and 39% declines in maximum load at six and 15 weeks, respectively); in the small-dose group, maximum load declined 27% at 15 weeks and remained near this level at one year. In the large-dose group, decreases in energy to failure were minimal at six weeks but showed a 43% decline at 15 weeks. In the small-dose group, a 27% decrease in energy to failure was found at both 15 and 52 weeks.[70] Noyes and associates[69] concluded that "a single intra-ligamentous or multiple intra-articular steroid injection has the potential to cause significant and longlasting deterioration in the mechanical properties of ligaments and collagenous tissues." They called attention to fibrocyte death within the ligament adjacent to the injection site and the delay of the reappearance of viable fibrocytes for as long as 15 weeks.

In an additional study, three intra-articular injections of methylprednisolone acetate were given at one-week intervals to the knee joints of rhesus monkeys. In load failure studies of bone-ligament-bone preparations, time-dependent and dose-related changes in mechanical properties were noted. After 15 weeks of a relatively high 6-mg/kg dose, tolerance to maximum load showed the greatest decline, with an 11% decline at six weeks and a 20% decline at 15 weeks in the large-dose group. However, when a 0.6-mg/kg dose was given for two weeks, the energy change was insignificant. In addition, there was no change at six weeks in the large-dose group. Although species variation makes drawing an analogy to human tissue difficult, a single intra-articular injection or repeated injections several months apart apparently produce minimal deleterious changes to exposed intra-articular ligament. Nonetheless, frequent administration of large intra-articular doses may alter the ligament's strength and function.[68] Cox[22] pointed out that Noyes and associates gave their large-dose group the equivalent of ten times the normal human dose (based on body mass). However, the small-dose group received approximately the equivalent of the normal human dosage, lending validity to the conclusions.

Because of problems such as modeling, species variation, dosage, and loading measures, it is not surprising that investigators have differed in their conclusions concerning the effects of injected corticosteroids on tendon. Matthews and associates,[61] using a rabbit patellar tendon model, injected methylprednisolone acetate (three or four 4-mg doses one week apart) and found no change in biomechanical properties (maximum load supported, stiffness, and mode of failure). However, the longest point of observation was 57 days, with an average of 33 days to the animal's death. They concluded that underlying degenerative abnormality contributed most significantly to tendon rupture after injection in athletes. Kapetanos[45] studied the Achilles tendon in rabbits. One of the three anatomically separate tendons forming the Achilles tendon complex was surgically transected, and then injected with 0.3 mg/kg of triamcinolone acetate on the second, eighth, 14th, and 20th days. The animals were killed on the 25th day after surgery. Microscopic examination showed that adequate healing had taken place in the tendons of both treated and untreated animals, but that the cortisone-treated tendon showed less peritendinous fibrous tissue than the controlled tendons. This correlated with the observations of Ketchum[50] and Wrenn and associates[83] regarding decreased fibrogenesis in cortisone-treated animals. Kapetanos[45] found a significant decrease in tendon weight (13%), the amount of adhesions (68%), load to failure (29.8%), and energy to failure (67.16%). Unverferth and Olix,[79] studying rabbit gastrocnemius tendons, found a lower modulus of elastic stiffness in tendons injected with steroids than in tendons injected with saline. If moduli of elastic stiffness are valid indicators of ultimate tensile strength, it can be assumed that steroid-injected tendons rupture at lower loads than saline-injected tendons. They were also concerned that suppression of symptoms in athletes with tenosynovitis would encourage a return to competition before adequate healing and recommended that local steroid injections not be used in the treatment of tenosynovitis.

Kennedy and Willis,[48] studying rabbit Achilles tendons treated with betamethasone sodium acetate, administered 25% to 50% of the usual adult dosage, and then killed the animals at five intervals between 48 hours and six weeks. They were able to correlate failure at a loading rate of 12.5 cm/min with underlying histologic changes. Large cystic spaces and collagen necrosis appeared as early as 48 hours. It is not clear whether these changes were the result of pressure necrosis secondary to the fluid volume of the injection or of carrier substances with toxic effects. Neutrophils and macrophages were present as early as seven days in a typical acute inflammatory and vascular response; their appearance was followed by the gradual appearance of acellular amorphous precursors of collagen (Fig. 1). Failing strengths at 48 hours were 35% lower than in controls and then progressively improved until failing strength returned to normal at 14 days. Electron micrographs demonstrated a partial return of the integrity of collagen fibrils at this stage and more complete restoration at six weeks (Fig. 2). Although it was not determined whether the observed weakening was a function of the steroid itself, of the inflammatory process, or of both, the authors recommended avoiding vigorous muscular activity for at least two weeks after injection. Repetitive local injections were also discouraged. Howes and associates[43] have shown that cortisone delays wound healing by retarding the formation of granulation tissue. Walter and Israel[80] showed that corticosteroids can prevent ground substance precursors of collagen from being sulfated.

Spontaneous tendon rupture has not undergone controlled study. Ford and DeBender[26] reported 15 ruptured tendons (eight biceps tendons, three Achilles tendons, two supraspinati, one anterior tibial tendon, and one lateral epicondylar attachment) in 13 patients. In most cases, triamcinolone acetonide mixed with procaine or lidocaine had been used. Kelly and associates,[47] in a discussion of patellar and quad-

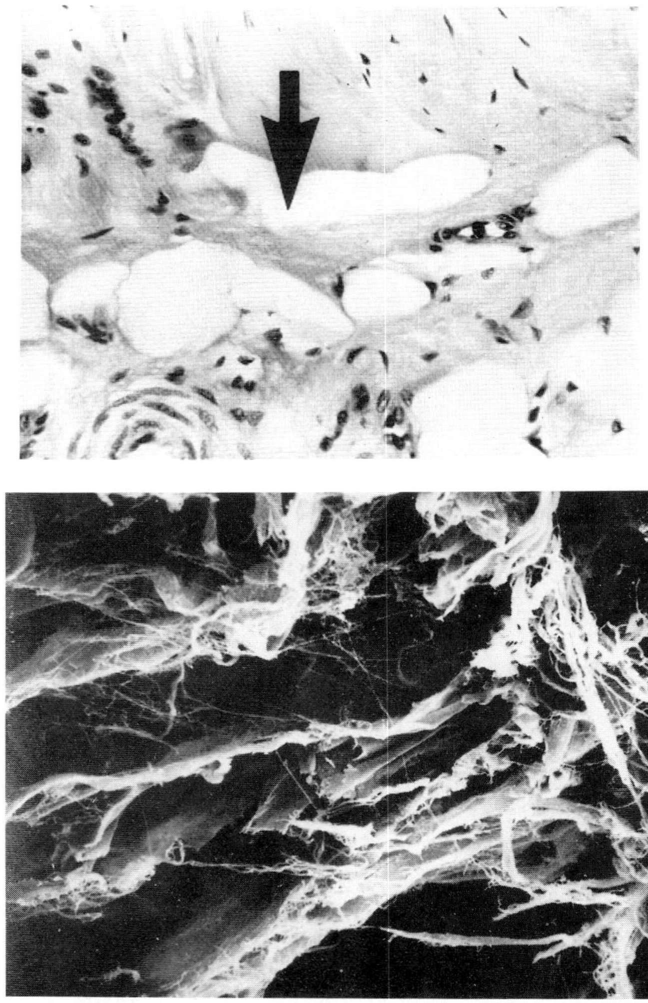

Fig. 1 *Effects of 0.25-ml steroid injection on tendon after 48 hours.* ***Top,*** *Light micrograph shows early collagen fiber necrosis.* ***Bottom,*** *Scanning micrograph shows collagen fiber disorganization. (Reproduced with permission from Kennedy JC, Willis RB: The effects of local steroid injections on tendons: A biomechanical and microscopic correlative study.* Am J Sports Med *1976;4:11–21.)*

riceps tendon ruptures, noted that eight knees had been injected with corticosteroids near the involved tendon at various times before rupture. Most patients had received an average of two to three injections; none had received more than 12. Four patients were professional basketball players, although it is not clear whether they were among the patients receiving injections. Kleinman and Gross[51] reported Achilles tendon ruptures in three patients within six weeks of their receiving

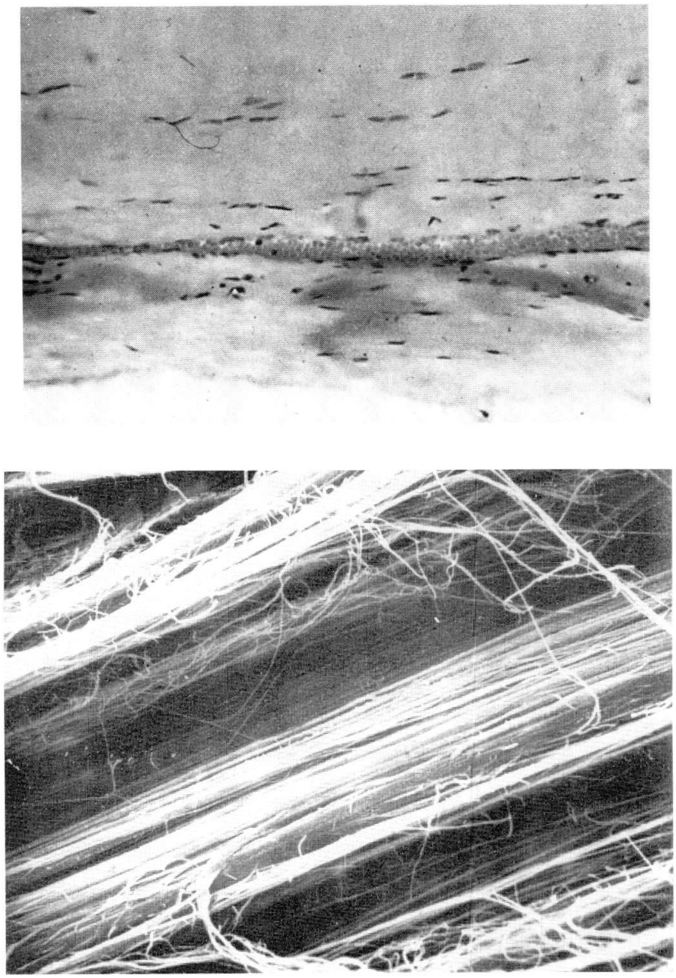

Fig. 2 *Effects of steroid injection on tendon after six weeks.* ***Top,*** *Light micrograph shows continued appearance of hyaline material at periphery.* ***Bottom,*** *Scanning micrograph shows normal parallel arrangement of collagen fibrils. (Reproduced with permission from Kennedy JC, Willis RB: The effects of local steroid injections on tendons: A biomechanical and microscopic correlative study.* Am J Sports Med *1976;4:11–21.)*

a single local steroid injection each. On the basis of rounding of the tendon ends and preexisting degenerative changes at the time of surgical repair, they concluded that it was not likely that the ruptures reflected a mere progression of existing tendinitis. It is not clear why the degenerative changes were ascribed to the effects of injection rather than other forms of microtrauma. However, such anecdotal reports are typical.[46,51]

In an editorial reply to Ford and DeBender, Neustadt[64] emphasized the increased risk of injecting the Achilles tendon in a patient with inflammatory arthropathy because to do so makes degeneration more likely. Beskin and associates,[7] in 42 patients with Achilles tendon ruptures, found the associated incidence of steroid injection to be 7.1%. The average age of their patients (mean, 39.4 years) called attention to other variables such as aging in the occurrence of spontaneous rupture. Pain was prodromal in 21% of cases, implying that suppression of pain would be particularly unwise. Similar clinical observations have been made by others.[56,62]

Spontaneous rupture of the plantar fascia was first described by Leach and associates[53] in 1978. They described six athletes, five runners and one basketball player, who had symptoms of plantar fasciitis. Five of the six had received local steroid injections before the rupture. In one case, the injection occurred one month before rupture, and in the others the interval between injection and rupture was not stated. Ahstrom[1] reported spontaneous rupture in five patients who had received local steroid injections.

Current Clinical Use of Parenteral Corticosteroids

Because there is no evidence that injected corticosteroid speeds the stages from inflammation to healing and repair (indeed, the opposite is likely to be true), the clinical application of these medications must be predicated on a different basis. Local corticosteroids are best indicated in chronic inflammatory processes, in which suppression of concentrations of inflammatory cells and increased concentrations of chemical mediators may prevent further tissue injury. They are contraindicated in acute macrotrauma because of their catabolic effects.[19,29] These medications are often given as a last resort before surgical intervention and after all other treatments, including exercise rehabilitation, have failed.[55,67]

Between 1979 and 1982, I administered corticosteroid injections to 124 of 2,200 athletes seen for various ailments, a rate of 5.7%. This group included 80 men and 44 women; five were children less than 16 years of age. There were 112 recreational, six varsity, five youth club, and six semiprofessional athletes. The average age was 43.3 years. The average duration of symptoms was 2.3 months and the average follow-up was 15 months. The majority received some type of additional therapy, such as ultrasound or galvanic stimulation and conditioning, either before or after the injection. However, in all cases, previous treatment had failed to improve or relieve the athlete's condition. An initial retrospective review showed excellent results (unrestricted play in two to six weeks) in 23%, good results (occasional symptoms, return to play in two to six weeks, minimal need for further care) in 63%, and poor results (pain unrelieved, inability to play, requiring prolonged rest or surgery) in 14%. At 15.3 months, however, the results had deteriorated: 22% were excellent, 53% good, and 25%

poor. The most common diagnoses treated were rotator cuff syndrome (9% excellent; 65% good; 26% poor), tennis elbow (13% excellent; 61% good; 26% poor); and plantar fasciitis (26% excellent; 50% good; 25% poor). The most responsive diagnoses were various bursitic inflammations, iliotibial band syndrome, ganglion cyst, tendinitis, and carpal tunnel syndrome. The least responsive were knee synovitis associated with internal derangements (75% poor); acromioclavicular joint arthritis (100% poor); and Morton's neuroma (66% poor). The experience with acromioclavicular joint arthritis paralleled that of Cox,[22] who encountered two cases of resorption of the distal clavicle after injection of the acromioclavicular joint with corticosteroids and therefore did not recommend steroid injection for this injury.

Bruno and Clarke,[15] in a recent review of usual and customary standards of care by 52 orthopaedic surgeons in Cincinnati, revealed a preference for injection in subacromial bursitis (34 of the 52), lateral epicondylitis of the elbow (24 of the 52), trigger finger (nine of the 52), and de Quervain's syndrome (eight of the 52).

Sports Involving the Upper Extremity

In overuse injuries of the shoulder, sustained in the throwing, swimming, lifting, and racket sports, there has been mixed testimony as to the efficacy of injection therapy. Norwood and associates[67] reported that injections did not relieve shoulder pain during throwing. Brunet and associates,[14] however, thought that one or two injections into the subacromial bursae might be helpful. Anderson[2] advocated corticosteroid injection when activity continues to be intolerable despite two decreases in workout intensity and trials of several different NSAIDs. A 2-ml solution of procaine hydrochloride and corticosteroid is injected into the site of maximal tenderness, with bursal tissue being the primary target. Rehabilitative therapy is continued on a protected activity basis. A second injection may be given two weeks later. If two injections of corticosteroid fail to provide long-term relief, an alternative treatment or surgery should be considered.[2]

Several authors have advocated lidocaine injections for a pain ablation test. Kerlan[49] noted:

> Once the inflamed area has been located, a therapeutic test with a mixture of Lidocaine and steroid administered with a 25-gauge, 5/8-inch needle is often useful. The steroid is added because it can provide significant anti-inflammatory action and treatment at the same time a diagnosis is confirmed. In addition, often this therapy allows the athlete to return to throwing while a long-term treatment regimen is still under consideration.

"Cuffitis," a somewhat imprecise term for what appears to be an inflammation of the rotator cuff caused by impingement, is the intended target of such treatment. In swimmer's shoulder, Pettrone[71] cautioned, steroid injection should be used infrequently because of the risk of "collagen breakdown" in the training athlete. A period of strict rest for ten days is advocated if injection is necessary.

As Leach and Schepsis[54] pointed out, "There are physicians who inject a great deal and there are those who do not." Although they placed themselves in the latter group, they advocated injections for subdeltoid bursa inflammation with a rest period of ten to 14 days and no more than three injections to a site. They also noted that shoulder "bursitis" during the 1950s and 1960s was frequently treated with steroid injection into the subdeltoid bursa, and that without a more refined diagnosis chronic disability and accumulative abuse often resulted.

Injection therapy has been widely accepted in tennis elbow and lateral epicondylitis. Nirschl and Pettrone[66] treated patients who had received four or five cortisone injections before surgery. Priest and Glick[73] were once willing to use three or four injections. However, since the 1970s there has been a quiet trend toward decreased use of local injection therapy and an increased focus on exercise rehabilitation and protective bracing. Today no more than three injections into a given site can be recommended (R.P. Nirschl, oral communication, May 23, 1989).

Sports Involving the Lower Extremity

Brubaker and James,[13] in treating running injuries, injected 8% but limited the injections to "tendinitis, bursitis and synovitis." Brody[12] thought steroid injections were helpful in "certain cases of greater trochanteric bursitis, iliotibial band friction syndrome, retrocalcaneal bursitis and plantar fasciitis." In their review of overuse injuries to the knee in runners, Newell and Bramwell[65] noted that most cases of iliotibial band syndrome respond to biomechanical control but that injecting the bursal area beneath the iliotibial band with corticosteroid offers an alternative. "This is one area we feel comfortable in injecting because it is into a bursa, not a tendon, and because the patient will usually experience good, long-term results as with the orthosis."

Franz[27] did not think injection necessary in iliotibial band syndrome and found that conservative therapy short of injection helped in more than 80% of cases. Although he advocated corticosteroids administered by phonophoresis or iontophoresis, he noted that 50% of the patients improved in three weeks or less with conservative therapy, which included rehabilitation and/or orthotic control. In patellar tendinitis and Achilles tendinitis, Stanish and associates[76] generally recommended against injection therapy because of the deleterious effects associated with steroid injections. Clancy and associates[20,21] were ambivalent, stating in 1976 that local steroids were not beneficial in the treatment of Achilles tendinitis but allowing in 1982 that "the judicious use of local steroid injection about the sheath but not directly into the tendon" might be considered in cases that failed to resolve by other means.

Blazina and associates[9] advocated injection of steroid for the patellar tendinitis known as "jumper's knee" but did not detail their dosage technique or injection frequency. Kelly and associates[47] and Martens and associates[60] have called attention to the temporal association of steroid injection with complete avulsion of the patellar tendon.

Williams,[82] in an exhaustive review of the pathophysiology of sports-related Achilles tendon lesions, identified the "non-role" of steroids in the management of Achilles tendon pain, noting the hazards of both intertendinous injection and paratendon bathing.[48,56,62,79] Ljungqvist[57] reported 24 instances of subcutaneous or partial rupture of the Achilles tendon. In ten cases, local steroid injections had been administered before the rupture. Two patients had each received one injection approximately a year before the rupture and had had no problems with the Achilles tendon during that period, despite intense activity. Therefore, it is difficult to attach any significance to the history of injection in these two cases. Six patients had received an injection two to four months before the rupture. Histologic tissue examination of the surgical cases showed no apparent difference between the steroid-treated and the untreated patients, with the exception of one case in which devitalized tendon tissue harbored a few small defined necrotic areas. Acute inflammatory cell infiltration was seen in seven cases and chronic cell infiltration in all 24 cases. Chronic changes, therefore, predominated over acute changes throughout the series. In at least four cases, symptoms at the time of injection were not at the site of rupture but elsewhere. Ljungqvist[57] concluded that pain relief permitted continued abusive overload with increased weightbearing, eventually leading to clinically manifest rupture. DaCruz and associates,[24] in a randomized, double-blind study of 28 patients with Achilles paratendinitis using peritendinous injections of 40 mg/g of methylprednisolone acetate, found no clinical improvement.

Refractory subcalcaneal pain or plantar fasciitis syndrome can be responsive to corticosteroid injection therapy.[11,12,22] The 20% or so of patients who do not respond to oral medication and orthotic measures are candidates for a single corticosteroid injection, especially if pain persists at a single point. Andrews[3] cautioned against local corticosteroid injection because of the possible, although uncommon, development of a local iatrogenic infection with calcaneal osteomyelitis.

Bursal and Lesser Tendon Sheath Injection

Weinstein and associates,[81] in a retrospective, nonrandomized comparison of patients with traumatic olecranon bursitis treated by aspiration alone or by aspiration with steroid injection, concluded that intrabursal steroid injection speeded recovery. Mysnyk and associates[63] reviewed prepatellar bursitis in wrestlers. Recurrence was prominent, despite injection therapy, which they concluded had no measurable effect. There was a 50% excision rate after injection of the prepatellar bursa. Both Weinstein and associates[81] and Boland[10] found frequent long-term complications, including infection, skin atrophy, and an increased incidence of localized chronic pain. Boland mentioned an 8% incidence of infection. This is doubly significant, in that diagnosis of septic bursitis can often be missed clinically, as was noted by Mysnyk and associates[63] in three of eight cases and Ho and associates[37] in eight of 25 cases of septic olecranon and prepatellar bursitis.

Stenosis tenovaginitis associated with de Quervain's stenosis tenosynovitis and trigger finger inflammations are appropriately treated by cortisone injection.[4] Gunther and associates,[33] in a series of 71 patients with trigger thumbs and fingers, reported that 90 of 104 injected digits (87%) remained asymptomatic for the duration of the study after only one injection (average follow-up, 42 months). Each injection used 0.6 ml of triamcinolone.

Neuropathy

In a prospective, randomized, double-blind study of epidural steroid use in lumbar radicular pain, Cuckler and associates[23] were unable to find a significant effect in either acute disk herniation or spinal stenosis. In addition, long-term follow-up averaging 20 months failed to demonstrate the efficacy of a second injection of epidural steroids administered to patients whose pain did not respond within 24 hours to an injection of either 80 mg of methylprednisolone acetate combined with 5 ml of 1% procaine or 2 ml of sterile saline combined with 5 ml of 1% procaine. Jackson and associates,[44] who used epidural cortisone injection in 32 young adult athletes, reported an efficacy rate of 44%. The proposed mechanisms of action were lysis of adhesions with volume injection and a direct anti-inflammatory effect. Takeuchi and associates[78] recently reported epineural compression injury prevention in an animal model after precompression intraperitoneal steroid administration. Phalen[72] reported that 24% of 215 cases of carpal tunnel syndrome resolved after one to five steroid injections; 38% showed moderate to marked improvement, 10% did not improve, and 28% required surgery. Local steroid injection was recommended as initial treatment for carpal tunnel syndrome unless marked sensory loss or thenar atrophy was present. However, Gray and associates,[32] after an exhaustive review of the literature, concluded that short-term symptomatic benefits may be achieved in most patients with carpal tunnel syndrome, but that a high relapse rate must be anticipated.

Complications and Adverse Effects

Both local and systemic complications of corticosteroid injection therapy have been described. Local complications include subcutaneous atrophy or fat necrosis, depigmentation or hyperpigmentation, tendon or ligament rupture, accelerated joint destruction or osteolysis, and flare reaction. Systemic complications include significant transient hyperglycemia in diabetics, vasovagal attack, psychological problems, and systemic allergic reaction.

In one review,[55] 116 athletes received only one injection and none received more than four injections in one site. The complications in-

Outline 2 Use of steroid injections

Proper use
- Six-week preinjection trial of rest, adjusted level of play, and conditioning
- Discrete, palpable site of complaint (avoid tendon)
- Peritendinous or inflammatory target tissue
- Limit of three injections, spaced weeks apart, given only if first led to demonstrated improvement
- Rest (protection) for two to six weeks after injection
- Avoidance of contributing mechanical cause (for example, equipment, conditioning)

Improper use
- Acute trauma
- Intratendinous injection
- Infection
- Multiple injections (>3)
- Injection immediately before competition
- Frequent intra-articular injections

cluded four cases of local skin depigmentation, four of intratendinous or intrabursal precipitates (documented at surgery), and one case of subcutaneous atrophy. No tendons ruptured, probably because injections of the Achilles or biceps tendon site were avoided.

Bruno and Clarke,[15] in a survey of 52 practicing orthopaedic surgeons, recorded the following percentages of surgeons encountering various complications: fat necrosis, 64% (most commonly at the elbow); skin depigmentation, 67%; tendon rupture, 17% (biceps, 4%; Achilles, 3%; patellar, 1%); accelerated joint destruction, 17% (knee, 7%); and systemic reactions, 60% (hyperglycemia, 10%; vasovagal reactions, 15%).

Factors contributing to the lack of response to injection therapy include those that are patient-related, that is, overuse, cyclic loading, faulty technique, evidence of advanced trauma and degenerative changes, and those that are physician-related, that is, improper diagnosis or inadequate injection technique.[55] Techniques for injections of specific joints have been described elsewhere.[17,28,31,75]

Conclusions

Strong statements regarding the efficacy of injection of corticosteroids are based primarily on experience with rheumatic disease. Such experience over 32 years, involving more than 400,000 injections in more than 12,000 patients, has led Hollander and associates[40] to conclude that, "No other form of treatment for *arthritis* has given such consistent local symptomatic relief in so many for so long with so few harmful effects." Another clinician, himself afflicted with rheumatoid arthritis, thought that steroid injections were poorly regarded "because of poor techniques and overuse."[49] It is my impression that there is indeed a "tissue responder," a person who seems uniquely predisposed to inflammatory reaction in soft-tissue microtrauma, and whose inflammatory cycle can be modified to allow cooperation with a rehabilitation program by the proper timing of corticosteroid injection. Judiciously used, this may be less expensive and offer less systemic risk than other treatments.

To remove the "fire alarm" of pain from the onset of tissue inflammation and injury clearly can place the athlete in great jeopardy. Paradoxically, the effect of injection therapy may be greatest in the inflammatory stages of the athletic injury (Outline 2). Until more is understood regarding the relative benefit of immediate inflammation suppression, steroid injection therapy must be used cautiously to avoid further harm, and it should remain an adjunctive therapy and not a sole means of treating sports-induced soft-tissue inflammation.

References

1. Ahstrom JP Jr: Spontaneous rupture of the plantar fascia. *Am J Sports Med* 1988;16:306–307.
2. Anderson TR: Rehabilitation of common shoulder injuries in athletes. *J Musculoskeletal Med* 1988;5:15–26.
3. Andrews JR: Overuse syndromes of the lower extremity. *Clin Sports Med* 1983;2:137–148.
4. Baker BE: Current concepts in the diagnosis and treatment of musculotendinous injuries. *Med Sci Sports Exerc* 1984;16:323–327.
5. Balch HW, Gibson JMC, El-Ghobarey AF, et al: Repeated corticosteroid injections into knee joints. *Rheumatol Rehabil* 1977;16:137-140.
6. Bentley G, Goodfellow JW: Disorganisation of the knees following intra-articular hydrocortisone injections. *J Bone Joint Surg* 1969;51B:498–502.
7. Beskin JL, Sanders RA, Hunter SC, et al: Surgical repair of Achilles tendon ruptures. *Am J Sports Med* 1987;15:1–8.
8. Bjork J, Smeadegar DG, Arfors KE: Methylprednisolone sets at the endothelial cell level reducing inflammatory responses. *Acta Physiol Scand* 1985;123:221–224.
9. Blazina ME, Kerlan RK, Jobe FW, et al: Jumper's knee. *Orthop Clin North Am* 1973;4:665–678.
10. Boland A: Soft-tissue injuries of the knee, in Nicholas JA, Hershman EB (eds): *Lower Extremity and Spine in Sports Medicine*. St. Louis, CV Mosby, 1986, pp 983–1012.
11. Bordelon RL: Subcalcaneal pain: A method of evaluation and plan for treatment. *Clin Orthop* 1983;177:49–53.
12. Brody DM: Techniques in the evaluation and treatment of the injured runner. *Orthop Clin North Am* 1982;13:541–558.
13. Brubaker CE, James SL: Injuries to runners. *J Sports Med* 1974;2:189–198.
14. Brunet ME, Haddad RJ, Polche EB: Rotator cuff impingement syndrome. *Phys Sportsmed* 1982;10:88–94.
15. Bruno LP, Clarke RP: The use of local corticosteroid injections in orthopaedic surgery. Presented at the 56th Annual Meeting of the American Academy of Orthopaedic Surgeons, Las Vegas, Feb 9–13, 1989.
16. Butler DL, Grood ES, Noyes FR, et al: Biomechanics of ligaments and tendon. *Exerc Sport Sci Rev* 1978;6:125–182.
17. Butters KP, Rockwood CA Jr: Office evaluation and management of the shoulder impingement syndrome. *Orthop Clin North Am* 1988;19:755–765.
18. Chandler GN, Jones DT, Wright V, et al: Charcot's arthropathy following intra-articular hydrocortisone. *Br Med J* 1959;1:952–953.
19. Chandler GN, Wright V: Deleterious effect of intra-articular hydrocortisone. *Lancet* 1958;2:661–663.

20. Clancy WG Jr: Tendonitis and plantar fasciitis in runners, in D'Ambrosia R, Drez D Jr (eds): *Prevention and Treatment of Running Injuries.* Thorofare, Charles B Slack, 1982, pp 77–82.
21. Clancy WG Jr, Newhart D, Brand RL: Achilles tendonitis in runners: A report of five cases. *Am J Sports Med* 1976;4:46–57.
22. Cox JS: Current concepts in the role of steroids in the treatment of sprains and strains. *Med Sci Sports Exerc* 1984;16:216–218.
23. Cuckler JM, Bernini PA, Wiesel SW, et al: The use of epidural steroids in the treatment of lumbar radicular pain: A prospective, randomized, double-blind study. *J Bone Joint Surg* 1985;67A:63–66.
24. DaCruz DJ, Geeson M, Allen MJ, et al: Achilles paratendonitis: An evaluation of steroid injection. *Br J Sports Med* 1988;22:64–65.
25. Fantone J, Ward P: Inflammation, in Rubin E, Farber JL (eds): *Pathology.* Philadelphia, JB Lippincott, 1988, pp 34–63.
26. Ford LT, DeBender J: Tendon rupture after local steroid injection. *South Med J* 1979;72:827–830.
27. Franz WB: Overuse syndromes in runners: Part II. Specific overuse injuries of runners, in Mellion MB (ed): *Office Management of Sports Injuries and Athletic Problems.* Philadelphia, Hanley & Belfus, 1988, pp 301–309.
28. Gatter RA: Arthrocentesis technique and intrasynovial therapy, in McCarty DJ (ed): *Arthritis and Allied Conditions: A Textbook of Rheumatology*, ed 11. Philadelphia, Lea & Febiger, 1989, pp 646–656.
29. Glick JM: Therapeutic agents in musculoskeletal injuries. *J Sports Med* 1975;3:136–138.
30. Goodwin JS: Mechanism of action of corticosteroids, in Goodwin JS (ed): *Mediguide to Inflammatory Diseases.* New York, Pfizer Laboratories, 1987, vol 16, pp 1–5.
31. Gray RG, Gottlieb NL: Corticosteroid injections in RA: How to get best results, in Dickson RA, Wright V (eds): *Musculoskeletal Disease.* London, Heinemann Medical Books, 1984, pp 48–60.
32. Gray RG, Tenenbaum J, Gottlieb NL: Local corticosteroid injection treatment in rheumatic disorders. *Semin Arthritis Rheum* 1981;10:231–254.
33. Gunther SF, Marks M, Gunther BB: The efficacy of cortisone injection for trigger fingers and thumbs. Presented at the 56th Annual Meeting of the American Academy of Orthopaedic Surgeons, Las Vegas, Feb 9, 1989.
34. Hench PS, Kendall EC, Slocumb CH, et al: The effect of a hormone of the adrenal cortex (17-hydroxy-11-dehydrocortisone; Compound E) and of pituitary adrenocorticotropic hormone on rheumatoid arthritis: Preliminary report. *Mayo Clin Proc* 1949;24:181–197.
35. Hernandez A, Dakezies EJ: Intra-articular steroid injection induced arthroscopy. *Orthopedics* 1983;6:1340–1343.
36. Hirata FE, Schiffmann E, Venkatasubramanian K, et al: A phospholipase A_2 inhibitory protein in rabbit neutrophils induced by glucocorticoids. *Proc Natl Acad Sci USA* 1980;77:2533–2536.
37. Ho G Jr, Tice AD, Kaplan SR: Septic bursitis in the prepatellar and olecranon bursae: An analysis of 25 cases. *Ann Intern Med* 1978;89:21–27.
38. Hollander JL: Arthrocentesis techniques and intrasynovial therapy, in McCarty DJ (ed): *Arthritis and Allied Conditions: A Textbook of Rheumatology*, ed 10. Philadelphia, Lea & Febiger, 1985, pp 541–553.
39. Hollander JL: Intra-articular hydrocortisone in arthritis and allied conditions: A summary of two years' clinical experience. *J Bone Joint Surg* 1953;35A:983–990.
40. Hollander JL, Brown EM Jr, Jessar RA, et al: Hydrocortisone and cortisone injected into arthritic joints: Comparative effects of and use of hydrocortisone as a local antiarthritic agent. *JAMA* 1951;147:1629–1635.

41. Hollander JL, Brown EM Jr, Jessar RA, et al: Local anti-rheumatic effectiveness of higher esters and analogues of hydrocortisone. *Ann Rheum Dis* 1954;13:297–301.
42. Hollander JL, Jessar RA, Brown EM Jr: Intra-synovial corticosteroid therapy: A decade of use. *Bull Rheum Dis* 1961:11:239–240.
43. Howes EL, Plotz CM, Blunt JW, et al: Retardation of wound healing by cortisone. *Surgery* 1950;28:177–181.
44. Jackson DW, Rettig A, Wiltse LL: Epidural cortisone injections in the young athletic adult. *Am J Sports Med* 1980;8:239–243.
45. Kapetanos G: The effect of the local corticosteroids on the healing and biomechanical properties of the partially injured tendon. *Clin Orthop* 1982;163:170–179.
46. Karpman RR, McComb JE, Volz RG: Tendon rupture following local steroid injection: A report of four cases. *Postgrad Med* 1980;68:169–174.
47. Kelly DW, Carter VS, Jobe FW, et al: Patellar and quadriceps tendon ruptures: Jumper's knee. *Am J Sports Med* 1984;12:375–380.
48. Kennedy JC, Willis RB: The effects of local steroid injections on tendons: A biomechanical and microscopic correlative study. *Am J Sports Med* 1976;4:11–21.
49. Kerlan RF: The treatment of common throwing injuries to the shoulder, in Zarins B, Andrews JR, Carson WG (eds): *Injuries to the Throwing Arm*. Philadelphia, WB Saunders, 1985, pp 112–127.
50. Ketchum LD: Effects of triamcinolone on tendon healing and function. *Plast Reconstr Surg* 1971;47:471.
51. Kleinman M, Gross AE: Achilles tendon rupture following steroid injection: Report of three cases. *J Bone Joint Surg* 1983;65A:1345–1347.
52. Kurihara A, Ohuchi K, Tsurufuji S: Reduction by dexamethasone of chemotactic activity in inflammatory exudates. *Eur J Pharmacol* 1984;101:11–16.
53. Leach R, Jones R, Silva T: Rupture of the plantar fascia in athletes. *J Bone Joint Surg* 1978;60A:537–539.
54. Leach RE, Schepsis AA: Shoulder pain. *Clin Sports Med* 1983;2:123–135.
55. Leadbetter WB: Corticosteroid injection for the treatment of athletic injury, abstract. *Med Sci Sports Exerc* 1983;15:103.
56. Lee HB: Avulsion and rupture of the tendo calcaneus after injection of hydrocortisone. *Br Med J* 1957;2:395.
57. Ljungqvist R: Subcutaneous partial rupture of the Achilles tendon. *Acta Orthop Scand* 1968;113(suppl):1–86.
58. Lundberg C, Gerdin B: The inflammatory reaction in an experimental model of open wounds in the rat: The effect of arachidonic acid metabolites. *Eur J Pharmacol* 1984;97:229–238.
59. Mankin HJ, Conger KA: The acute effects of intra-articular hydrocortisone on articular cartilage in rabbits. *J Bone Joint Surg* 1966;48A:1383–1388.
60. Martens M, Wouters P, Burssens A, et al: Patellar tendinitis: Pathology and results of treatment. *Acta Orthop Scand* 1982;53:445–450.
61. Matthews LS, Sonstegard DA, Phelps DB: A biomechanical study of rabbit patellar tendon: Effects of steroid injection. *J Sports Med* 1974;2:349-357.
62. Melmed EP: Spontaneous bilateral rupture of the calcaneal tendon during steroid therapy. *J Bone Joint Surg* 1965;47B:104–105.
63. Mysnyk MC, Wroble RR, Foster DT, et al: Prepatellar bursitis in wrestlers. *Am J Sports Med* 1986;14:46–54.
64. Neustadt DH: Tendon rupture and steroid therapy, letter. *South Med J* 1980;73:271–272.
65. Newell SG, Bramwell ST: Overuse injuries to the knee in runners. *Phys Sportsmed* 1984;12:80–92.

66. Nirschl RP, Pettrone FA: Tennis elbow: The surgical treatment of lateral epicondylitis. *J Bone Joint Surg* 1979;61A:832–839.
67. Norwood LA, Del Pizzo W, Jobe FW, et al: Anterior shoulder pain in baseball pitchers. *Am J Sports Med* 1978;6:103–105.
68. Noyes FR, Grood ES, Nussbaum NS, et al: Effect of intra-articular corticosteroids on ligament properties: A biomechanical and histological study in rhesus knees. *Clin Orthop* 1977;123:197–209.
69. Noyes FR, Keller CS, Grood ES, et al: Advances in the understanding of knee ligament injury, repair, and rehabilitation. *Med Sci Sports Exerc* 1984;16:427–443.
70. Noyes FR, Nussbaum NS, Torvik PJ, et al: Biomechanical and ultrastructural changes in ligaments and tendons after local corticosteroid injections, abstract. *J Bone Joint Surg* 1975;57A:876.
71. Pettrone FA: Shoulder problems in swimmers, in Zarins B, Andrews J, Carson WG (eds): *Injuries to the Throwing Arm*. Philadelphia, WB Saunders, 1985, pp 318–330.
72. Phalen GS: The carpal-tunnel syndrome: Seventeen years' experience in diagnosis and treatment of six hundred fifty-four hands. *J Bone Joint Surg* 1966;48A:211–228.
73. Priest J, Glick J: Prevention and treatment of tennis elbow. *Phys Sportsmed* 1977;5:33–49.
74. Roach JE, Tomblin W, Eyring EJ: Comparison of the effects of steroid, aspirin and sodium salicylate on articular cartilage. *Clin Orthop* 1975;106:350–356.
75. Rowe CR: Injection technique for the shoulder and elbow. *Orthop Clin North Am* 1988;19:773-777.
76. Stanish WD, Curwin S, Rubinovich M: Tendinitis: The analysis and treatment for running. *Clin Sports Med* 1985;4:593–609.
77. Steinbrocker O, Neustadt DH: *Aspiration and Injection Therapy in Arthritis and Musculoskeletal Disorders: A Handbook on Technique and Management*. Hagerstown, Harper & Row, 1972, p 2.
78. Takeuchi M, Lowdon IMR, Seaber AV, et al: Effect of steroid therapy on compression injury of peripheral nerves following epineurectomy. *Trans Orthop Res Soc* 1989;14:430.
79. Unverferth LJ, Olix ML: The effect of local steroid injections on tendon. *J Sports Med* 1973;1:31–37.
80. Walter JB, Israel MS: *General Pathology*. London, J & A Churchill, 1963, p 155.
81. Weinstein PS, Canoso JJ, Wohlgethan JR: Long-term follow-up of corticosteroid injection for traumatic olecranon bursitis. *Ann Rheum Dis* 1984;43:44–46.
82. Williams JG: Achilles tendon lesions in sport. *Sports Med* 1986;3:114–135.
83. Wrenn RN, Goldner JL, Markee JL: An experimental study of the effect of cortisone on the healing process and tensile strength of tendons. *J Bone Joint Surg* 1954;36A:588.

Chapter 36

Tissue Remodeling and Response to Therapeutic Exercise

Jesse C. DeLee, MD

Recent research has improved understanding of the biomechanics of and soft-tissue responses to therapeutic exercise. Experimental and chemical studies have examined the effects of tissue mobilization and immobilization on muscle, collagen, and ligament structures. These studies borrowed from studies of the response of bone to the application of stress in vivo to define what has been called "Wolff's law of soft tissues," a simplified concept of soft-tissue remodeling in response to therapeutic exercise.

However, little information exists on the use of specific types of therapeutic exercise and on the response of tendons and ligaments. This chapter evaluates current scientific data on the accuracy of "Wolff's law of soft tissues" by examining the responses of tendon, ligament, and skeletal muscle to various types of therapeutic exercise.

Tendon

The function of tendon is to transmit forces from a muscle to the skeleton with minimal elongation. Muscle and tendon are separate structures, but function as one unit—the "muscle-tendon unit." Tendons are composed of two proteins, collagen and elastin, embedded in a proteoglycan-water matrix. The collagen synthesizes into chains, forming a triple helix. These combine into fibrous structures and make up the primary tendon bundles.

Collagen and elastin are produced by the fibroblasts within the tendon's structure. The fibroblasts are more numerous during connective-tissue production, such as during development or repair after injury.

Tendons possess high tensile strength and minimum shear strength. They provide almost no resistance to compressive forces. These properties result from the structure of the collagen and elastin fibers in the tendons themselves. Most biomechanical studies of tendons have focused on their ultimate tensile strength and strain.[7,42] Large variations in the ultimate strain for tendons have been reported because different species and ages were studied. The stress-strain curve of a tendon begins in the "toe region," where tendon deforms easily, without much tensile force. Next, there is a fairly linear region, with the slope representing the elastic stiffness of the tendon. Finally, with additional tensile loading, the tendon fails and the stress-strain curve drops to zero.[15] Although tendons are viscoelastic materials, the rate of loading has only a slight effect on the stress-strain curve. If the loading rate increases, the curve shifts slightly to the left as the tendon stiffens.

Some research has examined the responses of tendons to applied mechanical stresses. Immobilization results in significant losses in water content, glycosaminoglycan concentration, and strength.[1-4,43,46] Exercise, however, increases fiber size, ultimate tendon strength, and stiffness.[7,26,28,42,45-47] Viidik[42] found that trained rabbits had increased tensile strength in their Achilles tendon mechanism compared with untrained rabbits. Woo and associates[45-47] found that these alterations in mechanical properties were more prevalent in extensor tendons, possibly because they have functional and anatomic requirements different from those of the flexor tendons.

The exercise-response mechanism of tendons is not clear. Some clues may be found in studies of flexor tendon repair. Duran and Houser[13] showed that limited motion during tendon repair prevents the tendons from adhering to the overlying sheath, perhaps because of the alternating stress and relaxation that occurs during movement. This may also induce a cellular response from both the tendon and the epitenon layer. Small loads and limited movement may stimulate cellular activity of the epitenon.

Hitchcock and associates[23] found that immediate, controlled tendon movement during repair did not prevent healing, but did eliminate the intervening phase of tendon softening. Controlling mobilization may induce a change in tendon healing by stimulating an intrinsic healing response.

These studies indicate that exercise, particularly to the point of fatigue, can damage the ultrastructure of the tendon units. This, combined with motion, triggers a healing response that repairs the ultrastructure, thereby increasing the tensile strength of the entire tendon unit.

Ligament

Ligament consists of a collagenous matrix interspersed with fibroblasts. The nuclei of the fibroblasts are elongated, basophilic structures that lie between the collagen bundles. Cellular density and nuclear shapes vary from one ligament to another. Light microscopy shows that the collagen in a ligament has an undulating appearance that produces a phenomenon known as "crimp." This "crimp" in the collagen matrix results in a degree of elasticity so that the ligament acts like a spring when load is applied and the crimp straightens.

The normal ligament is 90% fibrillar type I collagen and less than 10% type III collagen. This collagen is synthesized by the fibroblasts.

In the mature ligament, there is a balance between collagen synthesis and degradation. The half-life of the collagen in a ligament is thought to be between 300 and 500 days. Collagen turnover is probably stimulated by a number of factors that are not clearly understood.

Exercise increases strength at the ligament-bone junction.[10,33,37,38] Viidik[41] found that the junction of the anterior cruciate ligament with the tibia was stronger in exercised rabbits than in caged controls. The maximum tensile strength of the bone-ligament-bone preparation increased significantly in the exercised animals. The linear portion of the load deformation curve became steeper, indicating ligament stiffness. Tipton and associates[39] showed that treadmill exercise increased strength in anterior and posterior cruciate ligament complexes and decreased stiffness. Both Tipton and associates[39] and Viidik[41] used slow strain rates for failure testing and found that the bone-ligament-bone preparations failed by bony avulsion in all cases.

Cabaud and associates[10] used a strain rate of 95% per second and found significant increases in the strength and stiffness of the anterior cruciate ligament in exercised rats. Animals that were exercised daily had the greatest increase in strength. These authors concluded that endurance-type exercise increases the strength and stiffness of the anterior cruciate ligament but does not alter its functional capacity.

Oakes and associates[32] compared caged rats with rats in a four-week exercise program involving alternating daily periods of running and swimming. The anterior and posterior cruciate ligaments of the exercised rats had markedly increased numbers of small-diameter fibrils. The greater number of small-diameter fibrils may be responsible for the decreased elastic stiffness in the ligaments of exercised animals.[30] The number of large-diameter fibrils decreased in both the exercised and unexercised ligaments; the middle group of fibrils increased. This may explain the increase in tensile strength noted with training for longer periods.[44,47] Binkley and Peat[8] also showed that the number of small-diameter fibrils in rat medial collateral ligament diminished after six weeks of immobilization.

These studies support the concept that endurance-type exercise increases strength and stiffness of both the substance of the ligament and the bone-ligament junction.

Muscle

Skeletal muscle consists of muscle cells, a muscle-specific extracellular matrix, and a highly organized network of nerves and blood vessels. Muscle cells contain multiple nuclei, complex systems of intracellular membranes, and specific types of contractile protein. Normal muscle function depends on the integrity of the muscle cells and on the nerve and vessel networks that supply these cells. Different skeletal muscles exhibit significant histologic variations in their structure, based on compositional differences in the types of myofibrils present.

A generally accepted classification of fiber types includes types I, IIA, IIB, IIC, and IIM. Type I fibers are slow-twitch fibers, with the slowest contraction time and the lowest content of glycogen. These fibers are quite resistant to fatigue. The IIA fibers are fast-twitch oxidative fibers, with much faster contraction times than type I fibers. The IIA fibers are more resistant to fatigue than type IIB fibers. Type IIB fibers are fast-contracting fibers that rely on the glycolytic pathways for energy production. Type IIA fibers use fast red myosin, while type IIB fibers use fast white myosin. Type IIC fibers contain both types of fast myosin and are called intermediate fibers. Finally, type IIM fibers are the "superfast fibers." Type IIM fibers are found primarily in the jaw muscles and contain a myosin different from the myosins found in type I and other type II fibers. Much research on the effect of exercise on muscle fiber structure examined the specific effects of exercise on type I rather than type II fibers.

Faulkner[14] outlined principles of muscle training on the basis of overload, specificity, and reversibility. Skeletal muscle fibers respond to overloading by increasing their structure and functional capability. Specificity of training means that a specific stimulus elicits specific structural and functional changes in specific elements of the skeletal muscle. Because the muscle adapts in response to specific training, the rate of adaptation eventually levels off. Saltin and Gollnick[35] found that endurance training can double the oxidative capacity of whole-muscle homogenates and increase the percentage of fibers classified as high-oxidative in the limb muscles used. Finally, the effects of training are reversible; when training stops, detraining occurs and adaptive changes regress.[14]

Varnauskas and associates[40] and Morgan and associates[31] verified that skeletal muscle is responsive to changes in patterns of activity and inactivity. Gollnick and associates[18] studied persons who specialized in different athletic endeavors and found major differences in the oxidative potential of muscle groups. Endurance athletes had more than three times the concentrations of succinate dehydrogenase than individuals who were sedentary or who engaged in nonendurance sports such as weightlifting. Hoppeler and associates[24] believe this stems from an increase in total mitochondrial volume of the muscle fibers. In 1973, Gollnick and associates[17] demonstrated that the exceptionally high succinate dehydrogenase concentrations in the muscles of endurance athletes resulted from training, not genetics. The magnitude of the change in oxidative potential is a function of the type, duration, and intensity of the exercises used in training.

Muscle hypertrophy and increased muscle strength are produced by high-tension/low-frequency skeletal muscle contraction.[14] Strength-training programs increase the total muscle mass by increasing the number of myofibrils per fiber, resulting in an increase in the cross-sectional area of individual fibers. Type II fibers are generally more hypertrophic than type I fibers. Exercise programs designed to increase muscle strength do not alter the maximum blood flow, the oxidative capacity, or the mitochondrial density of skeletal muscle.[14]

Gollnick and associates[18] also showed that the composition of skeletal muscles in men varied among athletes who specialized in different events. Athletes in endurance events possessed high percentages of slow-twitch fibers (type I), whereas those in sprint events had greater numbers of fast-twitch fibers (type II). To determine whether these differences were inherited or the result of a given pattern of training, Gollnick and associates[17] placed sedentary persons with a high percentage of fast-twitch fibers in their muscles on an endurance program of training. Six months later, examination of muscle samples failed to show any major shift in the fiber population. Jansson and associates,[27] however, reported an interconversion in the fiber types in the leg muscles of endurance athletes after their training regimen changed. Because this study had no control values and the biopsy specimens contained only a small number of fibers, the results may not be valid.

In 1977, Saltin and associates[36] examined fiber-type distribution in the vastus lateralis of 16-year-olds of both sexes. The overall population appeared to have a normal distribution of fibers. A few individuals may have unusually high percentages of slow-twitch or fast-twitch fibers in their muscles, predisposing them to specific athletic endeavors. Komi and associates[29] tested monozygous and dizygous twins and found that the percentage of fibers in a given muscle is genetically determined and not influenced by training.

Capillary Supply

Andersen and Kroese[6] proved that the number of capillaries per fiber in human muscle is highest in oxidative fibers and lowest in anaerobic-type fibers. Endurance training increases the number of capillaries per fiber according to Hermansen and Wachtlova[22] and Andersen and Henriksson.[5]

Strength Training

There has been a major controversy about how skeletal muscle responds to strength training. That muscles enlarge as the result of hypertrophy of preexisting muscle fibers in response to functional overload is generally accepted. The controversy centers around the issue of hyperplasia of existing fibers vs fiber splitting. Reitsma[34] and Gonyea and associates[20,21] found branch muscle fibers in muscle enlarging in response to physiologic overload. This could mean that the fibers actively divided by longitudinal splitting. However, Gollnick and associates,[19] who dissected individual fibers from the muscles of rats, found that muscle growth was stimulated by a combination of ablation of synergistic muscle and high-intensity treadmill running. They concluded that hypertrophy of preexisting fibers caused muscle enlargement, not a proliferation of fibers resulting from fiber-splitting. The specific contributions to muscle enlargement of hyperplasia, fiber-splitting, and fiber-branching have not been definitively determined.[11]

Detraining of skeletal muscle has also been studied. When training stops, the number of oxidative fibers returns to the control value, and there is a compensatory reduction in the oxidative capacity of the muscle.

Whether the percentage of a given fiber type in an athlete's muscle is inherited or results from conversion of fiber types in response to training cannot be determined from current data. Blank and Puhl[9] were unable to demonstrate that training significantly altered muscle fiber composition, fiber area, or fiber diameter in either males or females subjected to isokinetic strength training.

Costill[12] found that patients with surgically treated limbs who did single-leg cycling developed significantly more endurance capacity in the treated limb than in the normal unexercised limb. However, these same patients had subnormal maximal leg-press power with the treated limb. This suggests that training adaptations are specific to the exercise used and do not carry over to other forms of exercise. Similarly, Houston and associates[25] demonstrated that the improvement in force production from strength training is related to increases in the cross-sectional area of type II muscle fibers, as well as to a learning or neural factor.

References

1. Akeson WH: An experimental study of joint stiffness. *J Bone Joint Surg* 1961;43A:1022–1034.
2. Akeson WH, Amiel D, LaViolette D: The connective-tissue response to immobility: A study of the chondroitin-4 and 6-sulfate and dermatan sulfate changes in periarticular connective tissue of control and immobilized knees of dogs. *Clin Orthop* 1967;51:183–197.
3. Akeson WH, Amiel D, LaViolette D, et al: The connective tissue response to immobility: An accelerated ageing response? *Exp Gerontol* 1968;3:289–301.
4. Akeson WH, Amiel D, Mechanic GL, et al: Collagen cross-linking alterations in joint contractures: Changes in the reducible cross-links in periarticular connective tissue collagen after nine weeks of immobilization. *Connect Tissue Res* 1977;5:15–19.
5. Andersen P, Henriksson J: Capillary supply of the quadriceps femoris muscle of man: Adaptive response to exercise. *J Physiol* 1977;270:677–690.
6. Andersen P, Kroese AJ: Capillary supply in soleus and gastrocnemius muscles of man. *Pflugers Arch* 1978;375:245–249.
7. Barfred T: Experimental rupture of the Achilles tendon: Comparison of experimental ruptures in rats of different ages and living under different conditions. *Acta Orthop Scand* 1971;42:406–428.
8. Binkley JM, Peat M: The effects of immobilization on the ultrastructure and mechanical properties of the medial collateral ligament of rats. *Clin Orthop* 1986;203:301–308.
9. Blank S, Puhl JL: Effect of isokinetic strength training on muscle fiber composition and fiber size in young men and women, abstract. *Med Sci Sports Exerc* 1982;14:112.
10. Cabaud HE, Chatty A, Gildengorin V, et al: Exercise effects on the strength of the rat anterior cruciate ligament. *Am J Sports Med* 1980;8:79–86.
11. Caplan A, Carlson B, Faulkner J, et al: Skeletal muscle, in Woo SL-Y, Buckwalter JA (eds): *Injury and Repair of the Musculoskeletal Soft Tissues.* Park Ridge, American Academy of Orthopaedic Surgeons, 1988, pp 213–291.

12. Costill DL: Muscle rehabilitation after knee surgery. *Phys Sportsmed* 1977;5:71–84.
13. Duran RJ, Houser RG: Controlled passive motion following flexor tendon repair in zones 2 and 3, in American Academy of Orthopaedic Surgeons *Symposium on Tendon Surgery in the Hand.* St. Louis, CV Mosby, 1975, pp 105–114.
14. Faulkner JA: New perspectives in training for maximum performance. *JAMA* 1968;205:741–746.
15. Gelberman R, Goldberg V, An K-N, et al: Tendon, in Woo SL-Y, Buckwalter JA (eds): *Injury and Repair of the Musculoskeletal Soft Tissues.* Park Ridge, American Academy of Orthopaedic Surgeons, 1988, pp 5–40.
16. Gelberman RH, Woo SL-Y, Lothringer K, et al: Effects of early intermittent passive mobilization on healing canine flexor tendons. *J Hand Surg* 1982;7:170–175.
17. Gollnick PD, Armstrong RB, Saltin B, et al: Effect of training on enzyme activity and fiber composition of human skeletal muscle. *J Appl Physiol* 1973;34:107–111.
18. Gollnick PD, Armstrong RB, Saubert CW IV, et al: Enzyme activity and fiber composition in skeletal muscle of untrained and trained men. *J Appl Physiol* 1972;33:312–319.
19. Gollnick PD, Timson BF, Moore RL, et al: Muscular enlargement and number of fibers in skeletal muscles of rats. *J Appl Physiol* 1981;50:936–943.
20. Gonyea WJ: Role of exercise in inducing increases in skeletal muscle fiber number. *J Appl Physiol* 1980;48:421–426.
21. Gonyea W, Ericson GC, Bonde-Petersen F: Skeletal muscle fiber splitting induced by weight-lifting exercise in cats. *Acta Physiol Scand* 1977;99:105–109.
22. Hermansen L, Wachtlova M: Capillary density of skeletal muscle in well-trained and untrained men. *J Appl Physiol* 1971;30:860–863.
23. Hitchcock TF, Light TR, Bunch WH, et al: The effect of immediate controlled mobilization on the strength of flexor tendon repairs. *Trans Orthop Res Soc* 1986;11:216.
24. Hoppeler H, Lüthi P, Claassen H, et al: The ultrastructure of the normal human skeletal muscle: A morphometric analysis of untrained men, women and well-trained orienteers. *Pflugers Arch* 1973;344:217–232.
25. Houston ME, Valeriote SP, Green HJ: Strength training and detraining: A one leg model, abstract. *Med Sci Sports Exerc* 1982;14:177.
26. Ingelmark BE: The structure of tendons at various ages and under different functional conditions: II. An electron-microscopic investigation of Achilles tendons from white rats. *Acta Anat* 1948;6:193–225.
27. Jansson E, Sjödin B, Tesch P: Changes in muscle fibre type distribution in man after physical training: A sign of fibre type transformation? *Acta Physiol Scand* 1978;104:235–237.
28. Kliskinen A: Physical training and connective tissues in young mice: Physical properties of Achilles tendons and long bones. *Growth* 1977;41:123–137.
29. Komi PV, Viitasalo JH, Havu M, et al: Skeletal muscle fibres and muscle enzyme activities in monozygous and dizygous twins of both sexes. *Acta Physiol Scand* 1977;100:385–392.
30. Larsen N, Parker AW: Physical activity and its influence on the strength and elastic stiffness of knee ligaments, in Howell ML, Parker AW (eds): *Sports Medicine: Medical and Scientific Aspects of Elitism in Sports.* Brisbane, Australian Sports Medicine Federation, 1982, vol 8, pp 63–73.
31. Morgan TE, Cobb LA, Short FA, et al: Effects of long-term exercise on human muscle mitochondria, in Pernow B, Saltin B (eds): *Muscle Metabolism During Exercise.* New York, Plenum Press, 1971, pp 87–95.

32. Oakes BW, Parker AW, Norman J: Changes in collagen fibre populations in young rat cruciate ligaments in response to an intensive one-month's exercise program, in Russo P, Gass G (eds): *Human Adaptation.* Williamsberg, Kentucky, Cumberland College of Health Sciences, 1981, pp 223–230.
33. Parry DA, Craig AS, Barnes GR: Tendon and ligament from the horse: An ultrastructural study of collagen fibrils and elastic fibres as a function of age. *Proc R Soc Lond* 1978;203:293–303.
34. Reitsma W: Skeletal muscle hypertrophy after heavy exercise in rats with surgically reduced muscle function. *Am J Physiol Med* 1969;48:237–258.
35. Saltin B, Gollnick P: Skeletal muscle adaptability: Significance for metabolism and performance, in Peachey LD, Adrian RH, Geiger SR (eds): *Handbook of Physiology: Section 10. Skeletal Muscle.* Bethesda, American Physiological Society, 1983, pp 555–631.
36. Saltin B, Henriksson J, Nygaard E, et al: Fiber types and metabolic potentials of skeletal muscles in sedentary man and endurance runners. *Ann NY Acad Sci* 1977;301:3–29.
37. Tipton CM, James SL, Mergner W, et al: Influence of exercise on strength of the medial collateral knee ligaments of dogs. *Am J Physiol* 1970;218:894–902.
38. Tipton CM, Matthes RD, Maynard JA, et al: The influence of physical activity on ligaments and tendons. *Med Sci Sports* 1975;7:165–175.
39. Tipton CM, Schild RJ, Tomanek RJ: Influence of physical activity on the strength of knee ligaments in rats. *Am J Physiol* 1967;212:783–787.
40. Varnauskas E, Björntorp P, Fahlén M, et al: Effects of physical training on exercise blood flow and enzymatic activity in skeletal muscle. *Cardiovasc Res* 1970;4:418–422.
41. Viidik A: The elasticity and tensile strength of the anterior cruciate ligament in rabbits as influenced by training. *Acta Physiol Scand* 1968;74:372–380.
42. Viidik A: Tensile strength properties of Achilles tendon systems in trained and untrained rabbits. *Acta Orthop Scand* 1969;40:261–272.
43. Woo SL-Y: Mechanical properties of tendons and ligaments: I. Quasi-static and nonlinear viscoelastic properties. *Biorheology* 1982;19:385–396.
44. Woo SL-Y, Amiel D, Akeson WH, et al: Effects of long term exercise on ligaments, tendons and bones of swine, abstract. *Med Sci Sports Exerc* 1979;11:105.
45. Woo SL, Gomez MA, Amiel D, et al: The effects of exercise on the biomechanical and biochemical properties of swine digital flexor tendons. *J Biomech Eng* 1981;103:51–56.
46. Woo SL, Gomez MA, Woo YK, et al: Mechanical properties of tendons and ligaments: II. The relationships of immobilization and exercise on tissue remodeling. *Biorheology* 1982;19:397–408.
47. Woo SL, Ritter MA, Amiel D, et al: The biomechanical and biochemical properties of swine tendons: Long term effects of exercise on the digital extensors. *Connect Tissue Res* 1980;7:177–183.

Chapter 37

Cellular Response to Loading

Cyril B. Frank, MD, FRCS(C)
David A. Hart, PhD

There is abundant experimental evidence suggesting that both the form and function of musculoskeletal soft tissues are influenced by mechanical loading.[41] While biomechanical, biochemical, morphologic, and other measurable changes in tissue matrix properties are clearly one manifestation of these influences, it could be argued that such matrix changes are really rather indirect measures of loading effects. Cells are thought to be the true transducers of load and thus should be studied more directly if these loading effects are to be defined more clearly. Cells in muscle, tendon, ligament, skin, and cartilage generally respond to "windows" of increased loading by increasing matrix synthesis, increasing metabolic activity, increasing their replication rates, and modifying their production of matrix components. Outside these physiologic windows are pathologic loading effects, such as excessive loads or no loads that lead either to reductions in cell synthesis and increases in degradative activity or to pathologic increases or decreases in both. These homeostasis-altering effects again seem to be load-, model-, and environment-specific and also seem to depend on some important interactions between cell, matrix, and environment.

Theories concerning how loads may influence cells can be classified into "indirect" (systemic, regional, and pericellular) and "direct" (the cell itself). While there is evidence that both indirect and direct mechanisms exist, the latter are generally perceived to be physiologically more important. Changes in pericellular pH values and in membrane ion permeabilities (affecting the second messenger systems) are the load-response mechanisms best defined thus far.

Evidence That Loading Influences Cells

Recent evidence indicates that mechanical stresses influence connective tissue cells themselves, and researchers have speculated about the mechanisms by which this may occur.[14,41] At the outset, though, it must be pointed out that while evidence for a link between mechanical stress and cellular processes is abundant and theories abound, the mechanisms by which tissue structure and function are related remain unclear and theories concerning these mechanisms are controversial. Many investigations have studied direct loading effects on soft connective tissue cells. Such studies are best grouped according to tissue of origin of the cells: muscle, skin, tendon, ligament, and cartilage.

Muscle

As reviewed recently by Booth,[11] muscle cells' responses to loading have probably been studied more extensively than any other cell. Myriad muscle-cell changes in response to exercise have been demonstrated, including changes in response to growth factors,[32] changes in insulin receptors[10,15] or β-adrenergic receptors,[33] increased mitochondria,[26,40] changes in facilitated glucose transport[8,47] and in proteins that control ion channels,[17] as well as in both direct and indirect effects on second messengers, such as Ca^{2+}, protein kinases, and phosphatidylinositol phosphates.[11] Collectively, these studies show that a cascade of events takes place in muscle cells both during and after muscle activity, resulting in measurable changes in cell metabolism and clearly altering muscle-cell character and reactivity. The exact details of these changes, their durations, and their significance in functional terms, however, remain controversial. The reader is referred to comprehensive sources of information on exercise (load)-induced changes in muscle,[11] as these studies are simply too voluminous to be noted here.

Skin and Tendon Fibroblasts

Fibroblasts' responses to loading appear to be the second most commonly studied soft tissue response.[4,20,21,50] While derived from a variety of sources, fibroblasts isolated from either skin or tendons have been investigated most often. These, along with fibroblasts studied in other models, will be discussed together, because they demonstrate the common finding that fibroblasts do respond to being loaded by changing shape, composition, and function (matrix metabolism and growth rates). Meikle and associates[37,38] in 1979 and 1980, for example, examined in vitro loading effects on newborn rabbit cranial sutures, and found that continuous stress led to an increase in collagen synthesis as part of a general increase in protein synthesis. In addition, they found simultaneous increases in matrix degradative enzymes that were apparently balanced by increases in enzyme inhibitors.[38] They thus explained a 1.5-fold to threefold increase in protein accumulation and a twofold collagen accumulation in the suture cells by the fact that both synthetic and degradative mechanisms had been "switched on" equally by the loading, but that the degradative pathway was being blocked by an inhibitor. This implies an interesting means by which matrix would accumulate and possibly subsequently be remodeled—simple removal or blocking of an inhibitor. At the very least, it implies that a cell product (the inhibitor) is being produced selectively during loading and represents evidence for a load-specific cell product. It also introduces the concept that matrix quality and quantity can be manipulated by means other than simple cellular synthetic and degradative pathways, potentially also being controlled by a subset of extracellular mediators (stimulators and inhibitors). Loading could clearly alter any of these. Brunette,[12] working with porcine epithelial cells grown on a stretched plastic substrate, found other evidence of fibroblast responses to loading. He showed that as little as 30 minutes of stretching led to a significant increase in the number of cells synthesizing DNA in vitro. He also made an observation of unknown significance: that such an effect was present only with high concentrations of serum. While this may imply some nutritive effect of movement (improved transport of nutrients to or into cells), it was not addressed in that study.

Kolega[34] in 1986 stretched mobile clusters of epithelial fibroblasts and found that microfilaments within the cells become aligned along the long axis of that tension, preventing cell protrusions away from that direction of tension and thus providing at least one clue toward a structural mechanism for fibroblast realignment with stress. Exactly how such an internal cellular rearrangement in response to tensile stress could occur, however, remains unknown. In a possibly related study, which also suggests a cellular reorganization in response to stress, Stockbridge and French[48] showed that stretch on a human fibroblast appears to open cation channels through its cell membrane.

Tendon fibroblasts have long been thought to respond to changes in tension by changes in their synthesis and degradation of matrix materials.[20] Gillard and associates[25] in 1979 demonstrated apparent cell-mediated changes in glycosaminoglycan contents of different areas of a tendon in response to both relief and return of compressive and tensile loading. Perhaps even more important than these changes in quantity, the authors found that there were measurable changes in the types of glycosaminoglycans in these different regions of the tendon, apparently in direct response to some qualities of the changing loading conditions. Much like the study by Meikle and associates,[37] this suggests a load-related alteration in matrix expression of fibroblasts, or perhaps the selection and differentiation of a specific subpopulation of cells. This demonstration of tendon matrix heterogeneity has been followed by several observations that cells, collagen, and matrix in tensile and pressure zones of different tendons are, in fact, different.[20,52]

In an attempt to show that such differences in tendon structure are more definitely load-dependent, Slack and associates[46] in 1984 studied a model of cyclic tensile loading of isolated embryonic chick tendons in vitro. In addition to the increased synthesis of proteins, glycosaminoglycans, and DNA by their fibroblasts, a selective increase in sulfated glycosaminoglycans was found. Again, some type of environment-specific fibroblast expression seems to have taken place. Vogel and associates[51] added another interesting piece to this puzzle by confirming that large proteoglycans are synthesized much more readily by fibroblasts isolated from within compressed regions of tendon than by fibroblasts in tensile regions,[52] and that this expression is preserved for significant periods in vitro. The subsequent slow "dedifferentiation" process of cells in culture in this and numerous other cell systems may also reflect an effect of loading; in this case, relative load deprivation.

Collectively, these studies support the observations made in skin that deformation can alter cell behavior. However, these tendon cell studies additionally suggest that certain qualities of the deformation (tensile, compressive) can cause selective alternations in expression by what may be the same population of cells. Alternatively, loading may be altering cell differentiation itself. These possibilities still require further definition.

Ligament

Ligament cells also appear to be responsive to their loading environments. Amiel and associates[2,3] reported that immobilization of the adult rabbit leg leads to early increases in the metabolic activity of cells in the medial collateral ligament. Increases in both synthesis and degradation of matrix occurred early after immobilization; after longer immobilization periods, degradative activity increased as a result of declining synthetic activity. Thus, immobilization results in a dysregulation of the balance between synthesis and degradation (remodeling) normally found in this tissue.

Recently, Hart and associates[31] and Walsh and associates,[53,54] using skeletally immature animals, investigated the effect of immobilization on ligament metabolism. Immobilization and confirmed disuse led to a rapid decline in metabolic activity along the entire length of the medial collateral ligament. There was coordinate loss of collagen synthetic activity and proteinase secretion. The decline in activity occurred in the midsubstance as well as at the growing tibial insertion. During more extended periods of immobilization there was an increase in degradative activity and a maintenance of the low level of matrix synthesis. Thus, immobilization of the growing ligament leads to a cessation of growth as well as to induction of a catabolic state. These biochemical alterations were correlated with a loss in the biomechanical maturation of this ligament. The medial collateral ligament of the contralateral leg in such immobilized animals exhibited enhanced levels of metabolic activity compared with the medial collateral ligament of age-matched untreated animals.

While our understanding of the mechanisms regulating growth (anabolic state) and atrophy (catabolic state) is incomplete, these investigations suggest that loading of the immature ligament is required for the continuation of the maturation process. Interruption of loading by immobilization therefore overrides the stimuli mediating growth. Such conclusions would have implications for the management and rehabilitation of young athletes requiring limb immobilization.

While this discussion has focused on the effect of loading on normal ligament maturation and homeostasis, an additional variable or set of variables is introduced during the inflammatory state. Recently, Hart and associates[31] (and unpublished data) indicated that exposure of ligaments to inflammatory mediators such as interleukin-1 in vitro can enhance proteinase secretion by the organ cultures. Whether such mediators, released as a consequence of direct injury to the ligament or through injury to another element within the joint, could influence ligament metabolism in a negative fashion in vivo remains to be proved but should not be ignored. Conversely, the same group found that exposure of ligaments to drugs frequently used for the treatment of sports injuries, such as steroids or nonsteroidal anti-inflammatory drugs in vitro, can down-regulate secretion of proteolytic enzymes capable of mediating matrix turnover. Thus, ligaments can respond to a number of endogeneous and exogenous stimuli that alter their metabolic activity. The outcome of the interaction between endogenous stimuli (loading, growth factors, inflammatory mediators) and between endogenous and exogenous stimuli (drugs) on the integrity of normal ligament and the ligament recovering from injury is of great interest and is the focus of current investigation.

Cartilage

Cartilage cell explants have been studied under various loading conditions in vivo and in vitro. De Witt and associates[16] in 1984 showed that cyclic stretching of chick epiphyseal chondrocytes led to increased label incorporation into newly synthesized glycosaminoglycans, along with a 2.4-fold increase of thymidine incorporation into DNA. They suggested that a 2.2-fold increase in cyclic AMP levels in these chondrocytes may have been involved in this mechanical effect. Tammi and associates[49] in 1988 showed that canine chondrocytes produce more prolyl 4-hydroxylase (PPH) in response to both excessive loading (increased by 11% to 13%) and stress deprivation (PPH increased by 53%) in vivo. On the basis of their additional observation that despite this excessive potential for cartilage collagen turnover, collagen contents were not altered, they concluded that collagen turnover in cartilage must be enhanced in load-bearing but that it must be increased even more during immobilization. Because inhibitors were not measured, however, this speculation may not be valid.[12] Gray and associates[28] have studied calf epiphyseal plates subjected to static compressive stresses from 0 to 3 mPa, and have found that proline and sulfate incorporations decreased monotonically with increased stress. On the basis of the other systems noted above, this is an unusual response that may, of course, be model-specific or tissue-specific. It is conceivable that excessive loading inhibits growth plates.[15] In related studies, Hall and Urban[30] found that low-level hydrostatic compressive effects actually stimulate both proline and sulfate incorporations by hyaline chondrocytes isolated from either bovine metacarpal joints or human femoral heads. Higher pressures for longer durations (eg, 50 mPA for two hours), on the other hand, inhibited incorporations by these cells as long as they were studied in their matrices. In contradistinction, all pressures from 5 to 50 mPA applied for durations from five minutes to two hours were found to inhibit isolated (extracted from their matrix) hyaline chondrocyte metabolism, suggesting that there is a crucial mediating effect of matrix on cell responses to such pressures.

Collectively, these studies suggest that both epiphyseal and hyaline cartilage cell metabolisms are responsive to compressive loading, but that the specific effects probably depend entirely on cell origins. Epiphyseal plate cartilage appears to respond differently from hyaline surface cartilage. In addition, the presence or absence of matrix around cartilage cells and the magnitudes of pressure that are applied very likely further modify these responses. As with all connective tissue cell types, there are almost certainly "physiologic windows of stress" that define synthetic, homeostatic, and degradative cell behaviors.[22–24] An additional variable, which should be emphasized in the context of cartilage, is that of tissue heterogeneity. Studies by Gravel and associates[27] and McAllister and associates[36] have indicated that articular cartilage explants derived from different anatomic areas within a joint and analogous areas from different joints appear to express and regulate the balance between anabolic and catabolic activity quite differently. On the basis of such findings, one may speculate that such differentiation (heterogeneity) is linked to the ability of the tissue to accommodate loading and maintain homeostasis. Such metabolic heterogeneity should also be considered when loading effects on articular cartilage are analyzed, as the tissue may also respond to loading in a heterogeneous fashion. Thus, one may not be able to generalize and consider cartilage as a uniform tissue.

Speculated Mechanisms Concerning How Loads May Affect Cells

Mechanical loading influences cell behavior in all soft tissues, but how it does so is not fully understood. No one experiment has differentiated cause and effect. We will attempt to classify existing theories about the causes of cell changes under loads in order to provide a framework for further thought and experimentation.

Basically, theories can be subdivided into those concerning direct causes (cell-related) and those concerning indirect causes (everything other than cells). "Indirect" theories are probably more common, but they seem to have been applied relatively rarely to the study of connective tissue other than muscle. It is commonly accepted, for example, that systemic release of hormones, growth factors, nutrients, and biochemical mediators[11] during exercise probably produces several modifying effects on peripheral cell behavior. These substances then rely on blood supply, the second potential indirect control mechanism for soft connective tissue. Bader and associates,[5] for example, demonstrated that a 10% strain in human skin can virtually obliterate capillary blood flow. Such an obliteration could then cause a cascade of events (changes in oxygen tensions, pH, pressures, supplies of ions and counter-ions to pumps, and a variety of other local phenomena) that would then almost certainly affect cells. At least for vascular tissues, therefore, the seemingly incidental effects of mechanical forces on rerouting blood may be a dramatic and not-so-incidental initiator of regional or even local changes. For less vascular tissues such as tendons or ligaments or an avascular tissue such as cartilage, these effects are probably negligible. Alternatively, it could also be speculated that cells in such hypovascular tissue may simply be exceptionally sensitive to small changes in local or regional conditions, a possibility that must certainly be considered in view of their in vitro sensitivities.[28,30]

A second subdivision of indirect theories involves effects that may involve more localized strain-induced biochemical events[35] in the tissues. These events may incite a chain of cellular or pericellular events, such as the apparently secondary increases in phospholipase A_2, arachidonic acid, and prostaglandin E_2 synthesis seen in loaded bone cells by Binderman and associates[6,7] and by Yeh and Rodan.[55] Cyclic AMP has also been found to be elevated[6,12] in loaded cells, probably merely as a later event in the biochemical pathway that has been activated.[7] Fatigue microdamage to matrix,[13,14] with subsequent matrix product breakdown, solubility, and local biochemical changes around cells is another possible explanation. A subset of this classification is the simple but intriguing possibility that the primary indirect local biochemical trigger may be the potential change in local pH induced by loading. Both Gray and associates[28] and Hall and Urban[30] found that changing counter-ion concentrations (eg, K^+, H^+) does mimic some of the cellular effects seen with chondrocytes under compression. This has led to the speculation that pericelluar pH values may simply be altered in some way by tension or compression, leading to the cascades of events seen. This clearly requires further investigation in situ.

The third subclassification of speculated indirect mechanisms involves a modification of the first two, in that no direct or significant deformation of the cell would necessarily be required. For these theories cell deformation would be an incidental event. Instead, deformation of matrix (water, collagen, proteoglycans) would be considered the primary event, leading somewhat indirectly to a local cellular response. The best example of this is the long-studied but unproven local "piezoelectric" effect of matrix on cells.[13,14] While apparently more relevant in bone,[9] the possibility that deformation of soft-tissue matrix or cells may also lead to functionally significant local electrical or vibrational signals cannot be ruled out.[9]

As the final indirect mechanism of loading, the consequence of innervation on the tissue response to loading should be considered. Fisher and Bray[19] reported that the rabbit anterior cruciate ligament and medial collateral ligament are more extensively innervated than previously thought. More thorough examination of other ligaments and connective tissue may also reveal patterns of innervation that could contribute to tissue responses to loading stimuli. Cartilage, on the other hand, is avascular and aneural, and loading stimuli may be translated via different mechanisms in such tissues. Therefore, one cannot assume that only "one" mechanism is operative in all tissues. Connective tissues such as muscle, ligaments, and articular cartilage vary quite dramatically in blood supply and innervation. Thus, specific tissues may also vary in the mechanisms by which the loading "stimulus" is translated to a biochemical response. Such variables should be considered when comparing loading effects on cell with effects on tissue in vitro or in vivo.

The most common "direct" theory for the effect of mechanical loading is some type of strain-induced "direct" effect on cells.[13,14,35,43–45,50] This could be caused by an actual deformation of the cell, physically reorganizing its cytoskeleton,[1,12,18,30,34] releasing membrane-bound vesicles into surrounding matrix or to other cells,[29,42] or changing (opening or closing) ion channels through the membrane.[48] It could also involve a direct effect on almost any other component of the cell, either internally (nuclear) or externally (membrane). The fascinating possibility that octahedral shear stresses and dilatational stresses[13,14,41] actually determine cellular deformation, and thereby become translated into specific matrix-producing signals, requires further investigation.

There seems to be little doubt that loading of soft connective tissues does play an important role in the cellular control of matrix. Loading, therefore, may represent a critical entity that may explain soft-tissue pathology in some circumstances, such as the "overuse injury" and may be the most controllable therapeutic modality available.

References

1. Albrecht-Buehler G: Role of cortical tension in fibroblast shape and movement. *Cell Motil Cytoskeleton* 1987;7:54–67.
2. Amiel D, Akeson WH, Harwood FL, et al: Stress deprivation effect on metabolic turnover of the medial collateral ligament collagen: A comparison between nine- and 12-week immobilization. *Clin Orthop* 1983;172:265–270.
3. Amiel D, Woo SL-Y, Harwood FL, et al: The effect of immobilization on collagen turnover in connective tissue: A biochemical-biomechanical correlation. *Acta Orthop Scand* 1982;53:325–332.
4. Arem AJ, Madden JW: Effects of stress on healing wounds: I. Intermittent noncyclical tension. *J Surg Res* 1976;20:93–102.
5. Bader DL, Barnhill RL, Ryan TJ: Effect of externally applied skin surface forces on tissue vasculature. *Arch Phys Med Rehabil* 1986;67:807–811.
6. Binderman I, Shimshoni Z, Somjen D: Biochemical pathways involved in the translation of physical stimulus into biological message. *Calcif Tissue Int* 1984;36(suppl):S82–S85.
7. Binderman I, Zor U, Kaye AM, et al: The transduction of mechanical force into biochemical events in bone cells may involve activation of phospholipase A2. *Calcif Tissue Int* 1988;42:261–266.
8. Birnbaum MJ, Haspel HC, Rosen OM: Transformation of rat fibroblasts by FSV rapidly increases glucose transporter gene transcription. *Science* 1987;235:1495–1498.
9. Black J: Electrical stimulation of hard and soft tissues in animal models. *Clin Plast Surg* 1985;12:243–257.
10. Bonen A, Clune PA, Tan MH: Chronic exercise increases insulin binding in muscles but not liver. *Am J Physiol* 1986;251:E196–E203.

11. Booth FW: Perspectives on molecular and cellular exercise physiology. *J Appl Physiol* 1988;65:1461–1471.
12. Brunette DM: Mechanical stretching increases the number of epithelial cells synthesizing DNA in culture. *J Cell Sci* 1984;69:35–45.
13. Carter DR: Mechanical loading histories and cortical bone remodeling. *Calcif Tissue Int* 1984;36(suppl):S19–S24.
14. Carter DR, Wong M: The role of mechanical loading histories in the development of diarthrodial joints. *J Orthop Res* 1988;6:804–816.
15. Crettaz M, Horton ES, Wardzala LJ, et al: Physical training of Zucker rats: Lack of alleviation of muscle insulin resistance. *Am J Physiol* 1983;244:E414–E420.
16. De Witt MT, Handley CJ, Oakes BW, et al: In vitro response of chondrocytes to mechanical loading: The effect of short term mechanical tension. *Connect Tissue Res* 1984;12:97–109.
17. Dolphin AC: Nucleotide binding proteins in signal transduction and disease. *Trends Neurosci* 1987;10:53–57.
18. Duke JC: Suppression of morphogenesis in embryonic mouse limbs exposed in vitro to excess gravity. *Teratology* 1983;27:427–436.
19. Fisher AW, Bray RC: Innervation patterns of the rabbit medial collateral ligament, abstract. *Br J Anat*, in press.
20. Flint M: Interrelationships of mucopolysaccharide and collagen in connective tissue remodelling. *J Embryol Exp Morphol* 1972;27:481–495.
21. Flint MH, Craig AS, Reilly HC, et al: Collagen fibril diameters and glycosaminoglycan content of skins: Indices of tissue maturity and function. *Connect Tissue Res* 1984;13:69–81.
22. Frost HM: A determinant of bone architecture: The minimum effective strain. *Clin Orthop* 1983;175:286–292.
23. Frost HM: *The Laws of Bone Structure.* Springfield, Charles C Thomas, 1964.
24. Frost HM: *The Physiology of Bone, Cartilage and Fibrous Tissues.* Springfield, Charles C Thomas, 1972.
25. Gillard GC, Reilly HC, Bell-Booth PG, et al: The influence of mechanical forces on the glycosaminoglycan content of the rabbit flexor digitorum profundus tendon. *Connect Tissue Res* 1979;7:37–46.
26. Gollnick PD, Armstrong RB, Saubert CW IV, et al: Enzyme activity and fiber composition in skeletal muscle of untrained and trained men. *J Appl Physiol* 1972;33:312–319.
27. Gravel C, McAllister D, Schachar N, et al: Non-uniform distribution of plasminogen activator expression and responsiveness to inflammatory mediators in bovine articular cartilage. *Trans Orthop Res Soc* 1989;14:534.
28. Gray ML, Pizzanelli AM, Grodzinsky AJ, et al: Mechanical and physicochemical determinants of the chondrocyte biosynthetic response. *J Orthop Res* 1988;6:777–792.
29. Grinnell F, Lamke CR: Reorganization of hydrated collagen lattices by human skin fibroblasts. *J Cell Sci* 1984;66:51–63.
30. Hall AC, Urban JPG: Responses of articular chondrocytes and cartilage to high hydrostatic pressure. *Trans Orthop Res Soc* 1989;14:49.
31. Hart DA, O'Brien MD, Walsh SL, et al: Plasminogen activators and inhibitors in rabbit connective tissues. *Fibrinolysis* 1988;2:171.
32. Jennische E, Hansson HA: Regenerating skeletal muscle cells express insulin-like growth factor I. *Acta Physiol Scand* 1987;130:327–332.
33. Ji LL, Lennon DL, Kochan RG, et al: Enzymatic adaptation to physical training under beta-blockade in the rat: Evidence of a beta 2-adrenergic mechanism in skeletal muscle. *J Clin Invest* 1986;78:771–778.
34. Kolega J: Effects of mechanical tension on protrusive activity and microfilament and intermediate filament organization in an epidermal epithelium moving in culture. *J Cell Biol* 1986;102:1400–1411.

35. Lanyon LE: Functional strain in bone tissue as an objective and controlling stimulus for adaptive bone remodelling. *J Biomech* 1987;20:1083–1093.
36. McAllister D, Gravel C, Schachar N, et al: Heterogeneity of metabolic activity and responsiveness to inflammatory mediators in bovine articular cartilage. *Trans Orthop Res Soc*, in press.
37. Meikle MC, Reynolds JJ, Sellers A, et al: Rabbit cranial sutures in vitro: A new experimental model for studying the response of fibrous joints to mechanical stress. *Calcif Tissue Int* 1979;28:137–144.
38. Meikle MC, Sellers A, Reynolds JJ: Effect of tensile mechanical stress on the synthesis of metalloproteinases by rabbit coronal sutures in vitro. *Calcif Tissue Int* 1980;30:77–82.
39. Merrilees MJ, Flint MH: Ultrastructural study of tension and pressure zones in a rabbit flexor tendon. *Am J Anat* 1980;157:87–106.
40. Morgan TE, Cobb LA, Short FA, et al: Effects of long-term exercise on human muscle mitochondria. *Adv Exp Med Biol* 1971;11:87–95.
41. Pauwels F: *Biomechanics of the Locomotor Apparatus.* Berlin, Springer-Verlag, 1980.
42. Poole CA, Flint MH, Beaumont BW: Morphological and functional interrelationships of articular cartilage matrices. *J Anat* 1984;138:113–138.
43. Rubin CT: Skeletal strain and the functional significance of bone architecture. *Calcif Tissue Int* 1984;36(suppl):S11–S18.
44. Rubin CT, Lanyon LE: Kappa Delta Award paper: Osteoregulatory nature of mechanical stimuli. Function as a determinant for adaptive remodeling in bone. *J Orthop Res* 1987;5:300–310.
45. Rubin CT, Lanyon LE: Regulation of bone formation by applied dynamic loads. *J Bone Joint Surg* 1984;66A:397–402.
46. Slack C, Flint MH, Thompson BM: The effect of tensional load on isolated embryonic chick tendons in organ culture. *Connect Tissue Res* 1984;12:229–247.
47. Sternlicht E, Grimditch GK, Barnard RJ: Combined effect of insulin and exercise on glucose transport in rat skeletal muscle sarcolemmal vesicles, abstract. *Med Sci Sports Exerc* 1987;19:S74.
48. Stockbridge LL, French AS: Stretch-activated cation channels in human fibroblasts. *Biophys J* 1988;54:187–190.
49. Tammi M, Kiviranta I, Peltonen L, et al: Effects of joint loading on articular cartilage collagen metabolism: Assay of procollagen prolyl 4-hydroxylase and galactosylhydroxylysyl glucosyltransferase. *Connect Tissue Res* 1988;17:199–206.
50. Urschel JD, Scott PG, Williams HT: The effect of mechanical stress on soft and hard tissue repair: A review. *Br J Plast Surg* 1988;41:182–186.
51. Vogel KG, Keller EJ, Lenhoff RJ, et al: Proteoglycan synthesis by fibroblast cultures initiated from regions of adult bovine tendon subjected to different mechanical forces. *Eur J Cell Biol* 1986;41:102–112.
52. Vogel KG, Thonar EJ: Keratan sulfate is a component of proteoglycans in the compressed region of adult bovine flexor tendon. *J Orthop Res* 1988;6:434–442.
53. Walsh S: *The Effects of Immobilization on the Growth and Maturation of the Rabbit Medial Collateral Ligament*, thesis. University of Calgary, 1988.
54. Walsh S, Frank C, Hart D: Immobilization alters cell function in growing rabbit ligaments. *Trans Orthop Res Soc* 1988;13:57.
55. Yeh CK, Rodan GA: Tensile forces enhance prostaglandin E synthesis in osteoblastic cells grown on collagen ribbons. *Calcif Tissue Int* 1984;36(suppl):S67–S71.

Future Directions

The study of the modification of soft-tissue inflammation has been frustrated by (1) a lack of precision in the definition of the site of injury, (2) a lack of quantification of inflammation and/or structural injury, and (3) a lack of tissue data in the early stages of sports-induced inflammatory injury because these conditions are not treated surgically. Further clinical study of modifiers demands better attention to study design.

The criteria established by Weiler and associates[1] for an ideal clinical study of the NSAIDs in sports trauma could well apply to the study of all modifiers of sports-induced soft-tissue inflammation and injury. They include (1) a double-blind, randomized, and placebo-controlled design; (2) rigid control of the time between injury and the onset of treatment; (3) randomization of types of injuries so that minor injuries, moderate injuries, and moderately severe injuries are equally likely to be in treatment and control groups; (4) comparison of specific injuries, such as knee injuries and ankle injuries, with each other; (5) control of variables such as age, race, size (height, weight, and surface area), and sex; (6) the study of athletes from a single sport as a group; (7) identification of level of performance; (8) application of a covariant test whenever concomitant therapy was employed; (9) definition of objective criteria for the signs of inflammation; (10) measurement of time until return to training, time until fit to return to competition, and time until full recovery; and (11) competent statistical analysis from the onset to determine whether statistically significant improvements were also important to performance, to weigh the risk-benefit ratio, and to assess the adverse effects of treatment by means of a two-tailed test.

In addition, the development of objective measures of functional outcome is needed. Subjective grading of pain by some type of rating scale would also be helpful.

An ideal experimental model of tendon injury might include characterization of the mechanical and histologic properties of the normal structure; creation of a controlled wound by a reproducible method; use of a previously studied model so that verification of data would be without controversy; and selection of a model that avoids testing difficulties. Although it is helpful to rely on previously established models when possible, spontaneous models of inflammation are not common.

The research challenges are extensive, but the following guidelines define the way in which these investigations can be conducted.

Define the Clinical Efficacy of NSAIDs

Adequate clinical studies of the efficacy of NSAIDs, especially in chronic overuse injury, are lacking. Among the unanswered questions are the following: Is there a size-adjusted dosage of NSAID that would be more efficacious than standard doses? Is there less long-term disability if NSAIDs are used? Is the return to performance quicker, yet safe? Are certain injuries more suitable for treatment with NSAIDs? Are certain tissues more suitable?

These studies are particularly pertinent in view of the early suppression of pain and the symptoms of inflammation promised by NSAID use. A database on coincident rates of structural healing and strength restoration is lacking. Quantifying the degree of trauma during the course of standard clinical treatment could clarify some of these issues. Newer imaging techniques such as computed tomographic scanning, magnetic resonance imaging, and magnetic resonance spectrophotometry may prove useful in overcoming quantification and definition difficulties.

Compare the Anti-inflammatory and Analgesic Effects of Aspirin and Nonacetylated Salicylates

The use of nonacetylated salicylates in acute sport injuries requires further study. This study would be aided by the definition of a homogeneous study group with one type of anatomic lesion, for example, trochanteric bursitis in runners or sprained lateral collateral ligaments in football players. Outcome measures would include assessment of pain by some type of standard scale, assessment of tenderness and swelling by volumetric data and clinical findings, assessment of warmth by thermography or temperature probe, and assessment of function by means of a rating system that takes into account the levels of performance before and after injury. Problems include the difficulty of defining the injury and the imprecision of subjective pain assessment. More objective criteria may be available in traumatic injuries such as lateral collateral ligament sprain (stress radiographs) and in bursitic lesions (injection of contrast material).

Study the Dose-Response Correlations for Oral Anti-inflammatory Drugs

In the triggering of inflammation, the critical issue is what cell populations are required to carry on the repair process. In this respect, the polymorphonuclear cells initially present at the site of injury may be less valuable in healing. If the triggering cells that initiate the harmful aspects of inflammation at the site of injury could be treated in the acute phase of inflammation, the second stage of repair and scar formation might be initiated earlier. This may explain the alleged improvement with oral medication. Possible experimental methods include the use of hamster cheek pouch, subcutaneous wound chamber, and rat paw models. Specific histochemical and immunofluorescent cellular techniques in cell culture may shed light on this issue.

Define the Mode of Influence and Characteristics of the Physical Modalities

Increasing attention has been paid to the efficacy of physical modalities in sports-induced injury. Thermotherapy, cryotherapy, high-voltage galvanic stimulation, and ultrasound all require extensive in vitro and in vivo experimentation to justify present utilization patterns. The role of these techniques in chronic inflammation has been almost totally neglected. Attention should be paid to controlling the mode of application, assessing anesthetic artifacts in subjective responses, quantifying the tissue penetration and tissue cellular response, and documenting any decrease in damage.

Creation of a controlled injury model may be difficult. The postulated physiologic tissue effects (such as changes in lymph flow, regional alterations in blood flow, and changes in cell nutrition) require further definition. Standardized animal models with various interventions can be used for analysis at the cellular level by means of selective staining, biologic markers, and more sophisticated techniques for identifying ultrastructural changes. Wound chamber, in vitro cell culture, and tensile strain models may be useful in assessing the chemical events affected by these therapies.

Investigate the Role of Electrical-Field Induction in the Stimulation of the Repair Cycle

Initial reports of direct electrical stimulation of tendon and ligament repair have been encouraging. The importance of variation in frequency, especially in the low range (1 to 1,000 Hz), has not been defined. A corollary issue is the level of stress-generated potentials derived from tendon compared with ligament and their stress-strain relationships. Further understanding of these relationships may prove helpful in predicting whether electrical- or electromagnetic-field induction will be useful. Phenomena analogous to the original piezoelectric findings in bone-bending experiments must be sought for soft-tissue models. Animal ligament studies involving cutting and repair with stimulation by different current frequencies under appropriate double-blind conditions and with various onsets of application are needed to judge the effects of timing of stimulation on early healing. Edema appears to retard healing and controlling edema may aid in tissue oxygenation and cellular repair. The effect of such variables as carrier frequency compared with modulated frequency in the control of edema is another area of potential interest. The correct timing and the threshold dose for a therapeutic response need definition. Problems of proper modeling exist, especially for the chronic inflammatory condition.

Define the Place of Low-Energy Laser Therapy in Clinical Treatment

Current experimental and clinical knowledge of low-energy laser therapy does not permit a balanced evaluation of the usefulness of this approach. However, such a wide variety of cellular tissues and immunologically based phenomena have been described that further efforts in this area are warranted.

Cellular, tissue, and in vivo human and animal studies are all needed. These should include careful, controlled tests of cell function after irradiation under conditions pertinent to soft-tissue injury and inflammation (for example, fibroblastic proliferation, proteolytic enzyme production, and lymphocytic function); studies of repair in appropriate target tissues (for example, tendon, ligament, and muscle) and other phenomena such as angiogenesis; and careful, comprehensive, masked studies of soft-tissue wounds and inflammation (for example, those in ankle sprains, lateral epicondylitis, Achilles tendinitis, and muscle contusions). Thermal and radiation effects should be controlled and separated in the study design.

The difficulties of evaluating low-energy laser therapy are the limitations of soft-tissue injury research in general, in that quantitative end points are difficult to establish in animal and human studies. In addition, even on the tissue and cellular levels, any end points such as cellular morphologic responses to radiation are semiquantitative in nature; thus, exquisite sensitivity to masking in laboratory animal studies and double-masking in human studies is essential.

Define the Rationale for and Efficacy of Corticosteroid Injections

The continued widespread use of steroid microcrystalline ester injection in sports trauma remains without proper substantiation even though such injection therapy has been advocated in both acute injuries such as intramuscular strain or acute ankle ligament injury and traditional chronic inflammatory overuse conditions such as epicondylitis or tendinitis. Such variables as solubility, pH, coincident injection of so-called inactive ingredients such as methylparaben and benzyl alcohol, and local tissue effects need further evaluation. Studies to date have centered primarily on the biomechanical and morphologic changes in rat or rabbit tendon models. Repeating these experiments with attention to changes in specific immunologic cell populations, changing enzyme production at the sites of injection, and selective matrix staining would permit a fuller evaluation of the ramifications of this modifier of inflammation.

Information about the intramuscular effects of injected corticosteroids after acute controlled trauma is lacking. The rabbit "pulled tendon junction" model may be useful for such studies. It should be noted that all studies of the potential soft-tissue effects of corticosteroid injection have used an animal model in which the tissue was essentially normal, without preexisting inflammation. This again points out the need for a chronic overuse tendinitis model from which to draw conclusions.

Further investigation is needed to clarify the effects of corticosteroid injection on the diseased tendon. In humans, the lack of biopsy-proven evidence of healing progression and failure to verify the presence of inflammation in the pretreated condition have been major obstructions.

Investigate the Roles of Overload and Overuse in the Initiation of Inflammation

Both overload and overuse affect matrix properties at the biomechanical, biochemical, and morphologic levels. In addition, connective-tissue cells are now recognized as potential transducers of load that may undergo dramatic changes in DNA synthesis with a subsequent impact on the surrounding matrix. There seems to be a "physiologic window of stress" that defines the conditions of synthetic, morphostatic, or degradative cell behavior. One critical need is to define the crossover zones from the positive cell response seen in the training effect to the triggering of a degradative response with so-called overload or overuse. A corollary would be the triggering of a disuse response by the absence of load or use. The theory of fatigue microdamage to matrix with subsequent matrix product breakdown and local biochemical changes around cells needs further clarification in the context of sports injuries. Does this type of process produce injurious mediators or a macromolecular trigger that incites degeneration? In this context, inflammation may be the secondary reaction in an initally cell- or matrix-mediated (piezoelectric) event. The possibility that octahedral shear stresses and dilational stresses determine cellular deformation and are thereby translated into specific matrix-producing signals requires further investigation.

Investigate the Initial Remodeling Response of Ligament, Muscle, and Tendon

Currently, scientific data are lacking as to the accuracy of "Wolff's law of soft tissue." Current research into the effects of therapeutic exercise should include an attempt to correlate specific exercise training programs, alterations in cross-sectional areas of specific muscle types, and improvement in functional capability. For example, it would be useful to study a specific training program that increases the cross-sectional area of fast-twitch muscle fibers and to note its effect on the performance of a series of functional exercise tests. Variables such as strain rate, direction, duration, pattern of load (that is, cyclic vs ballistic), and mode of muscle action (that is, isotonic, isometric, or isokinetic) should be correlated with patterns of induced changes in muscle cell behavior. Placing such observations in the context of inflammation remains difficult and requires the creation of controlled acute lesions and/or an induced chronic inflammatory animal model to assess the role of therapeutic exercise.

Reference

1. Weiler JM, Albright JP, Buckwalter JA: Anti-inflammatory agents in sports medicine, in Lewis AJ, Furst DE (eds): *Non-Steroidal Anti-inflammatory Drugs*. New York, Marcel Dekker, 1987, pp 71–88.

Section Four

Failed Healing Responses

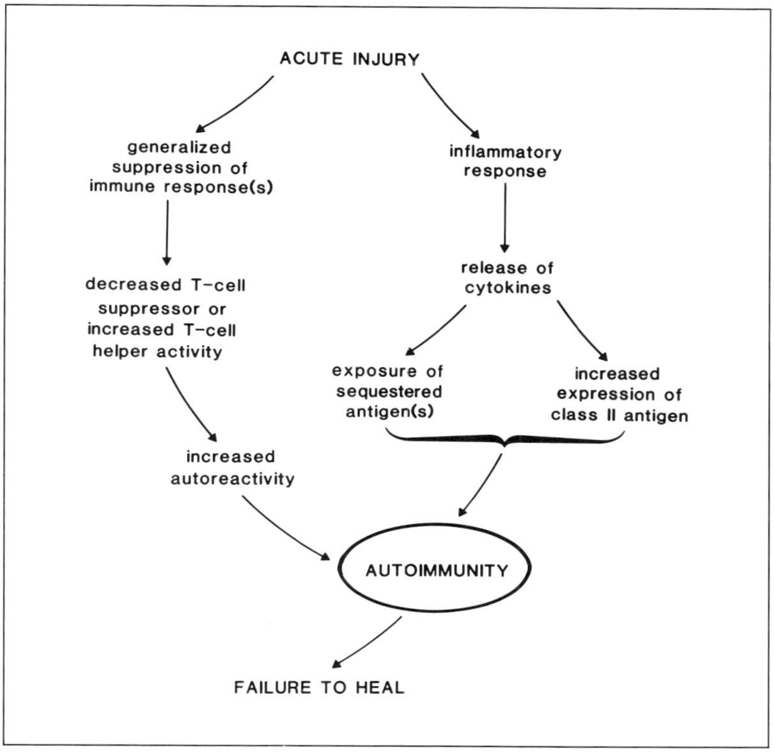

Group Leader

William Clancy, Jr., MD

Group Participants

Gary Friedlaender, MD
Peter Jokl, MD
Robert Nirschl, MD
Arnold Postlethwaite, MD
Per Renström, MD, PhD
Sharon Wahl, PhD

Overview

Little is known about the healing response in soft tissues injured as a result of overuse and/or overload. These injuries are common in all sporting activities, as well as in the workplace. Although these injuries are seldom permanently disabling, their symptoms are often severe enough to curtail or to prevent training or competition. Refraining from the inciting activity for several days to several weeks may be required before the symptoms resolve sufficiently to allow a return to participation without recurrence.

In some cases, several weeks or months of rest from the inciting activity may be required before performance can be resumed. In rare cases, symptoms and disability consistently recur despite discontinuation of the activity.

The tendon is often the soft tissue involved in these overload or overuse injuries, although cyclic loading of articular cartilage and frictional irritation in synovial structures (such as the bursa) also produce cellular and matrix changes that may be precursors of an inflammatory response. Present knowledge suggests that ligament is involved in these processes less often. Muscle tissue displays a unique inflammatory response to trauma, culminating in metaplasia and/or heterotopic bone formation.

Although most injuries resolve with appropriate nonsurgical treatment, what this section arbitrarily defines as "failed healing patterns" are encountered in both insufficient and excessive inflammation-repair processes. These lead to fibrosis and functional restriction. The key factors appear to be the type of tissue injured, the magnitude of the injury, the mechanism of the injury, individual variations and constitutional factors in healing (including age), and treatment variations.

In this section, tendon injuries constitute the starting point for discussion, as the best available clinical information concerning the progression of soft-tissue inflammation and injury is derived from sites of high tensile exposure and overload, such as the rotator cuff of the shoulder, the medial and lateral tendon origins of the elbow, the patellar tendon and quadriceps mechanism of the knee, and the Achilles tendon insertion and plantar fascia origin of the foot and ankle. Many of these areas have in common a fragile blood supply, a factor traditionally thought to be important in causing chronic inflammation and degeneration in these structures.

Although aging is known to play an important role in the reparative capacity of sports-injured soft tissue structures, younger, highly competitive, elite athletes, are also affected, calling attention to the multifactorial nature of chronic sports trauma. In addition, approximately 15% of patients have multiple sites of tendinitis despite relatively low exposure to load. This phenomenon has been dubbed the "mesenchymal syndrome," and may be related in women to diminished estrogen levels or possibly to a genetic link with the rheumatoid family of disorders. The causes of the mesenchymal syndrome as a clinical occurrence are otherwise unknown, but some form of collagen diathesis is theorized.

Grading systems for sports-related soft-tissue injury have become popular in an attempt to quantify a subjective pain complaint and relate it to the degree of acute injury and/or inflammation, as well as to the stage of structural healing. Such grading concepts lack a scientific basis. Although there is no consensus concerning the value of grading, the clinical application of such systems remains common. Factors that should be considered in applying current grading systems and in developing new systems include the tissue involved, the age of the individual, the chronicity of the problem, the degree of subjective and objective performance deficits, and the perception of pain intensity. Combining pain-measurement scales with measures of strength, endurance, flexibility, and range of motion may be the most effective means of developing valid and reliable grading systems.

At the crux of the clinical dilemma in the diagnosis of "tendinitis" is the question of whether inflammation is truly present. More acceptable nomenclature for the clinical entities observed includes peritendinitis, tendinitis, tendinosis, peritendinitis with tendinosis, partial rupture, and complete rupture. Within this scheme, tendinosis represents tendon degeneration without an inflammatory response. The progression of the injury may be related to a variety of changes in cell behavior, induced by load, which in turn lead to the production of matrix-altering mediators and eventual mechanical weakening. Inflammation in the classic sense of a round cell response within the tendon appears to occur most prominently and predictably with partial or complete tendon rupture.

A better understanding of the events triggering the observed changes in the microscopic and macroscopic architecture of the tendon after overuse or overload is essential to prevention and proper treatment. In the absence of obvious cell death to initiate a classic inflammatory response, proposed mechanisms for the observed clinical findings include diminished vascularity with subsequent decreased cellularity caused by attritional cell death, a failure of reparative cells to populate an area of tendon injury (a finding supported by biopsy data in younger patients with "chronic tendinitis" demonstrating no cellular activity other than a more metabolically active tenocyte), accelerated aging of the tenocyte, and age-dependent changes in the matrix that produce adverse biomechanical effects.

Although these findings have been documented primarily in the Achilles tendon, an angiofibroblastic hyperplasia response resembling classic granulation tissue has been found at the lateral epicondyle of the elbow. However, acute inflammatory cells are almost entirely absent in the tendon, with only a scattering of chronic inflammatory cells and then only in association with a traumatic degenerative tear.

A variety of medical conditions can lead to a frustrated healing response in tissue injury. Vascular insufficiency, malnutrition, corticosteroids, and radiation therapy have the potential to impair the repair process. Matrix components of connective tissue such as collagen, elastin, fibronectin, hyaluronic acid, and the like play important roles in inflammation and healing of injured tissues. Fragments released at the time of injury or subsequently by degenerative enzymes serve as chemoattractants and facilitate migration of reparative cells. Fibroblasts are influenced by local growth factors, cytokines, and matrix components in a complex interaction. Fibroblasts play a key role in both competence and progression. The change from inflammation to healing may involve the degradation of serum inhibitor of fibroblast migration. Any of the multitude of factors may be deficient (or excessive) and lead to failure to heal.

Both the healing response and the time required for healing have been well documented in the acutely lacerated and repaired tendon. It is the nondisrupted tendon injury resulting from overuse or overload that remains an enigma in that it may take a significantly longer period to resolve than seems to be indicated.

The concept of autoimmunity in the failure to heal of soft-tissue injuries has received little or no attention. A hypothesis of autoimmune pathophysiology may be more tenable in tissues with obvious immune potential, such as the synovium, or in cartilage in which sequestered chondrocytes may be exposed to new antigenic stimulation by attritional sports trauma. Autoimmunity as an explanation for the observed failed or refractory healing responses in joint, bursal, or tenosynovial inflammation is predicated on the theoretical traumatic induction of an antigenic protein such as a protein sequestered deep within the matrix. Some type of T-cell-mediated response would be expected at the site of inflammation if such a mechanism were operative, but this has not been studied as yet.

Hereditary constitutional variations in the human phenotype provide an intriguing and logical explanation for unusual susceptibility to "athletic trauma" and a retarded or failed healing response. In fact, the rigorous training required for athletic excellence may be linked to an internal capacity for rapid recovery from minor trauma. The occurrence of Achilles tendon rupture in the children of parents with similar conditions and the presence at an early age of classic overuse conditions in children of similarly affected parents call attention to what may be an intrinsically, genetically determined inequality. Several genetically determined diseases, such as osteogenesis imperfecta, Marfan's syndrome, and Ehlers-Danlos syndrome, offer a precedent for alterations in collagen type. The "mesenchymal syndrome" strengthens this theory and calls attention to the need for further research.

In acute traumatic sports injury, inflammation is the initial tissue response that sets the stage for proliferative and reparative processes. As such, it is required for the overall recovery of the athlete. Nevertheless, apparently inappropriate explosive inflammatory responses, such as acute traumatic bursitis and tenosynovitis, are common. Because of the associated pain, these are detrimental to athletic performance. The common end point for such inflammatory processes is the development of scar tissue and fibrosis. An excessive healing response can be as detrimental to athletic performance as insufficient repair. The sources and cellular and molecular mechanisms of the increase in proteoglycans and matrix during fibrogenesis are poorly understood. In persistent lesions, prolonged release of growth-promoting and matrix–inducing factors may escalate collagen deposition and displace functional soft tissue, changing the biomechanical properties of a structure in an adverse manner. Growth factors appear to play a prominent role in the determination of scar formation.

The process of fibrosis in soft-tissue injury may be the consequence of an imbalance between synthesis and degradation. The ability to regulate fibrogenesis and to limit inappropriate scar deposition has received little research attention.

Chapter 38

Patterns of Failed Healing in Tendon Injury

R. P. Nirschl, MD

In failed healing, a wide spectrum of issues must be considered. Key factors include the following: the type of tissue injured (ligament, tendon, synovium, muscle, articular surface); the magnitude of the injury (mechanical dissociation of infrastructure or suprastructure, either partial or total); type of injury (mechanical dissociation, vascular compromise, inflammatory process, or combinations); individual variations in healing (permanent, hereditary conditions vs temporary, reversible conditions, such as nutritional deficits); and treatment variations.

The clinical manifestations of failed healing are, of course, diverse; they usually include multiple variations of pain or deficiencies of function such as strength, endurance, flexibility, agility, and proprioception. Failed healing of suprastructure disruption usually results in primary functional deficits. Infrastructure disruption or alteration is more likely to result in chronic pain with associated secondary functional deficits resulting from the disuse caused by pain.

When a treatment scheme is being developed for soft-tissue injury, it must be remembered that mechanical deficits (except in certain knee ligaments and massive rotator cuff tears) respond reasonably well to surgical apposition of the disrupted tissues. The long-term ramifications of infrastructure distortion are more subtle and often more challenging when chronic pain enters the equation.

Although, as noted, a wide variety of soft tissues can be injured,[4,10,15,28,30] the focus of this chapter is on the failed healing of the internal tendon injury caused by repetitive overuse. The tendon is a complex tissue that includes the paratendinous sheath and the thin, synovial-type linings of epitenon and endotenon, as well as the infrastructure of collagen fascicles, matrix, fibroblasts, and neurovascular and connective support tissues.[11]

Common Sites of Persistent Tendon Pain

Overall, the human body is designed in such a way that tendon injuries occur in predictable areas.[5,23] The most common sites of injuries that result in chronic pain are listed in Outline 1.

Outline 1 Sites of injuries producing chronic pain

- Ankle
  - Achilles tendon 2 inches proximal to os calcis attachment and os calcis attachment point*
- Elbow
  - Lateral
    - Extensor aponeurosis*
    - Extensor carpi radialis brevis
  - Medial
    - Flexor carpi radialis
    - Flexor carpi ulnaris*
    - Flexor sublimis*
    - Pronator teres
  - Posterior
    - Triceps attachment to olecranon
- Foot
  - Plantar fascia attachment to medial os calcis
- Knee
  - Patellar tendon, midsubstance and attachment point at inferior pole of patella
  - Quadriceps (attachments of vastus intermedius to midsuperior pole of patellar and vastus lateralis to superior lateral pole)
- Leg
  - Posterior tibial tendon attachment to medial distal tibia
- Shoulder
  - Levator scapuli insertion to scapula; long head of the biceps*; supraspinatus section of rotator cuff

*To a lesser degree.

Many of these areas are at the apex of a convexity or concavity. In sports injuries, it is presumed that the already scant vascular supply characteristic of tendon tissue is further compromised by the tension overuse associated with the trauma. Other sites may also be stressed; these seem to be related to postural overload and include the midthoracic and posterior iliac crest areas of the spine. According to some theories, certain of these areas are affected as a result of focal electrical excitability or as part of the fibromyalgia syndrome. It is highly possible, however, that these areas may represent the phenomenon of tendinosis secondary to postural overload.

Typical Patient With Tendon Overload

Although the characteristics of the patient with chronic tendon pain are fairly consistent, wide variation does occur. In general, the underlying basis of the "tendinitis phenomenon" is repetitive overuse of the tendon or tendons in question.[3,6,7,13,18,25,26,32,33]

Another factor may be the patient's age; the physiologic age of the tendon, however, may be of even greater importance.[5,25] The typical recreational athlete is 35 to 50 years old.[5,26,29] One study on tennis elbow revealed an average age of 42.7 years.[27] Competitive athletes are usually much younger than recreational athletes but are likely to have subjected their tendons to greater physiologic demands. Thus, competitive athletes (such as swimmers, track athletes, baseball pitchers, and tennis players) in high-repetition sports often note symptoms when they are 15 to 17 years old.

Table 1 Characteristics of those most likely to sustain tendon overuse injuries

Characteristic	Recreational Athlete	Highly Competitive to Elite Athlete
Conditioning and fitness	Average	Superior
Age range (yr)	35 to 55	15 to 35
Sports participation		
Frequency (times/wk)	2 to 4	4 to 7
Intensity	Moderate	High
Technique	Above average	Superior
Other	Muscle weakness common	Muscle-tendon weakness with sports-imposed imbalances common

Although poor conditioning has been mentioned as a factor in tendon overuse injuries,[26,29] clinical experience suggests that such patients are less aggressive in regard to the frequency and duration of activity, so their cumulative overload is lower. The two groups most likely to sustain tendon overuse injuries are characterized in Table 1.

Systemic Considerations (Mesenchymal Syndrome)

The mesenchymal syndrome has been defined as multiple sites of tendon pain or alteration secondary to some systemic constitutional factor. It has long been known that tendinosis appears at multiple sites in approximately 15% of patients and that these sites were not necessarily subjected to obvious overuse. This phenomenon was initially reported in 1969 and named mesenchymal syndrome.[22] Mesenchymal syndrome appears to be more common in women and is often initially noted in those about 30 years of age. The typical patient seems to be susceptible to upper-extremity problems, including combinations of bilateral lateral tennis elbow, medial tennis elbow, ulnar nerve compression at zone 3 of the medial epicondylar elbow groove, rotator cuff tendinosis, carpal tunnel syndrome, de Quervains's syndrome, and trigger-finger tendinosis.

Laboratory test results, including rheumatologic tests, are characteristically normal in the patient with mesenchymal syndrome. In women, there is some suggestion that diminished estrogen levels, premature menopause, or premenopausal hysterectomy may be an associated problem. In these cases, tendon pain symptoms are often relieved by estrogen replacement therapy. It is clear that other factors are present, because the syndrome also occurs in men. The causes of the mesenchymal syndrome are otherwise unknown, but some form of collagen distortion has been theorized.

Other factors have been mentioned in regard to tendon pain. The most commonly cited include nerve compression in the same dermatome and gouty diathesis. There are no scientific data to confirm or deny these interrelationships.

Multiple Sites of Tendon Pain (Nonsystemic)

In certain patients the existence of multiple sites can be explained by mechanical overuse. Some patients merely compensate by switching the activity from one extremity to the other; in others, the activity is bilateral. For example, in golf, the leading elbow is susceptible to lateral tennis elbow, whereas the trailing elbow is susceptible to medial tennis elbow. In these situations overuse trauma is probably the key etiologic factor. There are, however, many clinical circumstances in which overuse traumas and mesenchymal syndrome appear to be acting in concert.[27]

Chronic "tendinitis" has been commonly theorized to be an inflammatory reparative process that follows mechanical microtrauma. Histologic examination of the tissue resected from pathologic tendons, however, often fails to reveal inflammatory cells, and the characteristic, consistent pattern of change appears to represent a degenerative process that is probably secondary to tensile overuse, fatigue, and weakness, and possibly to avascular changes.[19,20,25,31] Thus, the term tendinosis is a replacement term for the misnomer tendinitis.

The characteristic gross appearance of chronic tendinosis (angiofibroblastic tendinosis) differs from that of normal tendon in that it is dull, gray, friable, and often edematous. Microscopically, the normally orderly tendon fibers are disrupted by a characteristic invasion pattern of fibroblasts and vascular, atypical, granulation-like tissue that may be called angiofibroblastic tendinosis (Fig. 1).[23,25] The adjacent tendon appears to be hypercellular, degenerated, and microfragmented. The angiofibroblastic tissue insinuates itself through the abnormal hypercellular regions and extends focally into adjacent normal-appearing tendinous fibers.[12,24,25] In advanced lesions, the characteristic reaction occurs in supportive tissue as well as in the tendon itself. Acute inflammatory cells are almost always absent in the tendon, but a mild sprinkling of chronic inflammatory cells may be noted in the supportive fibroadipose, connective, and even skeletal muscle tissues.[25] If chronic inflammatory cells are evident in the tendon, they are those of traumatic repair rather than tendinosis and include either new or organizing granulation tissue and early-to-late cicatricial fibrous tissue (scar). The degree of angiofibroblastic infiltration appears to correlate with the clinical phases of pain and duration of symptoms.

Factors Leading to Failed Healing

Currently there is little information about the biochemical and physiologic factors concerning the infrastructural causes of chronic tendon pain. The same is true of the factors that lead to failed healing. Observations by patients, however, allow identification of some clinical factors.

Repetitive Overuse

Continuation of the abusive activities after the onset of symptoms is common in failed healing. It should be remembered when formu-

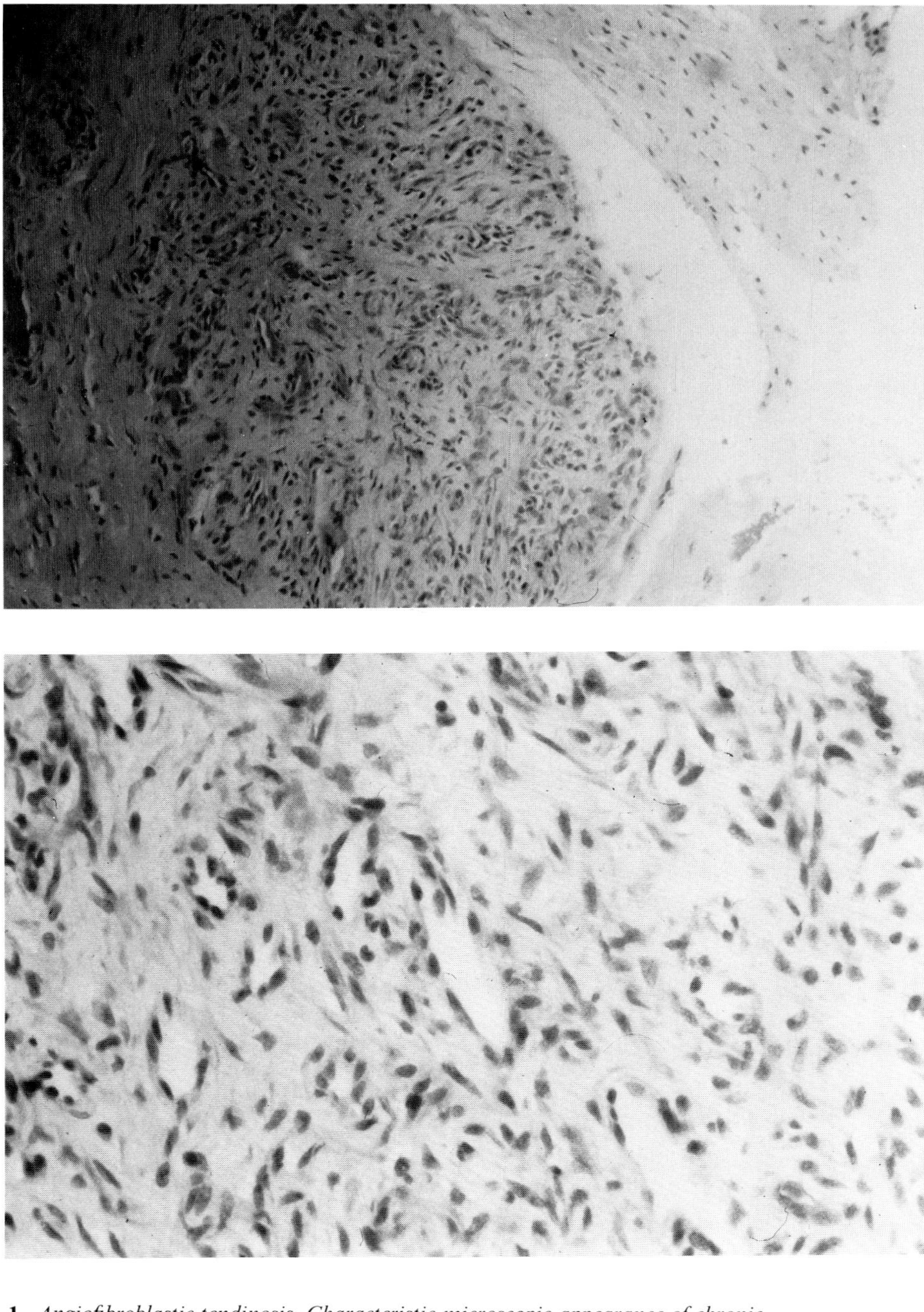

Fig. 1 *Angiofibroblastic tendinosis. Characteristic microscopic appearance of chronic tendinosis. Vascular and fibroblastic elements of typical pathologic change. Inflammatory cells are not present.* ***Top,*** *Low-power view (× 100).* ***Bottom,*** *Higher-power view (× 450).*

Outline 2 Pain phase scale

Phase 1:	Mild pain after activity, resolves within 24 hours
Phase 2:	Pain after activity, resolves with warm-up
Phase 3:	Pain on activity that does not affect exercise activity
Phase 4:	Pain on activity that does affect exercise activity
Phase 5:	Pain caused by the activities of daily living
Phase 6:	Constant pain (usually dull and aching) that does not disturb sleep
Phase 7:	Dull, aching pain that does disturb sleep

lating a treatment protocol, however, that abusive activities are distinct from normal activity. To be successful, the treatment protocol must address the abuses and muscle-tendon imbalances imposed by sport or occupational activities.

Tissue Age

The factors involved in age are twofold, both chronological and physiologic. Physiologic age is probably the predominant factor. In general, the aging process of tendon tissue is probably a predicated tissue response of cumulative overuse. The typical age range of highly competitive athletes is 15 to 35 years.

Constitutional Factors

The presence of mesenchymal syndrome correlates with an observed high failure rate of tendon healing by nonsurgical means. Surgical success does not appear to be affected, however, as long as the surgeon has located and excised the abnormal tissue.[24,27]

Duration of Symptoms

Pain symptoms that persist beyond six months have a much higher incidence of nonsurgical treatment failure.[18,23] Practical situations that reward a delayed clinical response (such as workman's compensation) may magnify the potential for failure. Longevity of symptoms does not appear to affect the surgical success of resection and repair techniques, however.[24,27]

Phases of Pain

The clinical character and phases of pain are germane to the identification of a failed healing response. Using the report of Blazina and associates[1] on the patellar tendon as a basis, I have developed a pain phase scale,[21] which has been helpful for formulating treatment protocols and predicting healing responses (Outline 2). Pain phases beyond phase 4 suggest significant pathologic alteration in the substance of the tendon. If pain phases 5, 6, and 7 fail to respond to medication and a quality rehabilitation program, a failed healing response is likely (especially if there are persistent functional deficits).

Persistent Functional Deficits

Objective measurements of strength, endurance, and flexibility are important to an accurate understanding of the clinical situation. Persistent deficits of these functions are hallmarks of a failed healing response, especially if they persist after a high-quality rehabilitation program.

Deficiencies of Treatment

The basics of a rehabilitative program for chronic tendinosis are (1) relief of pain; (2) promotion of healing (strength, endurance, flexibility programs); (3) enhancement of general fitness; and (4) control of abusive overloads.

In certain instances, the treatment protocol places undue priority on anti-inflammatory medication, including cortisone injections. It has been my observation that patients who receive more than three cortisone injections are at high risk for failure of healing. Whether a major pathologic change increases the need for cortisone or whether cortisone increases the pathologic change is not always clear, although I suspect the latter is true in the majority of cases.[14] I know of no evidence to suggest that anti-inflammatory medications actually promote healing. Clinical evidence suggests strongly that the lack of an appropriate rehabilitative exercise ensures failed healing in tendons with major pathologic changes.[5,25,33]

Imaging Techniques for Tendinosis

In addition to the clinical indicators for failed tendon healing, the contemporary imaging techniques of ultrasonography and magnetic resonance imaging appear to be helpful in preliminary observations.[2,8,9] These techniques are rapidly evolving and have a learning curve, and their accuracy varies among tendon sites. It has been suggested that ultrasonography is accurate in the diagnosis of rotator cuff disorders, but the evidence is controversial.[16] Conversely, others have reported that ultrasonography is indeed accurate in the diagnosis of patellar and Achilles tendinosis.[8,9] Preliminary data from one recent study indicate that magnetic resonance imaging is highly accurate in the diagnosis of rotator cuff abnormalities (G. Leather, M. Nelson, R. Nirschl, and associates, unpublished data).

As experience grows with these techniques, it is likely that failed healing responses will be identified more promptly.

Acknowledgment

Ellsworth Stay, MD, Department of Pathology, Arlington Hospital, Arlington, Virginia, described and categorized the pathologic tendon tissue.

References

1. Blazina ME, Kerlan RK, Jobe FW, et al: Jumper's knee. *Orthop Clin North Am* 1973;4:665–678.
2. Bodne D, Quinn SF, Murray WT, et al: Magnetic resonance images of chronic patellar tendinitis. *Skeletal Radiol* 1988;17:24–28.

3. Clement DB, Taunton JE, Smart GW: Achilles tendinitis and peritendinitis: Etiology and treatment. *Am J Sports Med* 1984;12:179–184.
4. Codman EA: *The Shoulder: Rupture of the Supraspinatus Tendon and Other Lesions in or About the Subacromial Bursa.* Boston, G Miller & Co, 1934.
5. Curwin S, Stanish WO: *Tendinitis, Its Etiology and Treatment.* Lexington, Collamore Press, 1984.
6. Ferretti A: Epidemiology of jumper's knee. *Sports Med* 1986;289–295.
7. Ferretti A, Puddu G, Mariani PP, et al: The natural history of jumper's knee: Patellar or quadriceps tendonitis. *Int Orthop* 1985;8:239–242.
8. Fornage BD: Achilles tendon: US examination. *Radiology* 1986;159:759–764.
9. Fornage BD, Rifkin MD, Touche DH, et al: Sonography of the patellar tendon: Preliminary observations. *AJR* 1984;143:179–182.
10. Frank C, Schachar N, Dittrich D: Natural history of healing in the repaired medial collateral ligament. *J Orthop Res* 1983;1:179–188.
11. Gelberman RH, Manske PR, Akeson WH, et al: Flexor tendon repair. *J Orthop Res* 1986;4:119–128.
12. Goldie I: Epicondylitis lateralis humeri (epicondylalgia or tennis elbow): A pathogenetical study. *Acta Chir Scand* 1964;339(suppl):1–119.
13. Gruchow HW, Pelletier D: An epidemiologic study of tennis elbow: Incidence, recurrence, and effectiveness of prevention strategies. *Am J Sports Med* 1979;7:234–238.
14. Kapetanos G: The effect of the local corticosteroids on the healing and biomechanical properties of the partially injured tendon. *Clin Orthop* 1982;163:170–179.
15. Kvist M, Józsa L, Järvinen MJ, et al: Chronic Achilles paratenonitis in athletes: A histological and histochemical study. *Pathology* 1987;19:1–11.
16. Mack LA, Nyberg DA, Matsen FA: Sonographic evaluation of rotator cuff. *Radiol Clin North Am* 1988;26:161–177.
17. Maffuli N, Regine R, Angelillo M, et al: Ultrasound diagnosis of Achilles tendon pathology in runners. *Br J Sports Med* 1987;21:158–162.
18. Martens M, Wouters P, Burssens A, et al: Patellar tendinitis: Pathology and results of treatment. *Acta Orthop Scand* 1982;53:445–450.
19. Mcnab I: Rotator cuff tendinitis. *Ann R Coll Surg Engl* 1973;53:271–287.
20. Moseley HF, Goldie I: The arterial pattern of the rotator cuff of the shoulder. *J Bone Joint Surg* 1963;45B:780–789.
21. Nirschl RP: *Arm Care: Relief and Prevention for Shoulder Tendonitis, Tennis Elbow, Wrist Sprain in Athletes and Other Activities.* Arlington Va, Medical Sports Publishing, 1981.
22. Nirschl RP: Mesenchymal syndrome. *Va Med Month* 1969;96:659–662.
23. Nirschl RP: Prevention and treatment of elbow and shoulder injuries in the tennis player. *Clin Sports Med* 1988;7:289–308.
24. Nirschl RP: Rotator cuff surgery, in Barr JS Jr (ed): American Academy of Orthopaedic Surgeons *Instructional Course Lectures, XXXVIII.* Park Ridge, American Academy of Orthopaedic Surgeons, 1989, pp 447–462.
25. Nirschl RP: Rotator cuff tendinitis: Basic concepts of pathoetiology, in Barr JS Jr (ed): American Academy of Orthopaedic Surgeons *Instructional Course Lectures, XXXVIII.* Park Ridge, American Academy of Orthopaedic Surgeons, 1989, pp 439–450.
26. Nirschl RP: Tennis elbow. *Orthop Clin North Am* 1973;4:787–800.
27. Nirschl RP, Pettrone FA: Tennis elbow: The surgical treatment of lateral epicondylitis. *J Bone Joint Surg* 1979;161A:832–839.
28. Perugia L, Ippolitio E, Postacchini F: A new approach to the pathology, clinical features and treatment of stress tendinopathy of the Achilles tendon. *Ital J Orthop Traumatol* 1976;2:5–21.

29. Priest JD, Branden V, Gerberich SG: The elbow and tennis: Part 1. An analysis of players with and without pain. *Phys Sportsmed* 1980;8:81–91.
30. Puddu G, Ippolito E, Postacchini F: A classification of Achilles tendon disease. *Am J Sports Med* 1976;4:145–150.
31. Rathbun JB, Mcnab I: The microvascular pattern of the rotator cuff. *J Bone Joint Surg* 1970:52B:540–553.
32. Schepsis AA, Leach RE: Surgical management of Achilles tendinitis. *Am J Sports Med* 1987;15:308–315.
33. Stanish WD, Rubinovich RM, Curwin S: Eccentric exercise in chronic tendinitis. *Clin Orthop* 1986;208:65–68.

Chapter 39

Clinical Staging Concepts in Sports Trauma

Wayne B. Leadbetter, MD

Clinical staging concepts are commonly used in assessing sports-induced soft-tissue inflammation and healing. They are a guide to recognizing the severity of the injury, judging its progression or resolution, and planning specific recommendations about activity levels and return to competition. The sports clinician must be familiar with both the usefulness and limitations of various staging concepts and grading systems.

Origin of a Concept

Staging is applied to both acute and chronic injuries in an attempt to describe a subjective or qualitative matter in quantitative or numerical terms. Grading of acute injuries originated in the traditional classification of ligament injury by the American Medical Association. This divided injuries into grade I (mild stretching with local tenderness, minimal swelling, no instability, and little disability), grade II (moderate with local tenderness, swelling, slight to moderate instability, and moderate disability), and grade III (severe with complete ligament disruption, swelling, hemorrhage, marked instability, and severe disability).[2] Blazina and associates[6] developed the first "phasing" concept of overuse injury with their description of "jumper's knee syndrome" or patellar tendinitis. The system was based on a correlation of symptoms and functional impairment. Phase I: Pain after activity only. No marked functional impairment. Phase II: Pain during and after activity. Performance still at a satisfactory level. Phase III: Pain during and for a prolonged period after activity. Satisfactory performance progressively more difficult to achieve. Phase IV, complete structural failure, was added later. Blazina and associates used this clinical guide to justify different treatment programs. Anti-inflammatory measures and nonsurgical care are emphasized in phase I, whereas phase III may involve surgical intervention.

This concept was later adapted to the injured runner by J. Henderson (unpublished data) and myself.[17] The prevalence of overuse and training abuse in runners[7,8,11,14] made such categorization attractive because preventive guidelines could also be provided. Three assumptions underlay these initial grading attempts: (1) There is a dose-related, graduated inflammatory response to soft-tissue injury. (2) The duration and subjective appreciation of the severity or type of pain correlates directly with the degree of tissue injury. (3) There is a consistent structural response such that a given level of pain correlates with a specific quality of tissue abnormality. Although clinical experience tends to validate these assumptions in individual cases, there is no scientific proof as to their reliability, and exceptions occur. The first assumption, that a dose-related response to trauma occurs in overuse injury, is supported by the linear relationship between the injury rate in runners and the miles run.[22] Powell and associates[22] also observed that once a training threshold of 30 miles per week was reached, yearly injury rates exceeded 20% per year for women and 15% per year for men. However, Puddu and associates[23] reported Achilles tendon rupture in patients with no history of pain. Kelly and associates[15] analyzed 13 cases of quadriceps and patellar tendon rupture and correlated them with Blazina and associates'[6] phases. They found that six patients in phase I and six in phase III sustained ruptures. The remaining patient was in phase II.

Pain and Its Occurrence in Sports Inflammation

Pain may simply be defined as the "hurt that we feel."[28] It is still unclear whether pain is a separate distinct sensation or just a feeling reaction. The specificity theory holds that the neural basis of pain involves unique anatomic and physiologic properties. The perception of threat or damage can be painful.[5] To the sports traumatologist, pain indicates that something is irritating the nerve's nociceptive sensors (Fig. 1).

In an attempt to categorize the clinical nature of pain, Nirschl[20] designated three types of pain. Benevolent pain is stiffness or mild soreness that usually lasts 24 hours or less after an activity. Semibenevolent pain is stiffness or mild soreness that can be relieved by warm-up exercises or protective equipment. Harmful pain interferes with activity or completely prohibits competition, disrupts sleep, and is present before and after activity. He recommended medical attention for semibenevolent and more severe pain that persists for more than one week.

The body's internal mechanisms may affect how much pain an individual feels. For example, endogenous opioids, such as beta-endorphin, leucine, enkephalin, and methionine, which are secreted by neurons in the brain and spinal cord, are more potent than morphine in inducing analgesia. Their overall effect is to inhibit transmission of pain during exercise. Armstrong[3] pointed out that this may modify pain perception during exercise in an injury such as delayed-onset muscle soreness.

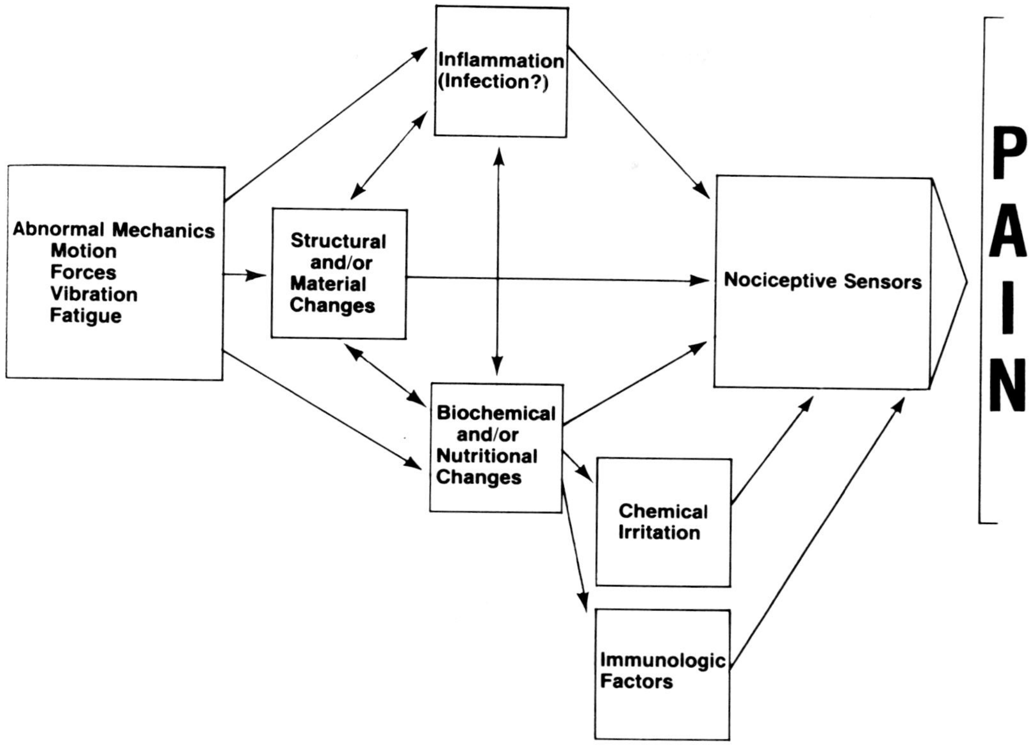

Fig. 1 *Possible mechanisms of pain. (Reproduced with permission from White AA III: The 1980 symposium and beyond, in Frymoyer JW, Gordon SL (eds):* New Perspectives in Low Back Pain. *Park Ridge, American Academy of Orthopaedic Surgeons, 1989, pp 3–17.)*

Such mechanisms may help explain Beecher's[4] observations of men wounded on the battlefield. Despite severe pain from their wounds, these soldiers were far less apt to ask for morphine than a matched group of civilians undergoing major surgery. Only 32% of the wounded patients requested narcotics, compared with 83% of the surgical patients.

However, Torgerson[29] noted that "pain is a subjective experience and any measure that is independent of the subjective experience is a measure of something else." Nonetheless, although pain, like light or odor, cannot itself be measured, certain aspects of pain or perceived light or odor can be measured. With pain, one can measure intensity, that is, how much it hurts.

Several scaling measures for assessing pain are used in clinical medicine. These techniques provide patients with a standardized way to tell or show a physician how intense, unpleasant, or bad the pain is.[29] These pain-measurement scales fall into two general classes—those with a response scale bounded at both ends and those with a response scale unbounded at the top. Examples of the first class include visual analog scales, numerical rating scales (0 to 10), and adjectival ratings (mild, moderate, severe). An example of the second class, described by Torgerson,[29] consists of subjecting the patient to a middle-level, pain-evolving standard stimulus. The patient assigns this stimulus a number and all subsequent stimuli (or episodes of clinical pain) are graded proportionately to the initial stimulus. Although both have some drawbacks, the results of different scaling procedures are usually highly correlated. Pain symptoms for individual patients can be calibrated by defining adjectives to describe the perceived intensity, and then providing controlled, pain-evoking stimuli that the patient can correlate with each of the adjectives. These methods can create a calibrated response to pain.

In the future, pain theory may provide a more reliable methodology for grading.

Specific Applications of Soft-Tissue Injury Staging

Soft-tissue injury grading, phasing, or staging can be specifically applied to four aspects of sports trauma—severity of injury, structural healing, rehabilitation and therapeutic recommendations, and return to activity guidelines.

Severity of Injury

Assessment of injury is exemplified by the standard AMA nomenclature,[2] but there are many other examples in both acute and chronic trauma. Jackson and Feagin's[13] classification of quadriceps contusion combines elements of subjective response (pain) and quantifiable objective reactions (swelling, loss of range of motion, and recovery time).

In ligament injury, Noyes and associates[21] emphasized that care must be taken with the concept of a partial tear or grade II injury. Present assessment methods are not reliable in quantifying partial injury in ligament. Significant decreases in strength, increases in length, or compromises in functional capacity depend on the amount of fiber disruption. Present methods provide only an arbitrary guess about the percentage of fiber disruption in ligament or muscle damage. Arthroscopy and arthrometric testing have been used to quantify partial tears of the anterior cruciate ligament more accurately. Direct vision remains unreliable in muscle tissue, but magnetic resonance imaging may prove to be helpful.

Overuse injury staging systems usually include four to six categories. The most severe category is characterized by severe daily activity pain, inability to perform sports, or complete tissue failure and rupture.[11,27] Severity of injury scales have also been developed for iliotibial band friction syndrome[18] and shin splints.[19]

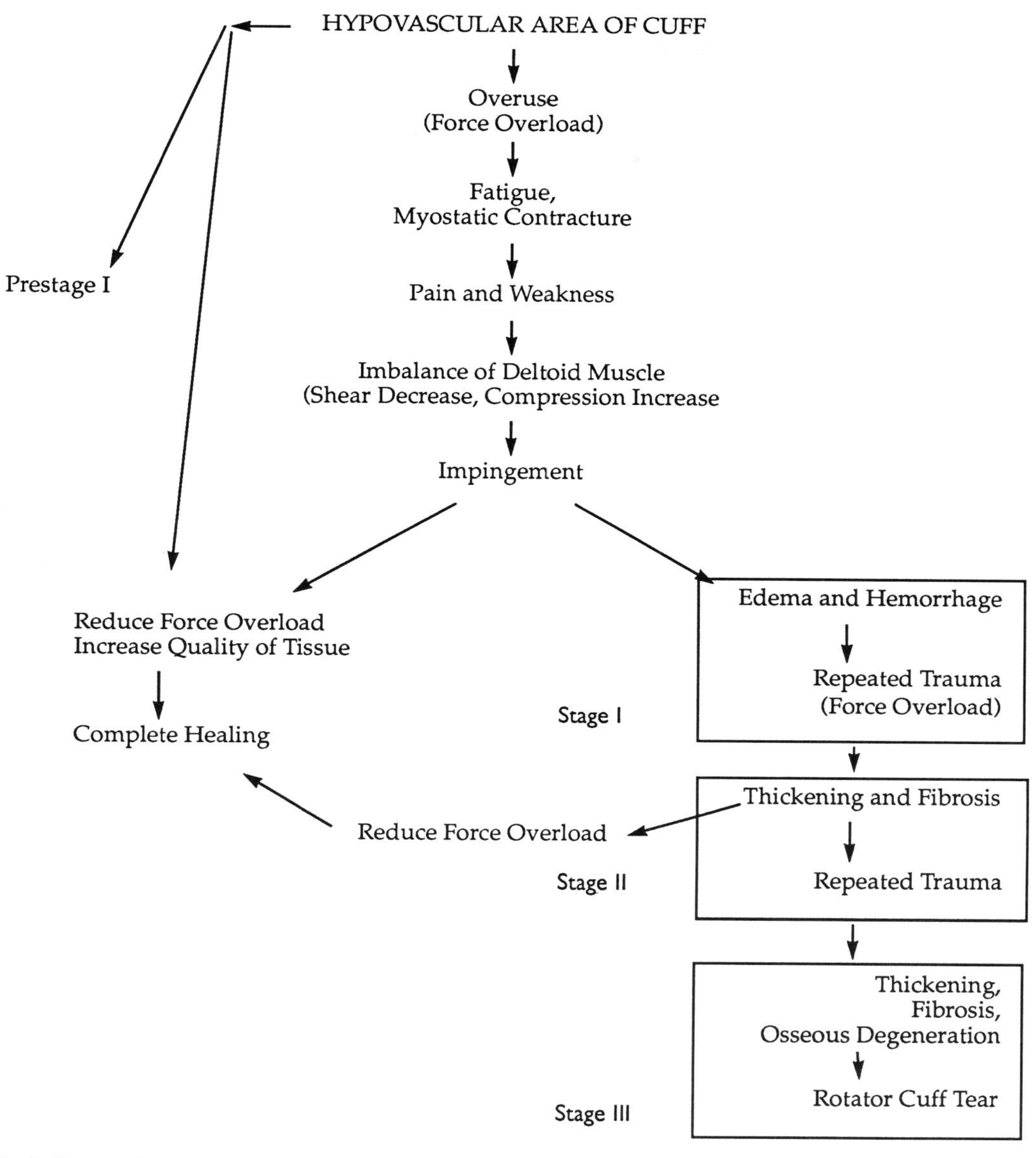

Fig. 2 *Stages of impingement lesions. (Reproduced with permission from Allman F: Impingement, biceps, and rotator cuff lesions, in Zarins B, Andrews JR, Carson WG (eds):* Injuries to the Throwing Arm. *Philadelphia, WB Saunders, 1985, pp 158–172.)*

Structural Healing

The concept of staging of structural healing was discussed by Allman[1] for subacromial impingement lesions of the shoulder (Fig. 2). In this

Table 1 Classification of patellar disorder*

Stage	Findings
1	Pain only after sports activity
2	Pain at the beginning of sports activity, disappearing with warm-up and reappearing with fatigue
3	Constant pain at rest and during activity; patient is unable to participate in sports at previous level
4	Complete rupture of patellar tendon

*Modified with permission from Curwin S, Stanish WD: *Tendinitis: Its Etiology and Treatment.* Lexington, Collamore Press, 1984. Based on data from Blazina and associates.[6]

scheme, the various stages of impingement are correlated with the evolution of soft-tissue abnormalities. Although advanced stages of this schema can be confirmed by biopsies when surgery is needed for a rotator cuff tear or impingement, the abnormality in pre-stage 1 and stage 1 lesions has been inferred from experimental models, because more than 90% of impingement lesions respond to conservative management with proper treatment.[1] Nevertheless, such classifications remain the rationale for advocating surgical treatment in refractory cases.

Roels and associates[24] found mucoid degeneration of tendon tissue in biopsy specimens from patients with patellar tendinitis but did not identify clinical symptoms that correlated with the biopsy samples. Leach and associates[16] studied a group of 11 competitive runners, one decathlete, one football player, one recreational jogger, and one tennis player. These 15 individuals had undergone a total of 20 Achilles tendon operations. Leach and associates found a variety of degenerative changes, including thickened tenosynovium, intratendinous calcification, inflamed retrocalcaneal bursa, and marked thickening of the Achilles tendon. A later description of these patients discussed various patterns of involvement of Achilles tendon, mesotendon, and retrocalcaneal bursa, but made no correlations on an increasing-severity basis.[26]

Rehabilitation and Therapeutic Recommendations

Stanish and associates,[27] Curwin and Stanish,[9] Nirschl,[20] Leadbetter,[17] Roy and Irvin,[25] and others have examined the implications of staging for therapeutic and rehabilitative guidelines (Tables 1 and 2). Stanish and associates'[27] conservative treatment program for patellar tendinitis correlated with Blazina and associates'[6] classification to provide a rationale for therapeutic measures. The pattern of pain response during an eccentric exercise program also shows how the subjective grading of pain by the patient can be used as a guide to adjust load and modify cellular stress responses to a directed therapeutic goal.[9] Roy and Irvin[25] based a complete rehabilitative program for an ankle sprain on five stages of inflammation and healing after ligamentous injury.

Return to Activity Guidelines

Grading of pain responses is also used to plan a return to sports activity. A typical example is Brody's[7] plan for a return to running

Table 2 Conservative treatment program for patellar tendinitis*

Stage	Treatment
1	Adequate warm-up (5 to 10 min of push-ups, sit-ups, etc); ice after activity; local anti-inflammatory treatment and anti-inflammatory drugs for several weeks; physiotherapy, including isometric quadriceps exercises; elastic knee support
2	Same as stage 1 plus some form of heat before activity and a period of rest
3	Same as stage 2 with rest period prolonged; abstention from sports
4	Primary repair of tendon

*Modified with permission from Curwin S, Stanish WD: *Tendinitis: Its Etiology and Treatment.* Lexington, Collamore Press, 1984. Based on data from Blazina and associates.[6]

Table 3 Return to running after injury*

The runner must be free of pain and tenderness, with normal daily activities before resuming his or her training program. (On a scale of 0 to 10, on which 0 is normal and 10 is the worst, the runner is asked to rate his or her pain with normal activities; they must be at 0.)

(A) If 0: Run every other day for two weeks, then a maximum of 5 days a week for the next four weeks. If the previous level was 4 to 6 miles per session, begin with 1 mile. (If previous level per session was less than 4, begin with 0.5 mile per session.) If no pain with running, follow the following weekly mileage schedule:

1	0	1	0	1	0	2
0	2	0	2	0	3	0
3	2	0	3	3	0	4
3	0	4	4	0	5	4
0	5	5	0	6	5	0 etc.

(B) If you have short intervals of pain with running:
- A. No running for two weeks.
- B. 10 minute total workout, alternating 4 minute run and 1 minute walk. If no pain, add 5 minutes every 3 days, working up to 30 minutes, then progress to the next step. If you experience pain, cut back 5 minutes and work up.
- C. 15 minutes total workout, alternating 4.5 minute run and 30 second walk. If no pain, add 5 minutes every 3 days, working up to 30 minutes, then progress to next step. If you experience pain, cut back 5 minutes and work up.
- D. Run steadily for 15 minutes, adding 5 minutes every 3 days. If you experience pain, cut back 5 minutes and work up.

(C) If you have pain after running:
- A. Cut your workout by 50%, and progress by adding 10% a week.
- B. If you cut your workout 50% and still have pain, cut it by 50% again and progress by adding 10% a week.

(D) Running routine:

moist heat (5 minutes) → stretch → run as prescribed → ice massage (10 minutes)

At night: moist heat (20 minutes) → stretch
weight lift
back exercises

*Slightly modified with permission from Brody DM: Techniques in the evaluation and treatment of the injured runner. *Orthop Clin North Am* 1982;13:541–558.

after injury (Table 3). The athlete bases the level of activity on the perceived pain intensity—a guiding principle in all grading systems. Current phasing systems for rehabilitation of an anterior cruciate ligament in a reconstructed knee typify the effort to combine subjective

Table 4 Grading of sports-induced soft-tissue inflammation*

Grade	Pain Pattern	Physical Signs	Relevant Therapeutic Measures
I†	Pain only after activity; duration of symptoms <2 wk	Generalized soreness	Proper warm-up and conditioning; avoidance of abrupt transition in activity level
II†	Pain during and after activity; no significant functional disability; duration of symptoms >2 wk	Localized pain; minimal or no other signs of inflammation	Analysis of technique and efficiency; decrease in abusive training; improve conditioning
III‡	Pain during and after activity; significant functional disability; duration of symptoms >6 wk	Intense point tenderness with prominent inflammation (edema, effusion, erythema, crepitus, etc)	Structural vulnerability; protected activity with sports modification; substitutions of sports activity to avoid excessive load
IV‡	Constant pain; significant functional disability; unable to train or compete; impending tissue failure	Grade III symptoms plus tissue breakdown, atrophy, etc	Surgery (fibrogenesis, repair, structural alteration); possible permanent withdrawal from activity (as in degenerative joint disease)

*Derived from data in Franz,[11] Leadbetter,[17] Nirschl,[20] and Roy and Irvin.[25]
†Benevolent or semibenevolent pain; also referred to as microinjury; self-help measures often effective.
‡Harmful pain; also referred to as macroinjury; medical diagnosis and opinion valuable.

clinical symptoms with progressive phases of wound repair and tissue remodeling.[10,12]

Conclusion

Grading systems for sports-related soft-tissue trauma, regardless of the exact schema, are attempts to quantify the subjective pain response as a characteristic of injury and inflammation and relate it to associated stages of structural healing. A unified grading system based on the current sports medicine literature can be postulated (Table 4). Higher grades are characterized by greater evidence of macrotrauma and a greater need for medical assistance. Although such efforts are unsupported by data confirmed by techniques such as biopsy in the early stages, there are strong clinical arguments for their use in both the diagnosis and the treatment of sports-related soft-tissue injuries. The grading or staging of an injured athlete's pain has useful pragmatic implications. In addition, it directs attention to the inflammation and repair cycle, thereby suggesting preventive and self-treatment measures to the injured athlete.

References

1. Allman F: Impingement, biceps, and rotator cuff lesions, in Zarins B, Andrews JR, Carson WG (eds): *Injuries to the Throwing Arm.* Philadelphia, WB Saunders, 1985, pp 158–172.
2. American Medical Association, Committee on the Medical Aspects of Sports. Subcommittee on Classification of Sports Injuries: *Standard Nomenclature of Athletic Injuries.* Chicago, American Medical Association, 1966, pp 99–101.
3. Armstrong RB: Mechanisms of exercise-induced delayed onset muscular soreness: A brief review. *Med Sci Sports Exerc* 1984;16:529–538.
4. Beecher HK: Relationship of significance of wound to pain experienced. *JAMA* 1956;161:1609–1613.

5. Bishop B: *Pain, Its Physiology and Rationale For Management.* Alexandria, American Physical Therapy Association, 1980.
6. Blazina ME, Kerlan RK, Jobe FW, et al: Jumper's knee. *Orthop Clin North Am* 1973;4:665–678.
7. Brody DM: Techniques in the evaluation and treatment of the injured runner. *Orthop Clin North Am* 1982;13:541–558.
8. Clement DB, Taunton JE, Smart GW, et al: A survey of overuse running injuries. *Phys Sportsmed* 1981;9:47–58.
9. Curwin S, Stanish WD: *Tendinitis: Its Etiology and Treatment.* Lexington, Collamore Press, 1984.
10. Fanton GS: Rehabilitation of the knee after anterior cruciate ligament surgery. *Phys Med Rehabil* 1987;1:639–648.
11. Franz WB III: Overuse syndromes in runners: Part I. Approaches to diagnosis and general treatment principles, in Mellion MB (ed): *Office Management of Sports Injuries and Athletic Problems.* Philadelphia, Hanley & Belfus, 1988, pp 289–300.
12. Huegel M, Indelicato PA: Trends in rehabilitation following anterior cruciate ligament reconstruction. *Clin Sports Med* 1988;7:801–811.
13. Jackson DW, Feagin JA: Quadriceps contusions in young athletes: Relation of severity of injury to treatment and prognosis. *J Bone Joint Surg* 1973;55A:95–105.
14. James SL, Bates BT, Osternig LR: Injuries to runners. *Am J Sports Med* 1978;6:40–50.
15. Kelly DW, Carter VS, Jobe FW, et al: Patellar and quadriceps tendon ruptures: Jumpers knee. *Am J Sports Med* 1984;12:375–380.
16. Leach RE, James S, Wasilewski S: Achilles tendinitis. *Am J Sports Med* 1981;9:93–98.
17. Leadbetter WB: Getting ahead of the injury. *Emerg Med*, June 15, 1979, pp 27–39.
18. Lindenberg G, Pinshaw R, Noakes TD: Iliotibial band friction syndrome in runners. *Phys Sportsmed* 1984;12:118–130.
19. Myburgh KH, Grobler N, Noakes TD: Factors associated with shin soreness in athletes. *Phys Sportsmed* 1988;16:129–134.
20. Nirschl RP: *Arm Care: Relief and Prevention for Shoulder Tendonitis, Tennis Elbow, Wrist Sprain in Athletes and Other Activities.* Arlington, Medical Sports, 1981.
21. Noyes FR, Keller CS, Grood ES, et al: Advances in the understanding of knee ligament injury, repair, and rehabilitation. *Med Sci Sports Exerc* 1984;16:427–443.
22. Powell KE, Kohl HW, Caspersen CJ, et al: An epidemiological perspective on the causes of running injuries. *Phys Sportsmed* 1986;14:100–114.
23. Puddu G, Ippolito E, Postacchini F: A classification of Achilles tendon disease. *Am J Sports Med* 1976;4:145–150.
24. Roels J, Martens M, Mulier JC, et al: Patellar tendinitis (jumper's knee). *Am J Sports Med* 1978;6:362–368.
25. Roy S, Irvin R: *Sports Medicine: Prevention, Evaluation, Management, and Rehabilitation.* Englewood Cliffs, Prentice-Hall, 1983.
26. Schepsis AA, Leach RE: Surgical management of Achilles tendinitis. *Am J Sports Med* 1987;15:308–315.
27. Stanish WD, Curwin S, Rubinovich M: Tendinitis: The analysis and treatment for running. *Clin Sports Med* 1985;4:593–609.
28. Sternbach RA: *Pain: A Psychophysiological Analysis.* New York, Academic Press, 1968.
29. Torgerson WS: What objective measures are there for evaluating pain? *J Trauma* 1984;24(suppl 9):S187-S197.

Chapter 40

Failed Healing Responses in Connective Tissue and a Comparison of Medical Conditions

Arnold E. Postlethwaite, MD

Introduction

Collagen, fibronectin, and hyaluronic acid facilitate the infiltration and accumulation of inflammatory cells and fibroblasts at sites of tissue injury. Fibroblasts responding to signals from cytokines and growth factors synthesize components of the reparative tissue. Deficiencies or excesses within this complex regulatory system may lead to failed healing. Several medical conditions may be associated with incomplete or failed healing.

Fortunately, most injuries to connective tissue components heal in a normal fashion. However, there are some medical conditions, such as advanced age, diabetes mellitus, hypertension, malnutrition, and therapies involving radiation, glucocorticoids, and chemotherapeutic drugs, that are associated with incomplete or failed healing of connective tissue. This chapter focuses on the factors that may be responsible for failed healing in these and other conditions.

Unique Qualities of Connective Tissue Inflammatory Processes

Traditionally, matrix components were thought simply to provide structural support for specialized cells of various organs of the body. In recent years, matrix components have also been shown to modulate the activities of a variety of cells, including component cells of the inflammatory and repair responses.

Collagen

Type I collagen, its constituent α chains, α_1 CB5 peptide, and types II, III, and IV collagen have the ability to induce platelet aggregation in vitro.[3,6] At sites of injury in vivo, these collagens can function to aggregate platelets released from damaged blood vessels. The interstitial collagens (types I, II, and III), their constituent α chains, and small peptides containing hydroxyproline are chemoattractants in vitro for human blood monocytes and for dermal fibroblasts.[28,34] This suggests that solubilized collagens and collagenous peptides generated as a result of the concerted action of collagenase and proteases at sites of tissue injury and inflammation may provide chemotactic signals that facilitate the accumulation of monocytes and fibroblasts.

Elastin

Tropoelastin and elastin peptides are chemotactic for fibroblasts in vitro, and Val-Gly-Val-Ala-Pro-Gly, a repeating peptide in elastin, is chemotactic for both monocytes and fibroblasts.[43,44] Like collagen, elastin fragments generated at sites of tissue injury in vivo could potentially function as fibroblast chemoattractants.

Fibronectin

The cellular and plasma forms of fibronectin have been shown to be potent fibroblast chemoattractants in vitro.[31,45] Fibronectin also induces epithelial cell migration, and fragments of fibronectin have been demonstrated to be chemoattractants for monocytes.[24,25] It has been known for more than a decade that fibronectin promotes cell attachment and spreading.[51] Fibronectin is a prominent constituent of dermal granulation tissue and, with fibrin, forms the initial meshwork that facilitates fibroblast invasion and attachment to type III collagen as well as growth of fibroblasts.

In addition to the chemotactic effect of certain fibronectin fragments for monocytes, fibronectin has nonspecific opsonic activity and can facilitate phagocytosis by macrophages, monocytes, and Kupffer cells and clearance of bacteria and cellular debris by the mononuclear phagocyte system. The nonspecific opsonic activity of fibronectin is extremely important in wound healing and probably results from the ability of fibronectin to bind to fibrin, the C1q component of complement, bacteria, actin, and DNA.[7,17,18,21,39,53] The ability of fibronectin to promote the adhesion and spreading of platelets on collagen fiber surfaces and the binding of circulating leukocytes to fibrin clots and exposed collagen are additional functions that are of immense importance in homeostasis and wound repair.

Hyaluronic Acid

The early production of large quantities of hyaluronic acid at the wound site in connective tissue is thought to facilitate the migration of inflammatory cells and fibroblasts by interfering with cell-cell and cell-substrate interactions. The ability of monocytes, macrophages, fibroblasts, and other cells to respond to growth factor, cytokine, and other protein mediator signals may also be modulated by hyaluronic acid through its ability to interfere with receptor-ligand binding.[12]

Role of Fibroblasts in Inflammation and Repair

In normal uninjured tissue, fibroblasts synthesize and maintain elements (collagens, fibronectin, proteoglycans, and other proteins) of the

Outline 1 Functions of fibroblasts

Self-replication

Synthesis of matrix components
- Collagen types I, III, V, VI, IX
- Fibronectin
- Other glycoproteins
- Proteoglycans and glycosaminoglycans

Migration
- Chemotactic (directed)
- Chemokinetic (nondirected)

Synthesis of enzymes
- Matrix-degrading enzymes (collagenases, proteoglycanases, nonspecific proteases)
- Plasminogen activator

Synthesis of cytokines
- Interleukin-1, interleukin-6, granulocyte colony-stimulating factor, granulocyte-macrophage colony-stimulating factor
- Growth factors
  - Platelet-derived
  - Transforming (alpha and beta)

Synthesis of other proteins
- Tissue inhibitor of metalloproteinase

connective tissue matrix. This matrix is continually being turned over and remodeled at a slow rate by fibroblasts and the various enzymes they synthesize (collagenases, proteoglycanases, glycosaminodases, and other proteases).

Injury (traumatic, surgical, chemical, thermal, or immunologic) to connective tissue evokes specialized reparative responses from resident connective tissue fibroblasts that result in the manufacture and deposition of new matrix at the injury site. In the normal healing response, all these functions of fibroblasts (Outline 1) are brought into play in a concerted and orderly fashion.

Inflammation

Fibroblasts residing in connective tissue that has sustained an injury are a ready source of several cytokines and growth factors, which play significant roles in the evolution of inflammatory and repair processes. Fibroblasts synthesize interleukin–6,[52] the major cytokine involved in stimulation of acute-phase protein synthesis by hepatocytes. It also stimulates immunoglobulin synthesis and enhances B cell growth.[52] Fibroblast interleukin–6 synthesis is stimulated by interleukin–1, tumor necrosis factor (TNF), and platelet-derived growth factor (PDGF).[52] Fibroblasts are also capable of synthesizing granulocyte colony-stimulating factor, granulocyte-macrophage colony-stimulating factor, interleukin–1, PDGF, and transforming growth factors alpha (TGF-α) and beta (TGF-β).[8,15] These fibroblast-derived cytokines and growth factors can exert effects on leukocytes that lead to stimulation of their growth and their release from bone marrow, chemotaxis, and accumulation of fibroblasts, neutrophils, monocytes, and T cells, and they may serve to recruit these cells to the site of injury, causing collagenase, proteoglycanases, and nonspecific proteases to be released from resident and recruited fibroblasts. These enzymes are responsible for degradation of connective tissue matrix components and solubilization of injured tissues, which may also aid in recruitment of monocytes and fibroblasts.

Repair

The major function of fibroblasts is repairing damage to tissue after injury and inflammation. As a result of investigations conducted during the last 15 years, it is now apparent that fibroblasts do not function autonomously but are subject to signals from matrix constituents, cytokine growth factors, and other agents derived from other cellular sources in addition to those elaborated by fibroblasts themselves.[30,33,35,49,50]

Chemotactic signals direct the migration of fibroblasts from neighboring connective tissue into the site of injury, where they further expand their numbers by proliferating in response to mitogenic signals from cytokines and growth factors. They then synthesize and remodel new matrix components that will compose the scar tissue that replaces the original normal connective tissue. Several fibroblast chemoattractants have been described since the original description of the application and modification of the Boyden technique to measure fibroblast chemotaxis.[37] Fibroblast chemoattractants include lymphocyte-derived chemotactic factor for fibroblasts (LDCF-F), an 80-kd serum-derived (C5) chemotactic factor for fibroblasts, collagen types I, II, and III and their constituent α chains and hydroxyproline-containing peptides, fibronectin and fibronectin peptides, tropoelastin and elastin peptides, PDGF, TGF-β, and leukotriene B_4.[29,31,32,34,36,37]

The host of chemoattractants for fibroblasts apparently ensures a great deal of redundancy so that the chemotactic signals will be adequate for fibroblasts to migrate to the site of tissue injury and inflammation.

Fibroblast populations are also increased at sites of tissue injury by replication. Many mitogenic and growth signals exist for fibroblasts and are able to stimulate their growth at sites of inflammation and injury. It is believed that there are at least two phases to the mitogenic response of fibroblasts and most growth factors are thought to work in one of two ways. The first phase is termed "competence" and occurs in the early G_1 phase of the cell cycle, rendering the cell "competent" to replicate its DNA, but does not result in DNA synthesis or the S phase.[47] The second phase, termed "progression," results in DNA synthesis, and occurs only in "competent" fibroblasts.[47] It has been possible to classify some polypeptide growth factors as competence or progression factors (Outline 2). Many of the mitogens listed in Outline 2 could stimulate fibroblast growth at sites of tissue injury. For example, platelets are a rich source of PDGF and TGF-β. Macrophages

Outline 2 Fibroblast mitogenic factors*

Competence factors
- Platelet-derived growth factor
- Fibronectin
- Acidic and basic fibroblast (transforming) growth factors
- Calcium-containing crystals
- Calcium phosphate precipitates

Progression factors
- Transforming growth factor alpha
- Epidermal growth factor
- Somatomedins A and C
- Insulin and insulin-like growth factor
- Alveolar macrophage-derived growth factor
- Multiplication-stimulating activity

Unclassified mitogens
- Interleukin-1α and interleukin-1β
- Interleukin-4
- Interleukin-2
- Bleomycin
- Transforming growth factor beta
- Vanadate
- Schistosomal granuloma macrophage-derived growth factor
- Tumor necrosis factor (alpha and beta)

*See Carpenter,[4] Cheung and associates,[5] Keski-Oja and associates,[16] Moses and associates,[22] Müller and associates,[23] Scher and associates,[40] Schilling,[41] Spencer and associates,[46] and Stiles and associates.[47]

produce interleukin–1α and interleukin–1β, TGF-β, TNF-α, PDGF, and other macrophage-derived growth factors. Fibroblasts produce PDGF, TGF-β, interleukin–1, and somatomedin C. T cells produce TGF-β, TNF-β, and T cell-derived fibroblast growth factor.

The increased numbers of fibroblasts at sites of tissue injury and repair probably contribute to the increased amount of new matrix synthesized at such sites. However, fibroblasts are also probably stimulated by cytokines and growth factors and perhaps other agents to increase synthesis of matrix components and tissue inhibitor of metalloproteinase (TIMP). TIMP inhibits collagenase and other metalloproteinases that can degrade newly synthesized collagen. Agents known to stimulate collagen and usually fibronectin production by fibroblasts include ascorbate, TGF-β, interleukin–1, hepatic fibrogenic factor, T cell-derived factor, bleomycin, γ-aminobutyric acid, and somatomedin C.[13,19,33,35,37,38] Hyaluronic acid synthesis has also been found to be stimulated by interleukin–1, TGF-β, and a 60-kd lymphokine. (Ehrlich[10] and A.E. Postlethwaite, J. Keski-Oja, H. Moses, and associates, unpublished data).

Fibroblasts in healing wounds exert a traction force on collagen fibers and bring about the organization of the new matrix and wound contraction. It appears that type III collagen can be organized more readily than type I collagen.[10] Ehrlich[10] suggested that the newly arrived fibroblasts, rather than older "myofibroblasts," produce the forces of wound concentration.

Granulation Tissue

The healing of open, gaping wounds that have lost tissue or of an infected closed wound is effected by the formation of highly vascularized tissue (granulation tissue) that grows from the base of the wound to fill the defect. Granulation tissue is also composed of newly arrived fibroblasts. The blood vessels at the base of the wound sprout new branches that grow upward to form loops and coils near the wound surface. Small hemorrhages occur from these vessels, and more neutrophils migrate into the granulation tissue, reinforcing those already present in the exudate on the wound surface and helping to minimize bacterial growth. The fibroblasts populating the early granulation tissue are at the base and along the walls of the wound and are usually oriented parallel to the new capillary walls, perpendicular to the wound surface. Some of the fibroblasts undergo mitosis. The granulation tissue continues to enlarge and grow until the wound space is filled and its surface is covered by epithelium. Fibroblasts then orient themselves parallel to the wound surface and begin synthesizing large amounts of collagen types III and V, hyaluronic acid, and fibronectin.[10] The collagen fibers are loosely formed and lack the birefringence characteristic of normal dermal collagen or mature scar collagen.[10] As healing progresses, there is gradual wound contraction and some of the new vessels disappear. Collagen is cross-linked and remodeled over several months, and the wound becomes progressively less cellular. The accumulation of fibroblasts and blood vessels that compose the early granulation tissue is facilitated by preexisting platelets and macrophages. The release of fibroblast chemoattractants and angiogenic factors (eg, PDGF, TGF-β) by these platelets and monocytes probably contributes to the process of vessel ingrowth, fibroblast accumulation, and growth. The migration of fibroblasts and new vessels is aided by the local increase in hyaluronic acid, which traps water and increases the volume of extracellular matrix. The fibronectin present in this early matrix influences cell adhesion and migration and, along with fibrin, forms a temporary scaffold to which migrating fibroblasts can adhere.

The vascular proliferation comes about by sprouting of capillaries from existing blood vessels at the wound margins; they advance along the line of least resistance into the wound. The capillary sprouts arise by rearrangement and migration of preexisting endothelial cells and by proliferation just behind the advancing tip of the sprout. The sprouts are solid at first but soon join one another or join a capillary carrying blood and develop a lumen. These new capillaries are delicate, lack a basement membrane, and leak protein-rich fluid, allowing the escape of some erythrocytes and neutrophils.

Conversion From Inflammatory Cycle to Repair Cycle

The inflammatory cycle of wounds is characterized by the presence of blood, fibrin, and dead cells. As monocytes phagocytose these elements and secrete degrading enzymes to clean up this debris, they clear the way for the ingrowth of blood vessels and inward migration of fibroblasts. Serum and plasma contain a potent inhibitor of fibroblast migration and chemotaxis called serum inhibitor of fibroblast migration (SIFM).[26] During the first few days, SIFM in the blood in the wound probably functions to exclude fibroblasts from the wound. As proteases from neutrophils and macrophages accumulate, they can degrade SIFM.[26] The removal of SIFM and the concomitant generation or presence of fibroblast chemoattractants (eg, collagen fragments, fibronectin fragments, PDGF, TGF-β, and leukotriene B_4) allow neighboring fibroblasts to migrate into the wound site, proliferate, and begin synthesis of matrix stimulated by cytokines, growth factors, and perhaps other agents discussed above. The rich ingrowth of blood vessels is essential for the rapid growth of the granulation tissue and provides substrates and nutrients for synthesis of new matrix.

States Characterized by Impaired Wound Healing

Vascular Insufficiency States

Impaired wound healing is associated with vascular insufficiency states such as occur in chronic lower-extremity venous stasis, diabetes mellitus, sickle cell disease, decubitus ulcers, peripheral vascular disease, and hypertension.[9] These conditions have in common microangiopathy and diminished blood supply to connective tissues. This contributes to defective capillary ingrowth in granulation tissue, because newly sprouted capillaries have a diminished blood supply, close their lumina, and are resorbed. This contributes to retarded and underdeveloped granulation tissue.

Malnutrition

Malnutrition is commonly encountered in the indigent population treated at most charity and public hospitals. There is a significant correlation between wound healing and nutritional status as judged by serum albumin levels and total lymphocyte counts in peripheral blood.[14] Generalized malnutrition can affect wound healing by several mechanisms. Generalized host defenses are lowered in malnourished persons. This results in decreased resistance to wound infections and diminished function of phagocytes and macrophages, and thus perhaps in decreased clearing of debris from wounds and retarding of the transition from the inflammatory to reparative cycles in wound healing. There is defective production of cytokines by macrophages in malnourished persons. There is a general deficiency of vitamins, especially vitamins A and C, and trace minerals important for matrix synthesis. The malnutrition state provides fewer of the substrates necessary for optimal matrix synthesis.

Glucocorticoids

Hypercortisolism is associated with impaired wound repair. At least two important alterations have been observed in hypercortisolism that may explain the adverse effects of corticosteroids on wound healing. Corticosteroids inhibit collagen synthesis by fibroblasts and inhibit wound contraction.[42,48] This results in an inhibition of conversion of granulation tissue to a collagen-rich tissue and defective maturation of the reduced matrix that is synthesized.

Aging

Patients of advanced age have poorer healing of soft-tissue injuries than younger persons.[9] This may be in part the result of defective microcirculation with resultant poor perfusion of the wound area. Other possible causes are related to diminished ability of aged fibroblasts to synthesize matrix components. Chemotaxis of aged fibroblasts does not appear to be decreased (personal observation). There may be diminished production of growth factors and cytokines by aged macrophages and monocytes.

Chemotherapy

Assessment of the effects of chemotherapy on healing surgical wounds has been hampered by the different ways that laboratory animals and humans metabolize chemotherapeutic drugs. It is difficult to do appropriately controlled studies on humans. In rats, cyclophosphamide has been shown to interfere with all three phases of wound healing (inflammation, proliferation, and maturation).[20] These effects are no doubt related to the ability of cyclophosphamide to inhibit DNA synthesis by cross-linking DNA strands and by transferring alkyl groups to various cellular components, thereby interfering with their function. Methotrexate and fluorouracil are antimetabolic drugs that interfere with DNA and RNA synthesis. They have milder and more transient effects on the inflammatory or proliferative phases of wound healing in rats.[20]

Radiation Therapy

Preoperative radiation therapy is detrimental to all phases of wound healing, and the degree of impairment is directly correlated with the radiation dosage. There are adverse effects on the inflammatory phase, with infections being more common and epithelialization, contraction, and fibroplasia diminished.[1,2,11,20,27]

References

1. Archer PR, Greenwell EJ, Ware T, et al: Irradiation effect on wound healing in rats. *Radiat Res* 1970;41:104–112.
2. Ariyan S, Marfuggi RA, Harder G, et al: An experimental model to determine the effects of adjuvant therapy on the incidence of postoperative wound infection: I. Evaluating preoperative radiation therapy. *Plast Reconstr Surg* 1980;65:328–337.
3. Beachey EH, Chiang TM, Kang AH: Collagen: Platelet interaction. *Int Rev Connect Tissue Res* 1979;8:1–21.
4. Carpenter G: Vanadate, epidermal growth factor and the stimulation of DNA synthesis. *Biochem Biophys Res Commun* 1981;102:1115–1121.

5. Cheung HS, Story MT, McCarty DJ: Mitogenic effects of hydroxyapatite and calcium pyrophosphate dihydrate crystals on cultured mammalian cells. *Arthritis Rheum* 1984;27:668–674.
6. Chiang TM, Beachey EH, Kang AH: Interaction of a chick skin collagen fragment (alpha 1-CB5) with human platelets: Biochemical studies during the aggregation and release reaction. *J Biol Chem* 1975;250:6916–6922.
7. Courtney HS, Simpson WA, Beachey EH: Binding of streptococcal lipoteichoic acid to fatty acid-binding sites on human plasma fibronectin. *J Bacteriol* 1983;153:763–770.
8. Deuel TF: Polypeptide growth factors: Roles in normal and abnormal cell growth. *Annu Rev Cell Biol* 1987;3:443–492.
9. Duncan HJ, Faris IB: Skin vascular resistance and skin perfusion pressure as predictors of healing of ischemic lesion of the lower limb: Influences of diabetes mellitus, hypertension, and age. *Surgery* 1986;99:432–438.
10. Ehrlich HP: The role of connective tissue matrix in wound healing, in Barbul A, Pines E, Caldwell M, et al (eds): *Growth Factors and Other Aspects of Wound Healing: Biological and Clinical Implications.* New York, Alan R Liss, 1988, pp 243–258.
11. Grillo HC, Potsaid MS: Studies in wound healing: IV. Retardation of contraction by local x-irradiation, and observations relating to the origin of fibroblasts in repair. *Ann Surg* 1961;154:741–750.
12. Heinegard D, Paulson M: Structure and metabolism of proteoglycans, in Piez KA, Reddi AH (eds): *Extracellular Matrix Biochemistry.* New York, Elsevier, 1984, pp 277–328.
13. Johnson RL, Ziff M: Lymphokine stimulation of collagen accumulation. *J Clin Invest* 1976;58:240–252.
14. Kay SP, Moreland JR, Schmitter E: Nutritional status and wound healing in lower extremity amputations. *Clin Orthop* 1987;217:253–256.
15. Kaushansky K: The molecular biology of the colony-stimulating factors. *Blood Cells* 1987;13:3–15.
16. Keski-Oja J, Leof EB, Lyons RM, et al: Transforming growth factors and control of neoplastic cell growth. *J Cell Biochem*, in press.
17. Keski-Oja J, Sen A, Todaro GJ: Direct association of fibronectin and actin molecules in vitro. *J Cell Biol* 1980;85:527–533.
18. Kuusela P: Fibronectin binds to *Staphylococcus aureus. Nature* 1978;276:718–720.
19. Mainardi CL: Localized fibrotic disorders, in Kelley WN, Harris ED Jr, Ruddy S, et al (eds): *Textbook of Rheumatology*, ed 3. Philadelphia, WB Saunders, 1989, pp 1245–1261.
20. McGonigal MD, Martin DM, Lucas CE, et al: The effects of breast cancer chemotherapy on wound healing in the rat. *J Surg Res* 1987;42:560–564.
21. Menzel EJ, Smolen JS, Liotta L, et al: Interaction of fibronectin with C1q and its collagen-like fragment (CLF). *FEBS Lett* 1981;129:188–192.
22. Moses AC, Nissley SP, Rechler MM, et al: The purification and characterization of multiplication stimulating activity (MSA) from media conditioned by a rat liver cell line, in Giordano G, Van Wyk JJ, Minuto F (eds): *Somatomedins and Growth.* London, Academic Press, 1979, pp 45–59.
23. Müller R, Bravo R, Burckhardt J, et al: Induction of c-fos gene and protein by growth factors precedes activation of c-myc. *Nature* 1984;312:716–720.
24. Nishida T, Nakagawa S, Awata T, et al: Fibronectin promotes epithelial migration of cultured rabbit cornea *in situ. J Cell Biol* 1983;97:1653–1657.
25. Norris DA, Clark RA, Swigart LM, et al: Fibronectin fragment(s) are chemotactic for human peripheral blood monocytes. *J Immunol* 1982;129:1612–1618.

26. Ochs ME, Postlethwaite AE, Kang AH: Identification of a protein in sera of normal humans that inhibits fibroblast chemotactic and random migration in vitro. *J Invest Dermatol* 1987;88:183–190.

27. Pohle EA, Ritchie G: Studies of the effect of roentgen rays on the healing of wounds: II. Histological changes in skin wounds in rats following post-operative irradiation. *Radiology* 1933;20:102–108.

28. Postlethwaite AE: Cell-cell interaction in collagen biosynthesis and fibroblast migration, in Weissmann G (ed): *Advances in Inflammation Research*. New York, Raven Press, 1983, vol 5, pp 27–55.

29. Postlethwaite AE, Kang AH: Fibroblast chemoattractants. *Methods Enzymol* 1988;163:694–707.

30. Postlethwaite AE, Kang AH: Induction of fibroblast proliferation by human mononuclear leukocyte-derived proteins. *Arthritis Rheum* 1983;26:22–27.

31. Postlethwaite AE, Keski-Oja J, Balian G, et al: Induction of fibroblast chemotaxis by fibronectin: Localization of the chemotactic region to a 140,000-molecular weight non-gelatin-binding fragment. *J Exp Med* 1981;153:494–499.

32. Postlethwaite AE, Keski-Oja J, Moses HL, et al: Stimulation of the chemotactic migration of human fibroblasts by transforming growth factor β. *J Exp Med* 1987;165:251–256.

33. Postlethwaite AE, Raghow R, Stricklin GP, et al: Modulation of fibroblast functions by interleukin 1: Increased steady-state accumulation of type I procollagen messenger RNAs and stimulation of other functions but not chemotaxis by human recombinant interleukin 1 α and β. *J Cell Biol* 1988;106:311–318.

34. Postlethwaite AE, Seyer JM, Kang AH: Chemotactic attraction of human fibroblasts to type I, II, and III collagens and collagen-derived peptides. *Proc Natl Acad Sci USA* 1978;75:871–875.

35. Postlethwaite AE, Smith GN, Mainardi CL, et al: Lymphocyte modulation of fibroblast function in vitro: Stimulation and inhibition of collagen production by different effector molecules. *J Immunol* 1984;132:2470–2477.

36. Postlethwaite AE, Snyderman R, Kang AH: Generation of a fibroblast chemotactic factor in serum by activation of complement. *J Clin Invest* 1979;64:1379–1385.

37. Postlethwaite AE, Snyderman R, Kang AH: The chemotactic attraction of human fibroblasts to a lymphocyte-derived factor. *J Exp Med* 1976;144:1188–1203.

38. Raghow R, Postlethwaite AE, Keski-Oja J, et al: Transforming growth factor-β increases steady state levels of type I procollagen and fibronectin messenger RNAs posttranscriptionally in cultured human dermal fibroblasts. *J Clin Invest* 1987;79:1285–1288.

39. Ruoslahti E, Vaheri A: Interaction of soluble fibroblast surface antigen with fibrinogen and fibrin: Identity with cold insoluble globulin of human plasma. *J Exp Med* 1975;141:497–501.

40. Scher CD, Shepard RC, Antoniades HN, et al: Platelet-derived growth factor and the regulation of the mammalian fibroblast cell cycle. *Biochim Biophys Acta* 1979;560:217–241.

41. Schilling JA: Wound healing. *Physiol Rev* 1968;48:374–423.

42. Oliver NA: Altered production of fibronectin and collagen in hypercortisolism may inhibit tissue repair, letter. *Arch Dermatol* 1987;123:570–571.

43. Senior RM, Griffin GL, Mecham RP: Chemotactic responses of fibroblasts to tropoelastin and elastin-derived peptides. *J Clin Invest* 1982;70:614–618.

44. Senior RM, Griffin GL, Mecham RP, et al: Val-Gly-Val-Ala-Pro-Gly, a repeating peptide in elastin, is chemotactic for fibroblasts and monocytes. *J Cell Biol* 1984;99:870–874.
45. Seppa H, Seppa S, Yamada KM, et al: The cell binding fragment of fibronectin and platelet derived growth factor are chemoattractants for fibroblasts, abstract. *J Cell Biol* 1980;87:323a.
46. Spencer EM, Skover G, Hunt TK: Somatomedins: Do they play a pivotal role in wound healing?, in Barbul A, Pines E, Caldwell M, et al (eds): *Growth Factors and Other Aspects of Wound Healing.* New York, Alan R Liss, 1988, pp 103–116.
47. Stiles CD, Capone GT, Scher CD, et al: Dual control of cell growth by somatomedins and platelet-derived growth factor. *Proc Natl Acad Sci USA* 1979;76:1279–1283.
48. Van Story-Lewis PE, Tenenbaum HC: Glucocorticoid inhibition of fibroblast contraction of collagen gels. *Biochem Pharmacol* 1986;35:1283–1286.
49. Wahl SM, Wahl LM, McCarthy JB: Lymphocyte-mediated activation of fibroblast proliferation and collagen production. *J Immunol* 1978;121:942–946.
50. Wyler DJ, Rosenwasser LJ: Fibroblast stimulation in schistosomiasis: II. Functional and biochemical characteristics of egg granuloma-derived fibroblast-stimulating factor. *J Immunol* 1982;129:1706–1710.
51. Yamada KM, Olden K: Fibronectins: Adhesive glycoproteins of cell surface and blood. *Nature* 1978;275:179–184.
52. Yihong Z, Lin J-X, Vilcek J: Synthesis of interleukin 6 (interferon β_2–1β cell stimulatory factor 2) in human fibroblasts is triggered by an increase in intracellular cyclic AMP. *J Biol Chem* 1988;263:6177–6182.
53. Zardi L, Siri A, Carnemolla B, et al: Fibronectin: A chromatin-associated protein? *Cell* 1979;18:649–657.

Chapter 41

Tendon Trauma and Overuse Injuries

William G. Clancy, Jr, MD

There is a significant amount of scientific data on the healing response of acutely traumatized tendon and ligament,[16] but little on nontraumatic injury to tendon and ligament. This chapter considers the possible causes and pathophysiologic features of a prolonged healing response or failure to heal response in nontraumatic injury to tendinous and ligamentous connective-tissue structures.

In most injuries to connective-tissue structures, no specific traumatic event can be associated with the onset of clinical symptoms. Symptoms begin gradually and become noticeable when the patient's activity level increases. Because these injuries often occur after repetitive, stressful loading of the tissue, they are called overuse injuries.

The most frequent tendon overuse problems in the upper extremity involve the supraspinatus tendon, with or without associated biceps tendinitis, in swimmers, throwers, and weightlifters. Similar overuse injuries occur in the proximal extensor carpi radialis brevis tendon in tennis players, and in the flexor/pronator tendon in throwers and tennis players. In sports such as crewing, various other tendon problems occur, including "crossover" tendinitis, consisting of abductor pollicis longus and extensor pollicis brevis tendinitis.

Tendon problems are more common in the lower extremity. Runners experience the most injuries, predominantly Achilles tendinitis and posterior tibial tendinitis with occasional involvement of the anterior tibial and peroneal brevis tendons.[20] Flexor hallucis longus tendinitis is frequent in ballet dancers, whereas infrapatellar tendinitis and, to a lesser degree, quadriceps tendinitis are seen in basketball and volleyball players, high and long jumpers, and weightlifters.

The clinical and pathologic findings of tendinitis are limited to two locations: the tendon and the tendon insertion into bone (insertional tendinitis). Rarely is tendinitis clinically evident at the musculotendinous junction, the predominant site of muscle strains.

Chronic overuse syndromes involving ligamentous tissue are far less common than those involving tendon. Usually, they are located in the ulnar collateral ligament of the elbow in throwers, the symphysis pubis in runners (osteitis pubis), the medial collateral ligament of the knee in swimmers (breaststroker's knee), and the plantar fascia in runners. These examples illustrate the body's failure to heal a chronic inflammatory state associated with repetitive strenuous activities in or about tendons or ligaments.

In most cases, the clinical symptoms subside, although prolonged rest from the initiating activity is frequently required. In a few cases, symptoms return when strenuous activity is resumed, necessitating additional rest before the patient can return to activities without recurrence of the injury.[7] In even fewer patients, symptoms persist despite prolonged conservative treatment when stressful activities are resumed. These patients have a failed healing response in the involved tissue and require surgical treatment.

The exact abnormality in these conditions is poorly understood, especially in patients with acute and subacute symptoms. The few reports of histologic findings in patients with tendinitis focus on those with chronic, unrelenting symptoms and may not truly reflect the condition of patients with acute injuries in whom symptoms resolve. Because pathologic specimens are from patients with chronic symptoms who have undergone surgery, there is significant confusion about the specific condition or conditions present and the appropriate terminology. For example, one report[39] called the state of chronic pain limited to the Achilles tendon "Achilles tenosynovitis." But the Achilles tendon has no synovial lining. Kvist and associates[21,22] used the term paratenonitis to describe patients with chronic Achilles tendon pain. Clement and associates[7] and Smart and associates[37] defined inflammation of the tendon sheath as peritendinitis. Puddu and associates[32] used the term tendinosis to describe the degenerative changes present in so-called spontaneous Achilles tendon rupture without previous pain symptoms. To further complicate matters, some descriptions of the pathologic findings in patients with chronic tendinitis are based on biopsy material from the tendon sheath only and not the tendon itself.[21,22,24,33,39]

Understanding an inflamed tendon depends on the use of consistent, defined anatomic terminology to describe the tendon and its surrounding tissue. The Achilles tendon is an excellent example to illustrate overuse injury because more information is available about it than about any other tendon.

Anatomy of the Tendon

Tendon joins muscle to bone and is an extremely strong structure with a tensile strength between 49 and 98 N/mm^2.[12] It is composed primarily of collagen fibers, which run the entire length of the structure, and a matrix of proteoglycans. Schneider,[35] Edwards,[11] and Schatzker and Brånemark[34] elucidated the macro structure of tendon. Collagen fibers group together to form primary bundles. These primary bundles are gathered in a hexagonal shape with a cross-sectional area of 0.125 to 0.375 mm^2 to form secondary bundles or fascicles. Edwards[11] con-

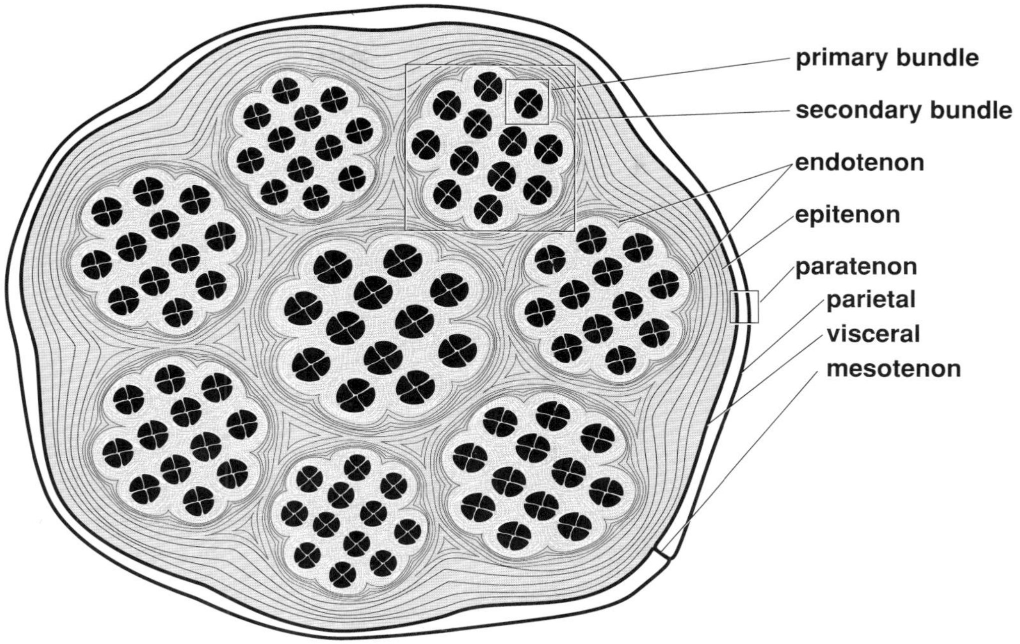

Fig. 1 *A cross section of a typical tendon. A double-layer tendon sheath called the paratenon surrounds the tendon. The outer or parietal layer is connected at points to the inner or visceral layer by bridges, the mesotenon. The tendon consists of primary collagen bundles grouped together to form secondary bundles. The secondary bundles are held firmly together by the intertwining connective tissue called the endotenon. All the secondary bundles are further surrounded circumferentially by connective tissue called the epitenon that lies adjacent to the visceral layer of the paratenon.*

sidered these the primary unit in the tendon structure. The secondary bundles then form tertiary bundles. A mesh of loose connective tissue containing elastin surrounds all the bundles and contains the vascular supply, lymphatics, and nerves. This interconnective, enveloping tissue is called the endotenon (Fig. 1). The elastin forms the wavy pattern of the tendon seen under light microscopy.

At the musculotendinous junction, the secondary bundles of the tendon are separate from the sarcomeres but are invaginated into the interstices of the sarcomeres. The perimysium of the muscle fibers blends into the endotenon. At the tendon-osseous junction, the collagen fibers pass through four zones described by Cooper and Misol.[8] Zone 1 consists of tenocytes with a normal collagen and proteoglycan matrix. In zone 2, the collagen fibers remain normal but the cell type gradually changes from tenocyte to chondrocyte, giving the matrix the appearance of fibrocartilage. The matrix in zone 3 is mineralized fibrocartilage; this transition from zone 2 is irregular but dramatic. The collagen fibers in zone 3 gradually blend into zone 4, which consists of typical bone matrix. The periosteum is contiguous with the endotenon.

The entire tendon is surrounded by a well-defined connective tissue layer called the epitenon, which is continuous on its inner surface with the endotenon. The paratenon surrounds the epitenon and is in immediate contact with it. The paratenon may vary considerably in structure, from a loose, fatty, areolar connective tissue to a well-defined, double-layer sheath, or even a bursa. Both inner surfaces of the double-layer sheath may be lined with synovial cells. The inner, or visceral, layer of the paratenon lies adjacent to the epitenon and is connected at intervals with the outer parietal layer by perpendicular connections called the mesotenon. When the paratenon forms a double-layered sheath lined by synovium, it is referred to as tenosynovium. When there is no synovial lining, it is called tenovagium. The flexor tendons of the forearm and hand are tenosynovia, whereas the Achilles tendon sheath is a tenovagium.

The tenocyte is the cellular component of tendon and produces collagen and the matrix proteoglycans. These tenocyte cells are elongated longitudinally, lie between the collagen fibrils, and contain numerous cellular filaments that extend among the fibrils. Tenocyte cells have a low respiratory quotient and a low rate of collagen turnover.[17]

The tendon receives its vascular supply in three ways. Although the capillaries on the muscle side of the musculotendinous junction are end loops and do not connect with those of the tendon, the larger vessels in the perimysium continue into the endotenon. At the tendon-osseous junction, the vessels in the outer periosteum continue into the endotenon. The main blood supply of tendon, however, is derived either from vessels in the paratenon that directly enter the epitenon and endotenon, or, if there is a doubled-layered sheath, from the vessels in the parietal layer that enter into the visceral layer through the mesotenon and then pass to the epitenon. Branches arise from the epitenon and radially enter the endotenon and tendon fascicles to anastomose with the internal vascular architecture.[34]

Schatzker and Brånemark[34] demonstrated that the blood supply and vascular complexities of tendon varied with the morphologic characteristics of the tendon. In flat tendons, most of the blood supply is arranged superficially in the epitenon. Thick rounded tendons have both superficial and deep internal arrangements. They suggested that the observed superficial and deep systems create a macrovascular unit that segments much of the tendon on the basis of differences in the vascular supply. They also showed that there was no circulation within the deep internal longitudinal vasculature when the paratenon was completely stripped. They concluded that the blood supply to the tendon was segmental, whether the tendon was surrounded by a single-layer paratenon or a double-layer tenosynovium, and that any surgery that freed the paratenon or mesotenon from the tendon devitalized that segment of the tendon.

Pathologic Conditions

I use terms based on the anatomy of the tendon and its surrounding tissues to describe possible pathologic conditions. These terms are paratenonitis, tendinitis, tendinosis, paratenonitis with tendinosis, partial rupture, and complete rupture.

The term paratenonitis describes an inflammation of the outer layer of the tendon (paratenon) alone. For example, if a tendon rubs over a bony exostosis or osteochondroma, the first structure to be irritated or injured is the paratenon, whether it is a single layer of areolar connective tissue or a more defined double-layer tendon sheath. The term paratenonitis includes the terms peritendinitis, tenosynovitis, and tenovaginitis.

Tendinitis describes any injury that produces an inflammatory response within the tendon. For example, if acute tendon injury occurs without injury to the sheath, a secondary inflammatory (repair) response would be expected to occur in the paratenon tissue, although this is unproven. The term tendinitis describes a condition in which the primary site of injury is the tendon, and there is an inflammatory response within the tendon with an associated reactive paratenonitis present.

A third pathologic condition consists of tendon degeneration without an inflammatory response. Puddu and associates[32] and others have histologic documentation that long-standing tendon degeneration can exist without clinical symptoms and without the presence of paratenonitis. Puddu and associates called this entity "tendinosis," referring to a tendon that has significant degenerative changes but no clinical or histologic signs of an inflammatory response within the tendon or paratenon tissue.

A fourth pathologic condition, previously called chronic tendinitis,[5,6] can be seen in tendon biopsy material from patients with chronic symptoms. These biopsy specimens reveal significant tendon degeneration and a definite inflammation of the paratenon, but no inflammatory cellular response in the tendon. Puddu and associates[32] called this entity peritendinitis with tendinosis, but a better name might be paratenonitis with tendinosis. The classic chronic inflammatory cellular response has been observed within tendon only in patients with grossly observable partial tendon rupture.[25]

A subcategory of paratenonitis with tendinosis includes the entity previously called insertional tendinitis. These patients experience pain at the bony insertion of the tendon and the adjacent tendon. Those with prolonged, significant symptoms frequently have positive findings on a bone scan. Although bone changes have been reported at the time of biopsy,[14] my colleagues and I have not been able to demonstrate any bony abnormalities on histologic evaluation in our patients. The proximal tendon shows evidence of collagen degeneration without any of the classic signs of an inflammatory response.

In both gross partial rupture[25] and "spontaneous" complete tendon rupture,[1,2] the characteristic pathologic findings consist of a chronic inflammatory response within the paratenon tissue and within the tendon itself, particularly around the ruptured fragments. There are, however, some features that are quite distinct from the histologic aspects of acutely lacerated tendons and the healing sequence after repair.

In partial and complete rupture, areas of marked tendon degeneration exist, separate from the rupture site and without the presence of acute or chronic inflammation or signs of a reparative process.[1,2,9,10,15,36] Biopsy samples taken within 24 hours of rupture confirm that these changes were present before the complete, spontaneous tendon rupture.[1] These findings are characteristic of the pathologic condition, tendinosis.

Tendinitis has been a catchall phrase used to define a symptom complex consisting of acute or chronic pain, with or without swelling, located in or about a tendon. The term has also been used to define any or all of the pathologic conditions already described. Significantly, a review of the reported histologic findings in biopsy specimens taken from patients with "chronic tendinitis syndrome" showed that they were all similar. All specimens contained demonstrated areas with various degrees of tendon degeneration, such as the loss of the normal collagen architecture, ranging from splaying of fibers to amorphic areas; the loss of cellularity in these areas; and the complete absence of the classic inflammatory response. Adolescent and young adult athletes showed a morphologic change in the fibroblasts adjacent to these areas of degeneration. The fibroblasts become more plump or rounded and granularity increased within the nucleus. These changes suggest an increased metabolic rate but there is no noticeable increase in collagen production.

Causes of Tendon Failure and Failure of Healing Response in Overuse or Overload

Histologic evaluation of chronic pathologic conditions that fail to respond to clinical treatment reveals no sign of a classic inflammatory or repair response within the tendon. There are also no significant signs of cell death, other than areas of decreased cellularity in some cases. Some cell death may have occurred, but it did not have significant magnitude to stimulate an inflammatory response.

The tendon is maintained by the tenocyte's production of collagen, which has a turnover time of 50 to 100 days.[17] The tenocyte must also be able to increase collagen and matrix production in response to increased loading. Additionally, there must be a blood supply adequate to maintain viability of the tenocytes, as documented in vascular studies.[38] Macnab[28] and Schatzker and Brånemark[34] have shown, however, that there is an area in both the supraspinatus tendon and the Achilles tendon that has a diminished blood flow. Blood flow to part of the supraspinatus tendon may be completely arrested during forceful abduction-circumduction-adduction rotation. Complete ruptures of the supraspinatus tendon and the Achilles tendon occur almost exclusively in these areas of diminished vascularity. With time, diminished vascularity may lead to decreased cellularity from attritional cell death. In areas of diminished cellularity, production of maintenance collagen may be limited and the response to increased tendon loading diminished.

Peacock and van Winkle[31] and others have theorized that the tenocyte is an end stage cell capable of limited mitosis and unable to produce increased amounts of collagen beyond maintenance. They observed that the ends of lacerated tendons isolated from the surrounding wound were "characterized by atrophy and resorption. There is no evidence of regeneration or synthesis of new protein." They theorized that the synovial cells of the paratenon did not have the potential for a repair response. Studies of intact digital flexor sheaths found no repair response when tendons within these intact sheaths ruptured. There was no mention of pathologic changes within these ruptured tendons.

Lundborg and Rank[26,27] found that when segments of freshly repaired rabbit flexor tendons were placed in the rabbit knee joint, there was an intrinsic tendon repair response with the proliferation of alleged tendon cells and the production of mature collagen. Manske and associates[29] hoped to eliminate the possibility of invasion of the repaired tendon by cells other than those of tendon origin. Rabbit flexor tendon with a 90% midsubstance laceration was placed directly into a tissue culture medium and evaluated at three, six, and nine weeks. Light and electron microscopic studies revealed that cells migrated from the epitenon to the site of laceration. These cells were phagocytic, removing cellular debris and collagen fragments. Cells within the endotenon demonstrated signs of increased cellular activity with secretions of filamentous material, although no mature collagen was found. Manske and associates[29] concluded that the phagocytic cells were a differentiation of fibroblasts in the epitenon.

There was no mention in this study as to whether the visceral paratenon was separated from the epitenon. If it was not removed, it is possible that cells from the paratenon layer differentiated and migrated to the site of injury. In a more recent study, Banes and associates,[4] using a cell-separation technique on avian flexor tendons removed from their sheaths, demonstrated two distinct cell populations. The cells from the superficial layer and epitenon area were found to be synovial cells. The cells found deep within the tendon endotenon were found to be fibroblasts. These studies suggest that tendons with a synovial layer adjacent to the epitenon and the endotenon may have some intrinsic repair response, and that cell death may not be necessary to initiate the classic inflammatory response. The role of the synovial cell layer or the epitenon fibroblast and the capacity of the endotenon fibroblast to produce mature collagen in this repair response are unknown at present.

A review of biopsy specimens from seven younger patients with "chronic tendinitis" found that tenocytes deep within the tendon and adjacent to the areas of collagen degeneration had changed shape from long, flattened spindle cells to round, plump cells with a more granular basophilic nucleus suggesting a more metabolically active cell. The area of degeneration had not been invaded, however, by any type of cell.

Another possible explanation of tendon failure and failure of the repair response is accelerated aging of the tenocyte. Ippolito and associates[18] made biochemical and morphologic evaluations of rabbit Achilles tendon at various ages and reported definite changes associated with aging. The tenocytes showed a marked decrease in the intracytoplasmic organelles responsible for protein synthesis. In newborns, the tenocytes demonstrated evidence of significant synthetic activity. With aging, the cytoplasmic organelles responsible for synthetic activity were greatly diminished or absent. Nagy and associates[30] also reported that DNA content decreased and the chromatin staining properties of the tenocyte were modified with aging. Laitenin[23] also described the metabolic inactivity of older tendon.

Ippolito and associates[18] noted that significant extracellular changes occurred with aging. The diameter of collagen fibers increased and there was an overall increase in insoluble collagen. Mucopolysaccharide content and water content decreased. Many investigators have found a marked increase in collagen cross-linking with aging.[3,13,40]

Ippolito and associates[19] evaluated human Achilles tendon tissues from a 6-month-old infant and 24-year-old and 60-year-old adults.[19] Water content decreased markedly between the infant and the young adult but there was little change between the young adult and the older adult. Collagen increased 50% between 6 months and 24 years of age, with minimal further decrease by 60 years. The amount of glycoprotein in the infant was reduced by one third at 24 years and remained essentially the same at 60 years. These results were compared biochemically and morphologically to tissue taken from an area of tendon degeneration in a 25-year-old adult with spontaneous Achilles tendon rupture.[18] When this area of tendon degeneration was compared with tissue from the normal 24-year-old, there was a 34% loss of collagen, an increase in mucopolysaccharides of more than 100%, and a significant increase in water and glycoprotein content. These changes indicate differences from normal tenocyte synthesis that adversely alter the biomechanical properties of the tendon.

Treatment

Surgical treatment is suggested if prolonged conservative treatment for chronic "tendinitis" is ineffective. Surgical treatment consists of an incision into the tendon sheath, followed by several longitudinal incisions that split the tendon at the site of the symptoms. There are two reasons for the longitudinal incisions into the tendon. (1) They enable the physician to explore the tendon and determine whether gross collagen degeneration or gross partial rupture is present. (2) These incisions may stimulate an acute, reparative inflammatory response.

This procedure has produced good-to-excellent overall results in more than 90% of treated patients.

References

1. Arner O, Lindholm Å: Subcutaneous rupture of the Achilles tendon: A study of 92 cases. *Acta Chir Scand* 1959;239(supp):1–51.
2. Arner O, Lindholm Å, Orell SR: Histologic changes in subcutaneous rupture of the Achilles tendon: A study of 74 cases. *Acta Chir Scand* 1958;116:484–490.
3. Bailey AJ, Robins SP, Balian G: Biological significance of the intermolecular crosslinks of collagen. *Nature* 1974;251:105–109.
4. Banes AJ, Donlon K, Link GW, et al: Cell populations of tendon: A simplified method for isolation of synovial cells and internal fibroblasts. Confirmation of origin and biologic properties. *J Orthop Res* 1988;6:83–94.
5. Clancy WG Jr, Neidhart D, Brand RL: Achilles tendonitis in runners: A report of five cases. *Am J Sports Med* 1976;4:46–57.
6. Clancy WG Jr: Tendinitis and plantar fasciitis in runners, in D'Ambrosia R, Drez D Jr (eds): *Prevention and Treatment of Running Injuries.* Thorofare, Charles B Slack, 1982, pp 77–87.
7. Clement DB, Taunton JE, Smart GW: Achilles tendinitis and peritendinitis: Etiology and treatment. *Am J Sports Med* 1984;12:179–184.
8. Cooper RR, Misol S: Tendon and ligament insertion: A light and electron microscopic study. *J Bone Joint Surg* 1970;52A:1–20.
9. Davidsson L, Salo M: Pathogenesis of subcutaneous tendon ruptures. *Acta Chir Scand* 1969;135:209–212.
10. DiStefano VJ, Nixon JE: Achilles tendon rupture: Pathogenesis, diagnosis, and treatment by a modified pullout wire technique. *J Trauma* 1972;12:671–677.
11. Edwards DAW: The blood supply and lymphatic drainage of tendons. *Anatomy* 1946;80:147–152.
12. Elliott DH: Structure and function of mammalian tendon. *Biol Rev* 1965;40:392–421.
13. Eyre DR, Paz MA, Gallop PM: Cross-linking in collagen and elastin. *Annu Rev Biochem* 1984;53:717–748.
14. Ferretti A, Ippolito E, Mariani P, et al: Jumper's knee. *Am J Sports Med* 1983;11:58–62.
15. Fox JM, Blazina ME, Jobe FW, et al: Degeneration and rupture of the Achilles tendon. *Clin Orthop* 1975;107:221–224.
16. Gelberman R, Goldberg V, An K-N, et al: Tendon, in Woo SL-Y, Buckwalter JA (eds): *Injury and Repair of the Musculoskeletal Soft Tissue.* Park Ridge, Illinois, American Academy of Orthopaedic Surgeons, 1988, pp 5–40.
17. Gerber G, Gerber G, Altman KI: Studies on the metabolism of tissue proteins: I. Turnover of collagen labeled with proline-U-C^{14} in young rats. *J Biol Chem* 1960;235:2653–2656.
18. Ippolito E, Natali PG, Postacchini F, et al: Morphological, immunochemical, and biochemical study of rabbit Achilles tendon at various ages. *J Bone Joint Surg* 1980;62A:583–598.
19. Ippolito E, Postacchini F, Ricciardi-Pollini PT: Biomechanical variations in the matrix of human tendons in relation to age and pathological conditions. *Ital J Orthop Trauma* 1975;1:133–139.
20. James SL, Brubaker CE: Injuries to runners. *Am J Sports Med* 1974;2:89–198.
21. Kvist H, Kvist M: The operative treatment of chronic calcaneal paratenonitis. *J Bone Joint Surg* 1980;62B:353–357.

22. Kvist M, Józsa L, Järvinen MJ, et al: Chronic Achilles paratenonitis in athletes: A histological and histochemical study. *Pathology* 1987;19:1–11.
23. Laitinen O: The metabolism of collagen and its hormonal control in the rat: With special emphasis on the interactions of collagen and calcium in the bones. *Acta Endocrinol* 1967;120(suppl):1–86.
24. Leach RE, James S, Wasilewski S: Achilles tendinitis. *Am J Sports Med* 1981;9:93–98.
25. Ljungqvist R: Subcutaneous partial rupture of the Achilles tendon. *Acta Orthop Scand* 1968;113(suppl):1–86.
26. Lundborg G, Rank F: Experimental intrinsic healing of flexor tendons based upon synovial fluid nutrition. *J Hand Surg* 1978;3:21–31.
27. Lundborg G, Rank F: Experimental studies on cellular mechanisms involved in healing of animal and human flexor tendon in synovial environment. *Hand* 1980;12:3–11.
28. Macnab I: Rotator cuff tendinitis. *Ann R Coll Surg Engl* 1973;53:271–287.
29. Manske PR, Gelberman RH, Vande Berg JS, et al: Intrinsic flexor-tendon repair: A morphological study in vitro. *J Bone Joint Surg* 1984;66A:385–396.
30. Nagy IZ, Von Hahn HP, Verzár F: Age-related alterations in the cell nuclei and the DNA content of rat tail tendon. *Gerontologia* 1969;15:258–264.
31. Peacock EE Jr, van Winkle W Jr: *Surgery and Biology of Wound Repair.* Philadelphia, WB Saunders, 1970, pp 334–336.
32. Puddu G, Ippolito E, Postacchini F: A classification of Achilles tendon disease. *Am J Sports Med* 1976;4:145–150.
33. Rais O: Heparin treatment of peritenomyosis (peritendinitis) crepitans acuta. *Acta Chir Scand* 1961;268(suppl):1–88.
34. Schatzker J, Brånemark PI: Intravital observation on the microvascular anatomy and microcirculation of the tendon. *Acta Orthop Scand* 1969;126(suppl):1–23.
35. Schneider H: *Die Abuntgungserkrankungen dersehnen und ibre therapic.* Stuttgart, George Thieme, 1959.
36. Skeoch DU: Spontaneous partial subcutaneous ruptures of the tendo achillis: Review of the literature and evaluation of 16 involved tendons. *Am J Sports Med* 1981;9:20–22.
37. Smart GW, Taunton JE, Clement DB: Achilles tendon disorders in runners: A review. *Med Sci Sports Exerc* 1980;12:231–243.
38. Smith JW: The blood supply of tendons. *Am J Surg* 1965;109:272–276.
39. Snook GA: Achilles tendon tenosynovitis in long-distance runners. *Med Sci Sports* 1972;4:155–158.
40. Torp S, Baer E, Friedman B: *Effects of Age and of Mechanical Deformation on the Ultrastructures of Tendon.* Bristol, University of Bristol, 1974, pp 223–249.

Chapter 42

The Autoimmune Nature of Sports-Induced Injury: A Hypothesis

Gary E. Friedlaender, MD
Peter Jokl, MD
Mark C. Horowitz, PhD

Specific immunologic responses, including autoimmunity, may contribute to the origins or pathophysiologic manifestations of some sports-induced disorders of the musculoskeletal system. Many overuse syndromes are characterized by inflammation, a nonspecific immune response, and can be identified by histologic, serologic, and physical examinations and frequently by evidence of mechanical disruption of tissue. Consequently, treatment may include surgical repair of injured parts and the use of anti-inflammatory approaches that combine rest, protected activity, or medications to block or diminish the nonspecific inflammatory response or its consequences. If, however, the immune response is directed against specific tissue antigens, then both our understanding of the pathogenesis and the recommended treatment must be revised.

The Nature of Autoimmune Responses

An extensive discussion of inflammation can be found elsewhere in this volume. A detailed review of specific immunity and its regulation is beyond the scope of this chapter, but a brief examination of the nature of the nonspecific inflammatory response, specific immunity, autoreactivity, and tolerance is necessary to support the proposition that some sports-induced disorders have an autoimmune component.

The immune system generates two broad categories of response, nonspecific (inflammation) and specific.

Nonspecific Inflammatory Response

The nonspecific inflammatory response is characterized by a complex but relatively predictable sequence of events that results in enhanced vascular permeability (edema and swelling), increased local blood supply (warmth), and the recruitment of acute and chronic inflammatory cells that release or induce a wide variety of mediators (pain, edema).[3,14] The inflammatory response can be triggered by foreign antigens, altered or cross-reactive endogenous proteins, inert stimuli, and tissue trauma. Humoral control of inflammation resides in histamine release and four interactive enzyme systems: clotting (initially factor XII), kinin (bradykinin induces pain), fibrinolytic (chemotaxis), and complement (vasodilation, chemotaxis, vascular permeability). In addition, leukotrienes and prostaglandins are synthesized and immunocompetent cells are recruited. Thus, the inflammatory response, if perpetuated, has the potential to cause considerable additional local "activity" and possible tissue damage.

In most cases, this local inflammatory response is characterized by a large influx of mononuclear cells, especially neutrophils, that release degradative proteins and produce high local concentrations of enzymes. This chronic enzymatic activity may include digestion of protein, ground substance, or matrix, as in immunologic vasculitis and nephritis. Thus, previously sequestered cells and potential antigens may be released. Cell surfaces are altered. Furthermore, hidden membrane proteins may be uncovered or the nature of exposed molecules changed so that they permit cross-reactivity with common antigens, or are perceived as foreign substances.

This scenerio of exposed antigens or altered native proteins supports, in theory, potential autoreactivity and the development of autoimmunity accompanied by tissue damage.

Specific Immunity

Specific immune responses are even more complex phenomena characterized by specificity for a particular antigen, a heterogeneous pool of immunocompetent cells, cell products, and interactions, and a memory that causes more rapid and increasingly intense responses to subsequent exposures to the antigen. Functionally distinct B and T lymphocytes,[7,10] macrophages,[9,12] cytokines,[11] reactive cell products, and genetically determined control mechanisms distinguish specific immunity from inflammation. The two types of responses are not, however, mutually exclusive; indeed, they may occur sequentially or in combination.

Tolerance

Tolerance is the antithesis of autoimmunity. In purely functional terms, tolerance is an apparent inability to respond to a specific antigen. This state can be achieved in various ways depending on the species, age, dose, method of administration, and nature of the antigen. Tolerance occurs naturally, but may sometimes be acquired through manipulation of the host. Both exogenous antigens and naturally occurring antigens that disappear during fetal development may be associated with a state of tolerance.

Because the immune system can, in theory, respond to any potential antigen, it is necessary to postulate a way for immunocompetent cells to recognize and ignore "self." T cells with the capacity to recognize "self" (autoreactive) start to develop in the thymus during fetal growth. These clones, however, are deleted by a strict, genetically controlled mechanism that is still poorly understood.[13] Consequently, the cells capable of recognizing "self" are removed on a continuous basis and are not available to respond.

In addition to a lack of reactivity, tolerance may also reflect the presence of active suppressor mechanisms, mediated by $CD8^+$ T lymphocytes.[4] Removing or deleting these T-suppressor cells, bypassing this activity by immunization, or exposing an individual to cross-reacting or altered antigens after trauma (including inflammation) may eliminate the "protection" of tolerance and produce a state of autoreactivity.

Autoreactivity

Autoreactivity is the generation of immunologic responses, specifically against normal, endogenous molecules. It occurs through a variety of mechanisms. As mentioned earlier, sequestered antigens may become exposed through trauma or through the digestion of a matrix that had hidden these cells from the afferent arm of the immune system. Molecules embedded in cell membranes may be forced to the surface by mediators, such as those found in inflammation or other posttraumatic responses. Or, existing molecules may be altered by enzymes or other humoral substances, be perceived as "foreign," and thereby induce an immune response. New antigens may arise or molecules normally expressed during fetal life may reappear. Humoral mediators associated with trauma or inflammation may evoke changes in protein (antigen) expression.

Ample evidence indicates that the presence of autoreactive cells is not common, and suggests that a major mechanism of tolerance is persistent suppression. Conversely, lack of necessary suppression may lead to autoreactivity and autoimmunity. Clones of suppressor cells may be deleted, depleted, neutralized, or destroyed. If some degree of suppression of specific T-helper cells reflects activity of an idiotype-specific nature alone, rather than antigen-specific T-suppressor activity, then altered expression of class II MHC antigens on an autoantigen presenting cell may be another way to bypass suppression and stimulate T-helper cells. This may result in B-cell activity and antibody production. Trauma (acute or chronic) or mediators associated with inflammation (acute or chronic) may participate in this type of autoreactivity. Cardiac autoantibodies appear after myocardial infarction,[2] but it is clear that autoantibodies are an uncommon consequence of trauma alone.

Autoimmunity

Immunity is the process of recognizing and reacting to foreign proteins, a physiologic condition that may or may not also harm the host. When the reaction is inappropriately intense or damaging, a state of hypersensitivity is created. If the specific antigen is autologous, the potential for immunologically mediated pathologic manifestations is readily apparent. This situation can be exemplified by a long list of autoimmune disorders, including Hashimoto's thyroiditis, pernicious anemia, some forms of male infertility, dermatomyocitis, scleroderma, systemic lupus erythematosus, rheumatoid arthritis, and many other diseases.

Before a case can be built for an autoimmune component to any disease, including sport-induced disorders, it is important to realize that the mere appearance of autoantibodies, even in the presence of disease, does not confirm an etiologic role. Indeed, the production of autoantibodies may actually be secondary to tissue damage caused by the primary process. Separate factors might be responsible for the underlying disease and the presence of autoantibodies. Thus, the role of autoreactivity in the pathogenesis of disease remains in doubt and requires the same careful approach to proof associated with bacteria and Koch's postulates.

The Potential Role of Autoimmunity in Sports-Related Disorders

With these caveats in mind, the potential etiologic or pathophysiologic role of autoimmunity in several sports-induced disorders can be suggested. There appear to be two general mechanisms for autoreactivity, each with several variations. First are those circumstances in which "new" antigens of endogenous origin are exposed to the immune system. Second is the modulation or abatement of a preexisting suppression of a specific response. Speculation on the role of autoimmunity in sports-induced disorders of the musculoskeletal system must address these mechanisms, and four separate scenarios will be described.

Overuse and Impingement Syndromes

Cumulative minor stress can lead to mechanical disruption of soft tissues, inciting an inflammatory response. These disorders, especially when chronic, are recognized as bursitis, tendinitis, and other "overuse" syndromes. Inflammatory cells are recruited, some of which also participate in the specific immune response, and numerous cell products and mediators are elaborated. Through digestion or altered cell membrane characteristics, some of this cellular activity may expose or directly change sufficient native proteins to express new (auto)antigens. Anticell surface antigen, antimatrix antibodies, and anticollagen antibodies are all possibilities. Some mediators, such as the cytokine interleukin–2, may be able to reduce the normal T-cell suppressor activity responsible for maintaining tolerance, leading to autoreactivity. Either mechanism may lead to specific immune responses and a state of hypersensitivity that could inflict further local tissue damage. Hypothetically automimmunity could be instrumental in weakening tendons, ligaments or other soft tissues, causing failure or rupture (Fig. 1).

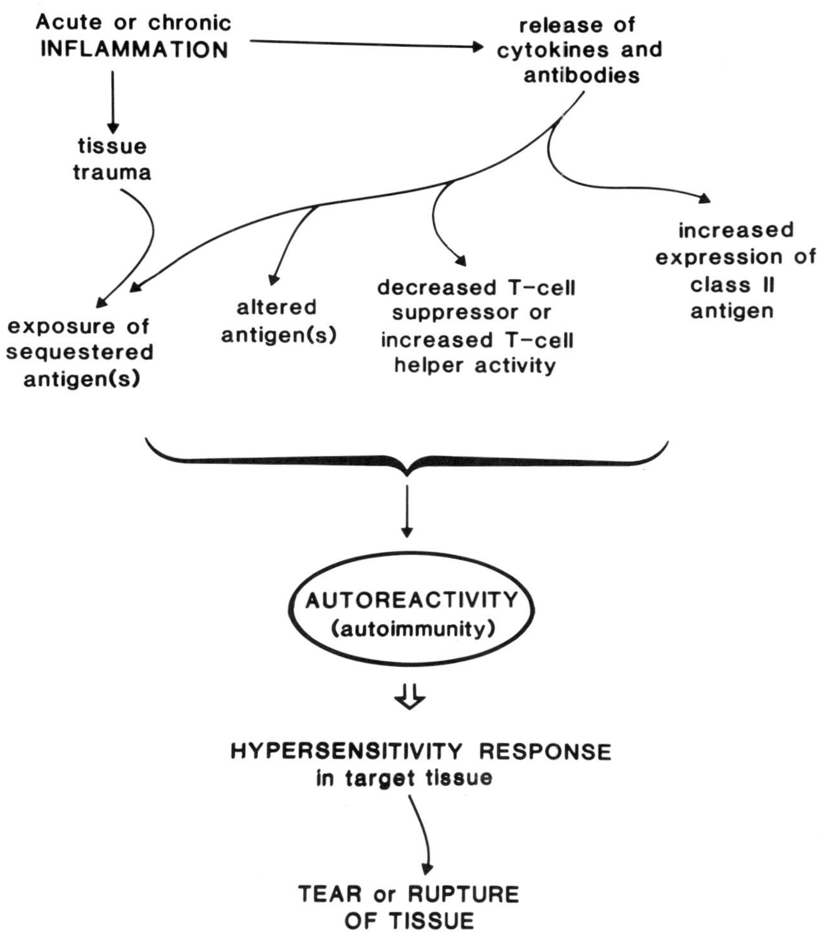

Fig. 1 *Hypothetical pathway for an autoimmune contribution to overuse or impingement syndromes.*

Chondromalacia

Although chondromalacia, particularly of the patella, is common in nonathletes as well as in athletes, it still deserves discussion as a model. Minor repetitive trauma from malalignment, excessive loading, and acute compression may all lead to mechanical disruption of cartilage matrix. Two events may proceed simultaneously. First, trauma leads to inflammation and the inflammatory response further digests matrix, thereby exposing previously sequestered chondrocytes or deep matrix antigens. Secondly, the mechanical damage alone uncovers these immunologically privileged sites. Cartilage matrix is an effective barrier to the ingress of immunoglobulin and immunologically competent cells

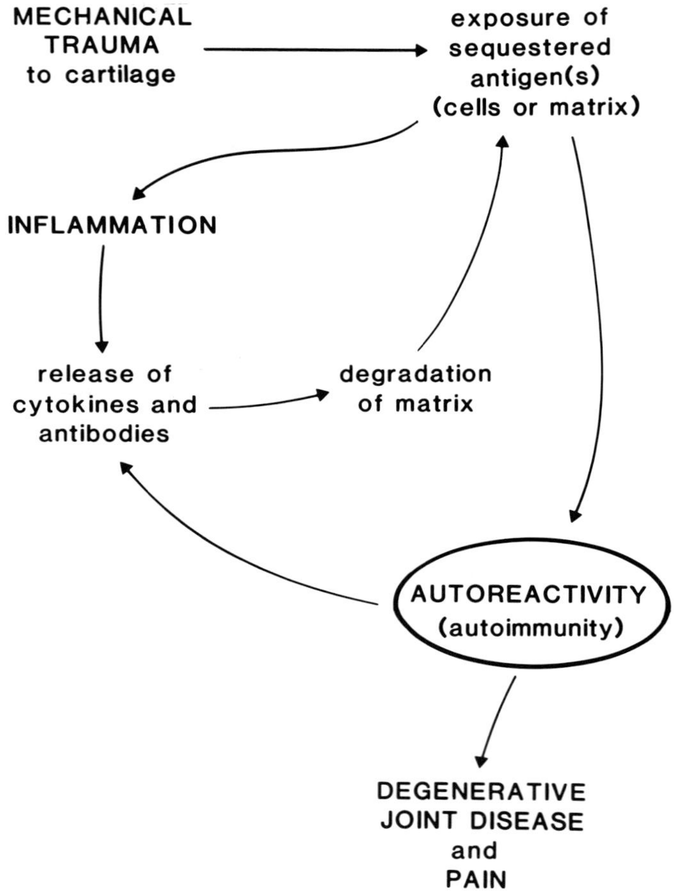

Fig. 2 *Hypothetical pathway for an autoimmune contribution to chondromalacia.*

(efferent response) as well as the egress of MHC cell-surface antigens (afferent arm).[8] The previously sequestered antigens, molecules which are not tolerated, may then stimulate a specific and, by definition, autoimmune response, resulting in further chondrocyte death, loss of matrix production, and additional chondocyte exposure. In extreme cases, this sequence of events produces pain, disruption of the articular surface, and eventually degenerative arthritis. These same events may result from a low-grade but persistent mechanical trauma, weakening the structural integrity of the meniscus cartilage and rendering it more vulnerable to further mechanical disruption (tear) (Fig. 2).

Acute Trauma

An acute disruptive injury occurs when a tissue's capacity to resist strain (ultimate stress point) is exceeded by the magnitude of load and

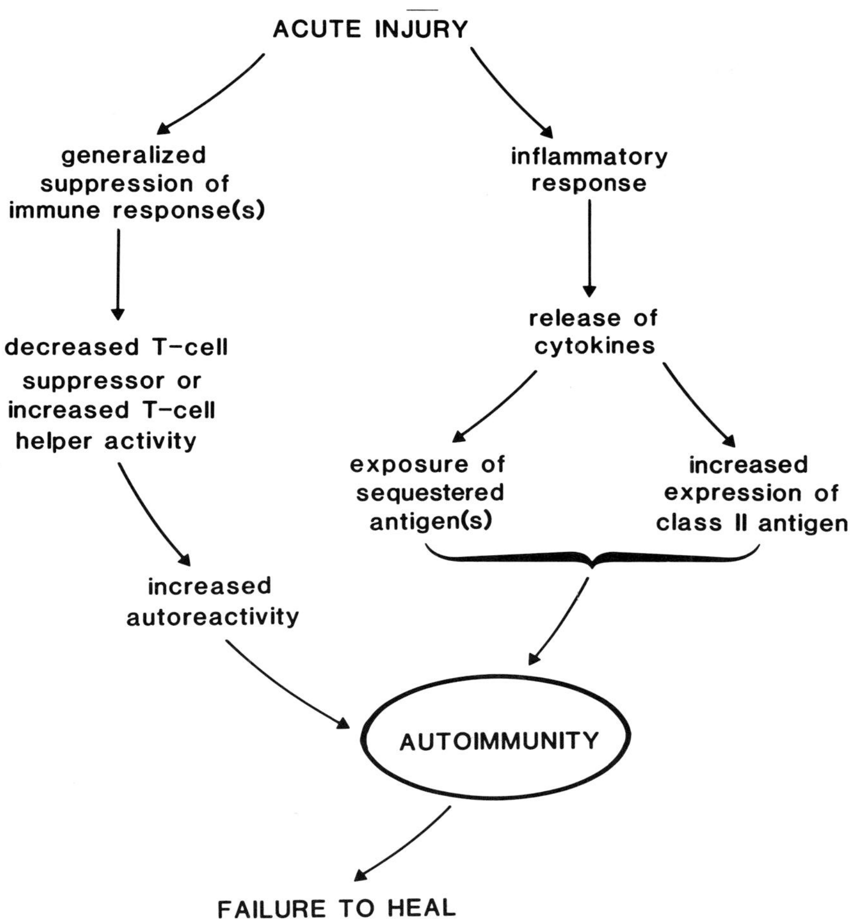

Fig. 3 *Hypothetical pathway for an autoimmune contribution to the response after acute trauma.*

its rate of application. Significant trauma (injury, surgery, burns), and the resultant physiologic stress cause generalized changes in the immune system that usually lead to hyporesponsiveness. Whether through clonal deletion, inability to maintain normal suppressor activities, or some other mechanism that bypasses the usual state of tolerance, autoimmunity may develop and interfere with a successful repair process (Fig. 3).

Stress Fractures

Stress fractures, a frequent sports-induced disorder, can be easily explained without mentioning the immune system. Repetitive trauma at inappropriate loads and/or rates for a particular bone can exceed

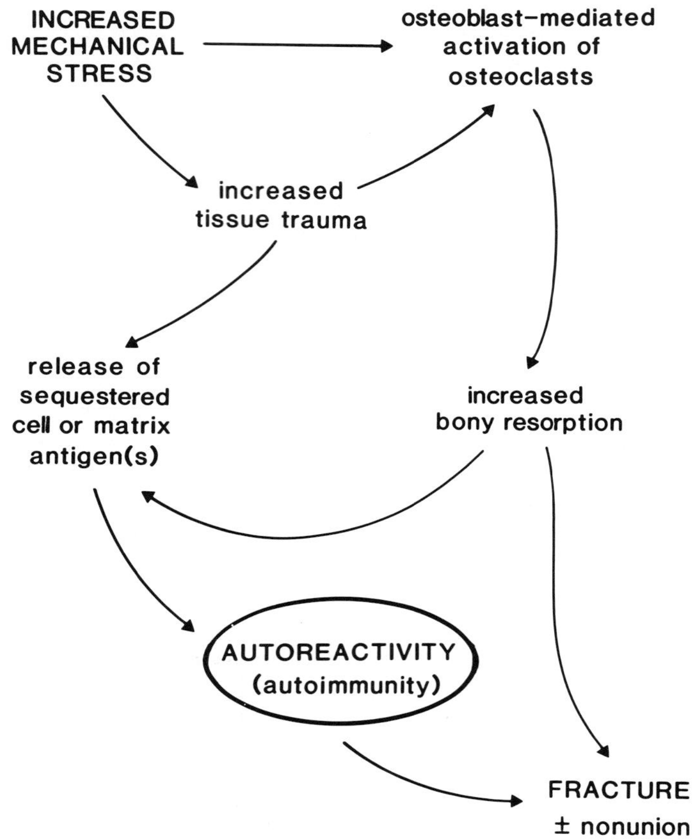

Fig. 4 *Hypothetical pathway for an autoimmune contribution to stress fractures.*

the tissue's ability to repair or remodel, producing a stress fracture. However, cells in bone remodeling (such as osteoclasts) and cells of the immune system (such as macrophages) share common precursors. Furthermore, immunocompetent cells and their lymphokines regulate osteoclastic activity directly and osteoblast function indirectly.[1,5,6] Increasing mechanical disruption of bone provokes an inflammatory response. The augmentation of blood flow, the influx of cells, and the elaboration of humoral factors contribute to enhanced osteoclastic resorption. Loss of bone mass further weakens the bone and gross fracture may result or union and healing may be retarded (Fig. 4). Although not classical autoimmunity, this sequence may represent an exaggerated immunologic response to endogenous cells responsible for tissue integrity and homeostasis.

Conclusions

Although these examples have been described separately, they may be more alike than distinct. More importantly, these descriptions draw heavily on conjecture and are meant to be provocative in a constructive sense. If the hypothesis is speculative, then diagnostic and, particularly, treatment implications move into the realm of fantasy. Nonetheless, it is important to test such imaginings because the results may be significant and useful.

References

1. Bertolini DR, Nedwin GE, Bringman TS, et al: Stimulation of bone resorption and inhibition of bone formation in vitro by human tumor necrosis factor. *Nature* 1986;319:516–518.
2. Denman AM: Immunological mechanisms and cardiovascular disease, in Lessof MH (ed): *Immunology of Cardiovascular Disease.* New York, Marcel Dekker, 1981, pp 1–73.
3. Fauve RM: Nonspecific immunity, in Bach J-F (ed): *Immunology.* New York, A Wiley, 1978, pp 395–409.
4. Gershon RK, Kondo K: Cell interactions in the induction of tolerance: The role of thymic lymphocytes. *Immunology* 1970;18:723–737.
5. Gowan M, Wood DD, Ihrie EJ, et al: An interleukin 1 like factor stimulates bone resorption in vitro. *Nature* 1983;306:378–380.
6. Horowitz MC, Coleman DL, Flood PM, et al: Parathyroid hormone and lipopolysaccharide induce murine osteoblast-like cells to secrete a cytokine indistinguishable from granulocyte-macrophage colony stimulating factor. *J Clin Invest* 1989;83:149–157.
7. Klein J: Cells of the immune system, in *Immunology: The Science of Self-Nonself Discrimination.* New York, A Wiley, 1982, pp 92–155.
8. Langer F, Gross AE: Immunogenicity of allograft articular cartilage. *J Bone Joint Surg* 1974;56A:297–304.
9. Mosier DE: A requirement for two cell types for antibody formation in vitro. *Science* 1967;158:1575–1576.
10. Mosmann TR, Cherwinski H, Bond MW, et al: Two types of murine helper T cell clone. *J Immunol* 1986;136:2348–2357.
11. Pick E: *Lymphokine.* New York, Academic Press, 1982.
12. Shevach EM, Rosenthal AS: Function of macrophages in antigen recognition by guinea pig T lymphocytes. *J Exp Med* 1973;138:1213–1229.
13. Von Boehmer H, Teh HS, Kisielow P: The thymus selects the useful, neglects the useless and destroys the harmful. *Immunol Today* 1989;19:57–61.
14. Ward PA: Inflammation, in Bellati JA (ed): *Immunology II.* Philadelphia, WB Saunders, 1978, pp 283–291.

Chapter 43

Genetic Predispositions to Traumatic Injury to the Musculoskeletal System

Reed E. Pyeritz, MD, PhD

Introduction

Genetic factors unquestionably contribute both to the development of the coarse phenotype "athletic performance" and to susceptibility to "athletic trauma." These conclusions are in part intuitive, in part derived from broad experience (genes play a role in every other human phenotype that has been examined closely, from metrical ones such as stature to ones difficult to quantify precisely such as personality and intelligence), in part suggested by anecdotes (think of the fathers and sons who play the same games well), and in part based on rare conditions caused by mutations at single genetic loci. Mendelian disorders of the skeletal, muscular, and neurologic systems are legion[7] but individually rare. If put to the test, essentially all would interfere with athletic performance, but, even in the aggregate, they do not contribute substantially to morbidity associated with athleticism. Nonetheless, having marshaled some support for the importance of genes in determining the ability to exercise and to compete (often two entirely different processes), it is diffcult to identify specific genetic factors that favor athletic performance.

The notions of performance and injury are intertwined. Everyone remembers many superb athletes whose careers were shortened by repeated injuries. If hard training is necessary for athletic excellence, and if the ability to train hard depends on prompt recovery from repeated minor traumas to muscles, joints, and bones, perhaps athletic "overachievers" are the best individuals to study for intrinsic resistance to athletic injury. In any event, the phenotype of "susceptibility to athletic injury" is broad and coarse, and not easily subjected to genetic epidemiologic scrutiny.

Many common phenotypes, including all of the diseases of middle age, share this failing. Still, ignorance is not readily tolerated these days, and consumers, health practitioners, and public health professionals are increasingly demanding information about genetic susceptibilities. After all, the human genome will be sequenced completely within the relatively near future, causes of mendelian diseases are being elucidated by "reverse genetics," gene probes by the dozen are being patented, and insurance companies are clamoring to screen potential policy-holders for inborn risk factors. Some day the awarding of an athletic scholarship may be contingent on passing a "gene screen" for the loci important in musculoskeletal strength and repairability. Until then, both the ethical consensus and science must advance far beyond current levels. The main goal of this chapter is to review the principles and clinical examples that underpin work in this field by reductionistic and synthetic approaches, in part to emphasize that both types of investigation are needed.

General Principles

Human health problems are multifactorial, and genes are almost always a part of the cause, the pathogenesis, or both. The importance of genetic factors can be seen as a broad continuum. At one end are diseases caused by mutations in single loci with phenotypes severe in any environment or genetic background. At the other end are environmental insults, such as severe trauma, that result in injury regardless of genetic constitution. Two corollaries are important. On the one hand, a lack of evidence of the contribution of genes to the cause and pathogenesis of a defect should only emphasize the need for more work. On the other, even overtly mendelian disorders (those usually thought of as "genetic diseases") may not be deleterious in a forgiving environment.

Next, three principles of clinical genetics deserve mention because they are pervasive concerns in classic hereditary disorders, and undoubtedly they are just as important in as yet unrecognized genetic susceptibilities. The actions of mutant genes are usually pleiotropic. In other words, a single genetic alteration usually affects more than one tissue or organ, often in diverse ways not immediately evident from biochemistry or cell biology.[12] Most mendelian conditions affect multiple organs,[4] with the musculoskeletal system among the more commonly involved. The phenotype of a given mutation usually reflects variable expression, even within the same family. At one extreme is nonpenetrance, in which an individual possesses a mutation but does not show it. As methods for detecting abnormal phenotypes become more sensitive (magnetic resonance and positron emission imaging are two examples), variability expands, and instances of true nonpenetrance decline. Genetic heterogeneity, or similar phenotypes caused by different genetic mutations, has been found in every human hereditary disorder that has been examined closely. Subtle differences are often evident only when phenotypes are defined at refined (and usually subclinical) levels. Thus, if the phenotype of interest is broadly expressed as susceptibility to musculoskeletal injury, or even narrowly expressed as, for example, damage to the lumbosacral spine, a diversity of genetic factors should be expected.

Familial aggregation of athletic injury should be used to advantage in identifying pedigrees worthy of close scrutiny, but the limitations of this method should be kept in mind. Relatives share a host of potential etiologic factors in addition to their genes—nutrition, education, interests, socioeconomic status, and so on. A variety of methods, such as examining twins reared apart, has been used in the study of other common phenotypes to separate familial environmental effects from genetic ones.

Finally, any analysis of susceptibility must recognize at least two major (but not unrelated) classes of athletic injury: acute trauma with immediate clinical problems, and repeated stresses and strains (microtrauma as well as more serious injuries) that lead to late sequelae. Some genetic factors may predispose more to one class than to the other but, in general, predisposition to major injury invariably also predisposes to chronic complications.

Typology of Genetic Influences on Connective Tissue

Following to an extent the traditional (but flawed) classification of genetic conditions, genetic effects on the extracellular matrix can be categorized as chromosomal, mendelian, and multifactorial. The limitations of this approach are well illustrated by a few examples: even a gene that has a major impact is influenced by the genetic background and the environment, and the phenotype is actually multifactorial; some "mendelian" conditions, once thought to be caused by single genes, are caused by minute chromosomal deletions, visible only after the development of high-resolution cytogenetics; and some chromosomal aberrations segregate in a family according to Mendel's laws, and the phenotypes thus appear to be autosomal dominant or X-linked. With these important caveats in mind, the rest of the discussion will use this typology.

Chromosomal Aberrations

Syndromes caused by chromosomal aberrations offer little insight into defects in extracellular matrix and their association with injury. This is not to deny their obvious clinical relevance. For example, people with the Down syndrome often have atlantoaxial instability, and their participation in certain sports must be restricted. Most other chromosomal anomalies cause, in addition to mental retardation that limits athletic pursuits, malformation of distinct regions of the skeleton. This observation says little more than that many genes spread throughout the genome contribute to skeletal development. The understanding of molecular rearrangements, deletions, and duplications of the human karyotype has improved greatly in the past few years, but we are still a long way from understanding how gene dosage and hemizygosity of particular loci produce clinical defects in complex systems.

Mendelian Disorders

Estimates place the total number of human genetic loci at 50,000 to 100,000. Nearly 2,000 have been located at specific sites on the gene map and 5,000 identified through the phenotypes that mutations produce.[7] Dozens of loci that encode components of the extracellular matrix have been mapped,[10] and hundreds of mendelian conditions affect the musculoskeletal system.[1] How much of this knowledge is relevant to the themes at hand was first emphasized in general terms by Harvey[4]: "nor is there any better way to advance the proper practice of medicine than to give our minds to the discovery of the usual law of Nature by careful investigation of cases of rarer forms of disease."

Many of the mendelian disorders are severe enough to preclude athletic activity. Some are either relatively mild or variable enough that patients can engage in normal activity. A partial list of these disorders is shown in Table 1. Clinical details of these disorders can be found in standard texts.[6,9,11,12]

The basic biochemical defects are unknown for most of these disorders, and it is, therefore, unclear how the intrinsic weakness in connective tissue can be explained in fundamental terms. The osteogenesis imperfecta syndromes are notable exceptions; most of these disorders are caused by mutations in the gene for either $alpha_1$ (I) or $alpha_2$ (I) procollagen. Because type I collagen is the major protein constituent of bone, susceptibility to fracture is readily apparent. Type I collagen is also a major component of tendon and ligament, yet dislocations and traumatic ruptures of these elements are uncommon in osteogenesis imperfecta. It may be that bones give way before the supporting structures of joints tear.

Predispositions Resulting From Heterozygosity for Genes of Major Effect

All humans are heterozygous at perhaps one third or more of all loci. A handful of these alleles are extremely deleterious if homozygous; fortunately, this fact is made evident only in the unlikely mating of two people, each carrying a rare mutant allele at the same locus, in which case there is a one-in-four chance that the offspring will inherit the two deleterious alleles and have a severe recessive hereditary disorder. Of course, the chance that two people are carrying the same mutant alleles is greatly increased if they are related, which accounts for the increased incidence of mendelian recessive phenotypes in consanguineous matings.

The high level of heterozygosity is important for maintaining population diversity, which serves as a reservoir for evolutionary response to environmental pressures. Many of the "mutant" alleles occur with relatively high frequency; if the population prevalence is greater than 1%, the allele is termed polymorphic. For example, alleles for cystic fibrosis occur in about 4% of whites of Northern European ancestry,

Table 1 Mendelian disorders that predispose to athletic injury*

Disorder	Entry No.†	Inheritance	Potential Injuries
Osteochondrodysplasias			
Achondroplasia	10080	AD	DJD of knees; spinal stenosis; disk herniation
Multiple epiphyseal dysplasia syndromes			
Fairbank disease	13240	AD	DJD of hips
Spondyloepiphyseal dysplasia syndromes			
Tarda form	31340	XLR	DJD of hips and shoulders; compression and DJD of spine
Heritable disorders of connective tissue			
Marfan's syndrome	15470	AD	Dislocations of patellas; joint hypermobility predisposing to DJD of knees, hips, and wrist; protrusio acetabuli; spontaneous pneumothorax; dissection of the aorta
Ehlers-Danlos syndromes			
Types I, II, III	13000 13001 13002	AD	Ecchymoses and soft-tissue hematomas; dislocations of any joint; hemarthroses
Type IV	13005	AD	Rupture of the bowel or major arteries
Stickler syndrome	10830	AD	Retinal detachment; DJD of hips, knees, and ankles
Osteogenesis imperfecta, types I, III, IV	16620 16622	AD, AR	Fractures
Familial articular hypermobility syndromes	14790	AD	Dislocations of appendicular joints
Lysosomal storage disorders			
Mucopolysaccharidoses			
Type IS (Scheie's syndrome)	25280	AR	DJD of hips; atlantoaxial instability
Type IIB (Hunter's syndrome)	30990	XLR	DJD of hands, hips; inguinal hernias
Mannosidosis	24850	AR	DJD of hips
Endocrine disorders			
Hyperparathyroidism, familial	14500	AD	Osteitis fibrosa; fractures; chondrocalcinosis
Hypoparathyroidism	24140 30770	AD XLR	Ectopic calcification
Pseudohypoparathyroidism	30080	XLR	Ectopic calcification
Hypophosphatemia	30780	XLR	Spinal stenosis; hastening of progressive ankylosis
Other disorders			
Articular chondrocalcinosis	11860	AD	Monoarticular and polyarticular arthropathy
Fibrodysplasia ossificans Progressiva form	13510	AD	Soft-tissue calcification, often secondary to minor trauma; ligamentous calcification

*AD, autosomal dominant; AR, autosomal recessive; XLR, X-linked recessive; DJD, degenerative joint disease.
†Entry number in McKusick.[7]

the allele for sickle cell anemia occurs in about 10% of blacks of Western African ancestry, and alleles for Tay-Sachs disease occur in about 3% of Ashkenazic Jews. Alleles for the recessive disorders listed in Table 1 are not this common, but nonetheless occur far more frequently than the overt phenotype. It is an open and important question as to whether some of these mutant alleles, when present in only one copy, interfere with the development or repair of the extracellular matrix. Given what is known about physiologic and developmental homeostasis, it is not surprising that some of these mutant alleles are deleterious, if only subtly so. As methods evolve for rapidly screening populations for heterozygosity at specific genetic loci and then determining the actual mutant or polymorphic alleles present, these important questions will be addressed.

For example, as more is learned about the components of cartilage and their genes are characterized, it will be possible to screen patients with chondromalacia patellae (and appropriate control subjects) for genetic variations. This common disorder clearly has many potential causes, including repeated athletic trauma, but it will be interesting to see if genetic variations in type II collagen, proteoglycan, or other cartilage constituents increase susceptibility to external causes.

Multifactorial Susceptibilities

This category subsumes a broad range of pathogenetic situations: from two or more genes with major effects interacting to produce a phenotype, to many genes with minor effects blending to produce a phenotype. Inheritance of the phenotype is not mendelian, although in a small family with several people affected, the pattern may simulate mendelism. An important practical point is that recurrence of the phenotype is not predictable (although empiric data can generate expectations, which can be useful in counseling patients).

A frequently encountered clinical example with great relevance to injury susceptibility is joint hypermobility. About 5% of whites can hyperextend their knees, elbows, or both beyond 10 degrees.[5] Some of these people may have mild varieties of a classic heritable disorder of connective tissue, some may be heterozygous for one of the recessive disorders as described, and some may have as yet undescribed mendelian disorders of the extracellular matrix. For example, it was recently shown that the phenotypic spectrum of the Marfan syndrome is impossible to distinguish (at the mild end) from an autosomal dominant syndrome that includes mitral valve prolapse, long limbs, striae atrophicae, and joint hypermobility.[3]

The majority of people with joint hypermobility probably do not have a recognized or unrecognized monogenic defect in connective tissue. Rather, their articular phenotype is probably the result of several, perhaps many, genes interacting. This notion is supported by racial differences in joint mobilities, that is, Asian Indians are more limber than European whites.[14]

Evidence is emerging for heritability of bone density.[2,13] Thus, genetic factors are important determinants of postmenopausal osteoporosis; perhaps earlier in life these same genetic factors increase susceptibility to fractures, slipped epiphyses, or other skeletal problems.

Spondylosis and spondylolisthesis are often familial. The proximate phenotype is not yet known; the clinical finding of slippage, even in the asymptomatic patient, may be the result of repetitive microtraumas to a susceptible vertebral column.

Osteochondritis dissecans is often but not invariably related to antecedent trauma. Consistent with a role for genetic factors is the observation that early osteochondritis dissecans in adolescents and young adults is more likely than the late-onset variety[8] to be familial.

References

1. Costa T, Scriver CR, Childs B: The effect of mendelian disease on human health: A measurement. *Am J Med Genet* 1985;21:231–242.
2. Evans RA, Marel GM, Lancaster EK, et al: Bone mass is low in relatives of osteoporotic patients. *Ann Intern Med* 1988;109:870–873.
3. Glesby MJ, Pyeritz RE: Association of mitral valve prolapse and systemic abnormalities of connective tissue: A phenotypic continuum. *JAMA* 1989;262:523–528.
4. Harvey W, quoted by Garrod A: The lessons of rare maladies. *Lancet* 1928;1:1055.
5. Kirk JA, Ansell BM, Bywaters EGL: The hypermobiliy syndrome. *Ann Rheum Dis* 1967;26:419–425.
6. McKusick VA: *Heritable Disorders of Connective Tissue*, ed 4. St. Louis, CV Mosby, 1972.
7. McKusick VA: *Mendelian Inheritance in Man: Catalogs of Autosomal Dominant, Autosomal Recessive, and X-Linked Phenotypes*, ed 9. Baltimore, Johns Hopkins University Press, 1990.
8. Phillips HO, Grubb SA: Familial multiple osteochondritis dissecans: Report of a kindred. *J Bone Joint Surg* 1985;67A:155–156.
9. Pyeritz RE: Pleiotropy revisited: Molecular explanations of a classic concept. *Am J Med Genet* 1989;34:124–134.
10. Pyeritz RE: Heritable defects in connective tissue. *Hosp Pract* 1987;22:153–168.
11. Pyeritz RE: Heritable and developmental disorders of connective tissue and bone, in McCarty DJ (ed): *Arthritis and Allied Conditions: A Textbook of Rheumatology*, ed 11. Philadelphia, Lea & Febiger, 1989, pp 1332–1359.
12. Pyeritz RE: Heritable disorders of connective tissue, in Schumacher HR, Klippel J, Robinson D (eds): *Primer on the Rheumatic Diseases*, ed 9. Atlanta, Arthritis Foundation, 1988, pp 230–235.
13. Seeman E, Hopper JL, Bach LA, et al: Reduced bone mass in daughters of women with osteoporosis. *N Engl J Med* 1989;320:554–558.
14. Wordsworth P, Ogilvie D, Smith R, et al: Joint mobility with particular reference to racial variation and inherited connective tissue disorders. *Br J Rheumatol* 1987;26:9–12.

Chapter 44

Fibrosis in Soft-Tissue Injuries

Sharon Wahl, PhD
Per Renström, MD, PhD

Humans and other vertebrates lack the ability to regenerate tissues or organs after injury. Thus, damaged tissue must be repaired by the synthesis of connective tissue. In tendons and other soft tissues, the healing process follows a common cellular and vascular pathway that consists of a series of events that occur simultaneously and interweave with each other, even many years after the initial injury. Hemostatic and inflammatory responses generally precede and influence the healing process. For example, the inflammatory cells modulate recruitment, proliferation, and matrix synthesis of mesenchymal cells responsible for restoring the integrity of the damaged tissue. This sequence of events normally repairs damage with minimal scar formation, but a persistent inflammatory response and continued release of inflammatory products can promote extended fibroplasia and fibrogenesis that can cause irreversible tissue damage.[45]

Fibrosis is a problem or an end result in several medical disorders such as pericardial and myocardial fibrosis and pulmonary fibrosis. In women, mammae may have localized fibrosis. Hepatic and pancreatic fibrosis may suppress normal organ functions. Interstitial renal fibrosis is common, and fibrosis can also occur in the bladder and ureter. Fibrosis has been described in corpus cavernosum, and there is also a post-priapism cavernosum fibrosis. Tumors of different kinds are associated with fibrosis. In the eyes, subretinal, posterior capsular, and ocular fibrosis can occur. Scleroderma produces fibrosis within the skin or internal organs. Radiation treatment can induce subcutaneous and muscular fibrosis. Wound healing can result in an excessive fibrotic reaction and cause keloid formation within the skin.

However, failure of the healing process and insufficient matrix generation is also detrimental. Thus, it is important to define the cellular and molecular mechanisms responsible for normal healing and fibrosis in order to devise rational approaches to augment or inhibit these processes in pathologic conditions.

The acute inflammatory response to injury, infection, or other foreign substances is characterized by increased vasodilation and vascular permeability with edema, hemorrhage, and creation of a fibrin meshwork connecting the margins of the wound. Inflammatory mediators are released, and circulating leukocytes infiltrate the area. At the inflammatory site, platelets adhere to the injured vessel surfaces, accelerate coagulation and fibrinolysis, and release factors to initiate homeostasis.[48] These factors include the eicosanoids, fibronectin, and other adhesion molecules that promote cell-to-cell interactions. Platelet-derived growth factor (PDGF) and transforming growth factors important in inflammation and tissue repair are also released.

Transforming growth factor beta (TGF-β) is a potent chemotactic signal for leukocyte recruitment.[46,50] In response to TGF-β and other chemotactic peptides, leukocytes move into the extravascular space and congregate in the damaged tissues. It is possible to identify T-lymphocyte subsets, monocytes, and other inflammatory cells as they move into the tissues by combining monoclonal antibodies to different leukocyte subsets with a sensitive immunoperoxidase staining procedure.[5] By isolating and culturing these cells, it is possible to analyze their level of activity and the products they generate that contribute to the inflammatory process. Phagocytic cells engulf debris and other foreign substances and release enzymes and inflammatory mediators. Recruited monocyte-macrophages phagocytize debris and generate numerous enzymes and cytokines to amplify and mediate the inflammatory response.[25] The release of reactive oxygen intermediates and hydrolytic enzymes, if not controlled, can degrade normal as well as injured tissue.

Among the macrophage enzymes, the neutral proteases, plasminogen activator, elastase, and collagenase, are central to matrix degradation. Collagenase catalyzes the initial, rate-limiting step in collagen degradation because it is the only enzyme that can cleave the triple-helix structure of collagen, making it susceptible to further nonspecific proteolysis. The ability of macrophages to synthesize and secrete collagenase is triggered by bacterial products, lymphokines, or other agents.[44] After stimulation, these cells produce prostaglandin E_2 to elevate intracellular levels of cyclic adenosine monophosphate (cAMP) and induce enzyme synthesis. Excessive or prolonged monocyte activation results in continued release of prostaglandin E_2 and enzymes such as collagenase and may contribute to a failed healing response. If cellular debridement is insufficient or inflammation persists, continued turnover, recruitment, and activation of mononuclear phagocytes may occur. To resolve such a localized persistent inflammatory response, the inflammatory stimulus must be eliminated and/or a fibrotic connective tissue barrier generated to inhibit access to the site or to modulate the host response.

Inflammatory cells also modulate the behavior of local endothelial cells to initiate an angiogenic response.[13] Angiogenesis includes the invasion of migration through soft tissues and the tube formation exhibited by microvascular endothelial cells in response to injury. The response of these vascular cells is partly modulated by the composition and organization of the surrounding newly synthesized matrix and by the various platelet factors and cytokines found at the site. TGF-β, a potent angiogenic agent in vivo, may exert this effect indirectly by its ability to recruit monocytes and to stimulate them to produce endothelial cell mitogenic and recruitment factors including PDGF, fibroblast growth factor, tumor necrosis factor, and TGF-β (N. McCartney-Francis, D. Mizel, H. Wong, and associates, unpublished data). Recruitment and proliferation of endothelial cells results in the formation of capillary sprouts that anastomose and form the capillary beds needed to establish blood flow in the developing granulation tissue.[13] This capillary network provides oxygen and other nutrients to support mesenchymal cell growth and matrix production.

Fibroblast recruitment depends on and accompanies neovascularization. Fibroblasts are critical to the outcome of the inflammatory process because matrix synthesis terminates the inflammation and heals the injury. Although fibroblast accumulation is most evident in the later stages of an inflammatory response, the reactions leading to it begin much earlier. Fibroblasts migrate to the injury site from neighboring connective tissue in response to chemotactic products of platelets, neutrophils, T-lymphocytes, and monocytes.[45] This repair process normally follows tissue injury, and includes recruitment of fibroblasts, their proliferation, collagen and matrix synthesis, and tissue remodeling. Mononuclear cells near active, proliferating fibroblasts produce polypeptide growth factors that regulate normal and/or pathologic repair responses. Each of these growth factors might be a target site for influencing the fibrotic response.

One of the most effective inducers of growth factor gene expression in monocytes is TGF-β, the 25-kd homodimer secreted by platelets and monocyte-macrophages.[6] The secretion of TGF-β by activated macrophages[6] and the ability of TGF-β to activate macrophages (McCartney-Francis and associates, unpublished data) implicate an important autocrine and/or paracrine loop regulating the monocyte-derived growth factor release essential for fibroblast proliferation and healing.

Among the macrophage-derived products regulated by TGF-β is interleukin–1, originally thought to stimulate fibroblast growth directly.[38] Recently, interleukin–1 has been shown to stimulate fibroblasts to generate PDGF. The PDGF then stimulates fibroblast growth.[34] Interleukin–1 also stimulates fibroblasts to produce granulocyte-macrophage colony stimulating factor[52] to augment monocyte interleukin–1 production[51] and provide a cycle of cellular activation and production of growth factors. Another monocyte product that shares many biologic activities with interleukin–1 is tumor necrosis factor. Tumor necrosis factor is also mitogenic for fibroblasts.[43]

PDGF released by activated macrophages[23,39] and platelets is a potent mitogenic signal for fibroblasts. Its presence in early and chronic stages of an inflammatory response may contribute to physiologic and/or overabundant tissue repair. Similarly, monocyte-derived fibroblast growth factor, which shares sequence homology with interkeukin–1 is an important promoter of endothelial cell and fibroblast proliferation.[9] Monocytes are important to this process, and interruption of normal monocyte recruitment and activation retards the healing process.[20] Macrophages may be a target for site-directed modulation of the fibrotic process.

A rapid deposition of connective tissue matrix is associated with fibroblast accumulation. Soft tissues are normally composed of various cell types organized on a scaffold of extracellular matrix. Many factors help maintain the proper equilibrium of matrix deposition and remodeling, but injury and inflammation alter this homeostatic system. Injury shifts the balance so there is an overabundance of fibrogenic factors favoring fibrosis. Recent evidence indicates that certain cytokines produced by inflammatory cells are among these fibrogenic factors.[33] If this is so, then failure to decrease their production in some individuals may lead to clinically significant fibrosis.

Tumor necrosis factor, interleukin–1, and TGF-β increase and regulate transcription and translation of collagen, proteoglycans, and the glycoproteins, fibronectin, laminin, and chondronectin, to form the ground substance of the extracellular matrix. In fibrotic lesions, there is a considerable increase and molecular rearrangement of proteoglycans and glycosaminoglycans with a prominent increase in hyaluronate, chondroitin sulfate, and dermatan sulfate.[33] Noncollagenous glycoproteins are important both as structural components of the extracellular matrix and as important elements for cell differentiation. Glycoproteins act as adhesion molecules, binding cells to themselves and influencing cell migration, polarization, proliferation, and gene expression. The sources and cellular and molecular mechanisms of the increase in proteoglycans in matrix during fibrogenesis are poorly understood. However, early increases in fibronectin synthesis have been implicated as important stimuli of subsequent fibrogenesis by mesenchymal cells. Interstitial collagens (types I and III) are predominantly synthesized in tissue repair. All of these changes result from the action of mediators on the mesenchymal cells and their genetic machinery.

In normal tissue repair, matrix generation is self-limiting and minimal scar formation occurs, but in a persistent lesion, the prolonged release of growth-promoting and matrix-inducing factors may escalate collagen deposition and replace the functional soft tissue.[45] Although the factors that determine whether synthesis of collagen and other matrix proteins continues are unknown, mononuclear cell products that suppress matrix synthesis have been identified and include interferon gamma.[14,36]

Under normal circumstances, many of the newly formed vessels disappear, the scar tissue contracts, and tissue remodeling occurs. Remodeling of scar tissue is important to restore normal function in tendons and other soft tissues. Adhesion inhibition or resorption also contributes to restored mobility. The turnover of matrix macromolecules depends on both fibroblasts and macrophages that secrete neutral and other proteases important in collagen resorption. The neutral metalloproteinase family that initiates degradation of the extracellular matrix consists of at least five structurally related members. They include fibroblasts, a macrophage collagenase that degrades interstitial collagens, a 72-kd type IV collagenase that cleaves basement membrane collagen and denatured collagens, a 92-kd type IV collagenase secreted by macrophages that also cleaves basement membrane and denatured collagens, and stromelysin, an enzyme that degrades proteoglycans and other extracellular matrix components.[42,49] Collagenase is the only enzyme that degrades collagen at physiologic pH, making it susceptible to degradation by additional proteases.

In inflammation, this process of remodeling may be heightened by the presence of PDGF, tumor necrosis factor, and interleukin-1. These not only affect growth and protein synthesis, but also increase the production of collagenase and other metalloproteinases.[33] In contrast, TGF-β inhibits the degradation of newly synthesized extracellular matrix by inhibiting enzyme synthesis. The expression pattern of the matrix-specific enzymes is clearly subject to the regulatory influences of both physiologic and pharmacologic agents and may be pivotal in determining the outcome of tissue repair. Activated fibroblasts and macrophages also release enzyme inhibitors, including a glycoprotein tissue inhibitor of metalloproteinases (TIMP) that inactivates collagenase and other enzymes.[33,42]

The accumulation of interstitial collagens in fibrosis may reflect alterations not only in matrix protein synthesis but also in matrix degradation. Enhanced degradation of interstitial collagens may be beneficial in fibrotic tissue injury, but further characterization of these processes is required before specific regulation of enzymatic matrix degradation can be attempted. Because alterations in the balance between enzyme and inhibitors contribute to the pathogenesis of fibrosis in abnormal healing syndromes, a shift to favor enzyme excess could result in a failed healing process. Insufficient levels of the relevant enzymes and/or excess matrix synthesis would create a fibrotic response. Regulating these proteolytic enzymes and inhibitors may be important in determining the extent of tissue deposition and destruction and the outcome and reversibility of fibrosis.

The process of fibrosis in soft-tissue injury may result from increased numbers (proliferation and recruitment) of collagen-synthesizing cells, increased matrix synthesis by existing cells, and/or deficient collagen degradation with continued collagen synthesis. An imbalance between synthesis and degradation leads to collagen accumulation. Studies on matrix abnormalities at the gene level may indicate ways to modulate these processes. Various immunochemical, biochemical, and molecular biologic techniques used to characterize fibrogenesis in specific types of fibrotic lesions provide complementary information, although each approach has advantages and limitations. Reversing the fibrotic process may be possible by inhibiting the inflammatory response (the source of the mediators and growth factors responsible for promoting fibroplasia and fibrogenesis), by inhibiting the angiogenesis essential for tissue repair and fibrosis, or by directly regulating mesenchymal cell function through inhibition of proliferation or matrix synthesis.

Clinical Occurrences of Fibrosis in Sports Medicine

Fibrosis in Synovial Structures

Frozen shoulder or idiopathic chronic adhesive capsulitis is characterized by a limited range of motion and the formation of adhesions in the bursae and joint. The joint capsule hypertrophy or fibrosis seems to be a response to increased stress levels and tissue remodeling, resulting in decreased extensibility.[19] The capsule is avascular, tense, and markedly adherent to the head of the humerus. Chronic inflammation with characteristic fibrosis and perivascular infiltration can be observed microscopically. Radiographs show that osteoporotic changes of the proximal humerus can last as long as two years after the syndrome has clinically subsided.[22] This condition is self-limited, although the joint does not always recover full range of motion. The cause of this syndrome is still unknown.

Intra-articular fibrosis (arthrofibrosis) has been recognized and analyzed more frequently during recent years. Intra-articular fibrosis is more likely to develop in the knee and other joints with abundant synovial tissue. Two factors that predispose a joint to arthrofibrosis are intra-articular surgery and prolonged postoperative immobilization. The joint capsule may become fibrous when the joint is immobilized after arthrotomy. Because of the lack of movement, the unorganized network of fibers forms adhesions and stiffens the capsule itself. Other factors that can contribute to the development of fibrosis include poor rehabilitation, sepsis, and fractures.

Knee ligament injuries are a common problem. The knee joint must be protected from stress and strain that exceeds the strength of the healing tissue but must also be mobilized as rapidly as possible to avoid excessive stiffening.

The deleterious effects of immobilization include loss of motion, muscle atrophy, loss of cartilage elasticity, and weakened periarticular bone and ligaments. Until recently, knee ligament injuries were treated with long-term immobilization that involved as much as six weeks in a cast and no vigorous activities for nine to 12 months after surgery.[18,28] The long-term immobilization resulted in the proliferation of fibrofatty connective tissue and eventual fibroankylosis.[1,2,10–12] Payr[30] studied the morbid anatomy of knee stiffness in detail and concluded that knee flexion loss started in the suprapatellar tissues and led to quadriceps sclerosis and patella-femur adhesions. The final stage was a fixed patella with patellar, femoral, and tibial articular cartilage destruction secondary to invasion by a fibrosclerotic pannus.

Severely restricted knee motion is a recognized complication of knee surgery or trauma and can result from intra-articular adhesion formation, contracture of the posterior capsule or collateral ligament, or shortening or adhesion of the quadriceps mechanisms.[26,40] Nicoll[26] identified four possible causes: fibrosis of the vastus intermedius and adjoining soft tissue just proximal to the suprapatellar pouch, intracapsular adhesions between the patella and the femoral condyles, fibrosis of the vastus lateralis with adhesions to the condyles, and shortening of the rectus femoris. Sprague and associates[41] arthroscopically evaluated 24 patients with restricted knee motion, categorizing them into three groups: those with discrete bands or a single sheet of adhesions, those with complete obliteration of the suprapatellar pouch and gutters with massive adhesions, and those with multiple bands of adhesions or obliteration of the suprapatellar pouch with an additional extracapsular band about 1 cm wide. This extra-articular fibrosis band is important in restricting motion.

The reported incidence of flexion contracture after knee ligament surgery is 32%. Noyes (personal communication, 1989) evaluated 237 patients with knee ligament reconstructions. He found that 10% had problems regaining motion and that 5% of these were caused by excessive scar formation. J.R. Steadman (personal communication, 1989) encountered more than 50 cases of restricted motion after knee ligament surgery. In most instances, the abnormal scar tissue involved the anterior and posterior medial aspect of the knee. Arthroscopic surgery of the lateral meniscus can initiate a hyperfibrosis reaction.

Paulos and associates[29] believe that 5% of patients undergoing knee surgery will have an abnormal fibrosclerotic healing response through the anterior retinacula and fat-pad tissues. A primary infrapatellar contracture syndrome will develop in a few patients regardless of the cause of injury or the treatment regimen. The contracture occurs primarily as an exaggerated pathologic fibrous hyperplasia of the anterior soft tissues of the knee. It can also be secondary to the prolonged immobility and lack of extension associated with intra-articular anterior cruciate ligament surgery.

This contracture syndrome has three stages. Stage 1, the prodromal stage, includes induration of the synovial fat pad and retinacular tissues. Motion is painful, patellar mobility is restricted, and quadriceps lag is present. Failure to improve with rehabilitation is an important clue to the presence of this syndrome. In stage 2, the active stage, there is continued peripatellar swelling and induration with severely restricted patellar motion. In stage 3, the burned-out stage, the development of patella infra is the key finding.

Paulos and associates[29] also found destructive changes in the articular surface of the tibia, femur, and patella associated with prolonged patellar entrapment. These changes had two origins. A pressure ulceration appeared wherever the fibrosclerotic fat pad impinged against a medial and/or lateral femoral condyle. A second cause appeared to be an infiltrating inflammatory pannus that extended from the medial and lateral gutters over the noncontact surfaces of the joint. This pannus was extremely adherent and the cartilage below was discolored, softened, and fibrillated. Microscopic sections of the cartilage revealed loss of glycosaminoglycans and subchondral bone atrophy. These changes were similar to those described by Waugh and associates.[47]

These clinical findings were supported by a cadaver study showing that fibrosclerosis in the fat pad results in a firm tissue block to normal knee extension.[29] Fibrous tissue bands passing through this area of inflammation and fibrosis create a nonextensible, rigid structure. Because the fat pad extends into the intracondylar notch through the ligamentum mucosum and is firmly attached to the anterior horns of the medial and lateral menisci, tibial impingement becomes prominent and locks extension.

Fibrosis in Extra-Articular Tissues

Use of the patellar tendon as a donor site in knee ligament surgery can result in peripatellar tendon fibrosis. A primary prerequisite for the occurrence of patella infra is a peritendinous inflammatory reaction that creates constricting scar tissue in the surrounding tissues of the patellar tendon. Extra-articular fibrosis may require open surgery. This is indicated whenever there is a persisting lack of extension that does not respond to usual rehabilitative techniques. The fibrosis surrounding the patellar tendon should then be resected. Postoperatively, continuous passive motion, anti-inflammatory medication, and supervised physical therapy are required.

Bursitis

The 150 bursae in the human body can be damaged by direct trauma or repetitive overuse. Direct trauma to the bursa may produce an acute hemorrhagic bursitis or hemobursa.[35] Hemorrhage within a bursa causes chemical irritation and, if severe enough, may clot, causing fibrosis and loose-body formation. The end result may be a dense fibrous scar, which can obliterate the entire bursa. This chronically fibrotic bursa may cause clinical problems for athletes severe enough to require surgical excision.

Chronic Muscle Problems

The repair of muscle injury includes two competing processes: the regeneration of muscle fibers and the simultaneous production of a connective tissue scar. If a large volume of muscle is devitalized by major trauma, proliferation of fibroblasts can rapidly lead to the formation of excessive scar tissue that may form a dense mechanical barrier to the regenerating muscle fibers.[24] Such scar tissue may then inhibit the complete regeneration of muscle fibers and may also disturb the proper orientation of the muscular elements.[3,4,7,8,17,21] Most muscle injuries heal well within a few weeks or months, but some, especially intramuscular fibrotic injuries, may cause long-lasting disability, including range of motion problems.

Old muscle ruptures can sometimes cause problems at late stages because of the scar tissue formed. A muscle with scar tissue consists of areas in which elasticity and capacity for contraction vary. These old ruptures may sometimes be mistaken for malignant tumors on palpation. Patients may also notice a growing mass.[31,32] This increase in size, however, may be the result of compensatory hypertrophy of the severed muscle caused by the shortened distance between its origin and new insertion.

Severe blunt or repeated trauma to a muscle can cause a muscle contusion and a hematoma that may contribute to the formation of myositis ossificans,[16] which is posttraumatic localized heterotopic bone formation in the muscle. The pathogenesis of heterotopic bone formation is poorly understood. The early treatment is traditionally extremely conservative and early surgery is not recommended.[15,27,37] A more aggressive approach in patients with severe knee motion problems caused by sports-induced myositis ossificans can, however, give successful results.[31] The surgery is usually done six to 12 weeks after the injury.

References

1. Akeson WH, Amiel D, LaViolette D: The connective tissue response to immobility: A study of the chondroitin-4 and 6-sulfate and dermatan sulfate changes in periarticular connective tissue of control and immobilized knees of dogs. *Clin Orthop* 1967;51:183–197.
2. Akeson WH, Woo SL-Y, Amiel D, et al: The connective tissue response to immobility: Biochemical changes in periarticular connective tissue of the immobilized rabbit knee. *Clin Orthop* 1973;93:356–362.
3. Allbrook D: Muscle regeneration. *Physiotherapy* 1973;59:240–247.
4. Allbrook D: Skeletal muscle regeneration. *Muscle Nerve* 1981;4:234–245.
5. Allen JB, Malone DG, Wahl SM, et al: The role of the thymus in streptococcal cell wall-induced arthritis and hepatic granuloma formation: Comparative studies of pathology and cell wall distribution in athymic and euthymic rats. *J Clin Invest* 1985;76:1042–1056.
6. Assoian K, Fleurdelys BE, Stevenson HC, et al: Expression and secretion of type β transforming growth factor by activated human macrophages. *Proc Natl Acad Sci USA* 1987;84:6020–6024.
7. Bailey AJ, Bazin S, Delaunay A: Changes in the nature of the collagen during development and resorption of granulation tissue. *Biochim Biophys Acta* 1973;328:383–390.
8. Bailey AJ, Shellswell GB, Duance VC: Identification and change of collagen types in differentiating myoblasts and developing chick muscle. *Nature* 1979;278:67–69.
9. Baird A, Mormede P, Bohlen P: Immunoreactive fibroblast growth factor in cells of peritoneal exudate suggests its identity with macrophage-derived growth factor. *Biochem Biophys Res Commun* 1985;230:358–364.
10. Burri C, Helbing G: Postoperative care after reconstructive and plastic surgery of the knee ligaments. *Monatschr Unfallheilkd* 1980;83:426–430.
11. Cooper RR: Alterations during immobilization and regeneration of skeletal muscle in cats. *J Bone Joint Surg* 1972;54A:919–953.
12. Enneking WF, Horowitz M: The intra-articular effects of immobilization on the human knee. *J Bone Joint Surg* 1972;54A:973–985.
13. Folkman J, Klagsbrun M: Angiogenic factors. *Science* 1987;235:442–447.
14. Granstein RD, Murphy GF, Margolis RJ, et al: Gamma interferon inhibits collagen synthesis *in vivo* in the mouse. *J Clin Invest* 1987;79:1254–1258.
15. Groh H: Sportverletzungen, in Groh H (ed): *Sportsmedizin*. Stuttgart, Ferdinand Enke Verlag, 1962.
16. Jackson DW, Feagin JA: Quadriceps contusions in young athletes: Relation of severity of injury to treatment and prognosis. *J Bone Joint Surg* 1973;55A:95–105.
17. Järvinen M: Healing of a crush injury in rat striated muscle: 4. Effect of early mobilization and immobilization on the tensile properties of gastrocnemius muscle. *Acta Chir Scand* 1976;142:47–56.

18. Johnson RJ, Pope MH: Knee joint stability without reference to ligamentous function, in Evarts CM (ed): American Academy of Orthopaedic Surgeons *Symposium on Reconstructive Surgery of the Knee*. St. Louis, CV Mosby, 1978, pp 14–25.
19. Kesseler R, Hersling O: *Management of Common Musculoskeletal Disorders*. Philadelphia, Harper & Row, 1983.
20. Leibovich SJ, Ross R: The role of the macrophage in wound repair: A study with hydrocortisone and antimacrophage serum. *Am J Pathol* 1975;78:71–91.
21. Lehto M, Järvinen M: Collagen and glycosaminoglycan synthesis of injured gastrocnemius muscle in rats. *Eur Surg Reg* 1985;17:179–185.
22. Lundberg BJ: The frozen shoulder: Clinical and radiographical observations. *Acta Orthop Scand* 1969;119(suppl):1–59.
23. Martinet Y, Bitterman PB, Mornex J, et al: Activated human monocytes express the c-*sis* proto-oncogene and release a mediator showing PDGF-like activity. *Nature* 1986;319:158–160.
24. McMinn RM: The cellular morphology of tissue repair, in Bourne GH, Danells JF (eds): *International Review of Cytology*. New York, Academic Press, 1967.
25. Nathan CF: Secretory products of macrophages. *J Clin Invest* 1988;74:2208–2218.
26. Nicoll EA: Quadricepsplasty. *J Bone Joint Surg* 1963;45B:483–490.
27. O'Donoghue DH (ed): *Treatment of Injuries to Athletes*, ed 2. Philadelphia, WB Saunders, 1970.
28. Paulos L, Noyes FR, Grood E, et al: Knee rehabilitation after anterior cruciate ligament reconstruction and repair. *Am J Sports Med* 1981;9:140–149.
29. Paulos L, Rosenberg T, Drawbert J, et al: Infrapatellar contracture syndrome: An unrecognized cause of knee stiffness with patella entrapment and patella infera. *Am J Sports Med* 1987;15:331–341.
30. Payr E: Zur operativen Behandlung der Kniegelenksteife. *Zentralbl Chir* 1917:44:809.
31. Peterson L, Renström P: *Sports Injuries: Their Prevention and Treatment*. London, Martin Dunitz, 1986.
32. Peterson L, Stener B: Old total rupture of the adductor longus muscle: A report of seven cases. *Acta Orthop Scand* 1976;47:653–657.
33. Postlethwaite AE, Kang AH: Fibroblasts, in Gallin JI, Goldstein IM, Snyderman R (eds): *Inflammation: Basic Principles and Clinical Correlates*. New York, Raven Press, 1988, pp 577–598.
34. Raines EW, Dower SK, Ross R: Interleukin-1 mitogenic activity for fibroblasts and smooth muscle cells is due to PDGF-AA. *Science* 1989;243:393–396.
35. Renström P, Peterson L: Groin injuries in athletes. *Br J Sports Med* 1980;14:30–36.
36. Rosenbloom J, Feldman G, Freundlich B, et al: Transcriptional control of human diploid fibroblast collagen synthesis by gamma interferon. *Biochem Biophys Res Commun* 1984;123:365–372.
37. Rothwell AG: Quadriceps hematoma: A prospective clinical study. *Clin Orthop* 1982;171:97–103.
38. Schmidt JA, Mizel SB, Cohen D, et al: Interleukin 1, a potential regulator of fibroblast proliferation. *J Immunol* 1982;128:2177–2181.
39. Shimokado K. Raines EW, Madtes DK, et al: A significant part of macrophage-derived growth factor consists of at least two forms of PDGF. *Cell* 1985;43:277–286.
40. Sisk TD: Ankylosis and deformity, in Crenshaw AH (ed): *Campbell's Operative Orthopedics*, ed 5. St. Louis, CV Mosby, 1971, vol 2, p 1205.

41. Sprague NF III, O'Connor RL, Fox JM: Arthroscopic treatment of postoperative knee fibroarthrosis. *Clin Orthop* 1982;166:165–172.
42. Strickland GP, Welgus HG: Human skin fibroblast collagenase inhibitor. *J Biol Chem* 1983;258:12252–12258.
43. Vilcek J, Palombella VJ, Henriksen-DeStefano D, et al: Fibroblast growth enhancing activity of tumor necrosis factor and its relationship to other polypeptide growth factors. *J Exp Med* 1986;163:632–643.
44. Wahl LM, Wahl SM: Inflammation, in Cohen IK, Diegelmann RF, Lindblad WJ (eds): *Wound Healing: Biochemical and Clinical Aspects*. Philadelphia, WB Saunders, 1990.
45. Wahl SM: Fibrosis: Bacterial cell wall induced hepatic granulomas, in Gallin JI, Goldstein IM, Snyderman R (eds): *Inflammation: Basic Principles and Clinical Correlates*. New York, Raven Press, 1988, pp 841–860.
46. Wahl SM, Hunt DA, Wakefield L, et al: Transforming growth factor beta (TGF-β) induces monocyte chemoaxis and growth factor production. *Proc Natl Acad Sci USA* 1987;84:5788–5792.
47. Waugh W, Newton G, Tew M: Articular changes associated with a flexion deformity in rheumatoid and osteoarthritic knees. *J Bone Joint Surg* 1980;62B:180–183.
48. Weksler BB: Platelets, in Gallin JI, Goldstein I, Snyderman R (eds): *Inflammation: Basic Principles and Clinical Correlates*. New York, Raven Press, 1988, pp 543–558.
49. Welgus HG, Campbell EJ, Bar-Shavit Z, et al: Human alveolar macrophages produce a fibroblast-like collagenase and collagenase inhibitor. *J Clin Invest* 1985;76:219–226.
50. Wiseman DM, Polverini PJ, Kamp DW, et al: Transforming growth factor beta (TGF-β) is chemotactic for human monocytes and induces their expression of angiogenic activity. *Biochem Biophys Res Commun* 1988;157:793–800.
51. Wong H, Hunt D, Dougherty S, et al: Colony stimulating factor (CSF)-induced gene expression in human monocytes. *FASEB J* 1988;2:A875.
52. Zucali JR, Dinarello CA, Oblon DJ, et al: Interleukin 1 stimulates fibroblasts to produce granulocyte-macrophage colony stimulating activity and prostaglandin E_2. *J Clin Invest* 1986;77:1857–1863.

Future Directions

Published reports and clinical observations have clearly established the fact that a great many overuse and overload soft-tissue injuries fail to heal. There is also much confusion and uncertainty regarding the abnormalities involved in these lesions and the terminology used to describe them. A great deal of in-depth research is needed to clarify the etiology, pathophysiology, and spectrum of symptoms associated with these injuries.

As a general recommendation, a classification scheme to define the clinical entities should be established, with universally accepted definitions and standardized diagnostic tests. Once unified criteria have been developed, natural history studies may help to define the progression of the healing failures. Histopathologic examinations of musculoskeletal tissues should be done whenever possible to provide precise information on the nature of defective healing. It may be valuable to create appropriate animal models to study the failed healing response.

Because future research must draw on solid knowledge in other fields, the following recommendations for future research are intentionally broad in nature.

Establish and Correlate Clinical Findings by Evaluating Injured Tissue

At present, most conclusions regarding the pathophysiology of failed healing responses in sports-induced soft-tissue injury, especially in tendon, are based on hematoxylin-eosin staining from standard hospital biopsy processing. More sophisticated analysis, using vital staining for matrix assessment and labeled and histochemical identification of products of cellular synthesis and rates of cell synthesis, would shed light on the presence or absence of inflammatory cell activity. Ultrastructural analysis of such conditions as the tendinosis lesion may help characterize both cellular and matrix changes induced by overload or overuse. A corollary of this recommendation is the thorough study of the microscopic and functional anatomy of the normal soft-tissue targets of sports-induced trauma. Unfortunately, biopsy material is rarely available in the early stages of sports-induced pathophysiology because these conditions do not require surgery. Access to a multidisciplinary team is implied in the pursuit of these questions.

Perform Natural History and Epidemiologic Studies of the Mesenchymal Syndrome

The patterns of occurrence of sports-induced soft-tissue trauma remain intriguing. The so-called "mesenchymal syndrome" is one example of an associated cluster of complaints that may or may not have statistical validity. Familial characteristics offer an opportunity to discover the real risk and exposure that possible hereditary determinants control. Clearly, if constitutional predispositions are statistically important, then steps could be taken to prevent injury. These studies would require carefully constructed criteria regarding definition of injury and onset of complaint, as well as close attention to epidemiologic and statistical verity. To achieve valid results, this form of study must have large-scale data collection, follow-up, and reexaminations.

Investigate the Reliability of Present Grading Schemes

Grading systems to measure pain and function seem to be gaining popularity in the assessment of sports-induced soft-tissue complaints. This popularity is propelled by the present lack of a pragmatic way of quantifying the early phases of sports trauma. Carefully constructed subjective criteria should be coupled with structural healing ratings that can be verified by newer techniques of soft-tissue assessment, such as nuclear magnetic resonance imaging and spectroscopy. Further work is required on the statistical validity of these subjectively based rating systems as they pertain to rehabilitation, therapeutic measures, and successful resumption of sports participation.

Investigate Factors Involved in the Occurrence of Arthrofibrosis

Excessive inflammatory response in scar formation represents a major disability in both posttraumatic and postsurgical healing. Determining statistically significant variables in a population of affected patients would help to further define groups at risk. Clinical investigation might also search for inappropriate concentrations of fibrosis-stimulating mediators in patients in whom such complications develop. Synovial fluid aspirates from postsurgical knees could be analyzed to evaluate growth factors such as fibronectin and interleukin-1. Factors that increase collagen synthesis or block collagen degradation should be sought. Treatment intervention experiments should center on at least three identifiable points of modulation: inhibition of the inflammatory cascade, inhibition of angiogenesis, and direct regulation of mesenchymal cell function by inhibition of cell proliferation or matrix synthesis.

Investigate the Genetic Predisposition to Failed Healing

Genetic factors, which play a role in human phenotype expression, are likely to influence both susceptibility to athletic trauma and the healing process. Any search for familial aggregations of cases of failed healing must separate common environmental factors from genetic factors. Studies of twins raised in different environments may provide an opportunity to distinguish these factors. Another approach is to study the prevalence of failed tissue healing in patients known to have inherited connective-tissue disorders. After general genetic associations are established, specific molecular defects can be investigated in affected individuals.

Elucidate the Mechanisms of Failed Healing

Biologic repair of injured connective tissue is a complex process. A study of normal repair might consider such issues as tissue specificity, severity of injury, and interaction with mechanical loading conditions. In any investigation of defective healing, efforts should be made to isolate specific components from the numerous interrelated factors. Development of appropriate animal models of failed healing would greatly facilitate research. Fluid and tissue samples from surgical patients may help to identify cytokines, local growth factors, and systemic cells and factors that are aberrant in individuals who failed to respond to conservative treatment. These observational studies may lead to a more detailed evaluation of specific defects in healing.

Study Failure of Fibrous Repair in Cell- and Tissue-Culture Models

Repair in soft-tissue injury depends on the formation of fibrous tissue and its remodeling to form tissues with structural integrity. Excessive tissue formation and scarring may produce strong but functionally painful connective tissues. The matrix produced by the healing process involves many complex cellular and molecular processes. Comparing the normal process with deficient or excessive modes of fibrous repair is the key to improving therapeutic practice. Modern molecular biology techniques, used to study factors that regulate fracture healing, can now be applied to the repair of soft connective tissues. Although powerful, these new technologies must be used with special caution because concentrations of growth factors and the presence of confounding agents can produce misleading results. It may be necessary to develop model systems before these culture studies can progress.

Investigate the Role of Autoimmune Mechanisms in Chronic Failed Healing Response

It is postulated that if autoimmune processes have a role in chronic soft-tissue breakdown and aborted healing, a protein produced at an initial traumatic event may be the inciting agent that triggers autoimmune activity. Conventional cell-culture technique offers a model for introducing various mediators and/or protein breakdown by-products. The immunologic staining of biopsy specimens involving inflammatory soft-tissue injury provides another opportunity to investigate the potential role of this mechanism.

Section Five

Protective Role of Training and Conditioning

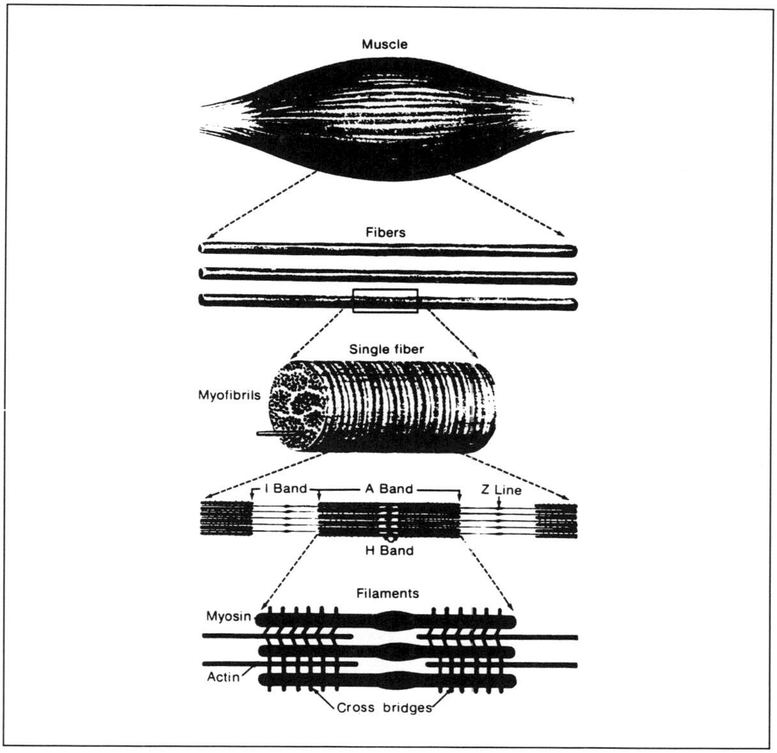

Group Leaders

Stephen Gordon, PhD
Frank Noyes, MD

Group Participants

David Butler, PhD
W. Ben Kibler, MD
William Kraemer, PhD
Arthur Siegel, MD
J. Richard Steadman, MD
Arthur Vailas, PhD
Ronald Watson, PhD
Ronald Zernicke, PhD

Overview

Training and conditioning programs are designed to enhance performance and prevent injuries. Direct correlations between training and acute or chronic inflammation from injury are not commonly available in the scientific literature. Most previous studies on training have focused on performance and injury, only indirectly indicating how these factors affect inflammation.

Sports-induced injuries and inflammation are related to certain clinical syndromes that are widely treated in sports-medicine clinics. Of particular concern are the effects of training, overtraining, and overuse conditions in inducing abnormally high or prolonged forces and deformations in musculoskeletal soft tissues. The importance of examining these sports-induced injuries and inflammatory states is related particularly to two objectives: (1) increased performance threshold and (2) knowledge of the role of chronic pain syndromes.

First, in terms of training, the goal is to increase the strength or endurance threshold of the particular soft-tissue structure. The hypothesis is that achieving a higher threshold will enable the soft-tissue part to function without failure. It is a given that sports involve the application of significant forces and deformations to soft tissues. The goal of a training program is to achieve a maximal physiologic state without inducing episodes of microtrauma or gross trauma that would induce inflammation, pain, swelling, and edema deleterious to sports performance. Training programs should maximize performance while inducing no unwanted inflammatory responses.

Second, this section critically examines the role played by the immune system in the chronic pain syndromes commonly seen in athletes. For example, a "shoulder impingement" has a significant inflammatory component that in many patients does not respond to treatment. It is perhaps more appropriate to label the clinical presentation as "anterior shoulder pain" and then look for the various etiologic factors (muscle and joint irregularities, abnormal motions and loads, immune components, tissue breakdown) that may be present.

In workshop discussions, overuse clinical syndromes were described as representing mechanical failure of a soft-tissue structure. From a biomechanical view, different mechanisms can cause structural failure. For example, failure can result from a single overload or from deformation beyond the normal elastic limit. Other failure mechanisms include fatigue, which involves repetitive loading and/or deformations at loads below ultimate failure. At present, the exact failure mechanism for most soft-tissue structures is not known. A useful label for these clinical states is "overuse injury," rather than "overload injury," which implies knowledge of a specific failure mechanism.

There is uncertainty as to the point in training when deleterious effects begin. Overuse injury may involve a single use or repeated use of an anatomic part, leading to structural changes that result in clinical symptoms or findings. Overtraining (or overconditioning) is a vaguely defined deterioration from baseline and threshold performance brought on by excessive training. Although it lacks generally accepted criteria or professional diagnoses, overtraining can cause a variety of musculoskeletal, systemic, or psychological alterations. Many athletes experience symptoms of overtraining. These responses to training (and overtraining) can affect various systems, such as the cardiovascular, endocrine, and immune systems, as well as local tissues, such as muscles, tendons, ligaments, and cartilage.

Endurance training decreases resting heart rate and increases baseline Vo_2max and heart-chamber volume. The improvement of Vo_2max involves both cardiac and peripheral muscle changes. Strength training leads to an increase in the thickness of the cardiac wall. Overtraining, on the other hand, increases the resting heart rate (compared with the trained level) and decreases Vo_2max. This decrease in oxygen delivery can conceivably lead to anoxia, cell death, and an inflammatory process.

After vigorous exercise (more than 70% of Vo_2max), there is an increase in corticosteroids followed, 30 minutes later, by a slow return to normal. Sprint training induces an increased response from baseline, while endurance training seems to have no effect. Corticosteroid production is particularly important because of its anti–inflammatory and protease activity. After rigorous activity (50% of Vo_2max), catecholamines have been shown to increase, as have enkephalins and endorphins. The response of trained individuals is somewhat stronger. In overtrained individuals, corticosteroid and catecholamine baseline levels appear to be increased.

The immune system's response to exercise and other factors that affect hormonal output is complex. With training, there is some evidence of a general increase in T cells, a decrease in interleukin-2 production, and a decrease in natural killer cell function. Overtraining may induce other modifications to the immune system.

The nervous system can enhance or inhibit musculoskeletal activity. In the first three to five weeks after weight training, there is an increase in strength with no increase in muscle fiber diameter. This change is attributed to a more efficient recruitment pattern. In an alternative fashion, pain or overtraining may induce central nervous system inhibition of performance.

Muscle responds to training by gaining efficiency and strength. There is little evidence of any significant degree of change in type of muscle fiber with training. Because muscles contain a mixture of fiber types, it is reasonable to assume that even the less prevalent types may play a role in the response to training. In overtraining, muscle degradation is marked by an increase in creatine kinase muscle isoenzyme and changes in calcium influx and intracellular pH.

With training, extensor tendons increase in size, ultimate load, and tensile strength. In flexor tendons, only the ultimate load increases. Collagen fiber size may decrease with training, but the number of fibers increases. Ligaments show small gains in ultimate load and modulus after a year of training. Life-long training induces no significant property changes, but ligaments in these individuals tend to fail in their substance rather than at the bone insertion. A decrease in tensile strength is noted in older animals.

Cartilage has a low annual turnover of extracellular matrix components (1% for collagen and 50% for proteoglycans). This implies a lower probability of tissue healing, although turnover rates may increase significantly in abnormal states. In general, a loss of proteoglycans, as occurs in disease, is a reversible condition. Disruption of the hyaluronic backbone of collagen, as occurs in injury, is a nonreversible event. Little is known regarding the effects of training on cartilage.

Flexibility, shoulder abnormalities, and knee disorders are also discussed in this section. Clinically relevant concepts related to flexibility may be based on anecdotal information describing the need for muscle flexibility of muscle-tendon units and the rather universal prescription of flexibility programs before participation in athletic activities. It is widely held that flexibility helps decrease failure or microfailure of the muscle-tendon unit, thereby decreasing a sports-induced inflammatory response. Despite increased understanding of muscle physiology, neurologic control of muscle tension, and the resting length of a muscle-tendon unit, there is no clinical evidence to support the idea that stretching and improved flexibility specifically prevent injury. Clinical data indicate that flexibility programs are important in preventing muscle soreness and microtraumatic episodes at the myotendinous junction. Flexibility programs are an important part of the warm-up program before athletic participation and are also prescribed for other effects. Their role in preventing episodes of sports-induced inflammation, however, awaits further scientific evidence.

Anterior shoulder pain and related syndromes are classified loosely as impingement problems and rotator cuff problems. Clinical evidence suggests that an overuse injury, caused either by abnormal forces on normal tissues or by normal forces on a degenerative tendon, may invoke an inflammatory response in a rotator cuff muscle-tendon unit. Clinical studies indicate that inflammation in these structures results in altered flexibility and motion of the shoulder, weakness and atrophy of various shoulder muscles and scapular muscles, altered patterns of muscle function during throwing, and the likelihood of inducing overload conditions in other structures about the shoulder, including the articular cartilage. Clinical evidence suggests that prevention of shoulder injuries involves the specific diagnosis of abnormal patterns of muscle function and muscle atrophy and attention to the dynamic stabilizing components of the glenohumeral joint.

Another example of sports-induced inflammatory mechanisms is related to inflammatory states present after surgery. For example, ligamentous reconstruction of the knee joint involves a surgically induced inflammatory response. This causes excessive edema, increased capillary permeability, and the release of inflammatory mediators that prolong the inflammatory response, all of which can have a deleterious effect on recovery. To what extent this release of inflammatory mediators is normal or excessive is yet to be defined, as is the variation in patient response to the release of excess inflammatory mediators. Also, it is unknown to what extent the inflammatory process aids the healing response. The problems the clinician faces are how to detect an unwanted inflammatory response that would delay functional recovery and what therapy to prescribe.

Chapter 45

Physiologic and Cellular Effects of Exercise Training

William J. Kraemer, PhD

Exercise training is a systematic process of creating an effective stimulus to elicit a physiologic adaptation over time. Endurance training and resistance training provide a continuum of modalities that affect various physiologic systems. The magnitude of change depends on the individual's pretraining level and the program's characteristics. Proper progression, variation, specificity and overload are needed to affect physiologic adaptations. An exercise training program can change every physiologic system of the body. Aerobic training adaptations improve maximal performance and the ability to perform prolonged exercise. A commonly measured change is an increase in maximal oxygen uptake associated with an increase in maximum cardiac output. Metabolic changes include increased respiratory capacity, lower blood lactate levels at a given exercise intensity, and increased mitochondrial density and enzyme activities. Conversely, heavy resistance training stimulates muscle hypertrophy and does not improve the body's ability to perform low-power-output endurance activities. It is an effective exercise modality and brings about a variety of functional changes in force-production capabilities. These changes are mediated by neural activity and subsequent increases in contractile protein content and enzymatic activities. Exercise training is an effective method of improving physical strength and high-intensity endurance.

In the evaluation of exercise physiology, considerable research is devoted to descriptions of the physiologic responses and adaptations with exercise training. Biologic microtechniques provide greater understanding of the underlying biochemical and cellular mechanisms that mediate exercise responses and adaptations. Biochemical and cellular techniques and advances in image analysis technology should enable future investigators to examine causal links between cellular tissue changes and improved physiologic function. Improved understanding of cellular mechanisms can lead to better exercise prescriptions. This chapter provides a basic overview of the exercise prescription process and the physiologic effects of exercise training.

Exercise Prescription Overview

The configuration of the exercise stimulus is vital to the body's adaptational responses. The level of the acute exercise stimulus determines the contributions of various physiologic systems in performing the exercise. The daily repeated exposure of this stimulus constitutes the training program. The effects of the training program depend on the individual's physiologic capabilities. Thus, the individual's genetic predisposition determines the adaptational responses and the magnitude of response.

Developing a training program involves many different variables. This makes it difficult to acquire complete data on the physiologic adaptations to training. Several factors affect the degree of adaptational responses, regardless of the training program used. These include the individual's genetic predisposition, pretraining status, and age.

The absolute performance abilities of an individual are genetically determined. Training improvements relate to the person's fitness level as the individual progresses from an untrained state to the genetic ceiling for a particular physiologic parameter. However, the magnitude of the performance gains lessens as the individual nears this theoretical ceiling. For example, an untrained individual may increase maximal aerobic capacity by 25% after 16 weeks of endurance training while an endurance athlete may have only a 5% increase.

The effects of gender have been examined,[20,24,38,44,67,109–111] and there seem to be no significant differences in the trainability of males and females. Differences exist primarily in the absolute physiologic levels of different variables and can often be attributed to the absolute differences in total body mass and/or fat-free mass.[12,28,79] Subtle gender differences may be found in the type of mechanisms that mediate various training adaptations, and these differences may have neurologic and neuroendocrine origins.

Progressive Overload and Variation in Training

As adaptation to exercise begins, the amount of exercise can be increased by modifying the variables, such as intensity, within the exercise program. Increases must be gradual and should match an individual's ability to tolerate exercise stress. Premature increases in an exercise program can lead to undue cardiovascular and musculoskeletal stress and possible injury, yet without adequate overload, physiologic adaptation does not occur. Thus, the program's effectiveness must be evaluated periodically and changes made if necessary.

In addition to progressive overload, a variation in the training stimulus must be provided to maintain the effectiveness of the exercise stimulus. Exercise programs ranging from running to weightlifting[76] can be divided into periods that allow for variation and rest within the context of the program's exercise demands. The training periods developed concentrate on the athlete's specific needs. Adjustments in the volume or intensity of exercise depend on the age and fitness level of the athlete. Thus, the preparatory phase of the training program may focus on low-intensity, high-volume exercise and gradually lead into the next phase of higher-intensity, lower-volume exercise protocols.

Variations in an exercise program may be observed within a week's routine. For example, an individual may schedule a high-intensity run for Monday, a low-intensity run for Wednesday, and a moderate-intensity run for Friday. Thus, the different exercise variables are modulated during the training program to vary the physiologic stress. Exercise stimulus, variation, and the need for rest are emphasized in theories of program periodization.[12,28,76]

Specificity

Exercise specificity is one of the basic concepts in exercise-training theory.[25,28] Adaptations achieved from training one muscle group are not made in other muscles in the body. For example, training adaptations from a leg-exercise program are not felt in the arms. Furthermore, exercise adaptations are also specifically related to the mode, velocity and metabolic demands of exercise and to the joint angles utilized.[7,12,81] Because the adaptations are directly related to the nature of the exercise stimulus, the exercise prescription must place physiologic demands on the specific components to be improved.

Aerobic Exercise Prescription

During the last 20 years a great deal of attention has been focused on endurance training. Individualization of training protocols is now widely accepted and implemented for all types of training, for cardiac patients as well as for elite endurance athletes.[2,5,6,25] The primary training variables in prescribing endurance exercise are exercise intensity, exercise duration, and training session frequency. In general, as an individual becomes more fit, the intensity, duration and frequency of training sessions must increase to improve physiologic function or performance. Elite endurance athletes require careful manipulation of training variables to avoid overuse or overtraining syndromes.[66] Fardy[25] described effective ranges for these variables on the basis of individual fitness levels. Effective ranges for a highly trained individual might be an intensity of 80% to 90% of maximum heart rate, a duration of one to two hours, and a frequency of five to seven days per week, whereas corresponding values for a beginner might be 60% to 85%, 15 to 45 minutes, and three to five days per week.

The training ranges may be modified to vary training and keep the adaptive stimulus high. Few exercise programs use the same protocol every day. Scientists need to examine more realistic training protocols that are not as constant.

Dynamic, rhythmic large-muscle-group exercises (such as cycling or running) are typically used to improve aerobic power. Both intermittent and continuous training techniques can improve aerobic fitness.[28,81,112]

Testing for Aerobic Power

Maximal aerobic power measures the body's ability to transport and extract oxygen for energy production. It can be used to assess levels of aerobic fitness and the effects of training because it is a reliable, reproducible measure.[7,25] Maximal oxygen uptake ($\dot{V}O_2max$) is "a measure of the maximal energy output by aerobic processes and the functional capacity of the circulation."[7] Oxygen consumption can be measured during any activity, but maximal or peak oxygen consumption is typically used to evaluate aerobic capabilities.

Testing for maximal or peak aerobic power usually uses open-circuit spirometry and exercise on a bicycle ergometer or motor-driven treadmill.[109] Graded-exercise protocols use either a continuous or discontinuous test format.[77] $\dot{V}O_2max$ can be quantitatively represented as the maximum amount (volume or V) of oxygen (O_2) consumed per unit of time by an individual during a graded-exercise test to voluntary exhaustion.[106] Oxygen consumption is usually reported as an absolute value ($L{\cdot}min^{-1}$) or relative to body weight ($ml{\cdot}kg{\cdot}min^{-1}$). Maximal oxygen consumption is typically determined by using the plateau criteria for certain tests (such as the treadmill) compared to a "peak $\dot{V}O_2$" measure for other tests (such as the cycle ergometer) in which there are typically no true plateaus.[12,106,109]

Exercise-treadmill protocols are individually designed to be completed in a reasonable amount of time (five to ten minutes after a warm-up).[106] Thus, the same exercise protocol would not be used for both a cardiac patient and a elite marathon runner. The test protocol developed by Costill and Fox[18] can be used to evaluate the aerobic capacity of both fit and unfit individuals if it is modified to the individual. A young, healthy, unfit individual not at risk for cardic problems might warm-up on the treadmill at a speed of 3.5 mph and a 0% grade for four minutes. On the basis of background information obtained from the subject before testing, loads can be developed for subsequent stages of the test. For example, if the person can run a nine-minute mile, the test could use a speed of 6 mph at 0% grade for the first four-minute stage with the treadmill grade increasing 2% for each subsequent three-minute stage until voluntary exhaustion. An elite runner who can run a five-minute mile might need a treadmill test speed of 10 mph.

Physiologic Effects of Endurance Training

Endurance training can improve an individual's aerobic power from 5% to 30%,[25,83,92] depending on the starting fitness level. Greater improvements can usually be attributed to exceptionally low starting levels.[19,25,92] Elite endurance athletes typically have the highest aerobic power capabilities,[7,42,93] exceeding endurance athletes without the same performance abilities.[99]

The intensity of training is one of the most important factors for improving and maintaining aerobic power.[19,32,51,68,84] Short, high-intensity bouts of interval sprints can improve maximal oxygen uptake if the interim rest period is also short.[34,61] Callister and associates[15] showed that sprint speed improves without significant increases in maximal aerobic power if a longer rest period (90 seconds) is taken after each 50-m and 100-m sprint. Duration and frequency are also important variables in endurance training. A number of studies show that duration[78,111] and frequency[84,85] of training can influence the increase in maximal aerobic power. Typically, longer, more frequent training sessions result in greater degrees of aerobic improvement.

Age and gender should also be considered. Maximal aerobic power decreases with age in adults.[5,6,108] Long-term adherence to an intense endurance-training program may alter this effect but this has not been directly demonstrated. On the average, the aerobic power values of women range from 73% to 85% of the values of men.[7,13,19,20,33,69,82,108] The physiologic response to training is similar in both men and women. The differences in aerobic power may be caused by several factors, including women's higher percentage of body fat and lower blood hemoglobin values, and men's larger heart size and blood volume.[7,12,81,108] Other cardiorespiratory changes occur in conjunction with an increase in maximal aerobic power. There are several published reviews on the cardiovascular changes associated with endurance exercise training.[10,11,16,48,53,58,88,95,97] Table 1 shows various physiologic changes that occur with short-term (three to six months) endurance training and compares the responses of typical untrained individuals with those of elite endurance athletes.

Cellular Changes With Endurance Training

High-level endurance performance capabilities are only achieved when oxygen utilization and oxygen transport capacities are balanced.[49,50,96] There are extensive published reviews on the biochemical and cellular changes associated with endurance training.[39,45–47,49]

Hormonal Influences

Other metabolic effects of training center on the hormonal enhancement of free fatty acid mobilization and utilization and on glycogen-sparing effects. Catecholamines, insulin, and glucagon are involved in regulating lipolysis, hepatic glycogenolysis, and gluconeogenesis.[35,36] During exercise, plasma and serum concentrations of hormones can increase ten to 20 times over their levels at rest. Several mechanisms contribute to these changes, including changes in hepatic and extrahepatic clearance rates and shifts in blood volume. Still, the increases are higher than can be explained by such mechanisms. Hormonal response is a function of both central and peripheral factors.[35] In both trained and untrained subjects, Galbo[35] reported, the hormonal response depends on the relative and not the absolute exercise intensity.

Endurance training seems to augment the absolute secretion rates of many hormones such as epinephrine in response to maximal exercise. Trained individuals appear to have blunted responses to sub-

Table 1 Composite physiologic profile

Variable	Subjects*		Elite Endurance Athletes
	Before Training	After Training	
HRrest (beats/min)	74	61	45
HRmax (beats/min)	194	190	185
SVrest (ml^2)	64	82	127
SVmax (ml^2)	122	142	201
COrest ($L \cdot min^{-1}$)	4.5	4.6	4.4
COmax ($L \cdot min^{-1}$)	22.3	25.8	34.9
Heart volume (ml)	750	823	1,250
Blood volume (L)	4.8	5.2	6.1
BPress (mm Hg)			
Systolic	130	124	105
Diastolic	80	78	65
BPmax (mm Hg)			
Systolic	206	202	209
Diastolic	85	82	69
VErest ($L \cdot m^{-1}$)	7	6	6
VEmax ($L \cdot m^{-1}$), BTPS	123	142	201
Breaths, BTPS (No./min)			
Resting	14	12	11
Maximum	42	47	59
TV_{rest}(L)	0.6	0.6	0.6
TV_{max}(L)	2.8	3.1	3.1
VC (L)	5.8	6.1	6.4
RV (L)	1.5	1.3	1.3
a-$\bar{v}O_2$ diff (ml/100 ml)			
Resting	6.1	6.1	6.1
Maximum	14.5	15.2	16.4
Blood HLa ($mmol \cdot L^{-1}$)			
Resting	0.4	0.4	0.4
Maximum	9.9	11.2	16.7
Vo_2max ($ml \cdot kg^{-1}min^{-1}$)	47	55	79
Weight (kg)	75	72	62
Relative % fat	16.0	14.9	5.7
Type I fibers (%)			
Fiber areas (μ^2)			
Type I	4,730	4,820	4,180
Type IIa	6,860	7,150	4,299
Type IIb	6,167	6,433	3,899
Capillaries			
No./mm^2	290	350	460
No./fiber	1.2	1.4	3.2
Citrate synthetase (activity units)	28	37	78
Hexokinase (activity units)	2.4	2.9	4.2
Lactate dehydrogenase (activity units)	580	654	629
Maximum fiber shortening velocity (fiber lengths$\cdot sec^{-1}$)			
Type I	0.86	?	1.10
Type II	4.85	?	1.74

*Previously untrained subjects who underwent short-term (three to six months) endurance training.

maximal exercise. Their hormone concentrations equal those of their untrained counterparts at the same relative exercise intensity, but they can exercise at much higher absolute exercise intensities.[54,64,70] They may have more effective mechanisms for receptor-binding interactions in the control and regulation of metabolic function. The greater hormonal response patterns to maximal and supramaximal exercise appear to augment the athlete's ability to tolerate and sustain prolonged high-exercise intensities.[64,65,70] When exercise duration is short (from five to 30 seconds), there are few changes in peripheral blood hormone concentrations.[65]

The neuroendocrine system also has a careful, balanced interaction with the immune system and inflammation.[9,37] For example, glucocorticoids interact with leukocytes and interleukin-1 interacts with the hypothalamic responses.

Responses of the Immune System

Little is known about the effects of exercise on the immune system. In general, exercise is associated with increased levels of lymphocytes, neutrophils, and interleukin-1.[98] Mononuclear phagocytes produce interleukin-1, so exercise may affect this component of the immune system. Exercise may also increase the development of natural killer cells, essential for resistance to tumor growth.[52]

For many of these immune factors, the increase is temporary and levels decrease within several hours after exercise.[98] Although lymphocyte levels sometimes increase after exercise, their effectiveness may decrease because of an altered ratio of T-helper to T-suppressor cells resulting in immune suppression. Another transient effect is a decrease in antibody levels.[75,107] Exercise decreases levels of IgA and IgM for as long as 24 hours. The response appears to be intensity-dependent. Few acute exercise protocols have been examined, so the interaction between training and the immune system responses remains unclear.

Body Composition

Endurance training is associated with alterations in body composition. Generally, endurance exercise training decreases the relative percentage of body fat and has little or no significant effect on fat-free mass.[85,86] Longer-term programs can result in greater decreases in the percentage of body fat.[17,18] When training intensity and volume balance anabolic and catabolic activities in muscle, the optimal prescription depends on the training level of the athlete and the variation in the exercise protocol. Excessive training might lead to a predominance of catabolic activity in the body.[61]

Neural Adaptations

Adaptations in the nervous system play a role in the early stages of endurance training. In the beginning, a person increases the efficiency and delays fatigue of the contractile mechanisms.[89] The motor unit activation in the prime movers needed to maintain a given submaximal force decreases as skill is acquired during training. Additionally, improved endurance performance may also result in a rotation of neural activity among synergists and among motor units within a muscle.[40,87,89] Thus, the individual produces more efficient locomotion during the activity with lower energy expenditure.

Resistance Training

Exercise Prescription

Professionals now have a greater understanding of the exercise prescription process in resistance training. There are published descriptions of these exercise prescription procedures.[28,57,60] A number of variables describe each resistance training workout, and the combination of variables in a workout determines the type of exercise stimulus and the body's adaptations.

Five basic variables describe a resistance training workout: choice of exercises; order of exercises; load used (intensity); length of the rest period between sets and exercises; and number of sets. These are called "acute program variables" and can be used to quantify any type of resistance exercise protocol. Choice of exercises refers to the mode of exercise, angle of exercise, and contraction type. The order of exercises indicates the progression through the chosen exercises (such as arm exercises followed by leg exercises or large muscle group exercises followed by small muscle group exercises). The load used refers to the magnitude of resistance used in a particular exercise. The lengths of the rest periods between sets and exercises must be quantified because they influence the physiologic stress imposed by the exercise protocol. The number of sets performed is important in an ongoing program to calculate volume of exercise.

Changing these variables results in changes over time (chronic programming) or periodization of resistance training. For example, exercise "volume" is determined by multiplying the number of sets by the number of repetitions performed in a workout. Volume and intensity of a workout change in different phases of training. A typical progression (that is, periodization) for improving muscle strength or power is to use high-volume, low-intensity exercise protocols in the initial phases and lower volumes and higher intensities as the individual peaks for a performance.[57,76] Any acute program variable, such as rest periods, can be altered during a training period, depending on the specific goals of the program.

Evaluation and Testing

Several variables are of primary interest in evaluating the effects of various resistance training programs. Strength is the maximal force produced at a specified velocity of movement.[55] Strength tests to determine functional changes in force production can be done on a variety of equipment, including isokinetic dynamometers with specific velocities, free weights and machines to determine repetition maximums (the maximal number of repetitions that can be performed with a given load or resistance), and isometric tests to find force production

Table 2 Comparative physiologic adaptations in response to resistance and endurance training

Variable	Resistance Trained	Endurance Trained
Muscle strength	Increased	No change
Muscle endurance	Increased for high power output	Increased for low power output
Muscle fiber size	Increased	No change/small increase
Capillary density	No change/decrease	Increased
Mitochondrial volume density	Decreased	Increased
Aerobic power	No change/slight increase	Increased
Creatine phosphokinase	Increased	Increased
Myokinase	Increased	Increased
Phosphofructokinase	Increased	Variable
Lactate dehydrogenase	No change	Variable
Stored ATP	Increased	Increased
Stored PC	Increased	Increased
Stored glycogen	Increased	Increased
Stored triglycerides	?/increased	Increased
Ligament strength	?	Increased
Tendon strength	?	Increased
Collagen content	?	Variable
Bone density	No change/increase	Increased
% body fat	Decreased	Decreased
Fat-free mass	Increased	No change

at zero velocity. Local muscular endurance (absolute and relative) can also be evaluated to determine the high-intensity endurance of various muscle groups.[4] Measures of muscular hypertrophy can be assessed by circumference tape measurements, thigh volumes, and image analysis procedures. Researchers have used percutaneous needle muscle biopsy techniques to obtain tissue samples for subsequent morphologic determinations of cellular hypertrophy.

Physiologic Effects

There are several extensive reviews of the physiologic effects of resistance training.[8,29–31,56,58,59,72,73,91,104] A comparison of the changes that occur in resistance and endurance training can be seen in Table 2.

Muscle Strength Increases in muscle strength from pretraining values can span a large range (7% to 45% increase).[28] Muscle strength gains may relate to the load used and the volume of exposure (sets times repetitions).[28] Studies commonly use multiple sets of an exercise and maximum voluntary contractions in the exercise protocol.[28,59] In a classic study, Anderson and Kearney[4] demonstrated that a repetition continuum exists. As the number of repetitions becomes higher, the return on strength gains decreases. Thus, heavier loads (six to eight repetition maximums) produce much larger gains in strength than lighter loads (30 to 40 repetition maximums). Differences among heavier loads (one to ten repetition maximums) appear irrelevant as they are all typically used in periodized training techniques to provide variation.

Neural Adaptations Initial gains in muscle strength during the first few weeks of training do not show a concomitant increase in muscle size or muscle cross-sectional area.[80,103] The correlations between increases in strength and increases in mass are weak. Factors other than muscle mass contribute to muscle force production.[80] This neural adaptation may mediate the initial improvements in strength.[90,91] Several mechanisms could contribute to increased force production, including increased inhibition of antagonists and better co-contraction of synergists, increased activation of synergists, inhibition of neural protective mechanisms, and increased motor neuron excitability.[89–91]

Muscle Size Increased muscle size from resistance exercise has been thought to occur through hypertrophy. At present, a training duration of six weeks or more appears necessary before significant changes in the ultrastructure of muscle can be seen.[71] Further study is needed to evaluate the time course of morphologic changes and how training status interacts with such adaptations. The increased cross-sectional area of muscle fibers may be caused by the greater number of actin and myosin filaments added to the myofibrils.[73] Heavy resistance training results in increased fiber cross-sectional area of both type I and type II fibers. Synthesis of contractile proteins appears greatest in type II fibers.[72,73] Differences among other fiber-type subgroups are not clear. Powerlifters and Olympic weightlifters have type II fiber areas almost twice the size of their type I fiber areas,[73,103,104] but bodybuilders do not. This suggests that the type of training protocols used may have a significant impact on the subsequent muscle fiber adaptations.[1,30,31] Fiber areas of lifters are significantly larger than those of runners and other control subjects.[101] Thus, resistance training is a more potent stimulus for cellular changes in hypertrophy than any other form of exercise.

Additional Cellular Adaptations Heavy resistance training reduces mitochondrial density in the trained muscles.[74] These changes in volume density of mitochondria parallel changes in muscle hypertrophy. Thus, the decreases in mitochondrial volume density may be attributed to increases in the total amount of protein in the contractile tissue.[104] An increase in the amount of contractile protein indicates decreased capillary density that parallels increases in muscle hypertrophy.[3] Powerlifters and Olympic weightlifters have significantly lower capillary densities when compared with control subjects.[104] Conversely, bodybuilders have more capillaries per fiber and capillary densities similar to nonathletes.[104] Kraemer and associates[63] demonstrated that bodybuilding workouts typically elevate blood lactate levels above 20 $mmol \cdot L^{-1}$, so tissue clearance mechanisms may depend on capillary supply. The type of exercise protocols used may influence cellular adaptations.

There are conflicting reports on enzyme changes with resistance training, which may stem from the exercise protocols and enzyme analysis techniques used. One study[21] showed that six months of heavy resistance training decreased activities of hexokinase, myofibrillar adenosine triphosphatase, citrate syntase, phosphofructokinase, myokinase, and creatine kinase but not lactate dehydrogenase. In this study, strength training associated with type II hypertrophy was not associated with increased enzymatic activities related to phosphagenic, glycolytic, or oxidative metabolism. Instead, the exercise-induced hypertrophy was associated with an attenuation of certain enzyme activities.[21,104] Another study[105] showed that citrate synthase activity in type I fibers was significantly lower in powerlifters and weightlifters than in bodybuilders and nonathletes. Thus, resistance training seems to result in decreased enzyme activities associated with aerobic and anaerobic metabolism. The key appears to be the exact nature of the exercise stimulus used during training.

Heavy resistance training induces increases in energy substrate levels in muscle.[21] After five months of training, adenosine triphosphate, creatine phosphate, creatine, and glycogen increased in the triceps brachii.[73] This is consistent with observations in bodybuilders. Prolonged heavy-resistance training may also increase capacity for intramuscular lipid storage.[104,105]

Cardiovascular Changes Increases ranging from an average of 5% to 8% in aerobic power result from resistance training.[38] Increases from circuit-weight training programs (light loads, short rests, and multiple exercises) are lower than those from conventional endurance training programs. Cellular changes such as decreased mitochondrial density probably influence the magnitude of cardiovascular changes. Conventional heavy resistance training programs do not increase aerobic power.[28]

Echocardiography can investigate morphologic changes of the left ventricle that occur as a result of resistance training. Cross-sectional studies show that highly weight-trained athletes have normal left ventricular systolic and diastolic internal dimensions and volumes,[26,27] whether judged as absolute values or as relative to body surface area. Short-term studies on left ventricular cavity changes are inconclusive, suggesting that longer training programs are needed to influence such changes.[26] The effects of resistance training on cardiac wall thickness is less clear because of discrepancies in control subjects, effectiveness of exercise program, and caliber of lifters.[26,31] Still, heavy resistance training may increase cardiac wall thickness but not equally for all individuals. The increased cardiac wall thickness causes the ratio of septum to free wall to exceed 1.3. This higher-than-normal ratio is usually associated with hypertrophic cardiomyopathy, but the competitive weightlifters and powerlifters had normal ratios of left ventricular mass to volume and normal wall thickness per body surface area, indicating normal hearts.[26,27]

No evidence suggests that heavy resistance training causes elevations in resting blood pressure.[26] Male bodybuilders have lower blood pressures than either recreationally trained or sedentary males while performing resistance exercises at the same relative load.[26,31] Although acute and dramatic elevations in blood pressure occur during heavy resistance exercise, there is no evidence that training elevates resting levels.

Body Composition Intense resistance training can cause changes in the body composition profile.[28] Resistance training can increase fat-free mass and decrease the percentage of body fat. Short-term resistance training programs have typically resulted in slight increases in fat-free mass.[110] The change in the percentage of body fat depends on caloric intake and the metabolic intensity of the resistance training program. Chronic adherence to a heavy resistance training program appears necessary to achieve optimal increases in fat-free mass and decreases in the percentage of body fat.[86]

Connective Tissue At present, little direct evidence exists on the effects of heavy resistance training on connective tissue changes.[100] Stone[102] pointed out that because of the nature of the exercise stimulus, resistance training may have a dramatic effect on the strength of ligaments and tendons. In trained bodybuilders, the absolute amounts of connective tissue in the muscle are greater than those in controls, but when corrected for muscle size, the relative amounts of connective tissue remain constant. Resistance exercise may act as a "growth promoter" mediated by growth-promoting peptides. Increases in insulin-like growth factor-1 have been observed with various heavy resistance exercise protocols.[62] A combination of tropic influences could mediate increased connective tissue growth and development resulting from heavy resistance exercise.

Hormonal Influences If the exercise protocol involves large muscle groups and is of adequate intensity, the exercise will stimulate the neuroendocrine system.[56] Hormonal influences may be involved with adaptations made to heavy resistance training. Changes in hormone concentrations are sensitive to the manipulation of the acute program exercise variables.[56,62] Furthermore, testosterone and cortisol changes are linked to maximal strength changes over training and detraining periods.[56] Resistance exercise produces significant increases in endogenous anabolic hormones such as testosterone and growth hormone. These hormones and growth factors influence the growth and development of muscle, bone, and connective tissue.

Compatibility of Strength and Endurance Training

Combining strength and endurance activities appears to interfere primarily with strength performances at high velocities of movement.[22] When strength and endurance training are done in excess (overtraining), maximal strength performance is blunted.[41] Possible explanations for this less-than-optimal strength development with concurrent training include overtraining and the transformation of fast-twitch to slow-twitch type muscle fibers.[23] No adverse effects on aerobic power have been observed, despite the expected cellular changes caused by heavy resistance exercise. Recently,[43] it has been shown that concurrent training improves the high-intensity muscle endurance that requires more fast-twitch muscle fiber recruitment patterns.[43] The proper combination of resistance and endurance training to induce optimal adaptations has not yet been found, and may be quite individualistic.

Recovery Detraining

Adequate recovery after exercise is needed for optimal adaptations to occur. Still, if inactivity occurs, a person loses training adaptations or experiences a "detraining" phenomenon. Little is known about detraining after various conditioning protocols.[28] Endurance adaptations are most sensitive to periods of inactivity,[14,28,94] because of the enzymatic basis of many endurance-training adaptations related to energy production. Conversely, strength changes appear more resistant to short periods of inactivity and decay over time at a much slower rate.[28] The exact cellular mechanisms that mediate these changes are unknown. Still, the differences in the adaptations to endurance and to strength training suggest some explanations. Further research is needed to clarify the underlying physiologic mechanisms of detraining.

Periodization training attempts to provide adequate recovery while preventing the athlete from becoming detrained.[76] Avoiding detraining phenomena is an important aspect of exercise training in its protective role in soft-tissue injury. With the use of proper exercise variation, maintenance programs, and active recovery periods (that is, the athlete remains active but participates in other physical activities), adequate protection against serious detraining effects is possible.[28]

References

1. Alway SE, MacDougall JD, Sale DG, et al: Functional and structural adaptations in skeletal muscle of trained athletes. *J Appl Physiol* 1988;64:1114–1120.
2. American College of Sports Medicine: The recommended quantity and quality of exercise for developing and maintaining fitness in healthy adults. *Med Sci Sports Exerc* 1978;10:vii–x.
3. Andersen P, Henriksson J: Capillary supply of the quadriceps femoris muscle of man: Adaptive response to exercise. *J Physiol* 1977;270:677–690.
4. Anderson T, Kearney JT: Effects of three resistance training programs on muscular strength and absolute and relative endurance. *Res Q Exerc Sport* 1982;53:1–7.
5. Astrand PO: Physical performance as a function of age. *JAMA* 1968;205:729–733.
6. Astrand I, Astrand PO, Hallbäck I, et al: Reduction in maximal oxygen uptake with age. *J Appl Physiol* 1973;35:649–654.
7. Astrand P-O, Rodahl K: *Textbook of Work Physiology: Physiologic Basis of Exercise.* New York, McGraw-Hill, 1986.
8. Atha J: Strengthening muscle. *Exerc Sports Sci Rev* 1981;9:1–73.
9. Bateman A, Singh A, Kral T, et al: The immune-hypothalamic-pituitary-adrenal axis. *Endocrine Rev* 1989;10:92–112.
10. Bevegård BS, Shepherd JR: Regulation of the circulation during exercise in man. *Physiol Rev* 1967;47:178–213.

11. Brooks GA: Anaerobic threshold: Review of the concept and directions for future research. *Med Sci Sports Exerc* 1985;17:22–34.
12. Brooks GA, Fahey TD: *Exercise Physiology: Human Bioenergetics and Its Applications*. New York, John Wiley & Sons, 1984.
13. Burke EJ: Physiological effects of similar training programs in males and females. *Res Q Am Assoc Health Phys Educ* 1977;48:510–517.
14. Brynteson P, Sinning WE: The effects of training frequencies on the retention of cardiovascular fitness. *Med Sci Sports* 1973;5:29–33.
15. Callister R, Shealy MJ, Fleck SJ, et al: Performances adaptations to sprint, endurance and both modes of training. *J Appl Sport Sci Res* 1988;2:46–51.
16. Clausen JP: Effect of physical training on cardiovascular adjustments to exercise in man. *Physiol Rev* 1977;57:779–815.
17. Costill DL: Metabolic responses during distance running. *J Appl Physiol* 1970;28:251–255.
18. Costill DL, Fox EL: Energetics of marathon running. *Med Sci Sports Exerc* 1969;1:81–86.
19. Daniels WL, Kowal DM, Vogel JA, et al: Physiological effects of a military training program on male and female cadets. *Aviat Space Environ Med* 1979;50:562–566.
20. Drinkwater B: Physiological responses of women to exercise. *Exerc Sport Sci Rev* 1973;1:125–153.
21. Dudley GA: Metabolic consequences of resistive-type exercise. *Med Sci Sports Exerc* 1988;20(suppl):S158-S161.
22. Dudley GA, Djamil R: Incompatibility of endurance- and strength-training modes of exercise. *J Appl Physiol* 1985;59:1446–1451.
23. Dudley GA, Fleck SJ: Strength and endurance training: Are they mutually exclusive? *Sports Med* 1987;4:79–85.
24. Falkel JE, Sawka MN, Levine L, et al: Upper to lower body muscular strength and endurance ratios for women and men. *Ergonomics* 1985;28:1661–1670.
25. Fardy PS: Training for aerobic power, in Burke EJ (ed): *Toward an Understanding of Human Performance*. Ithaca, Movement Publications, 1977, pp 10–14.
26. Fleck SJ: Cardiovascular adaptations to resistance training. *Med Sci Sports Exerc* 1988;20(suppl):S146-S151.
27. Fleck SJ, Bennett JB III, Kraemer WJ, et al: Left ventricular hypertrophy in highly strength trained males. Presented at the Second International Conference on Sports Cardiology, Sorrento, Italy, April 1987.
28. Fleck SJ, Kraemer WJ: *Designing Resistance Training Programs*. Champaign, Human Kinetics, 1987.
29. Fleck SJ, Kraemer WJ: Resistance training: Basic principles. *Phys Sportsmed* 1988;16:160–171.
30. Fleck SJ, Kraemer WJ: Resistance training: Physiological responses and adaptations. Part 2. *Phys Sportsmed* 1988;16:108–124.
31. Fleck SJ, Kraemer WJ: Resistance training: Physiological responses and adaptations. Part 3. *Phys Sportsmed* 1988;16:53–74.
32. Fox EL, Bartels RL, Klinzing J, et al: Metabolic responses to interval training programs of high and low power output. *Med Sci Sports* 1977;9:191–196.
33. Fox EL, Bowers RW, Foss ML: *The Physiological Basis of Physical Education and Athletics*, ed 4. Dubuque, Wm C Brown, 1988.
34. Gaesser GA, Wilson LA: Effects of continuous and interval training on the parameters of the power-endurance time relationship for high-intensity exercise. *Int J Sport Med* 1988;9:417–421.
35. Galbo H: Endocrinology and metabolism in exercise. *Int J Sports Med* 1981;2:203–211.

36. Galbo H: *Hormonal and Metabolic Adaptation to Exercise.* New York, Thieme-Stratton, 1983.
37. Garcia-Leme J: *Hormones and Inflammation.* Boca Raton, CRC Press, 1989.
38. Gettman LR, Pollock ML: Circuit weight training: A critical review of its physiological benefits. *Phys Sportsmed* 1981;9:44–60.
39. Gollnick PD: Relationship of strength and endurance with skeletal muscle structure and metabolic potential. *Int J Sports Med* 1982;3(suppl 1):26–32.
40. Hellsing G, Lindström L: Rotation of synergistic activity during isometric jaw closing muscle contraction in man. *Acta Physiol Scand* 1983;118:203–207.
41. Hickson RC: Interference of strength development by simultaneously training for strength and endurance. *Eur J Appl Physiol* 1980;45:255–263.
42. Hickson RC, Bomze HA, Holloszy JO: Linear increase in aerobic power induced by a strenuous program of endurance exercise. *J Appl Physiol* 1977;42:372–376.
43. Hickson RC, Dvorak BA, Gorostiaga EM, et al: Potential for strength and endurance training to amplify endurance performance. *J Appl Physiol* 1988;65:2285–2290.
44. Hoffman T, Stauffer RW, Jackson AS: Sex difference in strength. *Am J Sports Med* 1979;7:265–267.
45. Holloszy JO: Adaptation of skeletal muscle to endurance exercise. *Med Sci Sports* 1975;7:155–164.
46. Holloszy JO: Biochemical adaptations to exercise: Aerobic metabolism. *Exerc Sport Sci Rev* 1973;1:45–71.
47. Holloszy JO, Booth FW: Biochemical adaptations to endurance exercise in muscle. *Annu Rev Physiol* 1976;38:273–291.
48. Holloszy JO, Rennie MJ, Hickson RC, et al: Physiological consequences of the biochemical adaptations to endurance exercise. *Ann NY Acad Sci* 1977;301:440–450.
49. Howald H: Training-induced morphological and functional changes in skeletal muscle. *Int J Sports Med* 1982;3:1–12.
50. Jansson E, Sjödin B, Tesch P: Changes in muscle fibre type distribution in man after physical training: A sign of fibre transformation? *Acta Physiol Scand* 1978;104:235–237.
51. Karvonen MJ Kentala E, Mustala O: The effects of training on heart rate: A longitudinal study. *Ann Med Exp Biol Fenn* 1957;35:307–315.
52. Keast D, Cameron K, Morton AR: Exercise and the immune response. *Sports Med* 1988;5:248–267.
53. Keul J, Dickhuth HH, Lehmann M, et al: The athlete's heart: Haemodynamics and structure. *Int J Sports Med* 1982;3(suppl 1):33–43.
54. Kjaer M: Epinephrine and some other hormonal responses to exercise in man; with special reference to physical training. *Int J Sports Med* 1989;10:2–15.
55. Knuttgen HG, Kraemer WJ: Terminology and measurement in exercise performance. *J Appl Sports Sci Res* 1987;1:1–10.
56. Kraemer WJ: Endocrine responses to resistance exercise. *Med Sci Sports Exerc* 1988;20(suppl):152–157.
57. Kraemer WJ, Baechle TR: Development of a strength training program, in Allman FL, Ryan AJ (eds): *Sports Medicine*, ed 2. Orlando, Academic Press, 1989, pp 113–127.
58. Kraemer WJ, Daniels WL: Physiological effects of training, in Bernhardt DB (ed): *Sports Physical Therapy.* New York, Churchill-Livingstone, 1986, pp 29–53.
59. Kraemer WJ, Deschenes MR, Fleck SJ: Physiological adaptations to resistance exercise: Implications for athletic conditioning. *Sports Med* 1988;6:246–256.

60. Kraemer WJ, Fleck SJ: Resistance training: Exercise prescription. Part 4. *Phys Sportsmed* 1988;16:69–81.
61. Kraemer WJ, Fleck SJ, Callister R, et al: Training responses of plasma beta-endorphin, adrenocorticotropin, and cortisol. *Med Sci Sports Exerc* 1989;21:146–153.
62. Kraemer WJ, Marchitelli L, McCurry D, et al: Endogenous anabolic hormone responses to weight training protocols, abstract. *Med Sci Sports Exerc* 1988;20(suppl):S59.
63. Kraemer WJ, Noble BJ, Clark MJ, et al: Physiologic responses to heavy-resistance exercise with very short rest periods. *Int J Sports Med* 1987;8:247–252.
64. Kraemer WJ, Noble BJ, Culver B, et al: Changes in plasma proenkephalin peptide F and catecholamine levels during graded exercise in men. *Proc Natl Acad Sci USA* 1985;82:6349–6351.
65. Kraemer WJ, Patton JF, Knuttgen HG, et al: Hypothalamic-pituitary-adrenal responses to short-duration high-intensity cycle exercise. *J Appl Physiol* 1989;66:161–166.
66. Kuipers H, Keizer HA: Overtraining in elite athletes: Review and directions for the future. *Sports Med* 1988;6:79–92.
67. Laubach LL: Comparative muscular strength of men and women: A review of the literature. *Aviat Space Environ Med* 1976;47:534–542.
68. Lesmes GR, Fox EL, Stevens C, et al: Metabolic responses of females to high-intensity interval training of different frequencies. *Med Sci Sports* 1978;10:229–232.
69. Lortie G, Simoneau JA, Hamel P, et al: Responses of maximal aerobic power and capacity to aerobic training. *Int J Sports Med* 1984;5:232–236.
70. Luger A, Deuster PA, Kyle SB, et al: Acute hypothalamic-pituitary-adrenal responses to the stress of treadmill exercise: Physiologic adaptations to physical training. *N Engl J Med* 1987;316:1309–1315.
71. Lüthi JM, Howald H, Classen H, et al: Structural changes in skeletal muscle tissue with heavy-resistance exercise. *Int J Sports Med* 1986;7:123–127.
72. MacDougall JD: Adaptations of muscle to strength training; a cellular approach, in Saltin B (ed): *Biochemistry of Exercise VI: Metabolic Regulation and Its Significance*. Champaign, Human Kinetics, 1986, pp 501–513.
73. MacDougall JD: Morphological changes in human skeletal muscle following strength training and immobilization, in Jones NL, McCartney N, McComas, AJ (eds): *Human Muscle Power*. Champaign, Human Kinetics, 1986, pp 269–288.
74. MacDougall JD, Sale DG, Moroz JR, et al: Mitochondrial volume density in human skeletal muscle following heavy resistance training. *Med Sci Sports Exerc* 1979;11:164–166.
75. Mackinnon LT, Chick TW, VanAs A, et al: The effect of exercise on secretory and natural immunity. *Adv Exp Med Biol* 1987;216A:869–876.
76. Matveyev L: *Fundamentals of Sports Training*. Moscow, Progress Publishers, 1981.
77. McArdle WD, Katch FI, Pechar GS: Comparison of continuous and discontinuous treadmill and bicycle tests for max Vo_2. *Med Sci Sports Exerc* 1973;5:156–160.
78. Milesis CA, Pollock ML, Bah MD, et al: Effects of different durations of physical training on cardiorespiratory function, body composition, and serum lipids. *Res Q* 1976;47:716–725.
79. Moody DL, Wilmore JH, Girandola RN, et al: The effects of a jogging program on the body composition of normal and obese high school girls. *Med Sci Sports* 1972;4:210–213.

80. Moritani T, DeVries HA: Neural factors versus hypertrophy in the time course of muscle strength gain. *Am J Phys Med* 1979;58:115–130.
81. Noble BJ: *Physiology of Exercise and Sport*. St. Louis, Times Mirror/Mosby, 1986.
82. Patton JF, Daniels WL, Vogel JA: Aerobic power and body fat of men and women during army basic training. *Aviat Space Environ Med* 1980;51:492–496.
83. Pollock ML: The quantification of endurance training programs. *Exerc Sports Sci Rev* 1973;1:155–188.
84. Pollock ML, Broida J, Kendrick Z, et al: Effects of training two days per week at different intensities on middle-aged men. *Med Sci Sports* 1972;4:192–197.
85. Pollock ML, Cureton TK, Greninger L: Effects of frequency of training on working capacity, cardiovascular function and body composition of adult men. *Med Sci Sports Exerc* 1969;1:70–74.
86. Pollack ML, Jackson A: Body composition: Measurement and changes resulting from physical training, in Burke EJ (ed): *Toward an Understanding of Human Performance*. Ithaca, Movement Publications, 1977, pp 31–36.
87. Person RS, Kudina LP: Discharge frequency and discharge pattern of human motor units during voluntary contraction of muscle. *Electroencephalogr Clin Neurophysiol* 1972;32:471–483.
88. Rowell LB: Human cardiovascular adjustments to exercise and thermal stress. *Physiol Rev* 1974;54:75–159.
89. Sale DG: Influence of exercise and training on motor unit activation. *Exerc Sport Sci Rev* 1987;15:95–151.
90. Sale DG: Neural adaptation in strength and power training, in Jones NL, McCartney N, McComas AJ (eds): *Human Muscle Power*. Champaign, Human Kinetics, 1986, pp 289–307.
91. Sale DG: Neural adaptation to resistance training. *Med Sci Sports Exerc* 1988;20(suppl):S135-S145.
92. Saltin B: Physiological effects of physical conditioning. *Med Sci Sports Exerc* 1969;1:50–56.
93. Saltin B, Astrand PO: Maximal oxygen uptake in athletes. *J Appl Physiol* 1967;23:353–358.
94. Saltin B, Blomqvist G, Mitchell JH, et al. Response to exercise after bed rest and after training. *Circulation* 1968;38(suppl 7):1–78.
95. Schaible TF, Scheuer J: Response of the heart to exercise training, in Zak R (ed): *Growth of the Heart in Health and Disease*. New York, Raven Press, 1984, pp 381–419.
96. Schantz PG: Plasticity of human skeletal muscle with special reference to effects of physical training on enzyme levels of the NADH shuttles and phenotypic expression of slow and fast myofibrillar proteins. *Acta Physiol Scand* 1986;558(suppl):1–62.
97. Scheuer J, Tipton CM: Cardiovascular adaptations to physical training. *Annu Rev Physiol* 1977;39:221–251.
98. Simon HB: Exercise and infection. *Phys Sportsmed* 1987;15:135–141.
99. Sjödin B, Svedenhag J: Applied physiology of marathon running. *Sports Med* 1985;2:83–99.
100. Staff PH: The effects of physical activity on joints, cartilage, tendons and ligaments. *Scand J Soc Med* 1982;29(suppl):59–63.
101. Staron RS, Hikida RS, Hagerman FC, et al: Human skeletal muscle fiber type adaptability to various workloads. *J Histochem Cytochem* 1984;32:146–152.
102. Stone MH: Implications for connective tissue and bone alterations resulting from resistance exercise training. *Med Sci Sports Exerc* 1988;20(suppl):S162-S168.

103. Tesch PA: Acute and long-term metabolic changes consequent to heavy-resistance exercise, in Marconnet P, Komi PV (eds): *Muscular Function in Exercise and Training*. Basel, Karger, 1987, pp 67–89.
104. Tesch PA: Skeletal muscle adaptations consequent to long-term heavy-resistance exercise. *Med Sci Sports Exerc* 1988;20(suppl):S132-S134.
105. Tesch PA, Komi PV, Häkkinen K: Enzymatic adaptations consequent to long-term strength training. *Int J Sports Med* 1987;8(suppl 1):66–69.
106. Thoden JS, Wilson BA, MacDougall JD: Testing aerobic power, in MacDougall JD, Wegner HA, Green HJ (eds): *Physiological Testing of the Elite Athlete*. Canadian Association of Sport Sciences, 1982, pp 39–60.
107. Tomasi TB, Trudeau FB, Czerwinski D, et al: Immune parameters in athletes before and after strenuous exercise. *J Clin Immunol* 1982;2:173–178.
108. Vogel JA, Patton JF, Mello RP, et al: An analysis of aerobic capacity in a large United States population. *J Appl Physiol* 1986;60:494–500.
109. Wasserman K, Hansen JE, Sue DY, et al: *Principles of Exercise Testing and Interpretation*. Philadelphia, Lea & Febiger, 1987.
110. Wilmore JH: Alterations in strength, body composition, and anthropometric measurements consequent to a 10-week weight training program. *Med Sci Sports* 1974;6:133–138.
111. Wilmore JH, Royce J, Girandola PH, et al: Physiological alterations resulting from a 10-week jogging program. *Med Sci Sports Exerc* 1970;2:7–14.
112. Wilt F: Training for competitive running, in Falls HB (ed): *Exercise Physiology*. New York, Academic Press, 1968, pp 395–414.

Chapter 46

Physiologic and Cellular Basis of Overtraining

Arthur C. Vailas, PhD
William P. Morgan, EdD
James C. Vailas, MD

Introduction

Exercise scientists, coaches, and athletes agree that success in endurance events requires progressive increases in the training stimulus, and that a high level of physical activity is a prerequisite for peak performance.[9,23,34,44] Overtraining, however, can lead to staleness, which is characterized by (1) elevated resting and/or exercise heart rates; (2) hypertension; (3) reduced $\dot{V}O_2$ maximum; (4) elevated resting creatine kinase activity, perceived exertion during submaximal exercise, and resting cortisol level; (5) decreased muscle glycogen and testosterone; and (6) mood disturbances, such as depression and/or chronic anxiety. Research on elite distance runners shows that 60% of female and 66% of male athletes have experienced staleness during their competitive careers.[38,40,41,43] Although intense training sessions produce acute fatigue, the athlete can normally recuperate within 12 to 24 hours. For an overtrained athlete, performance in competition falls below expected or customary levels.[15,34,41,43,56]

Much early literature on overtraining syndromes investigated their underlying psychobiologic factors. These studies encouraged physiologists to investigate the underlying factors leading to or resulting from overtraining.[21,37,38,49] Research on swimmers showed that psychological distress (increased depression, anxiety, anger, fatigue, and confusion) and decreases in psychic vigor occur in a systematic and consistent manner during periods of increased training.[34] Thus, while vigorous exercise produces positive affective changes such as decreased anxiety and depression, overtraining leads to negative changes that affect performance and mood.[26,41–43] Mood disturbances occur in progressive direct proportion to increments in the training loads. In swimmers, a predictable, dose-response relationship was shown to exist between the global mood disturbance and the training distances swum.[26,47] Mood disturbances can be reduced by decreasing the training load, and the improvement is also in a direct proportional relationship. So, it is possible to increase and decrease mood disturbances by varying the training load.

The psychological manifestations associated with overtraining syndromes sometimes result from underlying alterations in the steady-state relationships of immune and endocrine interactions. Disturbing the hormonal and immune control of tissue homeostasis induces changes in tissue turnover (steady-state rate constants for anabolic and catabolic reactions) and potentially alters the morphologic, biomechanical, and biochemical properties of musculoskeletal tissues.

Interactions With Immune and Endocrine Systems

Overtraining changes the interactions between hormonal and immune mechanisms and thereby affects musculoskeletal homeostasis. Evidence suggests that hypothalamic dysfunction may develop in overtrained athletes.[1,5,15,19,22,25,46,63] Barron and associates[5] showed that pituitary hormone secretion in response to insulin-induced hypoglycemia was decreased in overtrained athletes. Overtrained athletes also maintain a higher level of plasma corticosteroids (cortisol and corticosterone) and a higher exercise-induced increase in plasma catecholamines.[17,25,30,31,46,48,63] High-intensity exercise increases sympathoadrenal activity.[19,25,30,48] Increases in plasma titers of catecholamines and glucocorticoids can cause immune suppression.[19,25] Recently, Gmünder and associates[19] studied immunologic parameters in those engaged in marathon training programs. He found a marked decrease in lymphocyte reactivity toward the mitogen, concanavalin A, and that leukocytosis increased 2.8 times. Other studies found a significant rise in lymphocytosis and neutrophilia.[19,25] Increases in adrenergic activity enhance the production of cyclic AMP, an inhibitor of both lymphocyte T- and B-cell responses to mitogens.[25]

Modification of endocrine-regulated immune responses associated with strenuous exercise becomes phasic at various stages during exercise and recovery.[19,25] For example, Gmünder and associates[19] showed that T-lymphocyte subsets (cytotoxic T cells, helper T cells, suppressor T cells), muscle soreness, and lymphocyte and leukocyte counts vary throughout the exercise-recovery cycle in opposite phase of the fluctuating plasma levels of cortisol and catecholamines. Blood analyses of B lymphocytes and T lymphocytes show increases 48 hours after a marathon race, compared with blood concentrations reported for the early postexercise recovery interval. In essence, strenuous exercise training programs modify cell-mediated and antibody-mediated immunity. Theoretically, sustained increases in basal plasma corticosteroids maintain some degree of immune suppression and enhance the susceptibility of overtrained athletes to low-grade infections, a frequent symptom associated with overtraining syndromes.[30]

Alterations in the endocrine and immune systems' control over tissue homeostasis has been described as the steady-state equilibrium between tissue anabolism and catabolism.[25,30] Overtraining and staleness are characterized by an increase in tissue catabolic activity.[30,43] Mechanisms associated with exercise-induced tissue catabolism are not well understood. Recent studies indicate that increased catabolic activity results partly from changes in immune and endocrine function.[25,30]

Catabolic Phase

Overtraining can increase catabolism,[3,30] which is manifested over time. For example, exercise alters many circulating hormones and affects the basal metabolism of musculoskeletal tissues.[3,7,58,59,61] The combined effects of cyclic mechanical stresses and variations in circulating hormones result in an increase in the overall basal metabolism of connective tissue cells.[7,50,58–62] Therefore, it is important to evaluate time-course alterations in connective tissue anabolism and catabolism during exercise and recovery periods. Overtraining syndromes could involve a progressive increase in the steady-state equilibrium between tissue anabolism and catabolism with a gradual shift toward more catabolic activity. This could increase the likelihood of symptoms developing and result in a net increase in the catabolism of many musculoskeletal tissues.[1,2,4,8,11–14,17,24,36,45,54,55,57]

Increases in tissue catabolism are often initiated by enhanced activity of tissue proteases.[6,19,35,54,55] One possible contributor to this activity involves the increased production of interleukin-1.[17,35] Evans and associates[17] studied the blood changes of interleukin-1 in highly trained and untrained men. They reported an increase in the interleukin-1 concentration of serum in trained athletes at rest compared with untrained subjects. They suggested that the increase in basal interleukin-1 activity of highly trained athletes may result from the progressive increase in muscle tissue catabolism associated with high-intensity exercise. They also reported a delayed increase in the ratio of urinary 3-methylhistidine to creatine after a single bout of strenuous exercise, occurring ten days after the exercise training period. This increase may be associated with the delayed onset of muscle soreness.[4,30]

Muscle soreness has a high correlation with increased muscle damage,[4,13,14,29,36,54,57] and several investigators have studied the effects of serum and tissue creatine kinase changes associated with strenuous exercise.[2,17,53] Increases in both tissue and serum creatine kinase activity have been used as clinical markers to indicate muscle injury.[2,8,17,53] Pronounced increases in creatine kinase activity are usually observed in the recovery phase after strenuous exerise.[2,8,17,53] The elevated levels of serum creatine kinase usually return to "normal" within 24 hours. However, in overtrained athletes, the serum creatine kinase levels do not return to baseline levels.[8] This indicates that high levels of strenuous exercise can increase the catabolism of musculoskeletal tissues.

Possible mechanisms associated with enhanced protease activity include: (1) macrophage induction of interleukin-1 production[6,17,19,25,35]; (2) induction of protease activity by increases in calcium influx across the membrane as a result of cycle strains imposed on tissue membranes[3,4,6,54,55,57]; and (3) cortisol binding to membrane receptors in gluconeogenesis.[3,19,25,31] No one has measured specific protease activities in connective tissues in animal models using strenuous exercise programs. However, indirect evidence suggests an increase in tissue protease activity for some dense fibrous connective tissues.[12,24,39,45,57] Recently, Curwin and associates[12] reported an increase in tendon collagen deposition and degradation in growing chickens as a result of high-intensity exercise. Others have used mice and rats to show that exercise increases turnover of tendon collagen and proteoglycans.[7,24,27,39,58–60] Both hormonal and mechanical factors may activate various inducers involved in the synthesis and degradation of connective-tissue matrix proteins.[58–60] Connective-tissue cells synthesize and secrete matrix metalloproteinases that can degrade the extracellular matrix.[6] Exercise increases musculoskeletal tissue cyclic AMP production, prostaglandin production (especially prostaglandin E_2), calcium influx, and hormone-mediated receptor activation of protease activity and decreases intracellular pH.[3] Variations of these homeostatic factors can activate a variety of cell proteases.

Most of the research on overuse and muscle injury associated with high levels of muscle activity has focused on skeletal muscle. The findings of these studies may have some relevance to overtraining, because overtrained athletes have a high probability of incurring muscle injuries. The possibility of connective tissue damage in overtrained athletes has received minimal attention.

High-intensity exercise induces muscle damage.[3,4,54,55] This rhabdomyolysis (degradation of muscle tissue) results from a number of possible mechanisms, including (1) an imbalance of calcium influx resulting in reduced mitochondral function and production of adenosine triphosphatase, (2) an increase in intracellular pH, which in turn destabilizes lysosomal membranes, and (3) macrophage induction of various lymphokines and monokines, enhancing protease activity. The observed rhabdomyolysis is often associated with degradation of proteoglycans and other basement membrane extracellular proteins.[3,4,54,55] Thus, overtraining results from a progressive increase in basal proteolytic activity of musculoskeletal tissues. All high-intensity exercise programs may not induce musculoskeletal tissue damage. According to some investigators, however, certain types of specific exercises have a higher probability of inducing tissue damage.[3,17,30]

Exercise Specificity

Recently scientists questioned the importance of exercise specificity and the overtraining syndrome.[3] Data from human and animal studies support the hypothesis of increased muscle damage with eccentric-type exercises.[3,4,17] The activation pattern of muscles during limb locomotion often includes eccentric contractions.[3,4]

The magnitude of an eccentric contraction may correlate with the incidence of muscle injury, as the greater the eccentric load imposed on muscle, the higher the probability of muscle damage. Eccentric exercises may also enhance the magnitude and frequency of cyclic strains. Increases in the strain environment imposed on connective tissues may subsequently induce a higher turnover of matrix components. For example, animal studies comparing swimming and treadmill exercise showed that ligament adaptation occurred in exercises that involved grade running but that little adaptation occurred with swimming.[58,59] These differences may be attributed to the differences in strain environments. Nevertheless, the soft-tissue load history is important for evaluating the adaptive response of connective tissues to exercise. Therefore, the criteria for evaluating the exercise stimulus must include the distribution of in vivo loads on various connective tissues and the resulting alterations in systemic markers.

A second evaluation criterion is the neuroendocrine response associated with the strenuousness of exercise. Different exercise intensities elicit different changes in the release of circulating hormones. For example, high-resistance weight training and sprinting elicit endocrine responses quite different from those elicited by prolonged high-intensity running.[1,5,22,46,48,63] Therefore, both the biomechanical modalities and the endocrine responses to a given type of exercise must be considered in evaluating an overtraining syndrome. More research is needed to develop uniform diagnoses of overtraining syndromes.

Clinical Assessment of Overtraining Syndromes

Proper clinical assessment of an overtraining syndrome requires a thorough understanding of the syndrome. However, many of the clinical criteria for the overtraining syndrome are unclear and have been extrapolated from anecdotal information. In addition, overtraining syndromes may be increasing as organized sports expand and the level of competition increases.

Some clinical manifestations include microtrauma to the various connective-tissue structures. During periods of excessive training (overtraining), these structures are stressed beyond their physiologic limits of adaptation. The result is structural damage, clinically known as injury. The biomechanics of injured tissue alter and these alterations are manifested clinically as a decrease in performance.

Athletes who want to be more competitive must train longer and more vigorously. Improper training with inadequate rest periods and excessive loads can lead to overtraining syndrome. Injuries are often reported in elite athletes between the ages of 20 and 29 years and in noncompetitive athletes between the ages of 30 and 49 years. Injuries are more prevalent in athletes who have been training regularly for at least two years.[51,52] The majority of the injuries, aproximately 80%, occur in endurance and one-person sports that require a specific skill technique for mastery.[28,51] For example, tennis players typically develop shoulder (rotator cuff tears) and elbow (tennis elbow) problems. In the general population, 80% of the injuries involve the lower extremities, with 28% involving the knees and 21% involving the feet.[51]

Among runners, 30% eventually suffer an overtraining problem of the patellofemoral joint.[56]

Overtraining injuries involving specific areas of the body are commonly sport-specific. For example, soccer players develop an adductor syndrome that involves a chronic strain of the adductor musculotendinous complex of the inner thigh, a muscle used repetitively for lateral movement and ball control. Competitive swimmers develop "swimmer's shoulder," a posterior instability of the glenohumeral joint as a result of increased ligamentous laxity, muscle imbalance, and anterior shoulder tightness.[18]

The clinical diagnosis of overtraining syndrome remains a challenge because of its broad definition. An athlete who demonstrates excessive soreness, decreased body weight, increased injury rates, plateaus in strengthening, or decreased performance may suffer from overtraining syndrome. In comparison, an athlete who continues to perform without any of these symptoms, but does have elevated plasma hydroxyproline levels during training may also have overtraining syndrome.[45] Overtraining syndromes follow a clinical spectrum ranging from the molecular level where asymptomatic biochemical changes in the form of specific protein abnormalities occur to the tissue level where symptomatic changes in the form of inflammation from musculoskeletal injury occur.

Most of the information for clinically diagnosing overtraining syndromes derives from detectable abnormalities at the tissue level that result primarily from the inflammatory process. Any major tissue becomes inflamed if it is subjected to repetitive excessive stress resulting in microtrauma. The process involves microbleeding, swelling, pressure, and necrosis.[51] The body's normal reaction to inflammation is increased temperature, redness, tenderness, and swelling.

Common clinical diagnostic techniques for evaluating overtraining injuries focus on the changes associated with inflammation. The simplest and most basic is the physical examination. The examiner looks for the common signs of swelling, tenderness, increased tactile temperature, and redness. In severe cases, all these signs are usually present, but less severe injuries may demonstrate only one or two. Another physical finding is an asymmetry in the musculoskeletal anatomy. For example, young runners may exhibit muscle imbalance with strong quadriceps and weak hamstring muscles, and gymnasts may develop hyperlordosis of the lumbar spine and tight hamstrings. These asymmetries may have been present before the injury and may have predisposed the athlete to the injury.

Other intrinsic factors associated with overtraining injuries in runners are patellofemoral malalignment, hyperpronation and flatness of the feet, and Achilles tendon tightness. Other factors to consider are skeletal maturity, diet, metabolic diseases, sex, and race.[51,56] The diagnostic challenge occurs in an athlete with normal physical findings but a history of exercise-induced pain or postactivity soreness. The clinician must rely on the history to support the diagnosis and look for extrinsic factors such as changes in training technique, equipment, and terrain that may contribute to the problem. The subjective symptoms of inflammation (stiffness, swelling, and soreness of the involved tissue) are also helpful. The athlete typically complains of difficulty in initiating movement, of early fatigue, of muscle spasms, or of recurrent injuries.

Technological Advances in Clinical Assessment

Technology can facilitate the diagnosis of injuries in overtrained athletes. Telethermography detects skin temperature changes that may occur if an underlying process alters the surrounding microvasculature and can be used to monitor the clinical response to treatment. A temperature difference must exist between the injured area and the matching normal area. The test is more sensitive in acute inflammation when the tissues are likely to be hyperemic. The technique may be more useful than subjective criteria in quantifying the injury. Proper testing requires special rooms for controlling temperature and air flow.[20]

Ultrasonography evaluates the echo images produced by tissues subjected to sound waves. It can demonstrate chronic changes in connective tissue that result in fibrosis or mucoid degeneration.[10,32] It is frequently used for injuries of the rotator cuff, Achilles tendon, and patellar tendon, and is being used more for musculoskeletal imaging because it is noninvasive and inexpensive and requires minimal testing time. However, this technique depends heavily on the experience of the technician and the sonographer.

Nuclear scanning with radioactive serum markers can be used for bone disturbances. Similar isotopes are used for detecting changes in nonosseous structures using SPECT imaging (serial image with coned views). Clinical enities such as enthesopathies, compartment syndromes, and muscle strains can be demonstrated scintigraphically because the involved tissue shows increased isotope uptake. However, during the chronic stages of the injury, this difference may not exist because vascularity changes as the injury moves from the acute to the chronic stage, and may seem normal. The test requires injection of a radioactive isotope, in addition to time-consuming serial scanning intervals.[16,33,36]

Magnetic resonance imaging is becoming popular because it is versatile and because several structures can be imaged at the same sitting. It does not expose the patient to ionizing radition but utilizes magnetic fields and reproduces near-anatomic images with high resolution. Changing the imaging sequences can show structural connective-tissue changes resulting from biochemical changes within the tissue (likely to be noted as a change in contrast of the image). Magnetic resonance imaging is commonly used for evaluating meniscal injuries, ligament tears, tendon tears, herniated intervertebral disks, and ischemic changes in tissues. It is expensive, however, and the limited availability of equipment has restricted its use.[10]

References

1. Adlercreutz H, Härkönen M, Kuoppasalmi K, et al: Effect of training on plasma anabolic and catabolic steroid hormones and their response during physical exercise. *Int J Sports Med* 1986;7(suppl 1):27–28.
2. Apple FS, Rogers MA, Casal DC, et al: Creatine kinase-MB isoenzyme adaptations in stressed human skeletal muscle of marathon runners. *J Appl Physiol* 1985;59:149–153.
3. Armstrong RB: Muscle damage and endurance events. *Sports Med* 1986;3:370–381.
4. Armstrong RB, Ogilvie RW, Schwane JA: Eccentric exercise-induced injury to rat skeletal muscle. *J Appl Physiol* 1983;54:80–93.
5. Barron JL, Noakes TD, Levy W, et al: Hypothalamic dysfunction in overtrained athletes. *J Clin Endocrinol Metab* 1985;60:803–806.
6. Bejarano PA, Noelken ME, Suzuki K, et al: Degradation of basement membranes by human matrix metalloproteinase 3 (stromelysin). *Biochem J* 1988;256:413–419.
7. Booth FW, Gould EW: Effects of training and disuse on connective tissue. *Exerc Sport Sci Rev* 1975;3:83–112.
8. Burke ER, Falsetti RD, Feld GS, et al: Creatine kinase levels in competitive swimmers during a season of training. *Scand J Sports Sci* 1982;4:1–4.
9. Costill DL, King DS, Thomas R, et al: Effects of reduced training on muscular power in swimmers. *Phys Sportsmed* 1985;13:94–101.
10. Crass JR, Craig EV: Non-invasive imaging of the rotator cuff. *Orthopedics* 1988;11:57–64.
11. Cundy T, Bartlett M, Bishop M, et al: Plasma hydroxyproline in uremia: Relationships with histologic and biological indices of bone turnover. *Metab Bone Dis Relat Res* 1983;4:297–303.
12. Curwin SL, Vailas AC, Wood J: Immature tendon adaptation to strenuous exercise. *J Appl Physiol* 1988;65:2297–2301.
13. Demos MA, Gitin EL, Kagen LJ: Exercise myoglobinemia and acute exertional rhabdomyolysis. *Arch Intern Med* 1974;134:669–673.
14. Dohm GL, Barakat H, Stephenson TP, et al: Changes in muscle mitochondrial lipid composition resulting from training and exhaustive exercise. *Life Sci* 1975;17:1075–1080.
15. Dressendorfer RH, Wade CE, Iverson D: Decreased plasma testosterone in overtrained runners, abstract. *Med Sci Sports Exerc* 1987;19(suppl):S10.
16. Ehman RL, Berquist TH, McLeod RA: MR imaging of the musculoskeletal system: A 5-year appraisal. *Radiology* 1988;166:313–320.
17. Evans WJ, Meredith CN, Cannon JG, et al: Metabolic changes following eccentric exercise in trained and untrained men. *J Appl Physiol* 1986;61:1864–1868.
18. Fowler P: Swimmer problems. *Am J Sports Med* 1979;7:141–142.
19. Gmünder FK, Lorenzi G, Bechler B, et al: Effect of long-term physical exercise on lymphocyte reactivity: Similarity to spaceflight reactions. *Aviat Space Environ Med* 1988;59:146–151.
20. Goodley: Musculoskeletal pain and thermography. *Acta Thermograph* 1980;5:1–3.
21. Griffith CR: *Psychology of Coaching.* New York, Charles Scribner's Sons, 1962.
22. Häkkinen K, Pakarinen A, Alén M, et al: Relationships between training volume, physical performance capacity, and serum hormone concentrations during prolonged training in elite weight lifters. *Int J Sports Med* 1987;8(suppl 1):61–65.
23. Harre D (ed): *Principles of Sports Training.* Berlin, Sportverlag, 1982.

24. Heikkinen E, Vuori I: Effect of physical activity on the metabolism of collagen in aged mice. *Acta Physiol Scand* 1972;84:543–549.
25. Keast D, Cameron K, Morton AR: Exercise and the immune response. *Sports Med* 1988;5:248–267.
26. Kereszty A: Overtraining, in Larson LA (ed): *Encyclopedia of Sport Sciences and Medicine.* New York, Macmillan, 1971, pp 218–222.
27. Kiiskinen A: Physical training and connective tissues in young mice: Physical properties of Achilles tendons and long bones. *Growth* 1977;41:123–137.
28. Kozar B, Lord R: Overuse injury in the young athlete. *Phys Sportsmed* 1983;11:116–121.
29. Kuipers H, Drukker J, Frederik PM, et al: Muscle degeneration after exercise in rats. *Int J Sports Med* 1983;4:45–51.
30. Kuipers H, Keizer HA: Overtraining in elite athletes. *Sports Med* 1988;6:79–92.
31. Kurowski TT, Chatterton RT Jr, Hickson RC: Countereffects of compensatory overload and glucocorticoids in skeletal muscle: Androgen and glucocorticoid cytosol receptor binding. *J Steroid Biochem* 1984;21:137–145.
32. Laine HR, Harjula AL, Peltokallio P: Ultrasonography as a differential diagnostic aid in achillodynia. *J Ultrasound Med* 1987;6:351–362.
33. Matin P: Basic principles of nuclear medicine techniques for detection and evaluation of trauma and sports medicine injuries. *Semin Nucl Med* 1988;18:90–112.
34. Matveyev L: *Fundamentals of Sports Training.* Moscow, Progress Publishers, 1981.
35. Mauviel A, Temime N, Charron D, et al: Interleukin-1 α and β induce interleukin-1 β gene expression in human dermal fibroblasts. *Biochem Biophys Res Commun* 1988;156:1209–1214.
36. McCully KK, Kent JA, Chance B: Application of ^{31}P magnetic resonance spectroscopy to the study of athletic performance. *Sports Med* 1988;5:312–321.
37. McNair DM, Lorr M, Droppleman LF: *Profile of Mood States Manual.* San Diego, Educational and Industrial Testing Service, 1971.
38. Mellerowicz H, Barron DK: Overtraining, in Larson LA (ed): *Encylopedia of Sport Sciences and Medicine.* New York, Macmillan, 1971, pp 1310–1312.
39. Michna H: Morphometric analysis of loading-induced changes in collagen-fibril populations in young tendons. *Cell Tissue Res* 1984;236:465–470.
40. Morehouse LE, Rasch PJ: *Scientific Basis of Athletic Training.* Philadelphia, WB Saunders, 1958.
41. Morgan WP: Affective beneficence of vigorous physical activity. *Med Sci Sports Exerc* 1985;17:94–100.
42. Morgan WP: Selected psychological factors limiting performance: A mental health model, in Clarke DH, Eckert HM (eds): *Limits of Human Performance.* Champaign, Human Kinetics, 1985, pp 70–80.
43. Morgan WP, Brown DR, Raglin JS, et al: Psychological monitoring of overtraining and staleness. *Br J Sports Med* 1987;21:107–114.
44. Morgan WP, Costill DL, Flynn MG, et al: Mood disturbance following increased training in swimmers. *Med Sci Sports Exerc* 1988;20:408–414.
45. Murguia MJ, Vailas AC, Mandelbaum B: Elevated plasma hydroxyproline: A possible risk factor associated with connective tissue injuries during overuse. *Am J Sports Med* 1988;16:660–664.
46. Näveri H, Kuoppasalmi K, Härkönen M: Metabolic and hormonal changes in moderate and intense long-term running exercises. *Int J Sports Med* 1985;6:276–281.

47. O'Connor PJ, Corrigan DL: Influence of short-term cycling on salivary cortisol levels. *Med Sci Sports Exerc* 1987;19:224–228.
48. Odink J, Van der Beek EJ, Van den Berg H, et al: Effect of work load on free and sulfate-conjugated plasma catecholamines, prolactin, and cortisol. *Int J Sports Med* 1986;7:352–357.
49. Parmenter DC: Some medical aspects of the training of college athletes. *Boston Med Surg J* 1923;189:45–50.
50. Pedrini-Mille A, Pedrini VA, Maynard JA, et al: Response of immature chicken meniscus to strenuous exercise: Biochemical studies of proteoglycan and collagen. *J Orthop Res* 1988;6:196–204.
51. Peterson L, Rendstrom P: General principles of sports injuries: Overuse syndromes, in Peterson L (ed): *Sports Injuries: Their Prevention and Treatment*. Chicago, Year Book, 1986.
52. Pollock ML, Cureton TK, Greininger L: Effects of frequency of training on work capacity, cardiovascular function and body composition of adult men. *Med Sci Sports Exerc* 1969;1:70–74.
53. Rogers MA, Stull GA, Apple FS: Creatine kinase isoenzyme activities in men and women following a marathon race. *Med Sci Sports Exerc* 1985;17:679–682.
54. Salminen A: Lysosomal changes in skeletal muscles during the repair of exercise injuries in muscle fibers. *Acta Physiol Scand* 1985;539(suppl):1–31.
55. Salminen A, Vihko V: Autophagic response to strenuous exercise in mouse skeletal muscle fibers. *Virchows Arch* 1984;45:97–106.
56. Stanish WD: Overuse injuries in athletes: A perspective. *Med Sci Sports Exerc* 1984;16:1–7.
57. Takala TE, Vuori J, Anttinen H, et al: Prolonged exercise causes an increase in the activity of galactosylhydroxylysyl glucosyltransferase and in the concentration of type III procollagen aminopropeptide in human serum. *Pflügers Arch* 1986;407:500–503.
58. Tipton CM, Matthes RD, Maynard JA, et al: The influence of physical activity on ligaments and tendons. *Med Sci Sports* 1975;7:165–175.
59. Tipton CM, Vailas AC, Matthes RD: Experimental studies on the influences of physical activity on ligaments, tendons and joints: A brief review. *Acta Med Scand* 1986;711(suppl):157–168.
60. Vailas AC, Pedrini VA, Pedrini-Mille A, et al: Patellar tendon matrix changes associated with aging and voluntary exercise. *J Appl Physiol* 1985;58:1572–1576.
61. Vailas AC, Tipton CM, Laughlin HL, et al: Physical activity and hypophysectomy on the aerobic capacity of ligaments and tendons. *J Appl Physiol* 1978;44:542–546.
62. Vailas AC, Zernicke RF, Matsuda J, et al: Adaptations of rat knee meniscus to prolonged exercise. *J Appl Physiol* 1986;60:1031–1034.
63. Vanhelder WP, Radomski MW, Goode RC, et al: Hormonal and metabolic response to three types of exercise of equal duration and external work output. *Eur J Appl Physiol* 1985;54:337–342.

Chapter 47

Myotendinous Adaptation to Conditioning

Ronald Zernicke, PhD
Barbara Loitz, PhD, PT

Muscle, tendon, and myotendinous junction constitute a unique functional unit among soft tissues because of their adaptability to various loading situations. During training and conditioning, skeletal muscles generate contractile forces with diverse rates of tension development, peak tension magnitudes, and durations. Tendons and myotendinous junctions must adapt to the contractile profile to transmit the developed tension and produce the intended movement safely and effectively. This chapter focuses on the morphology, the dynamic loading, and the functional adaptations that occur in muscles, tendons, and myotendinous junctions during training or injury. The morphologic and mechanical status of these tissues relates to their susceptibility to injury and subsequent tissue inflammation.

Morphology

Muscle

Skeletal muscle consists of two elements: contractile proteins and a viscoelastic network of connective tissue. The connective tissue forms the series- and parallel-elastic components of muscle. These components provide important functional stiffness to enhance the transmission of tension. There are important cellular interactions that direct muscle's physiologic responses, but the adaptation, or injury, of muscle can best be described by considering the mechanics of its functional units.

The myofibril is the contractile unit of muscle, with hundreds of myofibrils combining to form a single muscle fiber[5] (Fig. 1). Longitudinally, the myofibril has a striated appearance with transverse bands of repeating units called sarcomeres. The striations are created by the overlapping of the thick and thin contractile proteins, myosin and actin. Muscle shortening occurs when the myosin structure that allows interaction between the actin and myosin filaments changes, increasing the overlap between the fibers and decreasing sarcomere length. The

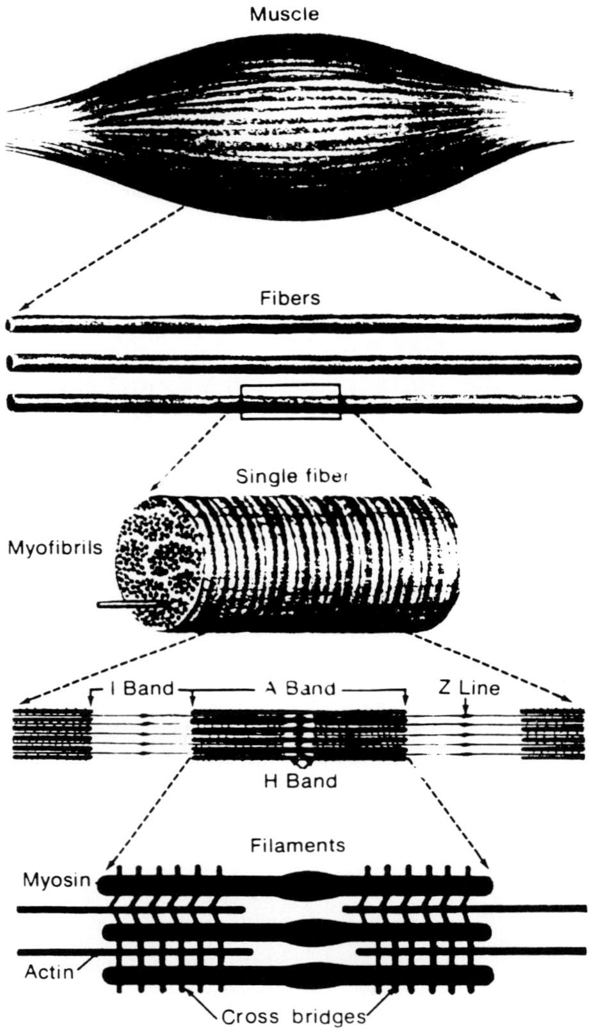

Fig. 1 *Diagrammatic dissection of a striated muscle. Each myofibril consists of alternating dark and light bands resulting from overlapping myosin and actin filaments. The sarcomere extends between Z lines and contains isotropic (I) and anisotropic (A) bands. (Reproduced with permission from Brooks SM, Paynton-Brooks N:* The Human Body: Structure and Function in Health and Disease, *ed 2. St. Louis, CV Mosby, 1980.)*

rate of actin-myosin interaction and the subsequent force developed depend on myosin's ability to hydrolyze adenosine triphosphate (ATP). Muscle fibers with greater myofibrillar adenosine triphosphatase (ATPase) activity are fast-twitch fibers, while those with less ATPase activity are slow-twitch fibers.[6,10]

Slow- and fast-twitch fibers differ not only in the rate of tension development, but also in the maximum tension that each fiber can produce and in the duration of tetanic tension that can be maintained. In humans, fast glycolytic fibers can develop a twitch tension of approximately 490 mN, but tetanic tension falls to less than 50% of maximum within two minutes. Slow oxidative fibers typically generate less than 49 mN of twitch tension, but can maintain more than 75% of tetanic tension for more than an hour. An intermediate group of fast-twitch oxidative fibers exists that can develop a peak twitch tension of about 200 mN and maintain 50% of peak tetanic tension for as long as five minutes and 25% of peak tetanic tension for an hour.[12] Although a muscle and its tendon are normally well matched,[13] these diverse contractile characteristics challenge muscle connective tissues, tendon, and myotendinous junction to respond to the variations in dynamics during training, without sustaining damage.

Collagen fibers in skeletal muscles provide structural support to assure proper muscle-fiber alignment. They also have an important role in transmitting contractile forces.[4] Muscle collagen is arranged in three layers: the epimysium surrounds the entire muscle, the perimysium separates muscle fascicles and offers structural support, and the endomysium surrounds individual muscle cells and links the myocytes to the numerous capillary beds. During muscle contractions, force transmission depends on the longitudinally arranged collagen bundles found primarily in the perimysium and epimysium. When a muscle is stretched, collagen helps distribute force across the entire muscle.

Borg and Caulfield[4] noted differences in the form and arrangement of connective-tissue layers among various skeletal muscles. Fast-twitch muscle contains well-developed perimysium with large collagen fiber bundles (1,500 to 1,800 nm in diameter); this may be important for efficiently transmitting rapidly developed contractile forces. Perimysium of slow-twitch, postural muscles tends to have smaller collagen bundles (800 to 1,000 nm in diameter) arranged both parallel and circumferential to the myocytes. Slow-twitch muscles contain more extensive endomysium and perimysium layers than fast-twitch muscles. This reflects the role of collagen in supporting the rich capillary supply of the slow-twitch fibers.[24]

Muscle connective tissue and contractile elements combine to form a dynamic system that performs movements with the lowest expenditure of energy by taking advantage of the viscoelastic characteristics of the tissues. Although concentric and eccentric contractions are often considered separate phenomena, each rarely occurs alone in normal movements. Instead, eccentric and concentric contractions follow one another, creating a stretch-shorten cycle that uses the elastic energy stored during the stretching to enhance the subsequent shortening contraction to optimize the force output of the final action (concentric contraction).[22] The increased tension does not come without a price, however, because exercise-related muscle damage is linked to repeated eccentric contractions.

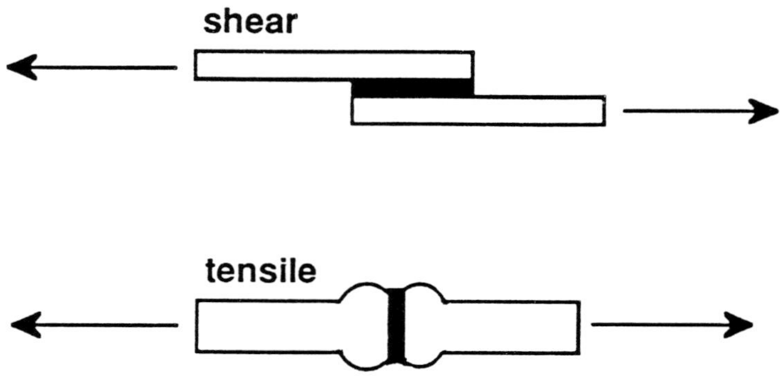

Fig. 2 *Schema of a joint loaded in shear and tension. Arrows indicate loading direction. (Adapted with permission from Tidball JG: The geometry of actin filament-membrane associations can modify adhesive strength of the myotendinous junction.* Cell Motil *1983;3:439–447.)*

Tendon

Tendon is a composite material containing collagen primarily and small amounts of mucopolysaccharides (primarily hyaluronic acid) and elastic fibers.[20] Under a light microscope, tendon appears crimped and wavelike because of the buckling phenomena created by the matrix impinging on collagen fibers.[7] Loading unfolds the crimped pattern and gives tendon a load-deformation curve with a characteristic "toe" region of low stiffness. This may protect the tendon from damage during rapid force development. As the crimping disappears and the collagen fibers transmit tension, tendon load and elongation retain a linear relationship until collagen exceeds its elastic limit. If the elongation continues, even with only small increases in load, microfailure and permanent deformation will result. Loads that exceed collagen's maximum strength will rupture collagen fibrils and, eventually, the tendon.

Myotendinous Junction

The myotendinous junction is a specialized region joining intracellular myofibrils to extracellular collagen fibers. The myotendinous junction is a four-layered region of longitudinal infoldings connecting the actin filament of a terminal sarcomere to tendon collagen fibers.[30,39,40] The membranous foldings increase the surface area and reduce stress on the junction during contractile-force transmission. In a circular paraboloid model, the surface area of the myotendinous junction is 22.2 times greater than the junctional area of a cell that ends as a right-circular cylinder.[36] Tidball[36] estimated that a fast-twitch myotendinous junctional membrane bears an average stress of 15 kPa. He also emphasized the significance of the infoldings relative to the

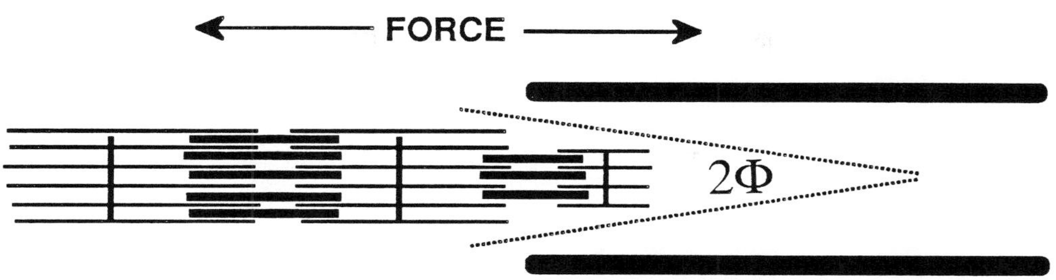

Fig. 3 *Diagram of a myotendinous junction. Muscle force is applied parallel to the longitudinal axes of the myofilaments and the collagen fibers. The junctional membrane lies at an angle relative to the myofilaments. (Adapted with permission from Tidball JG: The geometry of actin filament-membrane associations can modify adhesive strength of the myotendinous junction.* Cell Motil *1983;3:439–447.)*

angle between the sarcolemma membrane and the collagen fibril.[37] The strength of an adhesive junction such as the myotendinous junction depends both on the properties of the adjoining structures and on the orientation of forces across the junction. Junctions loaded in shear, where force is parallel to the membrane surface, are stronger than junctions with a large tensile component perpendicular to the membrane (Fig. 2). In a healthy fast-twitch cell, Tidball[36] estimated the angle to be 4.3 degrees with most of the force being a shear component (Fig. 3). Atrophied cells developed a junction angle of 9.1 degrees, with more than twice the tensile component of a healthy myotendinous junction. Tidball suggested that the increased probability of myotendinous junction failure among atrophied cells is related to the increase in tensile component at the junction.

Dynamic Loading

Muscle-Tendon Units

Knowledge of in vivo loads sustained by muscle-tendon units during movement provides important information about the neural control of movements and about muscle mechanics. In situ and in vitro muscle-tendon preparations describe components of muscle-tendon interactions, but in vivo recordings provide information about the neural modulation of muscle forces and about force magnitudes and durations.

Tendons in series with muscle fibers transmit the loads generated by the muscle's contractile elements.[31] When an active muscle is stretched, load distribution and elongation are determined by the stiffness of the respective tendinous and muscular components. Stretching isolated muscle fibers after isometric contraction shows an initial response of high short-range stiffness[32] from strains between actin-myosin crossbridges. As stretching continues, tension gradually increases, then plateaus. Tendon response to stretching differs from that of muscle, with an initial region of low stiffness until a strain of 2% to 4%. Above that, load and deformation increase on a linear basis until substantial damage to tendon fiber bundles occurs. Muscle-tendon stiffness, therefore, combines the responses of both the isolated myofibrillar and the tendinous components.[31]

Comparing the force and power output of muscles during locomotion and in related in situ experiments illustrates how the nervous system takes advantage of the short- and long-range stiffness characteristics of muscle. Gregor and associates[18] investigated output of cat soleus during treadmill locomotion and related isotonic loading conditions in situ. At the same shortening velocity, power generated during locomotion at 2.2 m/s was 2.6 times greater than the power generated in the isolated-muscle preparation. Recovery of strain energy stored in the active muscle-tendon unit during walking increased the muscle's subsequent mechanical output and may be a significant factor in magnifying the loading on muscle tissues during training. Gregor and associates[17] were also the first to report human in vivo muscle-tendon forces. A buckle transducer, surgically placed on the Achilles tendon, recorded forces generated by the triceps surae muscles during cycling. The peak Achilles tendon force of 660 N occurred as the stretch-shorten cycle augmented the force output of the ankle plantar flexors. Other studies inferred muscle stretch-shortening cycles from electromyography, but this was the first direct measurement of naturally occurring musculotendinous forces from the stretch-shorten phenomenon.

Myotendinous Junction

The myotendinous junction is viscoelastic, and mechanical behavior depends on load magnitude, frequency, and duration.[38] Such mechanical characteristics are important for comparing slow- and fast-twitch cells. Slow-twitch cells have loads of low amplitude and long duration, but fast-twitch cells generate high-amplitude, short-duration loads. These physiologic differences imply very different junctional loading conditions. Tidball and Daniel[38] suggested that duration of loading helps determine the degree of myotendinous membranous folding. Slow-twitch cells have a larger junctional surface area than fast-twitch cells. This prevents cell lysis under prolonged loading because the greater surface area reduces the stress across the membrane. Both peak force and rate of load application are important determinants of the myotendinous junction's characteristics.

Functional Adaptation and Injury

Muscle

Muscle adapts to endurance training by enhancing its oxidative potential[16] and to resistance training by increasing its myofibrillar diameter,[35] although muscle hypertrophy appears to occur most readily in untrained subjects rather than in athletes with previous strength training.[19] Evidence that muscle converts from one fiber type to another is limited. Schantz and associates[33] reported that the percentage of slow-twitch fibers in the human vastus lateralis does not change after long-duration endurance training. They noted only minimal (< 4%) conversion of one fast-fiber subtype to another in deltoid fibers. Muscle has the regenerative potential to repair myofibrillar damage sustained during most activities.[8]

Exercise can cause muscle injury and pain in several ways.[16,28,29] Direct trauma may cause obvious damage to the muscle and surrounding connective tissues and tendons. Decreased muscle pH or accumulation of metabolites such as lactate often result from sustained muscle contractions. Stopping the activity alleviates ischemic and metabolic-related pain. Prolonged eccentric contractions can cause myofibrillar tearing because the muscle develops excessive tension. The resulting pain differs from that caused by other factors; its onset is delayed until several hours after the activity and it lasts for several days. With the exception of direct trauma, muscle damage is related to overuse. Gollnick[16] stated that such muscle damage "... cannot be considered to be beneficial."

Armstrong[1] offered three explanations for exercise-induced muscle soreness: structural damage to muscle contractile or elastic elements caused by high tensile forces; cellular necrosis from cell-membrane damage and disruption of calcium homeostasis; and group IV sensory neuron stimulation as intracellular contents and byproducts of macrophage activity accumulate. No free nerve endings for pain exist in muscle fibers, so pain itself cannot be evidence of muscle fiber damage. In situ investigations reveal extensive muscle fiber damage after lengthening contractions and evidence supports damage induced by eccentric contraction, but isometric or shortening contractions do not cause fiber injury.[25,26]

Exercise-related muscle damage is linked to the mechanics of the eccentric contraction rather than to metabolic factors. Forced stretching of an actively contracting muscle produces greater tension than that generated by concentric or isometric contractions,[23] disrupts sarcomeres,[13] and damages the sarcolemma.[34] Severe damage of fibers occurs within the first five minutes of a repeated eccentric contraction, and then muscle fatigue prevents further injury. McCully and Faulkner[26] concluded that the fibers injured during long-term exercise are newly recruited fibers, rather than those fatigued by repeated contractions. Some studies found histologic evidence of injury in less than 5% of muscle fibers active during exercise,[2,41] but Fridén and associates[15] reported signs of injury in as much as 52% of muscle fibers in humans after exercise.

Fridén and associates[14] correlated morphologic changes in the muscle after eccentric contractions to intramuscular pressure readings taken before, during, and after exercise. After 400 submaximal eccentric contractions of ankle dorsiflexors (taking 20 minutes or less), biopsy specimens from the tibialis anterior showed no evidence of fiber necrosis and only limited inflammation.[14] Eccentrically contracted muscles had a significantly higher water content than concentrically contracted muscles, and their intramuscular pressure remained increased for a significantly longer period. This muscle fiber swelling may contribute to muscle soreness after eccentric contractions.

Eccentrically induced muscle pain rapidly diminishes or disappears with repeated activity. Serum creatine kinase, an indicator of myofibrillar damage,[21] peaks several days after exercise. When the same exercise is repeated one week later, however, there is minimal muscle pain and only slight increases in creatine kinase.[9] Newham[28] suggested that the first exercise bout damages or destroys a susceptible group of muscle fibers, perhaps those near the end of their life cycle. This leaves few susceptible fibers, limiting muscle soreness and creatine kinase release after repeated exercise.

Morphologic changes correlate with other indices of muscle damage after eccentric exercise.[21] Muscle biopsy specimens show little evidence of immediate cell necrosis, but within seven days, after the peak in serum creatine kinase, mononuclear cells infiltrate, and intracellular and extracellular acid phosphatase activity increases. This cellular infiltration appears to be in response to the muscle fiber damage[21] and unrelated to muscle degeneration. By day 21, biopsy samples show cell regeneration.

Tendon

Little quantitative information exists about exercise-related adaptations of tendon.[27,42] After one week of treadmill running, mice showed collagen fibril hyperplasia, hypertrophy, and larger cross-sectional areas in digital flexor tendons than did the sedentary controls.[27] After seven weeks of exercise, the mean fibril diameter was less in the test group, and signs of fibril splitting appeared. By the end of ten weeks, the flexor tendon cross-sectional areas were similar for both groups. Woo and associates[42] reported comparable results with immature swine flexor tendons. After one year of moderate exercise, there were no differences in mechanical properties or cross-sectional area between exercised and control animals. This indicates that flexor tendons may be able to adapt to exercise-induced changes in loading environment. There are no studies on how mature, weightbearing, extensor tendons adapt to exercise, but Curwin and associates[11] reported significant biochemical changes in immature tendon after strenuous exercise. High-intensity exercise delayed collagen maturation.[11] Labeled hydroxyproline activity, indicative of collagen synthesis, increased 46% in the Achilles tendon of immature chickens after eight weeks of exercise at 70% to 80% of maximum oxygen uptake. Tendon dry weight and collagen concentration did not change, however, suggesting that collagen degradation matched synthesis. However, mechanical tests are necessary to determine the exercise-related consequences of delayed collagen maturation and increased collagen turnover on immature tendon strength and stiffness.

Zamora and Marini[44] report marked changes in tendon morphology caused by compensatory overload in a rat plantaris tendon. Two weeks after removal of plantaris synergists, the plantaris tendon had replaced previously quiescent fibrocytes with active fibroblasts. The fibroblast cytoplasm contained many membrane-bound vacuoles, indicating active protein synthesis. Collagen bundles within the tendon were disrupted, leaving many empty longitudinal spaces. The overload-induced response did not appear to be inflammatory.

Changes in tendon morphology and mechanical properties caused by altered loading environments appear to be specific to the type and degree of load change. Although immobilization significantly diminishes tendon strength and stiffness,[43] exercise-related increases in loading cause temporary increases in cross-sectional area and collagen fibril numbers. Dramatic increases in tendon load after removal of a muscle's synergists result in enhanced collagen synthesis. Tendon possesses an adaptation specificity that obviates a simple relationship between load and adaptation.

There are few descriptions of the magnitudes of loads or loading rates during actual tendon injury in humans. Experiments cannot be performed that submit humans to maximum loading conditions, so data must be collected as an injury happens. Zernicke and associates[45] reported knee joint torques experienced by an athlete who ruptured his patellar tendon during weightlifting. They used inverse dynamics analysis to calculate the patellar-tendon tension at the time of rupture and found it to be 14.5 kN (more than 17.5 times the weightlifter's body weight). This provides a graphic example of the range of loads tendon could experience during training.

Barfred[3] summarized factors such as age and sex that appear related to human Achilles tendon ruptures. Men 30 to 50 years old are most susceptible to tendon rupture. Physical activity apparently maintains tendon strength and integrity and reduces the likelihood of rupture. With aging, calcaneal avulsions occur more frequently. Systemic or local disease does not contribute substantially to tendon injury, although reduced activity, such as bedrest associated with illness, may produce immobilization-like decrements. After surgical repair, a tendon may regain its preinjury strength.

Myotendinous Junction

Little is known about how the myotendinous junction adapts to training. Zamora and Marini[44] described morphologic changes in the plantaris myotendinous junction after two weeks of overload. Early changes include increased collagen synthesis and intensive membrane renewal and recycling. At first, with the compensatory hypertrophy of the plantaris, the sarcolemma of the projections of the muscle fibers shows many caveolae close to clusters of large subsurface vacuoles. The adaptive changes to overloading include a noninflammatory reaction of the tendon, consisting of enhanced collagen synthesis and intensive membrane renewal and recycling. Mechanically, this reaction may impair tendon resistance to stretch and increase the chance of injury.[44]

There is currently no evidence that the junctional angle between a myofibril and collagen changes with exercise. The relative magnitudes of the shear and tensile force components may provide optimal strength in the healthy myotendinous junction,[37] so there may be no need to change with training. Myotendinous junction adaptation manifests as changes in the quality of the collagen and sarcolemmal membrane rather than as changes in junction morphology. If or how maladaptive myotendinous junction changes occur with training overload is yet be determined.

References

1. Armstong RB: Mechanisms of exercise-induced delayed onset muscular soreness: A brief review. *Med Sci Sports Exerc* 1984;16:529–538.
2. Armstrong RB, Ogilvie RW, Schwane JA: Eccentric exercise-induced injury to rat skeletal muscle. *J Appl Physiol* 1983;54:80–93.
3. Barfred T: Achilles tendon rupture: Aetiology and pathogenesis of subcutaneous rupture assessed on the basis of the literature and rupture experiments on rats. *Acta Orthop Scand* 1973;152(suppl):1–126.
4. Borg TK, Caulfield JB: Morphology of connective tissue in skeletal muscle. *Tissue Cell* 1980;12:197–207.
5. Brooks SM, Paynton-Brooks N: *The Human Body: Structure and Function in Health and Disease*, ed 2. St. Louis, CV Mosby, 1980.
6. Burke RE, Edgerton VR: Motor unit properties and selective involvement in movement. *Exerc Sports Sci Rev* 1975;3:31–83.
7. Butler DL, Grood E, Noyes FR, et al: Biomechanics of tendons and ligaments. *Exerc Sports Sci Rev* 1978;6:125–183.
8. Carlson BM, Faulkner JA: The regeneration of skeletal muscle fibers following injury: A review. *Med Sci Sports Exerc* 1983;15:187–198.
9. Clarkson PM, Dedrick ME: Exercise-induced muscle damage, repair, and adaptation in old and young subjects. *J Gerontol* 1988;43:M91-M96.
10. Close RI: Dynamic properties of mammalian skeletal muscles. *Physiol Rev* 1972;52:129–197.
11. Curwin SL, Vailas AC, Wood J: Immature tendon adaptation to strenuous exercise. *J Appl Physiol* 1988;65:2297–2301.
12. Edington DW, Edgerton VR: *The Biology of Physical Activity*. Boston, Houghton Mifflin, 1976.
13. Elliott DH, Crawford GNC: The thickness and collagen content of tendon relative to the strength and cross-sectional area of muscle. *Proc R Soc London* 1965;162B:137–146.
14. Fridén J, Sfakianos PN, Hargens AR, et al: Residual muscular swelling after repetitive eccentric contractions. *J Orthop Res* 1988;6:493–498.
15. Fridén J, Sjöström M, Ekblom B: Myofibrillar damage following intense eccentric exercise in man. *Int J Sports Med* 1983;4:170–176.
16. Gollnick PD: Skeletal muscle morphology: Adaptation to altered demands, in Skinner JS, Corbin CB, Landers DM, et al (eds): *Future Directions in Exercise and Sports Science Research*. Champaign, Human Kinetics, 1988, pp 275–292.
17. Gregor RJ, Komi PV, Järvinen M: Achilles tendon forces during cycling. *Int J Sports Med* 1987;8(suppl 1):9–14.
18. Gregor RJ, Roy RR, Whiting WC, et al: Mechanical output of the cat soleus during treadmill location: In vivo vs in situ characteristics. *J Biomech* 1988;21:721–732.

19. Häkkinen K, Komi PV, Alen M, et al: EMG, muscle fibre and force production characteristics during a 1 year training period in elite weight-lifters. *Eur J Appl Physiol* 1987;56:419–427.
20. Hooley CJ, McCrum N, Cohen RE: The viscoelastic deformation of tendon. *J Biomech* 1980;13:521–528.
21. Jones DA, Newham DJ, Round JM, et al: Experimental human muscle damage: Morphological changes in relation to other indices of damage. *J Physiol* 1986;375:435–448.
22. Komi PV: Physiological and biomechanical correlates of muscle function: Effects of muscle structure and stretch-shortening cycle on force and speed. *Exerc Sport Sci Rev* 1984;12:81–121.
23. Komi PV, Buskirk ER: Effect of eccentric and concentric muscle conditioning on tension and electrical activity of human muscle. *Ergonomics* 1972;15:417–434.
24. Kovanen V, Suominen H, Heikkinen E: Connective tissue of "fast" and "slow" skeletal muscle in rats: Effects of endurance training. *Acta Physiol Scand* 1980;108:173–180.
25. McCully KK, Faulkner JA: Characteristics of lengthening contractions associated with injury to skeletal muscle fibers. *J Appl Physiol* 1986;61:293–299.
26. McCully KK, Faulkner JA: Injury to skeletal muscle fibers of mice following lengthening contractions. *J Appl Physiol* 1985;59:119–126.
27. Michna H: Morphometric analysis of loading-induced changes in collagen-fibril populations in young tendons. *Cell Tissue Res* 1984;236:465–470.
28. Newham DJ: The consequences of eccentric contractions and their relationship to delayed onset muscle pain. *Eur J Appl Physiol* 1988;57:353–359.
29. Newham DJ, Jones DA, Clarkson PM: Repeated high-force eccentric exercise: Effects on muscle pain and damage. *J Appl Physiol* 1987;63:1381–1386.
30. Ovalle WK: The human muscle-tendon junction: A morphological study during normal growth and at maturity. *Anat Embryol* 1987;176:281–294.
31. Proske U, Morgan DL: Tendon stiffness: Methods of measurement and significance for the control of movement. A review. *J Biomech* 1987;20:75–82.
32. Rack PM, Westbury DR: The short range stiffness of active mammalian muscle and its effect on mechanical properties. *J Physiol* 1974;241:331–350.
33. Schantz P, Billeter R, Henriksson J, et al: Training-induced increase in myofibrillar ATPase intermediate fibers in human skeletal muscle. *Muscle Nerve* 1982;5:628–636.
34. Schwane JA, Johnson SR, Vandenakker CB, et al: Delayed-onset muscular soreness and plasma CPK and LDH activities after downhill running. *Med Sci Sports Exerc* 1983;15:51–56.
35. Tesch PA: Skeletal muscle adaptations consequent to long-term heavy resistance exercise. *Med Sci Sports Exerc* 1988;20(suppl):S132-S134.
36. Tidball JG: Myotendinous junction: Morphological changes and mechanical failure associated with muscle cell atrophy. *Exp Mol Pathol* 1984;40:1–12.
37. Tidball JG: The geometry of actin filament-membrane associations can modify adhesive strength of the myotendinous junction. *Cell Motil* 1983;3:439–447.
38. Tidball JG, Daniel TL: Myotendinous junctions of tonic muscle cells: Structure and loading. *Cell Tissue Res* 1986;245:315–322.
39. Trotter JA, Eberhard S, Samora A: Structural connections of the muscle-tendon junction. *Cell Motil* 1983;3:431–438.

40. Trotter JA, Hsi K, Samora A, et al: A morphometric analysis of the muscle-tendon junction. *Anat Rec* 1985;213:26–32.
41. Vihko V, Salminen A, Rantamuäki J: Exhaustive exercise, endurance training, and acid hydrolase activity in skeletal muscle. *J Appl Physiol* 1979;47:43–50.
42. Woo SL, Gomez MA, Amiel D, et al: The effects of exercise on the biomechanical and biochemical properties of swine digital flexor tendons. *J Biomech Eng* 1981;103:5156.
43. Woo SL, Gomez MA, Woo YK, et al: Mechanical properties of tendons and ligaments: II. The relationships of immobilization and exercise on tissue remodeling. *Biorheology* 1982;19:397–408.
44. Zamora AJ, Marini JF: Tendon and myo-tendinous junction in an overloaded skeletal muscle of the rat. *Anat Embryol* 1988;179:89–96.
45. Zernicke RF, Garhammer J, Jobe FW: Human patellar-tendon rupture: A kinetic analysis. *J Bone Joint Surg* 1977;59A:179–183.

Chapter 48

Exercise, Hyperactivity, and Inactivity: Immune Cell Changes and Alterations in Pathogenesis

Ronald Ross Watson, PhD

Introduction

Exercise and fitness are significant modulators of the immune functions that are important components of inflammation and healing after sports injuries. Vigorous exercise generates diverse short-term changes, and fitness programs produce significant long-term changes. In many situations, exercise or conditioning activities can have a profound impact on the immune system.

Factors that can stimulate or suppress immune functions include age, malnutrition, nutrient supplementation, metabolic alteration, genetic factors, and changes in environment, anatomy, and physiology. Physical fitness, maturity, or vigorous activity modulate many body systems, including the lymphoid cells. Lymphoid cells, altered by exercise stress, may play important roles in inflammation, tissue damage, and disease resistance.

The immune system responds not only to antigens but also to neurologic and hormonal signals. The thymus gland's production of thymic factors is altered by the interleukins, by hormones such as corticosteroids, and by endorphins. Exercise or its lack should affect immune responses, but there are significant problems in assessing data from exercise-immunology studies. Many studies fail to mention the types of exercise used, the duration of the exercise program, or the degree of illness (chronic or severe). Detailed reviews of the effects of exercise on immune functions are helpful.[22,56]

Exercise and Disease

Exercise has beneficial effects in reducing the risk of cardiac disease. Moriguchi and Watson[32] reviewed the theory that immune functions can alter cardiovascular risk. However, detailed studies are needed to determine how exercise modulates immune function and subsequently affects cardiovascular disease development. Physical conditioning may improve health and immunomodulation, thus increasing resistance to disease. In addition, alterations in cell numbers and functions, even short-term ones from vigorous exercise, could affect inflammation or tissue damage.

A few clinical studies and case reports have suggested that athletes have an increased risk for infection.[2,3,56] Without adequate controls, however, it is almost impossible to identify a group of athletes who have an unusually low risk for infection. That is, outbreaks of infectious diseases in groups are recognized, but the absence of disease is rarely noted. However, immune changes caused by physical fitness or its lack can be studied and the effects on disease resistance or tissue damage can be inferred.

Exercise Stress and Immunoregulatory Hormones

Stress affects the immune response, but the individual's perception of and response to stress may be equally important.[1] Exercise-induced stress increases glucocorticoid production in sedentary people[58] but not in active people unless they are given high work loads. Dietary stress, such as starvation, has adverse effects associated in part with increased serum cortisol, which could explain malnutrition's effects on cellular immunity.[54]

Cortisol, the chief glucocorticoid in humans, is produced by the adrenal cortex under the direction of corticotropin.[55] Increased glucocorticoid levels cause lymphocytopenia and suppress T and B lymphocytes in humans and other animals.[14] The sensitivity of lymphocytes to glucocorticoids seems to depend on the cystolic glucocorticoid receptor concentration.[47] Stimulated lymphoblasts are more sensitive to glucocorticoids than resting lymphocytes, possibly because receptor concentration increases during transformation.[47] In experimental animals, plasma glucocorticoids increase soon after stress is induced, then gradually return to basal levels. The number of circulating lymphocytes inversely parallels the stress-related increases in plasma glucocorticoids before returning to normal levels.[20] Reducing stress with long-term exercise lowers corticosteroids levels. Other studies show that T-cell mitogenesis is suppressed after a single, vigorous exercise session.[55]

Plasma cortisol reaches its highest level ten minutes after vigorous exercise. In calves this level is seven times greater than the resting value.[25] These changes correlate with decreased percentages of T lymphocytes in the peripheral blood, decreased levels of secretory IgA, and slight decreases in lymphocyte mitogenesis.[21] Strenuous exercise is correlated with an increased incidence of poliovirus and coxsackievirus[21,40] and a decrease in tumor growth rate.[18,43] Corticosteroids regulate interleukin-1 production and, hence, immune functions. However, whether immunomodulation is directly related to or just associated with changes in disease or tumor resistance has not been clearly established in the few studies done.[22,56]

Moorthy and Zimmerman[31] found increased levels of cortisol and neutrophils, but not lymphocytes, after an endurance race. Short-term, vigorous exercise caused a temporary increase in cells other than T cells, with a rapid decline after exercise stopped.[59] This increase was reduced when prednisone (corticosteroid) was given five hours before the exercise.[59] A shorter exposure to steroids suppressed the expected increase in T cells only. T cells are readily mobilized,[46] and these results reflect this fact.

Physical activity on a bicycle ergometer increases the number of β-adrenoceptors per mononuclear leukocyte and alters the distribution of lymphocyte subsets in blood, increasing those that carry many high-affinity β-adrenoceptors.[27] This increase in β-adrenoceptors on mononuclear leukocytes, probably caused by the increase in the lymphocyte subsets carrying high numbers of β-adrenoceptors, may explain some lymphoid function changes.[27] Internalization of β-adrenoceptors accompanies reduced hormone responsiveness.

Stress is able both to suppress and to stimulate some immune reactions. Sympathetic nervous stimulation of the immune system may be a hidden component in changing immune functions (for example, if the athlete is under mental stress during competition).[17] For example, β-endorphin increases before a sporting event, with additional increases afterward. Thus, it is clear that some changes that influence lymphoid cell numbers and functions occur without exercise. Other hormones that change during exercise, such as epinephrine, norepinephrine, and other catecholamines, could help modify immune systems. Catecholamines increase exponentially with exercise duration or intensity. Catecholamines and norepinephrine injections increase the number of circulating lymphocytes. Both catecholamines and cortisol appear to affect the immune function adversely. A stress-induced increase in cortisol, however, tends to protect the organism from self-injury by reducing potentially destructive responses to stress. It may also prevent autoimmune disease and tissue damage from immune hyperactivity.

There are three possible mechanisms for exercise-induced granulocytosis. First, strenuous exercise produces shifts in extracellular fluids that commonly result in hemoconcentration. Second, exercise increases catecholamine levels and adrenalin to mobilize leukocytes from the marginal pool. Finally, cortisol mobilizes granulocytes from the marrow pool and slows their egress from the circulation. Cortisol levels are also increased by vigorous exercise. Immunomodulation accompanying the stress of long-term physical conditioning may well occur through interactions among the central nervous, endocrine, and immune systems.

Effects of Altered Diet and Nutrient Intake

The effects of nutrition on physically fit and unfit individuals relative to their immune functions have rarely been studied. Yet, nutrition is a significant variable associated with prolonged, regular exercise, because food consumption increases and vitamin and mineral supplements may be added to the diet. Deficiencies of some nutrients cause significant changes in immune function, as do high intakes of certain vitamins and minerals.[53] However, there is almost no information on relationships among nutrition, the modulation of immune function, the development or maintenance of physical fitness, and the changes associated with physical inactivity.

Recent Soviet studies indicate that high nutrient intakes can modify immune function during exercise and physical fitness development.[7,35] One report found that an amino acid supplement acted as a normalizer when given after a week of exercise.[7] Another study examined the effect of thiamine on the development of immune response during exercise.[35] A four-hour swimming regimen inhibited the development of the immune response to sheep erythrocytes in rats fed a high intake of thiamine. An additional dose of 100 g of thiamine increased the intensity of the response after exercise. The thiamine did not affect the exercise-induced synthesis and release of immunosuppressive factors, but it did reduce the sensitivity of effector cells of the humoral immune response to the action of these factors. A third study found that infecting rats with bacteria enhanced the suppressive effect of physical exercise on the development of antibody response to sheep erythrocytes.[36] Physical loading or stress may release factors that activate suppressor cells. The infection further enhanced this action. A combination of a modified high-fat diet and exercise changed immune functions in rats.[16]

These observations reinforce other studies[53] on the effects of deficient and high-nutrient intakes on immune functions and cell numbers. Vigorous, regular exercise can modify nutrient intakes and ultimately change immune systems.[56] Because both exercise and diet modify the cancer rate in animals,[51,56] the mechanisms of nutrient-cancer immunomodulation need further study.

Exercise and Natural Killer Cells

Natural killer (NK) cells are functionally identified by their ability to lyse a wide variety of target cells and are morphologically identified as large granular lymphocytes. Antibodies reactive with IgG-Fc receptors, such as Leu-11 ($CD16^+$), can identify essentially all NK cells. NK-cell activity is modulated by many agents of potential physiologic and pathophysiologic importance. Interferon and interleukin-2 stimulate NK-cell activity, whereas prostaglandins reduce their activity.

In one study, young, healthy, previously inactive men received aerobic training for 40 to 50 minutes each day, five days a week for 15 weeks. All lost weight, and body fat decreased as a result of the training. Submaximal steady-state heart rates dropped. Their improved physical fitness altered several cellular immune functions.[57] Training significantly decreased NK-cell activity. The men had 38.8% (± 3.8%) lysis of target cells by NK cells before training but only 29.3% (± 3.2%) afterward. The percentage of mature T lymphocytes and mitogenesis increased as NK-cell activity declined.[57] Immediately after exercise, peripheral blood NK-cell numbers and functioning decreased.[17] However, NK-cell activity on a per cell basis increased and returned to normal rapidly after exercise. This suggests that long-term physical conditioning can influence the maturation and functioning of cells in the cellular immune system.

Conversely, NK-cell activity (lysis per fixed number of mononuclear cells) increased during vigorous bicycle exercise, dropped to a minimum two hours later, and returned to pre-exercise levels within 24 hours.[2,38] Back-muscle exercise has no significant influence on NK-cell activity. Indomethacin fully restores suppressed NK-cell activity in vitro. The fact that the proportion of monocytes ($CD20^-$ cells) doubles two hours after work suggests that prostaglandins released by monocytes during heavy physical exercise may be responsible for down-regulation of NK cells.[24] Because the less vigorous back exercise has no effect on NK-cell activity, perhaps only exercise resulting in a major increase in stress hormones or oxygen consumption modulates NK-cell function.[39] This may be distinct from the effects of long-term training.[58]

In contrast to long-term exercise, a single exercise bout in conditioned runners[4,19,28,36] or bicycle exercise[38] increases NK-cell activity. NK-cell activity against K-562 cells declined over a 20-hour period after cessation of stress,[4] with no significant differences between sedentary and fit individals. NK cells increased immediately after exercise in physically fit athletes, but not in an untrained group.[36] There was a general decline in total T cells in both groups. Short-term physical exercise was used as a model for standardized sympathetic stimulation in vivo. Exercise produced lymphocytosis and monocytosis with a small increase in the number of total T cells, inducer T cells and B cells. However, NK cells with the Leu-7 phenotype doubled.[22]

Another study of physically fit cyclists showed that activated lymphocytes and NK, T-helper, and T-suppressor cells increased immediately after exercise and returned to normal in two hours.[28] Production of interleukin-1 temporarily increased and that of interleukin-2 decreased immediately after exercise.[28] Vigorous exercise decreased T-helper cells and increased T-suppressor-cytotoxic cells.[4] Serum factors seemed to have no effect on this process, and the source of serum for the assay did not affect the increase. Because NK-cells are refractory to corticosteroids, their secretion during exercise could lead to increases in NK-cell function but not number, as T-helper cells exit the blood and T-suppressor cells stay. Cattle without long-term endurance training had decreased T-cell mitogenesis.[2] Cortisol levels increased as much as 600% in these animals.[2]

Effects of Long-Term Conditioning

Various indicators can be used to measure cellular immunity. These include the release of signal or regulatory proteins such as interferon and interleukins from T cells and macrophages, mitogenesis, the killing

Table 1 Effects of vigorous short-term exercise on lymphoid cells

Cells	Effects	Studies
Natural killer cells		
No.	Increased	Keast et al[22]; Lewicki et al[28]
Rapid normalization of function	Increased	Blecha and Minocha[2]; Brahmi et al[4]; Hanson and Flaherty[19]; Lewicki et al[28]; Oshida et al[36]; Pedersen et al[38]
	Decreased	Gmünder et al[17]
Immunoregulatory hormones		
Catecholamines	Increased	Landmann et al[27]
No. of β-adrenoreceptors per cell	Increased	Watson[56]
Corticosteroids	Increased	Hefors et al[21]; Kuhlmann et al[25]; Moorthy and Zimmerman[31]; White et al[58]
Lymphocytes		
No.	Increased and no change	Yu et al[59]
T helper	Increased	Gmünder et al[17]; Keast et al[22]
T suppressor	Increased	Keast et al[22]
B cells	Increased and decreased	Gmünder et al[17]; Landmann et al[26]
Mitogenesis	Decreased	Gmünder et al[17]; Oshida et al[36]
Interleukin-1	Increased and decreased	Cannon and Kluger[6]; Fedde[15]

of tumor cells, and the numbers of T subsets identified by surface markers with fluorescent antibodies. The effects of long-term physical conditioning on T lymphocytes have not been investigated in great detail.[22,56]

Mitogens stimulate lymphocyte clones to proliferate, yielding a rapid increase in DNA synthesis.[22] Mitogens such as phytohemagglutinin and concanavalin A stimulate T cells, and lipopolysaccharide induces the proliferation of B cells. A decrease in concanavalin A-induced proliferation of lymphocytes in vitro is associated with a decline in cell-mediated immunity in vivo, and a decrease in lipopolysaccharide-induced proliferation is associated with a decline in antibody-mediated immunity. Therefore, the immunologic status of an organism can be assayed in vitro with these mitogens.[22] However, stimulation must increase 200% to 500% before significant differences appear. The effect of exercise on mitogenesis is still unclear; conflicting reports indicate that exercise has no effect, that it increases mitogenesis, and that it decreases mitogenesis.[22,56] T-cell mitogenesis significantly increases with long-term physical conditioning.[57]

Although various conditions can modify immune functions, studies, almost without exception, are done in young, healthy, physically active people or animals.[22,56] At the end of a six-month training period, spleen lymphocytes were isolated from exercised rats and from age-matched sedentary controls.[37] Although the age-related decline in mitogen-

Table 2 Effects of vigorous long-term conditioning on lymphocytes

Effects	Studies
T-cell mitogenesis	
Increased	Blecha and Minocha[2]; Watson[57]
Decreased	Pahlavani et al[37]
No. of T cells increased*	Watson[57]
Interleukin-2 production decreased*	Pahlavani et al[37]
Natural killer cell function decreased	Watson[57]

*No change in very old animals.

induced proliferation and interleukin-2 production was smaller in the exercised rats, this was the result of lower levels of mitogenesis and interleukin-2 production in young exercised rats. Exercise significantly decreased (by 23% to 32%) mitogen-induced lymphocyte proliferation and interleukin-2 production in 7-month-old exercised rats compared with sedentary rats of the same age. However, there was no significant difference in mitogen-induced lymphocyte proliferation and interleukin-2 production in 18- and 24-month-old exercised and sedentary rats.[37] This study concluded that exercise did not prevent the age-related decline in lymphocyte proliferation and interleukin-2 production, that exercise did reduce lymphocyte proliferation and interleukin-2 production, and that the degree of reduction in lymphocyte proliferation caused by exercise changed with age. Very little is known about lymphoid cells that are dysfunctional because of age when they are exposed to changes induced by physical conditioning.[22,56]

Training does not significantly change the percentage of total lymphocytes. The number of mature T lymphocytes (measured by the E-rosette technique) increased significantly after physical conditioning. T lymphocytes accounted for 65% (± 1.3%) of all lymphocytes before conditioning and 74% (± 1.4%) afterwards.[57] Although both B- and T-cell counts increased after exercise, T-cell counts were increased to a greater extent, possibly because they are the most readily mobilized class of human lymphocytes.[42] Although exercise produces granulocytosis, this does not have an important functional role in enhancing host defenses against infection. Tables 1 and 2 summarize the effects of exercise on lymphoid cells.

T-Cell Numbers and Functions

Short, vigorous exercise causes immediate changes in some lymphocyte functions.[2,4,11,18,19,21,28,31,36,40,42,43,50] For example, when Hefors and associates[21] compared samples of peripheral blood collected before and after a standardized cycle ergometer test, they found increased numbers of lymphocytes and changes in reactivity and composition. In another study,[26] the numbers of peripheral blood lymphocytes of various subsets were determined after a physical stress test with bicycle ergometry to evaluate short-term, maximal work capacity. In normal individuals, all subsets increased after ergometry. B cells and cells with suppressor or NK markers increased more than T-helper cells. In patients who had undergone splenectomy, the proportion of cellular changes was about one half of that in normal subjects, and the T-helper cells released into the peripheral blood did not increase. Both trained and untrained individuals had less phytohemagglutinin-induced mitogenesis after vigorous exercise.[36]

Gmünder and associates[17] assessed the response of critical immunologic characteristics to the sustained physical stress of marathon running in seven athletes. They analyzed mitogenic response to concanavalin A, the numbers of lymphocytes, lymphocyte subsets, and leukocytes, and determined blood levels of cortisol, epinephrine, and norepinephrine. After the run, lymphocyte responsiveness was severely depressed, although the lymphocyte count did not change. Leukocyte counts nearly tripled. No dramatic changes were found within the lymphocyte subsets, although there was a significant increase in pan-T cells and the helper-inducer subset two days after the run. The number of B cells decreased significantly. There was no change in the suppressor-cytotoxic subset. Cortisol levels more than doubled, epinephrine levels tripled, and norepinephrine levels nearly tripled. All returned to baseline values within two days. Thus, vigorous physical exercise may have a short-term effect on some lymphoid cells.

Exercise and Phagocytic Cells

Monocytes and macrophages play key roles in lymphocyte trafficking and stimulation, tissue damage, and destruction of pathogens and tumor cells by their engulfment and enzymatic dissolution, release of mediator, and/or direct contact killing. Limited evidence indicates that exercise affects disease resistance[15] and reduces tumor growth in animals. Robertson and associates[42] found that exercise-induced leukocytosis was short-lived, with granulocyte counts returning to normal within 45 minutes. In addition, the granulocytes of highly trained athletes were functionally indistinguishable from those of sedentary individuals. They suggested that nonspecific immune functions are suppressed by great physical exertion.[42]

Physical training may modify monocytes by increasing the number of their insulin receptors, producing more energy for phagocytosis.[30] However, phagocytosis and antigen processing are unchanged after extensive running, and neutrophil activity decreases.[22] Production of lymphokines during exercise or physical conditioning may be significant in immunomodulation and overall host defenses.[46] Monocytes produce various monokines, secreted proteins that have cytotoxic activity and modify functions of other cells.

A preliminary study suggested that plasma samples taken after exercise contained interleukin-1 because they enhanced mitogenic response to mouse thymocytes.[6] Increased interleukin-1 may account for the enhanced lymphocyte functioning seen after exercise. The effects of physical conditioning on interleukin-1 production must be determined before this hypothesis can be confirmed. A study on calves suggested that interleukin-1 produces an inhibitor. The calves were exercised at a medium trot. Serum from exercised calves was added to cultures containing lymphocytes from nonstressed calf and significantly suppressed the lymphocytes' response to a foreign substance. The suppressing mediator remained in the serum for 30 minutes but the cell response returned to normal within one hour. These results indicate that, when stressed by physical exertion, the calf produces a chemical mediator that depresses the immune response of its own lymphocytes. It may thus become more susceptible to microorganisms already present in low numbers in the respiratory tract.[15]

These results show that some cellular immune systems are modulated by the stress of long-term exercise and improvements in physical fitness and are in accord with a study of the neutrophils of youths who had undergone six years of physical conditioning through sports training.[49] However, T lymphocytes have been studied only after short-term vigorous exercise.[32] Physical conditioning with long-term vigorous exercise alters cellular immune functions by changing T cells, other effector cells (monocytes), and/or their signals (interleukins). This may have important implications for treating patients with immunosuppressive illnesses and individuals undergoing physical training.

Exercise and Immunoglobulins

The skin and secretory antibodies on mucosal surfaces protect the body from the external environment. The predominant immunoglobulin with antibody functions protecting the eye and the gut is IgA. Intense exercise temporarily suppresses salivary IgA and IgM but not nasal immunoglobulins.[29] During this period, the individual may be susceptible to upper respiratory diseases.[29] The functional activity of neutrophils decreases in response to exercise. This coincides with decreased serum and secretory immunoglobulins and lysozyme. Physical exercise affects salivary protein concentrations and the percentage of IgA binding to protein.[5,29] A study of the effects of competition on salivary IgA in professional skiers found some decreases,[50] but the reason for the decrease was not determined. The skiers' salivary IgA levels were lower than those of untrained controls before the competition, and they declined during the competition. Other information suggests that exercise does not influence antibody responses and serum immunoglobulin levels.[22]

Reduced secretory IgA in the gut could alter resistance to disease and permit entry of bacteria or their components. Large amounts of gram-negative bacteria and endotoxins are normally present in the intestines. Endotoxins, including lipopolysaccharides, form part of the outer cell wall of the gram-negative bacteria. A reduction in the splanchnic blood flow damages the intestinal wall and leads to excessive leakage of lipopolysaccharides into the portal circulation. This could overwhelm the liver's reticuloendothelial system, making it unable to remove the lipopolysaccharides from the circulation. Increased serum lipopolysaccharides in runners after a race seems to confirm increased endogenous pyrogen activity in human plasma after exercise.[22] It is possible that training-induced stress leads to some leakage of lipopolysaccharides into the circulation, perhaps by reducing secretory IgA in the gut. In turn, this results in self-immunization against lipopolysaccharides. Lipopolysaccharides activate macrophages to release interferon, tumor necrosis factor, and interleukin-1, resulting in immunoregulatory changes. Tumor necrosis factor is identical to cachexin, which causes tissue wasting. Whether exercise alters these modulators directly or indirectly is unknown.[22,56] The effects of athletic performance and exercise-induced changes in plasma lipopolysaccharides serum anti-lipopolysaccharides IgG levels, and IgA levels in the gut require further investigation.

Animal models are valuable in the study of exercise and immunology, because diet, genetics, age, and, to some degree, emotion can be controlled. For example, mice trained to run for ten minutes twice a day were immunized. Their levels of antibodies to a bacterial pathogen were higher than those in sedentary controls.[23] Similar results have been noted in humans immunized against tetanus.

Exercise-Induced Immunologic Diseases

It should be noted that inactivity and weightlessness have been shown to change some immue characteristics.[8,9,12,23,34,48,52] This topic was the subject of a recent review.[56]

Exercise is considered beneficial in reducing risk factors for several disease states. This may have an immunologic component.[32] Under selected conditions, however, exercise may alter immune function or cell location, leading to death or damage.[41]

For example, in mice infected with coxsackievirus B3, T cells migrate to the heart and produce myocardial calcification. Infected mice that were forced to swim had four times the number of T cells sensitized to the virus and redirected to the heart from other parts of the body than did control mice. When nonsensitized T cells were transferred to exercised mice, there was little cardiac calcification. Clearly, exercise alone can release T cells into the blood, and coxasackievirus virus B3 infection plus exercise increases the production of the virus in the heart. It is not clear why the virus multiplies more during exercise, but the increased cardiac antigen, increased T-cell traffic, and delayed turnoff of cell immune responses may all play roles. Enhanced T-cell circulation to the heart may indicate increased release of T cells from the thymus and other tissues rich in T cells.

The thymus glands of the infected animals that were forced to exercise were smaller than those of the control animals. The smaller thymus may have resulted in part from the increase in corticosteroids associated with stress. During exercise, epinephrine and norepinephrine are released into the plasma catecholamines. They act as neural hormones to regulate intercellular concentrations of cyclic adenosine phosphate and cyclic guanosine phosphate, which modulate hormonal and cellular immune responses. Increases in intracellular cGMP within B and T lymphocytes, leukocytes, and macrophages augment the functions of these cells. Hormone levels were enhanced in the thymus glands of infected, exercised animals. This finding correlated with the period of greatest T-cell-mediated myocardial toxicity and the release of cells from the thymus. Thus, exercise may have a significant controlling influence on the thymus and the release of its cells.

The fundamental question of whether habitual exercise training alters host resistance to infection remains unanswered. Clinical studies are needed.[46]

Exercise-Induced Asthma

In this condition, an asthmatic seizure occurs after exercise.[13] Patients with exercise-induced asthma have airway hyperreactivity. Sheffer and associates[45] suggested that a significant immunologic relationship exists between increased serum histamine levels and early clinical manifestations after experimental exercise. Exercise-induced asthma is associated with mast cell degranulation IgE-Fc-dependent activation secretion. The triggering mechanism responsible for mast cell degranulation in exercise-induced asthma is unknown.[10,44,45]

Exercise can induce albuminuria and erythrocyte cast formation in normal individuals. Cornacoff and associates[10] injected animals with bovine serum albumin and provided exercise stress. Exercise superimposed active immune-complex-mediated glomerular nephritis worsened the abnormal glomerular function. In humans, an increase in an antigen or host protein would be necessary. Exercise could cause this increase.

Acknowledgment

This study was supported by a grant from the Wallace Genetics Foundation.

References

1. Asgeirsson G, Bellanti JA: Exercise, immunology, and infection. *Semin Adolesc Med* 1987;3:199–204.
2. Blecha F, Minocha HC: Suppressed lymphocyte blastogenic responses and enhanced in vitro growth of infectious bovine rhinotracheitis virus in stressed feeder calves. *Am J Vet Res* 1983;44:2145–2148.
3. Bosenberg AT, Brock-Utne JG, Gaffin SL, et al: Strenuous exercise causes systemic endotoxemia. *J Appl Physiol* 1988;65:106–108.
4. Brahmi Z, Thomas JE, Park M, et al: The effect of acute exercise on natural killer-cell activity of trained and sedentary human subjects. *J Clin Immunol* 1985;5:321–328.
5. Bratthall D, Widerström L: Ups and downs for salivary IgA. *Scand J Dent Res* 1985;93:128–134.
6. Cannon JG, Kluger MJ: Endogenous pyrogen activity in human plasma after exercise. *Science* 1983;22:617–619.

7. Chogovadze AV, Shkrebko AN: Normalizatsiia immunologicheskoy reaktivnosti studentov-lyzhnikov belkovym preparatom [Normalization of the immunologic reactivity of student skiers with a protein preparation]. *Vopr Pitan* 1986;5:26–27.
8. Cogoli A, Tscopp A: Lymphocyte reactivity during spaceflight. *Immunol Today* 1985;6:1–4.
9. Cogoli A, Valluchi-Morf M, Mueller M, et al: Effect of hypogravity on human lymphocyte activation. *Aviat Space Environ Med* 1980;51:29–34.
10. Cornacoff JB, Hebert LA, Sharma HM, et al: Adverse effect of exercise on immune complex-mediated glomerulonephritis. *Nephron* 1985;40:292–296.
11. Douglas DJ, Hanson PG: Upper respiratory infections in the conditioned athlete. *Med Sci Sports* 1978;10:95.
12. Durnova GN, Kaplansky AS, Portugalov VV: Effect of a 22-day space flight on the lymphoid organs of rats. *Aviat Space Environ Med* 1976;47:588–591.
13. Eggleston PA: Exercise-induced asthma. *Clin Rev Allergy* 1983;1:19–37.
14. Fauci AS: Mechanisms of corticosteroid action on lymphocyte subpopulations: I. Redistribution of circulating T and B lymphocytes to the bone marrow. *Immunology* 1975;28:669–680.
15. Fedde F: The stress-respiratory disease link. *Feedlot Managememt* 1984;26:24–28.
16. Fernandes G, Rozek M, Troyer D: Reduction of blood pressure and restoration of T-cell immune function in spontaneously hypertensive rats by food restriction and/or by treadmill exercise. *J Hypertens* 1986;4(suppl):S469-S474.
17. Gmünder FK, Lorenzi G, Bechler B, et al: Effect of long-term physical exercise on lymphocyte reactivity: Similarity to spaceflight reactions. *Aviat Space Environ Med* 1988;59:146–151.
18. Good RA, Fernandes G: Enhancement of immunologic function and resistance to tumor growth in BALB/c mice by exercise. *Fed Proc* 1981;40:1040.
19. Hanson PG, Flaherty DK: Immunological responses to training in conditioned runners. *Clin Sci* 1981;60:225–228.
20. Hedman LA: The effect of steroids on the circulating lymphocyte population: IV. The effect of stress on the thoracic duct lymphocyte population in normal and neonatally thymectomized rats. *Lymphology* 1980;13:34–39.
21. Hefors E, Holm G, Ohnell B: Variations of blood lymphocytes during work studied by cell surface markers, DNA synthesis and cytotoxicity. *Clin Exp Immunol* 1976;24:328–335.
22. Keast D, Cameron K, Morton AR: Exercise and the immune response. *Sports Med* 1988;5:248–267.
23. Kimzey SL: Hematology and immunology studies, in Johnston RS, Dietlein LF (eds): *Biomedical Results From Skylab: NASA SP-377.* National Aeronautics and Space Administration, 1977, pp 249–283.
24. Konstantinova IV, Antropova YN, Legen'kov VI, et al: Izuchenie reaktivnosti limfoidnykh kletok krovi u chlenov ékipazha kosmicheskikh korableĭ "Soiuz-6", "Soiuz-7" i "Soiuz-8" do i posle poleta [Study of reactivity of blood lymphoid cells in crew members of the Soyuz-6, Soyuz-7 and Soyuz-8 spaceships before and after flight]. *Kosmi Biol Aviakosm Med* 1973;7:35–40.
25. Kuhlmann WD, Hodgson DS, Fedde MR: Respiratory, cardiovascular, and metabolic adjustments to exercise in the Hereford calf. *J Appl Physiol* 1985;58:1273–1280.
26. Landmann R, Dürig M, Gudat F, et al: Beta-adrenergic regulation of the blood lymphocyte phenotype distribution in normal subjects and splenectomized patients. *Adv Exp Med Biol* 1985;186:1051–1062.

27. Landmann R, Portenier M, Staehelin M, et al: Changes in beta-adrenoceptors and leucocyte subpopulations after physical exercise in normal subjects. *Naunyn Schmiedebergs Arch Pharmacol* 1988;337:261–266.
28. Lewicki R, Tchórzewski H, Majewska E, et al: Effect of maximal physical exercise on T-lymphocyte subpopulations and on interleukin 1 (IL 1) and interleukin 2 (IL 2) production in vitro. *Int J Sports Med* 1988;:114–117.
29. Mackinnon LT, Chick TW, van As A, et al: The effect of exercise on secretory and natural immunity. *Adv Exp Med Biol* 1987;216A:869–876.
30. Michael G, Vocke T, Fiehn W, et al: Bidirectional alteration of insulin receptor affinity by different forms of physical exercise. *Am J Physiol* 1984;246:E153-E159.
31. Moorthy AV, Zimmerman SW: Human leukocyte response to an endurance race. *Eur J Appl Physiol* 1978;38:271–276.
32. Moriguchi S, Watson RR: Nutrition, immune functions, and cardiovascular disease, in Watson RR (ed): *Nutrition and Heart Disease.* Boca Raton, CRC Press, 1987, vol 2, pp 111–118.
33. Oltras CM, Mora F, Vives F: Beta-endorphin and ACTH in plasma: Effects of physical and psychological stress. *Life Sci* 1987;40:1683–1686.
34. Omeliusik IL, Prokopenko LG: Ispol'zovanie tiamina dlia korrektsii immunnogo otveta pri fizicheskoĭ nagruzke [Use of thiamine for correcting the immune response during physical loading]. *Vopr Pitan* 1986;6:50–53.
35. Omeliusik IL, Prokopenko LG: Vliianie stafilokokkovoĭ infektsii na razvitie immunnogo otveta posle fizicheskoĭ nagruzki [Effect of a staphylococcal infection on the development of an immune response after physical loading]. *Zh Mikrobiol Epidemiol Immunobiol* 1986;4:44–49.
36. Oshida Y, Yamanouchi K, Hayamizu S, et al: Effect of acute physical exercise on lymphocyte subpopulations in trained and untrained subjects. *Int J Sports Med* 1988;9:137–140.
37. Pahlavani MA, Cheung TK, Chesky JA, et al: Influence of exercise on the immune function of rats of various ages. *J Appl Physiol* 1988;64:1997–2001.
38. Pedersen BK, Tvede N, Hansen FR, et al: Modulation of natural killer cell activity in peripheral blood by physical exercise. *Scand J Immunol* 1988;27:673–678.
39. Petrova IV, Kuz'min SN, Kurshakova TS, et al: Fagotsitarnaia aktivnost' neĭtrofilov i gumoral'nye faktory obshchego i mestnogo immuniteta pri intensivnykh fizicheskikh naguruzkakh [Neutrophil phagaocytic activity and the humoral factors of general and local immunity under intensive physical loading]. *Zh Mikrobiol Epidemiol Immunobiol* 1983;1:53–57.
40. Reyes MP, Lerner AM: Interferon and neutralizing antibody in sera of exercised mice with coxsackievirus B-3 myocarditis. *Proc Soc Exp Biol Med* 1976;151;333–338.
41. Reyes MP, Smith FE, Lerner AM: An enterovirus-induced murine model of an acute dilated-type cardiomyopathy. *Intervirology* 1984;22:146–155.
42. Robertson AJ, Ramesar KC, Potts RC, et al: The effect of strenuous physical exercise on circulating blood lymphocytes and serum cortisol levels. *J Clin Lab Immunol* 1981;5:53–57.
43. Rusch HP, Kline BE: Effect of exercise on growth of a mouse tumor. *Cancer Res* 1944;4:116–118.
44. Sheffer AL, Austen KF: Exercise-induced anaphylaxis. *J Allergy Clin Immunol* 1984;73:699–703.
45. Sheffer AL, Tong AK, Murphy GF, et al: Exercise-induced anaphylaxis: A serious form of physical allergy associated with mast cell degranulation. *J Allergy Clin Immunol* 1985;75:479–484.
46. Simon HB: The immunology of exercise: A brief review. *JAMA* 1984;252:2735–2738.

47. Smith KA, Crabtree GR, Kennedy SJ, et al: Glucocorticoid receptors and glucocorticoid sensitivity of mitogen stimulated and unstimulated human lymphocytes. *Nature* 1977;267:523–527.
48. Taylor GR, Dardano JR: Human cellular immune responsiveness following space flight. *Aviat Space Environment Med* 1983;54:S55-S59.
49. Tchórzewski H, Denys A, Zytkiewicz B: Sport training and some activities of human polymorphonuclear leukocyte lysosomes. *Zentralbl Bakteriol* 1976;162:402–407.
50. Tomasi TB, Trudeau FB, Czerwinski D, et al: Immune parameters in athletes before and after strenuous exercise. *J Clin Immunol* 1982;2:173–178.
51. Vorobyov EI, Gazenko OG, Genin AM, et al: Medical results of Salyut-6 manned space flights. *Aviat Space Environ Med* 1983;54:S31-S40.
52. Voss EW Jr: Prolonged weightlessness and humoral immunity. *Science* 1984;225:214–215.
53. Watson RR, Moriguchi S, Jackson JC, et al: Modification of cellular immune functions in humans by endurance exercise training during beta-adrenergic blockade with atenolol or propanolol. *Med Sci Sports Exerc* 1986;18:95–100.
54. Watson RR (ed): *Nutrition, Disease Resistance and Immune Function.* New York, Marcel Dekker, 1984, pp 1–399.
55. Watson RR: Disease, malnutrition and immunocompetence, in Watson RR (ed): *Nutrition, Disease Resistance and Immune Function.* New York, Marcel Dekker, 1984, pp iii–iv.
56. Watson RR: Exercise, weightlessness, and inactivity: Modifiers of immune functions, in Wolinsky I (ed): *Exercise and Sports Medicine.* Boca Raton, CRC Press, 1989, pp 385–395.
57. Watson RR: Stress caused by dietary changes: Corticosteroid production, a partial explanation for immunosuppression in the malnourished, in Watson RR (ed): *Nutrition, Disease Resistance and Immune Function.* New York, Marcel Dekker, 1984, pp 273–283.
58. White JA, Ismail AH, Bottoms GD: Effect of physical fitness on the adrenocortical response to exercise stress. *Med Sci Sports* 1976;8:113–118.
59. Yu DT, Clements PJ, Pearson CM: Effect of corticosteroids on exercise-induced lymphocytosis. *Clin Exp Immunol* 1977;28:326–331.

Chapter 49

Alterations in Tissue Response: Conditioning Effects at Different Ages

David L. Butler, PhD
Arthur Siegel, MD

Introduction

Conditioning (training) and aging affect musculoskeletal soft tissues in several ways. Athletic performance, tissue biomechanics, tissue structure, tissue chemistry, and cellular response can be used to assess training and aging effects on skeletal muscle, tendon, and ligament tissues.

Training especially affects skeletal muscle, and athletic activity alters tissue size and strength. Overtraining, however, can produce intramuscular fibrosis. Training also influences tendon and ligament properties by altering fibril size and chemistry. Changes in tissue biomechanics produced by training are more modest than the changes in skeletal muscle, and are still not well understood.

Aging reduces skeletal muscle performance and changes selected chemical measures, but clinical studies suggest that exercise conditioning may partially offset these declines. Aging dramatically affects ligament biomechanics, and the interactive effects of conditioning on aging tendons and ligaments need additional study.

Elderly individuals, a rapidly growing segment of the population, want to remain fit through a regular exercise program, but physicians and therapists are ill-equipped to outline appropriate programs. There is little current information on the interaction between aging and conditioning. The degree of activity necessary to promote increased fitness for the elderly without musculoskeletal soft-tissue injury has not been defined. Moreover, once a person has sustained an injury, the conditioning levels necessary for healing without reinjury are poorly understood. These conditioning levels or limits may change radically with age, but this is still unproven.

Results of the clinical studies on the effects of aging and conditioning on musculoskeletal soft tissues are difficult to interpret because of the number of uncontrolled variables that affect the responses of these tissues. Diet, general activity levels, and general state of health vary from subject to subject and are difficult to quantitate. Participants in such studies may represent the extremes of their age group and may be either healthier than their peers or more at risk for injury. In addition, tissue models subjected to different treatment levels can only undergo biopsy once or twice and cannot be evaluated in their entirety.

In animal studies, the extraneous variables of diet, activity levels, and general state of health can be controlled. Experiments can isolate and evaluate several levels of conditioning at different age levels. Animal tissues can be removed for comprehensive analyses at regular intervals. Nonetheless, these studies have drawbacks. Conditioning programs can be difficult to design and implement. Studies are often restricted to smaller, less expensive animals that can tolerate long-term treadmill experiments. The animals may resist these training regimens, and the results may be difficult or impossible to extrapolate to humans.

This chapter reviews the results of clinical, animal, and cell-culture studies on the physiologic and cellular responses of normal musculoskeletal soft tissues at different ages. It examines how different training regimens modulate tissue response at different ages and explores the differences between training and overtraining in tissues at different ages.

Three tissue models and several physiologic and cellular measures were used. The tissue models included skeletal muscle, tendon, and ligament. The physiologic measures included athletic performance and biomechanical, morphologic, and biochemical indices. Cellular measures included DNA content and activity, ultrastructural features of the cell, and replication rates.

Response of Normal Tissues at Different Ages

Skeletal Muscle

Skeletal muscle tissue adapts to exercise conditioning in a dynamic process involving biomechanical, anatomic, and biochemical changes. Alteration with aging is also a dynamic process and is the focus of recent specific studies. Understanding how these two dynamic processes—progressive conditioning and aging—interact and affect each other is important.

The rapid changes in peak athletic performance reflect changes in muscle physiology. High school track stars routinely break old world records for the mile. The 1913 world record holder for the marathon would not have qualified for the 1989 Boston Marathon, and the 1960 world record holder would not have qualified for the 1988 US Olympic trials. Women have shown even greater rates of improvement.

The impact of aging on skeletal muscle as shown by world record performance was studied in detail by Kavanagh and Shephard[42] at the World Master's Championships in August 1957. They asked middle-aged and elderly track competitors detailed questions about their training patterns and performance. They found that men 40 to 50 years old performed at roughly 80% of world record speeds. Performance declined with aging to the 70% range for sprints and middle-distance events but remained at the 80% level for long-distance events. Thus, aging slowly eroded maximal performance even among elite, highly selected athletes, but quality and capacity were still apparent.

A comparison of aerobic power (ml/kg·min [standard temperature and pressure, dry]) between this sample of elite competitors and other samples studied by Pollock[65] and Saltin and Grimby[68] shows that aerobic power declines only 4 to 5 ml/kg·min per decade between the ages of 35 and 65 years. In the absence of cardiovascular disease, aerobic power can be interpreted as a function of muscle performance. This comparison documents the gradual, moderate compromise of aerobic power with endurance training during aging. There are fewer data on elite female athletes, but extrapolation from the improvements in world records indicates that they also retain aerobic function and muscle performance during exercise conditioning.

The dynamic adaptation of skeletal muscle to aerobic conditioning involves changes in motor patterns, biomechanical response, and muscle biochemistry. In a runner, athletic performance depends on a combination of maximal flexibility and strength to obtain optimal speed. This involves the selection or recruitment of specific muscle fiber types that also develop with effort and training. Even within a single stride, a runner recruits different muscle fibers in actively contracting and relaxing opposing muscle groups. The process of training involves recruiting fiber groups and relaxing corresponding groups in opposing muscles. Maximal limb speed is attained through an appropriate, coordinated balance of relaxation and contraction between antagonistic muscle groups. Recruitment patterns within and among different muscles influence overall power, performance, and limb speed. Smooth acceleration and deceleration during a running stride depend on exercise conditioning to improve running efficiency.

Characteristics of aging human skeletal muscles have been studied from biomechanical, anatomic, and biochemical points of view. Skeletal muscle motor units and specific muscle fibers are divided into different types on the basis of physiologic, metabolic, and ultrastructural criteria. In humans, the pH sensitivity of the histochemical reactions of myofibrillar (actomyosin) adenosine triphosphatase is used to separate fiber types. Fibers are classified as type I and type II; there are three different subclasses of type II fibers. These fibers have different capacities for adenosine triphosphate hydrolysis and are selectively recruited according to the intensity of the overall physical effort. Type II fibers have approximately three times more capacity for adenosine triphosphate hydrolysis and are recruited for near-peak efforts. Type I fibers specialize in lower-intensity efforts and are recruited as muscle fatigue develops. There is only a small difference in size between the principal fiber types in young healthy adults.

In the untrained subject, most muscles contain a mixture of various types of motor units. Type I fibers are preferentially recruited at low force outputs while Type II fibers are progressively involved as higher force requirements develop. The hierarchy of recruitment thresholds may alter the phenotype of fibers so that more oxidative or type I fibers are recruited with aerobic conditioning. The sensitivity of muscle fibers to altered usage increases the difficulty of understanding the effects of the aging process itself.[38] Whether aging acts as an independent influence in altering human muscle structure and fiber composition or whether age-associated alterations are environmental or training-specific is unknown.

Muscle Fiber Characteristics in the Aging Adult Studies on aging human skeletal muscle find a progressive loss of total muscle fibers with advancing age.[24] Anatomic studies show a reduction in fiber numbers only after 60 years of age. After 70 years of age, fiber numbers are reduced approximately 25%. Studies on fiber-type distribution show that aging involves a specific loss of the high-performance or type II fibers. As many as 45% of these fibers may be lost between the ages of 30 to 70 years.[67] Physical activity has a mitigating effect on this loss, so exercise training during the middle and older years can help preserve muscle fibers and fiber-type distribution.

Exercise training can also help preserve youthful capillarization and energy metabolism.[24,67] Physical activity can also reduce the potentially deleterious effects of aging on the anatomic, physiologic, and metabolic attributes of skeletal muscle.[2] In summary, there is little evidence that muscle structure and composition in healthy humans are compromised until the age of 70 years. Exercise training can offset the atrophy of existing fibers and help preserve muscle structure, composition, and function.[41]

Tendon and Ligament

Mechanical Characteristics at Different Ages There have been studies to determine the changes in the mechanical properties of tendon and ligament with age.[5] Animal studies have concentrated on the effects of maturation and early skeletal maturity rather than on the effects of advancing age. Ligament[17,79,98] and tendon preparations[3,21,27,53,90] indicate that subfailure factors such as stiffness, modulus, and energy to the end of linear loading[17,21,53,89,98] as well as failure measures such as maximum load, maximum stress, failure energy, and strain-rate sensitivity[3,17,21,27,79,89,98] increase rapidly during the maturation phase but then stabilize (Fig. 1). The ligament-bone unit fails through the soft tissue-bone junction before epiphyseal closure and through the midsubstance after closure.[95] Few studies have evaluated the changes in mechanical properties with advancing age. Vogel[89] showed a decrease in strength and elasticity in rat-tail tendons with senescence, but skeletally mature littermates necessary for controlling animal-to-animal variability and large variances in mechanical characteristics are nearly impossible to obtain. Similar age-related changes were found when skin was tested.[88]

The mechanical properties of cadaveric tendons and ligament-bone units have also been measured.[43,55,77,100] Yamada's[100] compilation of tendon and ligament properties for the first two decades of life was similar to the results of the animal studies described above. After the

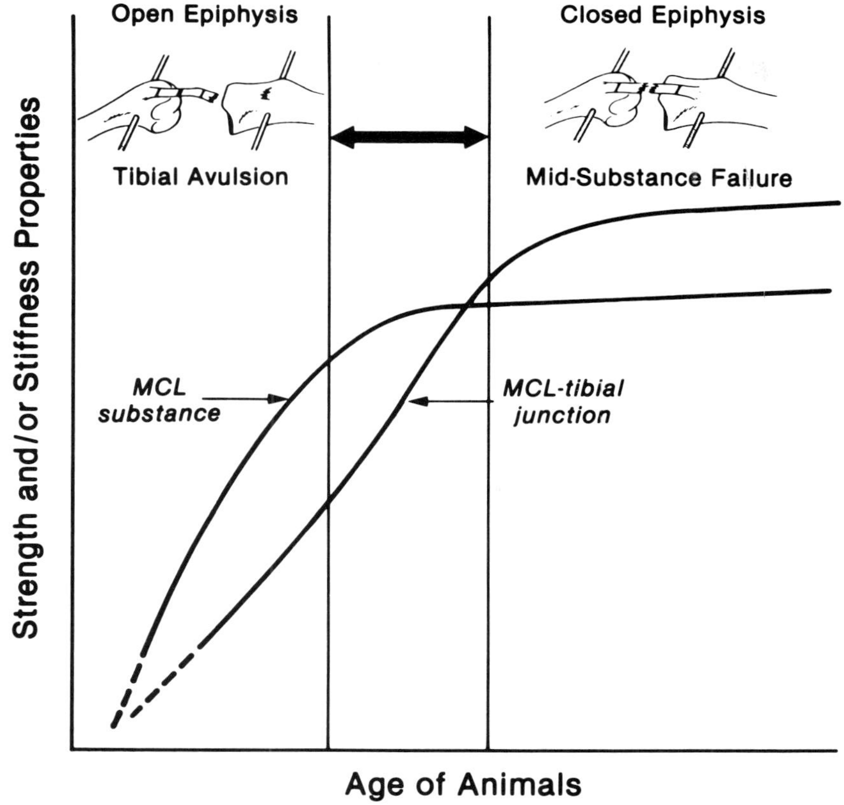

Fig. 1 *A diagram hypothesizing an asynchronous rate of maturation from both the structural characteristics of the femur-muscle-tibia complex and the mechanical properties of medial collateral ligament substance. (Reproduced with permission from Woo SL-Y, Orlando CA, Gomez MA, et al: Tensile properties of the medial collateral ligament as a function of age.* J Orthop Res *1986;4:133–141.)*

age of 50 years, however, load-related factors such as modulus and maximum stress decreased. Noyes and Grood[55] found significant decreases for the anterior cruciate ligament; there was a twofold decrease in modulus and a threefold decrease in maximum stress between the ages of 20 and 50 years (Fig. 2). The failure mode changed from soft tissue to bone avulsion at approximately 50 years, possibly because bone porosity beneath the insertion site increased. Other studies found no effect with age in this ligament model, although the tissue-testing methods and sample sizes preclude definitive conclusions.[43,77] The contradiction in the findings between the animal and human studies suggests that the animal studies may not be true "aging" studies.

Extracellular Morphologic and Biochemical Characteristics at Different Ages In tendon, collagen ultrastructure undergoes significant changes with increasing age.[7,26] The size of the fibrils increases after

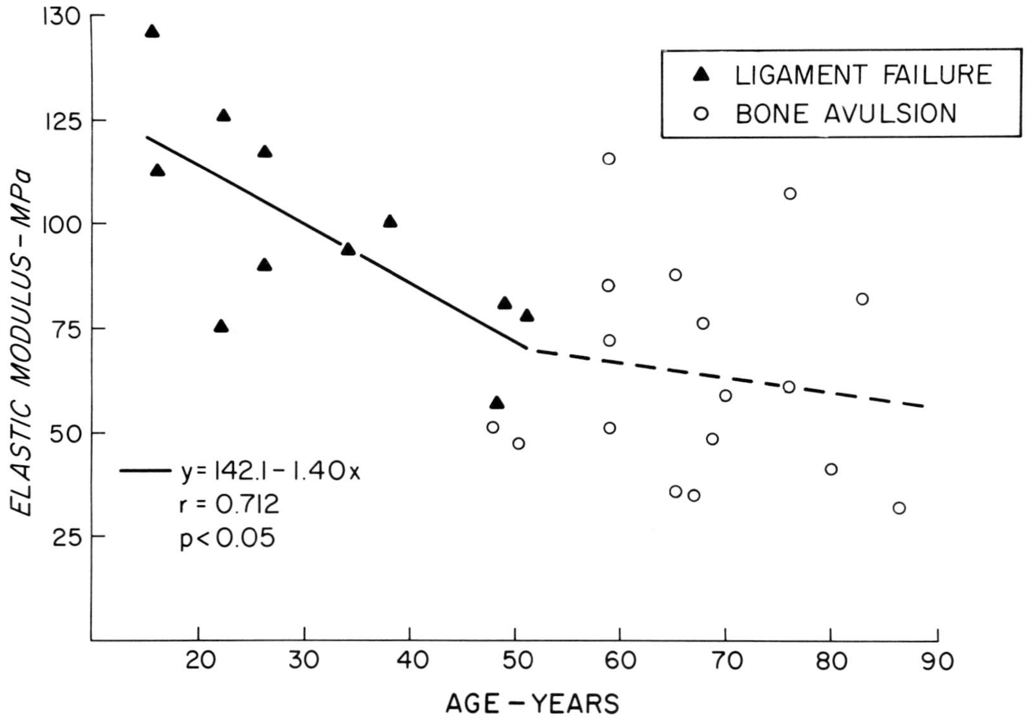

Fig. 2 *The correlation of ligament strength with age for femur-anterior cruciate-tibia preparations from humans. The solid lines represent the statistically significant correlation with age found in trauma and younger cadaveric preparations (triangles). All failures were through the body of the ligament. The broken lines represent the correlation (not statistically significant) found in amputation and older cadaver preparations (circles). These failed by avulsion fracture of the bone underneath the ligament insertion site. The equations of the solid lines and the correlation coefficients are also given.* ***Top,*** *Maximum stress.* ***Bottom,*** *Elastic modulus. (Reproduced with permission from Noyes FR, Grood ES: The strength of the anterior cruciate ligament in humans and rhesus monkeys: Age-related and species-related changes.* J Bone Joint Surg *1976;58A:1074–1082.)*

birth.[25,37,59,61] In the rat anterior cruciate ligament, fiber diameter increases during the maturation phase and plateaus until senility.[48] Similar results have been found in ligament and skin.[36,59,60,61,89,90]

Using a rat-tail tendon model, Vogel[89] found that changes in insoluble collagen correlated with mechanical changes during aging, but elastin and glycosaminoglycans did not. Water content in the ligament decreases with age.[79,83] This change may be associated with age-related decreases in chondroitin sulfate or hyaluronic acid.[75] The relative proportions of type III to type I collagen decrease with increasing age in rat skin,[51] but the age-related changes that occur in ligament or tendon collagen type are not known. Viidik[87] concluded that the stability of type I collagen in the musculoskeletal system and in skin is probably not a "true" aging phenomenon.

Cellular Characteristics at Different Ages There are extensive data on the aging of cells in vitro.[10] Early cell culture studies by Hayflick[31] and Hayflick and Moorhead[32] showed that diploid human embryonic fibroblasts lived for only a finite period but that their life span was not related to the culture conditions. Further, "the length of the life span varied inversely with donor age."[76] These results suggest that cellular senescence occurs as the cell's doubling capacity is exhausted. Generally, "cells aging in vitro and cells from aging organisms have many attributes in common."[23,76]

Cellular life span may be under genetic control and limited by the number of population doublings in vitro rather than by chronological time.[8,14] Embryonic cells double an average of 48 times in culture, but adult fibroblasts double only an average of 20 times.[31] Cells have four proliferative phases before senescence. Proliferation is rapid in the early phases and slows by phase 4. The proportion of the nonproliferating pool increases as age increases, but the cell's replicative ability shows no decrease. The cell size also increases[74] but without a dramatic increase in DNA content,[12] suggesting that growth and division are uncoupled in senescent cultures. The surface of the senescent fibroblasts shows a different set of surface glycoproteins and reduced amounts of fibronectin.[9,20,91] The fibroblast membrane shows increased permeability,[4,50] altered lipid composition,[45] and increased fluidity with age.[69] Mitochondrial mass increases with age.[22] The actin filaments within the cytoplasm form large bundles or sheets, creating a rigid structure that may contribute to the difficulty of replicating with age.[92] Protein content increases in vitro with increasing cell size,[11,34] but the rate of protein synthesis decreases.[35,40] Collagen synthesis has long been thought to decrease with age; however, this decrease may be overcome in the presence of ascorbic acid.[62] Fibroblasts appear to be capable of contracting a collagen lattice when seeded within one, regardless of cell type or donor ages.[93] These fibroblasts exhibit intertissue and intratissue differences in their properties. Young cells are spindle-shaped and older cells are flatter. There have been several recent reviews on cellular aging.[13,28–30]

How Different Training Regimens Modulate Tissue Response

Skeletal Muscle

The outstanding performances of older athletes show the profound mitigating effects of training on the aging process. The era of outstanding performance for midlife runners began with the 1984 Olympic Games in Los Angeles when a 37-year-old Portuguese runner, Carlos Lopes, won the men's marathon. Jack Foster of New Zealand set the world master's record for the marathon with a time of 2:11:19 in 1974, besting overall world records for men before 1967. At the 1988 Boston

Marathon, runners more than 40 years of age outnumbered younger runners for the first time.

Studies of skeletal muscle capillarity and enzyme activities in younger and older athletes show shifts consistent with attenuation of type II or low-oxidative fibers. This correlates with the relatively greater preservation of performance for older athletes in more aerobic or long-distance events.[42] Skeletal muscle fiber composition favors a predominance of oxidative fibers in older subjects that reflects the influence of training patterns and fiber recruitment in prolonged exercise. Mechanical efficiency may be reduced in older athletes, but this has not been systematically studied or proven.

Different Training Regimens Modulate Tissue Response at Different Ages The aging process imposes a slow onset of simple atrophy among existing muscle fiber types.[24] Most age-associated losses of performance or function are concentrated among the fast-twitch or high-oxidative fibers that specialize in power development. Recent studies of activity-induced transitions of fast- to slow-twitch fibers in mammalian muscle suggest that the emphasis on aerobic training and competition among older individuals might itself increase the predominance of high-oxidative fibers.[39,63] The phenotype of muscle fiber appears to be dynamic and modified by functional demand to favor a high-oxidative profile in older individuals.[64] This physiologic interpretation mirrors the performance records of older athletes, in whom performance is better preserved in endurance than in power-dependent events.[24] The decline in top performance is age-related but can be mitigated by training well into the sixth decade and beyond.[2] Longitudinal studies among older endurance athletes will continue to provide specific information on how much performance potential can be retained with endurance training.

Tendon and Ligament

Biomechanical Effects of Training Studies have assessed the effects of exercise on the biomechanical properties of tendon, ligaments, and their insertions.[1,6,47,48,56,78,80,81,85,86,95,96,97,99,102,103] Woo and associates[99] found positive effects on the tensile characteristics (modulus and maximum stress) of the extensor tendons of swine after 12 months of exercise training. Tipton and associates[81] showed that separation force and elongation in ligaments were unaffected by a single exercise bout but increased significantly with repeated periods of exercise. Cabaud and associates[6] also found that ligament-bone junction strength increased with exercise. However, these results reflect changes at the ligament-bone insertion rather than in the ligament midsubstance. Studies by Noyes and associates[56] concentrated on the effects of exercise on the anterior cruciate ligament in control limbs in primates. They found that an exercise program consisting of cyclic repeated limb loading against one-third body weight was required to maintain the mechanical properties of ligament with whole-body immobility.

Extracellular Morphologic and Biochemical Changes With Exercise After 12 months of moderate exercise training, swine tendons had significantly increased weight and total collagen content compared with sedentary controls.[99] Other studies using young rats showed that an intensive four-week exercise program produced a significant increase in the number of small-diameter fibrils of the anterior cruciate ligament compared with sedentary age-matched controls.[57,58] The number of large-diameter fibrils showed a corresponding decrease with exercise. The total cross-sectional area (and presumably weight) of the exercised ligaments was actually smaller than in the control tissues, contrary to the findings of Woo and associates.[99] Vailas and associates[83] compared skeletally mature 9-month-old and aging 28-month-old rats. They found that aging significantly decreased patellar tendon glycosaminoglycans and increased collagen concentration. They also found that moderate exercise increased glycosaminoglycan levels only at 9 months of age with no significant effect on collagen concentrations. Lapiere and associates[46] also suggested an interaction between collagen types I and III with conditioning.

Cellular Changes With Exercise No studies have documented cellular changes in tissues subjected to different levels of conditioning. If there were such studies, the cells extracted from tendon or ligament preparations in animals would probably have been exposed to one or more training regimens. Cell culture studies to evaluate various exercise programs would be difficult to design and nearly impossible to extrapolate to either the animal or human models.

Training vs Overtraining at Different Ages

Skeletal Muscle

Morphologic and biochemical studies of muscle soreness after exercise show evidence of anatomic and biochemical injury.[16,18] Exercise-induced skeletal muscle damage is particularly pronounced with eccentric exercise,[49] in which muscles produce force while lengthening, as in downhill running.[54] It may be several days before the damage peaks, and it may last for an extended period of time. Morphologic studies of delayed muscle soreness show subcellular injury with myofibrillar disruption and Z-band streaming.[19] Such morphologic evidence shows that the contractile structure of the muscle fiber has been overloaded and the contractile apparatus disrupted for periods of days to weeks. These morphologic findings correlate with quantitative peaks of creatine kinase release into the blood from injured muscle fibers, especially after eccentric exercise.[19]

The muscle overuse syndromes in long-distance runners have been especially studied in marathon competitions, in which demand for muscular work continues even after glycogen depletion. Runners experience moderate to severe stiffness in the quadriceps area with peak serum creatine kinase levels including the MM and MB isoenzyme fractions.

Elevated serum creatine kinase MB isoenzyme (CK-MB) activity in marathon runners after competition may arise from injury to skeletal muscle, myocardium, or a combined tissue source. Normal findings on radionuclide myocardial scintigraphy and the selective increase in skeletal muscle CK-MB reported in these runners suggest a peripheral source.[70–72] To explain this biochemical finding, an electron microscopy morphologic examination of gastrocnemius muscles was performed on 40 male marathon runners at intervals after competition.[33,94] Muscle samples showed ultrastructural changes characteristic of focal fiber injury and repair. In the first three days after the race, these changes included intracellular and extracellular edema with endothelial injury, myofibrillar lysis, dilation and disruption of the T-tubule system, and focal mitochondrial degeneration without inflammatory infiltrate.[94] The mitochondrial and myofibrillar damage showed progressive repair three to four weeks later. Biopsy specimens showed central nuclei and satellite cells characteristic of the regenerative response at eight to 12 weeks. Muscles from veteran runners showed intercellular collagen deposition that suggested a fibrotic response to repetitive injury. Control tissues from nonrunners showed none of these findings. Animal studies suggest the same changes occur with age and with endurance training.[44] The sequential morphologic changes in runners suggest that the increase in skeletal muscle CK-MB is a marker of cellular regeneration.

Some investigators have reported chronic muscular injury in ultra-long-distance runners, many of whom have engaged in endurance training and competition for many years.[73] Ultrastructural evidence of skeletal muscle injury and repair after competition may explain the persistent presence of regenerating muscle fibers that have a high concentration of MB subunits. Electron microscopy was used to assess skeletal muscle morphologic features in ultra-long-distance runners. Gastrocnemius muscle samples of five runners were taken 24 hours after a 100-mile run. The average age of the subjects was 44 years, and the mean finishing time of 26 hours included breaks for rest and nutritional repletion. These specimens showed a lesser degree of acute myofibrillar lysis, mitochondrial disruption, and endothelial injury than did specimens from marathon runners.[73] Four of the five specimens demonstrated evidence of chronic injury characterized by the presence of interstitial fibroblasts with collagen deposition (Fig. 3). Prominent numbers of satellite cells provided evidence of ongoing regenerative cell activity (Fig. 4). These findings suggest that the lower intensity level but increased duration of endurance activity in ultra-long-distance running leads to a balanced process of chronic muscular injury and repair. The increase in serum CK-MB after competition and in skeletal muscle tissue in ultra-long-distance runners may be a marker of this regenerative cell activity.

Studies in ultra-long-distance runners confirm a balanced presence of injury and repair with focal myofibrillar disruption and the com-

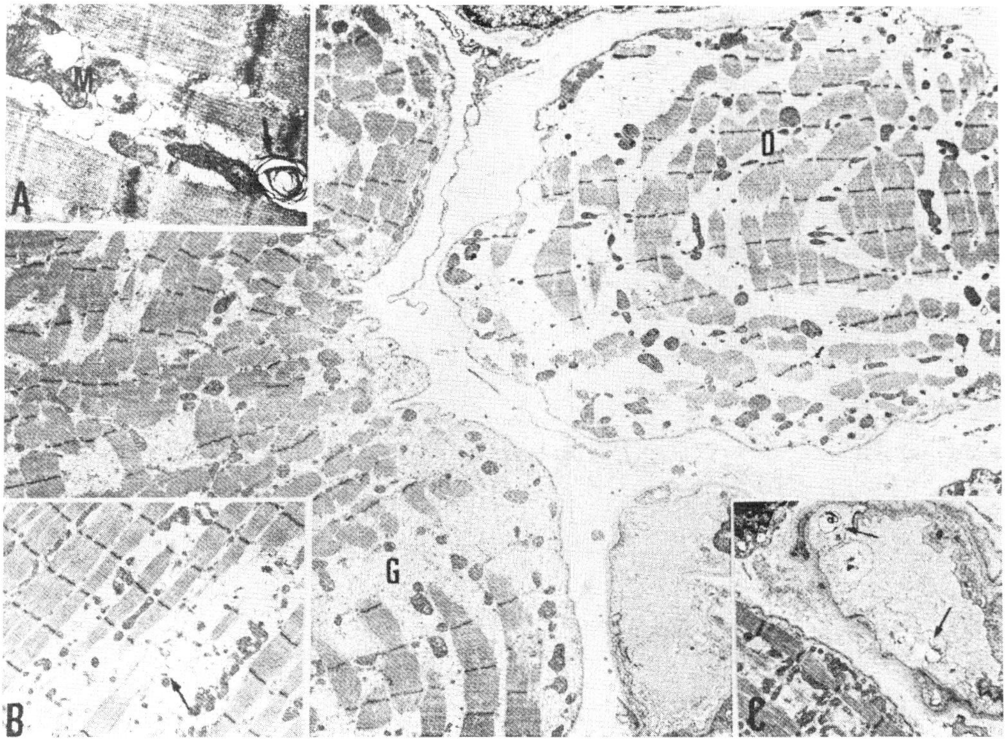

Fig. 3 *A low-power electron micrograph of two muscle fibers. One fiber (G) has a normal glycogen content and largely intact myofibrils. The other "pale" fiber (D) is depleted of glycogen and exhibits intracellular edema (×2,000).* ***Inset A,*** *Mitochondrial injury with both lysis of mitrochondral matrix (M), and the formation of intramitochondrial myelin fibers (×10,000).* ***Inset B,*** *A glycogen-depleted fiber with myofibrillar lysis and dilation of sarcoplasmic reticulum (arrow) (×2,000).* ***Inset C,*** *A capillary with injury to one endothelial cell characterized by loss of cytoplasmic density and the formation of intracellular myelin fibers (arrow) (×2,000). (Reproduced with permission from Siegel AJ, Warhol MJ, Lang G: Muscle injury and repair in ultra long distance runners, in Sutton JR, Brock RM (eds):* Sports Medicine for the Mature Athlete. *Indianapolis, Benchmark Press, 1986, pp 35–43.)*

pensatory appearance of satellite cells. Thus, selective glycogen depletion occurs in specific muscle fibers. This leads to focal injury, perhaps selective for newly recruited high-oxidative fibers,[15] leading in turn to a balanced process of chronic muscular injury and repair. The increase in skeletal muscle CK-MB with progressive training is a biochemical marker of the regenerative response to cellular injury. Some studies suggest that muscle fiber necrosis with an acute cellular inflammatory response can be associated with endurance-sports injuries, but this requires further study.[33] Prostaglandin A_2 may be a mediator of muscular repair, but research on the cellular mediators in inflammation and injury and the compensatory reparative response is needed.[66]

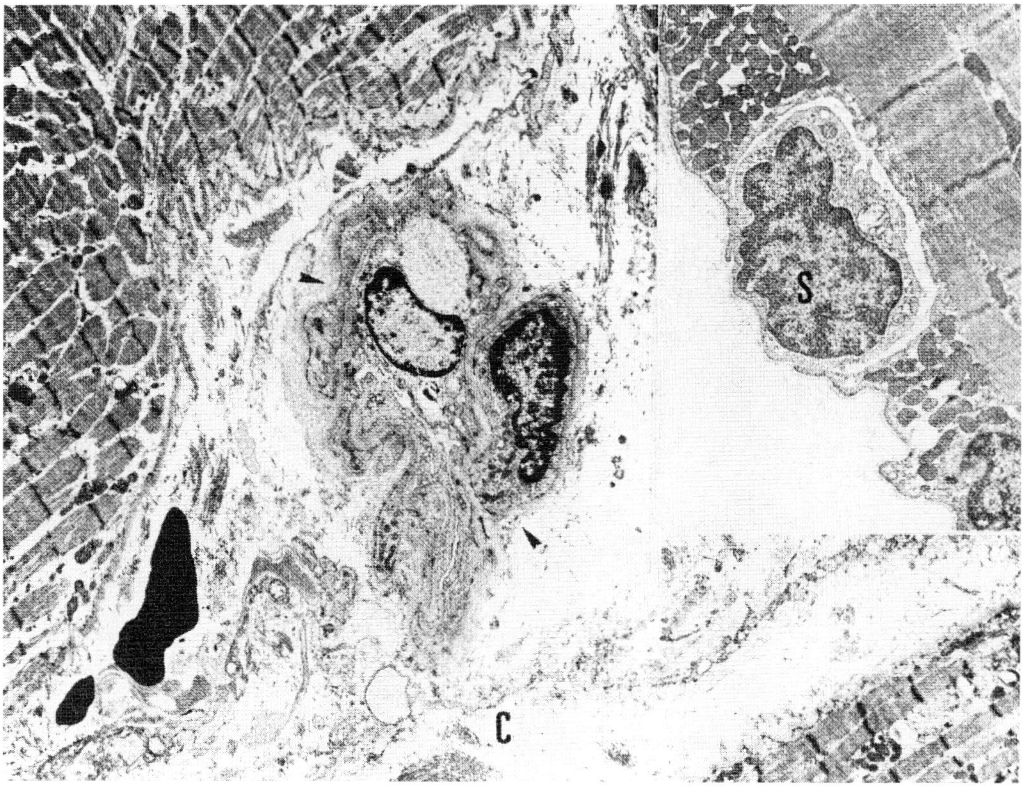

Fig. 4 *The changes in chronic injury. There are numerous collagen fibers (C) in the interspace. The capillary basal lamina is thickened and irregular (arrowheads) (×4,000). Satellite cells (S), located inside the basal lamina, were a prominent feature (×8,000). (Reproduced with permission from Siegel AJ, Warhol MJ, Lang G: Muscle injury and repair in ultra long distance runners, in Sutton JR, Brock RM (eds):* Sports Medicine for the Mature Athlete. *Indianapolis, Benchmark Press, 1986, pp 35–43.)*

Qualitative and quantitative degrees of myofibrillar injury result from overtraining in young, middle-aged, and older athletes alike. The chronic nature of intensive sports participation favors development of a chronic injury pattern in the older athlete. Glycogen-depleted muscle fibers incur mitochondrial injury, dilation of sarcoplasmic reticulum, and myofibrillar lysis. Capillary injury and endothelial disruption can also occur (Fig. 3).[72,94] The changes caused by chronic injury in older endurance athletes include deposition of numerous collagen fibers in the interstitial space and thickening of the capillary basal lamina (Fig. 4). Satellite cells located in the basal lamina are a prominent feature and show the reparative response to such cellular injury. The morphologic, biochemical, and inflammatory mediators of these injury and repair dynamics are still poorly understood, however.

Tendon and Ligament

Biomechanical, Morphologic, and Cellular Effects of Overtraining There is very little information on the effects of overtraining in tendons or ligaments. Spontaneous tendon rupture in competitive weightlifting has been reported, and the tissue forces at injury estimated[101] but significant amounts of connective tissue from patients who sustain overtraining injuries are obviously unavailable for direct mechanical evaluation. Biopsy specimens would provide some indication of overtraining effects, but regional variations in collagen or glycosaminoglycan concentrations could mask the effects of this variable, and the exact location of the injury site might be difficult to find. Animal studies may offer a way to assess overtraining effects, if exercise programs can be designed and instituted and if the animals can be made to engage in these regimens. However, no such studies are in progress. Animal studies in which a ligament or tendon was cut or torn[3,84] suggest tissue response to injury but may be inadequate simulations of repetitive damage caused by exercise.

Little data are available on the cellular changes in tendons or ligaments caused by overtraining. After a sheet of cells is wounded, the latent period before migration increases with in vivo donor age.[52] Although this study on cell motility in the presence of a wound is important, it did not simulate the repetitive damage stimulus that occurs with overtraining.

References

1. Adams A: Effect of exercise upon ligament strength. *Res Q Am Assoc Health Phys Educ* 1966;37:163–167.
2. Astrand PO: Exercise physiology of the mature athlete, in Sutton JR, Brock RM (eds): *Sports Medicine for the Mature Athlete.* Indianapolis, Benchmark Press, 1986, pp 3–13.
3. Barfred T: Experimental rupture of the Achilles tendon: Comparison of experimental ruptures in rats of different ages and living under different conditions. *Acta Orthop Scand* 1971;42:406–428.
4. Berumen L, Macieira-Coelho A: Changes in albumin uptake during the lifespan of human fibroblasts in vitro. *Mech Ageing Dev* 1977;6:165–172.
5. Butler DL, Grood ES, Noyes FR, et al: Biomechanics of ligaments and tendons, in Hutton RS (ed): *Exercise and Sports Sciences Reviews.* Washington DC, Franklin Institute Press, 1978, pp 125–181.
6. Cabaud HE, Chatty A, Gildengorin V, et al: Exercise effects on the strength of the rat anterior cruciate ligament. *Am J Sports Med* 1980;8:79–86.
7. Cetta G, Tenni R, Zanaboni G, et al: Biochemical and morphological modifications in rabbit Achilles tendon during maturation and ageing. *Biochem J* 1982;204:61–67.
8. Collins VP: The re-entry of long term density growth inhibited cells into the cell cycle. *Cell Biol Int Rep* 1983;7:1081–1089.
9. Courtois Y, Hughes RC: Surface labelling of senescent chick fibroblasts by lactoperoxidase-catalysed iodination. *Gerontology* 1976;22:371–379.

10. Cristofalo VJ (ed): *CRC Handbook of Cell Biology of Aging*. Boca Raton, CRC Press, 1985.
11. Cristofalo VJ, Howard BV, Kritchevsky D: The biochemistry of human cells in culture. *Res Prog Org Biol Med Chem* 1970;2:95–146.
12. Cristofalo VJ, Kritchevsky D: Cell size and nucleic acid content in the diploid human cell line WI-38 during aging. *Med Exp* 1969;19:313–320.
13. Cristofalo VJ, Stanulis-Praeger BM: Cellular senescence in vitro, in Maramorosch K (ed): *Advances in Cell Culture*. New York, Academic Press, 1982, vol 2, pp 1–68.
14. Dell'Orco RT, Mertens JG, Kruse PF Jr: Doubling potential, calendar time, and senescence of human diploid cells in culture. *Exp Cell Res* 1973;77:356–360.
15. Essén B: Glycogen depletion of different fibre types in human skeletal muscle during intermittent and continuous exercise. *Acta Physiol Scand* 1978;103:446–455.
16. Evans WJ: Exercise-induced skeletal muscle damage. *Phys Sportsmed* 1987;15:89.
17. Frank C, Woo SL-Y, Amiel D, et al: Medial collateral ligament healing: A multidisciplinary assessment in rabbits. *Am J Sports Med* 1983;11:379–389.
18. Fridén J, Sjöström M, Ekblom B: A morphological study of delayed muscle soreness. *Experientia* 1981;37:506–507.
19. Fridén J, Sjöström M, Ekblom B: Myofibrillar damage following intense eccentric exercise in man. *Int J Sports Med* 1983;4:170–176.
20. Fry M, Weisman-Shomer P: Surface proteins of young and senescent cultured avian fibroblasts. *Cell Biol Int Rep* 1977;1:399–407.
21. Galeski A, Kastelic J, Baer E, et al: Mechanical and structural changes in rat tail tendon induced by alloxan diabetes and aging. *J Biomech* 1977;10:775–782.
22. Goldstein S, Korczack LB: Status of mitochondria in living human fibroblasts during growth and senescence in vitro: Use of the laser dye rhodamine 123. *J Cell Biol* 1981;91:392–398.
23. Goldstein S, Singal DP: Senescence of cultured human fibroblasts: Mitotic versus metabolic time. *Exp Cell Res* 1974;88:359–364.
24. Green HJ: Morphological, ultrastructural, and functional characteristics of the aging human skeletal muscle, in Sutton JR, Brock RM (eds): *Sports Medicine for the Mature Athlete*. Indianapolis, Benchmark Press, 1986, pp 17–26.
25. Greenlee TK Jr, Ross R: The development of the rat flexor digital tendon: A fine structure study. *J Ultrastruct Res* 1967;18:354–376.
26. Hall DA: *The Ageing of Connective Tissue*. London, Academic Press, 1976, pp 13–67.
27. Haut RC: Age-dependent influence of strain rate on the tensile failure of rat-tail tendon. *J Biomech Eng* 1983;105:296–299.
28. Hayflick L: Cell aging. *Annu Rev Gerontol Geriatr* 1980:1:26–67.
29. Hayflick L: Intracellular determinants of cell aging. *Mech Ageing Dev* 1984;28:177–185.
30. Hayflick L: The cellular basis for biological aging, in Finch CE, Hayflick L (eds): *Handbook of the Biology of Aging*. New York, Van Nostrand Reinhold, 1977, pp 159–186.
31. Hayflick L: The limited in vitro lifetime of human diploid cell strains. *Exp Cell Res* 1965;37:614–636.
32. Hayflick L, Moorhead PS: The serial cultivation of human diploid cell strains. *Exp Cell Res* 1961;25:585–621.
33. Hikida RS, Staron RS, Hagerman FC, et al: Muscle fiber necrosis associated with human marathon runners. *J Neurol Sci* 1983;59:185–203.

34. Hildebran JN, Absher M, Low RB: Altered rates of collagen synthesis in in vitro aged human lung fibroblasts. *In Vitro* 1983;19:307–314.
35. Houck JC, Sharma VK, Hayflick L: Functional failures of cultured human diploid fibroblasts after continued population doublings. *Proc Soc Exp Biol Med* 1971;137:331–333.
36. Ingelmark BE: The structure of tendons at various ages and under different functional conditions: II. An electron-microscopic investigation of Achilles tendons from white rats. *Acta Anat* 1948;6:193–225.
37. Ippolito E, Natali PG, Postacchini F, et al: Morphological, immunochemical, and biochemical study of rabbit Achilles tendon at various ages. *J Bone Joint Surg* 1980;62A:583-598.
38. Ishihara A, Araki H: Effects of age on the number and histochemical properties of muscle fibers and motoneurons in the rat extensor digitorum longus muscle. *Mech Ageing Devel* 1988;45:213–221.
39. Järvinen M, Aho AJ, Lehto M, et al: Age dependent repair of muscle rupture: A histological and microangiographical study in rats. *Acta Orthop Scand* 1983;54:64–74.
40. Kaftory A, Hershko HA, Fry M: Protein turnover in senescent cultured chick embryo fibroblasts. *J Cell Physiol* 1978;94:147–160.
41. Karvonen MJ: Endurance sports, longevity, and health. *Ann NY Acad Sci* 1977;301:653–655.
42. Kavanagh T, Shephard RJ: The effects of continued training on the aging process. *Ann NY Acad Sci* 1977;301:656–670.
43. Kennedy JC, Hawkins RJ, Willis RB, et al: Tension studies of human knee ligaments: Yield point, ultimate failure, and disruption of the cruciate and tibial collateral ligaments. *J Bone Joint Surg* 1976;58A:350-355.
44. Kovanen V, Suominen H, Risteli J, et al: Type IV collagen and laminin in slow and fast skeletal muscle in rats: Effects of age and life-time endurance training. *Collagen Relat Res* 1988;8:145–153.
45. Kritchevsky D, Howard BV: The lipids of human diploid cell strain WI-38. *Ann Med Exp Fenn* 1966;44:343–347.
46. Lapiere CM, Nusgens B, Pierard GE: Interaction between collagen type I and type III in conditioning bundles organization. *Connect Tissue Res* 1977;5:21–29.
47. Laros GS, Tipton CM, Cooper RR: Influence of physical activity on ligament insertions in the knees of dogs. *J Bone Joint Surg* 1971;53A:275–286.
48. Larsen N, Parker AW: Physical activity and its influence on the strength and elastic stiffness of knee ligament, in Howell ML, Parker AW (eds): *Sports Medicine: Medical and Scientific Aspects of Elitism in Sports.* Brisbane, Australian Sports Medicine Federation, 1982, vol 8, pp 63–73.
49. Lieber RL, Friden J: Selective damage of fast glycolytic muscle fibres with eccentric contraction of the rabbit tibialis anterior. *Acta Physiol Scand* 1988;133:587–588.
50. Macieira-Coelho A, Taboury F: A re-evaluation of the changes in proliferation in human fibroblasts during ageing in vitro. *Cell Tissue Kinet* 1982;15:213–224.
51. Mays PK, Bishop JE, Laurent GJ: Age-related changes in the proportion of types I and III collagen. *Mech Ageing Dev* 1988;45:203–212.
52. Muggleton-Harris AL, Reisert PS, Burghoff RL: In vitro characterization of response to stimulus (wounding) with regard to ageing in human skin fibroblasts. *Mech Ageing Dev* 1982;19:37-43.
53. Nathan H, Goldgefter L, Kobyliansky E, et al: Energy absorbing capacity of rat tail tendon at various ages. *J Anat* 1978;127:589–593.
54. Newham DJ, Jones DA, Edwards RHT: Large delayed plasma creatine kinase changes after stepping exercise. *Muscle Nerve* 1983;6:380–385.

55. Noyes FR, Grood ES: The strength of the anterior cruciate ligament in humans and rhesus monkeys: Age-related and species-related changes. *J Bone Joint Surg* 1976;58A:1074–1082.

56. Noyes FR, Torvik PJ, Hyde WB, et al: Biomechanics of ligament failure: II. An analysis of immobilization, exercise, and reconditioning effects in primates. *J Bone Joint Surg* 1974;56A:1406–1418.

57. Oakes BW, Leslie J, Jacobsen J, et al: Mechanisms of connective tissue rehabilitation, in Howell ML, Parker AW (eds): *Sports Medicine: Medical and Scientific Aspects of Elitism in Sports*. Brisbane, Australian Sports Medicine Federation, 1982, vol 8, pp 39–62.

58. Oakes BW, Parker AW, Norman J: Changes in collagen fibre populations in young rat cruciate ligaments in response to an intensive one month's exercise program, in Russo P, Gass G (eds): *Human Adaptation*. Williamsberg, Kentucky, Cumberland College of Health Sciences, 1981, pp 223–230.

59. Parry DAD, Barnes GRG, Craig AS: A comparison of the size distribution of collagen fibrils in connective tissues as a function of age and a possible relation between fibril size distribution and mechanical properties. *Proc R Soc Lond* 1978;203:305–321.

60. Parry DAD, Craig AS: Growth and development of collagen fibrils in connective tissue, in Ruggeri A, Motta PM (eds): *Ultrastructure of the Connective Tissue Matrix*. Boston, Martinus Nijhoff, 1984, pp 34–64.

61. Parry DAD, Craig AS, Barnes GRG: Tendon and ligament from the horse: An ultrastructural study of collagen fibrils and elastic fibres as a function of age. *Proc R Soc Lond* 1978;203:293–303.

62. Paz MA, Gallop PM: Collagen synthesized and modified by aging fibroblasts in culture. *In Vitro* 1975;11:302–312.

63. Pette D: Adaptability of skeletal muscle to long-term use, in Sutton JR, Brock RM (eds): *Sports Medicine for the Mature Athlete*. Indianapolis, Benchmark Press, 1986, pp 27–34.

64. Pettigrew FP, Gardiner PF: Changes in rat plantaris motor unit profiles with advanced age. *Mech Ageing Dev* 1987;40:243–259.

65. Pollock ML: Physiological characteristics of older champion track athletes. *Res Q Am Assoc Health Phys Educ* 1974;45:363–373.

66. Rodemann HP, Goldberg AL: Arachidonic acid, prostaglandin E_2 and F_2 alpha influence rates of protein turnover in skeletal and cardiac muscle. *J Biol Chem* 1982;257:1632–1638.

67. Saltin B: Physiological characteristics of the masters athlete, in Sutton JR, Brock RM (eds): *Sports Medicine for the Mature Athlete*. Indianapolis, Benchmark Press, 1986, pp 59-80.

68. Saltin B, Grimby G: Physiological analysis of middle-aged and old former athletes: Comparison with still active athletes of the same ages. *Circulation* 1968;38:1104–1115.

69. Schroeder F, Goetz I, Roberts E: Age-related alterations in cultured human fibroblast membrane structure and function. *Mech Ageing Dev* 1984;25:365–389.

70. Siegel AJ, Silverman LM, Evans WJ: Elevated skeletal muscle creatine kinase MB isoenzyme levels in marathon runners. *JAMA* 1983;250:2835–2837.

71. Siegel AJ, Silverman LM, Holman BL: Elevated creatine kinase MB isoenzyme levels in marathon runners: Normal myocardial scintigrams suggest noncardiac source. *JAMA* 1981;246:2049–2051.

72. Siegel AJ, Silverman LM, Holman BL: Normal results of post-race thallium-201 myocardial perfusion imaging in marathon runners with elevated serum MB creatine kinase levels. *Am J Med* 1985;79:431–434.

73. Siegel AJ, Warhol MJ, Lang G: Muscle injury and repair in ultra long distance runners, in Sutton JR, Brock RM (eds): *Sports Medicine for the Mature Athlete*. Indianapolis, Benchmark Press, 1986, pp 35–43.
74. Simons JW: The use of frequency distributions of cell diameters to characterize cell populations in tissue culture. *Exp Cell Res* 1967;45:336–350.
75. Sinex FM: The role of collagen in aging, in Gould BS (ed): *Treatise on Collagen: Vol 2. Biology of Collagen, Part B*. London, Academic Press, 1968, pp 409–448.
76. Stanulis-Praeger BM: Cellular senescence revisited: A review. *Mech Ageing Dev* 1987;38:1–48.
77. Tipton CM, James SL, Mergner W, et al: Influence of exercise on strength of medial collateral knee ligaments of dogs. *Am J Physiol* 1970;218:894–902.
78. Tipton CM, Matthes RD, Martin RK: Influence of age and sex on the strength of bone-ligament junctions in knee joints of rats. *J Bone Joint Surg* 1978;60A:230–234.
79. Tipton CM, Matthes RD, Maynard JA, et al: The influence of physical activity on ligaments and tendons. *Med Sci Sports* 1975;7:165–175.
80. Tipton CM, Schild RJ, Tomanek RJ: Influence of physical activity on the strength of knee ligaments in rats. *Am J Physiol* 1967;212:783–787.
81. Tipton CM, Vailas AC, Matthes RD: Experimental studies on the influences of physical activity on ligaments, tendons and joints: A brief review. *Acta Med Scand* 1986;711(suppl):157–168.
82. Trent PS, Walker PS, Wolf B: Ligament length patterns, strength, and rotational axes of the knee joint. *Clin Orthop* 1976;117:263–270.
83. Vailas AC, Pedrini VA, Pedrini-Mille A, et al: Patellar tendon matrix changes associated with aging and voluntary exercise. *J Appl Physiol* 1985;58:1572–1576.
84. Vailas AC, Tipton CM, Matthes RD, et al: Physical activity and its influence on the repair process of medial collateral ligaments. *Connect Tissue Res* 1981;9:25–31.
85. Viidik A: Connective tissues: Possible implications of the temporal changes for the aging process. *Mech Ageing Dev* 1979;9:267–285.
86. Viidik A: Tensile strength properties of Achilles tendon systems in trained and untrained rabbits. *Acta Orthop Scand* 1969;40:261–272.
87. Viidik A: The effect of training on the tensile strength of isolated rabbit tendons. *Scand J Plast Reconstr Surg* 1967;1:141–147.
88. Vogel HG: Correlation between tensile strength and collagen content in rat skin: Effect of age and cortisol treatment. *Connect Tissue Res* 1974;2:177–182.
89. Vogel HG: Influence of maturation and age on mechanical and biochemical parameters of connective tissue of various organs in the rat. *Connect Tissue Res* 1978;6:161–166.
90. Vogel HG: Tensile strength, relaxation and mechanical recovery in rat skin as influenced by maturation and age. *J Med* 1976;7:177–188.
91. Vogel KG, Kelley RO, Stewart C: Loss of organized fibronectin matrix from the surface of aging diploid fibroblasts (IMR-90). *Mech Ageing Dev* 1981;16:295–302.
92. Wang E, Gundersen D: Increased organization of cytoskeleton accompanying the aging of human fibroblasts in vitro. *Exp Cell Res* 1984;154:191–202.
93. Wang SY, Merrill C, Bell E: Effects of ageing and long-term subcultivation on collagen lattice contraction and intra-lattice proliferation in three rat cell types. *Mech Ageing Dev* 1988;44:127–141.
94. Warhol MJ, Siegel AJ, Evans WJ, et al: Skeletal muscle injury and repair in marathon runners after competition. *Am J Pathol* 1985;118:331-339.

95. Woo SL-Y, Amiel D, Akeson WH, et al: Effects of long term exercise on ligaments, tendons and bones of swine. *Med Sci Sports* 1979;11:105.
96. Woo SL-Y, Gomez MA, Amiel D, et al: The effects of exercise on the biomechanical and biochemical properties of swine digital flexor tendons. *J Biomech Eng* 1981;103:51–56.
97. Woo SL-Y, Gomez MA, Woo YK, et al: Mechanical properties of tendons and ligaments: II. The relationships of immobilization and exercise on tissue remodeling. *Biorheology* 1982;19:397–408.
98. Woo SL-Y, Orlando CA, Gomez MA, et al: Tensile properties of the medial collateral ligament as a function of age. *J Orthop Res* 1986;4:133–141.
99. Woo SL-Y, Ritter MA, Amiel D, et al: The biomechanical and biochemical properties of swine tendons: Long term effects of exercise on the digital extensors. *Connect Tissue Res* 1980;7:177–183.
100. Yamada H: *Strength of Biological Materials.* Baltimore, Williams & Wilkins, 1970, pp 80–81.
101. Zernicke RF, Garhammer J, Jobe FW: Human patellar-tendon rupture. *J Bone Joint Surg* 1977;59A:179–183.
102. Zuckerman J, Stull GA: Effects of exercise on knee ligament separation force in rats. *J Appl Physiol* 1969;26:716–719.
103. Zuckerman J, Stull GA: Ligamentous separation force in rats as influenced by training, detraining, and cage restriction. *Med Sci Sports* 1973;5:44–49.

Chapter 50

The Use of Flexibility Exercises in Preventing and Treating Sports Injuries

William D. Stanish, MD, FRCS (C)
Sandra L. Curwin, PhD
Greg Bryson

Introduction

Flexibility exercises are widely used to prevent muscle overstretch injuries. The theoretical basis for this use is fairly well defined, but the epidemiologic and scientific evidence to support flexibility training is somewhat scanty. This chapter reviews the clinical and scientific evidence available to show how and why flexibility exercises can be used to prevent and treat sports injuries.

Physiology of Flexibility Without Injury

The muscle-tendon unit contains two basic components: a contractile or active element, and a noncontractile or passive element. The active component results from crossbridge interaction between the contractile proteins, rectin, and myosin within the muscle fibers. The noncontractile components include connective tissue elements within and around the muscle, the perimysium, epimysium, and endomysium; the sarcolemma; associated tendons and their insertions; and connections between the sarcolemma and the tendon.[8,24,60] To understand the physiology of flexibility, both neurophysiologic and mechanical aspects of muscle control and behavior must be examined.

Neurophysiology of Stretching

There are two types of muscle fiber, intrafusal and extrafusal. The extrafusal fibers are innervated by alpha motor neurons and are the main "motor" of the muscle. The intrafusal fibers are part of the muscle spindles, the sensory elements within the muscle that signal both length change and rate-of-change of length, are innervated by gamma and beta motor neurons (Fig. 1). Afferent signals from receptors in the muscle spindle travel to the central nervous system via Ia and II sensory nerves.[9] The spindle parallels the extrafusal fibers, so that increases in muscle length stretch it as well, causing depolarization and firing of the Ia and II endings.[56,78] This afferent signal activates the motor neurons

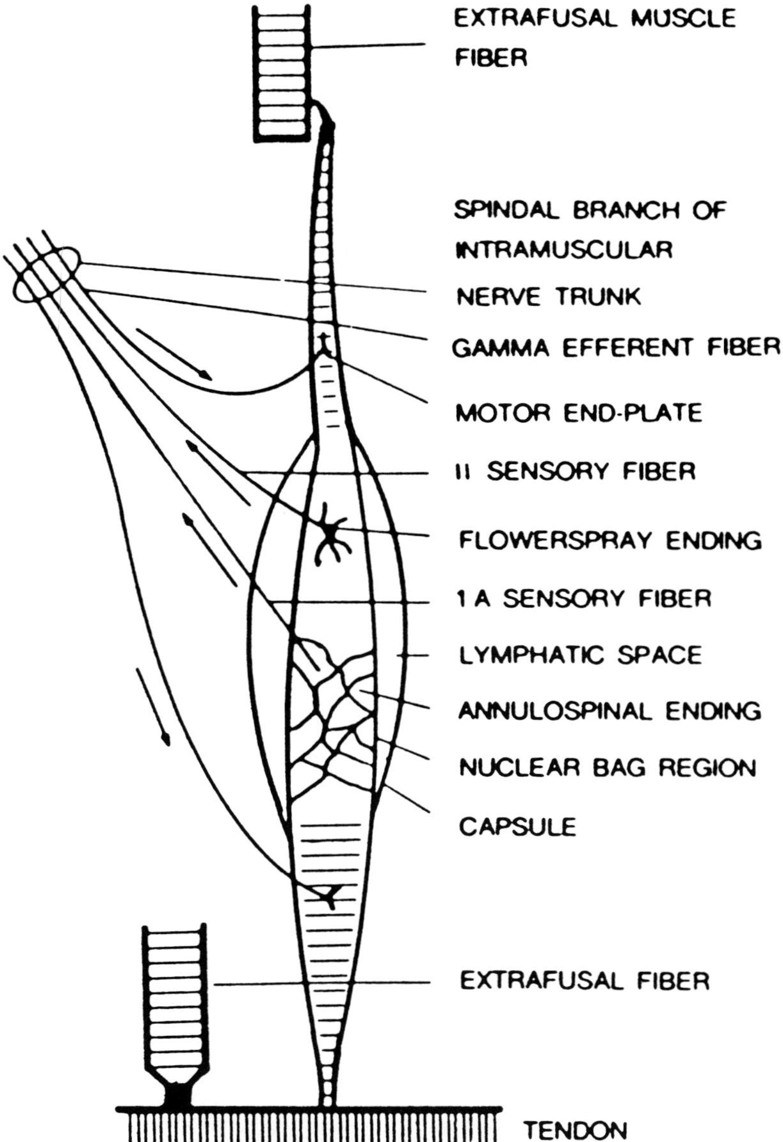

Fig. 1 *The muscle spindle. (Reproduced with permission from Stanish WD: Neurophysiology of stretching, in D'Ambrosia R, Drez D (eds):* Prevention and Treatment of Running Injuries. *Thorofare, Charles B Slack, 1982, pp 135–145.)*

that supply the stretched muscle through a monosynaptic stretch reflex and cause the muscle to contract.[15,26,56,57,78] Contraction relieves the stretch on the muscle spindles and decreases the activity of the static and dynamic receptors within it.

Afferent impulse rate depends on muscle length, movement, and efferent fusimotor activity, which can be modified by higher central nervous system commands or spinal activity. Fusimotor activity through γ-efferents resets the muscle spindle during muscle contraction so it can continue to signal length and velocity changes as the muscle shortens.

Sensors within the muscle-tendon unit are also sensitive to force production by muscle contraction. These receptors, the Golgi tendon organs, are located near the myotendinous junction and send afferent signals along Ib sensory neurons.[6] Their activity inhibits further motor neuron activity to the active muscle (the agonist), thus causing muscle relaxation. They also depolarize alpha motor neurons to the opposite muscle (the antagonist) and facilitate contraction.

Muscle contraction may modify reflex activity in various ways. Strong agonist contraction may inhibit monosynaptic reflex activity through recurrent inhibition of motor neurons,[21,42,43,63] and decrease the response of the agonist to subsequent stretching after relaxation.[21] However, other studies indicate that strong agonist contraction facilitates subsequent muscle contraction and increases the stretch reflex.[58] Contraction of the antagonist inhibits reflex activity in the agonist through reciprocal inhibition.

Mechanics of Flexibility

The mechanics of flexibility are governed by the collagenous tissues that make up most of the passive elements of the muscle-tendon unit. The response of these tissues has been well characterized.[11,45,47,76,80] From 0% to 4% elongation, little force is required as the crimped collagen fibrils straighten, and the tendon recovers its normal configuration immediately after the force is removed.[11,88] As the fibers straighten and then stretch, more force is required. Further application of force results in progressive fiber failure and eventual rupture. Although the best descriptions are for tendon and ligament, the same series of events applies to all collagenous tissues, including individual collagen fibrils.[11]

This typical behavior of connective tissue can be modified. Maintaining a fixed length results in relaxation of the tissue, and less force is required to stay at that same length. Conversely, if the force is constant, the tissue elongates, a process called creep. These properties depend on sustaining the mechanical disturbance. Rapid application of force to collagenous tissues results in increased stiffness. More force is required to achieve the same elongation that is possible when less force is used at slower rates of stretching. Thus, the ideal way to elongate these tissues is to apply force slowly and maintain it.[39]

Physiology of Flexibility With Injury

Indirect muscle injuries caused by excessive force or stress on a muscle include strains, muscle pulls, and muscle tears. These injuries

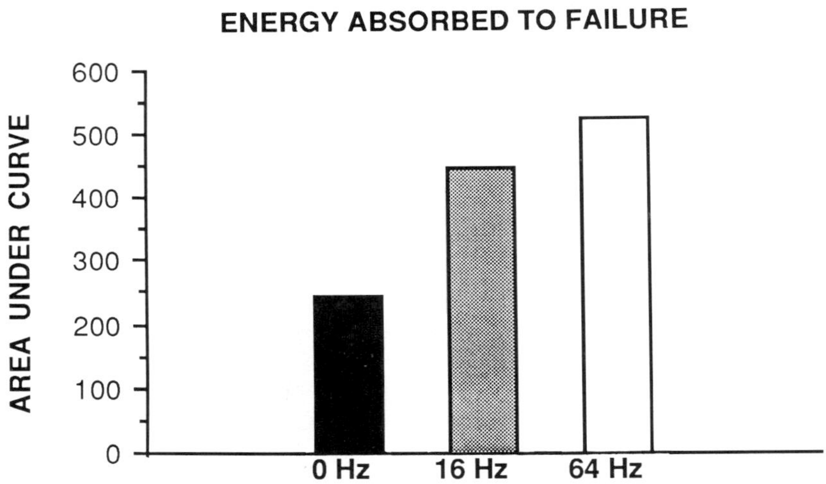

Fig. 2 *The energy absorbed by passive (0 Hz), slightly contracted (16 Hz), and maximally contracted (64 Hz) skeletal muscle while being pulled to failure. (Adapted with permission from Garrett WE Jr, Safran MR, Seaber AV, et al: Biomechanical comparison of stimulated and nonstimulated skeletal muscle pulled to failure.* Am J Sports Med *1987;15:448–454.)*

occur frequently in sports and result in lost training time or withdrawal from competition.[16,53] Overstretching the muscle-tendon unit causes injury, yet the nature, location, and healing of such injuries are still unclear. The general clinical thought is that torn muscle fibers are replaced by scar (connective tissue) that must not be allowed to heal in a shortened position, or muscle extensibility will be lost. However, new evidence suggests that muscle regeneration may be possible.[3]

Complete muscle-tendon unit tears occur almost exclusively at tissue junctions.[22–24,44,62] When a muscle is pulled to failure, rupture occurs through the muscle fibers near the myotendinous junction.[22] If the muscle is active and pulled to failure, injury occurs at the same location, but more energy is absorbed by the muscle before failure[23] (Fig. 2). Elongation at failure is the same in both cases (Fig. 3). This implies that a stiffer muscle may be more resistant to injury, because more energy is absorbed at a given amount of elongation before injury is produced.

The exact site of muscle rupture has not yet been examined thoroughly. Nikolaou and associates[62] showed that muscle fibers near the myotendinous junction are the site of injury, and that fibers a few millimeters long can still be attached to the tendon at failure. Sarcomeres in this region of the muscle are stiffer and less extensible than those in other parts of the muscle.[24] However, it is not clear how this finding relates to the fact that stiffer muscles overall may be more able to resist injury.

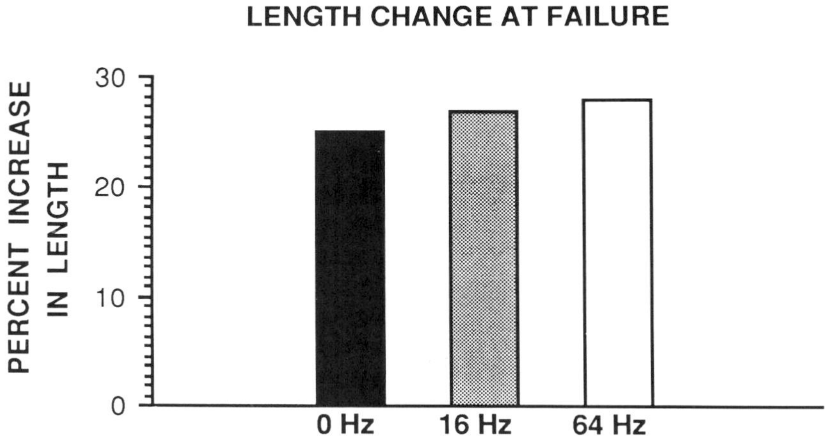

Fig. 3 *The changes in length passive (0 Hz), slightly contracted (16 Hz), and maximally contracted (64 Hz) skeletal muscle pulled to failure. (Adapted with permission from Garrett WE Jr, Safran MR, Seaber AV, et al: Biomechanical comparison of stimulated and nonstimulated skeletal muscle pulled to failure.* Am J Sports Med *1987;15:448–454.)*

Although studies of complete ruptures help clarify the mechanism of muscle injury, incomplete tears are more commonly seen. Nikolaou and associates[62] produced this type of injury in rabbit anterior tibial muscles by stretching the muscle to 80% of its maximum isometric tension. Initially, fiber disruption and hemorrhage were present (Fig. 4). During the next four days, a cellular inflammatory response occurred, and scar tissue was present by the seventh day. Also by this time, the muscle had regained normal tension production. This is similar to the pattern of force reduction and recovery after eccentric muscle injury.[32]

Unlimited physical activity early in healing may reinjure the tissue, causing the formation of more scar tissue. This would increase the barrier to regenerating muscle fibers,[48] yet exercise can also enhance soft-tissue healing.[76] Immobilization, on the other hand, increases joint stiffness[1,11] and decreases muscle strength by reducing the number of sarcomeres in series.[4,25] This creates a major problem in rehabilitation because the ideal combination of rest and exercise for optimal recovery has not been determined.

New research to define the injuries in muscle strains is promising, but few clinical studies have considered the pathophysiology of these injuries. Computed tomography, ultrasound, thermography, nuclear medicine techniques, or magnetic resonance imaging may be able to define and monitor these injuries in a clinical setting.[20,34,55] Furthermore, few animal studies have examined the effects on recovery of various stretching and flexibility protocols. Thus, the use of flexibility

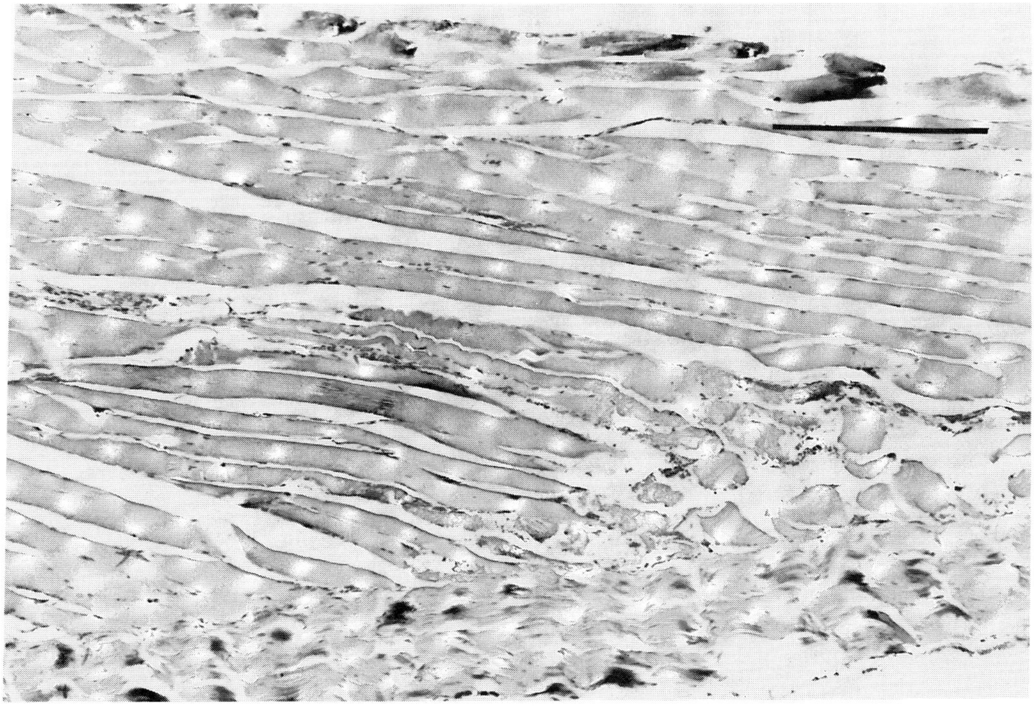

Fig. 4 *The location of fiber tearing in an incomplete muscle tear immediately after injury, with less than 1 mm of muscle fiber left attached to tendon (bottom and right). Bar = 0.5 mm. (Reproduced with permission from Garrett WE Jr, Tidball J: Myotendinous junction: Structure, function, and failure, in Woo SL-Y, Buckwalter JA (eds):* Injury and Repair of the Musculoskeletal Soft Tissues. *Park Ridge, Illinois, American Academy of Orthopaedic Surgeons, 1988, pp 171–207.)*

training in rehabilitation is determined only by the subjective complaints of the individual and the clinician's knowledge of the healing processes. Several questions about optimum rehabilitation of these injuries remain unanswered.

Assessment of Flexibility

Flexibility refers to the extensibility of a muscle-tendon unit and is correctly referred to as muscle flexibility. However, assessment techniques usually rely on measurements of the joint's range of motion. Zachazewski and Reischl[88,89] emphasized this point and stressed the need for both static and dynamic flexibility assessment.

Most assessment techniques for measuring flexibility elongate the muscle across the joint(s).[14,17,18,27,29,33,36,50–52,71,74] This angle can be measured with various types of goniometers or inclinometers[49] or on a photograph of the limb position. The patient's position should be carefully described so testing procedures can be reproduced.

Alternative methods of assessing flexibility rely on functional tests such as the sit-and-reach test. In this test, the person sits with knees straight or with one knee and hip flexed and bends at the hip to reach forward.[36] The distance between the tip of the middle finger and the knee or the second toe is usually the measured variable. This test is useful and functional, but can be affected by changes in trunk and upper-limb flexibility.

These methods assess static flexibility, yet the flexibility available to the person during activity may not match this measured variable. Thus, some means of measuring dynamic flexibility may be necessary. Dynamic flexibility could be measured by photographic methods or by electrogoniometry, which provides a record of the joint movements at the hip and knee. Speed measurement has not been considered but could be incorporated in film or electrogoniometry. Or, the time required to move a limb to a certain point could be measured. Which factor, range of motion or speed, is more important probably depends on the sport or activity involved. Dance requires great flexibility in some muscle groups and great control through the whole range of motion. Runners, conversely, may benefit more from the ability to move rapidly through an available range of muscle extension, a more ballistic type of movement. These issues have not yet been addressed in assessing flexibility or designing flexibility programs so their relative importance is unknown.

Factors Affecting Flexibility

Age and Sex

Joint range of motion and muscle flexibility decrease with age.[36,81] The shoulder joint's range of motion decreases approximately 15% to 20% between 20 and 60 years of age, and ankle motion declines by as much as 50%.[36,82] This decrease can be attributed to changes in periarticular tissue, such as increasing collagen content and cross-linking, that increase tissue stiffness.[1,2,80] Similar changes occur in these tissues during immobilization, suggesting an accelerated aging effect. Conversely, some forms of aerobic exercise decrease cross-linking and increase glycosaminoglycan concentration, which may indicate retardation of maturation or aging.[13,41,77,79]

Muscle flexibility also decreases with age, although the biochemical and ultrastructural changes that occur are largely unknown. Research has demonstrated that this flexibility can be regained with exercise programs 12 weeks and 25 weeks in duration.[65]

Females are generally more flexible than males,[7,37] at least in younger age groups. Whether these differences are maintained throughout aging is not known. Similarly, the quantitative responses of males and females to flexibility training programs have received little attention, although it appears that the two sexes are equally trainable.[74]

Thermal Effects

Increased temperatures has a considerable effect on collagen. Temperatures above 40 C relax collagen fibers, so that less force is required to produce deformation, or, alternatively, so that the same force produces more elongation.[47] The time required to deform collagen to failure decreases, and the force required increases, as the temperature increases. The most effective way to combine heat and deformation to achieve elongation is to apply them both simultaneously and to maintain the lengthened position after the heat is removed.[30,83]

These findings may be important in assessing the value of warm-up before stretching. Intramuscular temperature may increase to 39 C with active exercise,[70] which may influence collagen behavior. Golgi tendon organ sensitivity also increases with rising temperature and contributes to muscle relaxation. Most studies, however, report little or no effect of warm-up on muscle flexibility.[68,85,86] Hubley and associates[33] showed that both warm-up (cycling) and stretching increased muscle flexibility, but they did not examine the effects of warm-up plus flexibility. Small cyclic movements decrease muscle stiffness through a thixotropic effect[46] that may explain the benefits of cyclic movements on enhancing flexibility.

Cold appears to have no effect on collagen, and thus does not influence the mechanical components of muscle flexibility. Cold applications decrease muscle spasticity[35,58] and may decrease muscle spindle afferent activity, which may promote muscle relaxation. Combining cold and static stretching is more effective than combining heat and stretching in reducing muscle pain and electromyographic activity in an injured muscle within 24 hours of injury.[64] Cold may be applied via ice packs, cold-water immersion, or vapocoolant sprays. The effectiveness of vapocoolant sprays on flexibility is unclear; they may or may not have an effect.[27,40,61]

Specificity of Sport

Movement patterns are highly specific and there may even be task-specific groups of motor units within multifunctional muscles.[69] Joint range of motion and muscle flexibility also show sport specificity.[16,66] Gymnasts and ballet dancers are much more flexible in some movements than those who do not engage in these activities, but less flexible in others.[66] Pitchers show more lateral and less medial rotation of the shoulder than other baseball players.[10] This may result from sport-specific training or a natural selection process whereby individuals with these characteristics excel.

Reflex activity can also be altered with training. Volleyball players can adjust their response to drop jumps from a height so that quadriceps electrical activity increases during the eccentric phase of the jump, rather than decreases as it does in normal persons.[38,69]

Training Techniques for Improved Flexibility

In Health

Five types of stretching exercises advocated for general or clinical use are described in Table 1. The static stretching technique is generally most appropriate for regular use because it is simple and requires no assistance.[5,28,72,73] Body weight, other limbs, or external supports are used to stretch the muscle-tendon unit gently at the point of mild discomfort, and the stretch is maintained. During this time, spindle activity accommodates to the lengthened position and the muscle relaxes, enabling a further slight increase in length.

Ballistic stretching incorporates the same range of motion and movement pattern as static stretching, but short, bouncing movements are performed near the end of the available range. Such movements may facilitate the myotatic reflex by increasing both static and dynamic spindle activity[14] and muscle stiffness. These movements may potentially injure the muscle-tendon unit since stretch and muscle activity may occur simultaneously. However, they may be beneficial in certain preparatory phases for athletic activity,[89] because increased muscle stiffness may help prevent injury and enhance utilization of elastic energy.[75]

The hold-relax, contract-relax, and contract-relax-antagonist contract techniques are part of the proprioceptive neuromuscular facilitation method first described by Voss and associates[80] and popularized for athletes by Holt.[31] During the hold-relax and contract-relax techniques, agonist contraction causes Golgi tendon organ activity that promotes subsequent relaxation of the agonist and allows it to be stretched further. Muscle contraction also results in some extrafusal muscle fiber shortening that may decrease spindle firing even during the isometric contraction of the hold-relax technique. The contract-relax-antagonist contract technique incorporates all these features, as well as the principle of reciprocal inhibition, and may, in theory, be the most effective stretch.

Table 1 Types of flexibility training

Stretching Method	Description
Static	Stationary position with joints maintained in a position that stretches muscle
Ballistic	Quick, bobbing movements at the end of the available range of motion, produced by limb weight or contraction of muscle groups antagonist to those being stretched
Proprioceptive neuromuscular facilitation	
Contract-relax	Stretch statically at the end of range of motion; contract muscle slightly; relax as assistant gently pushes limb further
Hold-relax	Same as contract-relax, but emphasize isometric contraction
Contract-relax-antagonist contract	Same as contract-relax but antagonist muscles are contracted to assist in moving limb further.

Table 2 Routine for athletic participation*

Activity	Method and Purpose
General warm-up	Repetitive exercise of muscle groups to be stretched; warms up muscle and connective tissue before strain
Preparticipation stretching	Slow static stretching to elongate passive elements; ballistic stretching at the end of range of motion if there is no pain or injury
Neuromuscular warm-up	Simulate activities, slowly at first, then increasing speed under control; proprioceptive neuromuscular facilitation can be used to increase flexibility and improve motor learning
Postparticipation stretching	Static stretching while muscles are still warm; maintains flexibility and prevents muscle soreness

*Adapted with permission from Zachazewski JE: Improving flexibility, in Scully RM, Barnes MR (eds): *Physical Therapy*. Philadelphia, JB Lippincott, 1989, pp 698-738.

Experimental evaluation of these stretching techniques shows that the contract-relax-antagonist contract method is generally superior to the contract-relax or hold-relax techniques, but the differences are quite small.[18,29,54,67,74,75,87] Some studies found both contract-relax and hold-relax techniques to be more effective than static or ballistic stretching,[52] but other studies found no differences.[12,59] There is little difference between the static and ballistic methods.[14] The contract-relax-antagonist contract method may be more painful than other stretch methods, and it results in increased electrical activity in the stretched muscle, rather than the predicted electrical silence.[59] This finding has recently been questioned.[19] Intramuscular electrodes show electrical silence in the stretched soleus, while surface electrodes show activity. This suggests that crosstalk for tibialis anterior muscle activity may have been the source of the electrical activity observed by Moore and Hutton.[59]

The choice of stretching methods depends on a number of factors. Static stretching is recommended because it is an easy, safe, and appropriate means of maintaining flexibility. Proprioceptive neuromuscular facilitation methods are better for increasing flexibility and may be used when this is the primary aim. Their chief drawbacks are that a partner is usually required to perform the technique correctly and that both parties must be educated in the technique. However, these exercises can be adapted for a single person. Ballistic stretching is not recommended, but it may have a place in preparation for athletic activity.[88,89] Table 2 shows a suggested preparatory routine that illustrates the appropriate use of all these stretching techniques.

In Disease

Stretching techniques used after injury have different objectives, depending on the time elapsed after injury. During the first week after injury, gentle static stretching may be most appropriate, and the muscle-tendon unit should be maintained in a relatively lengthened position to prevent sarcomere loss.[4,48] Active techniques including the ballistic and proprioceptive neuromuscular facilitation methods are not recommended because of the potential for further injury. If muscle pain or increased reflex activity is present, perhaps caused by activation of other receptors in the muscle by chemical or pH changes, ice can be used to facilitate relaxation.[64]

Later in recovery, heat and stretching can be used to increase elongation of passive elements within the muscle,[84] and proprioceptive neuromuscular facilitation techniques can be employed to increase flexibility. Static stretching should be continued to maintain increases gained with proprioceptive neuromuscular facilitation, and active exercise can begin. Ballistic exercises are not appropriate at this time. Regular measurements of muscle length, joint range of motion, and strength of the affected muscle must be taken. When these are normal, controlled active movements through range and ballistic movements can be incorporated.

References

1. Akeson WH, Woo SLY, Amiel D, et al: The connective tissue response to immobility: Biochemical changes in periarticular connective tissue of the immobilized rabbit knee. *Clin Orthop* 1973;93:356–362.
2. Alnaqeeb MA, Al Zaid NS, Goldspink G: Connective tissue changes and physical properties of developing and ageing skeletal muscle. *J Anat* 1984;139:677–689.
3. Appell H-J, Forsberg S, Hollmann W: Satellite cell activation in human skeletal muscle after training: Evidence for muscle fiber neoformation. *Int J Sports Med* 1988;9:297–299.
4. Baker JH, Matsumoto DE: Adaptation of skeletal muscle to immobilization in a shortened position. *Muscle Nerve* 1988;11:231–244.
5. Beaulieu JE: Developing a stretching program. *Phys Sportsmed* 1981;9:59–69.
6. Bistevins R, Awad EA: Structure and ultrastructure of mechanoreceptors at the human musculotendinous junction. *Arch Phys Med Rehabil* 1981;62:74–83.
7. Boone DC, Azen SP: Normal range of motion of joints in male subjects. *J Bone Joint Surg* 1979;61A:756–759.
8. Borg TK, Caulfield JB: Morphology of connective tissue in skeletal muscle. *Tissue Cell* 1980;12:197–207.
9. Boyd IA: The action of the three types of intrafusal fibre in isolated cat muscle spindles on the dynamic and length sensitivities of primary and secondary sensory ending, in Taylor A, Prochazka A (eds): *Muscle Receptors and Movement.* New York, Oxford University Press, 1981, pp 17–32.
10. Brown LP, Niehues SL, Harrah A, et al: Upper extremity range of motion and isokinetic strength of the internal and external shoulder rotators in major league baseball players. *Am J Sports Med* 1988;16:577–585.
11. Butler DL, Grood ES, Moyes FR, et al: Biomechanics of ligaments and tendons. *Exerc Sport Sci Rev* 1978;6:125–182.
12. Condon SM, Hutton RS: Soleus muscle electromyographic activity and ankle dorsiflextion range of motion during four stretching procedures. *Phys Ther* 1987;67:24–30.
13. Curwin SL, Vailas AC, Wood J: Immature tendon adaptation to strenuous exercise. *J Appl Physiol* 1988;65:2297–2301.

14. de Vries HA: Evaluation of static stretching procedures for improvement of flexibility. *Res Q* 1962;33:222–229.
15. Edin BB, Vallbo AB: Stretch sensitization of human muscle spindles. *J Physiol* 1988;400:101–111.
16. Ekstrand J, Gillquist J: The frequency of muscle tightness and injuries in soccer players. *Am J Sports Med* 1982;10:75–78.
17. Ekstrand J, Wiktorsson M, Oberg B, et al: Lower extremity goniometric measurements: A study to determine their reliability. *Arch Phys Med Rehabil* 1982;63:171–175.
18. Ethnyre BR, Abraham LD: Gains in range of ankle dorsiflexion using three popular stretching techniques. *Am J Phys Med* 1986;65:189–196.
19. Ethnyre BR, Abraham LD: Antagonist muscle activity during stretching: A paradox re-assessed. *Med Sci Sports Exerc* 1988;20:285–289.
20. Fornage BD, Rifkin MD: Ultrasound examination of tendons. *Radiol Clin North Am* 1988;26:87–107.
21. Garland SJ, Garner SH, McComas AJ: Reduced voluntary electromyographic activity after fatiguing stimulation of human muscle. *J Physiol* 1988;401:547–556.
22. Garrett WE Jr, Nikolaou PK, Ribbeck BM, et al: The effect of muscle architecture on the biomechanical failure properties of skeletal muscle under passive extension. *Am J Sports Med* 1988;16:7–12.
23. Garrett WE Jr, Safran MR, Seaber AV, et al: Biomechanical comparison of stimulated and nonstimulated skeletal muscle pulled to failure. *Am J Sports Med* 1987;15:448–454.
24. Garrett W Jr, Tidball J: Myotendinous junction: Structure, function, and failure, in Woo SL-Y, Buckwalter JA (eds): *Injury and Repair of the Musculoskeletal Soft Tissues*. Park Ridge, Illinois, American Academy of Orthopaedic Surgeons, 1988, pp 171–207.
25. Gossman MR, Sahrmann SA, Rose SJ: Review of length-associated changes in muscle: Experimental evidence and clinical implications. *Phys Ther* 1982;62:1799–1808.
26. Guissard N, Duchateau J, Hainaut K: Muscle stretching and motoneuron excitability. *Eur J Appl Physiol* 1988;58:47–52.
27. Halkovich LR, Personius WJ, Clamann HP, et al: Effect of fluori methane spray on passive hip flexion. *Phys Ther* 1981;61:185–189.
28. Harris ML: Flexibility. *Phys Ther* 1969;49:591–601.
29. Hartley-O'Brien SJ: Six mobilization exercises for active range of hip flexion. *Res Q Exerc Sport* 1980;51:625–635.
30. Henricson AS, Fredriksson K, Persson I, et al: The effect of heat and stretching on the range of hip motion. *J Orthop Sports Phys Ther* 1984;6:110–115.
31. Holt LE: *Scientific Stretching for Sport*. Halifax, Sport Research Ltd, 1973.
32. Horswill CA, Layman DK, Boileau RA, et al: Excretion of 3-methylhistidine and hydroxyproline following acute weight-training exercise. *Int J Sports Med* 1988;9:245–248.
33. Hubley CL, Kozey JW, Stanish WD: The effects of static stretching exercises and stationary cycling on range of motion at the hip joint. *J Orthop Sports Phys Ther* 1984;6:104–109.
34. Kahn D, Wilson MA: Bone scintigraphic findings in patellar tendonitis. *J Nucl Med* 1987;28:1768–1770.
35. Kelly M: Effectiveness of a cryotherapy technique on spasticity. *Phys Ther* 1969;49:349–353.
36. Kendall HO, Kendall FP: Normal flexibility according to age groups. *J Bone Joint Surg* 1948;30A:690–694.
37. Kirby RL, Simms FC, Symington VJ, et al: Flexibility and musculoskeletal symptomatology in female gymnasts and age-matched controls. *Am J Sports Med* 1981;9:160–164.

38. Komi PV: Physiological and biomechanical correlates of muscle function: Effects of muscle structure and stretch-shortening cycle on force and speed. *Exerc Sport Sci Rev* 1984;12:81–121.
39. Kottke FJ, Pauley DJ, Ptak RA: The rationale for prolonged stretching for correction of shortening of connective tissue. *Arch Phys Med* 1966;47:345–352.
40. Koury S, Mamary M, Kagan R, et al: Effect of fluori-methane spray on hamstring extensibility during "contract/relax" and active stretching, abstract. *Phys Ther* 1986;66:806.
41. Kovanen V, Suominen H, Peltonen L: Effects of aging and life-long physical training on collagen in slow and fast skeletal muscle in rats: A morphometric and immuno-histochemical study. *Cell Tissue Res* 1987;248:247–255.
42. Kudina LP: Reflex effects of muscle afferents on antagonist studied on single firing motor units in man. *Electroencephalogr Clin Neurophysiol* 1980;50:214–221.
43. Kudina LP, Pantseva RE: Recurrent inhibition of firing motoneurones in man. *Electroencephalogr Clin Neurophysiol* 1988;69:179–185.
44. Kvist M, Järvinen M: Clinical, histochemical and biomechanical features in repair of muscle and tendon injuries. *Int J Sports Med* 1982;3(suppl 1):12–14.
45. LaBan MM: Collagen tissue: Implications of its response to stress in vitro. *Arch Phys Med Rehabil* 1962;43:461–466.
46. Lakie M, Robson LG: Thixotropic changes in human muscle stiffness and the effects of fatigue. *Q J Exp Physiol* 1988;73:487–500.
47. Lehmann JF, Masock AJ, Warren CG, et al: Effect of therapeutic temperatures on tendon extensibility. *Arch Phys Med* 1970;51:481–487.
48. Lehto M, Duance VC, Restall D: Collagen and fibronectin in a healing skeletal muscle injury: An immunohistological study of the effects of physical activity on the repair of injured gastrocnemius muscle in the rat. *J Bone Joint Surg* 1985;67B:820–828.
49. Leighton JR: An instrument and technic for the measurement of range of joint motion. *Arch Phys Med* 1955;36:571–578.
50. Leighton JR: Flexibility characteristics of four specialized skill groups of college athletes. *Arch Phys Med Rehabil* 1957;38:24–28.
51. Leighton JR: Flexibility characteristics of three specialized skill groups of champion athletes. *Arch Phys Med Rehabil* 1957;38:580–583.
52. Loudon KL, Bollier CE, Allison KA, et al: Effects of two stretching methods on the flexibility and retention of flexibility at the ankle joint in runners, abstract. *Phys Ther* 1985;65:698.
53. Lysholm J, Wiklander J: Injuries in runners. *Am J Sports Med* 1987;15:168–171.
54. Markos PD: Ipsilateral and contralateral effects of proprioceptive neuromuscular facilitation techniques on hip motion and electromyographic activity. *Phys Ther* 1979;59:1366–1373.
55. Matin P: Basic principles of nuclear medicine techniques for detection and evaluation of trauma and sports medicine injuries. *Semin Nucl Med* 1988;18:90–112.
56. McArdle WD, Katch FI, Katch VL: *Exercise Physiology: Energy, Nutrition, and Human Performance*, ed 2. Philadelphia, Lea & Febiger, 1986, pp 305–319.
57. McCrea DA: Spinal cord circuitry and motor reflexes. *Exerc Sport Sci Rev* 1986;14:105–141.
58. Miglietta O: Electromyographic characteristics of clonus and influence of cold. *Arch Phys Med* 1964;45:508–512.
59. Moore MA, Hutton RS: Electromyographic investigation of muscle stretching techniques. *Med Sci Sports Exerc* 1980;12:322–329.

60. Moore MJ: The dual connective tissue system of rat soleus muscle. *Muscle Nerve* 1983;6:416–422.
61. Newton A: Effects of vapocoolants on passive hip flexion in healthy subjects. *Phys Ther* 1985;65:1034–1036.
62. Nikolaou PK, MacDonald BL, Glisson RR, et al: Biomechanical and histological evaluation of muscle after controlled strain injury. *Am J Sports Med* 1987;15:9–14.
63. Pierrot-Deseilligny E, Bussel B: Evidence for recurrent inhibition by motoneurons in human subjects. *Brain Res* 1975;88:105–108.
64. Prentice WE Jr: An electromyographic analysis of the effectiveness of heat or cold and stretching for inducing relaxation in injured muscle. *J Orthop Sports Phys Ther* 1982;3:133–140.
65. Raab DM, Agre JC, McAdam M, et al: Light resistance and stretching exercise in elderly women: Effect upon flexibility. *Arch Phys Med Rehabil* 1988;69:268–272.
66. Reid DC, Burnham TS, Saboe LA, et al: Lower extremity flexibility patterns in classical ballet dancers and their correlation to lateral hip and knee injuries. *Am J Sports Med* 1987;15:347–352.
67. Sady SP, Wortman M, Blanke E: Flexibility training: Ballistic, static or proprioceptive neuromuscular facilitation? *Arch Phys Med Rehabil* 1982;63:261–263.
68. Safran MR, Garrett WE Jr, Seaber AV, et al: The role of warmup in muscular injury prevention. *Am J Sports Med* 1988;16:123–129.
69. Sale DG: Neural adaptation to resistance training. *Med Sci Sports Exerc* 1988;20(suppl):S135-S145.
70. Saltin B, Hermansen L: Esophageal, rectal, and muscle temperature during exercise. *J Appl Physiol* 1966;21:1757–1762.
71. Sapega AA, Quedenfeld TC, Moyer RA, et al: Biophysical factors in range-of-motion exercise. *Phys Sportsmed* 1981;9:57–65.
72. Schultz P: Flexibility: Day of the static stretch. *Phys Sportsmed* 1979;7:109–117.
73. Starring DT, Gossman MR, Nicholson GG Jr, et al: Comparison of cyclic and sustained passive stretching using a mechanical device to increase resting length of hamstring muscles. *Phys Ther* 1988;68:314–320.
74. Tanigawa MC: Comparison of the hold-relax procedure and passive mobilization on increasing muscle length. *Phys Ther* 1972;52:725–735.
75. Thys H, Faraggiana T, Margaria R: Utilization of muscle elasticity in exercise. *J Appl Physiol* 1972;32:491–494.
76. Vailas AC, Tipton CM, Matthes RD, et al: Physical activity and its influence on the repair process of medial collateral ligaments. *Connect Tissue Res* 1981;9:25–31.
77. Vailas AC, Pedrini VA, Pedrini-Mille A, et al: Patellar tendon matrix changes associated with aging and voluntary exercise. *J Appl Physiol* 1985;58:1572–1576.
78. Vallbo A: Basic patterns of muscle spindle discharge in man, in Taylor A, Prochazka A (eds): *Muscle Receptors and Movement.* New York, Oxford University Press, 1981, pp 263–275.
79. Viidik A: Connective tissues: Possible implications of the temporal changes for the aging process. *Mech Ageing Dev* 1979;9:267–285.
80. Voss DE, Ionta MK, Myers BJ: *Proprioceptive Neuromuscular Facilitation: Patterns and Techniques*, ed 3. Philadelphia, Harper & Row, 1985.
81. Walker JM, Sue D, Miles-Elkousy N, et al: Active mobility of the extremities in older subjects. *Phys Ther* 1984;64:919–923.
82. Wallin D, Ekblom B, Grahn R, et al: Improvement of muscle flexibility: A comparison between two techniques. *Am J Sports Med* 1985;13:263–268.

83. Warren CG, Lehmann JF, Koblanski JN: Heat and stretch procedures: An evaluation using rat tail tendon. *Arch Phys Med Rehabil* 1976;57:122–126.
84. Wiktorsson-Möller M, Oberg B, Ekstrand J, et al: Effects of warming up, massage, and stretching on range of motion and muscle strength in the lower extremity. *Am J Sports Med* 1983;11:249–252.
85. Williford HN: A comparison of proprioceptive neuromuscular facilitation and static stretching techniques. *Am Correct Ther J* 1985;39:30–33.
86. Williford HN, East JB, Smith FH, et al: Evaluation of warm-up for improvement in flexibility. *Am J Sports Med* 1986;14:316–319.
87. Wood TO, Cooke PH, Goodship AE: The effect of exercise and anabolic steriods on the mechanical properties and crimp morphology of the rat tendon. *Am J Sports Med* 1988;16:153–158.
88. Zachazewski JE: Improving flexibility, in Scully RM, Barnes MR (eds): *Physical Therapy*. Philadelphia, JB Lippincott, 1989, pp 698–738.
89. Zachazewski JE, Reischl SR: Flexibility for the runner: Specific program consideration. *Topics Acute Care Trauma Rehabil* 1986;1:9–16.

Chapter 51

Early Return to Function After Major Knee Injury or Surgery

J. Richard Steadman, MD
Russell J. Bodner, MD
William G. Rodkey, DVM

Introduction

In the Western world, the use of training and exercise as treatment for injuries and rehabilitation after surgery dates back to the Aesculapians of the Greek city-states of the fifth century BC.[7] These early physicians recognized that exercise would help wounded soldiers return to the ranks more rapidly. Exercise could also maintain and enhance the performance of competing athletes. Training regimens included exercise, diet, medications, and meditation and were gradually refined during the age of Hippocrates and the ancient games at Olympia.

Early return to competition after injury or surgery is a major consideration for both patients and physicians, especially for those in the Olympics, in professional athletics, and on athletic scholarships. Recent advances in sports medicine permit more aggressive treatment of serious athletic injuries. A rapid return to competition is aided by improved surgical techniques, more focused indications, increased understanding of cellular and physiologic responses to immobilization and exercise, and more sophisticated rehabilitation protocols. This chapter considers methods of helping an athlete return to competition after knee surgery. It examines the deleterious effects of injury and surgery, the techniques used to modify the inflammatory and healing response of the tissues during the recovery period, and a training program now in use.

Rationale and Principles

Early surgical repair and rehabilitation are needed to restore anatomic integrity and stability of injured tissues for immediate, controlled joint mobility. The various effects of joint immobilization are well documented.[2,3,5,27,29] Immobilization has adverse effects on articular cartilage,[33,92] ligaments,[97,100] periarticular and capsular structures,[1,4,101] insertion sites,[13,57,69,99] bone density,[30,41,43,55] muscle,[10,15,16,21,36,40,42,90] and neural[22,60,61] elements. It also decreases cardiovascular aerobic fitness and affects psychological equilibrium. Movement and weightbearing activities that apply controlled stress to the injured and repaired tissue, but avoid undue pain, inflammation, and excessive joint loads, are basic for early return to function.

Surgical techniques that help reduce postoperative bleeding, edema, and inflammation include arthroscopic procedures, pneumatic tourniquets, hemostasis, drains, and compressive stockings. Several therapies can be used to modify the inflammatory and proliferative stages of repair. They can be categorized as those that decrease pain, swelling, and joint effusion, such as various therapeutic agents and ice, and those that allow controlled mechanical motion of the joint, such as hinged braces.

Control of Pain and Inflammation

The loss of voluntary muscle activation from pain and injury is a major cause of muscle atrophy.[12] Slow-twitch type I motor fibers are high in oxidative enzymes such as succinate dehydrogenase and are especially sensitive to atrophy. Using continuous epidural analgesia after knee ligament surgery can improve quadriceps muscle function several thousand percent as measured by the integrated electromyographic technique.[28] After two or three days of continuous epidural analgesia, succinate dehydrogenase levels also decrease less than those of untreated control patients. However, patients given continuous epidural analgesia require extensive monitoring that may make this technique difficult to provide, despite the benefits of pain control.

Knee surgery inhibits reflex muscular action.[32,42,66] Immobilization and nonweightbearing alter tonic spinal arcs that must be relearned in order to regain strength and coordination.[14,24] The lost neuromuscular control results in rapid atrophy of surrounding muscles. Studies of weightlessness and prolonged bedrest show that the quadriceps and gastrocsoleus complex experience atrophy more than the hamstrings or the ankle and foot dorsiflexors.[36,37,58,75] These studies also found a loss of strength out of proportion to the loss of cross-sectional muscle area, a finding that indicates there is a significant neural component to atrophic weakness.

Electromyostimulation during the period of reflex inhibition and neural reeducation is a useful therapy. Studies of electromyostimulation use during or after immobilization show that patients have less atrophy, better strength, and higher levels of both oxidative and glycolytic enzymes.[9,28,34,35,67,87] The use of electromyostimulation is dictated by four principles: (1) the highest percentage of strength gains occurs in weakened muscles; (2) the position for greatest stimulus contraction of the quadriceps and hamstrings is at 30 degrees of knee flexion; (3) electromyostimulation combined with voluntary co-contraction results in greater use of muscular forces; and (4) larger electrodes placed directly over motor points are most effective.[59,66]

Co-contraction of hamstrings,"A," and quadriceps, "B," in sequential firing with a flexed position of more than 60 degrees may be used to protect an anterior cruciate ligament reconstruction from unacceptable strain.[25,50] That is, "A" fires first, followed by "B"; relaxation of "B" occurs first, followed by "A." Hence, the sequence is ABBA so that the hamstrings protect the anterior cruciate ligament. At the conclusion of the operation, low-intensity electrical stimulation, which produces an effect similar to that of transcutaneous electrical nerve stimulation, is used for pain control. Low-intensity stimulation does not cause muscle fasciculation or contraction, but has been described as closing the gate to the A-δ and C fiber afferents by stimulating large fibers within the dorsal horn of the spinal column.[64,88] It also stimulates the release of endorphins and enkephalins that may break down prostaglandin products at the injury site.[18,89] For example, Jensen and associates[48] found that postoperative use of transcutaneous electrical nerve stimulation decreased pain in 93% of patients and allowed a greater early range of motion after arthroscopic surgery.

The healing effects of nonsteroidal anti–inflammatory drugs (NSAIDs) have been studied in animal and human connective tissues.[6,11,17,23,74,94] Dahners and associates[23] found that treatment with piroxicam increased the rupture strength of rat medial collateral ligaments 42% one to six days postoperatively. In a double-blind study, Arvidsson and Eriksson[11] found that NSAIDs increased isokinetic muscle torque and improved range of motion seven days after open meniscectomies in humans. Ogilvie-Harris and associates[74] reported that NSAID administration after arthroscopic meniscectomy reduced pain, synovitis, and effusions. NSAIDs also enabled patients to return to sport function in 22.5 days compared with 56 days for patients taking a placebo. Others have reported similar experiences with NSAIDs.

Postoperatively, cryotherapy (ice packs or cooled thermal blankets) is used to relieve pain, to control swelling and edema, and to reduce muscular spasm caused by reflex arcs from cutaneous, muscle spindle, and stretch response afferents.[20,31,56,63] Farry and associates[31] found histologic evidence of decreased inflammation in experimentally induced ligament injuries in pigs treated with cryotherapy. However, a critical tissue temperature below 15 C may increase edema, lymphatic permeability, and inflammation and lead to superficial tissue damage or nerve palsy.[26,63] These complications can be avoided by using cooled thermal blankets. The blankets can also reduce narcotic requirements after anterior cruciate ligament reconstruction.[20]

Mechanical Control of Joint Motion

After surgery, the leg is placed in a long-leg hinged brace within demonstrated safe ranges of motion determined by biomechanical studies.[8,19,39,44,45,52,68,70–72,76] Exercises are performed within these protected ranges.

In the recovery room, the operated on limb is placed in a continuous passive motion machine to produce motion within the limits set by the brace. Continuous passive motion increases clearance of hemarthrosis and edema,[73] improves wound healing,[93] and increases ligament breaking force, tensile strength, strain at failure, stiffness, and rate of cartilage regeneration.[80–84] Consequently, there are fewer adhesions and stronger tissues. Some evidence indicates that important proprioceptive arcs may be stimulated to produce an effect on the patient's perception of pain like that of transcutaneous electrical nerve stimulation. For patients who have undergone knee ligament surgery, continuous passive motion can be maintained during the hospital stay. In those patients who have had procedures involving articular cartilage, continuous passive motion should be continued for at least eight hours daily for as long as eight weeks to help form fibrocartilage in chondral defects. This improvement in fibrocartilage formation in response to continuous passive motion has been observed (J.R. Steadman, unpublished data).

Rehabilitation Protocol

The patient can begin rehabilitative exercise protocols on the day of or the day after surgery. Restraints to rehabilitation are dictated only by the stability of the surgical repair. For example, rehabilitation after meniscal repairs should employ smaller ranges of motion than other soft-tissue repairs; and repairs involving subchondral drilling and abrasions should be kept nonweightbearing. The goals of this portion of the rehabilitation program are to achieve and increase neuromuscular control of the limb and to expose all tissues to physiologic stress so that they can adapt and respond. The healing area must be protected from mechanical and biologic insults.

Within 24 hours after surgery, the patient can begin therapy with quadriceps and hamstring isometrics and straight leg-raising exercises twice a day while wearing the hinged brace. The brace can be removed for active, assisted range-of-motion exercises. The patient can then return to the continuous passive motion machine for one hour at the achieved brace-free range. On the second day, crutch walking, double-leg one-third knee bends, and upper-extremity-supported deep knee bends are added, within the safe range of motion. Aerobic conditioning and cross-over effects are achieved with well-leg bicycling, rowing, and single-leg knee bends. These exercises provide concentric and eccentric muscular contractions of leg muscles with weightbearing, joint proprioception, and physiologic stress to the joint and myotendinous junctions. NSAIDs and ice or cooled thermal blankets are used to control swelling and minimize the painful by-products of the inflammatory response.

On the third or fourth day after surgery, resistive exercises with a cord of surgical tubing and attached handles can begin.[86] A warm-up of double-leg one-third knee bends is essential before resistive exercise. Warm-up activity increases muscle blood flow, tissue compliance and sensitivity, and speed of neural transmission.[85] Controlled double-leg one-third knee bends, seated hamstring, and leg-press exercises can be performed. The hip, ankle, and foot motor groups can then be included. Resting 30 to 60 seconds between sets builds endurance type I fibers. Electromyostimulation is used for the first eight weeks and patients can build up to maximal intensity with contraction.

Well-leg cycling, rowing, and cord exercises can be increased to one hour a day. Upper-body conditioning with the cord or weights should be stressed throughout rehabilitation. After eight weeks, the patient can usually bear full weight comfortably. When gait is painless with no noticeable limp, use of crutches can be discontinued.

As healing moves into the remodeling stages, fixation and the tensile strength of the repair increase to allow full range of motion. The protective brace can be reduced and hinges opened to accommodate the patient. Exercise repetitions and sets can be increased, and the operated on limb can be isolated with single-leg knee bends and incorporation into stationary cycling. A sequence of walking-through-jogging against the resistance cord can begin, and controlled concentric-eccentric low loading should be emphasized. A water workout with forward running, backward running, and flutter-kicking exercises may be used at this stage. Passive range-of-motion exercises should continue to be emphasized until full range of motion is achieved, about four months after surgery.

During the fourth month, the patient can begin slow side-to-side loading exercise against the cord and may bicycle without the brace. By then, the patient has usually regained most of his or her muscle mass and reflexes and is ready for jogging and sport-specific exercises. Attention to movement velocity, coordination, endurance, and flexibility is necessary to ensure overall readiness for competition. Most athletes can return to full activity with a lightweight fitted brace six to nine months after surgery. Cutting and jumping sports can be resumed after eight to 12 months.

Postoperative Progression

Mobilization has profound effects on many healing tissues. Cartilage nutrition, thickness, and healing are improved by cyclical loading and motion. Capsular and pericapsular connective tissues benefit from motion because edema is less and there is increased physiologic guidance for the deposition of newly made type III collagen and its replacement with cross-linked type I collagen and proper signals to produce non-collagenous matrix proteoglycans and proteins.[98] The bony insertion sites of ligaments, joint capsules, and tendons are extremely sensitive to applied stress, especially if they have indirect periosteal attachments.[102] Mobilization reverses the osteoclastic resorption of these bony insertions.[69,99] Myotendinous junctions respond to stress by incorporating new sarcomeres and adapting terminal junction properties to maintain homeostasis.[95,96] Stretching muscle to an elongated position reduces muscle atrophy, and increases the force and strain-to-failure of the muscles.[49]

As the tissue moves from the inflammatory phase to the proliferative phase, therapy should be less protective and should concentrate on building strength, with continued focus on both the joint and the neuromuscular units that serve the tissue. Resistance exercise stimulates neuromuscular adaptation and increases connective-tissue strength and mass, while well-leg and upper-body conditioning helps maintain aerobic fitness.

The increase in strength performance produced by training is determined by both muscular and neural factors. Every movement is specific in the activation of primary motor muscle groups, both for synergists and antagonists. The rate, peak, and duration of force development, and the interaction with each subsequent movement in time and space are also movement specific. Injury and surgery compromise the motor control of the limb, so many of the early gains in rehabilitation are from neural adaptations. These improvements include increased motor unit activation and rate of activation, facilitation and potentiation of reflex responses to voluntary contractions, and increases in recruitment and duration of high-threshold motor units.[79] Various reports show increases in voluntary strength without muscular hypertrophy as well as the "cross-training" effect that increases the strength of the untrained limb as the result of neural adaptations.[22,46,47,53,65,91,103]

There is great specificity to movement pattern, contraction type, and velocity in neural adaptation. It is better to train for those activities specifically needed by the patient, beginning with early weightbearing and gait training to the level of tolerance within a protective brace.[41,51,65,78] As strength and coordination return, the patient can begin exercises that are specific to muscle groups, movement, velocity, muscle and joint position, or sport.

Muscular adaptations include hypertrophy of type II and some type I fibers, changes in mitochondrial volume density, and increases in high-energy phosphate pools.[54,61] The contribution of fiber splitting, branching, or hyperplasia is not clear. However, the muscular adaptation in response to resistance exercises is specific to intensity, duration, frequency, and pattern. In the immediate postoperative period, such specificity may not be as important as the threshold for protein synthesis for maintenance.[38]

Complications

During the proliferative and cellular stages of healing, aberrant responses in the tissues may appear. Healing is controlled inflammation that gives way to the sequential deposition of cells and matrix. Increased production of inflammatory mediators, increased sensitivity of fibroblasts to humeral agents, or decreased collagen degradation may cause arthrofibrosis.[77] Histologic examination of tissue in these cases reveals continued inflammatory stimulation of synovial, capsular, and pericapsular tissues, without the normal progression to remodeling or maturation phases. The cause of this process is unknown, but it can be treated with dynamic motion exercises to free patellar entrapment and improve extensor coordination. Additionally, NSAIDs and manual patellar motion exercises are helpful. In recalcitrant cases, spring-loaded splints, manipulation, and surgical debridement and release are necessary.[70]

References

1. Akeson WH, Amiel D, LaViolette D: The connective-tissue response to immobility: A study of the chondroitin-4 and 6-sulfate and dermatan sulfate changes in periarticular connective tissue of control and immobilized knees of dogs. *Clin Orthop* 1967;51:183–197.
2. Akeson WH, Amiel D, Woo SL-Y: Immobility effects on synovial joints: The pathomechanics of joint contracture. *Biorheology* 1980;17:95–110.
3. Akeson WH, Woo SL-Y, Amiel D, et al: Biomechanical and biochemical changes in the periarticular connective tissue during contracture development in the immobilized rabbit knee. *Connect Tissue Res* 1974;2:315–323.
4. Akeson WH, Woo SL-Y, Amiel D, et al: Rapid recovery from contracture in rabbit hindlimb: A correlative biomechanical and biochemical study. *Clin Orthop* 1977;122:359–365.
5. Akeson WH, Woo SL-Y, Amiel D, et al: The connective tissue response to immobility: Biochemical changes in periarticular connective tissue of the immobilized rabbit knee. *Clin Orthop* 1973;93:356–362.
6. Almekinders LC, Gilbert JA: Biomechanical properties of muscle after experimental muscle strains and the role of non-steroidal anti-inflammatory medication. *Trans Orthop Res Soc* 1986;11:224.
7. Appelboom T, Rouffin C, Fierens E: Sport and medicine in ancient Greece. *Am J Sports Med* 1988;16:594–596.
8. Arms SW, Pope MH, Johnson RJ, et al: The biomechanics of anterior cruciate ligament rehabilitation and reconstruction. *Am J Sports Med* 1984;12:8–18.
9. Arvidsson I: *A Study of Rehabilitation After Knee Surgery With Special Emphasis on Pain Inhibition on Voluntary Muscle Activation*, thesis. Stockholm, Karolinska Institute, 1985.
10. Arvidsson I, Arvidsson H, Eriksson E, et al: Prevention of quadriceps wasting after immobilization: An evaluation of the effect of electrical stimulation. *Orthopedics* 1986;9:1519–1528.
11. Arvidsson I, Eriksson E: A double blind trial of NSAID versus placebo during rehabilitation. *Orthopedics* 1987;10:1007–1014.
12. Arvidsson I, Eriksson E, Knutsson E, et al: Reduction of pain inhibition on voluntary muscle activation by epidural analgesia. *Orthopedics* 1986;9:1415–1419.
13. Barfred T: Experimental rupture of the Achilles tendon: Comparison of various types of experimental rupture in rats. *Acta Orthop Scand* 1971;42:528–543.
14. Basmajian JV: *Muscles Alive: Their Functions Revealed by Electromyography*, ed 3. Baltimore, Williams & Wilkins, 1974, pp 1–139.
15. Booth FW: Effect of limb immobilization on skeletal muscle. *J Appl Physiol* 1982;52:1113–1118.
16. Booth FW, Gollnick PD: Effects of disuse on the structure and function of skeletal muscle. *Med Sci Sports Exerc* 1983;15:415–420.

17. Carlstedt CA: Mechanical and chemical factors in tendon healing: Effects of indomethacin and surgery in the rabbit. *Acta Orthop Scand* 1987;224(suppl):1–75.
18. Cheng RS, Pomeranz B: Electroacupuncture analgesia could be mediated by at least two pain-relieving mechanisms: Endorphin and non-endorphin systems. *Life Sci* 1979;25:1957–1962.
19. Clancy WG Jr, Narechania RG, Rosenberg TD, et al: Anterior and posterior cruciate ligament reconstruction in rhesus monkeys. *J Bone Joint Surg* 1981;63A:1270–1284.
20. Cohn BT, Draeger RI, Jackson DW: The effects of cold therapy in the postoperative management of pain in patients undergoing anterior cruciate ligament reconstruction. *Am J Sports Med* 1989;17:344–349.
21. Cooper RR: Alterations during immobilization and regeneration of skeletal muscle in cats. *J Bone Joint Surg* 1972;54A:919–953.
22. Costill DL, Coyle EF, Fink WF, et al: Adaptations in skeletal muscle following strength training. *J Appl Physiol* 1979;46:96–99.
23. Dahners LE, Gilbert JA, Lester GE, et al: The effect of a nonsteroidal antiinflammatory drug on the healing of ligaments. *Am J Sports Med* 1988;16:641–646.
24. Dehne E, Torp RP: Treatment of joint injuries by immediate mobilization: Based upon the spinal adaptation concept. *Clin Orthop* 1971;77:218–232.
25. Delitto A, Rose SJ: Electrical stimulation of hamstrings in a patient with anterior cruciate ligament insufficiency: A single case design, abstract. *Phys Ther* 1986;66:804.
26. Drez D, Faust DC, Evans JP: Cryotherapy and nerve palsy. *Am J Sports Med* 1981;9:256–257.
27. Enneking WF, Horowitz M: The intra-articular effects of immobilization on the human knee. *J Bone Joint Surg* 1972;54A:973–985.
28. Eriksson E, Häggmark T: Comparison of isometric muscle training and electrical stimulation supplementing isometric muscle training in the recovery after major knee ligament surgery: A preliminary report. *Am J Sports Med* 1979;7:169–171.
29. Evans EB, Eggers GW, Butler JK, et al: Experimental immobilization and remobilization of rat knee joints. *J Bone Joint Surg* 1960;42A:737–758.
30. Falch JA: The effect of physical activity on the skeleton. *Scand J Soc Med* 1982;29(suppl):55–58.
31. Farry PJ, Prentice NG, Hunter AC, et al: Ice treatment of injured ligaments: An experimental model. *NZ Med J* 1980;91:12–14.
32. Gerber C, Hoppeler H, Claassen H, et al: The lower-extremity musculature in chronic symptomatic instability of the anterior cruciate ligament. *J Bone Joint Surg* 1985;67A:1034–1043.
33. Ginsberg JM, Eyring EJ, Curtiss PH Jr: Continuous compression of rabbit articular cartilage producing loss of hydroxyproline before loss of hexosamine. *J Bone Joint Surg* 1969;51A:467–474.
34. Gould N, Donnermeyer D, Gammon GG, et al: Transcutaneous muscle stimulation to retard disuse atrophy after open meniscectomy. *Clin Orthop* 1983;178:190–197.
35. Gould N, Donnermeyer D, Pope M, et al: Transcutaneous muscle stimulation as a method to retard disuse atrophy. *Clin Orthop* 1982;164:215–220.
36. Greenleaf JE, Van Beaumont W, Convertino VA, et al: Handgrip and general muscular strength and endurance during prolonged bedrest with isometric and isotonic leg exercise training. *Aviat Space Environ Med* 1983;54:696–700.

37. Grigoryeva LS, Kozlovskaya IB: Effect of seven days without gravity load on velocity and strength of human skeletal muscles. *Kosm Biol Med* 1983;17:21–25.
38. Grimby G: Progressive resistance exercise for injury rehabilitation: Special emphasis on isokinetic training. *Sports Med* 1985;2:309–315.
39. Grood ES, Butler DL, Noyes FR: Models of ligament repairs and grafts, in Finerman G (ed): American Academy of Orthopaedic Surgeons *Symposium on Sports Medicine: The Knee.* St. Louis, CV Mosby, 1985, pp 169–181.
40. Häggmark T, Jansson E, Eriksson E: Fiber type area and metabolic potential of the thigh muscle in man after knee surgery and immobilization. *Int J Sports Med* 1981;2:12–17.
41. Häkkinen K, Komi PV: Training-induced changes in neuromuscular performance under voluntary and reflex conditions. *Eur J Appl Physiol* 1986;55:147–155.
42. Halkjaer-Kristensen J, Ingemann-Hansen T: Wasting of the human quadriceps muscle after knee ligament injuries. *Scand J Rehabil Med* 1985;13(suppl):5–55.
43. Hansson TH, Roos BO, Nachemson A: Development of osteopenia in the fourth lumbar vertebra during prolonged bed rest after operation for scoliosis. *Acta Orthop Scand* 1975;46:621–630.
44. Henning CE, Lynch MA, Glick KR Jr: An in vivo strain gage study of elongation of the anterior cruciate ligament. *Am J Sports Med* 1985;13:22–26.
45. Higgins RW, Steadman JR: Anterior cruciate ligament repairs in world class skiers. *Am J Sports Med* 1987;15:439–447.
46. Houston ME, Froese EA, Valeriote SP, et al: Muscle performance, morphology and metabolic capacity during strength training and detraining: A one leg model. *Eur J Appl Physiol* 1983;51:25–35.
47. Ikai M, Fukunaga T: A study on training effect on strength per unit cross-sectional area of muscle by means of ultrasonic measurement. *Int Z Angew Physiol* 1970;28:173–180.
48. Jensen JE, Conn RR, Hazelrigg G, et al: The use of transcutaneous neural stimulation and isokinetic testing in arthroscopic knee surgery. *Am J Sports Med* 1985;13:27–33.
49. Jones VT, Garrett WE Jr, Seaber AV: Biomechanical changes in muscle after immobilization at different lengths. *Trans Orthop Res Soc* 1985;10:6.
50. Kain CC, McCarthy JA, Arms S, et al: An in vivo analysis of the effect of transcutaneous electrical stimulation of the quadriceps and hamstrings on anterior cruciate ligament deformation. *Am J Sports Med* 1988;16:147–152.
51. Kanehisa H, Miyashita M: Effect of isometric and isokinetic muscle training on static strength and dynamic power. *Eur J Appl Physiol* 1983;50:365–371.
52. Kennedy JC, Weinberg HW, Wilson AS: The anatomy and function of the anterior cruciate ligament: As determined by clinical and morphological studies. *J Bone Joint Surg* 1974;56A:223–235.
53. Komi PV, Viitasalo JT, Rauramaa R, et al: Effect of isometric strength training of mechanical, electrical, and metabolic aspects of muscle function. *Eur J Appl Physiol* 1978;40:45–55.
54. Kraemer WJ, Deschenes MR, Fleck SJ: Physiological adaptations to resistance exercise: Implications for athletic conditioning. *Sports Med* 1988;6:246–256.
55. Krølner B, Tøndevold E, Toft B, et al: Bone mass of the axial and the appendicular skeleton in women with Colles' fracture: Its relation to physical activity. *Clin Physiol* 1982;2:147–157.

56. Laing DR, Dalley DR, Kirk JA: Ice therapy in soft tissue injuries. *NZ Med J* 1973;78:155–158.
57. Laros GS, Tipton CM, Cooper RR: Influence of physical activity on ligament insertions in the knees of dogs. *J Bone Joint Surg* 1971;53A:275–286.
58. LeBlanc A, Gogia P, Schneider V, et al: Calf muscle area and strength changes after five weeks of horizontal bed rest. *Am J Sports Med* 1988;16:624–629.
59. Lloyd T, DeDomenico G, Strauss G, et al: A review of the use of electromotor stimulation in human muscles. *Aust J Physiother* 1986;32:18–30.
60. MacDougall JD, Elder GC, Sale DG, et al: Effect of strength training and immobilization on human muscle fibres. *Eur J Appl Physiol* 1980;43:25–34.
61. McDonagh MJ, Davies CT: Adaptive response of mammalian skeletal muscle to exercise with high loads. *Eur J Appl Physiol* 1984;52:139–155.
62. McDonagh MJ, Hayward CM, Davies CT: Isometric training in human elbow flexor muscles: The effects on voluntary and electrically evoked forces. *J Bone Joint Surg* 1983;65B:355–358.
63. Meeusen R, Lievens P: The use of cryotherapy in sports injuries. *Sports Med* 1986;3:398–414.
64. Melzack R, Wall PD: Pain mechanisms: A new theory. *Science* 1965;150:971–979.
65. Moritani T, deVries HA: Neural factors versus hypertrophy in the time course of muscle strength gain. *Am J Phys Med* 1979;58:115–130.
66. Morrissey MC: Electromyostimulation from a clinical perspective: A review. *Sports Med* 1988;6:29–41.
67. Morrissey MC, Brewster CE, Shields CL Jr, et al: The effects of electrical stimulation on the quadriceps during postoperative knee immobilization. *Am J Sports Med* 1985;13:40–45.
68. Noyes FR, Butler DL, Grood ES, et al: Biomechanical analysis of human ligament grafts used in knee-ligament repairs and reconstructions. *J Bone Joint Surg* 1984;66A:344–352.
69. Noyes FR, DeLucas JL, Torvik PJ: Biomechanics of anterior cruciate ligament failure: An analysis of strain-rate sensitivity and mechanisms of failure in primates. *J Bone Joint Surg* 1974;56A:236–253.
70. Noyes FR, Mangine RE, Barber S: Early knee motion after open and arthroscopic anterior cruciate ligament reconstruction. *Am J Sports Med* 1987;15:149–160.
71. Noyes FR, Torvik PF, Hyde WB, et al: Biomechanics of ligament failure: II. An analysis of immobilization, exercise, and reconditioning effects in primates. *J Bone Joint Surg* 1974;56A:1406–1418.
72. Odensten M, Gillquist J: Functional anatomy of the anterior cruciate ligament and a rationale for reconstruction. *J Bone Joint Surg* 1985;67A:257–262.
73. O'Driscoll SW, Kumar A, Salter RB: The effect of continuous passive motion on the clearance of a hemarthrosis from a synovial joint: An experimental investigation in the rabbit. *Clin Orthop* 1983;176:305–311.
74. Ogilvie-Harris DJ, Bauer M, Corey P: Prostaglandin inhibition and the rate of recovery after arthroscopic meniscectomy: A randomised double-blind prospective study. *J Bone Joint Surg* 1985;67B:567–571.
75. Parker JF, Lewis CF, Christensen DG: *Conference Proceedings on Spaceflight Deconditioning and Physical Fitness: January 8–10, 1981, McLean, Virginia.* National Aeronautics and Space Administration, 1981, pp 13–81.
76. Paulos L, Noyes FR, Grood E, et al: Knee rehabilitation after anterior cruciate ligament reconstruction and repair. *Am J Sports Med* 1981;9:140–149.

77. Paulos LE, Rosenberg TD, Drawbert J, et al: Infrapatellar contracture syndrome: An unrecognized cause of knee stiffness with patella entrapment and patella infera. *Am J Sports Med* 1987;15:331–341.
78. Rösler K, Conley KE, Howald H, et al: Specificity of leg power changes to velocities used in bicycle endurance training. *J Appl Physiol* 1986;61:30–36.
79. Sale DG: Neural adaptation to resistance training. *Med Sci Sports Exerc* 1988;20(suppl):S135-S145.
80. Salter RB, Bell S: The effect of continuous passive motion on the healing of partial thickness lacerations of the patellar tendon of the rabbit. *Orthop Trans* 1981;5:209.
81. Salter RB, Bell RS, Keeley FW: The protective effect of continuous passive motion in living articular cartilage in acute septic arthritis: An experimental investigation in the rabbit. *Clin Orthop* 1981;159:223–247.
82. Salter RB, Hamilton HW, Wedge JH, et al: Clinical application of basic research on continuous passive motion for disorders and injuries of synovial joints: A preliminary report of a feasibility study. *J Orthop Res* 1984;1:325–342.
83. Salter RB, Minster RR: The effect of continuous passive motion on a semitendinosus tenodesis in the rabbit knee. *Orthop Trans* 1982;6:292–293.
84. Salter RB, Simmonds DF, Malcolm BW, et al: The biological effect of continuous passive motion on the healing of full-thickness defects in articular cartilage: An experimental investigation in the rabbit. *J Bone Joint Surg* 1980;62A:1232–1251.
85. Shellock FG, Prentice WE: Warming-up and stretching for improved physical performance and prevention of sports-related injuries. *Sports Med* 1985;2:267–278.
86. Silfverskiold JP, Steadman JR, Higgins RW, et al: Rehabilitation of the anterior cruciate ligament in the athlete. *Sports Med* 1988;6:308–319.
87. Sisk TD, Stralka SW, Deering MB, et al: Effect of electrical stimulation on quadriceps strength after reconstructive surgery of the anterior cruciate ligament. *Am J Sports Med* 1987;15:215–220.
88. Snyder SH: *Biological Aspects of Mental Disorder*. New York, Oxford University Press, 1980.
89. Spiegel EA: Relief of pain and spasticity by posterior column stimulation: A proposed mechanism. *Arch Neurol* 1982;39:184–185.
90. Stillwell DM, McLarren GL, Gersten JW: Atrophy of quadriceps muscle due to immobilization of the lower extremity. *Arch Phys Med* 1967;48:289–295.
91. Thorstensson A: Observations on strength training and detraining. *Acta Physiol Scand* 1977;100:491–493.
92. Troyer H: The effect of short-term immobilization on the rabbit knee joint cartilage: A histochemical study. *Clin Orthop* 1975;107:249–257.
93. van Royen BJ, O'Driscoll SW, Dhert WJ, et al: A comparison of the effects of immobilization and continuous passive motion on surgical wound healing in mature rabbits. *Plast Reconstr Surg* 1986;78:360–368.
94. Vogel HG: Mechanical and chemical properties of various connective tissue organs in rats as influenced by non-steroidal antirheumatic drugs. *Connect Tissue Res* 1977;5:91–95.
95. Williams PE, Goldspink G: Connective tissue changes in immobilised muscle. *J Anat* 1984;138:343–350.
96. Williams PE, Goldspink G: The effect of immobilization on the longitudinal growth of striated muscle fibres. *J Anat* 1973;116:45–55.
97. Woo SL-Y, Amiel D, Akeson WH, et al: Effects of long term exercise on ligaments, tendons and bones of swine, abstract. *Med Sci Sports Exerc* 1979;11:105.

98. Woo SL-Y, Buckwalter JA (eds): *Injury and Repair of the Musculoskeletal Soft Tissues.* Park Ridge, Illinois, American Academy of Orthopaedic Surgeons, 1988, pp 114–117.
99. Woo SL-Y, Gomez MA, Seguchi Y, et al: Measurement of mechanical properties of ligament substance from a bone-ligament-bone preparation. *J Orthop Res* 1983;1:22–29.
100. Woo SL-Y, Gomez MA, Sites TJ, et al: The biomechanical and morphological changes in the medial collateral ligament of the rabbit after immobilization and remobilization. *J Bone Joint Surg* 1987;69A:1200–1211.
101. Woo SL-Y, Matthews JV, Akeson WH, et al: Connective tissue response to immobility: Correlative study of biomechanical and biochemical measurements of normal and immobilized rabbit knees. *Arthritis Rheum* 1975;18:257–264.
102. Woo SL-Y, Ritter MA, Amiel D, et al: The biomechanical and biochemical properties of swine tendons: Long term effects of exercise on the digital extensors. *Connect Tissue Res* 1980;7:177–183.
103. Yasuda Y, Miyamura M: Cross transfer effects of muscular training on blood flow in the ipsilateral and contralateral forearms. *Eur J Appl Physiol* 1983;51:321–329.

Chapter 52

Concepts in Exercise Rehabilitation of Athletic Injury

W. Ben Kibler, MD

Basic Concepts

Proper rehabilitation of an athletic soft-tissue injury, after the injury itself or after necessary surgery or immobilization, requires understanding and clinically applying the consequences of inflammation and healing of the tissues. Although these consequences are varied when viewed at a cellular or subcellular level, involving many organelles, enzyme systems, anatomic locations, and metabolic systems, only a few basic concepts are involved (Outline 1).

First, tissue inflammation invariably accompanies tissue injury. The inflammatory cycle is initiated as a result of tissue injury, whether the injury is major, extremely symptomatic, and disabling[13] or relatively minor, subclinical, and capable of asymptomatic healing.[1] The same process occurs whether the injury is acute,[13] an acute exacerbation of a chronic condition,[4] or chronic,[16] and the process is similar regardless of the anatomic site, whether it be the plantar fascia,[4] Achilles tendon,[7] elbow,[16] or lateral patellar retinaculum.[5] In each case, microscopy shows vascular congestion, inflammatory cell infiltration, edema, chronic fibrosis, and deposition of scar tissue.

This tissue inflammation alters the ability of the tissues to function maximally in an athletic setting. This occurs in both the acute inflammatory process, in which edema, pain, and muscle inhibition alter athletic function,[8] and in chronic inflammation, in which pain, weakness, and inflexibility alter athletic function.[7,16,18]

This alteration in function of the tissues can alter athletic performance. This alteration can be divided into two general types—performance cessation or performance modification. Performance cessation occurs in overt clinical "injury" and accompanies clinical symptom complexes such as hamstring muscle tear, Achilles tendinitis, ruptured biceps tendon, or acute rotator cuff tendinitis. In these situations, performance must be stopped because of inability to initiate and implement athletic activities. Performance modification is more common, and is a response to minor, usually subclinical, alterations in function caused by mild or chronic inflammation. In these situations, perform-

Outline 1 Basic concepts

Tissue inflammation accompanies tissue injury
Tissue inflammation alters athletic function
Altered function leads to altered performance
  Cessation—clinical symptoms
  Modification—subclinical symptoms
Rehabilitation must consider functional alterations as well as clinical symptoms

ance can be continued but only at a lower level of muscle efficiency because of inability to sustain normal athletic activities. This situation is best described in the context of a disability, or inability to function in an entirely normal pattern.[8]

Finally, the goal of sports medicine rehabilitation is to restore athletic function to as normal a level as possible. In this context, all the ways in which the soft-tissue inflammatory process affects tissue function and performance must be understood. This includes both symptoms (for example, pain, swelling, and edema) and functional alterations (muscle weakness, imbalance, or inflexibility). Proper rehabilitation results from the recognition that functional alterations as well as the symptoms must be corrected.

Functional Alterations as a Result of the Inflammatory Process

Studies of athletes with injury-induced inflammation have shown that clinical function is altered by several consequences of the inflammatory cycle (Outline 2). Pain, whether induced by direct tissue damage, histamine or other peptide release, edema, or intra-articular fluid, is a potent inhibitor of soft-tissue function. It plays a major role by itself, or as a contributor to other problems, such as reflex muscle weakness or alteration in the linked sequence of extremity activities called the kinetic chain.[15]

Muscle strength is decreased as a result of the inflammatory cycle. This may be the result of direct tissue damage, with intrafibrillar,[1] myotendinous junction,[6] or intramuscular[12] lesions. It also results from disuse because of the injury or subsequent surgery and/or immobilization. The rate of muscle strength decrement may approach 1% per day in immobilized muscles.[7] Finally, muscle strength may be decreased secondary to neurologic deconditioning as a result of pain inhibition or alteration in proprioceptive feedback.[19]

Closely accompanying a change in muscle strength, but separate in significance, is an alteration of the normal balance between muscle groups that couple to control force production around joints and efficiently transfer this force to the next link in the kinetic chain.[15] For each coupled muscular activity, one group can be considered prime movers, or agonists, and the reciprocal group can be considered regulators. In most circumstances, the term antagonists is not appropriate

Outline 2 Consequences of the inflammatory cycle that alter athletic function

Pain
Decreased muscle strength
Alteration of strength balance
Inflexibility
Substitute muscle activities

for this group, as it does not accurately describe the proper function of this group. The quadriceps muscle is the prime mover at the knee in jumping, with the hamstrings and gastrocnemius as regulators, controlling the rate of rotation and transferring the rotational torque into linear acceleration.[14,17] The roles are reversed at the hip, with the hamstrings, acting in concert with the gluteals, as the prime movers, and the quadriceps acting as a regulator.[17] In throwing motions at the shoulder, the prime movers in the acceleration phase are the pectorals, latissimus dorsi, anterior deltoid, and supraspinatus,[9] while the posterior deltoid, infraspinatus, and trapezius act as regulators.[10] As a result of clinical and subclinical inflammation, scar, inflexibility, neurologic alteration, and weakness, strength imbalances can be created in the force couples. This has been demonstrated in the ankle in plantar fasciitis,[11] the knee in anterior cruciate ligament deficiency,[19] the shoulder in shoulder pain,[10] and in the elbow after injury.[20] The resulting disruption in normal force production and force transfer leads to decreased function as the mechanical efficiency of the joint-muscle complex is decreased because of increasing shear forces.[2]

Inflexibility, or decreased ability to lengthen without symptoms or further damage, of myotendinous units results from the intramuscular or myotendinous[6] scar that follows tensile overload and subsequent inflammation-based healing. This should be distinguished from joint tightness secondary to capsular or ligamentous contractures that may or may not be present. In the shoulder, both are present, and they significantly alter the normal rotational process of the scapuloglenohumeral complex. Scar tissue and the resulting muscle inflexibility may alter the degree to which the muscle can lengthen in an eccentric contraction, causing pain or changing the force-velocity curve of a muscle, or can alter the length-tension curve of force production by interfering with normal concentric contraction. In either case, functional alteration results.

Because these major or minor functional alterations decrease efficiency of performance, the athlete tries to maintain optimal performance by substituting or recruiting other muscles or muscle patterns. In early plantar fasciitis, foot strike is sustained on the metatarsal heads rather than the heels,[11] and runners shorten their stride length and stance time because of the symptoms. In "tennis elbow," the position of the elbow alters in the backhand stroke, so that as the elbow leads, forearm pronation increases.[16] In rotator cuff tendinitis, alterations occur in the throwing position of the shoulder, so that the arm "drops down" to a more sidearm position; alterations also occur in timing

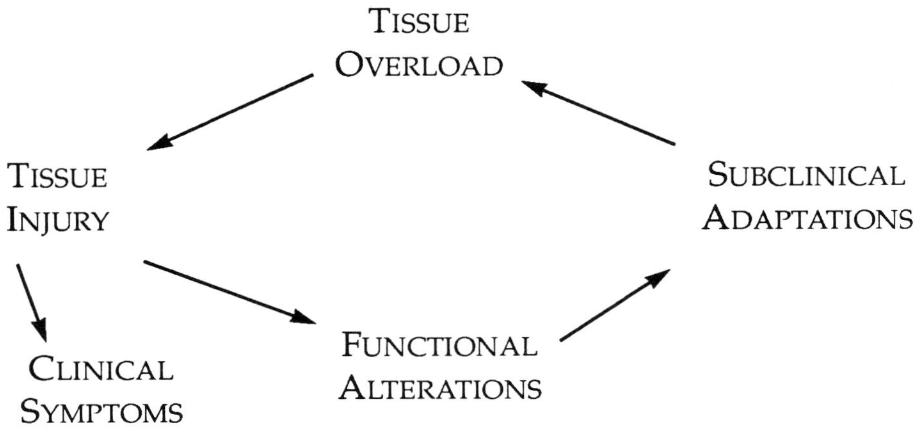

Fig. 1 *Negative-feedback cycle.*

and recruitment of muscle firing.[9,10] Each of these alterations, while compensatory, is less efficient than the original function. These alterations may lead to further injury from more local tissue tensile overload secondary to altered biomechanics resulting from muscle fatigue, or alterations in other components of the kinetic chain. For example, "dropping down" of the shoulder may injure the rotator cuff further, but can also overload the medial elbow area or the back and trunk muscles.

Tissue injury and the inflammatory cycle have wide ranging effects on both clinical and subclinical aspects of muscle function and performance. In addition, the interplay of these effects can exacerbate already existing functional deficits. Not all these effects are symptomatic in the usual sense. The rest are relatively asymptomatic in mild forms, but are still capable of causing functional alteration if the right combination of athletic stresses is present. For example, an athlete may be able to throw easily for 20 to 30 minutes, or to throw hard for five to ten throws, but not be able to throw at maximum speed and accuracy for very long. These varied effects can be linked to show their interaction. This linkage can also be used as a schema by which each injury can be evaluated in terms of extent of athletic disability, assignment of proper rehabilitation modalities, and completeness of athletic rehabilitation. Finally, it can be used as a tool to understand the difference between symptom-based rehabilitation and function-based rehabilitation.

In its most basic form, this framework can be depicted as a negative-feedback cycle (Fig. 1). In this cycle, each stage of soft-tissue injury can lead to further problems if the tissue continues to be used. Tissue injury leads to either clinical symptoms or subclinical alterations. Further use of these altered tissues can lead to functional adaptations that may impose intolerable overloads on the tissues, leading to more injury and thus closing the circle.

Each of these stages is composed of a complex of symptoms and anatomic alterations that result from inflammation and further use. The more detailed framework is shown in Figure 2. The tissue injury complex consists of macrotears of the muscular, myotendinous, ligamentous, or capsular soft tissues, secondary to repetitive overload trauma, as demonstrated by Nirschl[16] and Garrett,[6] by direct trauma, or by surgical intervention. As far as can be determined, the nature or amount of inflammatory response is not related to the injurious agent, only the amount of tissue injury. Caplan[20] determined that skeletal muscle tears involving less than 3 g of tissue heal with normal results, but tears involving more tissue do not. This amount probably defines the line between "microtears" and "macrotears." The absolute amount of tissue damage necessary to distinguish between "large" macrotears and "medium" macrotears is not known. As a working definition, "large" macrotears result in clinical symptoms, whereas "medium" macrotears result in functional alterations.

The clinical symptom complex consists of the findings normally associated with a muscle injury. These include pain, alteration of muscle strength, localized tenderness, localized edema, and perhaps a palpable mass. In addition, there is usually decreased athletic performance secondary to alteration in tissue function. Athletes in this situation of necessity decrease or cease athletic participation, and most seek medical help.

For every athlete who has "large" macrotears and overt clinical symptoms as a result of tissue injury and inflammation, many more sustain "medium" macrotears that reduce the efficiency of muscle function. In a United States Tennis Association study (unpublished data) and an international study of elite junior tennis players,[12] there were six athletes with subclinical alterations in strength, strength balance, or inflexibility for every athlete with overt clinical symptoms. In a study of athletes who put tensile stress on the lower extremity,[11] the ratio was approximately the same. As has been shown, these alterations impose an inefficiency of muscle action that can be best described as a functional biomechanical deficit.

This deficit can be seen as a result of tissue inflammation and repair of "large" or "medium" macrotears. The fact that alterations represented by this deficit are present is the major reason why symptom-based rehabilitation that depends on rest and is not performance-oriented rarely results in normal performance.

Therefore, sport-specific, performance-oriented, function-based rehabilitation is necessary to eliminate this deficit, which impedes progress toward normal function and predisposes to injury. The functional biomechanical deficit is a deviation from normal muscle strength, balance, or flexibility and may be asymptomatic or mildly symptomatic. However, when optimal or competitive function is required, the athlete must adapt either by changing performance mechanics (altering the normal sequence of the kinetic chain, increasing recruitment of motor

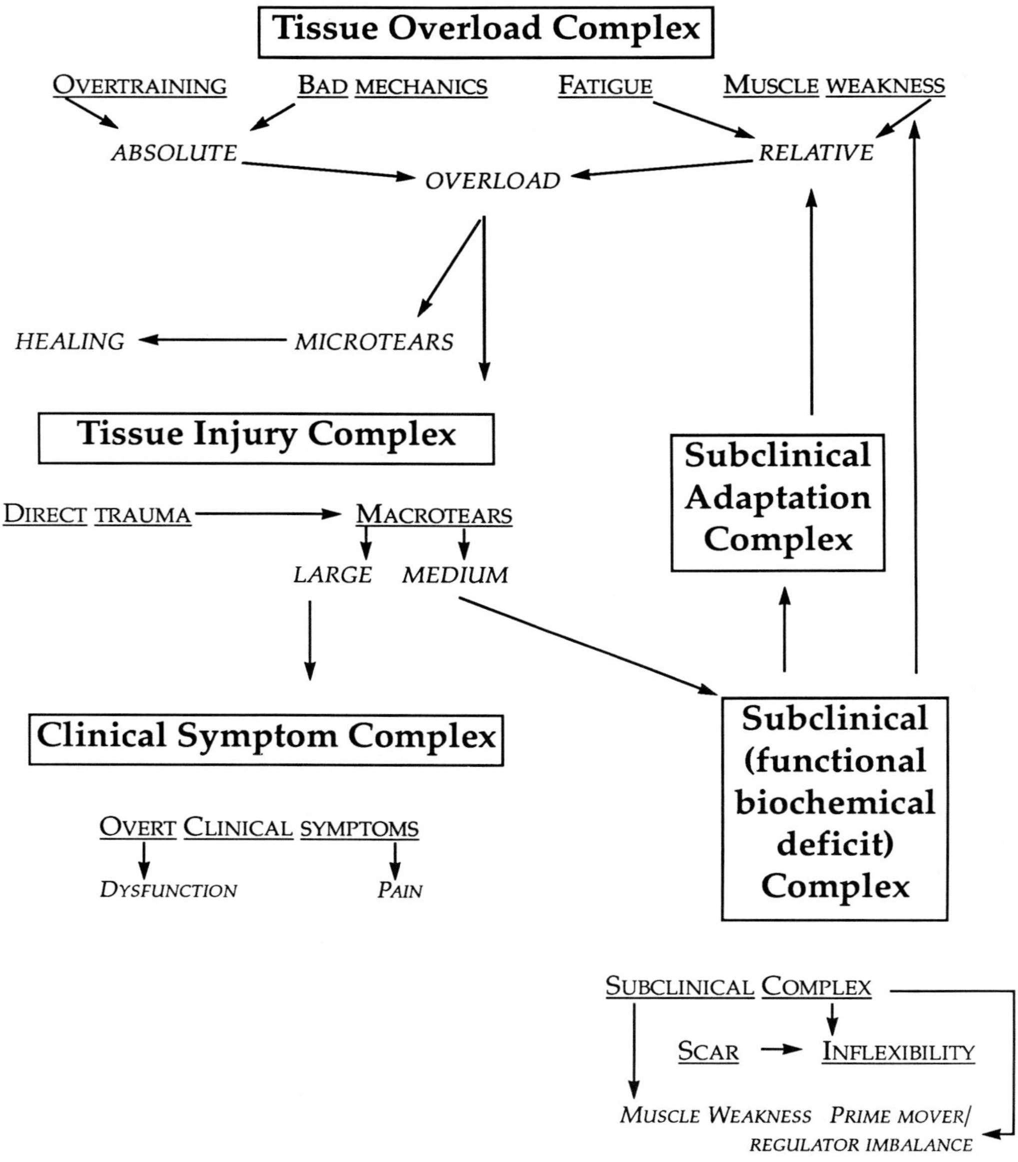

Fig. 2 *Complex of symptoms and anatomic alterations that result from inflammation and further use.*

units, or using other physiologic parameters to accomplish the same function[2]) or by decreasing performance to stay within functional limitations.

This substitute activity complex can be illustrated by the runner

Table 1 Ankle sprains

Complex	Findings	
	Acute Sprains	**Acute-on-Chronic Sprains**
Tissue injury complex	1st-, 2nd-, or 3rd-degree lateral or anterior ligamentous sprain	1st-, 2nd-, or 3rd-degree lateral or anterior ligamentous sprain
Clinical symptom complex	Pain with or without instability; inability to run or jump; swelling	Pain with or without instability; inability to run or jump; swelling
Functional biomechanical deficit	None	Ligamentous instability; Achilles tendon inflexibility; peroneal and/or gastrocnemius weakness; hip abductor and quadriceps weakness; gastrocnemius-tibialis anterior muscle imbalance; loss or proprioception
Substitute activity complex	None	Pronation of foot on jump; functional Trendelenburg position of hip; shortened stance time
Tissue overload complex	None	Gastrocnemius and peroneal muscles; anterior capsular tissues

with mild plantar fasciitis who changes stride length to hit more on the metatarsal heads, experiences more muscle fatigue when running the same distance because of increased energy expenditure, and who eventually increases the time needed to run a mile.

Continued athletic activity will put more load on the weakened, tight, and/or fatigued muscle. This load is in the form of a tensile stress overload, with the muscle-tendon-bone unit unable to protect itself from the stresses. As a result, further tissue overload stress occurs, thus closing the circle and setting the stage for further inflammation and further functional performance alterations, which can eventually lead to overt clinical symptoms.[6]

There are many clinical examples of this process. Acute ankle sprain (Table 1) is a traumatic event that produces immediate pain and disability. The clinical symptom complex is secondary to a well-defined tissue injury. Prompt treatment diminishes symptoms, with minimal inflexibility or other deficits. However, if the injury is ignored, or rehabilitation is incomplete, alterations in flexibility and/or strength will occur and substitute activities will develop. If this occurs, as many as 80% of athletes will reinjure the ankle within three months[8] and will have acute symptoms exacerbating a chronic condition (Table 1).

Rotator cuff impingement (Table 2), although usually considered an acute traumatic event, in most cases is actually the culmination of many revolutions of the vicious cycle. Studies have demonstrated the overload in the posterior shoulder complex consisting of the scapular stabilizers, posterior musculature, and posterior capsule.[9,10,12] This biomechanical deficit can then lead to substitute activities. Pain is not usually present, but functional alteration is. Continued use can then lead to anatomic rotator cuff changes secondary to mechanical im-

Table 2 Rotator cuff impingement

Complex	Findings
Tissue overload complex	Tensile load on posterior shoulder capsular structures; tensile load on posterior shoulder muscles; tensile load on scapular stabilizers
Tissue injury complex	Tears in posterior capsule; rotator cuff impingement; glenoid labral attrition
Clinical symptom complex	Rotator cuff impingement; pain; anterosuperior glenohumoral instability; decreased ball or service velocity
Functional biomechanical deficit	Internal-rotation inflexibility; external-rotation strength
Substitute activity complex	Alteration of shoulder throwing position or motion; decreased velocity

Table 3 Plantar fasciitis

Complex	Findings
Tissue overload complex	Tensile load on gastrocnemius muscle-tendon and tendon-bone units; tensile load on planter fascia
Tissue injury complex	Gastrocnemius myotendinous junction; planter fascia attachment to calcaneus
Clinical symptom complex	Point-tender pain over fascia-calcaneus junction; decreased running ability
Functional biomechanical deficit	Dorsiflexion inflexibility; planter flexor strength deficit; functional pronation
Substitute activity complex	Shortened stride length; running on metatarsal heads

pingement, or to clinical symptoms secondary to attritional tears of the anterior superior glenoid labrum.

Plantar fasciitis (Table 3) is a classic overload injury in which a tensile overload occurs at the insertion of the plantar fascia on the calcaneus. It has been shown[11] that long-distance running imposes tensile loads on the gastrocnemius-Achilles tendon complex that create muscle weakness and imbalance. Symptoms develop because of increased inflexibility in the plantar flexor and tensile strain on the mechanically disadvantaged plantar fascia.[11]

These examples show that soft-tissue injury can affect performance not only overtly, but on a subclinical level and may set the stage for the development of additional symptomatic conditions if the early functional alterations are not recognized and properly rehabilitated.

Rehabilitation

The traditional goals of rehabilitation of any type of athletic musculoskeletal injury have been (1) to establish an accurate and complete diagnosis of all the anatomic and functional deficits resulting from the injury, (2) to minimize the deleterious local effects of the acute injury,

(3) to allow anatomic healing of the injury, (4) to maintain other components of athletic fitness, and (5) to regain previous athletic function.[8]

The methods by which these goals can be accomplished include (1) adequate tissue protection during healing, (2) proper sequence and use of therapeutic techniques, (3) proper rehabilitation of muscular flexibility, strength, and balance; (4) proper rehabilitation of all the links in the kinetic chain that include the injured part, and (5) establishment of sport-specific or activity-specific criteria for return to play, backed up by a complete assessment of the ability of the athlete to function normally in the sport or activity.

The rehabilitative process can be broken down into three phases. Acute-phase rehabilitation is concerned with protection of the injured tissues by splinting, bracing, or other support to allow healing and control of the early inflammatory process to reduce the clinical symptoms. This phase blends into the recovery phase, in which efforts are directed toward return to normal flexibility and strength of the injured tissues and gradual controlled physical activities, usually with the aid of braces or supports. At the end of this phase, the athlete usually has no clinical symptoms and may have no flexibility defects. The final phase of rehabilitation is the maintenance phase. This is the most important phase for restoring maximal performance and minimizing the risk of reinjury. During this phase, maximal flexibility, strength, and balance are achieved, exercises are done to ensure that these levels are maintained, and sport-specific testing is conducted to ensure that the athlete can compete with safety. Only then should unrestricted return to play be allowed.

The schema of the tissue injury cycle can be used in decision-making about the goals of rehabilitation, to guide proper implementation of the methods of rehabilitation, and to recognize the phases of rehabilitation.

A complete and accurate diagnosis can be made by establishing which of the various stages of the cycle are present. In acute injuries to previously normal tissues, some stages may never appear. However, treatment confined to pain relief and initiation of healing without functional restoration by other rehabilitation methods may result in development of biomechanical deficits.

The tissue overload cycle is particularly useful in defining the rehabilitation problems in the athlete with mild symptoms but with performance dysfunction or disability. All the stages of tissue dysfunction can be clearly defined, so appropriate treatment of the deficits can be begun. The progress of rehabilitation in the recovery phase can be monitored by improvement in flexibility and strength and restitution of balance in both the injured tissues and in the rest of the kinetic chain.

In the maintenance phase, the schema allows the development of specific criteria for return to play. Only after all the clinical symptoms and biomechanical deficits have resolved, or are no longer causing subclinical adaptations in the specific tasks related to the sport, should the athlete return to uncontrolled play. Thus, the rehabilitation process

Table 4 Flow chart of the rehabilitation cycle

Goal	Method	Result
Acute phase		
Accurate and complete diagnosis	Listing of all abnormalities in each stage of injury cycle	Complete assessment of all functional and anatomic alterations
Minimizing acute injury	Tissue protection	Initiation of anatomic healing
Recovery phase		
Anatomic healing	Tissue protection during mobilization; respect biologic healing rate	Complete anatomic healing
Recovery of muscle strength and tissue flexibility	Sequential initiation of mobilization and strength; start kinetic chain rehabilitation	Relief of clinical symptoms of pain, swelling, and/or weakness; symptom-based rehabilitation
Maintenance phase		
Maintain other components of athletic fitness	Cross-training; splinted use of involved part	Maintain kinetic chain and cardiovascular fitness
Rehabilitation of injured part to normal function	Full range-of-motion; symmetric muscle strength and balance; no biomechanical deficits	Normal function of injured part
Return to play	No subclinical adaptations; sport-specific and activity-specific testing in controlled situations; continuation of preventative exercise program	Return to athletic activity at maximal level; function-based rehabilitation.

can be organized around a flow chart based on the tissue injury cycle (Table 4).

In acute ankle sprain, for example, initial treatment, based on accurate diagnosis of the injury complex and resulting muscle weakness, is directed toward reducing the clinical symptoms and maintaining flexibility and strength. In the recovery phase, any residual imbalances or deficits are assessed and restored. In the maintenance phase, functional evaluation of jumping, cutting, running, and kicking is done under controlled circumstances to ensure that function has been maximized. Only then are actual play situations allowed.

In chronic rotator cuff impingement, the tissues subject to overload (that is, the supraspinatus, infraspinatus, posterior capsule, and scapular stabilizers) are examined for inflexibility or weakness and appropriate physical therapy is undertaken. If acute clinical symptoms are superimposed, physical therapy is begun during the acute phase. Once the symptoms have resolved, recovery-phase rehabilitation includes correction of rotational inflexibilities and strength imbalances that were part of the biomechanical deficit that led to functional alterations. Once these have been resolved, maintenance rehabilitation includes continued exercises to maintain posterior muscle balance and appropriate flexibility. Criteria for return to play include serving or throwing with normal motion and speed.

References

1. Armstrong RB: Cellular aspects of muscle overload injury. *Med Sci Sports Exerc*, in press.
2. Baratta R, Solomonow M, Zhou BH, et al: Muscular coactivation: The role of the antagonist musculature in maintaining knee stability. *Am J Sports Med* 1988;16:113–122.

3. Caplan A, Carlson B, Faulkner J, et al: Skeletal muscle, in Woo SL-Y, Buckwalter JA (eds): *Injury and Repair of the Musculoskeletal Soft Tissues.* Park Ridge, Illinois, American Academy of Orthopaedic Surgeons, 1988, pp 213–291.
4. Clancy WG Jr: Tendinitis and plantar fasciitis in runners, in Drez D Jr, D'Ambrosia R (eds): *Prevention and Treatment of Running Injuries.* Thorofare, New Jersey, Charles B Slack, 1982, pp 77–87.
5. Fulkerson JP: The etiology of patellofemoral pain in young, active patients: A prospective study. *Clin Orthop* 1983;179:129–133.
6. Garrett WE Jr: Injuries to the muscle tendon unit, in Bassett FH III (ed): *Instructional Course Lectures, XXXVII.* Park Ridge, Illinois, American Academy of Orthopaedic Surgeons, 1988, pp 275–282.
7. Gilstrom P, Ljunquist R: Long term results after operation for partial rupture of Achilles tendon. *Acta Chir Scand* 1978;482(suppl):78.
8. Herring S: Rehabilitation from muscle injury. *Med Sci Sports Exerc*, in press.
9. Jobe FW, Moynes DR, Tibone JE, et al: An EMG analysis of the shoulder in pitching: A second report. *Am J Sports Med* 1984;12:218–220.
10. Kibler WB: Lateral scapular slide in throwing athletes. Presented at the annual meeting of the American Orthopaedic Society for Sports Medicine, Traverse City, Michigan, June 19, 1989.
11. Kibler WB: Strength and flexibility findings in athletes with plantar fasciitis. *Am J Sports Med*, in press.
12. Kibler WB, McQueen C, Uhl T: Fitness evaluations and fitness findings in competitive junior tennis players. *Clin Sports Med* 1988;7:403–416.
13. Krejci V, Koch P: *Muscle and Tendon Injuries in Athletes.* Chicago, Year Book Medical, 1970, p 5.
14. Mann RA, Hagy J: Biomechanics of walking, running, and sprinting. *Am J Sports Med* 1980;8:345–350.
15. Marino M: Current concepts on rehabilitation in sports medicine research and clinical interrelationships, in Nicholas JA, Hershman EB (eds): *The Lower Extremity and Spine in Sports Medicine.* St. Louis, CV Mosby, 1986, vol 1, pp 117–193.
16. Nirschl RP, Pettrone FA: Tennis elbow: The surgical treatment of lateral epicondylitis. *J Bone Joint Surg* 1979;61A:832–839.
17. Peterson L, Frankel H: Biomechanics of the knee in athletes, in Nicholas JA, Hershman EB (eds): *The Lower Extremity and Spine in Sports Medicine.* St. Louis, CV Mosby, 1986, vol 1, pp 695–726.
18. Renström P, Johnson RJ: Overuse injuries in sports: A review. *Sports Med* 1985;2:316–333.
19. Solomonow M, Baratta R, Zhou BH, et al: The synergistic action of the anterior cruciate ligament and thigh muscles in maintaining joint stability. *Am J Sports Med* 1987;15:207–213.
20. Solomonow M, Guzzi A, Baratta R, et al: EMG-force model of the elbows antagonistic muscle pair: The effect of joint position, gravity and recruitment. *Am J Phys Med* 1986;65:223–244.

Future Directions

Clinical Studies

Investigation of a broad range of clinical research issues may provide more information on the interaction of training, sports-induced injury and inflammation, and healing and help to improve current training and conditioning programs. The availability of new bioassays and such nondestructive tissue tests as magnetic resonance imaging and magnetic resonance spectroscopy should contribute to the success of these projects. These studies may involve both humans and appropriate animal models.

Determine the Probability of Injury in a Given Population

With ever-widening participation in sports activities, prevention and early intervention are needed to reduce the risk and impact of sports-induced injuries. Prospective, longitudinal studies are required to determine accurately the risk factors for injury. Parametric statistical techniques can screen large populations for predisposition and measurable factors, to be followed by smaller-scale studies of individuals with a high probability of injury. A broad range of anatomic, physiologic, biochemical, and functional assessments should be considered in early screening. The specificity and accuracy of measurements must be well defined in order to establish uniform clinical criteria for injury that can be applied to all subjects. The time and expense of such studies suggest the desirability of a series of pilot (screening) tests of increasing scope to justify the next level of complexity. One possible focus would be a specific sport or activity with a generally high incidence of injury.

Study the Long-Term Effects of Lower-Extremity Alignment, Anatomy, and Form

Clinical experience in treating runners and joggers indicates that certain lower-limb malalignments are related to overuse injuries. With 15 to 20 million joggers, these injuries are frequent and the need for preventive measures clearly justifies attempts to determine their causes.

A select population of runners should be chosen and given a comprehensive physical examination before a running program is initiated. The examination should include determination of lower-limb anatomy, alignment, and muscle strength, a video analysis of running style, and clinical determination of knee joint, patellofemoral, and foot and ankle abnormalities. Controlled variables would include running distance, shoes, jogging terrain, and training history. Participants would be required to refrain from other sports activities to avoid variables that would affect the analysis. Any strength and flexibility defects would be corrected before the study began. The lower-limb analysis would be repeated after one to two years of running. Potential problems include the difficulty of obtaining a uniform population of joggers who would follow the prescribed exercise program, potentially high participant drop-out rates, and injuries to test subjects caused by other sports.

Establish the Relationship of Anterior Shoulder Pain to Abnormal Patterns of Muscle Contraction and Upper-Extremity Kinematics During Throwing

Clinical studies have shown that weaknesses of rotator cuff muscles and/or scapular muscle stabilizers can cause abnormal shoulder kinematics in throwing. The alterations in patterns of muscular contraction and motion may increase loads in shoulder capsular and joint structures and may be significant factors in microtrauma, shoulder tendon degeneration, and sports-induced inflammatory states.

The study population could comprise a select group of injury-free baseball and tennis players. Shoulder kinematics and electromyographic patterns of muscle contraction would be determined. This population would be followed longitudinally with repeat evaluations at any time an injury occurred and at the conclusion of the study. Although it is expensive to perform a comprehensive shoulder analysis in a large number of athletes, it is important to determine that a specific overload injury is caused by differences in joint kinematics and not by preexisting in vivo tissue degeneration.

Identify Physiologic Responses to Different Exercise Protocols

It is clear that training programs (both endurance and strength) cause major changes in systemic factors and musculoskeletal tissues. Clinicians and sports scientists are often asked to recommend training regimens; however, the lack of rigorous studies means that generalizations are of limited value to specific individuals. Factors to be studied include growth, repair, remodeling, and functional performance. It is extremely important to consider and control all possible variables. Subject selection and characterization are also critical. To ensure meaningful results, assays should be specific and sensitive.

A broad range of possible experiments can fit within this general concept. Discrete and focused questions should be addressed to limit the scope of research protocols. Each project needs careful consideration of factors such as nutrition that can have an impact on the results. A sophisticated statistical design is required.

Characterize Chronic Aspects of Overtraining Syndromes by Serum Markers

Preliminary data suggest that levels of isoenzymes and isoforms for muscle are increased in basal resting states in overtrained athletes. In large study groups, it is important to compare overtrained, trained, and sedentary individuals. Serum samples and microbiopsy samples from muscle could be collected during rest, during exercise stress-tests, and during recovery. Creatine kinase in serum and muscle tissue would be one significant assay. It is critical to establish uniform and objective criteria for identifying and classifying the overtraining syndrome.

Establish the Immunologic Response to Training

The immune system may be an important central control system involved in inflammation and healing of microinjuries and macroinjuries. Therefore, the relationship between training and the immune system may affect the response to any level of injury. Training can be assessed in both human and animal studies. It would be valuable to measure circulating immunologic mediators, such as interleukin, tumor necrosis factor, T cells, and macrophages, and to correlate these factors with the local immune environment in which the inflammation and healing occur. Many factors, including nutrition, previous state of training, and level of training stimulus, can influence the immune response, and these variables must be carefully controlled. The interaction of endocrinologic agents such as corticosteroids may be critical in determining the response to training.

Determine the Appropriate Recovery Period Between Exercise Events

Training activities are separated by periods of rest and recovery. It would be valuable to understand the impact of a recovery period at fundamental mechanistic and practical performance levels. The results of such studies could help athletes improve training and performance and avoid injury and overtraining.

The wide range of recovery duration (time) and recovery intensity (rest vs alternative activities) requires a study design that focuses on a limited number of well-controlled variables. Outcome measures of tissue properties, serum markers, and performance must be uniformly applied. Both animal and human studies are possible.

Basic Science Studies

There is much to be learned about how training influences musculoskeletal tissues and their inflammatory response to injury. In a correlative sense, the response of these tissues to inflammatory agents requires further study. A broad range of fundamental questions should be investigated to help form the basis for additional clinical studies.

Identify the Effects of Inflammation on Ligaments

Clinical evidence suggests that inflammatory states induced by sports injury are characterized by an immune response, including inflammatory cell migration, release of inflammatory mediators, and development of an inflammatory response. It is not known if this inflammatory response has a deleterious effect on ligament tissue homeostasis defined by material and structural mechanical properties and matrix components.

An animal model of anterior cruciate deficiency that invokes a well-defined inflammatory response may be used. Mechanical loading studies of the posterior cruciate ligament and medial collateral ligament may allow determination of material and structural mechanical properties in response to the induced inflammatory process. Biochemical studies should determine collagen cross-linking, collagen type, and matrix composition. It will be difficult to develop a similar inflammatory response in all animals and to characterize inflammatory mediators. It is important to be able to compare sports-induced inflammatory responses, which are usually low-grade inflammatory reactions, with the acute reactions normally seen in inflammation.

Study the Effect of Exercise on the Aging of Tendon and Ligament

The elderly segment of our population is becoming increasingly active, indicating a need for exercise programs specific to this age group that will not induce injury. Decreases in musculoskeletal tissue function previously ascribed to the aging process may actually represent disuse and atrophy and might be prevented by maintaining activity and exercises with advancing age.

It is important in selecting an animal model to choose one that can be controlled to determine the effect of age on tendon and ligament properties. A specific exercise stimulus may be induced during the aging process. The imposition of a well-defined exercise program means that it would be necessary to measure the specific in vivo forces on the ligament and tendon structures to characterize precisely the local forces induced by the exercise program. Variables other than age must be carefully controlled. Ensuring appropriate levels of exercise in the experimental animal may be difficult. The ability to measure in vivo tissue forces requires the development of new in vivo measuring devices.

Determine the Effects of NSAIDs on the Healing Response of Ligaments

Many clinical questions exist about the unknown effects of nonsteroidal anti-inflammatory drugs (NSAIDs) on the healing of knee ligament repairs. Ligament surgery involves a significant inflammatory response, which is commonly treated with NSAIDs. Indomethacin has been reported to alter bone healing in experimental animals, leading to recommendations that this agent be avoided in fractures. The extent to which the common postoperative use of NSAIDs has a deleterious effect on soft-tissue healing has not been determined.

The study should use a known experimental model of ligament healing in animals, perhaps an anterior cruciate or medial collateral ligament. A known surgical insult should be applied to the ligament, followed by postoperative treatment for four weeks with a NSAID (and placebo control). Material and structural mechanical properties should be determined under in vitro loading conditions. Biochemical analyses may include collagen matrix constituents, cross-linking, and fibril organization. Problems include the difficulty of developing a uniform surgical injury to the ligament and the need to ensure the same level of activity in all animals studied.

Study the Role of Repetitive Microtrauma in Training-Induced Injuries

One important theory of injury in an individual who trains regularly is that microtraumas accumulate and eventually produce a clinically significant injury. This area of research has both basic and clinical interest. It appears that the turnover of musculoskeletal tissue in normal physiologic states is probably accelerated during exercise training. A fundamental question relates to whether inflammatory processes are always involved in this turnover or only arise in response to repeated microtrauma. Topics for possible research in this area are very broad. Because many tissues and many systemic factors may be involved, it is important to control as many variables as possible and to focus on clear, answerable questions.

Determine How Myotendinous Junctions Adapt to Training

Because the myotendinous junction has been implicated as the primary site of injury in the muscle-tendon complex, establishing specific training benefits would make it possible to avoid injury. It is possible to study the morphologic, biochemical, and strength changes in the myotendinous junction in relation to specific training and detraining regimens. It would be valuable to use sophisticated methods to establish a mechanistic interrelationship between form and function applied to the training response. One possible problem may be performing multiple tests on small tissue samples. The exercise program must be specific to avoid potentially confounding variables such as intensity, duration, and frequency.

Study the Local Mechanical Environment During Training Activities

The mechanical and failure properties of musculoskeletal tissue have been studied in isolated tissues from various animals and from cadavers. A relationship should be established between nontraumatic (but repeated) loading in training activities and the actual mechanical forces delivered to local tissues. Such research could enhance understanding of the microinjury concept. Measurement and understanding of local loads will require miniature force or strain transducers (with minimal invasion of the tissue itself) coupled with sophisticated mathematical models. When appropriate, the biochemical structure of tissue may be assessed.

Determine the Effect of Increased Loads on Tendon

The purpose of training programs is to increase the threshold and baseline of tissue strength, thereby preventing or lessening the chance of failure under the high tissue loads that occur during athletic activities. The specific adaptation of tendon as a structure is unknown, and controversy exists as to the manner in which mature collagenous structures respond to increased loading states.

An animal model such as the rabbit gastrocnemius muscle-tendon unit should be selected for study. An exercise state should be achieved and the imposed in vivo loads measured. Material and structural mechanical properties may be studied under in vitro loading conditions. Biochemical determinations include tendon cross-linking, fibril organization, and matrix constituents. It is important to impose a uniform exercise input to provide a significant loading response to the tendon. It may be possible to use native goats, sheep, or other animals to avoid an experimental model that depends on inbred animals.

Determine the Effect of Mechanical Deformation on Aging Fibroblasts

Altered cellular processes observed in cultured fibroblasts (decreased collagen and matrix production) have been ascribed to cellular senescence or aging. Similar changes caused by cellular senescence are proposed as an explanation for incremental decreases in tissue strength with advancing age. Clinical evidence suggests that maintenance of an active lifestyle and an exercise program can lessen age-related atrophy. The development of tissue models allows the response curve of loading and its effect on cellular functions to be determined in a manner more precise than that available in clinical studies.

Recently developed culture systems allow a predetermined deformation to be applied to fibroblasts. Various deformation histories can be correlated with cellular functions, including DNA synthesis, protein synthesis, and matrix component synthesis. It may be difficult to obtain a fibroblastic culture system that phenotypically remains the same. It is important to select deformation histories that impose a natural "cell signal" to activate a cellular response.

Section Six

Provocative Issues

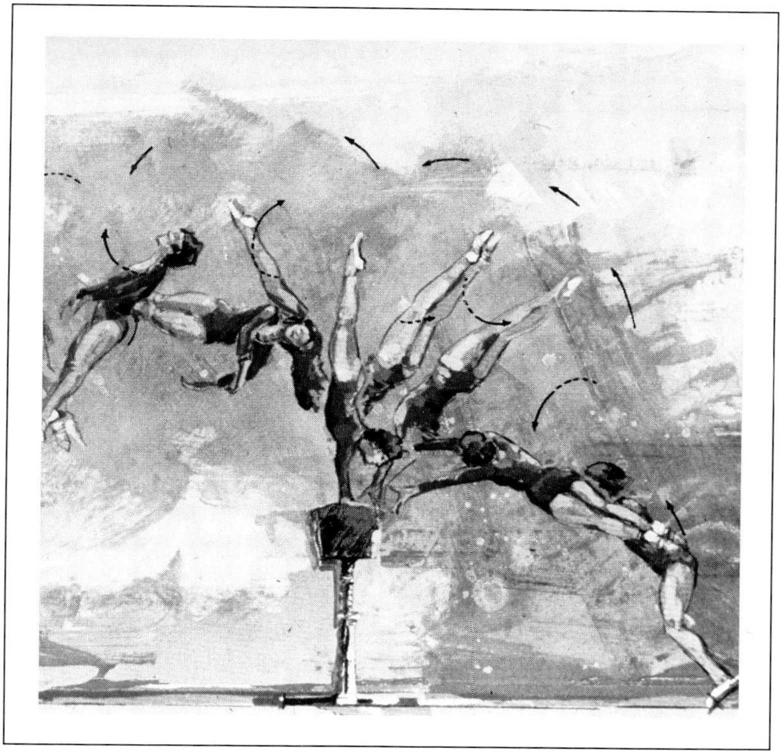

Group Leader

James Farmer, Jr, EdD

Group Participants

All participants

Overview

This workshop was the third sponsored by the American Orthopaedic Society for Sports Medicine to address anomalous topics in orthopaedic sports medicine. An anomaly is an issue that is puzzling or problematic because it deviates from or is inconsistent with normal expectations.

Although many aspects of sports-induced soft-tissue inflammation generated lively, interdisciplinary discussions, this final section focuses on eight provocative and controversial issues related to sports-induced soft-tissue inflammation.

Workshop leaders noted main issues from the daily presentations and discussions and presented these lists at the evening meeting of the leaders. Four issues, selected as particularly provocative and important to the main topic, were then discussed during the two-hour session. The essence of those discussions appears in the next chapter.

Several participants in the workshop correctly noted that it did not conform exactly to what are traditionally considered the main purposes of "continuing professional education," which are to update professionals about a body of knowledge and to contribute to their competence performance through education.

Although considerable learning occurred in preparation for and during the workshop, its purpose was not only to update knowledge about sports-induced soft-tissue inflammation but also to encourage and promote professional and scientific inquiry and the creation of a body of knowledge about the subject. The workshop sought to inform participants about specific aspects of the topic, to encourage interdisciplinary discussion of important relevant issues, and to suggest promising directions for further clinical and scientific inquiries.

A survey of 450 professionals in five fields (including orthopaedics) asked what they considered to be their most meaningful work-related learning experiences. The responses indicated that the most meaningful experiences tended to occur in specialty workshops that had a relatively small number of participants, focused on an area that was important for their practice but was also anomalous to them, and combined knowledge update with inquiry. Some of these workshops were composed of homogeneous groups, whereas others were heterogeneous. Some sought to contribute to understanding at the clinical level, others at the basic science level, and some at both levels. Workshops were typically designed and implemented from a critical viewpoint, because they valued the contributions of basic science research and encouraged the application of knowledge gained through research to fields such as orthopaedic sports medicine. In other words, such workshops sought to encourage and promote research resulting in both scientific and "situated" knowledge. This is potentially useful to a particular applied field such as orthopaedic sports medicine.

This workshop met all these criteria for specialty workshops. It was attended by orthopaedic sports-medicine physicians and basic scientists from various fields engaged in research relevant to the topic. It sought to contribute to understanding at the clinical and basic science levels, and to further the understanding of the relationship between the two.

A strength of the provocative issues discussions was the nature and extent of participation by both clinicians and basic scientists. At times, clinicians asked for specific information from a particular scientist or from any scientists present who wished to respond. At times, the basic scientists asked clinicians for specific information. No attempt was made to determine the nature or extent of agreement among the participants on any of the provocative issues discussed. Rather, participants were invited to come to their own conclusions on the basis of what they brought to and heard in the discussions.

Chapter 53

Provocative Issues

James A. Farmer, Jr, EdD
Arthur C. Pearl, MD

Through a process described in the Overview to this section, eight questions pertaining to sports-induced soft-tissue inflammation were identified as being provocative:

(1) Does suppression of acute inflammation impair healing?

(2) How can pain be graded, and is pain associated with acute inflammation beneficial?

(3) Is tissue injury necessary to produce acute sports-induced soft-tissue inflammation?

(4) Should clinical, animal, and mathematical studies of sports-induced soft-tissue inflammation be conducted in isolation, parallel to one another, or in sequence?

(5) Does Wolff's law apply to soft tissue?

(6) When is conservative treatment of sports-induced soft-tissue inflammation considered to be a failure?

(7) Are there diagnostic screening procedures and/or tissue markers for soft-tissue inflammation and/or destruction?

(8) Is there a syndrome of excessive fibroblastic hyperplasia?

No attempt was made to resolve these issues or produce a definitive statement about them. Rather, each was presented in the provocative issues session for interdisciplinary discussion. This chapter presents the results of those discussions. Participants were invited to arrive at their own conclusions about each of the issues, on the basis of their previous learning, research, and/or experience. The readers of this chapter are invited to do the same. It is hoped that some participants in the workshop or readers of this book will be stimulated to conduct clinical and/or basic science research on one or more of these provocative issues.

Does Suppression of Acute Inflammation Impair Healing?

The discussion of this issue was relatively brief. It began by considering the distinction between purposeful and purposeless inflammation. One participant suggested that it might be useful to think of soft tissues as having or not having useful functions relative to sports-induced inflammation.

Participants noted that suppression of acute inflammation may relate to healing in various ways. Their questions or conjectures can be summarized in the following statements:

Nonsteroidal anti–inflammatory drugs (NSAIDs) prescribed for specific inflammatory events do not seem, for the most part, to influence later events. Therefore, the use of NSAIDs is probably acceptable.

If there is no cell death, there may be no need for inflammation.

Corticosteroids appear to block all inflammatory responses.

Hyaluronate may have an increasingly identifiable role in mediating synovial joint repair.

Inflammation may be necessary to recovery from injury, but it is not part of good joint functioning.

Masking pain may suppress warning mechanisms.

How Can Pain Be Graded, and Is Pain Associated With Acute Inflammation Beneficial?

In discussing these issues, participants made the following comments:

There are various systems of grading pain. A dose-response (injury-pain) relationship is assumed. The upper and lower ends of a subjective scale are not particularly problematic, but the middle is a gray zone.

It seems important to treat pain to maintain control of vulnerability.

Residual pain may not be related to the primary injury.

Pain has a role in neuromuscular feedback.

Generally, pain should be treated as a beneficial warning.

Pain is closely related to function.

Functional changes in kinetic mechanisms of sports movement or protective equipment may remove pain.

It is important to specify the type of pain to avoid.

During the discussion, additional questions were raised as follows: When is pain associated with structural alteration? Can pain by itself cause abnormalities? How can pain associated with serious disturbance be identified?

One participant noted that pain cannot be both functional and non-functional. This comment generated further discussion on the use of the term functional. Another participant proposed considering pain that is associated with structural alteration and pain that is not. All pain affects function, and may be either benevolent or nonbenevolent. The physician's role is to eradicate the effects of pain on function and to determine whether or not a structural deficiency exists. If there is no structural deficiency, there is no risk involved in an athlete's returning to activity even though pain relief is only temporary.

Another participant asked if pain by itself could cause abnormalities. Others pointed out that pain could alter performance in a minor way and thus lead to problems. An athlete who does not feel pain should not necessarily be allowed to play, especially if performance has been altered.

One participant noted that steroids can mask pain and impair the healing response because they interfere with the inflammatory cascade. Other participants observed that steroids should almost never be used and asked if NSAIDs used to mask pain inhibit healing. Perhaps masking pain interferes with the healing process.

Another participant pointed out that pain is more encompassing than injury and asked how one could tell when pain in a runner reflects an injury. Other participants responded that there is no way of telling when pain in a runner reflects injury. Persistence, severity, and pattern of pain and response to activity are variables by which injury is assessed. In the prestage or early stages of injury there are no obvious pathologic findings that can be correlated with the clinical findings, as there are in stage-three or stage-four injuries. Pain is not pathognomonic for injury. There is a correlation between acute pain and injury but not between minor or moderate pain and injury. Pain may or may not be associated with structural disturbances.

The association between pain and serious or potentially serious tissue disturbance was also discussed. Pain can alter performance but may not necessarily be associated with tissue disturbance.

Participants recommended several steps, beginning with an examination of the tissue. If it is disrupted and there is pain, the disturbance is likely to be serious. Another step would be to determine the length of time pain continues after injury, and to determine if the pain is reproduced when the action is repeated. A physical examination is most useful, but new kinds of imaging studies might be used to develop better methods of identification.

Is Tissue Injury Necessary To Produce Acute Sports-Induced Soft-Tissue Inflammation?

This session began by discussing whether there were ways other than tissue injury to produce acute sports-induced inflammation. Participants thought that tissue injury could result from internal stresses, metabolic causes, or chemical causes, as well as from structural stress or strain.

A participant noted that a whole realm of cellular activity can be defined that is sports-induced but does not relate to the classic inflammatory response. This activity can cause disability but not be part of an inflammatory response.

Participants asked if there are inflammatory responses that are lacking in one or more aspects of the classic response and yet are important to consider. If these responses exist, is the physician dealing with the inflammatory response or something else? Participants noted that physicians conclude that inflammation is necessarily present if there is swelling, heat, and pain. However, there is both a classic and nonclassic inflammatory response, and people respond differently to injury in this regard.

In discussing the definitions of injury and inflammation, participants observed that there may be a spectrum of tissue activity from homeostasis through injury and inflammation. If so, inflammation would be a quantitative change rather than a qualitative change, as the body constantly repairs itself.

A participant asked what inflammation is and what the *sine qua non* and the characteristics of inflammation are. Are cell death, swelling, pain, or other factors necessary for inflammation? Another participant noted that there are three main components of the cascade: vascular permeability, cellular exudate, and a trigger event. All induce a cellular response, but all may not be necessary for such a response. However, healing without a cellular response does not occur. One attendee expressed the opinion that an inflammatory response is so-called if it produces a cellular response.

The discussion continued by considering the end of the inflammatory spectrum at which injury repairs itself before cell death occurs. Can there be a pure fibroblastic response without the other aspects of classic inflammatory response?

A participant asserted that cells are the key to the inflammatory response. It may be useful to break out of the classic way of viewing inflammation and to consider other forms of inflammatory response under a quantitative spectrum. Healing cannot occur without inflammation or hyperplasia.

This discussion ended with the following comments:

Different tissues may respond differently to inflammation. A true injury may not be necessary to trigger an inflammatory response.

In sports, increased loading of a tissue can affect response.

There may be a beneficial threshold, but more basic scientific research is needed to define this point.

Should Clinical, Animal, and Mathematical Studies of Sports-Induced Soft-Tissue Inflammation Be Conducted in Isolation, Parallel to One Another, or in Sequence?

Given limited resources, which research strategy should be employed and should single studies, a concentration of studies, or a sequence of studies be emphasized? The assumption is that a better understanding of the underlying mechanisms would lead to more effective prevention and treatment of sports injuries. Research choices include clinical, animal, and mathematical studies.

Clinical models to define specific sports-induced soft-tissue injuries rigorously in clinical terms would develop strategies, possibly through the use of imaging studies and others, to help understand such injuries, their healing processes, and effective clinical treatment. Animal models would reproduce similar injuries in animals and extrapolate from the findings. Mathematical and/or computer-based models would explore how changes in these tissues occur.

One suggestion was that clinical studies could be done first. On the basis of the results, animal studies could be devised. From these findings, computer models could be developed. Another suggestion was to identify priority areas and to encourage tandem studies in them. Researchers could determine what was needed to support the best investigator with the best testable hypothesis and the young investigator as well.

One participant said that tendon injury is the biggest problem, so therefore it should receive the highest priority for investigation and extensive focus. In discussing that comment, participants noted that there is a lack of understanding about tendons. The entity needs to be carefully defined and studied in all feasible ways to determine normal versus abnormal. The whole unit should be included—muscle, tendon, and bone. Animal studies on tendons have not reproduced human-type injuries. Most animal studies have been done on immature animals rather than on mature ones. They have not reproduced the mechanism of injury, and more objective studies are needed.

One participant found a "catch-22" in such research because the development of a good hypothesis and the use of a well-tested model precedes work. He favored a sequential, rather than a parallel, approach. In this system, the first step would be to show clinical relevance. The second step would be to undertake animal or culture studies. The results could be taken back to the clinical setting to see how the injury reacts and how beneficial interventions can be done. Participants also suggested that the definition of sports injuries be broadened to include capsule, tendon, and cartilage.

Discussion continued on an informal basis among participants even after the sessions concluded. One basic scientist later noted that sound and useful research requires that clinicians and basic scientists interact in an interdisciplinary manner, sometimes working alone and sometimes together. The clinician needs to describe the injury. For example, the clinician must specify the extent of trauma necessary to classify an injury as an overuse injury. The pathology associated with this injury must be described. The best situations for healing and the effects of various modalities, treatments, and conditions must be determined. The function of pain and the effects of preconditions must also be determined. Finally, implications for the prevention, diagnosis, and treatment of the specific type of sports-induced soft-tissue inflammation need to be determined. Clinicians or clinical researchers and basic scientists have different roles to play at various stages of such an inquiry.

Does Wolff's Law Apply to Soft Tissue?

Of the eight provocative issues, the question on Wolff's law generated the longest discussion. The effects on muscle, tendon, and cartilage were all considered separately. Finally, the application of Wolff's law to soft tissues in general was considered.

One participant observed that a normal remodeling process is assumed for bone formation and removal, as well as for muscle, tendon, ligament, and cartilage. Another participant suggested that there may be a spectrum of remodeling that affects the training response, that an applied force will result in an increase in strength in soft tissues such as tendon, ligament, and muscle.

Is remodeling associated with an inflammatory aspect? Which aspect is a normal part of remodeling? Is there a separate mechanism, a mechanism of microtrauma, an inflammatory mechanism, in relation to sports? With the limited turnover of articular cartilage (only 1% turnover in a year in the collagen fraction), is a microtraumatic episode necessary to increase tissue strength in remodeling? What is the effect of normal remodeling in these tissues? What are the effects of training or overtraining?

Does Wolff's Law Pertain to Muscle?

One participant asked what, in essence, is Wolff's law? Another responded that Wolff's law is the normal in vivo response of a biologic system to stress and deformation in order to maintain homeostasis in the system. This implies a change in architecture at both the structural and material levels. Some of the response in bone seems to apply to soft tissues. Wolff's law was originally postulated to describe changes in bone in response to increasing load. Muscle changes in response to the amount of work that it is expected to do.

Another participant commented that bone is peculiar as an entity because it replaces itself virtually anew through remodeling. The product is similar to the antecedent organ in matrix, cell population, and structure. In fact, bone responds to mechanical stress by producing more bone in those areas of greatest force. A stress-generated potential also plays a role in bone remodeling. With respect to muscle, the issue is whether or not it changes under stress and, if so, what cellular and mechanical events signal it to change? Specific aspects of Wolff's law must be precisely considered in this matter.

A participant stated that hyperpolarization may be a key factor in muscle response. When a muscle is stretched, it hyperpolarizes in much the same way as it does when insulin is applied to it: the muscle grows. However, its shape and other characteristics are not changed as in bone because of the high protein content in muscle.

One participant said that if a muscle was given a certain amount of inertia to overcome, the muscle would adapt through hyertrophy with a somewhat proportional increase in mass. This provides a rudimentary analogy to Wolff's law.

Muscle responds not only to intermittent exercise but also to extremes such as immobilization in a stretched position. A muscle immobilized in a stretched position undergoes histologic changes (hyperfocy).

Another participant stated that bone, tendon, ligament, and cartilage are not active tissues. Bones respond to forces on them, but they cannot generate force. Muscle generates force. With exercise, muscle mass increases, and there is a physiologic response to the increased mass that is fundamentally different from Wolff's law, although there may be a biologic reaction.

One participant asked about muscle turnover. Turnover can occur with reduced use, disuse, or immobilization. Under certain conditions, 60% of muscle can atrophy in seven days. This happens in spaceflight as well. Even if the muscles are active, if there is no load, they can atrophy. Scientists are trying to determine what triggers the controlling transduction.

Participants also commented that it may be advisable to refer to "generalized Wolff's law," so it can be applied to both active and nonactive tissues. Wolff talked about load being the cause of deformation; thus the question makes more sense if it is worded: How do these tissues respond to load?

Muscle is more dependent than the other soft tissues on innervation for hypertrophy and atrophy. It requires an intact nerve supply to function. It has a dynamic component, but it also changes if it is held static.

Does Wolff's Law Apply to Tendon and Ligament?

One participant postulated that muscle hypertrophy is attended by tendon hypertrophy. This may or may not pertain to ligament. There are no studies in which ligament length has been changed. The tension on these tissues must be measured. Unless these tissues are immobilized in a shortened position, the loads on them during the remodeling process cannot be determined.

Another participant noted the potential benefits of strengthening ligaments with exercise without damaging them. This would require carefully designed studies. In one study, when ligament and tendon were notched out in primates, each of the notched-out tissues produced a very large callus deposit in the notch in eight to nine weeks. Each tissue showed a marked disuse effect both above and below the notch that suggested a response to the change in load on the tissue and the effects of the injury.

In another study, rats made to run on a 30% grade were compared with those that ran on a level surface. There was a significant increase in ligament mass in the rats that ran the 30% grade. The change in the locomotive pattern may have stimulated ligamentous sufficiency. Other studies found that strain history correlates to the amount of matrix produced. However, the in vivo strains in the tissues are not known and can only be estimated.

Participants also commented on the following:

It is a clinical impression that highly trained athletes have a better quality of cruciate ligament. But the quality of the ligament may be part of their physiologic make-up.

A generalized Wolff's law would imply that soft tissue responds to outside force, and appears to remodel over time. However, ligaments and tendons turn over slowly.

Mass and the level of organization of the tissue both pertain in repair. However, load may not be equally important for both of them.

Studies show that a change in alignment can create considerable differences in response, so one participant wondered whether transecting an Achilles tendon with a square and replacing the plug at a 90-degree rotation would cause the fibers to realign with those in distress. An answer was not forthcoming.

How Does Cartilage Respond?

One participant noted that when the meniscus is removed, there may be attempts to remodel or regenerate it. The vascular zone created can be quite thick.

Another participant believed that because cartilage responds similarly to bone, Wolff's law may be quite applicable. Whether this response is age-dependent is unknown. It is difficult to describe the nature of cartilage remodeling. Such changes may be short-term and may revert over longer periods, or with greater or lesser loads, or with the application of external forces.

Conclusions

According to one participant, Wolff was referring to compressive rather than tensile forces. The structures of ligament and muscle are active, while those of tendon and bone are not. The literature is not clear whether tendon growth is hypertrophic or hyperplastic. A similar phenomon may also occur in muscle. What happens in ligament is unclear; there may be hypertrophy or a shift in mass of the articular surface. There is a definite response in all the tissues.

A second participant agreed that although there is a definite response in all these tissues, especially muscle, he would not apply Wolff's law to all soft tissues. Some of the bone repair and remodeling processes do not occur in soft-tissue repair.

A third participant concluded that studies show a dramatic resorption rate in soft tissues, but the resorption phenomenon has not yet been identified. By asking how soft tissue and muscle respond to increased loads from exercise, researchers may be able to find the threshold limit for injury.

When Is Conservative Treatment of Sports-Induced Soft-Tissue Inflammation Considered To Be a Failure?

In the opinion of one participant, conservative treatment of sports-induced soft-tissue inflammation is considered a failure when the patient is not improving and wants further treatment. The physician must decide if the patient's frustration is justified. When the patient and the physician agree that an appropriate amount of time and effort has been spent on conservative treatment, and the patient still cannot engage in activities that are an integral part of his or her lifestyle, conservative treatment has failed.

Another participant considered conservative treatment a failure when progress is unsatisfactory. He noted, however, that the circumstances must be carefully considered. There may have been an incorrect or inadequate protocol.

The failure of a particular conservative treatment plan does not necessarily indicate that surgery is necessary. The patient must meet the following criteria:

(1) The patient has an unacceptable loss of quality of life.

(2) The patient's pain indicates a permanent, pathologic change inside the affected soft tissue.

(3) The patient has night pain that disturbs his or her sleep but that does not necessarily imply tumor or infection.

(4) The patient has pain when active or at rest.

(5) The patient no longer wants to live with the symptoms.

(6) Surgical treatment is likely to improve the condition.

One participant asked if surgery is indicated when the patient experiences pain only when participating in sports. Another participant answered that the patient has to make that decision. The physician can tell the patient that he or she meets the criteria for surgery, but that it is elective. Both the physician and the patient must consent to surgery.

One participant gave his clinical impression that a positive bone scan does not bode well for conservative treatment. A bone scan or magnetic resonance imaging complements objective evidence of a permanent, pathologic condition.

According to another participant, patient history, presence of pain, loss of function, physical examination, and tissue examination to determine the extent of damage are all important in deciding the success or failure of conservative treatment. New tissue-imaging techniques may enable a physician to do a better job of diagnosis.

A participant added that there are a number of factors that are difficult to determine and deal with satisfactorily. For example, if an elite athlete is under external or self-imposed pressure to return to participation, the physician may promote surgery more aggressively than otherwise.

Participants questioned the role of behavior modification in treating sports-induced soft-tissue inflammation. If an athlete cannot return to the same sport, is participation in a less demanding sport during treatment a viable option? In response, another participant noted that the affected movement, not the sport, is the issue.

Are There Diagnostic Screening Procedures and/or Tissue Markers for Soft-Tissue Inflammation and/or Destruction?

This discussion concerned the possible existence of markers that could be used to trace developments during the early stages of sports-induced soft-tissue inflammation. One participant believed that both tissue markers and inflammation markers exist. Some collagen markers may be markers for all of the tissues.

Another participant noted that although these markers are being used in research, their potential clinical value is undetermined. Collagen propeptide type III is being studied, but whether it is a measure of new synthesis or a degradation of old type III collagen is unknown. Propeptides are retained in tissue structure for a considerable time. According to a Finnish study, some or all elements of the muscle-tendon unit resulted from rapid collagen increase.

One participant noted that keratan sulfate is often used as a marker but that levels vary from individual to individual, so the practical use of keratan sulfate at this time is as a longitudinal marker for the individual. In orthopaedics, keratan sulfate can be used before surgery and at six-month intervals after surgery to measure changes in level of articular cartilage synthesis or degradation.

A participant observed that the most difficult problem may be to identify tissue-specific markers that differentiate the various types of soft tissues. Basic scientists should be encouraged to investigate specific soft tissues such as ligaments, capsules, and bursae to identify tissue-specific or cell-surface markers. Isoenzymes, cell-surface markers such as antigens, inflammatory mediators, and differentiating markers could all be investigated.

Participants also observed that type I and type III collagen exist in all these types of soft tissues; that there is considerable variation among types of tendons; and that the use of markers with muscles is somewhat promising.

One participant concluded that any injury capable of causing significant, persistent pain probably produces a marker that correlates with the process and can be used in diagnosis and treatment. He predicted that this marker will be found.

Is There a Syndrome of Excessive Fibroblastic Hyperplasia?

This discussion began with the suggestion that there are persons whose presenting problem after injury or surgery is excessive fibroblastic hyperplasia that cannot be identified in advance.

Another participant contended that there has to be a syndrome of excessive fibroblastic hyperplasia, which is an inability of the body to break down the scar and can be seen in tissues that do not have surgical or any other obvious injury. It is easier to identify in the knee, but it can occur in other areas as well.

Participants also observed that the frozen shoulder is similar, that excessive fibroblastic hyperplasia may be the upper end of a spectrum of response on the part of individuals to injuries, and that the problem may be associated with diabetes and is a hormonal issue.

According to one participant, the syndrome exists in about 5% of patients who have knee surgery. It seems to occur when the joint is immobilized. Another participant concluded that the stimulus for excessive fibroblastic hyperplasia is unknown and is a significant problem that needs further investigation.

Index

X